DISCARD

Nutrition
and
Diet Therapy

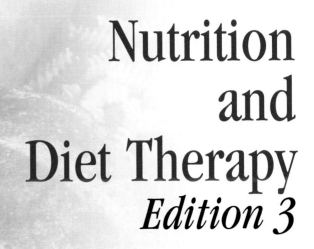

Nutrition
and
Diet Therapy
Edition 3

Carroll A. Lutz, MA, RN
Associate Professor Emerita
and Adjunct Professor
Jackson Community College
Jackson, Michigan

Karen Rutherford Przytulski, MS, RD
Director of Dietary
Doctors Hospital of Jackson
Jackson, Michigan

F. A. DAVIS Company • Philadelphia

F. A. Davis Company
1915 Arch Street
Philadelphia, PA 19103
www.fadavis.com

Printed in the United States of America

Last digit indicates print number: 10 9 8 7 6 5 4 3 2 1

Acquisitions Editor: Melanie Freely
Developmental Editor: Tom Lochhaas
Cover Designer: Louis J. Forgione
Cover and Unit opener art: Helen Uger

As new scientific information becomes available through basic and clinical research, recommended treatments and drug therapies undergo changes. The author(s) and publisher have done everything possible to make this book accurate, up to date, and in accord with accepted standards at the time of publication. The author(s), editors, and publisher are not responsible for errors or omissions or for consequences from application of the book, and make no warranty, expressed or implied, in regard to the contents of the book. Any practice described in this book should be applied by the reader in accordance with professional standards of care used in regard to the unique circumstances that may apply in each situation. The reader is advised always to check product information (package inserts) for changes and new information regarding dose and contraindications before administering any drug. Caution is especially urged with using new or infrequently ordered drugs.

Library of Congress Cataloging-in-Publication Data

Lutz, Carroll A.
   Nutrition and diet therapy / Carroll A. Lutz, Karen Rutherford
Przytulski.—3rd ed.
      p. cm.
   Includes bibliographical references and index.
   ISBN 0-8036-0804-7
   1. Dietetics.   2. Diet therapy.   3. Nutrition.   I. Przytulski,
Karen Rutherford. II. Title
   RM217 .L88 2001
   613.2—dc21

                         2001017385

Dedications

I would like to thank the following professors at Michigan State University for teaching me:

- Food is supposed to be enjoyable. Never take that away from someone you are trying to help. (Jean McFadden)
- Just take one step at a time. Be persistent. (Burness Wenberq)
- Most people can achieve excellence. Those people who have achieved it just kept doing the same work over and over again until it was correct. (Rachel Schemmel)
- There are only two things you can say about the future. It won't be like the past and it won't be what you think it will be. Accept change with dignity. (Katherine Hart)

Karen Rutherford Przytulski

To:

- My grandchildren, whose photographs illustrate some of the concepts presented in the book, with the hope that they will find career satisfaction similar to that which nursing has given me over a lifetime.
- All who read this book, especially those who thereby enhance their own or assist others to improve their nutrition.
- Everyone who is working to alleviate hunger on this continent, in this hemisphere, and in the world. Thank you for the example and your dedication.

Carroll A. Lutz

Preface

The third edition of *Nutrition and Diet Therapy* is designed to provide the beginning student with an understanding of the fundamentals of nutrition related to the promotion and maintenance of optimal health. Practical applications and treatment of nutrition-related pathologies are emphasized. In addition, basic scientific knowledge is introduced to enable students to begin to evaluate nutritional issues discussed in the mass media. The sequential introduction of material is a unique feature of this text. The authors resisted the temptation to introduce concepts and examples of applications before the underlying basic science and vocabulary were discussed. The third edition has been extensively updated and contains one new chapter entitled Complementary Therapy: Botanical Remedies and Ergogenic Aids. Although this information may not always be taught in an introductory course, the authors believe it to be of use for readers who utilize the text as a reference. All healthcare workers receive many questions about these subjects.

This book was written to meet the educational needs of nursing students, dietetic assistants, diet technicians, and others. Support materials for the nursing student include case studies with examples of care plans presented throughout the text as well as clinical analysis study questions. This edition incorporates the standardized nursing terminology of NANDA, NIC, and NOC into each chapter's nursing care plans to show its usefulness in many different settings. Critical Thinking Questions have been added following the Care Plans and are designed to provoke imaginative thought and to foster discussion. An information explosion exists related to the science of nutrition. As researchers discover new and more effective treatments for nutrition-related disorders and health maintenance, the ability to think critically becomes increasingly important for professional growth and development. Students need not only to grasp the facts but also to apply the information in a clinical environment. This text has been developed to facilitate acquiring these skills.

This text can be used to teach a complete course in nutrition or as a desk reference for practitioners. The student using this book needs no previous exposure to anatomy, physiology, or medical terminology. Subjects are fully supported by diagrams, illustrations, figures, or tables. Depending on the curriculum, chapters may be omitted or presented in a different sequence. We recognize that this text contains an immense amount of data and information. We hope that this rich store permits instructors to adapt the text to the objectives of their courses while at the same time serving as a reference and directory for students to satisfy their curiosity or to complete solo or group projects.

Nutrition and Diet Therapy, ed. 3, is organized into three units:

Unit I, **The Role of Nutrients in the Human Body**, covers basic information on nutrition as a science and how this information is applied through the nursing process. A thorough discussion of all the essential nutrients includes definitions and descriptions of functions, effects of excesses and deficiencies, and food sources. Information on the use of food in the body and how the body maintains energy balance completes the unit. The RDAs and DRIs current as of press time are incorporated in this edition. Instructors and students will want to be alert for additional updates because all of the recommendations are no longer published simultaneously.

Unit II, **Family and Community Nutrition**, provides an overview of topics such as nutrition in the life cycle, food management, complementary therapy (botanical remedies and ergogenic aids), and nutrient delivery.

Unit III, **Clinical Nutrition**, focuses on the care of clients with pathologies caused by or causing nutritional impairments. Pathological conditions include diabetes mellitus and hypoglycemia, cardiovascular disease, renal disease, gastrointestinal disease, cancer, and AIDS. Other topics discussed include interactions among foods, nutrients, and drugs; weight control; nutrition during stress; and care of clients with terminal illness.

Special features are used throughout the text to facilitate the teaching and learning process. The chapters include the following:

Study Aids: Chapter Review Questions and Clinical Analysis Questions that are similar to those on the NCLEX examination. Answers to the Study Aids questions are contained in Appendix M.

Case Studies, each with a proposed **Nursing Care Plan**, allows the student to see how the nutrition principles described in the chapter are applied in a specific clinical situation. The case studies were written to incorporate elements that are likely to recur in practice. One of the new case studies focuses on community practice.

Clinical Applications stimulate the interest of the beginning student by showing how the information might be used in practice. These cover a variety of topics that emphasize application to clinical practice or current use in the healthcare professions.

Clinical Calculations isolate and explain many of the mathematical calculations that are used in the nutritional sciences.

Critical Thinking Questions invite the student to think holistically with compassion and creativity. They can be used as a basis for class discussion.

Web Sites: Each chapter includes Web sites and Web sources of cited references. Note that a Web site is not a library. Unlike a library, a Web site may be available one day but not the next day. Anyone can open a Web site, even people with limited financial resources and no credentials. Information obtained from a Web site must be read critically. Even academic Web sites have been found to contain outdated information. If this is the case, why does this text publish Web sites in each chapter? Web sites, especially those from governmental agencies and professional organizations, are usually considered credible, and information can be retrieved from them instantaneously. To disregard the vast communication potential of the Internet would be to ignore reality. We hope the solid scientific foundation of the text encourages students to carefully critique their sources of information, whether electronic, printed, or word of mouth.

Undoubtedly, when the student attempts to access them, some of the Web sites listed will be unavailable. This may be the result of a permanent change or a revision of the pages at the site. We often list the complete address or Uniform Resource Locator (URL) to a specific page at a site. If the particular page cannot be accessed, the user is advised to try the basic address and then search for the desired link. For example, the Web site page http://www.eatright.org/womenshealth/diabetes.htm/ may be unavailable, but the information on diabetes possibly could be accessed by using http:/www.eatright.org and then searching for the link to the desired information.

This text also includes the following aids:

Glossary includes over 800 entries.

Appendices: This edition contains two additions: a table on nutritional supplements and client teaching aids that may be copied and distributed as needed.

Accompanying the text for instructors who adopt it for their classes are:

Teaching Aids: An Instructor's Guide that includes transparency masters and classroom or student activities. Ideas for teaching the material as a stand-alone course or integrated into other courses in the curriculum are also presented.

Cybertest: An electronic testbank containing more than 700 questions arranged by chapter.

We believe that *Nutrition and Diet Therapy*, ed. 3, provides the clinical information necessary for a fuller understanding of the relationship between knowledge about nutrition and diet and its clinical application. This text balances direct explanations of the underlying science with the clinical responsibilities of the health-care professional.

Acknowledgments

A project as mammoth as the writing of a book, even a third edition, requires the assistance of many people. We thank all the organizations and publishers that gave permission for the use of their materials. John and Judy Przytulski deserve special commendations for the many clerical tasks they completed and the computer skills they taught us. Joe and Leah Lutz advised on the contributed photographs. Dr. Russell Tobe again graciously provided us with expert consultation, diagnostic images, and technical support. The staff at the Jackson Comunity College Learning Resource Center—Cliff Taylor, Marion VanLoo, and Hope Friedland—obtained voluminous literature through interlibrary loans. Likewise, the Medical Library staff at Foote Hospital, especially Janet A. Zimmerman and Mabel Hill, shared their resources generously. Special thanks go to Bob Weber for technical advice and expert counsel. The editorial and production staff at F. A. Davis Company shared their knowledge and expertise in our joint project. Our developmental editor, Tom Lochhaas, served admirably as the reader's advocate and as the authors' watchdog.

Many of our colleagues contributed to this project. In particular, we would like to thank Betty Ackley, Stevie Huffman, Lisa Lazarus, Diane Morris, Connie O'Connor, and Jim Reynolds. Betty Ackley is particularly noteworthy as the developer of an online nutrition course at Jackson Community College that used the second edition of the text. Aside from Betty and Dr. Rachel Schemmel, all the reviewers listed are strangers to us who favored us with their time and expertise in an effort to create the best nutrition book possible.

Last on the page, but first in understanding the time and effort that writing a textbook entails, are our husbands, Bob Lutz and Paul Przytulski. They have learned to adapt their lives to our long hours at our desks. Many thanks.

Consultants for the Third Edition

Betty Ackley, RN, BSN, MSN
Professor of Nursing
Jackson Community College
Jackson, MI

Evelyn Burruss, RN, BSN
Public Health Nurse, Technical Writer
Fresno County Human Services System
Fresno, CA

Rhonda Comne, RN, BSN
Director of Undergraduate Nursing Program
Southern Illinois University
Edwardsville, IL

Colleen Duggan, RN, BSN, MSN
Professor of Nursing
Johnson County Community College
Overland Park, KS

Laura A. Filippelli, MS, RD, LDN
Instructor
St. Joseph Hospital School of Nursing
North Providence, RI

Bernadine Fitzloff, RN, BSN, MSN
Assistant Professor
Concordia University West Suburban College of Nursing
Oak Park, IL

Jean A. Foote, RN, BSN, MS
Associate Professor
Grand Canyon University
Phoenix, AZ

Julie Marie Goyette, MS, RD
Instructor
Wenatchee Valley College
Omak, WA

Marinell F. Guild, MS, RDLD, FADA
Program Director, Coordinated Program in Clinical Dietetics
University of Oklahoma Health Sciences Center
Oklahoma City, OK

Theresa Isom, RN, BSN, MS
Nursing Director
Tennessee Technology Center
Memphis, TN

Meri Beth Kennedy, RN, BSN, MS
Director of Nursing
Dakota County Technical College
Rosemount, MN

Mary Delia Linthacum, RN, BSN, MSEd, MSN
Assistant Professor
Del Mar College
Corpus Christi, TX

Joy A. Price, RN, BSN, MSM
Nursing Instructor
Northeast Mississippi Community College
Booneville, MS

Gail Janet Smith, RN, BSN, MSN
Associate Professor
Miami Dade Community College
Miami, FL

Virginia Teel, RN, BSN, MSN, MS
Instructor
Huthinson Community College
Hutchinson, KS

Susanne M. Tracy, RN, MS, MA
Associate Professor of Nursing
Rivier College
Nashua, NH

Contents

Preface   vi

Acknowledgments   ix

Consultants for the Third Edition   xi

Unit I   The Role of Nutrients in the Human Body   1

1. Evolution and Science of Nutrition   3
2. Individualizing Client Care   11
3. Carbohydrates   35
4. Fats   45
5. Protein   59
6. Energy Balance   75
7. Vitamins   87
8. Minerals   111
9. Water and Body Fluids   141
10. Digestion, Absorption, Metabolism, and Excretion   163

Unit II   Family and Community Nutrition   181

11. Life Cycle Nutrition: Pregnancy and Lactation   183
12. Life Cycle Nutrition: Infancy, Childhood, Adolescence   203
13. Life Cycle Nutrition: The Mature Adult   235
14. Food Management   255
15. Nutrient Delivery   273
16. Complementary Medicine: Botanical Remedies and Ergogenic Aids   293

Unit III   Clinical Nutrition   309

17. Food, Nutrient, and Drug Interactions   311
18. Weight Control   327
19. Diet in Diabetes Mellitus and Hypoglycemia   349
20. Diet in Cardiovascular Disease   373
21. Diet in Renal Disease   403
22. Diet in Gastrointestinal Disease   421
23. Diet and Cancer   449
24. Nutrition During Stress   469
25. Diet in HIV and AIDS   483
26. Nutritional Care of the Terminally Ill   497

Appendices   509

A   Exchange Lists of the American Dietetic and Diabetes Associations   510
B   Nutritive Value of Foods   518
C   Nutritional Assessment Tools   583
D   Growth Charts for Boys and Girls 0–18   589
E   Body Fat and Skinfolds of Adults and Children   594
F   Dietary Reference Intakes: RDAs and AIs   598
G   Tolerable Upper Intake Levels (UIs) for Certain Nutrients   602
H   1989 Recommended Dietary Allowances (RDAs)   604
I   Estimated Safe and Adequate Daily Dietary Intakes of Selected Minerals   605
J   Estimated Sodium, Chloride, and Potassium Minimum Requirements of Healthy Persons   606
K   Medical Nutritional Formulas   607
L   Client Teaching Aids   610
M   Answers to Questions   623
N   Glossary   626

Index   649

The Role of Nutrients in the Human Body

CHAPTER 1

Evolution and the Science of Nutrition

LEARNING OBJECTIVES

After completing this chapter, the student should be able to:

1. Discuss the relationship between the biologic evolution of the human body and present-day nutritional concerns.
2. State the three functions of nutrients.
3. Identify the six classes of nutrients.
4. Discuss the effects of malnutrition on health and provide examples.
5. Describe the relationship between nutrition and health.

Food and health have always been connected. In this chapter, we compare food habits and their effect on the health of our ancestors with those of present-day people. The chapter highlights past and present views about health and health care and discusses the effect of these views on the role of health-care professionals. It also examines the science of nutrition and introduces some basic terminology.

Evolution of the Human Body and Emergence of Health Issues

Throughout history our ancestors survived on a variety of diets (Fig. 1–1). What prehistoric humans (prehistoric refers to the period in time before humans were able to write) ate in any particular geographic area depended in large part on the climate in which they lived, their hunting and gathering skills, their food-processing technology, and available foods. Clues from pictures painted on cave walls, artifacts, and fossils suggest that the earliest humans were hunter-gatherers: people who ate wild game and any plants, fish, seeds, and honey they could find (Bednarz, 1997). Stone tools excavated from sites suggest that the use of tools accompanied a big increase in meat consumption.

The human body evolved the capability to subsist on a wide variety of foodstuffs of both plant and animal origin. The traditional diet of

Eskimos, for example, consists of mostly fish, whereas some other native American tribes subsist mostly on fruit (Bednarz, 1997). Humans' ability to adapt makes it possible for them to survive for long periods on inferior diets.

Effect of Agriculture

Early Mexican farmers began to grow crops about 8000 years ago. Evidence suggests they started growing corn about 3000 years ago. The Egyptians grew wheat, dates, and chickpeas more than 5000 years ago. About 4800 years ago, the Chinese began to grow rice (Bednarz, 1997).

The emergence of agriculture led to population expansion. Individuals learned to work together to grow crops and began to live together in larger groups to protect their cultivated fields and harvested food stores. The formation of such communities led to the development of villages and towns. Food distribution systems for the rationing of the harvest from one growing season to the next evolved to help ensure an adequate food supply in the event of a poor harvest or natural disaster.

Agriculture, however, especially single-crop agriculture, limited the variety of foods available to a given community. Today we understand that growth deficiencies can result from a diet based on single-crop agriculture; no single food can furnish all the raw materials necessary for optimal human growth and health maintenance. Variety, moderation, and balance in the diet are all necessary for health (Wellness Tip 1–1).

Adaptation to Feast and Famine

Seasonal and cyclical variations in food availability affected our ancestors. An example of a seasonal variation is an abundance of food during summer and fall compared with a scarcity of food late in winter. A cyclical variation is a recurring series of events such as a period of drought and famine followed by a period of plentiful rainfall.

Biologically, the human body adapted to such feast-or-famine conditions by developing the capacity to store energy as fat. This adaptation enabled human beings to survive famine, but it did not ensure optimal nourishment. The situation is much the same today. Famine still exists in many countries in the world, and even in developed countries some popu-

Wellness Tip 1-1

- Variety, moderation, and balance promote good health.

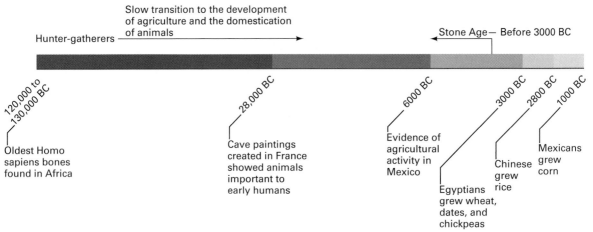

Figure 1–1:
Timeline from the discovery of the oldest *Homo sapiens* bones to 1000 BC, when Mexican farmers grew corn. Humans evolved slowly and adapted to be able to survive on a wide variety of foodstuffs.

lation groups—notably, poor, very young, and elderly people—suffer from malnutrition. For other population groups—those with unlimited access to food—the human body's capacity to store fat in unlimited amounts has lead to an epidemic of chronic disease related to overnutrition.

Food Safety Issues

Many people like to imagine the so-called natural man or woman who lived a healthy, happy life on unprocessed foods. Although the food our ancestors ate may have been free of pesticides and additives, it was not always safe. Meat, for example, could turn rancid and harbor parasites; fungal infestations could contaminate both stored grain and grain in the fields; and heavy metals (lead, for example) leached out of utensils into food, often with fatal effects.

Our Ancestors' View of Health

In the past, it was commonly held that health was subject to supernatural laws. For example, the recurrent epidemics of bubonic plague that swept Europe in the Middle Ages (between 1340 and 1660 AD) were thought to result from witchcraft and the work of the devil. The discovery of bacteria in the late 1880s and the subsequent development of antibiotics in the 1940s rendered many diseases treatable.

Until recent decades, health care focused mainly on curing disease. Slowly, in part because of scientific progress, the impetus behind health-care delivery has shifted to disease prevention. The use of vaccines is one form of prevention. The consumption of certain food substances that can help prevent certain diseases is another.

Current Attitudes toward Health and Health Care

Today many diseases are known to be linked to lifestyle behaviors such as smoking, lack of adequate physical activity, and poor nutritional habits. Health-care providers emphasize the relationship between lifestyle and the risk of disease. Many people, at least in industrialized countries, are increasingly managing their health problems and making personal commitments to lead healthier lives.

Nutrition is, in part, a preventive science. Given sufficient resources, how and what one eats is a lifestyle choice. Health is defined as a state of complete physical, mental, and social well-being, and not just the absence of disease or infirmity.

The ability to detect disease early using highly sophisticated technology is another major focus of the health-care system. Early disease detection not only often reduces suffering and mortality but also enables people to alter the behaviors, including food habits, that affect disease progression. Early identification of disease frequently results in a cost saving to individuals. Although educating and screening clients for disease is expensive for society as a whole, society has increasingly come to realize that it is less costly than treating disease. For this reason, all health-care providers should take advantage of each encounter with clients to educate them.

The Changing Role of Health-Care Professionals

Changing attitudes about health have altered the role of health-care professionals. No longer are clients totally reliant on physicians; their care is now in the hands of a multidisciplinary team.

Clients are the focus of the health-care team. It is a fact that clients who participate in their own care are more likely to achieve the set goals or objectives. Family members, caregivers, or designated guardians who care for clients who are unable to care for themselves need to be involved with the health-care team.

An institutionalized client's health-care team may include more than 15 members. The respective titles and responsibilities of the major members of the health-care team are outlined in the following sections.

REGISTERED NURSES Registered nurses (RNs) are responsible for clients' daily health care, including their nutritional care. RNs communicate with physicians and dietitians regarding clients' response to food, including intake and tolerance. They also provide nutrition education, if needed, and record information on clients' charts. Box 1–1 discusses in more detail nursing roles pertinent to nutrition.

LICENSED PRACTICAL NURSE/LICENSED VOCATIONAL NURSES Licensed practical nurses and vocational nurses (LPNs/LVNs), supervised by RNs, feed clients, monitor food consumption, measure intake and output, and record data.

CLINICAL PHARMACISTS Pharmacists (RPhs) prepare, preserve, and compound medicines and dispense them according to the prescriptions of physicians. They counsel clients about food–drug and drug–drug interactions and function as valuable resources for all team members.

PHYSICIANS Physicians are responsible for the diagnosis and treatment of medical conditions. They manage medical care, order laboratory tests, prescribe medications and diet, and explain treatment plans to clients.

REGISTERED DIETITIANS Registered dietitians (RDs), together with physicians, have the responsibility to meet clients' nutritional needs. This responsibility includes interpreting the physician's diet order in terms of clients' food habits and food choices, evaluating clients' response to

therapeutic diets, and providing nutrition education and counseling for clients.

DIETETIC TECHNICIANS Dietetic technicians (DTs) assist dietitians by taking nutrition histories and body measurements, reviewing records, and monitoring clients' food intake.

OTHER HEALTH-CARE PERSONNEL Other health-care personnel who may be involved in client care include licensed social workers, medical technologists, nurse practitioners, and physical and occupational therapists.

Nutrition Is a Science

Stated simply, nutrition is the science that studies the relationship of humans to food. The discussion of nutrition in this text involves the following topics:

- The chemical content of food
- The body's use of food
- The relationship of food to health
- Selection of food
- Techniques to modify food habits

Box 1–1 Nursing Roles Pertinent to Nutrition

Nurses classify their functions by role. Although we divide them here for purposes of discussion, the roles often all come into play in a single client interaction.

Care Providers

Nurses monitor clients' food intake and report and record deficits. Nurses coordinate clients' diagnostic tests and promote compensatory food and fluid intake when tests are completed. Nurses prepare clients and their surroundings for meals, prepare food served for self-feeding, and feed clients who are unable to feed themselves.

Teachers

Nurses provide information and coach clients in required skills to maximize nutritional care. To accomplish this end, the nurse may have to assess feelings and motor skills. Nurses tailor the educational materials used to clients' reading levels. A general rule for health education is that printed materials should be written at a maximum of the eighth-grade reading level. Pilot testing material on intended audience will reveal weaknesses. Self-paced learning programs have been effective in guiding clients, even children, to acquire necessary information (Shannon et al, 1994). Because the learning takes place over an extended time, the program provides its own reinforcement.

The desired outcome of health education is behavior, not increased knowledge. A prerequisite to making a behavior change, however, is the knowledge necessary to make the change. An objective measure to evaluate if a change in behavior has occurred is helpful. For example, blood cholesterol levels can be used to evaluate instruction. Multiple teaching sessions produced better results than a single lesson (Byers et al, 1995).

Counselor

Nurses assist clients in making decisions affecting their health. A counselor focuses on attitudes, feelings, and behaviors to encourage the client in achieving self-control. Especially when the client displays self-destructive behaviors, the nurses may need special training to remain nonjudgmental and to avoid speculating on reasons for the client's behavior (Sutherland, 1995). The nurse needs to ensure that clients receive a diet that they are willing to follow and adapted to their home situation. Studies have shown that facilitation skills of customizing, adapting, and including the client in decision making exert the strongest force on client satisfaction and intention to comply with dietary counseling (Trudeau and Dube, 1995). An imperfect diet that is followed is preferable to a perfectly designed one that is ignored. The role of counselor contrasts with that of teacher who helps the client to acquire new knowledge and skill.

Client Advocate

Nurses act to protect and support the client's rights. Basic to these rights is the client's right to choose being informed of treatment options, risk, and expected outcomes.

Health Team Member

Modern health care requires the cooperation of many individuals of varied professions, and the nurse is part of this multidisciplinary team. Nutrition instruction can be provided by anyone on the health-care team including physicians, nurses, pharmacists or dietitians. Sometimes the nurse may have the knowledge, interest, and time to provide nutrition instruction. When the nurse is unable to teach the client, it is important to refer the client to another team member. Nurses are often responsible for coordinating the care among members of the multidisciplinary team.

- Diet as treatment for disease
- The relationship between medications and food intake

As this list suggests, the science of nutrition encompasses ideas from many other sciences: biology, chemistry, economics, educational theory, nursing, medicine, pharmacology, physiology, psychology, and sociology. This connection with other disciplines suggests the far-reaching implications of good nutrition.

Nutrients

The science of nutrition has historically been based on the nutrients found in food. Nutrients are the chemical substances supplied by food that the body needs for growth, maintenance, and repair. Nutrients can be divided into six groups:

1. Carbohydrates (often abbreviated as CHO)
2. Fats (lipids)
3. Proteins
4. Minerals
5. Vitamins
6. Water

Each group is discussed in a separate chapter.

Nutrients are considered either **essential** or nonessential, depending on whether the body can or cannot manufacture them. When the body requires a nutrient for growth or maintenance but lacks the ability to manufacture it in amounts sufficient to meet bodily needs, this essential nutrient must be supplied by foods in the diet. Vitamin C, vitamin A, and calcium are three of the more than 40 essential nutrients. Nutrients not needed in the diet because the body can make them are called nonessential. For example, the amino acid alanine is a nonessential nutrient because the body can manufacture it from other raw materials.

Functions of Nutrients

All nutrients perform one or more of the following functions:

1. Serve as a source of energy or heat
2. Support the growth and maintenance of tissue
3. Aid in the regulation of basic body processes

These three life-sustaining functions collectively are part of **metabolism**, the sum of all physical and chemical changes that take place in the body. Nutrients have specific metabolic functions and interact with one another to maintain the body.

Source of Energy

Energy is defined in the physical sciences as the capacity to do work. Energy exists in a variety of forms: electric, thermal (heat), chemical, mechanical, and others.

All food enters the body as chemical energy. The body processes the chemical energy of food and converts it into other energy forms. Chemical energy is transformed into electric signals in nerves, for example, and mechanical energy in muscles.

Carbohydrates, fats, and proteins, the nutrients that supply energy, are referred to as the **energy nutrients**. The energy both in foods and in the body is measured in kilocalories, abbreviated kcal (see Glossary). Because energy cannot be seen, heard, or felt, it is one of the most diffi-

cult biological concepts to understand. For this reason, it warrants an entire chapter of its own in this book (see Chapter 6).

Growth and Maintenance of Tissues

Some nutrients provide the raw materials for building the body structures and participate in the continued growth and maintenance of necessary tissues. Water, proteins, fats, and minerals are the nutrient classes that contribute in a major way to building body structures.

Regulation of Body Processes

Some nutrients control or regulate chemical processes in the body. For example, certain minerals and proteins help regulate how water is distributed in the body. Vitamins are necessary in the series of reactions involved in generating energy. Vitamins themselves are not energy sources, but if the body lacks a particular vitamin, it will not produce energy efficiently.

Malnutrition

Ingesting too much or too little of a nutrient can interfere with health and well-being. There is a beneficial range of intake for any nutrient; an intake below or above that range is incompatible with optimal health. Thus, malnutrition (poor nutrition) occurs when body cells receive too much or too little of one or more nutrients. For example, a single-food diet, such as a grapefruit diet to lose weight, will result in malnutrition if followed for an extended period.

Undernutrition

Malnutrition includes undernutrition, the result of a deficiency of one or more nutrients. Undernutrition may be related to:

- An individual's inability to obtain foods that contain the essential nutrients
- An individual's failure to consume essential nutrients
- The body's inability to use the nutrients in food
- Disease conditions that increase the body's need for nutrients
- A disease process that causes nutrients to be excreted too rapidly from the body.

Undernutrition occurs in many different circumstances. For example, stress from trauma, surgery, or burns frequently produces a state of undernutrition. People exposed to such severe and prolonged stressors may be undernourished even if they consume an apparently normal diet. Prolonged physical stress causes the body to break down internal protein stores, and protein is excreted as a result.

Although undernutrition is not widespread in the United States, it does exist as a result of poverty, illness, neglect, poor dietary planning, or environmental hazards. It can occur as well in institutional settings if caregivers fail to provide adequate nourishment, monitor clients' food intake, and make sure they have help eating. Groups especially vulnerable to undernutrition are children, pregnant women, and elderly people. Malnourished children grow at a slower rate than adequately nourished ones, and they are prone to infections and are more likely to have mental and developmental problems.

Overnutrition

Overnutrition, which is an excessive intake of nutrients, is another form of malnutrition. Overnutrition often results from the use of self-prescribed

Table 1–1 Selected Functionsl foods, Phytochemicals, and Reported Health Benefits

Functional Foods	Phytochemical(s) Identified	Reported Health Benefit
Tomatoes, grapefruit	Lycopene	Decreased risk of prostate and stomach cancer
Garlic, onions, chives	Allyl sulfides	Lower risk of stomach and colon cancer
Soy products, legumes, peanuts	Isoflavones: genistein and diadzein	May reduce risk of breast, prostate, and endometrial cancer May decrease risk of heart disease May reduce risk of osteoporosis May assist in the treatment of menopausal symptoms
Whole flaxseed	Lignans and phytoestrogens	Increase laxation (increased frequency and bulk of feces) May protect against heart disease, cardiac arrhythmia, and stroke May prevent cancer of the hormone-sensitive cancers Favorably affects the immune system by reducing inflammation May prevent retinopathy in premature infants
Green tea	Polyphenols	May reduce risk of skin, lung, and stomach cancers
Broccoli, cabbage, Brussels sprouts, cauliflower, kohlrabi, watercress, turnips	Sulforaphanes, indoles, isothiocyanates	May reduce risk of breast, stomach, and lung cancers May protect the retina from light induced oxidative damage May be responsible for reversing eye damage or macular degeneration in very early stages
Fruits, vegetables, nuts, tea, wine, and oregano	Flavonoids	May reduce cancer risk; acts as an antioxidant

over-the-counter vitamin and mineral supplements. For example, when ingested in very high doses once or habitually, preformed vitamin A can cause headache, vomiting, bone abnormalities, and liver damage. Vitamin D toxicity can lead to the deposit of calcium in soft tissues and irreversible kidney and cardiovascular damage. Overnutrition is associated also with eating too much food and hence having an excessive intake of many nutrients rather than of a single one.

Phytochemicals

The prefix phyto- comes from the Greek word for "plant." Phytochemicals are nonnutrient food components (food chemicals) that provide medical or health benefits, including the prevention or treatment of a disease (Table 1–1). Large studies that examined the dietary patterns among different cultures have revealed the first clues about fruits' and vegetables' protective role against heart disease and cancer (Kendall, 1998).

Recent advances in research techniques have allowed scientists to study the functions of such plant constituents in the laboratory as well as in animals and humans. Phytochemicals appear to be able to stop a cell's conversion from healthy to cancerous at many different stages of cell division and growth. Phytochemicals also may decrease risk for chronic diseases, such as cardiovascular disease, cancer, and diabetes (Slavin, 1999). This is an area of active research.

It is not known whether each of the more than 400 phytochemicals produces its reported health benefits by functioning alone or in combination with others. Most experts advise eating a wide variety of fruits and vegetables (Figure 1–2) and not narrowing intake to particular foods.

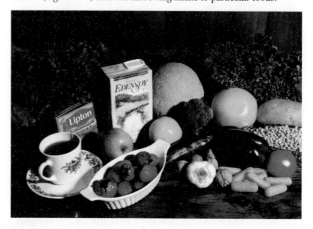

Figure I–2:
Eating a wide variety of fruits, vegetables, whole grains, tea, soy, and flaxseed is an excellent way to obtain a natural supply of phytochemicals.

Nutrition and Health

Good nutrition is essential for good health and important for physical growth and development, good body composition, and mental development. People's nutritional state can protect them from or predispose them toward chronic disease. Medical treatment for many diseases includes diet therapy. Nutrition is thus both a preventive and a therapeutic science.

Physical Growth and Development

Although heredity determines much of individual growth patterns and genetic potential, malnutrition can delay or prevent individuals from achieving that potential. Without enough calcium, phosphorus, and protein, for example, bones cannot grow properly. Children who are malnourished may never reach their genetic potential for height.

Slowed growth is of the first clinically measurable indicators of inadequate dietary intake in children. For this reason, health-care providers measure an infant's height and weight and record them on growth charts on each visit. Examples of growth charts for the height and weight of infants and children are in Appendix D.

Body Composition

Nutrient intake can affect body composition, which in turn can affect health. The human body is composed of four main types of substances (water, fat, ash, and protein) and one minor substance (carbohydrate) (Fig. 1–3). One-half to three-quarters of the body is made up of water. A normally active woman has a body fat content between 18 and 22 percent. A normally active man has a body fat content between 15 and 19 percent. Body ash, which accounts for approximately 6 percent of body weight, is the body's mineral content. It includes, for example, the calcium and phosphorus that are constituents of the human skeleton.

About 15 percent of the body's weight is protein; the male body contains more protein than the female body. With age body composition typically becomes higher in fat and lower in protein. Protein is stored

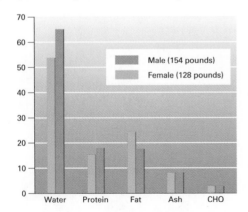

Figure 1–3:
Approximate body composition of a typical 25-year-old man (154 lb.) and woman (128 lb.). Note that the typical woman has a higher percentage of body fat than does the typical man. The man has a higher percentage of lean body mass. The percentage of ash content is equal in both sexes. The human body has minimal carbohydrate content.

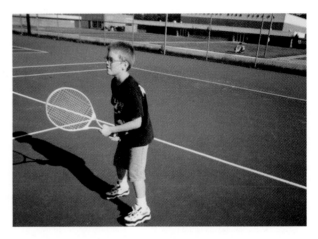

Figure 1–4:
A young man developing muscle tissue while enjoying a sport.

primarily in muscle tissue, organs, and certain body chemicals. When the body loses protein, it is losing muscle tissue, organ mass, the protein stored in body substances, or combinations thereof. Preservation of body protein is necessary for optimal health. A loss of structural body content (heart muscle, kidney, liver, blood proteins) is undesirable and leads to illness.

A person's body fat and protein content can be modified by food intake, exercise, or both. Exercise increases body protein content by increasing muscle content (Fig. 1–4). Eating too much food (ingesting more calories than the body expends) increases the fat content of the body because fat is stored for future use.

Mental Development

Research continues on the relationship between undernutrition and brain development in the child. It has been found that undernourished babies have smaller and fewer brain cells, but the relationship between intelligence and the size and number of brain cells is not clear. There is some evidence that the mental development of infants younger than 6 months of age is particularly vulnerable to the effects of malnutrition. Some nutritional deficiencies may cause permanent impairment of the central nervous system (CNS) in young infants.

Some conditions that affect the CNS may be reversible through diet. Nutrition plays an important role, for example, in the prevention and management of some forms of dementia. Dementia is an impairment of intellectual function that is usually progressive and interferes with normal social and occupational activities (impairment refers to any condition that causes a person to deteriorate; progressive means it becomes more severe or spreads to other parts). Excessive alcohol intake or nutritional deficiencies may result in dementia. Correcting the deficiency or eliminating alcohol from the diet may improve intellectual function. Not all forms of dementia are directly related to poor nutrition.

Diet As Therapy

A modified diet is often an important component of a client's total health care. A modified diet is one that has been altered to include more or fewer nutrients, to effect a change in the texture or consistency of what is ingested, or to restrict the intake of any substance. For example, diet is an important part of the treatment for clients with a metabolic disease such as diabetes. Special dietary measures are often required to maintain the lives of patients who have chronic heart, kidney, liver, and gastrointestinal diseases. These diets must also take into consideration the effects of medications on nutrients. Adjustments in diet are also necessary in other situ-ations, such as after highly stressful or traumatic events, including severe burns, broken bones, and surgery.

Although deficiency of a single nutrient is rare, it is seen in some clients. In such cases, adding foods to the diet that contain the missing nutrient is often sufficient to solve the problem. The last section of this book describes various diets for specific clinical situations.

Summary

Nutrition is the science of food and its relation to people. The human body evolved by adapting to a wide variety of diets. Although survival is possible on an inferior diet, optimal health is not. Health is a state of complete physical, mental, and social well-being, not just the absence of disease or infirmity. Nutrition is vital to optimal health. The principles of nutrition are applied by the health care team to promote health and treat many dis-eases. The science of nutrition is based on chemical constituents of foods called nutrients, which function to provide fuel, support tissue growth and maintenance, and regulate body processes. A nutrient is called essential if the body requires it and cannot manufacture it in sufficient amounts to meet bodily needs. A balanced nutrient intake is vital for physical growth and development, optimal body composition, mental development, and disease prevention.

 ## Study Aids

Subjects	Internet Sites
Phytochemicals	.http://www.flaxcouncil.ca
	http://www.peanut-institute.org
	http://www.soytalk.com
American Dietetic Association	.http://www.eatright.org
U.S. Department of Health and Human Services	.http://www.healthfinder.gov
Society for Nutrition Education	.http://www.sne.org
Tufts University Nutrition Navigator	.http://www.navigator.tufts.edu
National Cattlemen's Beef Association	.http://www.beef.org
National Dairy Council	.http://www.nationaldairycouncil.org
International Food Information Centers	.http://www.ificinfo.health.org
Food andNutrition Education	.http://www.nalusda.gov/fnic
Food Marketing Institute	.http://www.fmi.org
Nutritional Evolution	.http://www.ag.arizona.edu/nsc/courses/104nsck/ch0s/sld028.htm

Chapter Review Questions

1. Women's bodies normally contain more _____ and less _____ than men's bodies.
   a. Carbohydrate, protein
   b. Fat, protein
   c. Protein, ash
   d. Water, fat
2. The human body has adapted to feast-or-famine conditions by developing the capacity to store:
   a. Fluid
   b. Carbohydrate
   c. Fat
   d. Protein
3. Which of the following is not one of the traditional groups of nutrients?
   a. Phytochemicals
   b. Vitamins
   c. Minerals
   d. Proteins

4. An example of an energy nutrient is:
   a. Water
   b. Carbohydrates
   c. Vitamins
   d. Minerals
5. Malnutrition always occurs as a result or part of:
   a. The aging process
   b. A low income
   c. Infirmity
   d. Overnutrition

Clinical Analysis

1. Mrs. A believes she can cleanse her body of toxic compounds by abstaining from all food for 10 days. You should:
   a. Tell Mrs. A she needs to drink extra fluids for this approach to succeed.
   b. Ignore Mrs. A because you think she will not listen to you.
   c. Pretend to agree with Mrs. A. because you do not want to make her angry.
   d. Explain to Mrs. A the importance of variety, balance, and moderation in the diet.

2. Mr. and Mrs. J are members of a local fitness club and have recently had their body fat content analyzed. Mr. J expresses concern because his wife's body fat content (20%) is higher than his body fat content (15%). He asks, "Why is there a difference?" An appropriate response would be:
   a. A normally active woman has a body fat content between 18 and 22 percent.
   b. A normally active woman has a body fat content between 15 and 19 percent, so his wife should exercise more.
   c. A person's body fat content is not that important.
   d. If his wife would increase her protein intake, her body fat content would decrease.

3. Billie is an 18-month-old boy who weighs 25 lb and is 32-1/2 in long. His mother asks you to evaluate his growth. (Hint: Use the growth chart in Appendix D for boys, birth to 36 months.) You should tell her:
   a. Billie weighs too much for his height.
   b. Billie weighs too little for his height.
   c. Billie is in the 90th percentile.
   d. Billie is in the 50th percentile, or about average.

Bibliography

American Dietetic Association: Position paper of the American Dietetic Association: Phytochemicals and functional foods. J Am Diet Assoc 95:493, 1995.

Bednarz, S: Discover Our Heritage. Houghton Mifflin, Boston, 1997.

Buyers, T, et al: The costs and effects of a nutritional educational program following on-site cholesterol screening. Am J Public Health 85:650, 1995.

Clark, N (ed.): Should we be getting more garlic? Environmental Nutrition 21:9, 1998.

Clinton, SK: Lycopene: Chemistry, Biology, and Implications for Health and Disease. Nutr Rev 56:2 (Part I); Feb. Tufts University, Boston 1998.

Dao, T: Taking a closer look at phytochemicals. VHL Family Alliance Home Page 1999 April (accessed 1999 April 4): Available from URL: http://www.VHL.org/newsletter/VIII1999

Hasler, CM: Functional foods: Their role in disease prevention and health promotion. Institute of Food Technologists' Expert Panel on Food Safety and Nutrition 52; Nov. 1998.

Kendall, P: Phytochemicals in disease prevention, Part 1.Colorado State University Cooperative Extension, August 19, 1998. Available from URL: (accessed 1999 April 5).

King, AK, and Young, G: Characteristics and occurrence of phenolic phytochemicals. J Am Diet Assoc 99:227, 1999.

Peiss, B, Kurlets, B, and Rubenfire, M: Physicians and nurses can be effective educators in coronary risk reduction. J Gen Intern Med 10:77, 1995.

Subcommittee on the Tenth Edition of the RDAs. Food and Nutrition Board. Commission on Life Sciences. National Research Council: Recommended Dietary Allowances. National Academy Press, Washington, DC, 1989.

Trudeau, E, and Dube, L: Moderators and determinants of satisfaction with diet counseling for patients consuming a therapeutic diet. J Am Diet Assoc 95:34, 1995.

CHAPTER 2

Individualizing Client Care

LEARNING OBJECTIVES

After completing this chapter, the student should be able to:

1. Define the terminology used in the nursing process and in nutrition assessment.
2. Describe methods of nutrition assessment.
3. Demonstrate the use of three techniques to analyze dietary status.
4. Describe the dietary exchange system and identify the exchange lists of foods.
5. Identify components of the health belief systems of large cultural groups that affect their nutrition.
6. Explain the components of various religious customs that affect individual food intake.
7. Discuss strategies to provide culturally competent nutritional care.

This chapter introduces the steps of the nursing process as they apply to nutrition, as well as the terminology and methodology used for measuring and evaluating nutritional status. Because cultural traditions influence the way people regard certain foods and the effects of those foods on health, the last section of this chapter discusses culturally competent care. Students will become aware of the influence of cultural, religious, educational, and economic backgrounds on clients' nutrition and health care.

The **nursing process** is a systematic method of planning, delivering, evaluating, and documenting care; it is used by nurses throughout the world (Akiwumi, 1994). The nursing process serves also as part of the organizing framework of the licensing examinations for registered nurses and licensed practical/vocational nurses. The nursing process is summarized in Box 2–1.

Fictional case studies throughout this book integrate the steps of the nursing process: **assessment** or data collection, **analysis** yielding a nursing diagnosis, **planning** for desired outcomes, **implementation** of nursing actions, and **evaluation**.

Terminology

Nurses and dietitians have defined the terminology used in the practice of their professions. Knowledge of this terminology will help students understand the clinical examples in the following chapters.

Standardized Nursing Language

Computerized information systems hold great potential for collecting and analyzing data pertaining to health care. For them to work most efficiently, however, the data must be in an appropriate form. Words must have standardized meanings regardless of the health-care setting.

North American Nursing Diagnosis Association

To facilitate agreement on nursing terminology, since 1982 the North American Nursing Diagnosis Association (NANDA) has worked to define and clarify the client problems nurses are licensed to treat. This work is proceeding on an international level and encompasses all of nursing, not just client problems related to nutrition. The nursing diagnoses developed thus far (North American Nursing Diagnosis Association, 1999) have been arranged in patterns and assigned code numbers within the patterns. The codes permit computerization of client records, comparison of client outcomes, and validation of nursing's contribution to health care.

Nursing Interventions Classification

In 2000, the third edition of Nursing Interventions Classification (NIC) was published, listing interventions and definitions, each followed by many nursing activities that a nurse could select to treat the client's problem (McCloskey and Bulechek, 2000). To retain the standardized language, the interventions and the definitions are used as written, but the nursing activities may be changed to fit each situation. This work carefully distinguishes the ongoing assessment activities that are part of the intervention by using the words "monitor" or "identify" to denote this use, rather than the term "assess," which is the first step in the nursing process. Linkages to nursing diagnoses by NANDA are also suggested.

Nursing Outcomes Classification

In 2000, the second edition of Nursing Outcomes Classification (NOC) was published. It includes nursing-sensitive outcomes with definitions, indica-

---

Box 2–1 Steps in the Nursing Process

ASSESSMENT

Assessment, or data collection, is an organized procedure to gather facts necessary to help the client. A physical examination of the client follows the taking of his or her history. The two types of data pertinent to the nursing process are subjective data and objective data.

The symptoms the client recounts are subjective data and not verifiable by another. Objective data can be observed and verified by someone other than the client. These data are called signs, obtainable by physical examination or through laboratory tests and diagnostic studies.

ANALYSIS

Analysis of the data involves comparing it against standards to identify problem areas. The assessment findings are shared with the client (and family or caregiver as appropriate), and the problem is defined using input from the client or his or her representative.

In many areas of health maintenance the client's active participation is essential. Often clients must learn about their diseases and treatments. If clients do not participate in the nursing diagnostic process and their priorities are not respected, they may not cooperate with treatment plans. When the treatment plan includes diet change, the client elects to follow it or not. The analysis of the client's subjective and objective data leads to a nursing diagnosis, a statement of a client's nursing problem that the nurse is licensed to treat.

PLANNING

Planning the care appropriate for the client's nursing problems encompasses two parts: a desired outcome or goal and the actions necessary to achieve it. The desired outcome describes a successful resolution to (or a significant improvement in) the nursing problem. To facilitate later evaluation of the nursing process, desired outcomes are most useful when they are client-centered, realistic, and measurable and contain a desired deadline for completion.

IMPLEMENTATION

Implementation of the plan of care includes directions for the health-care providers to produce a unified effort on behalf of the client. These nursing actions or interventions should be clear and specific so that a new person assigned to care for a client can proceed without hesitation. A correct nursing action is one that is likely to produce the desired outcome. The reason for selection of a nursing action to produce a certain outcome is called a rationale. The nursing care plans in this text contain statements of rationale to demonstrate the logical connection between desired outcomes and nursing actions.

EVALUATION

Evaluation is the process of comparing the client's status after the nursing implementation has been completed with the stated desired outcome. The nurse and client judge whether the problem has been resolved. If not, the nursing process is again set in motion beginning with an assessment.

Table 2–1 Examples of Nursing Diagnoses, Nursing-Sensitive Outcomes, and Nursing Interventions Pertinent to Nutrition

Nursing Diagnosis (Client states identified for improvement or retention)	Nursing-Sensitive Outcome (Variable client or caregiver state, behavior, or perception that is responsive to a nursing intervention)	Nursing Intervention (Nurse behavior or activity)
NANDA terminology (North American Nursing Diagnosis Association, 1999, with permission.)	NOC terminology (Johnson, Maas, and Moorhead, 2000, with permission.)	NIC terminology (McCloskey and Bulechek, 2000, with permission.)
Altered nutrition: More than body requirements	Nutritional status: nutrient intake	Weight reduction assistance
Altered nutrition: Less than body requirements	Nutritional status: food and fluid intake	Eating disorders management
Altered nutrition: Risk for more than body requirements	Nutritional status: body mass	Nutrition management
Fluid volume excess	Electrolyte and acid/base balance	Fluid management
Fluid volume deficit	Hydration	Hypovolemia management
Risk for fluid volume deficit	Fluid balance	Electrolyte management
Feeding self-care deficit	Self-care: eating	Feeding
Impaired swallowing	Self-care: eating	Swallowing therapy

Table 2–2 Admission Nutrition Screening Tool

A. Diagnosis
  If the patient has at least ONE of the following diagnoses, circle and proceed to section E to consider the patient AT
      NUTRITIONAL RISK and stop here.
    Anorexia nervosa/bulimia nervosa
    Malabsorption (celiac sprue, ulcerative colitis, Crohn's disease, short bowel syndrome)
    Multiple trauma (closed-head injury, penetrating trauma, multiple fractures)
    Decubitus ulcers
    Major gastrointestinal surgery within the past year
    Cachexia (temporal wasting, muscle wasting, cancer, cardiac)
    Coma
    Diabetes
    End-stage liver disease
    End-stage renal disease
    Nonhealing wounds

B. Nutrition intake history
  If the patient has at least ONE of the following symptoms, circle and proceed to section E to consider the patient AT
      NUTRITIONAL RISK and stop here.
    Diarrhea (>500 mL × 2 days)
    Vomiting (>5 days)
    Reduced intake (<1/2 normal intake for >5 days)

C. Ideal body weight standards
  Compare the patient's current weight for height to the ideal body weight chart on the back of this form. If at <80%
      of ideal body weight, proceed to section E to consider the patient AT NUTRITIONAL RISK and stop here.

D. Weight history
  Any recent unplanned weight loss? No _____ Yes _____ Amount (lbs or kg) _____
  If yes, within the past _____ weeks or _____ months
  Current weight (lbs or kg) _____
  Usual weight (lbs or kg) _____
  Height (ft, in or cm) _____
  Find percentage of weight lost: $\dfrac{\text{usual wt} - \text{current wt}}{\text{usual wt}} \times 100 =$ _____ % wt loss
  Compare the % wt loss with the chart values and circle appropriate value

Length of time	Significant (%)	Severe (%)
1 week	1–2	>2
2–3 weeks	2–3	>3
1 month	4–5	>5
3 months	7–8	>8
5+ months	10	>10

  If the patient has experienced a significant or severe weight loss, proceed to section E and consider the patient AT
      NUTRITIONAL RISK.

E. Nurse assessment
  Using the above criteria, what is this patient's nutritional risk? (check one)
    _____ LOW NUTRITIONAL RISK
    _____ AT NUTRITIONAL RISK

---

tors, and measurement scales (Johnson, Maas, and Moorhead, 2000). The scales have yet to be tested for validity and reliability but are a beginning step to measure progress toward a goal rather than determining only whether or not a goal has been achieved.

Even though many disciplines contribute to health-care outcomes, nursing care is a major component to the outcomes included in NOC. Here, too, the outcomes and definitions are to be used as written. The selection of outcomes depends on the nurse's clinical judgment. The outcomes are not designed to be used as goals, but an individual indicator at a specified level of attainment may serve as a goal. Linkages to nursing diagnoses by NANDA are suggested as in the NIC volume.

Examples of some of the nursing diagnoses, nursing outcomes, and nursing interventions pertinent to nutrition are listed in Table 2–1. Neither the interventions (NIC) nor the outcomes (NOC) are prescriptive. Nurses are free to select any outcomes or interventions they believe to be appropriate. The selections in Table 2–1 illustrate a variety of outcomes and interventions. Some of this standardized terminology is used in the case studies and care plans in this text.

Nutritional Terms

Nutritional terminology also involves specific meanings. Nutritional status refers to the body's condition as it relates to the intake and use of nutri-

Table 2–3 Sample Subjective and Objective Nutritional Data

Subjective	Objective
Usual diet and fluid intake	Accurate actual height and weight
Number of meals per day	
Last meal: time, foods, and amounts	Body build or frame
	Skin turgor and/or dryness
Food and nutrient supplements	Condition of teeth and gums
Appetite	
Problems with digestion and/or elimination	Hair quantity and quality
Allergies or food intolerances	Body fat measurements
	Complete blood count
Chewing and/or swallowing problems	Serum albumin
	Serum electrolytes
Use of dentures	
Usual weight and recent changes	
Likes and dislikes	

ents. All members of the health-care team have roles in the effective evaluation of a client's nutritional status. Dietary status describes what a client has been eating. Although a client's dietary status may be adequate, his or her nutritional status may nevertheless be poor. An evaluation of a client's dietary status can help to determine the reason for this poor nutritional status, or it may rule out poor diet as the source of the client's problem.

Two levels of methodology are commonly used to identify clients at nutritional risk. Table 2–2, a validated screening tool, is an example of the first level of nutritional care, *screening*. A nutritional screening should be brief enough that the information can be gathered in a short time. The time to administer the tool presented in Table 2–2 may be extremely brief; if one factor is found to be present, the screening is stopped and the client is declared at nutritional risk and referred to a dietitian.

The second level of care is a nutritional assessment. The phrase *nutritional assessment* is used differently by physicians and dietitians than by nurses. A nutritional assessment is the evaluation of a client's nutritional status (nutrient stores) based on a physical examination, anthropometric measurements, laboratory data, and food intake information. Many members of the health-care team are involved in a comprehensive nutritional assessment, including the physician, dietitian, nurse, social worker, and laboratory staff.

Because it requires many resources, this second level of nutritional care is usually completed only in the case of clients at a high nutritional risk. For example, a surgeon may order a comprehensive nutritional assessment before surgery to determine whether the client could tolerate a procedure better after nutritional rehabilitation.

The Nursing Process — Assessment

The first and most basic step of the nursing process is assessment. An organized and systematic search for pertinent subjective and objective data (Table 2–3) creates a sound foundation upon which to build health care.

Subjective Data

Subjective data as they relate to nutrition include the client's history from an interview or questionnaire. When more detailed food intake information is required, the five techniques listed in Table 2–4 may be used; some of the advantages and disadvantages of each are given.

It is interesting to note that not every technological change has an immediate benefit. Computerized programs for taking diet histories, for example, have been evaluated and judged to be adequate for epidemiological studies but not for assessment of individuals (Landig et al., 1998).

Neither reported dietary intake nor any other item of assessment data is suitable as the sole criterion of nutritional status.

Objective Data

A physical examination can include general appearance, anthropomorphic measurements, and laboratory or other diagnostic tests. Table 2–3 lists objective data relevant to a nutritional assessment.

General Appearance

Well-nourished people generally look healthy and usually have an optimistic perspective. Table 2–5 compares the appearance of a well-nourished individual with one less well nourished. A person need not display all the abnormal signs listed in Table 2–5 to be regarded as malnourished.

Anthropometric Data

For clinical purposes, body size, weight, and proportions are determined by anthropometry, the science of measuring the body. Such measurements are used to determine growth, body composition, and nutritional status. The body's energy and protein stores can be determined by these measurements.

The collection of anthropometric data on height and weight, triceps skinfold, midarm circumference, abdominal circumference, and waist and hip measurements is described briefly in the following sections. Other measurements, too, may be selected.

HEIGHT AND WEIGHT Height may be measured in inches or centimeters. Adults and older children are measured standing with head erect; infants and young children, lying on a firm, flat surface.

Weight may be recorded in pounds or kilograms. The agency policy regarding calibration of the scale should be followed. Each time the client is weighed, it should be on the same scale, at the same time of the day, and the client should be wearing the same kind of clothing.

TRICEPS SKINFOLD The measurement of subcutaneous tissue over the triceps muscle in the upper arm provides an estimate of the amount of body fat. The triceps skinfold measurement helps to differentiate between a person who is heavy because of muscle mass and one who is heavy because of excess fat.

The ability to take accurate measurements requires practice. Often research designs require the same researcher to take all measurements and record the average of two or three values at each site. Body areas other than the triceps can also be used to measure skinfolds. Although nurses usually do not make skinfold measurements, they do need to be able to answer clients' questions regarding the procedure and the information derived from it.

MIDARM CIRCUMFERENCE Because 50 percent of the body's protein stores are located in muscle tissue, the circumference (circumference is the outside edge of a circle) of the midarm provides information about

Table 2–4 Commonly Used Techniques to Obtain Food Intake Information

Technique	Comments
Comparison with the Food Pyramid Model Health care provider asks client what he or she eats and compares this reported food intake with the Food Pyramid Model.	Can be used to screen many clients quickly. Does not require a trained interviewer. Is not comprehensive. May overlook some clients who would benefit from nutritional care.
Food Frequency Health care provider requests client to fill out a questionnaire asking about usual food intake during specified times such as "What do you usually eat for breakfast?" mation collected.	Questionnaire can be tailored to particular nutrients of interest (e.g., lactose, gluten). May assess food usage for any length of time: day, week, month, weekends versus weekdays, summer versus winter, etc. Initial client contact does not require a trained interviewer. May require special resources (e.g., computer database) to evaluate the information collected. Provides limited information on a client's food behaviors such as meal spacing, length of usual mealtime, etc.
Food Records Health care provider asks client to record his or her food intake for a specified length of time (1 or 3 or 7 days).	A motivated client will provide reasonably accurate information. A less highly motivated client will "forget to keep" part or all of the food record. Research shows some clients will change their food habits while keeping a food record; therefore, this technique works poorly to assist in determining a client's dietary and/or nutritional status. This technique works well when a behavior change is desired. May require special resources (e.g., a computer database) to evaluate the information obtained. Client needs to be available for a follow-up visit to review the evaluated food records. Analysis of results is time-consuming.
24-h Dietary Recall Health care provider asks client what he or she has eaten during the previous 24 h.	Is a fairly simple technique. Interviewer should be trained not to ask leading questions. Yields limited information only about the kinds of foods and beverages consumed within the previous 24 h. The previous 24 h may not have been usual for the client. Frequently clients may not remember what they ate and the amounts they ate.
Diet History A diet history is an in-depth interview that yields information about the usual food intake, drug and medication usage, alcohol and tobacco use, financial ability to obtain food, special dietary needs, food allergies and intolerances, weight history, cultural and religious preferences that may influence food selection, ability to chew and swallow foods, previous dietary instructions received, client knowledge about nutrition, and elimination patterns.	Is comprehensive. Requires a trained interviewer who is usually a dietitian. An analysis of the results obtained can usually be provided on the same day the information is collected. Is a good technique for high-risk clients when information is needed to evaluate the need for nutritional support. Is highly dependent on the willingness of the client to reveal information to the interviewer. Client must be a good historian. Is time-consuming.

SOURCE: Adapted from Moore, MC: Pocket Guide, Nutrition and Diet Therapy. Mosby, St. Louis, 1993, p. 10, and from Mason, M, Wenberg, BG, and Welsch, PK: The Dynamics of Clinical Dietetics, p. 10. John Wiley & Sons, New York, 1982.

Table 2–5 General Appearance as an Indicator of Nutritional Status

	Normal	Abnormal
Demeanor	Alert, responsive Positive outlook	Lethargic Negative attitude
Weight	Reasonable for build	Underweight Overweight, obese
Hair	Glossy, full, firmly rooted Uniform color	Dull, sparse, Easily, painlessly plucked
Eyes	Bright, clear, shiny	Pale conjunctiva Redness, dryness
Lips	Smooth	Chapped, red, swollen
Tongue	Deep red Slightly rough One longitudinal furrow	Bright red, purple Swollen or shrunken Several longitudinal furrows
Teeth	Bright, painless	Cavities, painful, mottled, or missing
Gums	Pink, firm	Spongy, bleeding, receding
Skin	Clear, smooth, firm, slightly moist	Rashes, swelling light or dark spots Dry
Nails	Pink, firm	Spoon shaped, ridged spongy bases
Mobility	Erect posture Good muscle tone Walks without pain or difficulty	Muscle wasting Skeletal deformities Loss of balance

body protein stores. The upper arm is measured between the shoulder and the elbow. Because bone mass variations, age, and gender are not considered in this measurement (Flanigan, 1997), the midarm circumference measurement must be interpreted as part of a complete assessment.

BODY FRAME SIZE Wrist measurement is one method of categorizing a person's frame. It requires no tools or references. Have the client wrap the thumb and middle finger of one hand around the smallest part of the opposite wrist (Feldman, 1988). The body frame size is as designated below. If the thumb and middle finger:

Overlap by 1 cm or more = small frame
Meet = medium frame
Cannot meet by 1 cm or more = large frame

An alternative method is shown in Clinical Calculation 2–1. Elbow width has also been used as an indication of frame size and is the measure used in the 1983 Metropolitan Height–Weight tables (Shils, 1999).

ABDOMINAL CIRCUMFERENCE (GIRTH) The measurement of the abdomen, in inches or centimeters, is often taken at the umbilicus. **Abdominal circumference (girth)** provides information when an indi-

vidual is accumulating fluid in the abdominal cavity, a condition called **ascites**. Girth measurements are also taken to monitor growth of a fetus or of abnormal tissue within the abdomen.

WAIST AND HIP MEASUREMENTS Within an agency, a standard procedure should be used for waist and hip measurements. At one clinic the most accurate waist measurement was taken at the smallest dimension with clients lying on their backs (Jensen, 1992). The hips are measured at the largest dimension as clients stand with the feet together.

BODY DENSITY MEASURES Muscle and fat tissue have different rates of metabolism. Therefore, the proportions of each in the body influence whether a person is overweight. These proportions can be determined by several techniques, including underwater weighing, dual-energy x-ray absorptiometry, and bioelectrical impedance.

Underwater weighing (hydrodensitometry) compares the person's scale weight with his or her weight underwater. After correcting for lung volume, the examiner calculates the proportion of body fat. Underwater weighing provides the most accurate assessment of the amount of fat in the body. It is not easily determined, however. Even in research studies, several measurements must be taken and averaged to obtain a value that minimizes error. Because the technique is cumbersome and time consuming and requires special equipment, its main use is in research.

In dual-energy x-ray absorptiometry (DEXA) two x-ray beams are passed through the body. The amount of energy detected after the beams pass through the body varies with bone, fat, and muscle tissue. DEXA has been validated against underwater weighing and is another research tool (Daniels, Khoury, and Morrison, 1997). In clinical practice, DEXA is used to measure bone mineral density as an indicator of conditions marked by bone loss such as osteopenia and osteoporosis (Chapter 8). A screening test to determine a person's level of risk for those conditions can be conducted with an **ultrasound bone densitometer** that requires no radiation exposure.

In the **bioelectrical impedance test**, the greater electrolyte content and conductivity of the body's fat-free mass is compared with that of fat or bone (Baumgartner, Chumlea, and Roche, 1990). Tissues rich in water and electrolytes allow an electrical current to pass with greater ease than do denser fat and bone (Heymsfield, Nunez, and Pietrobelli, 1997). Measurements are not painful and usually are not felt at all because the frequencies used do not stimulate nerves and muscles (Jacobs, 1997). Many health-care providers commonly perform bioelectrical impedance testing.

Body composition is predicted in the bioelectrical impedance test from a measure of total body water. The client's fat-free mass is predicted, and his or her percentage of body fat is determined by comparing body weight with the predicted fat-free mass (Baumgartner, Heymsfield, and Roche, 1995). The measurements obtained are percentage of body water, percentage of lean body mass, and percentage of body fat.

These procedures were validated on adults and are not necessarily applicable to dissimilar groups of adults (Jacobs, 1997), children (Wu, et al, 1993), or athletes (Oppliger et al., 1992). A reference group whose race, age, gender, or degree of obesity are different from that of the person being measured may produce an inaccurate result (Jacobs, 1997). Prediction equations developed on healthy adults may not apply to critically ill adults or surgical clients (Jacobs, 1997). Because bioelectrical impedance is based upon total

Clinical Calculation 2–1
Determining Body Frame Type

Measure the smallest part of the wrist between the wrist bones and the hand. If the person's height is not known, measure him or her, in feet and inches, without shoes. Taking that information, look at the chart below. Find the: person's height on the left and wrist size at the bottom, and compare the shaded area with the boxes at the bottom. As an example, find the frame size of a person who is 5 ft 4 in and has a wrist circumference of 6 1/4 in. (The person has a medium frame.)

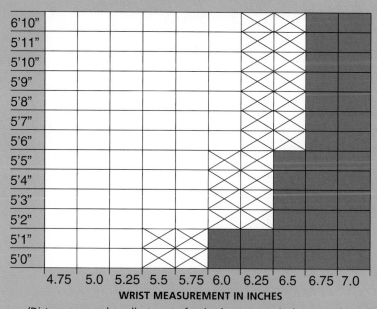

WRIST MEASUREMENT IN INCHES
(Distance around smallest part of wrist, between wrist bones and hand)

☐ = Small frame

☒ = Medium frame

■ = Large frame

body water, any factors disturbing water balance may alter the results. Examples are diuretic use, excessive sweating, hemodialysis, premenstrual edema, and alcohol consumption within the 24 hours before the test.

Laboratory Tests

Body fluids and excretions are analyzed by laboratory tests. These data include results from blood, urine, and stool tests. From these tests, much information can be obtained concerning what a person has eaten, what his or her body has stored, and how the body is using nutrients. Blood can be analyzed for glucose, protein, or fat content. Vitamin and mineral status can be determined directly by examining the blood or indirectly by examining enzymes related to the vitamin or mineral. Many experts doubt, however, that vitamin or mineral body stores can be accurately determined by blood samples. The uncertainty lies in whether the nutrient in the blood reflects body stores, a transport form of the nutrient, or the amount in one specific body compartment.

Good clinical judgment must be used in selecting tests and interpreting results. Reliance upon a single test or single reading is not recommended. Several studies have shown a thorough nutritional history and physical examination are as effective in identifying malnutrition as a battery of laboratory tests (Moore, 1993).

The Nursing Process—Analysis

The health-care provider uses subjective or objective data or both to identify the level of the client's wellness as regards nutrition. The client's data are compared with standard nutritional parameters. Those in common use include height-weight tables, body mass index, waist-to-hip ratio (WHR), the Dietary Guidelines from the U.S. Departments of Agriculture and Health and Human Services, the Food Pyramid, the Food and Nutrition Board of the Institute of Medicine's Recommended

Table 2–6 Metropolitan Life Insurance Company Height-Weight Table

Height (in Shoes*)			Men (Indoor Clothing†)						
			Small Frame		Medium Frame		Large Frame	
Feet	Inches	Centimeters	Pounds	Kilograms	Pounds	Kilograms	Pounds	Kilograms
5	2	157.5	128-134	58.2-60.9	131-141	59.5-64.1	138-150	62.7-68.2
5	3	160.0	130-136	59.1-61.8	133-143	60.4-65.0	140-153	63.6-69.5
5	4	162.6	132-138	60.0-62.7	135-145	61.4-65.9	142-156	64.5-70.9
5	5	165.1	134-140	60.9-63.6	137-148	62.3-67.2	144-160	65.5-72.7
5	6	167.6	136-142	61.8-64.5	139-151	63.2-68.6	146-164	66.4-74.5
5	7	170.2	138-145	62.7-65.9	142-154	64.5-70.0	149-168	67.7-76.4
5	8	172.7	140-148	63.6-67.2	145-157	65.9-71.4	152-172	69.1-78.2
5	9	175.3	142-151	64.5-68.6	148-160	67.2-72.7	155-176	70.5-80.0
5	10	177.8	144-154	65.5-70.0	151-163	68.6-74.1	158-180	71.8-81.8
5	11	180.3	146-157	66.4-71.4	154-166	70.0-75.5	161-184	73.2-83.6
6	0	182.9	149-160	67.7-72.7	157-17()	71.4-77.3	164-188	74.5-85.5
6	1	185.4	152-164	69.1-74.0	160-174	72.7-79.1	168-192	76.4-87.3
6	2	188.0	155-168	70.5-76.4	164-178	74.5-80.9	172-197	78.2-89.5
6	3	190.5	158-172	71.8-78.2	167-182	75.9-82.7	176-202	80.0-91.8
6	4	193.0	162-176	73.6-X0.0	171-187	77.7-85.0	181-207	82.3-94.1

			Women (Indoor Clothing†)					
			Small Frame		Medium Frame		Large Frame	
			Pounds	Kilograms	Pounds	Kilograms	Pounds	Kilograms
4	10	147.3	102-111	46.4-50.0	109-121	49.5-55.0	118-131	53.6-59.5
4	11	149.9	103-113	46.8-51.4	111-123	50.0-55.9	120-134	54.5-60.9
5	0	152.4	104-115	47.3-52.3	113-126	51.4-57.2	122-137	55.5-62.3
5	1	154.9	106-118	48.2-53.6	115-129	52.3-58.6	125-140	56.8-63.6
5	2	157.5	108-121	49.1-55.0	118-132	53.6-60.0	128-143	58.2-65.0
5	3	160.0	111-124	50.5-56.4	121-135	55.0-61.4	131-147	59.5-66.8
5	4	162.6	114-127	51.8-57.7	124-138	56.4-62.7	134-151	60.9-68.6
5	5	165.1	117-130	53.2-59.0	127-141	57.7-64.1	137-155	62.3-70.5
5	6	167.6	120-133	54.5-60.5	130-144	59.0-65.5	140-159	63.6-72.3
5	7	170.2	123-136	55.9-61.8	133-147	60.5-66.8	143-163	65.0-74.1
5	8	172.7	126-139	57.3-63.2	136-150	61.8-68.2	146-167	66.4-75.9
5	9	175.3	129-142	58.6-64.5	139-153	63.2-69.5	149-170	67.7-77.3
5	10	177.8	132-145	60.0-65.9	142-156	64.6-70.9	152-173	69.1-78.6
5	11	180.3	135-148	61.4-67.3	145-159	65.9-72.3	155-176	70.5-80.0
6	0	182.9	138-151	62.7-73.6	148-162	67.3-73.6	158-179	71.8-81.4

*Shoes with 1-in heels.
†Allow 3 lb.
SOURCE OF BASIC DATA: Build Study, 1979, Society of Actuaries and Association of Life Insurance Medical Directors of America, 1980. ©1983 Metropolitan Life Insurance Company.
NOTE: The weights presented are those associated with the lowest mortality. They are not necessarily the weights of which people are healthiest, perform their jobs optimally, or even look their best. From Metropolitan Life, Warwick, RI, with permission.

Dietary Allowances (RDAs) and Adequate Intakes (AIs), and the ADA Exchange Lists. Making a judgment on the basis of a single parameter is not recommended.

Basic Nutritional Parameters

The data collected from the client are compared with various norms and recommendations to determine an appropriate nursing diagnosis (see Table 2–1). The parameters commonly used for comparison are discussed in the next section.

Height-Weight Tables

Many height-weight tables are currently in use, each based on a different underlying assumption (see Chapter 18). Table 2–6 shows the Metropolitan Life Insurance Table, which lists weights for height based on the lowest mortality (note that it is by no means certain that the specified weights in this table are equated with maximum health). A reliable height-weight table should stipulate allowable shoe heel height and the weight of clothing. The information from height-weight tables is used to calculate a person's percentage of healthy body weight (HBW). If a range of weights is given, the midpoint of the range is used. Clinical Calculation 2–2 illustrates the process.

Body Mass Index (BMI)

The body mass index (BMI), also called **Quetelet's Index** (Keys et al., 1972), is derived from weight and height (weight in kilograms divided by the square of height in meters). It can also be calculated using common American measures as shown below.

Clinical Calculation 2–2
Percent Healthy Body Weight

The formula for calculating percent healthy body weight is:

$$\frac{\text{Client's weight}}{\text{Weight from table}} + 100 = \begin{array}{c}\text{Percent healthy}\\\text{body weight}\end{array}$$

For example, according to the height-weight table (Table 2-6), a 5 ft 5 in woman with a medium frame has a range of 130 to 144 lb, including 3 lb of clothing. Assuming she is 5 ft 5 in, barefoot, the table is entered at 5 ft 6 in, to allow for 1-in heels. The midpoint of the range is 137 lb.

If the woman weighed 137 lb, her HBW would be 100 percent. If she weighed 159 lb, her HBW would be 116 percent, calculated as follows:

$$\frac{159 \text{ lb}}{137 \text{ lb}} \times 100 = 116 \text{ percent}$$

A person at 111 to 119 percent HWB is overweight. One at 120 percent or more is obese.

1. Multiply weight in pounds by 705.
2. Divide the result by height in inches.
3. Divide the second result by height in inches.

Body mass index was designed to provide a measure of weight independent of height. Although the body mass index has been used as an indicator of obesity, it fails to distinguish adipose from muscle or water weight. Gallagher et al. (1996) determined that the BMI varied with age and gender but not with ethnicity in their sample of healthy adults who did not engage in extensive physical activity or exercise training. They concluded that BMI cannot be used as a comparable measure of fatness in men and women, because women have significantly more body fat than men for equal BMIs for all age groups. Daniels, Khoury, and Morrison (1997) documented that BMI varies with gender, race, stage of maturation, and waist-to-hip ratio in 7- to 17-year-olds. Figure 2–1 shows weight classifications using body mass indices, but as suggested earlier, clinical judgment is required to apply these classifications to individuals.

Waist-to-Hip Ratio (WHR)

To attain waist-to-hip ratio (WHR), the waist measurement is divided by the hip measurement. A WHR greater than 0.85 in women and greater than 1.0 in men indicates increased risk of problems related to obesity.

Dietary Guidelines for Americans

The U.S. Departments of Agriculture and Health and Human Services have jointly published Dietary Guidelines for Americans every five years since 1980. This publication can be read or downloaded from their Web site (Fig. 2–2). The ten guidelines for health promotion and some of the rationale for each can be found in Clinical Application 2–1.

These guidelines target the healthy general population to assist in the prevention of chronic and degenerative diseases. They do not apply to

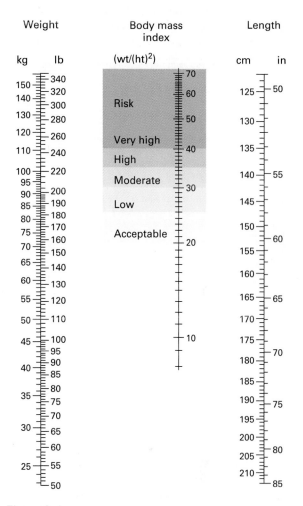

Figure 2–1:
The BMI (weight for height ranges) for adults are not exact ranges of healthy and unhealthy weights. They do show, however, that health risk increases at higher levels of overweight and obesity. Even within the healthy BMI range, weight gains can carry health risks for adults. (United States Department of Agriculture, 2000 Dietary Guidelines for Americans)

individuals who have diseases or conditions that alter normal nutritional requirements.

The guidelines are intended to be applied to several days' intake; it is inappropriate to use them to evaluate individual food items, a single meal, or one day's intake (Callaway, 1997). Wellness Tips 2–1 suggests ways to incorporate the Dietary Guidelines into a person's life.

The Food Pyramid

The U.S. Department of Agriculture created the Food Pyramid, which illustrates healthful diet choices (Fig. 2–3). Foods are grouped into categories—(1) bread, cereal, rice, and pasta; (2) vegetable; (3) fruit; (4) meat, poultry, fish, dry beans, eggs, and nuts; (5) milk, yogurt, and cheese; (6) fats, oils, and sweets—on the basis of similar nutrient con-

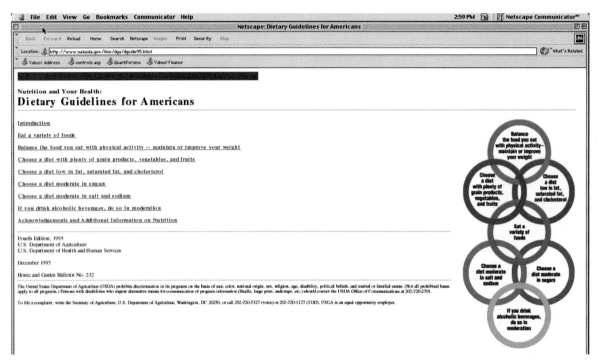

Figure 2–2:
The web site Nutrition and Your Health: Dietary Guidelines for Americans includes a comprehensive overview of nutrition for healthy living (Home and Garden Bulletin, ed 5, No. 232) by the U.S. Departments of Agriculture and Health and Human Services. The figure shows the basic structure of the new Guidelines. Much more detail on the Guidelines can be accessed at http://www.ars.usda.gov/dgac

tent. For example, foods in the milk, yogurt, and cheese group are high in calcium, riboflavin, and protein. Each of the food groups supplies some but not all of the essential nutrients, and some servings from each of the groups should be eaten daily.

Serving size (individual portion) is specified. For example, one slice of bread or 1 ounce of ready-to-eat cereal is a grain serving. A vegetable serving is one-half cup of cooked or raw vegetables or 1 cup of leafy vegetables. One medium-sized fresh fruit (apple, banana, orange), one-half cup of cooked fruit, or one-fourth cup of dried fruit is a serving. Meat group servings would be 2 to 3 ounces of lean cooked meat, poultry, or fish or 2 to 3 eggs. One cup of milk or yogurt or 1.5 ounces of cheese constitutes a serving.

In terms of quantity, the group at the base of the pyramid (bread, cereal, rice, and pasta) should be the foundation of the diet and supply the most servings eaten. The group at the top of the pyramid (fats, oils, and sweets) should provide the least number of daily servings.

Tools for Analysis of a Client's Situation

A client's reported or recorded food intake must be analyzed to reach a conclusion. The foods can be grouped according to the classifications in the Food Pyramid, or individual foods can be analyzed using a table of food composition or a computerized diet analysis program.

Tables of Food Composition

Food composition tables list foods and the amounts of selected nutrients for a specified volume or weight of the food. The U.S. Department of

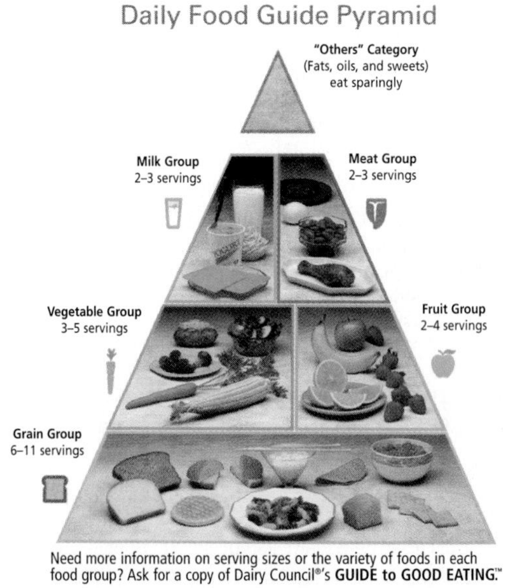

Daily Food Guide Pyramid

"Others" Category
(Fats, oils, and sweets)
eat sparingly

Milk Group
2–3 servings

Meat Group
2–3 servings

Vegetable Group
3–5 servings

Fruit Group
2–4 servings

Grain Group
6–11 servings

Need more information on serving sizes or the variety of foods in each food group? Ask for a copy of Dairy Council®'s **GUIDE to GOOD EATING.**™

Figure 2–3:
The Food Pyramid is commonly used to evaluate the dietary status of individuals and to educate clients about food choices. (Daily Food Guide Pyramid Guide to Good Eating, courtesy of National Dairy Council,® with permission.)

CLINICAL APPLICATION 2–1

Dietary Guidelines

Eat a variety of foods.
Benefits of eating a wide variety of food include increasing assurance of adequate nutrient intakes, avoiding deficiencies or excesses of any single nutrient, ensuring an appropriate balance of trace minerals, and reducing the likelihood of exposure to contaminants in any single food.

Balance the food you eat with physical activity. Maintain or improve your weight.
The chances of developing health problems are increased when a person is overly fat. Excess body fat is connected with high blood pressure, stroke, heart disease, the most common form of diabetes, certain cancers, and other types of illness.

Choose a diet with plenty of grain products, vegetables, and fruits.
Healthy adults need at least 3 servings of vegetables, 2 servings of fruits, and 6 servings of starches (preferably whole-grain) each day. These foods contain complex carbohydrates, dietary fiber, and other components that are linked to good health.

Choose a diet low in fat, saturated fat, and cholesterol.
Populations like ours with diets relatively high in fat tend to have more obesity and certain types of cancers. A high intake of saturated fat and cholesterol is linked to our increased risk of heart disease.

Choose a diet moderate in sugars.
A significant health problem from eating too much sugar is tooth decay. Contrary to widespread belief, too much sugar in the diet does not cause diabetes or hyperactivity. Sugar provides kilocalories (fuel) but few other nutrients. Thus, diets with large amounts of sugar should be avoided because they often displace other, more healthful foods in the diet.

Choose a diet moderate in salt and sodium.
A high sodium intake may predispose a person to high blood pressure. In populations with low salt intakes, high blood pressure is less common than in populations with diets high in salt. Other factors besides salt intake affect blood pressure. At present there is no way to predict who might develop high blood pressure and who will benefit from reducing dietary salt and sodium. However, most experts consider it wise for most people to eat less salt and sodium than they now eat. Such reduction will benefit those people whose blood pressure rises with salt intake.

If you drink alcoholic beverages, do so in moderation.
People who should **not** drink are children and adolescents, persons who cannot moderate their consumptions, and women who are or want to become pregnant. Alcoholic beverages are high in calories and low in nutrients. Even moderate drinkers who are overweight should decrease their intake of alcohol. Heavy drinkers often develop nutritional deficiencies as well as more serious diseases, such as cirrhosis of the liver and certain forms of cancer. Consumption of alcohol by pregnant women may cause birth defects or other problems during pregnancy; there is no known "safe" level of alcohol intake in pregnancy.

Wellness Tips 2-1

- Adding a healthy behavior is easier than eliminating a less healthy one. With the establishment of the healthy behavior, the unhealthy one may diminish.
- Eating five servings of fruits and vegetables every day would provide many nutrients known to affect health for the better.
- If milk intake is low, selecting equivalent items from this food group would also improve long-term health.
- Small increases in physical activity can help to start a person on the path to recommended levels of exercise.
- Keep score. Add one additional serving of desirable food or ten minutes of physical activity every week or two.
- Keep at it. Instant success at anything is rare; it seems to occur only because outsiders just don't see the work that preceded the success or the restarts after failure.
- Evolutionary changes in lifestyle are more likely to be lasting than revolutionary ones.

Agriculture (USDA) publishes a food composition table entitled "Nutritive Values of the Edible Part of Foods" (Appendix B). Tables of food composition serve as a practical reference in which to look up the nutritive content of a particular food or ingredients in a recipe.

Because of changes in food fortification orders (see Folic Acid, Chapter 7) and modifications in recipes or formulations of prepared foods, Tables of Food Composition must be updated periodically. Consequently, caution is urged in interpreting information from food composition tables.

Computerized Diet Analysis

Many computer software programs are available to compare an individual's intake with the RDA. Table 2–7 shows an analysis of the food intake data given in Case Study 2–1 obtained from a free website. Dietary allowances necessitate updating the software. Even before the easy availability of computer software, some nutrient databases contained blank spaces for one or more nutrient values for a given food item, and such missing data affect the final value obtained for the nutrient.

Computerized diet analysis programs can save time, but to use them correctly you must be careful when inputting data. For example, selection of "orange juice concentrate" instead of "orange juice" will skew the analysis. Even with excellent databases, the information gained from such a program needs interpretation. The only scientifically correct statement is that the intake for a given period does or does not meet the RDA. It is inappropriate to base a judgment of nutritional or dietary status solely on a comparison to the RDA.

The Nursing Process—Planning

Having assessed and analyzed a client's nutritional status, the nurse's next step is to plan a strategy that addresses any identified problems or strengths to reinforce. The Nursing Outcomes Classification lists indicators that can then be used to track progress toward a particular outcome.

In addition to traditional library sources, the Internet can deliver much information. To help evaluate the wealth of material available in

Table 2–7 Diet Analysis Web Page

VIEW INTAKE

Your Intake So Far

Food	# Units	Amount Unit Measure
Orange juice, frozen concentrate, unsweetened, diluted with 3 volume water	12	1 fl oz
Coffee, instant, regular, prepared with water	12	1 fl oz
Yogurt, fruit, low fat, 9 grams protein per 8 oz	1	1 cup (8 fl oz)
Cookies, graham crackers, plain or honey (includes cinnamon)	4	1 cracker (2½" square)
Candies, Hershey Krackel Chocolate Bar	1	1 bar (1.5 oz)
Pork, fresh, loin, sirloin (chops), boneless, separable lean only, cooked, braised	1	3 oz
Peppers, sweet, green, raw	0.5	1 cup, chopped
Broccoli, raw	1	1/2 cup chopped or diced
Celery, raw	0.5	1 cup diced
Lettuce, iceberg (includes crisphead types), raw	1.5	1 cup, shredded or chopped
Salad dressing, French, diet, low fat, 5 calories per teaspoon, without salt	2	1 tablespoon
Carbonated beverage, low calorie, cola, with aspartame and sodium saccharin, contains caffeine	1	1 can (12 fl oz)

ANALYSIS OF INTAKE

Females 19–24 years

Nutrient	Intake Amt.	RDA	% RDA
Energy	1002.364 kcal	2200 kcal	45.562%
Protein	43.912 g	46 g	95.460%
Vitamin A	211.328 mcg_RE	800 mcg_RE	26.416%
Vitamin E	3.047 mg_ATE	8 mg_ATE	38.096%
Vitamin C	262.363 mg	60 mg	437.273%
Thiamin	1.192 mg	1.1 mg	108.450%
Riboflavin	1.002 mg	1.3 mg	77.117%
Niacin	7.500 mg	15 mg	50.003%
Vitamin B-6	0.990 mg	1.6 mg	61.898%
Folate	314.266 mcg	180 mcg	174.592%
Vitamin B-12	1.528 mcg	2.0 mcg	76.41%
Calcium	557.957 mg	1200 mg	46.496%
Phosphorus	631.784 mg	1200 mg	52.648%
Magnesium	147.260 mg	280 mg	52.593%
Iron	4.675 mg	15 mg	31.168%
Zinc	4.985 mg	12 mg	41.546%

Here the food intake in Case Study 2–1 is displayed. It is compared to the RDAs for 19- to 24-year-old women (col. 3). The percentage of the RDAs for the day is reported (col. 4) and graphed (Table 2–7 (b)). The Diet Analysis Web Page was accessed at http://dawp.anet.com on 7/8/99. (Reproduced with permission.)

cyberspace, Tufts University's website, listed in the Study Aids at the end of the chapter, rates nutrition sites for content (accuracy, depth of information, and last update) and for usability. In evaluating literature, also, it is wise to regard findings cautiously, especially those of a single study, until the study has been replicated (repeated with similar results). Often findings related to health and nutrition are publicized in the general press before being critiqued by the scientific community. In general, good advice for clients is to avoid extremes of dietary practices in favor of balance, moderation, and variety.

A fundamental decision in planning client care is whether to treat the client's nutritional problems within the nursing department or to refer the client to the dietary department. Many factors affect this decision. A nurse is likely to refer the client to a dietitian if the nutritional problem is severe or complex. A lack of nursing time and resources also may necessitate a referral.

The referral system has two functions. First, it ensures that the client and his or her family receive comprehensive care. Second, it arouses clients' and families' awareness of their needs for and the benefits of nutritional services.

If the nurse decides to treat the client directly, an efficient approach is to use the same nutritional parameter to educate the client as used during the assessment. When the nurse chooses to treat the client's nutritional problems, it is crucial to prioritize the problems with the client and to select acceptable interventions. One or two changes may be easier for the client to sustain than a complete dietary overhaul. For that reason, it is important to select those interventions most likely to make a major difference in the client's health status.

The **Recommended Dietary Allowances (RDAs)** and **Adequate Intakes (AIs)** can be used to establish dietary goals for individuals.

Table 2–7(b) Diet Analysis Web Page

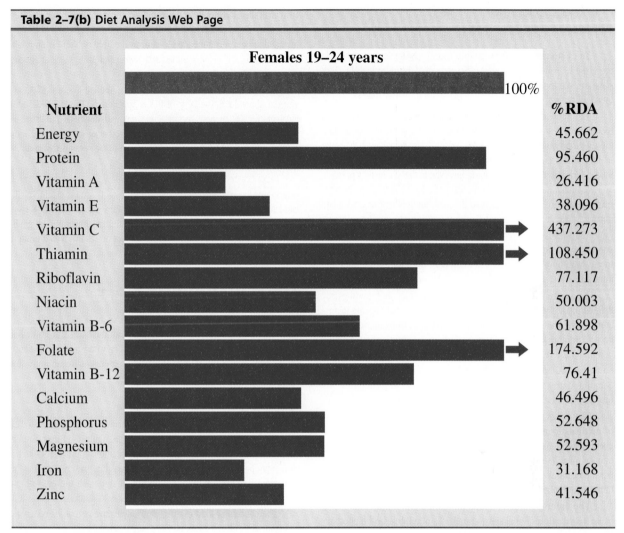

Nutrient	%RDA
Energy	45.662
Protein	95.460
Vitamin A	26.416
Vitamin E	38.096
Vitamin C	437.273
Thiamin	108.450
Riboflavin	77.117
Niacin	50.003
Vitamin B-6	61.898
Folate	174.592
Vitamin B-12	76.41
Calcium	46.496
Phosphorus	52.648
Magnesium	52.593
Iron	31.168
Zinc	41.546

RDAs and Estimated Safe and Adequate Daily Dietary Intakes (ESADDI)

Although the term "RDA" has been in use for decades, the concept is being given a new meaning and a different process to derive its values is under way. Under the system used since 1941, RDAs were defined as the levels of essential nutrients that, on the basis of scientific knowledge, were judged by the Food and Nutrition Board of the National Research Council as adequate to meet the known nutrient needs of practically all healthy people (Subcommittee on the 10th Edition of the RDAs, 1989).

RDAs were designed to be used to plan and evaluate diets for groups of people such as school children and people living in institutions. Other governments published standards appropriate to their populations. The Canadian Council on Nutrition's standards were somewhat different from those of the United States. Information was judged insufficient to list RDAs for two vitamins and five minerals. For these nutrients, only an **Estimated Safe and Adequate Daily Dietary Intake (ESADDI)** was set by the Food and Nutrition Board.

Dietary Reference Intakes

A new system of dietary reference values is gradually replacing the old system of RDAs and ESADDIs. Since 1993 the Food and Nutrition Board of the Institute of Medicine has worked to re-evaluate the RDAs, which originally focused on preventing deficiency diseases. Recent research findings support a role for certain nutrients in reducing the risk of chronic diseases. This information is evaluated as part of the process of establishing the new standards. The effort, in collaboration with Canada, has produced nutrient recommendations for North America. It is hoped that Mexico will participate in future meetings.

Dietary Reference Intakes (DRIs) are composed of four nutrient-based reference values that can be used for assessing and planning diets. The DRIs include new RDAs for some nutrients. As with the old RDAs, the DRIs are intended to apply to the healthy general population.

All DRIs refer to average daily intakes for one or more weeks. The four components of the DRIs are:

• Estimated Average Requirements (EARs)
• Recommended Dietary Allowances (RDAs)

- Adequate Intakes (AIs)
- Tolerable Upper Intake Levels (ULs)

The **Estimated Average Requirement (EAR)** is the intake that meets the estimated nutrient need of 50 percent of the individuals in a life-stage and gender group. It is used to set the RDA and to assess or plan the intake of groups.

The newly defined **Recommended Dietary Allowance (RDA)** is the intake that meets the needs of 97 to 98 percent of the individuals in a life-stage and gender group. It is intended for use as a goal for daily intake by individuals, not for assessing the adequacy of an individual's nutrient intake. It does serve as a benchmark, however, in that if a healthy person's average intake meets or exceeds the RDA, the intake is likely to be adequate. If average intake is less than the RDA, there is risk of inadequate nutrient intake.

The RDA is expressed as a single absolute value and does not take into account a person's height or weight. One might expect nutrient need to vary with body size, but present knowledge does not permit finer distinctions.

Adequate Intake (AI) is the average observed or experimentally defined intake by a defined population or subgroup that appears to sustain a defined nutritional state, such as normal circulating nutrient values, growth, or other functional indicators of health. Information on the reduction of disease risk is incorporated into the setting of AIs.

If an EAR or RDA cannot be set because of the scarcity of information, the AI may be used as a goal for an individual's nutrient intake. AIs may also be used to set tentative goals for group intakes.

The values listed for EARs, RDAs, and AIs represent the quantities of nutrients found in typical diets in the United States and Canada. If clients take supplements for the sources of nutrients or if they follow very unusual diets (such as diets consumed by individual ethnic groups), it may be necessary for caregivers to make adjustments in planning clients' nutritional intakes.

The **Tolerable Upper Intake Level (UL)** is the maximum intake by an individual that is unlikely to pose risks of adverse health effects in 97 to 98 percent of individuals in specified life-stage and gender groups.

TABLE 2–8 Correctly and Incorrectly Stated Desired Outcomes

Correct	Incorrect	Critique of Incorrect
Client will lose 2 lb per week for the next 4 weeks.	Client will lose 20 lb in 2 weeks.	Not realistic
	Client will lose 20 lb.	No deadline
Client will consume a vegetable rich in vitamin A every other day for the next 6 weeks.	Client will increase intake of vitamin A.	Not measurable
	Teach client to consume vegetables rich in vitamin A.	Not client centered

Ordinarily the UL refers to intake from food, fortified food, water, and supplements; exceptions are noted in the listing (see Appendix G). UL is not intended to be a recommended level of intake because there is no established benefit for healthy individuals associated with nutrient intakes above the RDA or AI levels.

The Dietary Reference Intakes showing AIs and the new RDAs are given in Appendix F. The table of ULs is Appendix G. The 1989 RDAs for nutrients for which new recommendations had not been published at press time appear as Appendix H. Other groups of nutrients and food components are scheduled for review as part of the revamped system.

Desired Outcomes/Evaluation Criteria

Clearly worded outcome and evaluation statements are essential to facilitate later evaluation of a client's progress toward a goal. Table 2–8 gives several examples of statements describing desired outcomes or goals. Correctly and incorrectly formulated outcomes are shown with a critique of the faulty ones.

The Nursing Process— Implementation

Once the nurse has developed a care plan with the client and his or her family, putting it into effect is the next step. It may take time and patience on the nurse's part to select appropriate interventions for an individual client or family.

Nursing Interventions

For clients requiring basic nutritional information, the activities listed as part of Nursing Interventions Classification (see Table 2–1) may simplify the task of implementing and documenting the nursing process. Complex cases may be referred to a dietitian. A given diet prescription may be implemented in various ways, but finding the approach a client will use faithfully is not only a challenge but also the key to success.

The concept of food exchanges is an effective system for educating and counseling clients about nutrition and meal planning.

American Dietetic and Diabetes Associations Exchange Lists

A food guide called the ADA Exchange Lists is published jointly by the American Dietetic Association and the American Diabetes Association. The ADA Exchange Lists are used for some clients with diabetes (discussed in Unit III) and also with clients interested in maintaining a balanced diet while modifying their food intake, such as those who are attempting to achieve a healthier body weight (Unit III). Exchange lists are used to calculate a client's food intake, to educate the client about nutrition and meal planning, and to counsel the client about food choices.

The system is composed of six lists of foods grouped by nutrient composition. For example, corn is on the starch list because it is closer in composition to a slice of bread than to green beans. It is possible to approximate a client's carbohydrate, fat, protein, and kilocalorie intake with exchange lists.

There are six basic exchange lists: (1) starch; (2) fruit; (3) milk in three groups: skim, low fat, and whole; (4) vegetable; (5) meat in

TABLE 2–9 Typical Foods in Each Exchange List

Exchange List	Food Items
Starch	Cereals, grains, pasta, dried beans, peas, lentils, starchy vegetables, bread, crackers
Meat	Beef, pork, veal, poultry, fish, wild game, cheese, eggs, tofu, peanut butter
Fruit	Fresh, frozen, or unsweetened canned fruit; dried fruit; fruit juice
Vegetable	Raw or cooked nonstarchy vegetables, vegetable juices
Milk	Milk, yogurt, evaporated milk, powdered milk
Fat	Avocado, margarine, mayonnaise, nuts, seeds, oil, salad dressing, bacon, coconut, powdered coffee whitener, cream, sour cream, whipped cream, cream cheese, salt pork

TABLE 2–10 Energy Composition of the Six Exchange Lists

Exchange List	CHO (g)	Protein (g)	Fat (g)	Calories
Starch	15	3	0-1	80
Meat				
Very lean	0	7	0-1	35
Lean	0	7	3	55
Medium fat	0	7	5	75
High fat	0	7	8	100
Vegetable	5	2	0	25
Fruit	15	0	0	60
Milk				
Skim	12	8	0-3	90
2 percent	12	8	5	120
Whole	12	8	8	150
Fat (all)	0	0	5	45

SOURCE: The exchange lists are the basis of a meal planning system designed primarily for people with diabetes and others who must follow special diets. The exchange lists are based on principles of good nutrition that apply to everyone. © With permission 1995 American Diabetes Association and American Dietetic Association.

four groups: very lean, lean, medium fat, and high fat; and (6) fat in three groups: monounsaturated, polyunsaturated, and saturated. Table 2–9 identifies typical foods in each exchange list. In addition, some foods are considered "free" and are permitted in large amounts because they contain little energy (few calories). Free foods are on a separate list. Note that some free foods have limitations on the amount to be consumed in a day or at one time. The complete exchange lists appear in Appendix A.

Table 2–10 shows the amount of carbohydrate, protein, fat, and kilocalories (energy) in one exchange on each list. As you can see from the table, one exchange on the fruit list is not equal to one exchange on the starch list. To correctly use this method of meal planning, it is necessary for clients to choose the appropriate number of items from each appropriate list.

Understanding the meaning of the term exchange is important. In this context, it means only and precisely a defined quantity of food within an exchange list. For example, one bread exchange is a single slice (a defined quantity). Individual food items within an exchange list are essentially equal to each other in nutrient composition and can thus be exchanged or "swapped" for each other. Portion sizes for various items have been adjusted to make each exchange approximately equal. For example, Table 2–11 shows items equal to one starch exchange.

Using the Exchange Lists

Exchange lists can be adapted for any prescribed kilocalorie, protein, fat, or carbohydrate level. A specific meal plan for the client to follow should be given with the exchange lists.

A meal plan is a food guide that shows the number of choices or exchanges the client should eat at each meal or snack. Table 2–12 illustrates two different meal plans for two different kilocalorie levels. One example is provided for distributing the various exchanges among meals. It is also possible to calculate different meal plans for the same kilocalorie level. Table 2–13 illustrates two 1200-kilocalorie meal plans.

Exchange lists and meal plans give clients a selection of food choices that necessitates minimal calculation. This method can also be used to control the distribution of nutrients throughout the day. For clinical reasons, many clients need to modify meal frequency.

The Nursing Process—Evaluation

At the time of the deadline stated in the desired outcome, the nurse and the client decide whether or to what degree the objective has been met. If the progress has been unsatisfactory, they explore the reasons such as unrealistic expectations, not enough time elapsed, or nursing actions not appropriate or not implemented.

A diet can be measured against three criteria: balance, moderation, and variety. A balanced diet includes foods from each of the five major food groups daily. The five major food groups are those in the Food Pyramid with the exception of fats, oils, and sweets. Moderation means avoiding too much or too little of any one food or food group. Variety means eating many different foods within each food group.

Impact of Culture on Nutrition

Culture comprises the learned, shared, and transmitted values, beliefs, and norms of a particular group that guide their thinking, decisions, and actions in patterned ways (Leininger, 1991). Although nation of origin, ethnic identity, and religious affiliation are prime examples of culture, other alliances such as colleges, corporations,

TABLE 2–11 Examples of One Starch Exchange

Puffed cereal	1 1/2 cups
Bread	1 slice
Corn, whole kernel	1/2 cup
Rice, cooked	1/3 cup

TABLE 2–12 1500- and 1800-kcal Meal Plan Using Exchanges for 1 Day

	1500 kcal	1800 kcal
Starch	7	7
Meat, lean	1	3
Meat, medium	3	3
Vegetable	4	5
Fruit	3	5
Milk, skim	2	2
Fat	6	7

DISTRIBUTION OF EXCHANGE THROUGHOUT THE DAY
1500-kcal Meal Plan

	Breakfast	Lunch	Dinner	Snack
Starch	2	2	2	1
Meat, lean	0	1	0	0
Meat, medium	0	0	3	0
Vegetable	0	2	2	0
Fruit	1	1	1	0
Milk, skim	1	0	0	1
Fat	2	2	2	0

TABLE 2–13 Two 1200-kcal Meal Plans Using Exchanges for 1 Day

Exchanges	Meal Plan 1	Meal Plan 2
Starch	5	6
Meat, lean	4	1
Meat, medium	1	3
Vegetable	2	4
Fruit	3	2
Milk, skim	2	1
Fat	4	4

individual's food choices. Figure 2–4 shows a multigenerational birthday party shaped in part by culture.

Even among individuals of similar cultural heritage, differences exist. Dietary preferences, for example, differ among people of Hispanic descent from such diverse places as Cuba, Puerto Rico, and Mexico (Loria et al., 1995). Just because a person belongs to a certain ethnic or religious group does not mean that he or she has adopted its traditional lifestyle and practices.

Ethnocentrism

The belief that one's own group's view of the world is superior to that of others is **ethnocentrism**. The dominant cultural group in the United States has been white descendants of northern Europeans who are middle class and Protestant. Education, work, punctuality, independence, and a future orientation—important values of this dominant culture—are reflected in the health-care system.

Health-care providers have tried, often unsuccessfully, to deliver this version of health care to clients without regard to the clients' cultures. Clients who failed to achieve goals that were imposed on them were labeled "noncompliant" (Wuest, 1995). Clients unable to communicate in the dominant culture's language were defined as having "altered communication" (Eliason, 1993; Levine, Ortmann, and Lunney, 1994).

The validity of a single standard of health regardless of ethnicity is questionable, because even research involving health care has systematically excluded large subgroups of the population. For example, Caucasians tend to excrete caffeine faster than Asians (Kudzma, 1992); thus standards of health related to caffeine intake that were set for Caucasians may not apply equally to Asians. Because waist-to-hip ratio norms used to identify high risk for cardiovascular disease are based on white populations, they may not be appropriate for other racial groups (Croft et al., 1995).

Acculturation

The process of adopting the values, attitudes, and behavior of another culture, **acculturation**, often puts people at risk in their overall health. For example, Latino women most acculturated into norms of the United States were least likely to initiate and to continue breastfeeding (Rassin et al., 1994).

Another adverse effect of acculturation is seen in the increase in diabetes in native populations. The major disease affecting widely scattered indigenous populations undergoing acculturation is Type II diabetes mellitus, also called noninsulin-dependent diabetes mellitus (NIDDM). The Pima Indians in Arizona have the highest reported prevalence of the dis-

professions, political parties, and service clubs also imbue people with values and norms.

Health practices draw together people of similar habits, such as athletes or vegetarians. Thus some aspects of culture are passed on from birth, but other aspects are voluntarily selected. All aspects of culture, including the family's food ways, ethnicity, and religion, may influence an

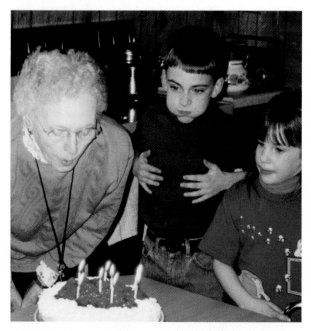

Figure 2–4:
Many cultures have their own ways to observe life's milestones: births, birthdays, weddings, deaths. These children are sharing a birthday tradition with their 88-year-old great-grandmother.

CLINICAL APPLICATION 2–2

Using Ojibway Mythology in Diabetic Teaching

The Native American adage to walk in another's moccasins offers insight into culturally competent care. A program in Toronto capitalized upon Ojibway mythology to provide instruction on the self-care of diabetes. The program was organized at the request of Native Canadians and included daylong educational workshops. These sessions were conducted by an elder, and all participants sat in a circle. The circle confers equal status on every individual and represents harmony with nature. The beginning focus was on Nanabush, a legendary teacher of the Ojibway who symbolizes moderation and balance. Traditional narratives show him conversing with Diabetes. The moral of the story is to learn about "Diabetes," to live with him, and to control one's life through spiritual strength. Workshop activities included exercise breaks and a buffet lunch that allowed participants to choose their meals. Practitioners learned that avoiding a rigid diet prescription would enhance the individual's freedom, which was highly valued among the Ojibway (Hagey, 1984).

ease (McCance, et al., 1994). In native residents of Canada and Australia the incidence of Type II diabetes is higher than in the general population of those regions (Daniel and Gamble, 1995; D'Alessio, 1995). The death rate from diabetes for native Hawaiians is more than three times that of the general U.S. population, and their mortality from heart disease is 44 percent higher (Mokuau, Hughes, and Tsark, 1995).

Culturally Competent Care

Knowledge of, acceptance of, and respect for other cultures are necessary to provide culturally competent care. The goal is a treatment plan that successfully blends the client's cultural beliefs with the practices of modern medicine. Clinical Application 2–2 illustrates the adaptation of diabetic teaching to Native American mythology.

Food Preferences of Ethnic Groups

Food items considered appropriate for human consumption vary widely by culture, and are influenced by economic and geographic constraints. The Seminole language, for instance, has no word for "vegetables," for which the word "weeds" is substituted (Nelson, et al., 1993).

Rituals of preparation may be culturally determined. Ethnic identity is important in determining staple foods, meal structure, and traditional holiday feasts.

Foods may be culturally endorsed treatments for disease. Certain foods traditionally given to children when they are sick may also bring comfort to adults. The following brief summaries describe traditional foods of five cultural groups and suggest possible applications for adapting nutritional needs to accommodate these preferences.

African-Americans

The traditional African-American cuisine features meat and greens that are cooked together as one-pot dinners to tenderize the meat and flavor the vegetables. These stews often contain pork and greens such as dandelion, turnip, and collard. Other foods often served are dried beans,

sweet potatoes, rice, grits, cornbread, and specialty gravies (red-eye, sausage, or cream).

African-Americans who choose this type of food should be encouraged to use beans, rice, and sweet potatoes but to cook without a lot of fat, such as by steaming. Traditional foods can be prepared to decrease fat consumption by baking, braising, broiling, or grilling instead of frying. Fat-free broths can be substituted for rich gravies.

Hispanic Americans

The dietary pattern we discuss here is that of Mexican Americans. Table 2–14 lists characteristic foods consumed by Puerto Rican and Cuban people as well as other ethnic groups.

Corn is the staple crop of Mexico. When corn is served with beans, the combination provides adequate protein. Vegetables and meat often are incorporated into a main dish and served with salsa. Foods are often stewed or fried in oil or lard. Fruits are popular. Sweet foods, such as yeast pastries, are common in the traditional Mexican diet, and sugar is often added to foods.

A health belief that may influence a Mexican American's food choices is the "hot-cold" system. Illness and physiological conditions are categorized as "hot" or "cold." Foods of the opposite category are eaten in an attempt to return balance to the body. Because these categories vary widely from region to region, it is best simply to ask clients what foods they would like to eat.

The traditional Mexican diet can be adapted to the recommendations of the Food Pyramid with some changes in preparation. Beans can be boiled, for example, instead of refried; beef can be grilled instead of fried; diet drinks can be substituted for lemonade or soda. The starches and fruits that are part of the Mexican American diet can be used within the Food Pyramid guidelines.

Native Hawaiians

Before the arrival of Westerners, native Hawaiians consumed a diet based on taro (a starch root similar to potato), sweet potatoes, breadfruit, fruit, greens, and seaweed. Fat content was about 10 percent of kilocalories. Foods were eaten raw or steamed.

Adopting a Western diet has been detrimental to native Hawaiians' health. The prevalence of obesity among native Hawaiians is second only to that of the Pima Indians of all the population groups in the United States. Longevity is greater in Hawaii than in any other state, except among native Hawaiians, who have the shortest lifespan of the ethnic groups.

An experimental diet was introduced to native Hawaiians to determine whether short-term diet changes could alter their risk factors for cardiovascular disease. At the start these individuals had an average BMI of 39.6. All the food was provided in two on-site meals and take-home snacks. The evening meal included a cultural or health education session. During the 3-week experiment the participants were encouraged to eat as much they wanted of traditional Hawaiian foods but limited amounts of fish and chicken. Average energy intake decreased 41 percent. Average weight loss was 17.1 pounds (7.8 kilograms). Serum cholesterol decreased 14 percent (Shintani, et al., 1991).

As discussed in later chapters, total fat and cholesterol intakes are connected to an increased risk of chronic disease. Adopting a diet that resembled that of their ancestors dramatically altered risk factors for dia-

TABLE 2–14 Characteristic Eating Patterns of Selected Cultural Groups

Group	Grains and Starches	Fruits	Vegetables	Meat and Meat Substitutes	Milk and Milk Substitutes	To Decrease Fat
Latinos Mexicans	Tortillas, corn products, potatoes, corn		Chili peppers, tomatoes, onions, beets, cabbage, pumpkins, string beans	Meat, poultry, eggs; pinto, calico, garbanzo beans	Cheese (milk seldom consumed)	Encourage: • Salsa as dip or topping • Baked corn tortillas, especially stuffed with chicken to make tamales, tostados, or enchiladas
Puerto Ricans	Platanos (starchy vegetable that looks like a large banana), Puerto Rican bread (resembles Italian bread), rice, viands (starchy vegetable whose roots and tubers are peeled, boiled, and eaten as a side dish)	Guava, canned peaches, pears, fruit cocktail	Beets, eggplant, carrots, green beans, onions	Legumes (especially red kidney beans), eggs, pork, chicken, cod, fish, pigeon, peas, garbanzo beans	Milk seldom consumed, flan (custard)	• Rice with chicken or beans • Reduced-fat cheeses Discourage: • Fried tortillas • Sour cream and regular cheese as toppings • Refried beans that are cooked in lard • Deep-fried foods such as chimichangas
Cubans	Rice		Green peppers, onions, tomatoes	Black beans, pork, chicken, chorizo, (a highly seasoned sausage)	Milk seldom used	
Italians	Pasta, yeast breads, starchy root vegetables		Green peppers, onions, tomatoes	Spiced sausages, fish, tomato-based meat sauces	Cheese (milk seldom consumed—high incidence of lactose intolerance in Italians)	Encourage: • Salad with no-fat dressing • Minestrone soup • Pasta with tomato or clam sauce • Grilled meat or seafood Discourage: • White sauces made with cream, butter, cheese • Breaded and fried meats and vegetables • Sausages and other fatty meats such as prosciutto (spiced ham)
Southern Black Americans	Cornbread, biscuits, white bread, butter beans, corn, sweet potatoes, grits, rice, white potatoes, corn, yams	Melons, bananas, peaches	Kale, collards, and mustard greens, okra, tomatoes, cabbage, summer squash	Catfish, pork, chicken, black-eyed peas, other dried beans and peas	Buttermilk, evaporated milk, ice cream (high incidence of lactose intolerance in blacks)	Encourage: • Baked fish and chicken • Steamed vegetables • Fresh melon • Grilled foods
Asians Southern Chinese	Rice	All	Mushrooms, bean sprouts, Chinese greens, bok choy	Beef, pork, poultry, seafood	Limited except for ice cream	Encourage: • Hot and sour soup; wonton soup • Steamed (not fried) dumplings
Northern Chinese	Wheat, millet seed used in noodles, bread, dumplings		Chinese greens, bamboo, alfalfa sprouts, bok choy	Beef, poultry, seafood, eggs, tofu, soybeans	None (high incidence of lactose intolerance among all Chinese)	• Lightly stir-fried chicken or seafood • Steamed whole fish • Steamed vegetables; steamed rice

TABLE 2–14 Characteristic Eating Patterns of Selected Cultural Groups (continued)

Group	Grains and Starches	Fruits	Vegetables	Meat and Meat Substitutes	Milk and Milk Substitutes	To Decrease Fat
Japanese	Rice, most other complex carbohydrates		All	Fish, beef, pork, eggs, poultry, shellfish, soybean products	None (high incidence of lactose intolerance among all Japanese)	Discourage: • Egg rolls • Crispy fried noodles • Fried rice • Deep-fried entrees • Spareribs • Tempura
Middle Eastern	Pita bread		Grape leaves	Lamb, chicken, goat, legumes	Yogurt	Encourage: • Lean beef, pork, poultry
Europeans	Bulgar, dark breads, wheat breads, potatoes	All	All, especially, onions, carrots, beans	Beef, pork, poultry, fish, shellfish, eggs, sausages	All cheese and milk products	• Broiled, poached, or steamed meats • Wine- and tomato-based sauces • Consomme Discourage: • Creamed soups and sauces • Sausages • Whole milk and whole-milk products • Fried potatoes • Sour cream

TABLE 2-15 Selected Religious Customs that Affect Food Intake

Religious	Restricted Food and Beverages
Buddhism	1. All meat.
Catholicism	1. Meat prohibited by some denominations on holy days such as Good Friday and Ash Wednesday. 2. Alcoholic beverages by some denominations.
Hinduism	1. Beef, pork, and some fowl.
Islam	1. All pork and pork products. 2. All meat must be slaughtered according to ritual letting of blood. 3. Coffee and tea. 4. All alcoholic beverages.
Orthodox Judaism	1. All pork and pork products. 2. All fish without scales and fins. 3. Dairy products should not be eaten at the same meal that contains meat and meat products. 4. All meat must be slaughtered and prepared according to Biblical ordinances. Since blood is forbidden as food, meat must be drained thoroughly. 5. Bakery products and prepared food mixtures must be prepared under acceptable kosher standards. 6. Leavened bread and cake are forbidden during Passover.
Seventh-Day Adventist	1. All pork and pork products. 2. Shellfish. 3. All flesh foods (some members). 4. All dairy products and eggs (some members). 5. Blood. 6. Highly spiced foods. 7. Meat broths. 8. All alcoholic beverages. 9. Coffee and tea.

betes mellitus and heart disease in these native Hawaiians. Some of the success was attributed to the stimulation of pride in their heritage.

Chinese Americans

Chinese cooking is based on either northern or southern traditions. Wheat is produced in northern China, where noodles and dumplings are part of the cuisine. Southern China produces rice, the staple grain for southern Chinese.

Cooking technique involves cutting meats into bite-sized pieces in the kitchen. Experience with diseases resulting from poor sanitation led to avoidance of cold water and raw fruits and vegetables. Fruits and vegetables are quickly cooked to retain a crisp texture.

Chinese medicine views sickness as an imbalance between *yin* and *yang* forces, a system that some compare to the parasympathetic and sympathetic nervous systems. Certain illnesses, foods, and medicines are categorized as *yin* or *yang*. *Yin*, or "cold," foods include pork, most vegetables, boiled foods, foods served cold, and white foods. *Yang*, or "hot," foods include beef, chicken, eggs, fried foods, foods served hot, and red foods. Noodles and soft rice are neutral, neither *yin* nor *yang*.

To maintain fluid intake, Chinese Americans prefer hot tea to ice water. Dairy products are rarely used. A caregiver interested in increasing a Chinese American's calcium intake would probably achieve better results advocating green leafy vegetables or tofu than milk. Family members may cook food at home to provide the hospitalized client with hot or cold foods (Chan, 1995). Because *yin* and *yang* cover various categories of foods, cooking methods, and colors, the perceptive nurse or dietitian can suggest items or procedures that also fit the diet prescribed by Western medicine. Clinical Application 2–3 relates such a case.

Jewish Americans

Orthodox Jews interpret dietary laws stringently. There are three key characteristics of strict kosher food preparation: (1) only designated animals can be eaten, (2) some of those animals must be ritually slaughtered and dressed, and (3) dairy products and meats must not eaten at the same meal. Separate cooking and serving utensils are used for dairy meals and meat meals. Fruits, vegetables, and starches need no special preparation and can be served with either meat or dairy meals.

> ### CLINICAL APPLICATION 2–3
>
> **Bridging *Yin* and *Yang* Beliefs and the Germ Theory of Disease**
>
> A Chinese infant was experiencing repeated bouts of diarrhea. Several tests were performed, and changes were made in the child's formula to no avail. Finally a nurse made a home visit. She discovered several bottles of home-prepared formula on the windowsill, while others were in the refrigerator. The family lived in an apartment in New York without air-conditioning, and it was midsummer. When she was asked about the procedure used to store the formula, the mother stated that because childbirth is regarded as a cold condition and she should therefore avoid cold, her husband was taking the day's bottles from the refrigerator before he left for work in the morning so they would be "warm." The nurse explained that storage at room temperature permitted bacteria to grow in the formula, which was the cause of the baby's diarrhea. Together, the mother and nurse searched for another procedure to bridge the cultural belief and the germ theory of disease. The mother decided to don a coat, hat, and gloves before opening the refrigerator to retrieve each bottle. The nurse wisely guided the mother to a solution that left her belief system intact. The infant suffered no further episodes of diarrhea (Jackson, 1993).

When a preplanned kosher meal is unavailable, a cottage cheese fruit plate is a good choice for an orthodox Jew. The cottage cheese should be transferred to a paper plate with new disposable plastic utensils because neither the plate nor the utensils used can have ever touched meat. If bread or crackers are served, labels must indicate that they contain no meat products.

Table 2–14 lists the characteristic eating patterns of selected cultural groups with suggested means of decreasing fat intake. Table 2–15 lists selected religious customs that affect food intake.

- -

Summary

The assessment of a client's nutritional status includes subjective data (knowledge of nutrition, usual intake) and objective data (general appearance, anthropometric data, body density measures, and diagnostic tests). Nursing diagnoses are derived by comparing the client's data with nutritional parameters (height–weight tables, body mass index, U.S. Dietary Guidelines, the Food Pyramid, and Recommended Dietary Allowances). Diet prescriptions and instructions may use the American Dietetic Association and American Diabetes Association Exchange Lists.

To avoid stereotyping individuals because of their ethnic or religious affiliations, the best practice is to ask clients to describe their dietary preferences. Nurses can then design nursing actions that will be meaningful to the client.

Case Study 2–1

A student in a beginning nutrition course is showing a friend the textbook. "You could help me improve my diet," the friend says. "I know I am not eating right." At the time the friend was eating a chocolate bar. The student asks the friend to list what he has eaten during the past 24 hours. From the friend's list, the student gathers the following data:

Breakfast: Orange Juice, black coffee
Lunch: Yogurt and graham crackers
Midafternoon snack: Chocolate bar
Dinner: Pork chop, green salad, French dressing, diet cola

Comparing the friend's intake to the Food Pyramid, the student finds the following:

	Number of Servings	
	Friend's Intake	*Food Pyramid*
Fats, oils, sweets	2	Use sparingly
Milk, yogurt, cheese	1	2–3
Meat, poultry, fish, dried beans, eggs, nuts	1	2–3
Vegetables	1	3–5
Fruits	1	2–4
Bread, cereal, rice, pasta	1	6–1 1

In this situation the student may not formalize a nursing care plan for the friend. The following plan illustrates the thought process involved in developing a nursing care plan for this case..

....

Nursing Care Plan

Subjective Data	Client expresses need for instruction in healthy diet. A 24-hour recall shows fewer than the recommended Food Guide Pyramid servings in all food groups except fats, oils, and sweets.
Objective Data	Client is observed eating a chocolate bar at 3 P.M

Desired Outcomes Evaluation Criteria	*Nursing Actions/ Interventions*	*Rationale*
NOC: Health Seeking Behavior (Johnson, Mass, and Moorhead, 2000)	NIC: Nutrition Management (McCloskey and Bulechek, 2000)	
Friend will keep a food record for 3 days.	Instruct friend to list everything he eats or drinks for 3 days.	Food record will gather facts about the friend's food intake to use as an instructional tool.
Friend will read the section on the Food Pyramid in student's textbook by this evening.	Lend friend textbook to read.	Providing literature utilizes expert opinion to reinforce student's teaching. Reading and seeing illustrations elicits active participation and employs senses other than hearing.
Friend will meet with student in 4 days to compare food record to Food Pyramid and design a plan of action.	Meet with friend in 4 days to sort and analyze food record data. Provide apples at meeting to model healthy snack food.	Setting follow-up visit just after food record is completed will maintain the friend's interest. Modeling desirable behavior is a technique to encourage change.

....

Critical Thinking Questions

1. When the student meets with the friend 4 days later, the friend says she has not been keeping the requested food diary. "I'm hopeless. I'll never be able to control my eating," she moans. What steps might be taken to refocus her attitude?

2. You have a friend or relative who displays food intake similar to that described in Case Study 2–1. You care deeply for this person. How might you approach the subject of healthy eating if the person does not ask for assistance?

3. Which of the nutrient groups listed in Chapter 1 is missing from the Food Pyramid? If the person in Case Study 2–1 followed the minimum Food Pyramid recommendations, to what extent would the need for this nutrient be met?

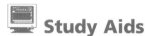

Study Aids

Subjects	Internet Sites
On standardized nursing languages	http:// www.nanda.org
	http:// www.nursing.uiowa.edu/search/index.htm
To calculate Body Mass Index	http:// www.nhlbisupport.com/bmi
On dietary guidelines	http:// www.usda.gov/cnpp/DietGd.pdg
	http:// www.nic.ca
On the Food Pyramid	http:// www.nal.usda.gov:8001/py/pmap.htm
	http:// www.usda.gov/cnpp
On Dietary Reference Intakes and other health subjects	http://www2.nas.edu/subjectindex/health.html
For cultural customs and foreign language educational materials	http://www.eatethnic.com
	http://monarch.gsu.edu/nutrition
	http://www.fcs.uga.edu/
	http://www.cdc.gov/spanish
	http://ohioline.ag.ohio-state.edu/lines/food.html
	(Scroll to cultural diversity)
For ratings of Web sites on nutrition	http://www.navigator.tufts.edu
For diet analysis	http://www.ag.uiuc.edu/~food-lab/nat/
	http://dawp.anet.com
	http://www.nal.usda.gov/fnic/foodcomp/
	http://63.73.158.75

Chapter Review

1. Which of the following statements about a nutrient analysis calculated by a computer is correct:
   a. The results obtained will not vary from one nutrient database to another.
   b. Nutrient databases using the RDA to compare and analyze results may be outdated.
   c. The results obtained are self-explanatory and need not be explained to the client.
   d. The results are always more accurate than those obtained from manual calculations using a table of food composition.
2. Which of the following is not a part of the U.S. Dietary Guidelines?
   a. Choose a diet low in fat, saturated fat, and cholesterol.
   b. Eliminate salt and sugar from the diet.
   c. Maintain a healthy weight.
   d. Vary the foods you consume.

3. Which statement about the use of the ADA Exchange Lists is true?
   a. Two starch exchanges can be substituted for two meat exchanges.
   b. Exchange lists are used to calculate an individual's RDA.
   c. An exchange is a defined quantity of food on a particular exchange list.
   d. All 1200-kilocalorie meal plans contain six starch exchanges and only lean meat exchanges.
4. Which of the following is true of the traditional Chinese yin and yang health belief system?
   a. A cold, or yin, condition is balanced by consuming hot, or yang, foods.
   b. A hot condition is flushed with large quantities of cold water.
   c. Rice is considered magical and is consumed at every meal.
   d. Yang, or hot, foods include only foods served hot.
5. Adherents to strict kosher regulations:
   a. Avoid cheese and cheese products.
   b. Eat only certain cuts of pork.
   c. Keep separate utensils and dishes for meat and dairy meals.
   d. Serve lobster, clams, and shrimp only on festive occasions.

Clinical Analysis

1. Ms. G has just been diagnosed with Type II diabetes (NIDDM). She is a Native American who has left her reservation for employment in town. Which of the following actions by the nurse shows respect for Ms. G's culture?
   a. Instructing her to increase her intake of vegetables.
   b. Telling her to lose weight and avoid alcohol and fast-food restaurants.
   c. Giving Ms. G an instruction sheet based on the ADA exchange system.
   d. Asking Ms. G how she "sees" or perceives diabetes in her life.
2. Mr. P is a 65-year-old man, recently widowed, whose physician is recommending weight loss. Mr. P has had little experience with grocery shopping or cooking. Which of the following systems for instructing Mr. P would the nurse select to offer the best chance of success?
   a. A computerized diet analysis program
   b. The Food Pyramid
   c. The ADA Exchange Lists
   d. The RDA/AI and RDA/ESADDI tables
3. Ms. E attended a community health fair where she entered her recalled intake for the previous 24 hours into a computer for analysis. On the basis of the printout she was given, she now thinks she should begin taking vitamin and mineral supplements. A friend who is a nurse correctly bases her advice on the following:
   a. A 1-day diet recall is an inadequate base to begin the supplementation.
   b. A hand recalculation should be done to verify the accuracy of the computer printout.
   c. The RDAs on which computer programs are based are intended for only the 50 percent of the population who are obsessed with health.
   d. Undoubtedly, the operators of the computer at the fair had a product to sell: "Let the buyer beware."

Bibliography

Akiwumi, A: In search of the 21st century nurse for Ghana. Int Nurs Rev 41:118, 1994.

American Dietetic Association and American Diabetes Association: Exchange Lists for Meal Planning. American Dietetic Association and American Diabetes Association, Chicago and Alexandria, VA, 1995.

Baumgartner, RN, Chumlea, WC, and Roche, AF: Bioelectric impedance for body composition. Exerc Sport Sci Rev 18:193, 1990.

Baumgartner, RN, Heymsfield, SB, and Roche, AF: Human body composition and the epidemiology of chronic disease. Obes Res 3:73, 1995.

Broderick, E, et al: Baby bottle tooth decay in Native American children in Head Start Centers. Public Health Rep 104:50, 1989.

Callaway, CW: Dietary guidelines for Americans: an historical perspective. J Am Coll Nutr 16:510, 1997.

Chan, JYK: Dietary beliefs of Chinese patients. Nursing Standards 9:30, 1995.

Cook, L: The value of lab values. Am J Nurs 99:66, 1999.

Croft, JB, et al: Waist-to-hip ratio on a biracial population: Measurement, implications, and cautions for using guidelines to define high risk for cardiovascular disease. J Am Diet Assoc 95:60, 1995.

D'Alessio, V: Running a Band-aid service. Nursing Standards 9:22, 1995.

Daniel, M, and Gamble, D: Diabetes and Canada's aboriginal peoples; the need for primary prevention. Int J Nurs Stud 32:243, 1995.

Daniels, SR, Khoury, PR, and Morrison, JA: The utility of Body Mass Index as a measure of body fatness in children and adolescents: differences by race and gender. Pediatrics 99:804, 1997.

Devine, CM, et al.: Life-course influences on fruit and vegetable trajectories: qualitative analysis of food choices. J Nurs Educ 30:361, 1998.

Diabetes Care and Education Dietetic Practice Group of the American Dietetic Association: Chinese American Food Practices, Customs, and Holidays. The American Dietetic Association and American Diabetes Association, Chicago and Alexandria, VA, 1990.

Diabetes Care and Education Dietetic Practice Group of the American Dietetic Association: Jewish Food Practices, Customs, and Holidays. The American Dietetic Association and American Diabetes Association, Chicago and Alexandria, VA, 1989.

Diabetes Care and Education Dietetic Practice Group of the American Dietetic Association: Mexican American Food Practices, Customs, and Holidays. The American Dietetic Association and American Diabetes Association, Chicago and Alexandria, VA, 1989.

Diabetes Care and Education Dietetic Practice Group of the American Dietetic Association: Soul and Traditional Southern Food Practices, Customs, and Holidays. The American Dietetic Association and American Diabetes Association, Chicago and Alexandria, VA, 1995.

Eliason, MJ: Ethics and transcultural nursing care. Nurs Outlook 41:225, 1993.

Feldman, EB: Essentials of Clinical Nutrition. FA Davis, Philadelphia, 1988.

Flanigan, KH: Nutritional Aspects of Wound Healing. Advances in Wound Care 10:48, 1997.

Gallagher, D, et al: How useful is body mass index for comparison of body fatness across, age, sex and ethnic groups? Am J Epidemiol 14:143, 1996.

Grootenhuis, PA, et al: A semiquantitative food frequency questionnaire for use in epidemiologic research among the elderly: Validation by comparison with dietary history. J Clin Epidemiol 48:859, 1995.

Hagey, R: The phenomenon, the explanations and the responses: Metaphors surrounding diabetes in urban Canadian Indians. Soc Sci Med 18:265, 1984.

Heymsfield, SB, Nunez, C, and Pietrobelli, A: Bioimpedance analysis: What are the next steps? Nutr Clin Prac 12:201, 1997.

Jackson, LE: Understanding, eliciting and negotiating clients' multicultural health beliefs. Nurse Pract 18:30, 1993.

Jacobs, DO: Bioelectrical impedance analysis: Implications for clinical practice. Nutr Clin Prac 12:204, 1997.

Jensen, M: Research techniques for body composition assessment. J Am Diet Assoc 92:454, 1992.

Johnson, M, Maas, M, and Moorhead, S: Nursing Outcomes Classification (NOC), ed 2. Mosby, St. Louis, 2000.

Keys, A, et al.: Indices of relative weight and obesity. J Chron Dis 25:329, 1972.

Kovacevich, DS, et al: Nutrition risk classification: A reproducible and valid tool for nurses. Nutr Clin Prac 12:20, 1997.

Kudzma, EC: Drug response: All bodies are not created equal. Am J Nurs 92(12):48, 1992.

Landig, J, et al.: Validation and comparison of two computerized methods of obtaining a diet history. Clin Nutr 17:113, 1998.

Larson, E: Exclusion of certain groups from clinical research. Image 26:185, 1994.

Leininger, M: The theory of culture care diversity and universality. In Leininger, M (ed): Culture Care Diversity and Universality: A Theory of Nursing. National League for Nursing Press, New York, 1991.

Levine, MA, Ortmann, D, and Lunney, M: Nursing diagnosis in crosscultural settings. Nurs Diag 5:158, 172, 1994.

Loria, CM, et al: Macronutrient intakes among adult Hispanics: A comparison of Mexican Americans, Cuban Americans, and mainland Puerto Ricans. Am J Pub Health 85:684, 1995.

Mason, M, Wenberg, BG, and Welsch, PK: The Dynamics of Clinical Dietetics. John Wiley & Sons, New York, 1982.

McCance, DR, et al: Birthweight and non-insulin dependent diabetes: Thrifty genotype, thrifty phenotype, or surviving small baby genotype? Br Med J 308:942, 1994.

McCloskey, JC, and Bulechek, GM: Nursing Interventions Classification (NIC), ed 3. Mosby, St. Louis, 2000.

Metropolitan Life Insurance Company Height-Weight Table. Metropolitan Life, Warwick, RI, 1983.

Moggatt, MEK: Current status of nutritional deficiencies in Canadian aboriginal people. Can J Physiol Pharmacol 73:754, 1995.

Mokuau, N, Hughes, CK, and Tsark, JAU: Heart disease and associated risk factors among Hawaiians: Culturally responsive strategies. Health Soc Work 20:46, 1995.

Moore, MC: Pocket Guide, Nutrition and Diet Therapy. Mosby, St Louis, 1993.

National Academy of Sciences: Dietary Reference Intakes. Nutr Rev 55:319, 1997.

National Academy of Sciences: Origin and framework of the development of Dietary Reference Intakes. Nutr Rev 55:332, 1997.

National Academy of Sciences: Uses of Dietary Reference Intakes. Nutr Rev 55:327, 1997.

National Research Council: Diet and Health: Implications for Reducing Chronic Disease Risk. Report of the Committee on Diet and Health, Food and Nutrition Board, Commission on Life Sciences. National Academy Press, Washington, DC, 1989.

Nelson, M, et al: Problem of changing food habits: Reaching disadvantaged families through their own food cultures. In Karp, RJ (ed): Malnourished Children in the United States. Springer, New York, 1993.

North American Nursing Diagnosis Association: NANDA Nursing Diagnoses: Definitions and Classification, 1999–2000. North American Nursing Diagnosis Association, Philadelphia, 1999.

Opplinger, RA, et al: Body composition of collegiate football players: Bioelectrical impedance and skinfolds compared to hydrostatic weighing. J Orthop Sports Phys Ther 15:187, 1992.

Pacy, PJ, et al: Body composition measurement in elite heavyweight oarswomen: A comparison of five methods. J Sports Med Phys Fitness 35:67, 1995.

Rassin, DK, et al: Acculturation and the initiation of breastfeeding. J Clin Epidemiol 47:739, 1994.

Reimers, KJ, and Lind, R: Making the most of diet analysis software. Strength and Conditioning 19:72, 1997.

Rooubenoff, R, Dallal, GE, and Wilson, PWF: Predicting body fatness: The body mass index vs estimation by bioelectrical impedance. Am J Public Health 85:726, 1995.

Shils, ME, et al (eds): Modern Nutrition in Health and Disease, ed 9. Williams and Wilkins, Baltimore, 1999.

Shintani, TT, et al: Obesity and cardiovascular risk intervention through the ad libitum feeding of traditional Hawaiian diet. Am J Clin Nutr 53:1647S, 1991.

Stolarczyk, LM, et al: The fatness-specific bioelectrical impedance analysis equations of Segal et al: are they generalizable and practical? Am J Clin Nutr 66:8, 1997.

Subcommittee on the Tenth Edition of the RDAs. Food and Nutrition Board. Commission on Life Sciences. National Research Council: Recommended Dietary Allowances. National Academy Press, Washington, DC, 1989.

United States Departments of Agriculture and Health and Human Services: Dietary Guidelines for Americans, ed 5. Washington, DC, 2000. Accessed 6/26/2000 at http://www.usda.gov/cnpp/DietGd.pdf

Wu, Y, et al: Cross-validation of bioelectrical impedance analysis of body composition in children and adolescents. Phys Ther 73:320, 1993.

Wuest, J: Removing the shackles: A feminist critique of noncompliance. Nurs Outlook 41:217, 1993.

Yates, AA, Schlicker, SA, and Suitor, CW: Dietary Reference Intakes: the new basis for recommendations for calcium and related nutrients, B vitamins, and choline. J Am Diet Assoc 98:699, 1998.

Carbohydrates

Carbohydrates, fats, and proteins all meet the body's basic energy needs. Carbohydrates, however, are recommended as the major source of energy because they break down rapidly and are therefore readily available for use by the body. This chapter discusses the body's use of carbohydrates and the way carbohydrates relate to the other energy nutrients.

Carbohydrates are manufactured by green plants during photosynthesis, a complex process in which sugars and starches are formed in the plant from the combination of carbon dioxide from the air and water from the soil. Sunlight and the green plant pigment chlorophyll are necessary for this conversion. Through photosynthesis the sun's energy is transformed into food energy in the form of carbohydrates.

Carbohydrates may be divided into two major groups: sugars and starches. The chemical structure of each carbohydrate determines whether it is a sugar or starch. Sugars have a simple chemical structure whereas starches are more complex. Therefore sugars are often called simple carbohydrates and starches complex carbohydrates. The terms sugar, starch, simple, and complex all refer to the intricacy of the chemical structure of the carbohydrate.

Composition of Carbohydrates

Understanding the composition of carbohydrates involves understanding three structures: molecule, element, and atom. A **molecule** is the smallest quantity into which a substance may be divided without loss of its characteristics. For example, water's formula is H_2O. If the hydrogen atoms are pulled apart from the oxygen atom, the resulting products are hydrogen and oxygen, which bear no resemblance to water. Molecules are made of elements. In the case of water, H_2O, the elements are hydrogen and oxygen. An **element** is a substance that cannot be separated into simpler parts by ordinary means. An **atom** is the smallest particle of an element that retains its physical characteristics.

Classification of Carbohydrates

Carbohydrates are composed of the elements carbon, hydrogen, and oxygen. The ratio of hydrogen to oxygen is the same as that for water, two parts of hydrogen to one part of oxygen. The simplest carbohydrates have the formula $C_6H_{12}O_6$. Carbohydrates in general are frequently abbreviated CHO.

Simple carbohydrates, sugars, include monosaccharides and disaccharides (mono means "one," di means "two," and saccharide means "sweet"). Starches are also called polysaccharides.

Simple Carbohydrates

A **monosaccharide** contains one molecule of $C_6H_{12}O_6$. A **disaccharide** is composed of two molecules of $C_6H_{12}O_6$ joined together (minus one unit of H_2O). When the body joins two molecules of monosaccharides together, a molecule of water is released in the process. Both monosaccharides and dissacharides are classified as simple carbohydrates.

Monosaccharides

The monosaccharides are the building blocks of all other carbohydrates. The three monosaccharides of importance in human nutrition are *glucose, fructose,* and *galactose.* Note the ose ending in the name of each of these sugars. All monosaccharides and disaccharides end with the letters "ose."

GLUCOSE The monosaccharide glucose in the body is commonly called the blood sugar. It is the major form of sugar in the blood. Normal fasting blood sugar (FBS) is 70 to 100 milligrams per 100 milliliters of serum or plasma. Regardless of the form of sugar consumed, the body readily converts it to glucose. Glucose is present in only small amounts in some fruits and vegetables and is moderately sweet.

Another name for glucose is dextrose. In all health care facilities some clients are on intravenous feedings (intravenous simply means "within or into a vein"). The most common intravenous feeding is D5W, used primarily to deliver fluids to the client. The abbreviation D5W means that the solution contains 5 percent dextrose (glucose) in water.

FRUCTOSE Found in fruits and honey, fructose is commonly referred to as the honey sugar. It is the sweetest of all the monosaccharides. Relatively new on the list of food sweeteners is high-fructose corn syrup. Fructose is used extensively in soft drinks, canned foods, and various other processed foods. The human body readily converts fructose to glucose after ingestion.

GALACTOSE The monosaccharide galactose comes mainly from the breakdown of the milk sugar lactose. Yogurt and unaged cheese may contain free galactose. It is the least sweet of all the monosaccharides. The body converts galactose into glucose after ingestion.

Disaccharides

When two monosaccharides are linked together, a disaccharide is formed. The three disaccharides of importance are sucrose, lactose, and maltose.

SUCROSE The most prevalent disaccharide, sucrose, is ordinary white table sugar made commercially from sugar beets and sugar cane. Brown, granulated, and powdered sugars are all forms of sucrose. Sucrose is also found in molasses, maple syrup, and fruits. The two monosaccharides joined together to form sucrose are glucose and fructose. The average American's total daily intake of both sucrose and fructose is considered

excessive and has been estimated at 84 grams a day (Guthrie and Morton, 2000). See Clinical Calculation 3–1 for an explanation of converting grams of simple sugars to teaspoons of sugar. This calculation is designed to help you learn to read and interpret food labels.

LACTOSE Because it occurs naturally only in milk, lactose is commonly referred to as the milk sugar. Lactose is the least sweet of the disaccharides. The two monosaccharides that make up lactose are glucose and galactose.

MALTOSE The disaccharide maltose is produced when starches are broken down by the body into simpler units. This disaccharide is present in malt, malt products, beer, some infant formulas, and sprouting seeds. Maltose consists of two units of glucose joined together.

SUGAR ALCOHOLS Food labels use the term "sugar alcohols" (Figure 3–1). Sugar alcohols have various names such as sugar replacers, "polyols," "nutritive sweeteners," and "bulk sweeteners." Lactitol, maltitol, isomalt, sorbitol, xylitol, and mannitol are all sugar alcohols (also called sugar replacers) and currently are approved for use in the United States. Sugar alcohols are commonly used on a one-for-one replacement basis for sugars in recipes. For example, one cup of sugar would be replaced with one cup of isomalt in a recipe. Sugar alcohols add not only sweetness but also bulk to recipes. Sugar alcohols have these characteristics (www.caloriecontrol.org/isomalt).

- Generally do not promote tooth decay
- Commonly have a cooling effect on the tongue
- Are slowly and incompletely absorbed from the intestine into the blood
- May have a laxative effect for some people if consumed in excess.

Generally sugar alcohols provide a sweet taste in the mouth without being absorbed in the body. They exit the body in the feces. Sugar replacers have been known to cause diarrhea. If a patient who previously has not

---

Clinical Calculation 3–1 Converting Grams of Sugar into Teaspoons of Sugar

The average American's intake of sugar is considered excessive and has been approximated to be 80 g of sugar per day and 18 percent of kcal (National Research Council, 1989).

The expression "eighty grams of sugar" does not mean much to the average American consumer, since most Americans are unfamiliar with the metric system. Many food labels use the metric system to list the nutritional content of a product. To convert grams of sugar to its equivalent in teaspoons, remember one teaspoon of sugar contains 4 g of carbohydrate.

$$\frac{80 \text{ g of sugar}}{4 \text{ g of sugar per tsp}} = 20 \text{ tsp of sugar}$$

Eighty grams of sugar is equal to 20 tsps. Table 3–1 lists sweeteners that also contain 4 g of carbohydrate per tsp. Figure 3-I provides another opportunity to convert grams of sugar to teaspoons of sugar.

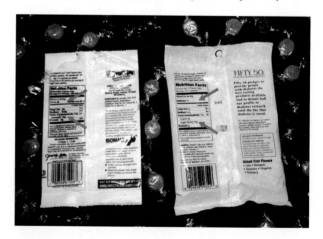

Figure 3–1:
The sugar replacement isomalt is displayed on the candy label on the left. Note that the product contains 15 grams of isomalt and 15 grams of carbohydrate. This means that the sole source of carbohydrate in this product is isomalt. The label on the left is another example of a sugar replacement. This product contains 16 grams of a sugar alcohol.

Box 3–1 Artificial Sweeteners

Artificial Sweetener	Trade Name	Comments
Aspartame Http://www.aspartame.org	Nutrasweet Equal	Used in sweetened products such as puddings, gelatins, frozen desserts, yogurt, hot cocoa mixes, powdered soft drinks, carbonated beverages, teas, breathe mints, chewing gums, some vitamins and cold preparations. Also used as a table-top sweetener. Reviewed by such regulatory agencies as the Centers for Disease Control (CDC) and Food and Drug Administration (FDA) and found to be safe. Should not be used by individuals with a rare genetic disease called Phenylketonuria (PKU). Artificial sweetener.
Saccharin	Sweet N Low Sugar Twin	Carbonated beverages, toothpaste, cold remedies, dietetic puddings, cakes, cookies, etc. Saccharin was banned in Canada in 1977. The U.S. Food and Drug Administration also proposed a ban on saccharin but Congress passed a moratorium on the ban until 2002. Although high doses of saccharin were shown to cause bladder cancer in male rats, numerous human studies have shown no association between saccharin and cancer at human levels of consumption.
Sucralose	Splenda	Only noncaloric sweetener made from sugar. Approved for use by the Food and Drug Administration (FDA).
Stevia	Stevia	Natural alternative sweetener which is classified as an herb. It is sold as a dietary supplement. Stevia has not gone through the FDA approval process as a sweetener.

had diarrhea and after the introduction of a new medication or oral food supplement develops loose stools, check the label of the product to see if sorbitol is one of the ingredients.

Intense Sweeteners

Intense sweetener is the new terminology for "non-nutritive sweeteners" or artificial sweeteners (Box 3–1). Note that intense sweeteners are not sugar replacers. They do not add bulk or volume to a food product, only sweetness. They are 150 to 500 times sweeter than sugar and are mostly artificial/synthetic.

Complex Carbohydrates (Polysaccharides)

More chemically complex carbohydrates are called polysaccharides. Poly means many, and polysaccharides are many molecules of $C_6H_{12}O_6$ joined together, with many molecules of water released. Polysaccharides can be com-

Table 3–1 Composition of Carbohydrates

Elements	C (carbon)
	H (hydrogen
	O (oxygen)
Molecule	$C_6H_{12}O_6$
Monosaccharide (simple)	One unit of $C_6H_{12}O_6$
Disaccharide (simple)	Two units of $C_6H_{12}O_6$ minus one unit of H_2O
Polysaccharide (complex)	Many units of $C_6H_{12}O_6$ minus many units of H_2O

posed of various numbers of monosaccharides and disaccharides. The three types of complex carbohydrates of nutritional importance are starch, glycogen, and fiber. Table 3–1 summarizes the composition of carbohydrates.

Starch

Starch, the major source of carbohydrate in the diet, is found primarily in grains, cereals, breads, pasta, starchy vegetables, and legumes. Legumes include dried peas and beans such as black beans, pinto beans, kidney beans, navy beans, soybeans, black-eyed peas, split green or yellow peas, chick peas (garbanzo beans), and lentils. Many consumers erroneously believe that complex carbohydrate foods are fattening. In fact, gram for gram, fat has more than twice the kilocalories of carbohydrates. Strictly speaking, all starches yield simple sugars on digestion; starchy foods are mostly low in fat and high in carbohydrates, and some starchy foods have the advantage of containing much fiber (discussed in a later section).

Glycogen

The polysaccharide glycogen is commonly called the animal starch. It is a starchlike substance stored in the liver and muscle tissues that is changed to glucose as needed for muscular work and for conversion to heat. Glycogen represents the body's carbohydrate stores. Liver glycogen helps sustain blood glucose levels during sleep.

The typical human body has an available store of glucose in the form of glycogen for about one day's energy needs. Because the body's ability to store carbohydrate in the form of glycogen is limited, an adequate intake of dietary carbohydrates is essential. When glycogen is stored, water is also stored. Each glycogen molecule attracts many molecules of water because of the way the elements are arranged. With glycogen stores completely filled, the average person weighs about 4 pounds more than when glycogen stores are empty.

Dietary Fiber

Dietary fiber refers to food constituents, mostly from plants, that the human body cannot break down or digest. Fiber is eliminated from the body in the form of fecal material. Sometimes called roughage or bulk, fiber adds almost no fuel or energy value to the diet, but it does add volume.

Experts recommend that a healthy adult eat 20 to 35 grams of dietary fiber a day. Among the reported benefits of fiber are that it promotes regularity, may reduce risk of cancer and diverticular disease, may reduce cholesterol levels, may assist in the control of blood sugar, and may promote weight loss. In the United States the average person consumes only about 11 grams of dietary fiber per day, and few people ingest the recommended levels (Slavin, 1995).

Eating too much fiber can also cause problems. Much evidence suggests that eating more than 50 grams of fiber a day can interfere with mineral absorption, which can lead to problems like anemia and osteoporosis. Healthy people should achieve a desirable fiber intake not by adding fiber concentrates (like Metamucil) to the diet but by eating fruits, vegetables, legumes, and whole-grain cereals, excellent sources of fiber that also provide minerals and vitamins.

Fiber is classified as either soluble or insoluble. **Solubility** is the ability of one substance to dissolve in another. For example, oil does not dissolve in water, so oil is insoluble in water. Insoluble fiber does not dissolve in water, whereas soluble fiber does. Soluble and insoluble fiber react differently in the body and are needed for different reasons (Wellness Tip 3–1).

SOLUBLE FIBER Sources of soluble fibers include beans, oatmeal, barley, broccoli, and citrus fruits; oat bran is a particularly good source of soluble fiber. Soluble fiber dissolves in water and thickens to form gels. The reported health benefits of soluble fibers include reduced cholesterol levels, regulated blood sugar levels, and weight loss (by helping dieters control their appetites).

INSOLUBLE FIBER Examples of sources of insoluble fibers include the woody or structural parts of plants, such as fruit and vegetable skins, and the outer coating (bran) of wheat kernels. Insoluble fibers have been reported to promote regularity of bowel movements and reduce the risk of diverticular disease and some forms of cancer. Table 3–2 lists the food sources of each type of fiber and their reported health benefits.

Functions of Carbohydrates

Carbohydrates play the following roles in the body:

1. Provide fuel
2. Spare body protein
3. Help prevent ketosis
4. Enhance learning and memory processes.

Wellness Tip 3-1

- Include foods that contain both soluble and insoluble fiber in the diet.

TABLE 3–2 Food Sources and Reported Benefits of Fiber

	Insoluble Fiber	Soluble Fiber
Solubility	Does not dissolve in water	Dissolves in water
Food Sources	Wheat bran Corn bran Vegetables Nuts Fruit skins Some dry beans*	Oatmeal Oat bran, barley Some fruits such as apples, oranges Broccoli Some dry beans*
Reported Benefit	Promotes regularity May help reduce risk of some forms of cancer May reduce risk of diverticular disease	May help reduce cholesterol levels May assist in regulating blood sugar levels May promote weight loss by Increasing satiety†

*Current laboratory methods to assay soluble fiber content of individual foods are imprecise. This is the subject of much research.
†Satiety is defined as the sensation of fullness aster eating.

Provide Fuel

Just as gasoline is a car's fuel, so carbohydrates, proteins, and fats are the human machine's fuel. The brain, other nervous tissue, and the lungs use carbohydrate as a primary source of fuel. Because the brain cannot store carbohydrate, it must have an uninterrupted, ongoing source of carbohydrate. This need has many clinical implications, which will be discussed throughout this book.

Spare Body Protein

When we eat an inadequate amount of carbohydrates, our bodies suffer. We must have a continuous supply of glucose for all cells to function, particularly those of the central nervous system. Remember that our glycogen stores are limited. But the body can convert protein to glucose. Therefore, the body will break down internal protein stores (muscle tissue) before fat stores if carbohydrate intake is inadequate. An adequate supply of dietary carbohydrates spares body protein stores from being partially converted into glucose and allows protein to be used for growth and repair of body tissue. This principle has important ramifications for human nutrition, which will be discussed throughout the text

Help Prevent Ketosis

A balanced intake of energy nutrients is vital. If a person's carbohydrate intake is too low, the body will break down both stored fat and internal protein stores to meet its fuel needs. The human machine cannot optimally handle the excessive breakdown of stored body fat because it lacks the necessary equipment. As a result, partially broken-down fats accumulate in the blood in the form of ketones, and the person is said to be in a state of ketosis. Survival is possible on a very low carbohydrate diet but good health is not (Wellness Tip 3–2).

Fatigue, nausea, and lack of appetite are some of the undesirable consequences of ketosis. Coma and death have occurred in severe cases.

Wellness Tip 3-2

- Include adequate carbohydrate in the diet to spare body protein stores and prevent ketosis.

The presence of ketosis is easily determined by testing for the presence of acetone or diacetic acid in the urine. Acetone and diacetic acid are ketone bodies. A minimum of 50 to 100 grams of carbohydrate each day is usually enough to prevent ketosis.

Enhance Learning and Memory

Considerable evidence exists that blood glucose concentrations regulate several brain functions. Glucose enhances learning and memory in healthy, aged humans. In one study, subjects were asked to recall information from a previously read short story. Glucose improved by approximately 17 to 34 percent the performance expected of age-matched healthy subjects (Gold, 1999). Another study showed that glucose enhanced retention in or retrieval from long-term memory (Foster, Lidder, and Sunram, 1997). The process by which memory formation is regulated involves glucose.

Consumption Patterns

Most of the world's population subsists primarily on carbohydrates. Foods rich in carbohydrates are easily grown in most climates, are low in cost, and are easily stored. Many carbohydrates do not require refrigeration or electricity, and their shelf life may stretch to years. In Asia, where rice is a dietary staple, carbohydrates provide as much as 80 percent of the fuel in the diet.

In 1909 Americans obtained about 66 percent of their total carbohydrate intake from starches such as corn, potatoes, wheat, and beans, and about 33 percent from sugars such as table sugar, maple sugar, molasses, jelly, and jam. By 1980, sugars furnished more than 50 percent of the carbohydrates in the food supply. Between 1994 and 1996, Americans aged 2 years and older consumed 20-1/2 teaspoons per day of added sugar (Guthrie and Morton, 2000). The largest source of added sweeteners was regular soft drinks, which accounted for one-third of intake.

The United States government has monitored food consumption trends since 1971. The surveys are known as National Health and Nutrition Examination Surveys NHANES. NHANES I was conducted between 1971 and 1974, NHANES II between 1976 and 1980, the Hispanic HANES (HHANES) between 1982 and 1984, and NHANES III between 1988 and 1994.

A comparison of data from NHANES II to NHANES III shows an increase in amount of carbohydrate average Americans consume (Rolls and Hill, 1998), not so much from starch but from sugar. Excessive sugar intake has replaced dietary constituents such as fiber and other nutrients. For example, one study showed children who habitually consumed soft drinks had lower intakes of milk and fruit juices (Harnack, Stang, and Story, 1999) (Wellness Tip 3-3).

Wellness Tip 3-3

- Be careful that regular soft drinks do not displace milk and fruit juices in the diet.

Relationship to Dental Health

Several studies have shown a relationship between carbohydrate consumption and dental caries, the gradual decay of the teeth. A dental cavity is a hole in a tooth caused by dental caries. The interaction of four factors is necessary to cause dental caries: a genetically susceptible tooth, bacteria, carbohydrate, and time (Figure 3-2).

Genetic Susceptibility

Genetic susceptibility is an individual's likelihood of developing a given trait as determined by heredity. Genetics is one reason each client must be evaluated as unique.

Other Factors Related to Cavity Formation

Bacteria, carbohydrate-containing foods, and the length of time that teeth are exposed to sugars influence cavity formation. Bacteria normally present in the mouth interact with dietary carbohydrates and produce acids. The acids, not the sugar, cause decay. All types of sugars can promote cavity formation, including fructose, glucose, maltose, lactose, and sucrose.

A strong relationship exists between the length of time sugars are actually present in the mouth and the development of caries. For example, sticky foods like caramels and raisins, which adhere to the tooth surface for longer periods, are more likely to lead to tooth decay in susceptible people. Sipping sweetened beverages continually throughout the day can also lead to tooth decay. Clinical Application 3-1 discusses a common health care problem known as nursing-bottle syndrome.

Certain foods may help counteract the effects of the acids produced by oral bacteria. Aged cheese (cheddar, Swiss, blue, Monterey jack, Brie, gouda), as well as processed American cheese, may inhibit tooth decay. Cheese stimulates the production of saliva. Chewing fibrous foods such as apples or celery stimulates the production of generous amounts of saliva. Saliva helps clear the mouth of food and counteracts acid production. Because saliva production is increased during a meal, sugars eaten with a meal are less likely to cause decay than those eaten between meals.

Food Sources

As indicated earlier, carbohydrates fall into two general groups: sugars and starches. All starches contain fiber; however, all starches do not provide equal amounts of fiber.

CLINICAL APPLICATION 3-1

Nursing-Bottle Syndrome

Nursing-bottle syndrome is a dental condition caused by the frequent and prolonged exposure of an infant or young child to liquids containing sugars. Milk, formula, fruit juice, or other sweetened drinks can all cause rampant dental caries.

Typically, nursing-bottle syndrome occurs when a caretaker habitually puts a baby to bed with a bottle of milk, juice, or other sweetened liquid. During sleep the flow of saliva decreases, which allows the liquids from the nursing bottle to pool around the teeth, undiluted, for extended periods. Mothers need to be cautioned against this practice.

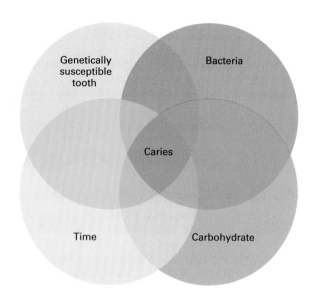

Figure 3–2:
Interactions necessary for dental caries formation. Each of these four variables is necessary for a cavity to form. We cannot control our genetic susceptibility for cavities, and bacteria are always present in our mouths and difficult to eliminate. However, we can control the length of time foods containing carbohydrates are in our mouths and the kinds of carbohydrates we eat.

Sugars

Sugar, as mentioned in Clinical Calculation 3–1, contains 4 grams of carbohydrates per teaspoon. When determining a person's sugar consumption, we consider not only the simple sugars such as honey, jam, and jelly but also the sugars present in carbonated beverages, ice cream, sherbet, cakes, pies, cookies, and donuts. Tables of food composition may be used to approximate the actual intake a person may have from combination foods (see Appendix B). Simple sugar intake can be estimated using the value of 4 grams of carbohydrates per teaspoon (see Table 3–3). The new sugar replacers contain on the average about 2 grams of carbohydrate per teaspoon.

Starches

Starches are complex carbohydrates and are important sources of fiber and other nutrients. Figure 3–3 illustrates a typical cereal grain. Its main parts, the germ, bran, and endosperm, are labeled. Most of the nutrients in cereal are in the bran and germ.

Emphasis on Whole Grain

During the milling of grain, the germ and bran from the grain kernel are removed. Products made from the milling process are said to be refined. White flour results from the milling of wheat, white rice from the milling of rice. Oat products are not normally milled. Refined cereals and bread products are not as nutritious as their whole-grain counterparts because the bran and germ contain appreciable vitamins, minerals, and fiber. The

Table 3–3 Sweeteners that Contain 4 Grams of Carbohydrates per Teaspoon
Molasses
Granulated sugar
Powdered sugar
Syrup
Brown sugar
Jam
Marmalade
Honey
Jelly
High fructose corn syrup

nutritive value of cereal depends on the amount of bran and germ retained during the milling process. For this reason, the use of whole grains should be encouraged whenever possible.

Enrichment

The addition of nutrients that were previously present in a food but were removed during food processing or lost during storage is called enrichment. Enrichment of bread and white flour is mandatory in about two-thirds of the United States, but in fact nearly all white bread in the United States is enriched with certain B vitamins and iron (National Research Council, 1989). Other enriched products include macaroni, noodles, spaghetti, and ready-to-eat cereals.

Enriched products are not nutritionally equal to their whole-grain counterparts, however, because not all of the nutrients, such as fiber, lost during the milling process are replaced. If a person will not eat

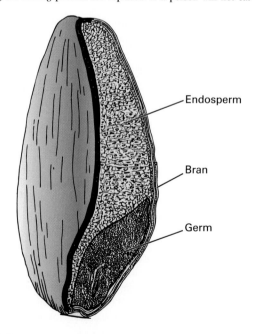

Figure 3–3:
A grain of wheat. The most nutritious parts of this grain are the bran and germ, which are removed during the milling of grain. For this reason, the use of whole-grain products should be encouraged.

whole grains, encourage him or her at least to select enriched grain products.

Exchange List Values

Exchange lists were introduced in Chapter 2. This section focuses on exchange lists that contain carbohydrates. A complete copy of the exchange lists is included in Appendix A. Exchanges that include carbohydrates are the starch/bread, vegetable, fruit, and milk lists.

Starch/Bread Exchange List

One American Dietetic Association/American Diabetes Association (ADA) exchange of starch contains approximately 15 grams of carbohydrate. For example, each of the food items in Figure 3–4 is equal to one starch exchange. Whole-grain products average about 2 grams of fiber per serving. Some foods are higher in fiber (Table 3–4). As a general rule, 1/2 cup of cooked cereal, grain, or pasta or 1 ounce of a bread product is one starch exchange.

Vegetable Exchange List

Raw and cooked vegetables are also good sources of carbohydrates. Vegetables contain between 2 and 3 grams of fiber per serving. One vegetable exchange contains approximately 5 grams of carbohydrate. Table 3–5 defines one vegetable exchange. Vegetables also contribute vitamins and minerals to the diet.

Fruit Exchange List

Fruits are another source of carbohydrates. One ADA exchange of fruit contains approximately 15 grams of carbohydrate (Table 3–6). Many fruits are excellent sources of fiber and contain vitamins and minerals.

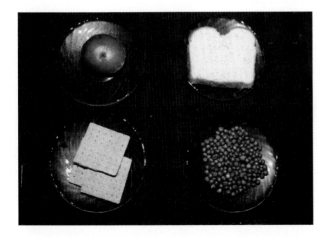

Figure 3–4:
Each of these foods is equal to one starch/bread exchange. An exchange is a defined quantity of a food item. One small potato, one slice of bread, three graham crackers, and one-half cup of peas are all defined quantities (amounts of food). One starch/bread exchange contains 15 grams of carbohydrate.

TABLE 3–4 Selected Starch Exchanges

Bran cereals*	1/2 cup
Cooked cereal	1/2 cup
Ready-to-eat, unsweetened cereals	3/4 cup
Sugar-frosted cereal	1/2 cup
Beans and peas (cooked)*	1/3 cup
Corn, whole kernels	1/2 cup
Potato, baked	1 small (3 ounces)
Whole wheat bread	1 slice (1 ounce)

General rule: 1/2 cup of cereal, grain, or pasta or 1 oz of a bread product is equal to one starch exchange.
*Higher in fiber.

TABLE 3–5 Vegetable Exchanges

1/2 cup of cooked vegetables
1/2 cup of vegetable juice
1 cup of raw vegetables

TABLE 3–6 Selected Fruit Exchanges

Apple (raw 2 in across)	1 apple
Banana (small)	1 banana
Blueberries*	3/4 cup
Grapefruit (medium)	1/2 grapefruit
Nectarine (1 1/2 in across)*	1 1/2 nectarine
Strawberries (raw whole)*	1 1/4 cup
Prunes (dried)*	3 medium
Orange (2 1/2 in across)	1 orange
Orange juice	1/2 cup

*Contain 3 or more g of fiber.

Milk Exchange List

Milk, with its lactose content, is an important source of carbohydrates. One cup of milk contains 12 grams of carbohydrates. Skim, whole, and 2 percent milk all contain approximately the same amount of carbohydrates. Eight ounces of plain low-fat yogurt (with added nonfat milk solids), 1/3 cup dry nonfat milk, 1/2 cup evaporated milk, and 1 cup of buttermilk are each equal to one exchange.

Estimating the Fiber Content of Foods

Table 3–7 lists the carbohydrate and approximate fiber content in one serving from each of the carbohydrate-containing exchange lists. Because the fiber content of starches, fruits, and vegetables is highly variable, using the exchange list to approximate a client's fiber intake provides only an estimate. For example, 1/3 cup of All-Bran cereal contains 10 grams of fiber, several more grams than the exchange list value of 2 grams would suggest.

The fiber values given in Table 3–7 may be useful to screen large numbers of clients to identify individuals with a potential fiber deficiency. If a more accurate intake of a client's fiber intake is necessary, other techniques include using a computerized nutritional analysis or looking up individual food items in a table of food composition (Appendix C).

TABLE 3–7 Carbohydrate and Fiber Content of ADA Exchanges

	Carbohydrate (g)	Fiber (g)
Milk	12	0
Fruit	15	2*
Starch	15	2*
Vegetable	5	2–3

*Unless identified as a food with 3 or more g of fiber per serving.

Dietary Recommendations

There is no recommended dietary allowance for carbohydrates. The United States Department of Health and Human Services published the following national objectives in "Healthy People 2010" for improving health (www.health.gov/healthypeople).

1. Increase the numbers of people age 2 and older who consume at least two daily servings of fruit
2. Increase the numbers of people age 2 and older who consume at least 3 servings daily of vegetables
3. Increase the numbers of people age 2 years and older who consume at least 6 daily servings of grain products, with at least 3 being whole grain.

Someone who consumes the recommended number of servings of fruits, vegetables, and starches most likely is taking in the recommended amount of dietary fiber. Additionally, using the Food Pyramid guide, the total carbohydrate intake should approximate 50 percent of kilocalories with no more than 10 percent of kilocalories from sugar.

Summary

Carbohydrates are comprised of sugars and starches. All carbohydrates are composed of $C_6H_{12}O_6$ in single units or joined together. The average American's intake of sugars is considered excessive, whereas the intake of starches is considered low. Many Americans would also benefit by increasing their fiber intake through the consumption of more starches, fruits, and vegetables. The consumption of whole-grain starches should be encouraged. Dietary carbohydrates promote tooth decay in susceptible individuals. The ADA Exchange Lists that contain carbohydrates are the starch, vegetable, fruit, and milk lists.

Adverse consequences follow inadequate carbohydrate consumption. The human body must have a continuous source of glucose for proper central nervous system function, but its glycogen stores are limited. Therefore, when there is no carbohydrate in the diet and the body uses protein or fat for a fuel source, the body in effect cannibalizes itself for glucose. Muscle and organ mass are lost in the process. A minimum of 50 to 100 grams of carbohydrate a day is usually adequate to prevent these consequences.

Case Study 3–1

KL is a 19-year-old college student. He is interested in body building and spends much of his time on strength conditioning. He lifts weights or uses the Stairmaster (an aerobic conditioning machine) daily. He is 6 feet tall and weighs 175 lb. For the past 3 weeks, he has been drinking a powdered protein supplement (that contains no carbohydrate) instead of eating the dorm food, which he claims "isn't any good anyway." He also takes a high-stress vitamin and mineral tablet. He arrived at the clinic today with complaints of fatigue, nausea, a lack of appetite, light-headedness, and memory loss. His urine tested positive for ketones.

Nursing Care Plan

Subjective Data: Client has chosen not to eat any foods that contain carbohydrates for approximately 3 weeks.

Objective Data: Urine positive for ketones

Nursing Diagnosis: NANDA: Nutrition, altered: Less than body requirements (North American Nursing Diagnosis Association, 1999, with permission) for CHO, related to knowledge deficit as evidenced by verbal statements that he has not been eating CHO-containing foods and by urine positive for ketones.

Desired Outcomes Evaluation Criteria	Nursing Actions/ Interventions	Rationale
NOC: Nutritional Status (Johnson, Maas, and Moorhead 2000)	NIC: Nutrition Management (McCloskey and Bulechek, 2000)	
Client will state one reason why he needs CHO by the end of the appointment	Encourage client to consume foods from the Food Pyramid, including milk, starches, fruits, and vegetables. Refer to the dietitian for instruction on normal nutrition and protein needs for athletes.	Explaining why carbohydrates are necessary in the diet may motivate the client to eat carbohydrates. Milk, vegetables, fruits, and starches are all good sources of CHO. The nurse may need to educate the client about dietary sources of carbohydrates.
Schedule the client for a return visit in one week. Client will keep a food record until next visit.	On next visit, ask client to demonstrate knowledge gained. (For example, How many servings of starch, fruits, and vegetables do you need daily?)	
	Test the urine for ketones at the next visit.	
	Review the client's food record and determine if he is eating at least 50 to 100 grams of CHO each day.	The minimum recommended intake to prevent ketosis is 50 to 100 grams of CHO per day.

Critical Thinking Questions

1. At the client's next visit, what would you do if the food records showed a recorded carbohydrate intake of only 30 grams for most days? What if the client said, "I don't want to eat any more because I feel better"?

2. At the next client visit, what would you do if the food records showed that the client ate only sugar to increase his carbohydrate intake because "Sugar is a quick energy food"?

Study Aids

Subjects	Internet Sites
Sweeteners defined	www.sugars.com/sweetterms.html
Multiple carbohydrate topics	http://www.healthletter.tufts.edu
Food/sugar comparison chart	http://www.naturalland.com/nv/nn/swtable.htm
Sugar substitutes	http://www.asparatame.org
Genetic susceptibility	http://www.niehs.nih.gov/dert/programs/special/genesusc.htm
Provides a link to grain products	http://www.healthchecksystems.com/grains1.htm
Multiple carbohydrate topics	http://www.heartinfo.com/nutrition/wholegrains100998.htm
Health People 2010	http://www.health.gov/healthypeople/Document/default.htm
British Medical Journal	http://www.bmj.com
Sugar replacers	http://www.caloriecontrol.org
Glucose and memory	http://www.people.virginia.edu/~ecm5f/afargrnt.html

Chapter Review

1. Which of the following is a disaccharide?
   a. Glucose
   b. Lactose
   c. Fructose
   d. Galactose
2. A healthy adult needs _____ grams of fiber each day.
   a. 5 to 10
   b. 11 to 19
   c. 20 to 35
   d. More than 50
3. Twelve grams of simple carbohydrate is equal to _____ teaspoon(s) of sugar:
   a. 1
   b. 2
   c. 3
   d. 8
4. One slice of bread contains approximately _____ grams of carbohydrates:
   a. 5
   b. 8
   c. 10
   d. 15
5. Which of the following may cause diarrhea?
   a. A medication that contains sorbitol
   b. A lack of dietary fiber
   c. A lack of exercise
   d. An insufficient fluid intake

Clinical Analysis

1. Ms. C is concerned about the dangers associated with the consumption of artificial sweeteners and wants to know if they are safe. As a health-care worker, it is appropriate for you to:
   a. Ignore Ms. C's comments because you think she is overly concerned
   b. Assure her that the government wouldn't allow a food or herbal product to be sold if they were hazardous to her health
   c. Explain to her that no food is guaranteed to be 100% safe and it is best to avoid artificial sweeteners if she is not comfortable with these products
   d. Refer her to the local health food store
2. Mr. J claims he is trying to lose weight and his urinalysis shows that there are ketones in his urine (ketonuria). You should ask him:
   a. When he ate last
   b. How much milk, fruit, and starch he usually eats
   c. What else he usually eats
   d. All of the above
3. Mr. P complains of constipation. As his nurse, you would like to teach him to eat more insoluble fiber to help alleviate his discomfort. You should encourage the intake of:
   a. Wheat and corn bran, nuts, fruit skins, and dried beans
   b. Eggs, cheese, and chicken
   c. Milk, yogurt, and ice cream
   d. Oatmeal, barley, and broccoli

Bibliography

American Dietetic and Diabetic Associations: Exchange Lists for Meal Planning. The American Dietetic Association, Chicago, 1995.

Benton, D, et al: Breakfast improves memory. Am J Clin Nutr 772S-8S (supp), 1998.

Forman, A: Sugar substitutes have sour image: Safety issues simmer. Environ Nutr 21:9, Sept. 1998.

Foster, JK, Lidder, PG, and Sunram, SI: Glucose and memory fractionation of enhancement effects? Depart of Psychology, University of Manchester. Oxford Rd. M 139 P1, UK, October, 1997. (http://springer-ny.com/link/service/journals/00213/bibs/8137003/8130259.htm) accessed, March, 2000

Gold, PE: Role of glucose in regulating the brain and cognition. Am J Clin Nutr 61(Suppl): 9875–9955, 1995.

Guthrie, JF, and Morton, JF: Food sources of added sweeteners in diets of Americans. J Am Diet Assoc 100:43, 2000.

Harnack, L, Stang, J, and Story, M: Soft drink consumption among US children and adolescents: Nutritional consequences. J Am Diet Assoc 436–441, 1999.

Johnson, M, Maas, M, and Moorhead, S: Nursing Outcomes Classification (NOC), ed 2. Mosby. Philadelphia, 2000

Low-Calorie Sweeteners: Sucralose. Accessed December 2000 at www.caloriecontrol.org.

McCloskey, JC, and Bulechek, GM: Nursing Intervention Classification (NIC), ed. 3. Mosby, Philadelphia, 2000.

National Heart, Lung, and Blood Institute: Healthy People 2010. Accessed December 2000 at www.health.gov/healthypeople

National Research Council, 1989.

North American Nursing Diagnosis Association: Nursing Diagnoses: Definitions and Classification 1999-2000, North American Nursing Diagnosis Association, Philadelphia, 1999.

Pennington, JA, and Church, HW (eds): Food Values of Portions Commonly Used, ed 17. Lippincott, Williams & Wilkins, Philadelphia, 1997.

Rolls, BJ, and Hill, JO: Carbohydrates and Weight Management, ILSI North American Technical Committee on Carbohydrates. ILSI Press, Washington, DC, 1998.

Slavin, JL: Health benefits of soy fiber, the soy connection 2:1. United Soybean Board, Chesterfield, MD, 1995.

Subcommittee on the Tenth Edition of the Recommended Dietary Allowances: National Research Council: Recommended Dietary Allowances, ed 10. National Academy Press, Washington, DC, 1989.

Thomas, CL (ed): Taber's Cyclopedic Medical Dictionary, ed 18. FA Davis, Philadelphia, 1997.

United Dairy Industry of Michigan: Tooth decay: Protective effect of certain cheeses. Nutrition Reports 1:3, 1995.

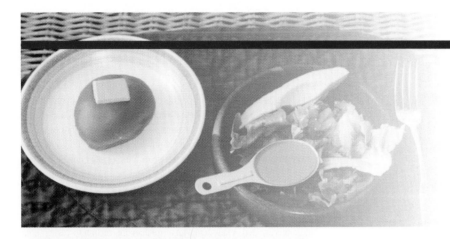

Fats

LEARNING OBJECTIVES
After completing this chapter, the student should be able to:
1. Identify how fats are classified and discuss their physical properties.
2. List the major functions of fats both in the diet and in the body.
3. Discuss the relationships to health of cholesterol, saturated fat, polyunsaturated fat, and monounsaturated fat.
4. List three current recommendations of the Food and Nutrition Board of the National Research Council that pertain to fats.
5. Correctly read food labels and identify the amounts and kind of fats in foods.

The descriptive name for fats of all kinds, lipids, is used in client's medical records. The lipids include true fats and oils as well as related fat-like compounds such as lipoids and sterols. Fats and oils are present in the body and in foods. Fats are typically thought of as solids, whereas oils are regarded as liquids. For example, the body produces oil adjacent to hair. Not as readily apparent to some people is the layer of fat beneath the skin, which is solid. At room temperature, dietary fats such as lard and butter are solid, whereas corn and olive oils are liquid.

Lipids are insoluble in water and are greasy to the touch. When two insoluble substances are mixed together, they separate readily, such as vinegar and oil. You can shake the vinegar and oil combination repeatedly but it will still separate after the agitation stops.

Composition of Fats

Lipids are composed of the elements carbon, hydrogen, and oxygen. These are the same three elements that make up carbohydrates, but the proportion of oxygen to carbon and hydrogen is lower in fats (the implications of which are discussed later). The basic structural unit of a true fat is one molecule of glycerol joined to one, two, or three fatty acid molecules. Glycerol is thus the backbone of a fat molecule.

A fatty acid is composed of a chain of carbon atoms with hydrogen and a few oxygen atoms attached. The fatty acid chains joined to the glycerol molecule vary in length (depending on the number of carbon atoms present) and composition. The different taste, smell, and physical appearance of each fat results from the variety of fatty acids and their physical arrangement in the fat molecules. Beef tastes, smells, and looks different from chicken mostly because of the difference in fatty acid composition. All fats contain fatty acids.

A fat can have from one to three fatty aids. As you will see, the number of fatty acids a fat contains has important implications for both diet and health.

Monoglycerides and Diglycerides

When a single fatty acid is joined to a glycerol molecule, the resulting fat is called a monoglyceride. When two fatty acids are joined to a glycerol molecule, the fat is called a diglyceride. The terms monoglyceride and diglyceride are commonly seen on food labels.

Triglycerides

When three fatty acids are joined to a glycerol molecule, a triglyceride is formed. Most of the fat found in our diets and in the body is in the form of triglycerides. Excess triglycerides are stored in the specialized adipose cells that make up adipose tissue. The human body has a virtually unlimited capacity to store fat. Figure 4–1 illustrates the structure of monoglycerides, diglycerides, and triglycerides.

Length of Fatty Acid Chain

Fatty acids vary in the length of their fatty acid chains. The length of each fatty acid chain is determined by the number of carbon atoms present and can vary from 2 to 24 carbons. The length of the fatty acid chain determines how the body transports the fat in the body, since fatty acid chains of short length (<6 carbon atoms) and medium length (8 to 12 carbon atoms) are processed differently than from longer chains. This is a fact that has implications for diet in many diseases. For example, in certain

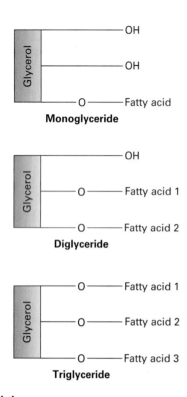

Figure 4–1:
Monoglycerides, diglycerides, and triglycerides. A monoglyceride has one fatty acid attached to the glycerol molecule, a diglyceride has two fatty acids attached to the glycerol molecule, and a triglyceride has three fatty acids attached to the glycerol molecule.

diseases of malabsorption, the client cannot tolerate foods with long-chain fatty acids. This problem is discussed in more detail in later chapters.

Degree of Saturation

The terms saturated, unsaturated, monounsaturated, and polyunsaturated have become household words. Consumers and clients ask sophisticated questions about fats and often expect health-care professionals to define and explain the terminology. Technically, all of these terms refer to the chemical structure of fatty acids, based on the degree of hydrogen atom saturation.

The degree of saturation of a fatty acid depends on the extent to which hydrogen is joined to the carbon atoms present. A saturated fatty acid is

Wellness Tip 4–1

- Read food labels. Some products (those with health claims) will list the % of saturated, mono-unsaturated, and polyunsaturated fat in the item. Avoid saturated fat.

filled with as many hydrogen atoms as the carbon atoms can bond with and has no double bonds between carbons. In this case, a double bond describes the type of chemical connection between two neighboring carbon atoms, each lacking one hydrogen atom. In an unsaturated fatty acid, the carbon atoms are joined together by one or more of such double bonds.

Wherever a double bond occurs, another hydrogen atom could potentially "join" the chain. In other words, the fatty acid chain is lacking hydrogen atoms and is thus less saturated than a chain that is completely filled. A fatty acid with only one carbon-to-carbon double bond is monounsaturated. A fatty acid with more than one carbon-to-carbon bond is polyunsaturated. See Figure 4–2 for a structural comparison of saturated, monounsaturated, and polyunsaturated fatty acids.

In addition to the fats in the body, the fats found in foods are combinations of saturated and unsaturated fatty acids. They are designated as follows:

- Saturated fat: Composed mostly of saturated fatty acids
- Unsaturated fat: Composed mostly of unsaturated fatty acids
- Monounsaturated fat: Composed mostly of monounsaturated fatty acids
- Polyunsaturated fat (PUFA): Composed mostly of polyunsaturated fatty acids

Figure 4–3 graphs the concept that dietary fats contain mixtures of fatty acids. See Wellness Tip 4–1.

Physical Properties and Food Sources

Saturated Fats

Saturated fats are likely to be solid at room temperature. and They are usually found in animal products such as meat, poultry, and whole milk. The exceptions are tropical coconut and palm-kernel oils and cocoa butter, which are vegetable sources of saturated fat. See Tables 4–1 and 4–2 for a more complete list of foods containing saturated fat.

Saturated fats become rancid very slowly because the chemical bond between carbon and hydrogen is very stable. A rancid fat has an

Table 4–1 Food Sources of Saturated Fats	
Meat products	Visible fat and marbling in beef, pork, and lamb, especially in prime-grade and ground meats, lard, suet, salt pork
Processed meats	Frankfurters
	Luncheon meats such as bologna, corned beef, liverwurst, pastrami, and salami
	Bacon and sausage
Poultry and fowl	Chicken and turkey (mostly beneath the skin), cornish hens, duck, and goose
Whole milk and whole-milk products	Cheeses made with whole milk or cream, condensed milk, ice cream, whole-milk yogurt, all creams (sour, half-and-half, whipped)
Plant products	Coconut oil, palm-kernel oil, cocoa butter
Miscellaneous	Fully hydrogenated shortening and margarine, many cakes, pies, cookies, and mixes

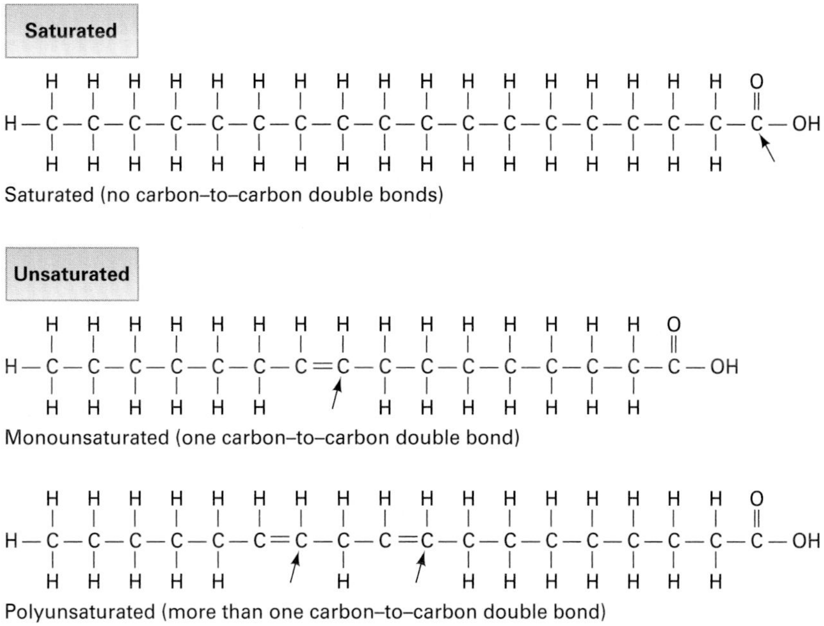

Saturated

Saturated (no carbon–to–carbon double bonds)

Unsaturated

Monounsaturated (one carbon–to–carbon double bond)

Polyunsaturated (more than one carbon–to–carbon double bond)

Figure 4–2:
Saturated, monounsaturated, and polyunsaturated fatty acids. A saturated fatty acid has no carbon-to-carbon double bonds. A monounsaturated fatty acid has one carbon-to-carbon double bond. A polyunsaturated fatty acid has more than one carbon-to-carbon double bond.

offensive odor and taste caused by the partial chemical breakdown of the fat's molecular structure. Consumers usually discard rancid foods because of the highly offensive odor. Products made with saturated fats have a longer shelf life (the time a product can remain in storage without deterioration) because the fat in the product is more stable. Saturated fats have been targeted for reduction in the average American's diet by health authorities because of their unhealthful effects when ingested in excess of the body's needs.

Unsaturated Fats

Unsaturated fats are likely to be liquid at room temperature and of plant origin; they tend to become rancid more quickly than saturated fats. The double carbon bonds in unsaturated fatty acids are very unstable and therefore easily broken. For this reason, many convenience products have traditionally been made with saturated fats to lengthen their shelf life. The food industry is slowly changing this practice; increasingly, more convenience products are made with unsaturated fats. Examples of unsaturated fats are corn, cottonseed, safflower, soybean, and sunflower oils. See Table 4–3 for a more complete list of unsaturated fats.

Hydrogenation

Commercial food processing frequently involves hydrogenation—adding hydrogen to a fat of vegetable origin (unsaturated) to either extend the fat's shelf life or make the fat harder. This process of adding hydrogen to a fat is called hydrogenation. If only some of the fat's double bonds are broken by the hydrogenation, the product becomes "partially hydro-

Table 4–2 Selected Foods High in Cholesterol and/or Saturated Fat

Foods	Amount	Cholesterol (mg)	Saturated Fat (mg)
Liver	3 oz	410	2.4
Cream puff	1	228	10.0
Baked custard	1 cup	213	7.0
Egg, hard cooked	1	215	5.0
Waffles, homemade	2	204	8.0
Coconut custard pie	1 pce	183	8.0
Cheesecake	3.25 oz	170	10.0
Shrimp, boiled	6 lg	167	0.2
Eggnog, commercial	1 cup	149	11.0
Bread pudding/raisins	1 cup	142	4.5
Whole milk	1 cup	124	5.0
Ground beef, 21 percent fat	3 oz. cooked	76	7.0

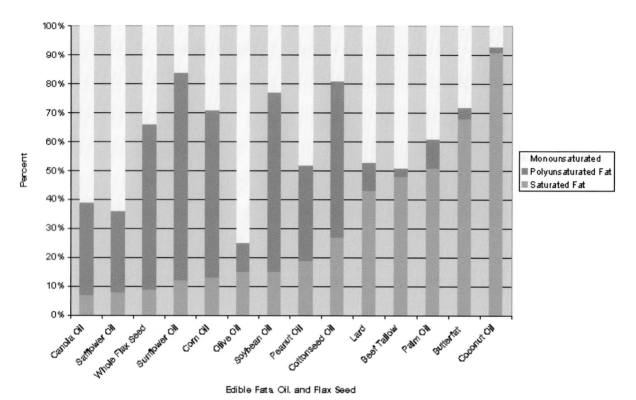

Figure 4–3:
Comparison of fatty acid composition of edible fats, oils, and flax seed. The oil with the highest monounsaturated fat content is olive oil. The oil with the lowest saturated fat content is canola.

genated." If all of the double bonds are broken, the product becomes "completely hydrogenated." Completely hydrogenated fats are highly saturated fats, that is, they have no carbon-to-carbon double bonds. For example, a completely hydrogenated corn oil is closer to lard in saturation than a partially hydrogenated corn oil. All vegetable spreads, such as corn oil margarine, have been hydrogenated to some extent. If these spreads had not been hydrogenated, they would be liquids (except for the saturated tropical oils). Clients are usually advised to avoid products that contain completely hydrogenated fats when the therapeutic goal is to decrease saturated fat intake.

Classification

Lipids can be classified according to three criteria: whether the fat is either emulsified or nonemulsified, whether the fat is visible or invisible, and/or whether the fat is simple or compound.

Emulsified or Nonemulsified Fats

Fats can be classified as emulsified or nonemulsified. Fat does not mix with water because fat is less dense than water and will rise to the surface of any water and fat mixture. An emulsion is a mixture in which the fat and water molecules are evenly dispersed throughout. An emulsifier is an agent that prevents fat from rising to the surface of any fat and water mixture. This is possible because an emulsifier has a molecule with two different kinds of ends. One end attracts one molecule of fat and the other end attracts one molecule of water. Whole milk is an example of a food that is naturally emulsified. Egg yolk is an example of a natural emulsifier.

Visible or Invisible Fats

Dietary fat can be is classified as either visible fat or invisible fat according to whether if it can or cannot be seen. About 40% of dietary fat is ingested as visible fat. This 40% includes vegetable oils, butter, mar-

Table 4–3 Food Sources of Unsaturated Fats	
Foods High in Monounsaturated Fatty Acids	**Foods High in Polyunsaturated Fatty Acids**
Canola, olive, peanut oils	Corn, cottonseed, mustard seed, safflower, sesame, soybean, and sunflower seed oils
Almonds, avocados, cashews, filberts, olives, and peanuts	Halibut, herring, mackerel, salmon, sardines, fresh tuna, trout, whitefish

garine, lard, mayonnaise, salad dressings, visible fat on meats, and shortening. People trying to decrease the fat content of their diets should try to eliminate visible fats first.

Invisible fats cannot be identified as readily. These fats are present in egg yolks, poultry, emulsified milk and milk products, the marbling in meat, and many baked goods and snacks. Invisible fat accounts for the remaining 60% of fat in the American diet. Even if clients eliminate all visible forms of fat from their diet, large amounts of invisible fat may be present. Clients should be taught to identify the invisible forms of fat. Food labels and a knowledge of food composition help teach clients the many sources of invisible fat. Exchange lists can be used to increase knowledge of food composition. See Wellness Tip 4–2.

Simple or Compound Fats

Fats are also classified as simple or compound. Simple fats are lipids that have only fatty acids or a hydroxyl molecule joined to glycerol. Think of the hydroxyl molecule as being just a simple chemical "filler." Monoglycerides, diglycerides, and triglycerides are all simple fats.

When one of the fatty acid chains joined to the glycerol molecule is replaced by a protein, the result is a compound fat. This structure is then called a lipoprotein. Lipoproteins are composed of fat, protein, and fat-related components. They transport fat in the blood stream. The human body makes four types of lipoproteins: chylomicrons, very low-density lipoproteins (VLDL); low-density lipoproteins (LDL); and high-density lipoproteins (HDL). As is evident by their names, the lipoproteins vary in density. The higher the protein content of the lipoprotein, the greater the density. Lipoproteins also vary in the proportional amounts of fat and protein each contains. The type and amount of lipoproteins in people's blood can protect them or predispose them to, heart disease. Lipoproteins are discussed further in Chapter 20 on cardiovascular disease.

Wellness Tip 4–2

- Serving sizes are important. A one tablespoon servings has three times the amount of fat as a one teaspoon serving.

Functions of Fats

Lipids are important in the diet and serve many functions in the human body.

Fats in Food

Fats serve several functions in food. Fats in food serve as a fuel source and act as a vehicle for fat-soluble vitamins.

FUEL SOURCE Fats are the major dietary source of fuel. Because fats have proportionately more carbon and hydrogen and less oxygen than carbohydrates, fats have a greater potential for the release of energy. In practical terms, this means that fats are a concentrated source of fuel or kilocalories. Fats furnish more than twice as many kilocalories, gram for gram, as carbohydrates. Each gram of fat yields 9 kilocalories, so 1 teaspoon of fat, which is equivalent to 5 grams of fat, yields 45 kilocalories. Compare these numbers with those for with carbohydrates, each gram of which yields only 4 kilocalories. A teaspoon of sugar contains 4 grams of carbohydrate and therefore yields therefore only 16 kilocalories.

VEHICLE FOR FAT-SOLUBLE VITAMINS In foods, fats act as a vehicle for vitamins A, D, E, and K. In the body, fats assist in the absorption of these fat-soluble vitamins.

SATIETY VALUE Fats also contribute flavor, satiety value, and palatability to the diet. They supply texture to food, trap and intensify its flavor, and enhance its odor. Satiety is defined as a person's feeling of fullness and satisfaction after eating. Fat contributes to the sensation of satisfaction after consumption because it leaves the stomach more slowly than carbohydrates. Consider for a moment the difference sensations felt when between eating 2 cups of ice cream versus eating 2 cups of chopped apples. Ice cream has a high fat content and apples have no fat. The individual may feel full after eating 2 cups of apples but complain of a bloated feeling and a lack of gratification. Satiety is feeling full and completely satisfied and the feeling that enough or too much food has been eaten.

SOURCES OF ESSENTIAL FATTY ACIDS An essential nutrient is one that must be supplied by the diet because the body cannot manufacture it in sufficient amounts to prevent disease. Fat contains the essential fatty acids linoleic, arachnidonic, and linolenic. Linolenic acid is subdivided into two groups the alpha and gamma. Box 4–1 diagrams the pathways of these fatty acids.

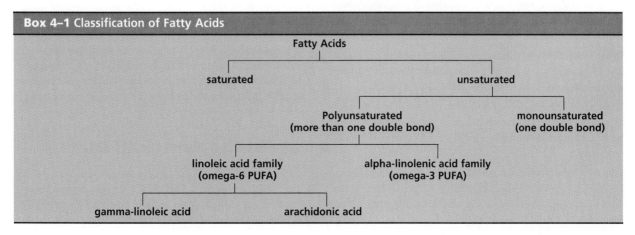

Box 4–1 Classification of Fatty Acids

Although the body can manufacture gamma-linoleic (γ-linolenic) acid and arachidonic acid from linoleic acid, all three of these fatty acids are now considered essential. Linoleic is called an omega-6 fatty acid. Omega is the last letter in the Greek alphabet and is used by chemists for naming fatty acid classes by their chemical structure. The six designation means that the first double bond is located six carbons down the chain (counting from the omega end).

Linoleic acid strengthens cell membranes and has a major role in the transport and metabolism of cholesterol. The omega-6 fatty acids together prolong blood-clotting time, hasten fibrolytic activity, and are involved in the development of the brain. Prostaglandins, compounds with extensive hormone-like actions, require arachidonic acid for synthesis.

Another name for alpha-linolenic fatty acid is omega-3 polyunsaturated fatty acid (PUFA). The omega-3 PUFA have a variety of biological effects that may influence the risk of cardiovascular disease (Harris, 1997). This area of research is discussed further in Chapter 20 on cardiovascular disease.

A deficiency of linoleic acid can occur in infants and hospitalized clients under certain conditions. Linoleic acid deficiency was first observed in infants fed formulas deficient in linoleic acid; drying and flaking of the skin has been observed (Wiese, Hansen, and Adam, 1958). This deficiency was again observed in the early 1970s in hospitalized clients fed exclusively with intravenous fluids containing no fat. The symptoms included scaly skin, hair loss, and impaired wound healing. Linoleic acid deficiency is still seen occasionally with intravenous feeding.

Fats in the Body

Fat serves six major functions in the body, as described in the following sections. Fats in the body supply fuel to most tissues, function as an energy reserve, insulate the body, support and protect vital organs, lubricate body tissues, insulate the body and nerve fibers, and form an integral part of cell membranes.

FUEL SUPPLY Fat serves as a fuel that supplies body tissues with needed energy.

FUEL RESERVE Fat also functions as the body's main fuel or energy reserve. Excess kilocalories consumed are stored in specialized cells called adipose cells. When an individual does not eat enough food to meet the energy demands of the body, the adipose cells release fat for fuel.

ORGAN PROTECTION Fatty tissue cushions and protects vital organs by providing a supportive fat pad that absorbs mechanical shocks. Examples of organs supported by fat are the eyes and kidneys.

LUBRICATION Fats also lubricate body tissue. The human body manufactures oil in structures called sebaceous glands. Secretions from the sebaceous glands lubricate the skin to retard loss of body water to the outside environment.

INSULATION The subcutaneous layer of fat beneath the skin helps to insulate the body by protecting it from excessive heat or cold. A sheath of fatty tissue surrounding nerve fibers provides insulation to help transmit nerve impulses.

CELL MEMBRANE STRUCTURE Fat serves as an integral part of cell membranes and in this capacity plays a vital role in drug, nutrient, and metabolite transport and provides a barrier against water-soluble substances.

Cholesterol

Cholesterol is not a true fat but belongs to a group called sterols. Cholesterol is a component of many of the foods in our diet. In addition, the human body manufactures about 1000 milligrams of cholesterol a day, mainly in the liver. The liver also filters out excess cholesterol and helps to eliminate it from the body.

Functions

Cholesterol has several important functions: it is a component of bile salts that aid digestion; it is an essential component of all cell membranes; it is found in brain and nerve tissue and in the blood. Cholesterol is necessary for the production of several hormones, including cortisone, adrenaline, estrogen, and testosterone. A hormone is a substance produced by the endocrine glands and secreted directly into the bloodstream. Hormones stimulate functional activity of organs and cells or stimulate secretion of other hormones to do so.

Blood Cholesterol Levels

An elevated level of cholesterol in the blood is a major risk factor for coronary artery disease. Lowering blood cholesterol levels reduces the risk of heart attacks due to coronary disease. Individuals with cholesterol levels of 200 to 239 milligrams per deciliter have a borderline to high risk of coronary heart disease (CHD). A cholesterol level over 240 milligrams per deciliter places the individual at a high risk.

Food Sources

Cholesterol is present in the foods we eat. In fact, many of the products sold in supermarkets are targeted to shoppers interested in controlling their blood cholesterol levels through diet. Cholesterol occurs naturally in all animal foods and is produced only in liver tissue. When we ingest animal products, we also ingest the cholesterol the animal made. For this reason, The American Heart Association recommends that a healthy woman eat no more than 6 ounces of lean meat per day and a healthy man no more than 7 ounces of lean meat per day.

Table 4–2 lists selected foods high in cholesterol. Note that one egg supplies about 215 milligrams of cholesterol. Eggs are the major contributor of cholesterol into the average American's diet. The American Heart Association recommends that consumers limit their intake of egg yolks to no more than four per week.

Fats in the American Diet

Fat available in the national food supply increased from an average of 124 grams per day per person in 1909 to 172 grams per day per person in 1985. There are approximately 5 grams of fat in a teaspoon; therefore, 124 grams converts to 25 teaspoons of fat and 172 grams to 34 1/2 teaspoons. Thus, as of 1985, Americans were eating about 9 1/2 more teaspoons of fat per day than they did in 1909. The relative proportion of fat from saturated versus polyunsaturated sources has also changed. The intake of animal fat from red meat has declined whereas that of vegetable fat has risen. Americans are also consuming less whole milk and more low-fat milk, but fat intake in the average American diet is still considered excessive. Recent estimates indicate that Americans derive approximately 37% percent of their total caloric intake from fat, whereas most experts agree that less than 30% percent of total caloric intake should derive from fat.

Calculating the amount of fat as a percentage of total kilocalories is a convenient way of evaluating the level of fat in a food item. Clinical Calculation 4–1 demonstrates how to calculate the percent of kilocalories from fat in a food item. If a food item contains more than 30 percent fat, it should be balanced with other items that contain less fat, such as fruits and vegetables. What is important is the concept of balance. The main objective is to reduce overall fat intake.

Dietary Recommendations Concerning Fat

There is no RDA for fat. Most government health authorities and professional groups recommend that the fat content of the U.S. diet not exceed 30% percent of kilocaloric intake. They also recommend that less than 10% percent of kilocalories should be provided from saturated fatty acids and that dietary cholesterol should be less than 300 milligrams per day.

Table 4–4 Recommended Maximum Fat Intake at Selected Kilocalorie Levels

Kilocalorie Level	Total Fat (g)
1200	40
1500	50
1600	53
1800	60
2000	67
2200	73
2400	80
2500	83

Some fat is needed to provide the essential fatty acids. The Food and Nutrition Board of the National Research Council recommends a minimum adequate intake of linoleic acid as opposed to a set amount. The minimum adequate amount of linoleic acid is 1 to 2 percent of total dietary kilocalories. The healthy adult can obtain this amount from about 1 teaspoon of oil per day. For infants consuming 100 kilocalories per kilogram, this percentage would correspond to a daily intake of 0.2 grams per kilogram of body weight.

Dietary Fat Intake and Health

Dietary Fat

Excessive dietary fat has been associated with an increased risk of cardiovascular disease, the development of obesity, and an increased risk of certain cancers, especially cancers of the prostate. Although it is difficult to predict exactly what factors will lead to a disease in a particular individual, scientists have been able to develop a list of factors closely associated with particular diseases in large population groups. These factors are called risks. Saturated fat increases the risk of coronary heart disease independent of other factors. High dietary cholesterol also contributes to the development of atherosclerosis and increased coronary heart disease risk in the population, but to a lesser extent. Table 4–4 shows the maximum recommended grams of fat an individual should consume at selected kilocaloric levels.

Some experts argue that it is far from proven that eating low-fat foods automatically help individuals keep off excess weight. The food industry has cut the amount of fat in foods such as reduced-fat cakes, cookies, ice cream, luncheon meats, salad dressings, and other foods. Yet Americans are still getting heavier. Many experts attribute this weight gain to the substitution of sugar and refined carbohydrates for fat. A healthier choice would be to substitute vegetables and whole grains for fat. This is an area of current research.

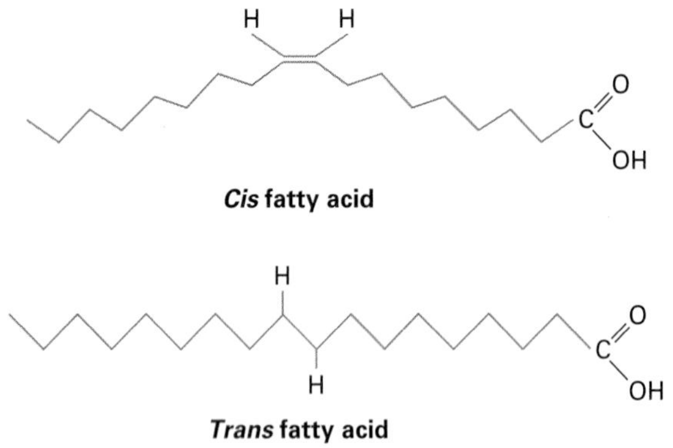

Cis fatty acid

Trans fatty acid

Figure 4–4:
A *cis* fatty acid and a *trans* fatty acid. Whenever there is a change from *cis* to *trans* configuration in a fatty acid, the three-dimensional shape of the molecule is altered.

Monounsaturated Fats

The health benefits of monounsaturated fatty acids have been a better understood phenomenon. Most health educators recommend that the average American increase his or her intake of monounsaturated fats intake while decreasing his or her intake of saturated and polyunsaturated fats.. There is some evidence that individuals with a high intake of monounsaturated fats, a low intake of saturated fats, and a low total fat intake may have a decreased risk of and prostrate cancer.

Polyunsaturated Fats

The Committee on Diet and Health of the National Research Council does not recommend that the average American increase his or her intake of polyunsaturated fat. At very high levels of polyunsaturated fat intake, animal studies consistently show an increase in colon and mammary cancers. Observations in humans have shown that a polyunsaturated fat intake of less than 10 percent of kilocalories does not increase the population's risk of cancer. Box 4-2 discusses researchers' renewed interest in one type of polyunsaturated fatty acid.

Body Fat

Both the amount of body fat a person carries as well as its distribution on the body are related to health risk. Many experts feel that the ratio of body fat to total weight is more important than total weight. Healthy ranges for body fat are 15 to 19 percent for men and 18 to 22 percent for women. A high percentage of body fat has been associated with increased risk of disease, even when total body weight is normal.

The location of excess body fat is also important. Excessive fat on the lower body, specifically on the hips and thighs, appears to be less dangerous than excessive fat on the abdomen and upper body, which is associated with a much higher risk of diseases such as cancer, heart disease, and diabetes. The exchange lists in the next section can be used to assist in planning meals low in fat and teach clients about food composition.

Wellness Tip 4–3

- Choose nonfat or reduced- fat dairy products such as nonfat milk and yogurt and reduced-fat cheese

Table 4–5 Grams of Fat in One Milk Exchange

Type	Fat (g)	Percent Kilocalories From Fat
Whole milk	8	48
2 percent (low fat)	5	38
Skim milk	Trace	<1

Exchange Lists

Exchange lists can be used to assist in planning meals low in fat and teach clients about food composition. Exchange categories that include fat are the milk, meat, and fat lists. The amount of fat in one exchange of meat or milk varies within the list. Some foods not listed on the exchange lists are also high in fat. Many of these foods may be found in the Nutritive Values of Edible Parts of Food Tables (see Appendix B).

Milk Exchange List

The fat content of milk varies according to the type of milk—whole, 2%, 1%, skim. Table 4–5 shows the grams of fat and percent of kilocalories from fat in one milk exchange for each kind of milk. Although whole milk and 2% milk contain saturated fat and cholesterol, the protein, carbohydrate, vitamin, and mineral content of whole, 2%, 1%, and skim milk are comparable. Skim milk contains only a trace of fat and is thus a nutritional bargain. See Wellness Tip 4–3.

Meat and Meat Substitute Exchange List

The meat exchange list is divided into four subgroups: one very lean meat exchange contains less than 1 gram of fat; one lean meat exchange contains 3 grams of fat; one medium-fat meat exchange contains 5 grams of fat; and one high-fat meat exchange contains 8 grams of fat. Table 4–6 lists selected food examples from each of these meat exchanges.

Many clients have misconceptions about meat. Some clients avoid all red meat because they believe that all red meat contains excessive fat. In fact, some beef and pork products are not excessively high in fat. Not all fish and poultry items constitute lean meat exchanges. Nurses can help clients by giving them this kind of information.

Figure 4–5 compares meat animals in the prized 1940s hogs with with those from the 1990s hogs, and Figure 4–6 compares 1940s steers with 1990s steers. In both figures, note how much leaner the 1990s animals appear than the 1940s animals.

Many consumers are not aware of the lean cuts of beef or pork. Conversely, not all fish and poultry items are lean meat exchanges.

Different methods of food preparation can greatly influence the fat content of these foods (Wellness Tip 4–4). Some clients have the misconception that if they eat only lean meats; they can eat as much as they like. This is not true because all meat contains fat, not to mention calories. The maximum amount of meat any healthy individual should eat each day is about 6 to 7 ounces. The American Cancer Society recom-

Wellness Tip 4–4

- Bake, boil, broil, grill, or roast meat and poultry.

Table 4–6 Examples of Very Lean, Lean, Medium-Fat, and High-Fat Meat Exchanges

Each of the Following is 1 Very Lean Meat Exchange and Contains Less Than 1 g of Fat:

Poultry:	Chicken or turkey (white meat, no skin)	1 oz
Fish:	Fresh or frozen cod, flounder, haddock	1 oz
Game:	Venison	1 oz
Cheese:	Nonfat cottage cheese	1/4 cup
	Fat-free cheese	1 oz
Other:	Egg whites	2
	Hot dogs with less than 1 g of fat	1 oz
	Egg substitute	1/4 cup

Each of the Following is 1 Lean Meat Exchange and Contains 3 g of Fat:

Beef:	Round, sirloin, or flank steak	1 oz
Fish:	Salmon (fresh or frozen)	1 oz
Pork:	Tenderloin	1 oz
Veal:	Lean chop or roast	1 oz
Poultry:	Chicken, dark meat, no skin	1 oz
Game:	Goose, no skin	1 oz
Cheese:	4.5 percent fat cottage cheese	1/4 cup
	Cheeses with less than 3 g of fat per oz	1 oz
Other:	Hot dogs with less than 3 g of fat per oz	1 oz
	Processed lunch meat with less than 3 g of fat per oz	1 oz

Each of the Following is 1 Medium-Fat Meat Exchange and Contains 5 g of Fat:

Beef:	Ground beef, corned beef	1 oz
Pork:	Chops	1 oz
Poultry:	Chicken, dark meat, with skin	1 oz
Fish:	Any fried fish product	1 oz
Cheese:	Mozzarella	1 oz
Other:	Egg (high in cholesterol)	1
	Tofu	1/2 cup

Each of the Following is 1 High-Fat Meat Exchange and Contains 8 g of Fat:

Pork:	Spareribs, pork sausage	1 oz
Cheese:	All regular cheeses such as cheddar, Swiss, and American	1 oz
Other:	Bologna	1 oz
	Knockwurst, bratwurst	1 oz
	Bacon	3 slices

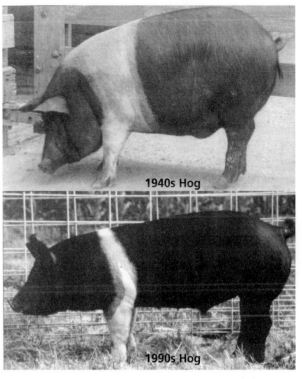

1940s Hog

1990s Hog

Figure 4–5:
The fat content of hogs has decreased during the last 50 years. Consumers are increasingly demanding leaner red-meat products, and farmers are responding. (From National Live Stock and Meat Board, 444 North Michigan Ave., Chicago, IL 60611, with permission.)

Whether the meat is classified as a very lean, lean, medium-fat, or high-fat meat exchange, the grams of fat in each exchange are calculated based on the following assumptions:

- Visible fat on meat is not consumed.
- Meat is weighed after cooking.
- Meat is cooked by a low-fat method—baked, boiled, broiled, grilled, or roasted (unless otherwise indicated).

Since 1994 food-labeling regulations have become more comprehensive. Regarding the fat content labeling of meat, poultry, seafood, and game meats, two terms now have legal definitions: "lean" and "extra lean." The term "lean" can be used on meat, poultry, seafood, or game meat products only if the product contains less than 10 grams of fat, less than 4 grams of saturated fat, and less than 95 milligrams of cholesterol per 100-gram serving (3 1/2 ounces). The legal term "lean" thus equals the ADA exchange list definition for a lean meat exchange. The term extra lean can be used only if the product contains less than 5 grams of fat, less than 2 grams of saturated fat, and less than 95 milligrams of cholesterol per serving and per 100 grams (3 1/2 ounces) (U.S. Food and Drug Administration, 1992).

Clients may choose for many reasons not to eat animal products. Health-care workers should always accommodate their client's religious,

mends only 2 to 3 ounces of cooked lean meat, poultry, and fish per day (www2.cancer.org/prevention).

Meat exchanges are usually 1 ounce, but a usual portion is 3 ounces. For example, half a chicken breast is 3 ounces. Table 4–7 totals the fat content of three meat exchanges. Typically, Americans eat large amounts of meats such as prime rib (from 6-ounce to 16-ounce servings). Teaching clients about meat portion sizes is usually indicated when the goal is to decrease fat intake.

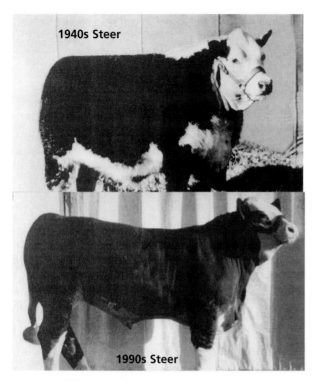

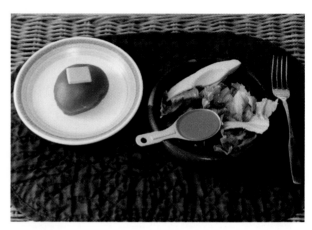

Figure 4–7:
One teaspoon of margarine, one teaspoon of regular French dressing, and 1/8 of an avocado are each equal to one fat exchange.

rated fats (monounsaturated and polyunsaturated) and saturated fats. Table 4–8 lists selected exchanges from each group.

Additional Food Sources of Fat

It is important to advise clients that snack foods including crackers, cakes, pies, donuts, and cookies may be high in fat. Often potato chips, gravies, cream sauces, soups, pizza, tacos, and spaghetti are high in fat. Microwave popcorn is higher in fat than air-popped popcorn (without added fat).

Consumers who desire low-fat foods need not avoid eating out, but they do need to make wise food choices. It is possible to eat a low-fat meal at a fast-food restaurant. However, many of the specialty fast-food hamburgers are high in fat. A small hamburger is the best burger choice. A small side salad with low-fat dressing is a better low-fat choice than French fries. Skim milk is lower in fat than either a milk shake or whole milk. Consumers who desire low-fat foods need not avoid eating out, but they do need to make wise food choices.

Food labeling regulations spell out what terms may be used to describe the level of fat in a food and how they can be used. "Fat-free" on a food label means that the food contains no more than 0.5 grams of fat per serving. Synonyms for "free" include "without," "no," and "zero," and "nonfat." These terms can legally be used on a food label only if the product contains no amount of—or only trivial or "physiologically inconsequential" amounts of—fat, saturated fat, and cholesterol.

Figure 4–6:
For beef, the ideal 1940s market animal was short legged, short and deep in body, and exhibited good evidence of body fat. By the 1980s and 1990s, improved breeding techniques and animal nutrition resulted in a dramatic change in the characteristics of the typical animal. Muscle now replaces much of the fat in today's beef animals. (From National Live Stock and Meat Board, 444 North Michigan Ave., Chicago, IL 60611, with permission.)

ecological, and ethical beliefs and values. Appendix A lists details the Exchange Lists of the American Dietetic And American Diabetes Associations, which include meat substitutes in detail. Many low-fat meat substitutes are not derived from animals, including dried beans, peas, and lentils. Medium-fat vegetarian meat exchanges include soymilk, tempeh, and tofu. Peanut butter, which contains 8 grams of fat per exchange (2 tbsp), and thus is a high-fat meat exchange.

Fat Exchange List

Each fat exchange provides 5 grams of fat. Figure 4–7 illustrates three fat exchanges. The fat list is subdivided into comprises two groups: unsatu-

Table 4–7 Total Fat in Three Meat Exchanges			
Meat	**Subgroup**	**Grams of Fat/Exchange**	**Grams of Fat Per Serving**
Cod	Very lean	1	3
Sirloin steak	Lean	3	9
Hamburger patty, broiled*	Medium fat	5	15
Spareribs†	High fat	8	24

*About 4 oz raw
†Boneless

Box 4–3 Fat Replacers

Some fat replacers are made from ingredients commonly found in food. Some are made from chemically synthesized ingredients. They can be protein-based, carbohydrate-based, or fat-based. Each type of fat replacer has uses, advantages, and limitations.

Protein-based

Using whey (an ingredient in milk), egg, or sometimes corn protein, protein-based fat replacers are made by special cooking and blending processes. Among the uses for protein-based fat replacers are cheese, mayonnaise, butter, salad dressings, sour cream, spreads, dairy products, ice cream, baked goods, and yogurt. Protein-based fat replacers are suitable for use in many food products and are often used with a carbohydrate-based fat replacer in frozen products and baked goods. One limitation of protein-based fat replacers is that they cannot be used in high-temperature applications.

Carbohydrate-based

Carbohydrate-based fat replacers are made of modified food starch, gums, and grain or fruit-based fiber. They are used in dairy products, sauces, frozen desserts, salad dressings, baked goods, confections, meat products, chewing gum, dry cake, cookie mixes, and frostings. A carbohydrate-based fat reducer retains moisture and adds texture to foods. One limitation of this type of replacer is that it can not be used for frying.

Fat-based

A fat-based fat-replacer is made from various fats and oils, like soybean oil, and linked to another compound such as sugar (sucrose). Examples of fat-based fat replacers are Olestra and Salatrim. These products work well in savory and salty snacks, chocolate, confections, and baked products. A fat-based fat replacer can partially or fully replace fats and/or oils in all typical consumer and commercial uses. They provide the same mouth-feel and flavor as fat in foods. They can be used in high-temperature cooking and frying. With some fat-based fat replacers, a few individuals may experience digestive changes similar to those people experience when eating many common foods like some types of fruit and high-fiber foods. The fat-soluble nutrients, vitamins A, D, E, and K are not absorbed as readily when eaten with fat replacers.

Source: International Food Information Council and the Food and Drug Administration

---

"Low-fat" is legally defined as a food that contains no more than 3 grams of fat in a serving. "Low saturated fat" is legally defined as a food that contains no more than 1 gram of saturated fat per serving. "Low cholesterol" is defined as a food that contains less than 20 milligrams of cholesterol per serving.

Table 4–8 Examples of Monounsaturated, Polyunsaturated and Saturated Fat Exchanges

Each of the Following is 1 Fat Exchange High in Monounsaturated Fatty Acids and Contains 5 g of Total Fat:	
Olives	10 large
Canola oil	1 tsp
Peanut butter	2 tsp
Pecans	4 halves

Each of the Following is 1 Fat Exchange High in Polyunsaturated Fatty Acids and Contains 5 g of Total Fat:	
Margarine; stick or tub	1 tsp
Mayo, regular	1 tsp
Corn oil	1 tsp
English walnuts	4 halves

Each of the Following is 1 Fat Exchange High in Saturated Fatty Acids and Contains 5 g of Total Fat:	
Bacon	1 slice (20 slices/lb)
Butter, stick	1 tsp
Cream cheese, regular	1 tbsp (1/2 oz)
Cream cheese, reduced-fat	2 tbsp (1 oz)
Sour cream, regular	2 tbsp
Sour cream, reduced-fat	3 tbsp

Synonyms for low include "little," "few," and "low source of." Additionally, serving sizes listed on food labels are standardized to make nutritional comparisons of similar products easier.

Fat Replacers

Consumers demand food products that are both low in fat and taste good. Fat helps determine texture and taste of food. For example, fat adds the smooth texture in salad dressings, the mouth feel of ice cream, the moist and tender texture of cake, and the consistency of cheese. Fat contributes to satiety. The ideal fat replacers would be able to fulfill all of these roles.

The Food and Drug Administration approved the use of fat replacers in January of 1996. A fat replacer is a nonabsorbable calorie-free fat substitute. Initially these products were approved for use in savory snack foods such as potato chips, corn chips, and crackers. The use of fat replacers such as Olestra in food has been controversial. Olestra is one example of a noncalorie fat replacer. Olestra remains inside the gastrointestinal tract after consumption and exits the body in the fecal material. It is not absorbed.

Some consumer groups object to FDA approval of a food product that may produce abdominal cramping, diarrhea, and loose stools. Any food that is not absorbed and exits the body in fecal material can produce side effects in susceptible people. The FDA studied Olestra extensively before approving its use. Several studies have shown that modest portions of salty foods made with fat replacers are no more likely to result in diarrheas, loose stools, or abdominal cramping than the consumption of snacks with conventional fats (Zorich et al., 1997; Cheskin et al., 1999).

Summary

The group name for all fats is lipids. Lipids include true fats and oils and related fat-like compounds such as lipoids and sterols. Lipids are insoluble in water and greasy to the touch. Hydrogen, oxygen, and carbon are the primary elements in fats. Gram for gram, fats contain more than twice the kilocalories of carbohydrates.

All fats contain fatty acids. The number of fatty acids in a fat determines whether it is a monoglyceride, a diglyceride, or a triglyceride. Most fats in foods and in body stores are triglycerides. The length of a fatty acid chain determines how the body transports a fat. The degree of hydrogen atom saturation or the presence or absence of carbon-to-carbon double bonds determines whether a fatty acid is saturated or unsaturated.

Fats are labeled according to the amount and type of fatty acids they contain as saturated, unsaturated, monounsaturated, or polyunsaturated. Fats can also be classified as emulsified or nonemulsified, visible or invisible, and simple or compound. Fats serve many important functions in our diets and our bodies.

Americans currently derive about 37 percent of their kilocalories from fat. Many experts consider this excessive. Excess fats in our diets are associated with cardiovascular disease, obesity, and some types of cancer. Cholesterol is a fat-like substance that is present in animal food sources and produced by the human body. Many Americans would benefit from decreasing their intake of cholesterol and saturated fat intake. The ADA exchanges that contain fat are the milk, meat, and fat lists. The current recommendations are that the fat content of the diet should not exceed 30 percent of kilocaloric intake, less than 10 percent of kilocalories should be provided from saturated fats, and dietary cholesterol should be less than 300 milligrams per day.

Case Study 4–1

Mr. D had his cholesterol level analyzed during a routine physical examination. The nurse employed in the office of Mr. D's doctor is responsible for the following:
1. Scheduling the patient for follow-up with the physician
2. Developing a nursing care plan that addresses the patient's nursing problem to complement the medical diagnosis

Mike Rod, the nurse, scheduled the appointment. Mr. D was instructed by the nurse to write down all food he consumed for 1 day prior to the appointment. The client was advised to choose a typical day to record his food intake to provide a more accurate analysis of his usual diet. Mr. D arrived on the appropriate day and handed his food record to the nurse for review. Mike calculated the grams of fat in Mr. D's food record based on a combination of ADA exchanges and a table of food composition similar to the table in the Appendix. Mr. D's food record and Mike's calculations are as follows:

11 :00 AM Restaurant	
Food	*Grams of Fat*
Salad bar:	
Assorted vegetables and lettuce	0
2 tbsp blue cheese dressing	10 (2 fats)
1 oz shredded cheese	8 (1 high-fat meat)
1 oz diced ham	3 (1 lean meat)
1/2 cup potato salad	108*
Dinner roll	0
1 tsp butter	5 (1 fat)
1 cup clam chowder	78*

7:00 PM Restaurant	
Food	*Grams of Fat*
4 oz hamburger, ckd. weight	20 (4 medium-fat meats)
1 oz cheese	8 (1 high-fat meat)
1 tbsp mayo	15 (3 fats)
Bun	0
6 onion rings	15*
Tossed salad	0
2 tbsp blue cheese dressing	10 (2 fats)

11:00 PM Home	
Food	*Grams of Fat*
1 cup 2% milk	5
1 orange	0
Total fat for the day	116g of fat

*Values obtained from a table of food composition

The physician has just seen the client, reviewed Mr. D's food record and Mike's calculations, and determined that the client's elevated cholesterol level is secondary to his dietary habits. Mr. D.'s cholesterol level was 225 mg/dL, he weighed 135 lb and is 5 feet, 6 inches tall. Mr. D stated, "I cannot understand why my cholesterol is elevated. My weight is stable. I always select the salad bar for lunch, avoid sweets, and drink low-fat milk."

Nursing Care Plan

Subjective Data	Admitted knowledge deficit. Food record for 1 day contained 116 grams of fat.
Objective Data	Cholesterol level: 225 mg/dL Height: 5 ft, 6 in Weight: 135 lb
Nursing Diagnosis	NANDA: Knowledge: Diet (North American Nursing Diagnosis Association, 1999, with permission) more than body requirements related to admitted lack of understanding and a cholesterol level of 225 mg/dL.

Desired Outcomes Evaluation Criteria	Nursing Actions/ Interventions	Rationale
Treatment Behavior: Illness (NOC) (Johnson, Maas, and Moorhead, 2000)	(NIC): Nutrition Counseling (McCloskey and Bulechek, 2000, with permission.)	
Client will decrease his visible fat intake	Instruct the client on efficient means of recording. Review food records with him at 6-week intervals.	Keeping food records will remind the client of the importance of decreasing his or her fat intake. Reviewing them with the nurse permits positive reinforcement and correction of misperceptions.
Client will keep a diary over the next 3 months	Review visible dietary sources of fat with the client; concentrate on blue cheese dressing, butter, and mayonnaise. Suggest alternatives to using visible fats. Review the diet selected by the physician with the client.	It is prudent to eliminate visible fats first from an individual's diet as they are easily identifiable.
	Tell client to call the nurse if he is having trouble interpreting dietary instructions at home.	Offers the client support between visits.

Critical Thinking Questions

1. Although this client is likely to respond to diet therapy, many clients do not. What would you do if after 3 months a client's food diary shows greatly reduced dietary fat but his or her cholesterol has not dropped? The physician would probably decide to prescribe medication to lower the cholesterol. How would you explain this therapy to the client?

2. What would you do if, at the following visit, the food diary shows that the client has returned to his former eating habits thinking fat consumption no longer matters because he is on medication?

Chapter Review

1. Monoglycerides and diglycerides are names of lipids commonly seen:
   a. In clients' medical records
   b. On laboratory reports
   c. On food labels
   d. On clients' skin
2. Cholesterol is found: _____:
   a. only in saturated fats
   b. only in foods of animal origin
   c. mostly in eggs
   d. only in triglycerides
3. Saturated fats are:
   a. Liquid at room temperature
   b. More likely to become rancid than other types of fats
   c. Primarily of animal origin
   d. Composed of many double carbon bonds

4. According to most health authorities, the average American would benefit by increasing his or her intake of which of the following fats while decreasing intake of other fats?
   a. Corn oil
   b. Canola oil
   c. Safflower oil
   d. Lard
5. One ounce of very lean meat contains 1 gram of fat and 35 kilocalories. What percent of kilocalories come from fat?
   a. 9
   b. 20
   c. 26
   d. 49

Clinical Analysis

1. Mrs. S, 50 years old, has a cholesterol level of 233 milligrams per deciliter. She weighs 125 pounds and is 5 feet, 5 inches tall. The dietitian has approximated estimated her body fat content to be 35 percent. When taking a nursing history, the nurse asks Mrs. S if she eats any foods that may be related to her elevated cholesterol level. Which of the following groups of foods are most related to an elevated cholesterol level?

   a. Vegetable oils such as corn, cottonseed, and soybean
   b. Fruits and vegetables
   c. Starches such as bread, potatoes, rice, and pasta
   d. Animal fats such as butter, meats, lard, and bacon

2. Mr. B buys as many low-fat foods as possible. He eats fat-free muffins for breakfast, eats low-fat brownies or cookies for lunch each day, uses only fat-free ice cream, and buys fat-free salad dressings. He eats very little meat and chooses fat-free dairy products. He wonders why he hasn't lost more weight. The best advice is to encourage him to:

   a. Eat more whole grains and vegetables in place of the fat-free desserts because these foods also contain fiber and other ingredients
   b. To eat even less meat
   c. To consume less dairy products
   d. To quit trying to lose weight

3. When Mrs. L describes her regular intake of foods, you observe that her diet is especially low in monounsaturated fats. Which of the following oils would you recommend be used in place of corn oil to increase her intake of monounsaturated fats?

   a. Sunflower seed
   b. Soybean
   c. Olive
   d. Cottonseed

Bibliography

American Dietetic and Diabetic Associations: Exchange Lists for Meal Planning. American Dietetic Association, Chicago, 1995.

Blumberg, JB: Should you be eating more fat and fewer carbohydrates? Tufts University Health and Nutrition Letter V. 16; No. 12:1. Boston, MA, February 1999.

Cheskin, IJ, et al: Gastrointestinal symptoms following consumption of olestra or regular triglyceride potato chips. JAMA 279 No. 2: 150–152, 1998.

Etherton-Kris, PM, and Nicolosi, RJ: Trans Fatty Acids and Coronary Heart Disease Risk. International Life Sciences Institute, Washington, DC, 1995.

Harris, W: Fish oils, omega-3 polyunsaturated fatty acids, and coronary heart disease. Background. Roche Vitamins, Inc., Paramus, New Jersey, 07652, July, 1997.

International Food Information Council (IFIC) and The Food and Drug Administration (FDA): The Benefits of Balance: Managing Fat in Your Diet. IFIC and FDA, 1100 Connecticut Avenue, NW, Suite 430, Washington, DC 20036, February, 1998.

Johnson, M, Maas, M, and Moorhead, S: Nursing Outcomes Classification (NOC), ed 2. Mosby, Philadelphia, 2000.

Kendler, BS: Recent nutritional approaches to the prevention and therapy of cardiovascular disease. Progress in Cardiovascular Nursing. 12(3) 3-22, summer, 1997.

Lichtenstein, AH: Trans fatty acids and hydrogenated fat—What do we know? Nutrition Today 30:102, 1995.

Lichtenstein, AH,: et al: Dietary fat consumption and health. Nut Rev 56:53-19, May, 1998.

McCloskey, JC, and Bulechek, GM: Nursing Interventions Classification (NIC), 3 ed. Mosby, Philadelphia, 2000.

National Cholesterol Education Program. Step by Step: Eating to lower your high blood cholesterol. Washington DC: NIH. 1994.

National Institutes of Health, National Heart, Lung, and Blood Institute: Clinical Guidelines on the Identification and Treatment of Overweight and Obesity in Adults. Bethesda, MD. U.S. Department of Health and Human Services, 1998.

National Research Council: Recommended Dietary Allowances. National Academy Press, Washington, DC, 1989.

North American Nursing Diagnosis Association: Nursing Diagnoses: Definitions and Classification 1999-2000. North American Nursing Diagnosis Association, Philadelphia, 1999.

U.S. Department of Agriculture (USDA): The food guide pyramid. USDA Home and Garden Bulletin No. 252, Washington DC, 1992.

U.S. Department of Agriculture (USDA) and US Department of Health and Human Services. Dietary Guidelines for Americans. 4th ed. USDA Home and Garden Bulletin No. 232. Washington, December, 1995.

U.S. Department of Health and Human Services: The Surgeon General's Report on Nutrition and Health. DHHS Publication No. (PHS) 88-55 210, Washington, DC, 1988.

Wiese, HF, Hansen, AE, and Adam, DJD: Essential fatty acids in infant nutrition. J Nutr 58:345, 1958.

Willett, WC: Diet, Nutrition, and the Prevention of Cancer. In Shils, ME (ed): Modern Nutrition in Health and Disease. ed 9. Williams and Wilkins, Baltimore, 1999.

Zorich, N et al: Randomized double-blind, placebo-controlled, consumer rechallenge test of Oolean salted snacks. Regulatory Toxicology and Pharmacology 26: 200-209, 1997.

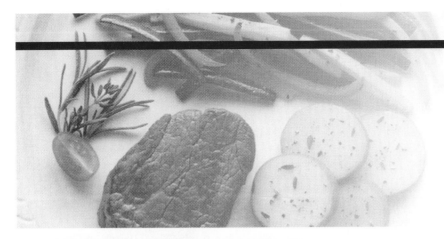

CHAPTER 5

Protein

LEARNING OBJECTIVES

After completing this chapter, the student should be able to:

1. Discuss the functions of protein for humans in health and in illness.
2. Explain the difference between complete and incomplete proteins and give examples of food sources of each.
3. Define anabolism and catabolism and list possible anabolic and catabolic conditions.
4. List the grams of protein in each exchange list containing significant amounts of protein.
5. Calculate the protein allowance for a healthy adult, given the person's healthy body weight.
6. Design a daily meal plan with adequate protein intake for a healthy adult.
7. Design a daily meal plan with adequate protein intake for a healthy adult on an ovolactovegetarian diet.

The importance of protein in nutrition and health was first emphasized by an ancient Greek who called this nutrient "proteos," meaning primary or taking first place. Protein is essential for body growth and maintenance. If kilocaloric intake is inadequate to support fuel requirements, dietary protein may be used for energy rather than for tissue growth and maintenance. As is true of carbohydrates and fats, protein eaten in excess can contribute to body fat stores.

Proteins are the building blocks of the body's tissues and organs. Almost half the dry weight of the body's cells is protein. It is second only to water in amounts present in the body. A description of some of the tissues composed of protein appears in Box 5–1.

Composition of Proteins

To understand the functions of protein in the body, it is necessary first to comprehend their basic structure: their chemical elements and how those elements are arranged.

Proteins are composed of carbon, hydrogen, oxygen, and nitrogen. Phosphorus, sulfur, iron, and iodine often form part of the protein molecule, but nitrogen is the element that distinguishes proteins from carbohydrates and fats. These elements are arranged in building blocks called amino acids.

The importance of a balanced diet and correct food processing techniques can be illustrated by the occurrence of an irreversible paralytic disease called konzo, which affects tens of thousands of women and children in Africa. Faulty food processing and a deficient diet combine to produce the paralysis. Konzo is caused by the consumption of inadequately processed cassava roots along with insufficient sulfur-based amino acids in the diet. The cassava roots contain cyanide, which could be detoxified by sulfur-based amino acids if contained in the diet (Boivin, 1997).

Amino Acids

The amino acids are linked in an exact order to make a particular protein. Amino acids are linked together by peptide bonds. A chain of two or more amino acids joined together by peptide bonds is called a polypeptide. A single protein may consist of a polypeptide of from 50 to thousands of amino acids. Scientists have estimated that the body contains up to 50,000 different proteins, of which only about 1000 have been identified. Thus, an enormous variety of combinations is possible.

To visualize these combinations, examine Figure 5–1, a schematic representation of the beef insulin molecule. It might also help to think of the elements as the letters of the alphabet and amino acids as words. There are countless ways to make words (amino acids) from the 26 letters (the elements). Words put into a certain order make up sentences that have a specific and unique meaning. In this comparison, a sentence is a protein. Each protein has a specific and unique sequence of amino acids. To complete the analogy of language to anatomy, see Table 5–1.

Animal proteins that we eat are disassembled in the digestive process into component amino acids. They are then reassembled to form human proteins (see Chapter 10, "Digestion, Absorption, Metabolism, and Excretion").

Precision is necessary to manufacture proteins. A slight error in the construction of a protein, such as occurs in sickle-cell disease, can have severe consequences (Clinical Application 5–1).

Box 5–1 Examples of Protein in the Human Body

Most of the cells of the body require periodic maintenance or replacement. Even bone tissue undergoes change in the healthy adult. However, the body cannot repair tooth enamel that is destroyed by decay, hence the need for dental fillings.

Scar Tissue
The healing of the simplest wound requires proteins. Many blood clotting factors, such as the protein prothrombin, form a blood clot. The fibrin threads that form the mesh to hold the scar tissue in place are composed of protein. The white blood cells which dispose of the waste products of the injury and the healing process are also proteins.

Hair Growth
Hair cells are dead. Hence, haircuts do not hurt. The new growth of hair does require protein building blocks, however. One sign of malnutrition is hair that can be easily and painlessly plucked.

Blood Albumin
Albumin is a transport protein that carries nutrients or elements to where they are needed. Albumin plays a significant role in medication absorption and metabolism (see Chapter 17). In addition to transporting substances to all the cells of the body, albumin also has functions relating to water balance.

Hemoglobin
Another transport protein, hemoglobin, is the oxygen-carrying part of the red blood cell. The globin part of this molecule is a simple protein.

Small wonder, then, that people need a steady intake of protein for normal maintenance of the body. When the person is growing or has diseased or injured tissue to repair, the need for protein is even greater.

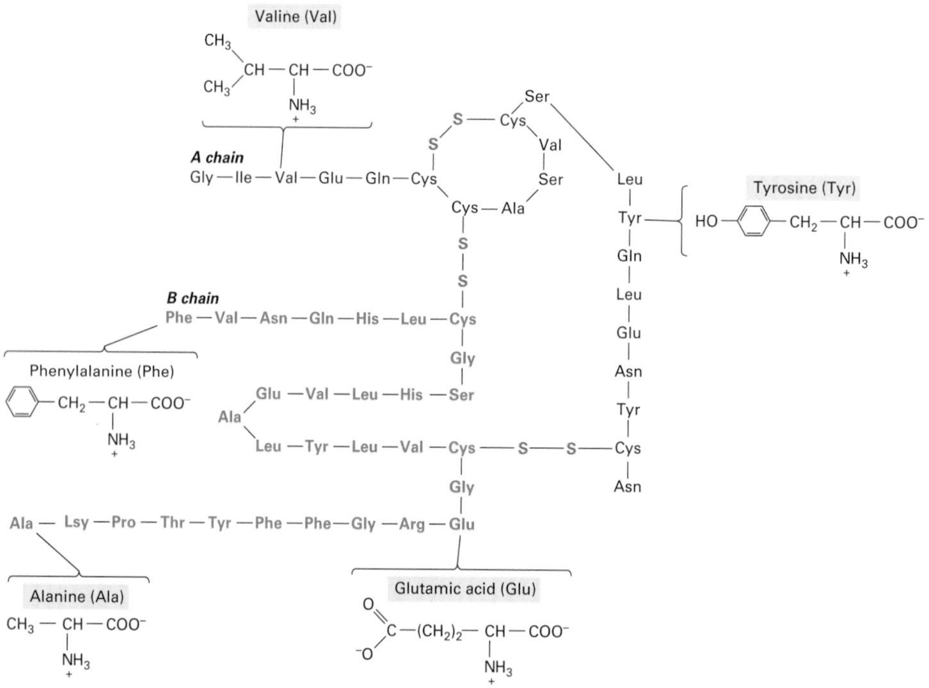

Figure 5–1:
Beef insulin molecule. The central core represents the amino acids in correct sequence. The six exploded views depict the composition of the individual amino acids. (Adapted from Solomons, TWG: Fundamentals of Organic Chemistry, ed 4. John Wiley & Sons, New York, 1994, and Schumm, DE: Essentials of Biochemistry. FA Davis, Philadelphia, 1988. Reprinted by permission.)

Table 5–1 Comparison of Language and Anatomy

Component of Language	Component of Anatomy
Letters	Elements such as carbon, hydrogen, oxygen, nitrogen, sometimes sulfur
Word	Amino acid
Sentence	Protein
Paragraph	Cell
Chapter	Tissue
Book	Organ
Books on a given subject	System
Library	Human body

Twenty-three amino acids have been identified as important to the body's metabolism. These amino acids are classified as essential, conditionally (or acquired) essential, or nonessential.

Essential Amino Acids

As is true of other nutrients, an amino acid is classified as essential if the body is unable to make it in sufficient amounts to meet metabolic needs.. All essential amino acids must be available in the body simultaneously and in sufficient quantity for the synthesis of body proteins (Fig. 5–2). These amino acids may come from recently ingested food or from the body's own cells as they age and are broken down and replaced. Approximately 340 g of amino acids enter the free pool each day, but only about 90 g are derived from the diet (Matthews, 1999).

A person's physiologic state influences the need for essential amino acids. Thus, for infants and young children, 30 percent of protein should be constituted of essential amino acids. That figure drops to 20 percent in later childhood and to 11 percent in adulthood (Matthews, 1999).

Conditionally (Acquired) Essential Amino Acids

Other amino acids are conditionally essential or can become essential, depending on the biochemical needs of the body. Such situations include prematurity, immaturity, genetic disorders, disease states, and severe stress. A very high intake of particular amino acids can alter the need for other amino acids. For example, cysteine and tyrosine become indispensable in immaturity, in metabolic disorders, and during severe stress. A high intake of cysteine and tyrosine can reduce the requirements for the essential amino acids methionine and phenylalanine.

Nonessential Amino Acids

Nonessential amino acids are those that the body can build in sufficient quantities to meet its needs. Often they are derived from other amino acids. Nonessential amino acids are necessary for good health, but under normal conditions adults do not have to obtain them from food. Table 5–2 lists the amino acids that have been classified as essential, conditionally and/or acquired essential, and nonessential.

CLINICAL APPLICATION 5–1

Sickle Cell Disease

Hemoglobin (Hgb) is an important blood protein consisting of 146 amino acids combined in a specific order. In the hemoglobin of a person with sickle cell disease, one amino acid, glutamic acid, has been replaced by valine at one specific location on the protein chain. In sickle cell disease the body has 99.3 percent of the amino acids in the correct sequence in the red blood cell, but early death results from the 0.7 percent error.

Sickle cell disease, an autosomal recessive disease, is common among black people of equatorial Africa but also occurs in people in Greece, Saudi Arabia, and India (Serjeant, 1997). In sickle cell disease the red blood cells have a lifespan of 10 to 12 days compared with the normal 120 days (Serjeant, 1997). Additionally, they become rigid and crescent-shaped. These abnormal cells tend to clump together and block small blood vessels in many different organs.

Among the effects of sickle cell disease are recurrent painful episodes in 70 percent of clients, acute chest syndrome in 40 percent of clients, strokes in 10 percent of affected children, septicemia from various infections (Steinberg, 1999), and impaired growth (Singhal et al., 1997).

No cure is known, but research is continuing, including investigations of gene therapy (Steinberg, 1999). About 120,000 babies with sickle cell disease are born annually (1,000 in the United States). Fewer than 2 percent live to the age of 5 years (Steinberg, 1999), but in the United States mean survival ages are 42 years for males and 48 years for females (Platt, Brambilla, and Ross, 1994). Comprehensive care includes antibiotic treatment, use of pneumococcal vaccines, and newborn screening programs which in 1992 evaluated 99 percent of black newborns in 43 states (Davis et al., 1997). Marked differences in mortality across the United States have been documented, indicating a need to improve access to medical care, parents' health care-seeking behavior, and adherence to antibiotic prescriptions (Davis, Gergen, and Moore, 1997). Techniques to diagnose the disease in a fetus in the first three months of pregnancy are available (Serjeant, 1997).

Functions in the Body

Protein serves five major functions in the body:

- Growth and maintenance of tissue
- Regulation of body processes
- Development of immunity
- Circulation of blood and nutrients
- Backup of source energy

Table 5–3 lists examples of each function.

Maintenance and Growth

Because protein is a part of every cell (half the dry weight), adults as well as growing children require adequate protein intake. As cells of the body wear out, they must be replaced.

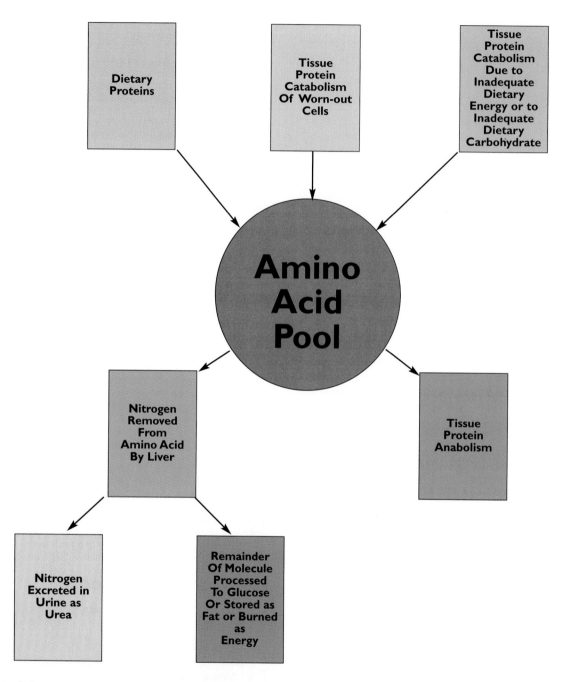

Figure 5–2:
Anabolism/Catabolism of Protein. The body obtains amino acids from dietary protein and the catabolism of body tissue. The body uses amino acids to build new tissue or for immediate or future energy use. Every meal or snack does not have to contain every essential amino acid to permit anabolism. To maximize health, all essential amino acids should be supplied in adequate amounts by diet daily or at least every two to three days.

TABLE 5–2 Essential, Conditionally and/or Acquired Essential, and Nonessential Amino Acids

Essential	Conditionally and/or Acquired Essential	Nonessential
Histidine	Arginine	Alanine
Isoleucine	Carnitine[1]	Asparagine
Leucine	Citrulline[2]	Asparticacid
Lysine	Cysteine[3]	Glutamicacid
Methionine	Taurine[4]	Glutamine[5]
Phenylalanine	Tyrosine	Glycine
Threonine		Proline
Tryptophan		Serine
Valine		

[1] In newborns, can enhance the use of fat as an energy source; can be made from lysine and methionine in adults.
[2] Not used in protein synthesis, but critical in the urea cycle.
[3] Also called cystine.
[4] Not used in protein synthesis, but essential in retinal functioning, especially in young children.
[5] Antonio and Street, 1999.

Anabolism versus Catabolism

Two processes of building up or breaking down of body tissues are anabolism and catabolism. **Anabolism** is the building up of tissues as occurs in growth or healing. **Catabolism** is the breaking down of tissues into simpler substances that the body can use or eliminate.

Both processes occur simultaneously in the body. For example, tissue proteins are constantly being broken down into amino acids, which are then reused for building new tissue and repairing old tissue. Anabolism and catabolism, however, are not always in balance; at times, one process may dominate the other.

Nitrogen Balance

Foods containing protein are the body's only external source of nitrogen. Nitrogen is excreted in the urine, feces, and sweat and is sometimes lost through bleeding or vomiting. A person is in nitrogen equilibrium or nitrogen balance when the amount of nitrogen eaten is equal to the amount excreted (Clinical Calculation 5–1). A healthy adult at a stable body weight is usually in nitrogen equilibrium. Under certain circumstances, however, nitrogen balance may be either positive or negative.

POSITIVE NITROGEN BALANCE **Positive nitrogen balance** is positive when a person consumes more nitrogen than he or she excretes. In other words, the body is building more tissue than it is breaking down. This state is desirable during periods of growth such as infancy, childhood, adolescence, and pregnancy.

NEGATIVE NITROGEN BALANCE Nitrogen balance is negative when a person consumes less nitrogen than he or she excretes. Such a person is receiving insufficient protein, and the body is breaking down more tissue than it is building. Situations marked by negative nitrogen balance include undernutrition, illness, and trauma.

Although skipping food for one day may create a temporary negative nitrogen balance, noticeable physical signs are not likely to occur. A prolonged negative nitrogen balance, however, can adversely affect children's growth rate and diminish a person's capacity to resist infections.

Clinical Calculation 5–1: Nitrogen Balance Studies

To calculate an individual's nitrogen balance, the amount of nitrogen in the foods he or she consumes is compared with the amount of nitrogen excreted in the urine. (Other potential losses are estimated.) Protein is approximately 16 percent nitrogen, so to calculate the nitrogen content in the foods, the amount of protein consumed (in grams) is multiplied by 0.16. Thus, a person who ingests 50 g of protein has a nitrogen intake of 8 g. To be in nitrogen equilibrium, he or she would therefore by expected to excrete or lose 8 g of nitrogen.

Disruption of body integrity by surgery, burns, or fractures causes an acute protein loss. It is estimated that bed rest alone causes a loss of 8 grams of protein per day. People who are well nourished before the disruption are better prepared to weather the resulting catabolism. Poorly nourished people are at increased risk for weight loss, anemia, and infection.

Some individuals may be undernourished even when their total food intake is sufficient. Public health studies from Asia and Latin America describe economic and cultural factors within households that produce a relative deprivation of women and children. Women and girls in some parts of India may receive sufficient kilocalories in staple foods but not enough sources of animal protein, fruits, and vegetables.

In some African societies, women don't eat because it is believed to interfere with fertility. In Nepal, some adolescent and adult women deprive themselves in order to follow cultural "hot—cold" food rules for reproductive-aged women, avoiding nutrient-rich fruits and vegetables (Messer, 1997). In the United States, the unwise and constant dieting practiced by some women and girls determined to achieve the cultural ideal of a slim body deprives them of nutrients necessary for good health.

Severe undernutrition results in specific clinical pictures. Starvation in poor countries may be due to famine, but the term is also used to describe clients who receive inadequate food, sometimes for days, because of treatments or diagnostic tests. The alert nurse intervenes as client advocate or coordinator of care in such cases to rearrange meal schedules or obtain food supplements.

Clients in institutions are also susceptible to **protein–calorie malnutrition (PCM)** or **protein–energy malnutrition** when they are unable to feed themselves. In the developed world, PCM most often

Table 5–3 Functions of Protein in the Body, with Examples

Function	Example
Maintenance and growth	Hair growth
Regulation of body	Glucagon (actions opposite those of insulin)
Immunity	Antibodies against measles
Energy source	If adequate carbohydrate and fat are lacking
Contribution to fluid	Albumin draws fluid back into capillaries from between the cells

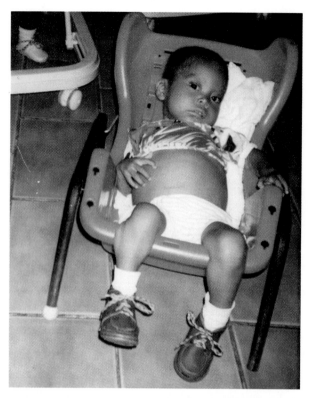

Figure 5–3:
A child with kwashiorkor at the Nutrition Rehabilitation Center in San Carlos, Bolivia.

accompanies a disease process. Surveys of hospitalized children in this country found PCM in 20 to 40 percent of them (Baker, 1997).

Individuals with wasting diseases may suffer from PCM. Two types of PCM are **marasmus** and **kwashiorkor**. Marasmus occurs when the victim consumes too few kilocalories and insufficient protein. The person appears to be wasting away. Marasmus is often seen in children in developing countries, but also occurs in debilitating diseases such as cancer or AIDS.

Kwashiorkor classically occurs in a child shortly after weaning from breast milk. The child receives more kilocalories than one with marasmus but not enough protein to support growth. Clinically, he or she may look chubby, especially in the abdominal area, but the cause of this swelling is fluid retention, not fat (Fig. 5–3). Kwashiorkor is endemic in areas where the staple diet has a low protein–energy ratio. It seems to disrupt the slowing of metabolism that would normally be expected in response to inadequate diet (Lunn, Morley, and Neale, 1998).

Clinical Application 5–2 presents a firsthand account of the desperate situation of people in a developing country. Although rare, kwashiorkor also occurs in industrialized nations, not because of lack of food but because of parental ignorance about nutrition (Buno, Morelli, and Weston, 1998; Lunn, Morley, and Neale, 1998).

Regulation of Body Processes

Protein contributes to the regulation of body processes and is necessary for the regulation of hormones, enzymes, and the nucleus of every

---

CLINICAL APPLICATION 5–2

Letters From Valle de Sacta, Bolivia

By Constance O'Connor BSN, RN

Your letter arrived January 17th, the first mail since a week before Christmas. Mail here is an event . . . no TV, no newspapers. Shortwave BBC is about it for input. Much of what I do is aimed at keeping us healthy, such as ironing all line-dried clothes to get rid of any tiny insects or larvae. All fruits and vegetables are washed in chlorine bleach solution before use. We have gotten so used to the taste we may have to put a bottle on the table like a condiment when we get back home. Water we consume is either bottled or boiled for twenty minutes.

The people here are very poor, most living out in the bush, clearing land to grow bananas, pineapples, oranges, lemons, and coca. They usually construct a two-story hut on stilts so they can get out of the water with the rains. There are half-walls, if any, no screens, no toilets, rarely a well. It is a hard life. Few people survive past 55 and many children die at birth or in the first year.

Statistics are hard to obtain, as reporting even of births and deaths is minimal. A WHO report for 1963 to 1973 estimated there were 9.5 million children aged 0 to 5 years in Latin America affected by protein–energy malnutrition. A study done in our area in 1998 found 38.9% of children under 5 years of age suffering from chronic malnutrition, and 0.6% with acute malnutrition.

One acute case we saw, an 18-month-old boy, was so jaundiced and had such swelling in his lower extremities, we thought he had a kidney or liver problem. We did get care for him and learned the doctors here call that edema "the edema of hunger." These parents were motivated to get treatment as their first child died at eighteen months with same symptoms.

We took a 3-year-old girl to an ophthalmologist because she had a whitish membrane over one eye and could not see well. She was known to be anemic, but the eye doctor said her main problem was kwashiorkor. Sadly, the family refused placement in a hospital, a center for disnutrition, or even the orphanage run by our nuns. We thought this was unusual until we visited a center for disnutrition about 50 miles from us. Of the 54 children, all under three years old, 21 had kwashiorkor.

Today I am taking a 3-year-old child to a malnutrition center about a three-hour drive from us, hoping that it is not too late to save her life. The parents refused care for her up to this point though our pueblo elders, neighbors, and other family members pleaded with them. She has protein-energy malnutrition with kwashiorkor syndrome.

We personally pay for the children we send to these centers. Obviously, if the parents had money their children would not be starving. Most poor parents just accept that the children will die. They will dress them in their nicest clothes, hold them almost constantly during this dying process, and bury them soon after death. No funeral, no coffin.

Malnutrition is a factor in many of the measles, pneumonia, shigellosis, staphylococcal disease, and of course, tuberculosis cases Jim and I care for here. On our first Christmas here we were in the middle of a yellow fever outbreak. I have had to cope with children dying from malnutrition, dehydration, infections that did not get treated in time. I think I will always see their faces.

I hope to see you in March when I'm home begging for medicines and supplies. Many thanks for your letters.

Table 5–4 Examples of Regulators of Body Processes

Regulator	Examples
Hormones	Insulin, thyroid hormone
Enzymes	Lactase, Sucrase
Nucleoproteins	DNA, RNA

cell. Table 5–4 lists the three kinds of regulators and gives examples of each.

Hormones

Hormones are chemicals secreted by various organs to regulate body processes. Hormones are secreted directly into the bloodstream rather than within an organ. Insulin and glucagon are two important protein hormones that help control glucose metabolism.

Enzymes

The body makes specialized proteins called enzymes. Enzymes are crucial to many body processes, such as digestion. The breakdown of foods in the stomach and small intestine involves enzymes, which act as catalysts (chemicals that influence the speed at which a chemical reaction takes place but do not actually enter into the reaction). Without the aid of enzymes, many of the processes in the body would proceed too slowly to be effective.

An enzyme provides a place (its surface) for two substances to meet and react with each other. If it were not for enzymes, these two substances would be less likely to encounter one another, and basic body functioning would be impossible.

The lack of a specific enzyme can have devastating effects on health, even on life itself (Clinical Application 5–3).

Nucleoproteins

Nucleoproteins are the third example of regulatory proteins. The center or nucleus of every cell contains nucleoproteins. Their function is to direct the maintenance and reproduction of the cell. Two well-known nucleoproteins are DNA and RNA.

Deoxyribonucleic acid (DNA) is present in all body cells of every species. It is the basic component of **genes**, which serve as patterns to guide reproduction. **Ribonucleic acid (RNA)** is another nucleoprotein present in all living cells. It controls the manufacturing of cellular protein. Each of the common amino acids has its own RNA to transport it to the correct location in the protein chain.

Immunity

A specific protein called an **antibody** is produced in the body in response to the presence of a foreign substance or a substance that the body senses to be foreign. Antibodies provide **immunity** to certain diseases and other toxic conditions. A specific antibody is created for each foreign substance.

If a person is exposed to a certain kind of disease-producing bacteria, the body creates an antibody that neutralizes the harmful effects of only that particular species or strain of bacteria. For some diseases, once the body has produced antibodies, it can respond quickly to another attack, making the individual immune to that disease. All antibodies belong to a group of blood proteins called **immunoglobulins**.

CLINICAL APPLICATION 5–3

Phenylketonuria (PKU)

PKU is the most common of all amino acid pathologies (de Freitas et al., 1999). About 1 in 60 Caucasians, mostly of Northern European ancestry, is a carrier for this autosomal recessive disorder, which occurs once in 10,000 to 25,000 live births. Clients with **phenylketonuria** are unable to convert the essential amino acid phenylalamine to tyrosine because the enzyme phenylalanine hydroxylase is lacking or defective.

Phenylalanine occurs in all protein foods, including milk. Affected infants are immediately at risk of accumulating high blood levels of phenylalanine with consequent mental retardation. Impaired intellectual functioning has been documented even in children receiving standard treatment (Medical Research Council, 1993).

In the United States, screening tests, using a few drops of blood from the infant's heel, are mandated by all states. The test is highly accurate when performed 24 hours after birth through the 7th day of life (PKU, 1999). With mothers and infants discharged from the maternity unit within 24 hours, efforts must be made to ensure proper timing of the screening test. The American Academy of Pediatrics recommends that infants tested when they are less than 24 hours old be re-screened at 1 to 2 weeks of age (Sinai et al., 1995).

The devastating effects of this deficiency can be avoided if strict regulation of the proteins the client consumes is begun in the first three weeks of life (PKU, 1999) and blood levels are monitored weekly for the first four years of life (Medical Research Council, 1993). A great majority (87%) of PKU centers in the United States and Canada favor life-long dietary control of phenylalanine intake (Fisch et al, 1997). Until the 1980s, restrictions were relaxed as the client grew, so that new concerns have arisen that women who ceased treatment for PKU may harm their unborn children because phenylalanine crosses the placenta (Acosta and Wright, 1992; Bowe, 1995) such that the fetus is exposed to higher phenylalanine concentrations than the mother (Medical Research Council, 1993). Careful history-taking may tease out the fact that a woman was on a special diet as a small child and thus may need to have phenylalanine levels tested and to resume the diet before attempting pregnancy. An alert nurse could identify this situation before any damage is done.

The artificial sweetener aspartame (Equal, NutraSweet), which is composed of aspartic acid and phenylalanine, bears a warning label regarding PKU. Clients with PKU and their families may have to be reminded regularly of the importance of dietary compliance.

Ongoing research is focusing on timing of feedings and blood levels of phenylalanine (MacDonald et al., 1998), feeding practices (MacDonald et al., 1997), adequacy of nutrition (Acosta et al., 1999; Acosta and Yannicelli, 1999), more palatable PKU formulas, and gene therapy to provide a cure (PKU, 1999). Also needed are improved methods of ascertaining blood levels of phenylalanine, revamping of the phenylalanine food exchanges, and reformulation of special foods for phenylketonuria treatment (Medical Research Council, 1993).

Circulation

The main protein in the blood is albumin. It helps to maintain blood volume by drawing fluid back into the veins from body tissues. Thus it plays a major role in maintaining blood pressure.

Some proteins serve as transport vehicles for nutrients or drugs, such as the proteins that attach to fats to become lipoproteins. Drugs bind with albumin in the bloodstream. The term protein-bound refers to the portion of a dose of a drug that is inactive because it is attached to albumin. This process has implications that are discussed in Chapter 17.

Energy Source

Glucose is the most efficiently used source of energy, but fat and protein can be adapted as backup sources. Most other body systems utilize fat for energy more readily than the nervous system. When the body has insufficient glucose available for nervous system energy needs (as in a carbohydrate dietary deficit of longer than 12 hours), the body will utilize body protein tissue to meet the energy needs of the brain and spinal cord. Thus, adequate carbohydrate intake is necessary to (1) spare protein for its unique contribution to tissue building and (2) avoid the undesirable consequences—ketosis and muscle loss—of obtaining energy from the less efficient sources—fat and protein. The amount of energy obtained from a gram of protein is the same as the amount obtained from a gram of carbohydrate: 4 kilocalories.

Loss of about 30 percent of body protein is likely to be fatal. Contributing to the outcome is reduced muscle strength for breathing, impaired immune function, and decreased organ function (Matthews, 1999).

Classification of Food Protein

Few foods contain only protein. The white of an egg comes close, deriving 80 percent of its kilocalories from protein. Most foods embody various combinations of protein, fat, and carbohydrates. Some foods, however, are better sources of protein than others.

Protein foods are classified by the number and kinds of amino acids they contain. **Complete proteins** are foods that supply all nine essential amino acids in sufficient quantity to maintain tissue and support growth. **Incomplete proteins** lack one or more of the essential amino acids.

Scoring systems have been devised to rate the quality of proteins on the basis of their amino acid composition. The reference foods often used are eggs and cow's milk.

It is difficult to compare foods in this way because certain factors intervene between the test situation and the family table. Some plants, for example, contain substances that inhibit digestion of protein. These inhibitors can be destroyed by heat processing, but so can amino acids (Matthews, 1999).

Complete Protein

With few exceptions, single foods containing complete protein come from animal sources such as meat, poultry, fish, eggs, and cheese. Gelatin, an animal product, is an incomplete protein because it lacks the essential amino acid tryptophan.

Meat and milk products are both good sources of complete protein. An adult following the guidelines of the food pyramid would consume two or three servings from the meat group and two or three servings from the milk group daily. The USDA Food Pyramid categorizes cheese with milk, whereas the exchange-group system places it with meat.

Each exchange of meat contains 7 grams of protein regardless of the amount of fat. All beef is not high in fat, just as all fish and poultry are not low in fat. Figure 5–4 shows a 3-ounce portion of beef tenderloin equal to 3 lean meat exchanges providing 21 grams of protein.

Each milk exchange furnishes 8 grams of protein. Examples of one milk exchange are 1 cup of milk, buttermilk, or yogurt; 1/2 cup of canned evaporated milk; or 1/3 cup of dry skim milk. All of these milk products offer equal protein nutrition, but all are not nutritionally equivalent because their fat content varies.

Incomplete Protein

Plant foods that contain protein lack sufficient amounts of one or more of the essential amino acids. Thus, the protein of plants is called incomplete. But the term "incomplete" does not mean these foods should be avoided. Grains, vegetables, legumes, nuts, and seeds are valuable sources of incomplete protein.

Plant proteins are valuable because they supplement the animal proteins in the diet. Several different types of plant protein sources can be eaten to obtain all the essential amino acids. The plant foods deficient in some amino acids can be complemented by one or more of the other plant foods.

The vegetable and starch/bread exchanges are sources of incomplete protein. Some vegetables such as corn, peas, and dried beans are closer in energy content to a slice of bread than to most vegetables. For this reason they appear on the Starch/Bread Exchange List. A vegetable exchange contains 2 grams of protein. One vegetable exchange would be 1/2 cup of asparagus or 1/2 cup of chopped broccoli. One starch/bread exchange would be 1/2 cup of corn, 1 small potato, 1/2 cup of winter squash, 1 slice of bread, 1/2 bagel or 1/2 English muffin, or 3 square graham crackers.

It is important to note the size of the item; specialty bagels and muffins may be much larger than the referenced item on the exchange list. A starch/bread exchange contains 3 grams of protein (Table 5–5).

Limiting Amino Acids and Complementation

Plants are classified as incomplete protein sources because they lack one or more essential amino acids. This undersupplied amino acid is called the **limiting amino acid**. In cereal grains the limiting amino acid is lysine; in legumes, it is methionine.

Based upon animal studies, the principle of **complementation** was promulgated. It stated that plant foods should be combined to provide all the essential amino acids in a given meal. There are two major flaws in projecting the results of these animal studies to humans. Animals have greater protein needs than humans. Also, the experimental animal diets were completely lacking in the amino acid being studied, a situation not likely to occur with selection of whole foods (Johnston, 1999).

Adult humans can derive adequate nutrition when they consume a balanced selection of plant protein throughout the day. As shown in Figure 5–2, supplying the amino acid pool is a dynamic process. Young children did show less effective use of protein if the complementary protein was fed at intervals greater than 6 hours, but this is an

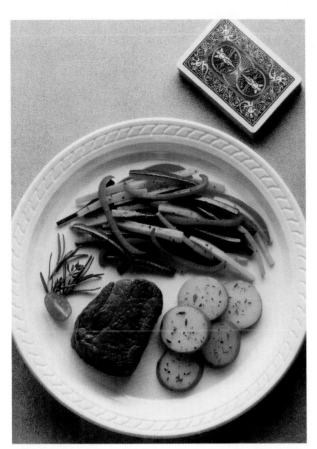

Figure 5–4:
The 3-oz. beef tenderloin pictured equals 3 lean meat exchanges. The standard deck of playing cards is shown for size comparison. (From the National Live Stock and Meat Board, 444 North Michigan Ave., Chicago, IL 60611, with permission.)

unusually long time between meals or snacks for young children (Johnston, 1999).

Vegetable Sources of Protein

For vegetarians or other individuals who limit their intake of animal foods, **legumes** are an important protein source. Legumes are plants having roots containing nitrogen-fixing bacteria that "lock" nitrogen into the plant's structure, thus increasing its nitrogen content. Legumes contain two to three times as much nitrogen as most other vegetables.

Commonly consumed legumes are peas, beans, lentils, and peanuts. Not all peas and beans are legumes. Figure 5–5 compares the protein content of peas, beans, and nuts. Examples of one exchange of legumes are

Table 5–5 Grams of Protein per Exchange

Exchange	Grams of Protein
Milk	8
Meat	7
Starch/Bread	3
Vegetable	2

1/2 cup of peas, 1/3 cup of kidney beans, or 1/4 cup of baked beans. On the exchange lists, these legumes are classified as starch/bread. Because many legumes are not only low in fat but also high in fiber, they are valued by health-conscious people.

Nuts appear on the fat exchange list. One tablespoon of cashews or 20 small peanuts is one exchange. Peanut butter is on the high-fat meat list; 1 tablespoon equals 1 exchange.

Textured vegetable protein products made from soybeans, peanuts, and cottonseed can enhance the vegetarian diet. The protein is spun into fibers and flavored, colored, and shaped for use as a meat substitute. In their natural form, plant proteins are less digestible than animal proteins, but well-processed soybean isolates are as digestible as egg protein (Johnston, 1999).

Vegetarianism Can Be a Healthy Lifestyle

There are many degrees of vegetarianism, depending upon the beliefs of the individual or family. Some people eat animal products such as milk and eggs but not animal flesh. Others eat only plant foods. Some eat only fruits. The more restrictive the diet, the more care required in monitoring intake for adequacy of protein and other nutrients.

Embracing a healthful vegetarian lifestyle encompasses more than just eliminating foods derived from animals. It is necessary to find substitutes for the nutrient-dense animal products. Many traditional regional or ethnic dishes call for a combination of a grain with a legume; the two incomplete proteins eaten together serve to complement each other and provide adequate protein. Some favorite combinations such as a peanut butter sandwich or baked beans with brown bread are grain-and-legume combinations. The Mexican burrito, a thin cornmeal bread filled with beans, is another example. Clinical Application 5–4 distinguishes various vegetarian diets.

Health-conscious vegetarians must read labels carefully. Eliminating meat does not automatically decrease a person's fat intake, especially when prepared meals are used (Vegetarian Fare, 1997). Vegetable oils and cheeses used in sauces to enhance flavor increase the number of kilocalories.

CLINICAL APPLICATION 5–4

Vegetarian Diets

Vegetarians practice different degrees of strictness. From most liberal to most restrictive, the vegetarian diets are ovolactovegetarian, lactovegetarian, ovovegetarian, and strict vegetarian or vegan. The prefixes ovo- and lacto- mean eggs and milk. So an ovovegetarian will consume eggs, a lactovegetarian milk, and an ovolactovegetarian both. A vegan eats no animal products.

Foods Permitted in the Various Vegetarian Diets

	Meat, Fish, Poultry	Dairy Products	Eggs
Ovolactovegetarian	No	Yes	Yes
Lactovegetarian	No	Yes	No
Ovovegetarian	No	No	Yes
Strict Vegetarian (vegan)	No	No	No

Adequate assessment of the client's physiological state, knowledge, and values will enable the nurse to provide appropriate nutritional care for vegetarian clients.

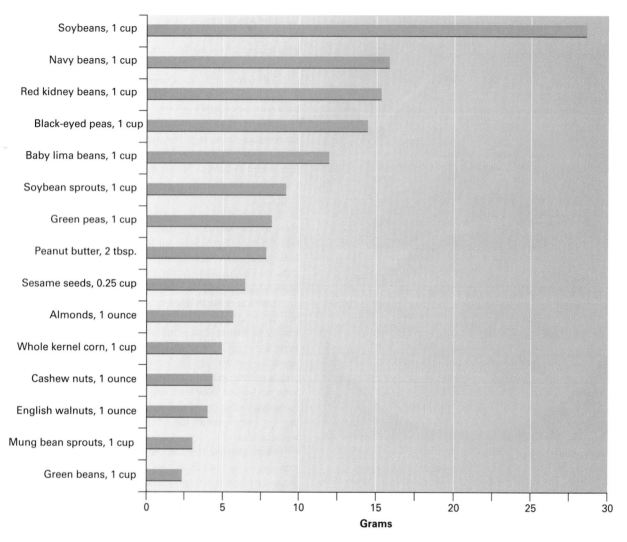

Figure 5–5:
Protein content of selected food plants. Notice that all foods named peas or beans are not legumes. Green beans offer just 2 g of protein compared to navy beans that contain 16 g.

Vegetarian diets can be healthful as long as appropriate foods are selected and prepared in various ways. Pregnant women, infants, children, and elderly people who are vegetarians in particular need special attention.

Usually hospital or care facility dietitians can provide a balanced vegetarian diet. It is much better, when a nurse encounters a vegetarian client, to inform the dietitian rather than expect the client to select items from a general menu. Figure 5–6 illustrates a vegetarian food pyramid.

Recommended Dietary Allowances

The adult RDA for protein is 0.8 gram of protein per kilogram of body weight. Clinical Calculation 5–2 shows the procedure for calculating this

amount based on a person's healthy body weight. Pregnancy and lactation increase the need for protein, as do periods of growth.

During pregnancy and breast-feeding, the mother requires additional protein to build new tissue. The "eating for two" advice for pregnant women refers to the quality of foods eaten, not the quantity. Infants up to the age of 6 months have the greatest protein requirement in proportion to their body size: 2.2 grams per kilogram.

Overeating protein foods can adversely affect a person's health. Excess dietary protein taxes the kidneys, which must excrete the surplus nitrogen. The Committee on Diet and Health (National Research Council, 1989) recommends that protein intake be no more than twice the RDA. If individuals follow the guidelines of the Food Pyramid, protein should account for 12 to 20 percent of kilocalories (Table 5–6).

Clinical Calculation 5–2:
RDA for Protein

To determine a person's daily protein allowance, first determine his or her healthy body weight, as explained in Chapter 2. Taking the body weight in pounds, convert the pounds to kilograms. There are 2.2 lb/kg. Consider a 5 ft 4 in. woman, whose healthy body weight is 131 lb.

$$\frac{\text{Weight in pounds}}{2.2 \text{ pounds in kilogram}} = \text{Weight in kilograms}$$

$$\frac{131 \text{ lbs}}{2.2 \text{ pounds in kilogram}} = 59.5 \text{ kilograms}$$

The adult RDA for protein is 0.8 g of protein per kg of healthy body weight. So multiply the weight in kg by 0.8 g/kg.

59.5 (weight in kilograms) × 0.8 (grams per kilogram) = 47.6 grams of protein daily

Thus the daily protein allowance for our sample woman is 47.6 g.

Choosing Protein Foods Wisely

Producing meat is expensive. For every 5 pounds of vegetable or fish protein fed to livestock, only 1 pound of meat protein is produced. In the United States, the consumption of animal protein between 1910 and 1991 nearly doubled. Now, meat, fish, and poultry contribute 42 percent of the protein intake, dairy products 20 percent, and grains 18 percent (Smit et al., 1999).

In Third World countries, the search for cost-effective means to provide adequate amounts of protein for large populations has scientists researching microorganisms as an alternative source of protein as animal feed or human food. Like plants, microorganisms use nitrogen to produce protein, but because microorganisms can be grown artificially, they are not subject to the vagaries of weather the way plant crops are. Among the microorganisms under study are bacteria, yeasts, fungi, and algae (Kuhad, et al, 1997).

Table 5–6 RDA for Protein for Healthy Individuals

Age In Years	Grams of Protein per Kilogram of Healthy Body Weight
0–1/2	2.2
1/2–1	1.6
1–3	1.2
4–6	1.1
7–14	1.0
15–18 (Males)	0.9
15–18 (Females)	0.8
19 and older	0.8
Pregnant	Nonpregnant RDA + 10 g
Lactating	
First 6 months	Nonpregnant RDA + 15 g
Remainder	Nonpregnant RDA + 12 g

Nurses can help clients who have limited funds and those who wish to decrease their meat intake. Table 5–7 lists equivalent sources of 10 grams of protein. The regular prices of nationally advertised brands were used, except for bread, cottage cheese, eggs, milk, and steak. Peanut butter provided 10 grams of protein for 11 cents. Water-packed tuna has the most protein per kilocalorie of the foods listed and was the least expensive complete protein food. The most expensive source in the list was bologna. The nurse could make similar calculations for clients' favorite foods or frequently purchased foods to assist them to choose wisely. Wellness Tips 5–1 list other general principles nurses can teach clients.

Wellness Tips 5–1

- Note portion size to avoid overconsumption of protein. Occasionally measure amounts that are served.
- Replace less-liked items with others in the same category: substitute yogurt or cheese for milk, eggs or legume–grain casseroles for meat or fish.
- Try to incorporate meatless meals or ethnic dishes into your eating pattern regularly.

Table 5–7 Comparative Sources of 10 Grams of Protein with Kilocalories and Costs

Food	Portion	Kilocalories	Cost/Amount	Cost/Portion
Peanut butter	2 tbsp	190	$3.19/28 oz	$0.11
Tuna, canned in water	1 oz	45	$0.73/6 oz	$0.12
Large eggs, poached	1.7	126	$0.89/doz	$0.13
2% milk	1.25	110	$1.89/gal	$0.15
Cottage cheese, 2% low fat	1/3 cup	68	$2.09/1.5 lb	$0.23
American cheese	1.7 oz	175	$4.49/2 lb	$0.24
Boneless sirloin steak	1.1 oz	66	$4.28/lb	$0.29
Bean soup, condensed	1.25 cups	213	$0.99/11.5 oz	$0.43
Cracked wheat bread	5 slices	325	$1.19/24 oz	$0.44
Bologna	2.9 oz	261	$2.79/lb	$0.51

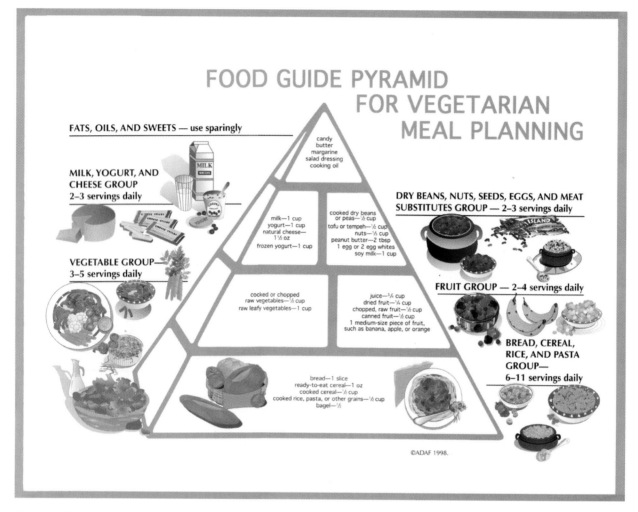

Figure 5–6:
An adaptation of the food guide pyramid for vegetarians. (From the National Center for Nutrition and Dietetics, American Dietetic Association, 1998, with permission.)

Summary

Protein is necessary for tissue maintenance and growth, the regulation of body processes, the development of immunity, the circulation of blood and nutrients, and as a backup source of energy. The element that distinguishes protein from carbohydrates and fats is nitrogen. The body combines carbon, hydrogen, oxygen, and nitrogen in certain ways to form amino acids, which then become the building blocks of various proteins.

Complete protein foods contain all essential amino acids in amounts sufficient to support growth. Complete protein foods usually come from animal sources, especially the meat and milk groups.

Incomplete protein foods are grains, vegetables, legumes, nuts, and seeds. A person who eats a grain product and a legume at the same meal, however, is likely to receive all essential amino acids.

A normal healthy adult should consume 0.8 gram of protein per kilogram (2.2 pounds) of healthy body weight. A simple method of estimating protein intake uses the exchange list system. Milk exchanges provide about 8 grams of protein, meat exchanges 7 grams, bread/starch exchanges 3 grams, and vegetable exchanges 2 grams.

Case Study 5–1

Mrs. F is a 72-year-old widow who eats independently in her family homestead. Her usual meals are tea and toast for breakfast, canned fruit and a muffin for lunch, and frozen potpie or canned hash for dinner. She complains that she has been having trouble chewing and has not been eating as much food as she usually does. She does not like milk.

Nursing Care Plan

Subjective Data	Food deficit as evidenced by usual food intake information
	Has trouble chewing
	Does not like milk
Objective Data	Height: 5 ft 4 in.
	Weight: 106 lb
	Wrist circumference: 5.75 in.
Nursing Diagnosis	NANDA: Altered nutrition: less than body requirements (North American Nursing Diagnosis Association, 1999, with permission) for protein and kilocalories, related to difficulty chewing, as evidenced by stated usual intake of 28–32 g of protein per day and body weight 7 percent under minimum for height and frame

Desired Outcomes Evaluation Criteria	Nursing Actions/ Interventions	Rationale
NOC: Nutritional Status: Nutrient Intake (Johnson, Maas, and Moorhead, 2000, with permission.)	NIC: Nutritional Counseling (McCloskey and Bulechek, 2000, with permission.)	
Client will gain 1 lb per week during the next 2 weeks.	Encourage easily chewed sources of complete protein: cheese, eggs, ground meat, fish.	Complete protein foods contain all essential amino acids necessary for tissue building.
Client will increase her total protein intake by 9–13 g per day	Create a model meal plan with Mrs. F using the Exchange Group system to count grams of protein.	Mrs. F requires 41 g of protein for her healthy body weight. The meal plan she described in her history contains only 28 to 32 g depending on dinner selection.
Client will call for dental appointment within next 2 weeks	Explore sources of financial assistance for dental care if necessary.	Better fitting dentures would permit Mrs. F a wider variety of foods.

Critical Thinking Questions

1. What other food groups are lacking in Mrs. F's usual diet? Would you have given any of them a higher priority than protein? Why or why not?
2. Speculate on the reasons Mrs. F has developed her present meal pattern. What additions could you make to the care plan to improve her nutritional intake?
3. When following up after 2 weeks, the nurse finds that Mrs. F has gained one-half pound instead of 2 as set in the desired outcome. She has increased her intake of eggs and cheese as instructed but says she feels full before finishing her meal. What additional information should the nurse obtain? What modifications to the nursing care plan might she and Mrs. F institute?

 Study Aids

Subjects . . . . .Internet Sites	
Complete Protein Foods	.http://www.canadaegg.ca
	http://www.beefnutrition.org
	http://www.nppc.org
Incomplete Protein Foods	.http://www.peanutbutterlovers.com
	http://www.soyfoods.com
	http://www.spcouncil.org/contents.htm
Multi-lingual Teaching Aids	.http://mhcs.health.nsw.gov.au/health-public-affairs/mhcs/publications/nutri.../BHC-3340.htm
PKU	.http://www.noah.cuny.edu/pregnancy/march_ofdimes/birth_defects/pkuinfo.html
	http://www.wolfe.net/~Kronmal/
Sickle Cell Disease	.http://www.umc.rochester.edu/smd/genetics/brochures/sc.htm
	http://text.nlm.nih.gov/ahcpr/sickle/www/scdctxt.html
	http://www.healthy.net/hwlibrarybooks/healthyself/sickle.htm

Chapter Review

1. For which of the following functions of protein can other nutrients be substituted?
   a. Energy source
   b. Immunity
   c. Maintenance and growth
   d. Regulation of body processes
2. Which of the following foods is a complete protein?
   a. Baked beans
   b. Broccoli
   c. Beef kabobs
   d. Bread sticks
3. If a person had difficulty purchasing meat to serve every day, which of the following foods should the nurse suggest as offering the best source of protein?
   a. Bran muffins with raisins
   b. Red beans and rice
   c. Green bean, onion, and mushroom casserole
   d. Sweet potatoes and cornbread
4. How much protein should a normal healthy adult consume each day?
   a. 0.8 gram per kilogram of actual body weight
   b. 0.8 gram per kilogram of healthy body weight
   c. 0.8 gram per pound of actual body weight
   d. 0.8 gram per pound of healthy body weight
5. Which of the following people would the nurse treat as being in a catabolic state?
   a. Adolescent boy who is into bodybuilding
   b. Lactating mother
   c. Pregnant woman in the second trimester
   d. Surgical patient, first day after a stomach resection

Clinical Analysis

Mr. P, a 65-year-old man, widowed for 6 months, has been referred to your home health agency for assistance in managing his nutritional intake. He has lost 10 pounds over the past 6 months. A physical examination within the past month revealed no disease processes requiring treatment.

1. In assessing Mr. P, which of the following data would the nurse gather first?
   a. List of current medications the client takes.
   b. Blood protein levels analyzed during the recent physical examination.
   c. A description of the procedure Mr. P uses to weigh himself.
   d. Dietary recall of Mr. P's food and fluid intake.
2. Which of the following plans would be most appropriate to increase Mr. P's protein consumption immediately?
   a. Refer client to nutrition education program.
   b. Have Mr. P apply for home-delivered meals.
   c. Recommend that Mr. P supplement his meals with one of the milk-based liquid breakfast products.
   d. Suggest to Mr. P that he sign up for cooking lessons at the local high school or community college.
3. Which of the following outcomes would indicate achievement of the nutritional objective for Mr. P?
   a. A gain in weight of 2 pounds in 2 weeks.
   b. An invitation to the nurse to join him for a dinner he has learned to cook.
   c. A report by Mr. P that he is eating better.
   d. A visual inspection of Mr. P's refrigerator revealing fresh meat and milk products in abundance.

Bibliography

Acosta, PB and Wright, L: Nurses' role in preventing birth defects in off-spring of women with phenylketonuria. JOGNN 21:270, 1992.

Acosta, PB and Yannicelli, S: Plasma micronutrient concentrations in infants undergoing therapy for phenylketonuria. Biol Trace Elem Res 67:75, 1999.

Acosta, PB, et al: Protein status of infants with phenylketonuria undergoing nutrition management. J Am Coll Nutr 18:102, 1999.

Antonio, J, and Street, C: Glutamine: a potentially useful supplement for athletes. Can J Appl Physiol 24:1, 1999.

Baker, SS: Protein-energy malnutrition in the hospitalized pediatric patient. In Walker, WA and Watkins, JB (eds): Nutrition in Pediatrics. BC Decker, Inc. Publisher, Hamilton, Ontario, 1997.

Boivin, MJ: An ecological paradigm for a health behavior analysis of "konzo," a paralytic disease of Zaire from toxic cassava. Soc Sci Med 45:1853, 1997.

Bowe, K: Phenylketonuria: An update for pediatric community health nurses. Pediatr Nurs 21:191, 1995.

Buno, IJ, Morelli, JG, and Weston, WL: The enamel paint sign in the dermatologic diagnosis of early-onset kwashiorkor. Arch Dermatol 134:107, 1998.

Davis, H, Gergen, PJ, and Moore, RM Jr: Geographic differences in mortality of young children with sickle cell disease in the United States. Public Health Reports 112:52, 1997.

Davis, H, et al: National trends in the mortality of children with sickle cell disease, 1968 through 1992. Am J Public Health 87:1317, 1997.

de Freitas, O, et al: New approaches to the treatment of phenylketonuria. Nutr Rev 57:65, 1999.

Fisch, RO, et al: Phenylketonuria: current dietary treatment practices in the United States and Canada. J Am Coll Nutr 16:147, 1997.

Johnson, M, Maas, M, and Moorhead, S: Nursing Outcomes Classification (NOC), ed 2. Mosby, Philadelphia, 2000.

Johnston, PK: Nutritional implications of vegetarian diets. In Shils, ME, et al (eds): Modern Nutrition in Health and Disease ed 9. Lippincott Williams and Wilkins, Philadelphia, 1999.

Kuhad, RC, et al: Microorganisms as an alternative source of protein. Nutrition Reviews 55:65, 1997.

Lunn, PG, Morley, CJ, and Neale, G: A case of kwashiorkor in the UK. Clinical Nutrition 17:131, 1998.

MacDonald, A, et al: Abnormal feeding behaviors in phenylketonuria. Journal of Human Nutrition and Dietetics 10:163, 1997.

MacDonald, A, et al: Does a single plasma phenylalanine predict quality of control in phenylketonuria? Arch Dis Child 78:122, 1998.

Matthews, DE: Proteins and amino acids. In Shils, ME, et al (eds): Modern Nutrition in Health and Disease ed 9. Lippincott Williams and Wilkins, Philadelphia, 1999.

McCloskey, JC, and Bulechek, GM: Nursing Interventions Classification (NIC), 3 ed. Mosby, Philadelphia, 2000.

Medical Research Council: Recommendations on the dietary management of phenylketonuria. Arch Dis Child 68:426, 1993.

Messer, E: Intra-household allocation of food and health care: current findings and understandings—introduction. Soc Sci Med 44:1675, 1997.

National Live Stock and Meat Board, 444 North Michigan Ave., Chicago, IL 60611.

National Research Council: Diet and Health: Implications for Reducing Chronic Disease Risk. Report of the Committee on Diet and Health, Food and Nutrition Board, Commission on Life Sciences, National Academy Press, Washington, DC, 1989.

North American Nursing Diagnosis Association: Nursing Diagnoses: Definitions and Classification 1999–2000, North American Nursing Diagnosis Association, Philadelphia, 1999.

PKU Public Health Education Information Sheet. Accessed Jun 21, 1999, at http://www.noah.cuny.edu/pregnancy/march_of_dimes/birth_defects/pkuinfo.html.

Platt, OS, Brambilla, DJ, and Ross, WF: Mortality in sickle cell disease: life expectancy and risk factors for early death. N Engl J Med 330:1639, 1994.

Schumn, DE: Essentials of Biochemistry. FA Davis, Philadelphia, 1988.

Serjeant, GR: Sickle-cell disease. Lancet 350:725, 1997.

Sinai, LN, et al: Phenylketonuria screening: effect of early newborn discharge. Pediatrics 96:605, 1995.

Singhal, A, et al: Is there an energy deficiency in homozygous sickle cell disease? Am J Clin Nutr 66:386, 1997.

Smit, E, et al: Estimates of animal and plant protein intake in US adults: results from the Third National Health and Nutrition Examination Survey, 1988–1991. J Am Diet Assoc 99:813, 1999.

Solomons, TWG: Fundamentals of Organic Chemistry, ed. 4. John Wiley & Sons, New York, 1994.

Steinberg, MH: Management of sickle cell disease. N Engl J Med 340:1021, 1999.

Vegetarian fare: fat chance of a lean meal? Consumer Reports on Health 9:20, 1997.

Energy Balance

In approximately half the U.S. population, the human body regulates energy intake and expenditure automatically to maintain an energy balance. This balance occurs even when the amount of energy needed varies and food intake is erratic. The body can also compensate during food restriction or starvation by conserving energy. The energy balance system in the rest of the U.S. population has a malfunction.

This chapter focuses on energy balance (Chapter 18 on weight control focuses on energy imbalance), the effect of energy intake and energy expenditure on energy balance. Topics include energy measurements, factors that can influence the body's need for energy, energy consumption patterns, the kilocaloric content and nutrient density of foods, energy allowances, and current recommendations concerning energy consumption. A basic understanding of the energy balance system in the human body is a necessary foundation for understanding energy imbalance.

Homeostasis

The human body seeks homeostasis—that is, equilibrium or balance. Homeostasis, in terms of energy balance, occurs when the number of kilocalories eaten equals the number used to produce energy. An individual who maintains a stable body weight is usually in energy balance.

Energy Intake

The typical adult eats 500,000 to 850,000 kilocalories per year. Eating an excess of only 1 percent or 15 extra kilocalories per day would result in a weight gain of 1.5 pounds per year—the kilocalories in 1/3 teaspoonful of butter or a quarter of a small apple. Individuals at a stable, healthy weight give little thought to the amount of food that they eat each day, yet their body weight remains constant.

Eating appears to be a voluntary act influenced by the external environment, but it is regulated internally as well. The internal regulation of energy balance involves the gastrointestinal tract, the endocrine system, the brain, and body fat stores. Physiologic regulation is evidenced by the constancy of body weight in adults and the fact that after weight gain or loss this constant body weight is reestablished. Over the long term, food energy intake is regulated to balance energy expenditure.

Energy Expenditure

Energy expenditure, which varies daily, is measured by the number of kilocalories an individual uses to meet the body's demand for fuel. A person uses many more kilocalories to run a marathon than to sleep all day. Physical activity expends energy.

Adaptive Thermogenesis

Energy expenditure frequently adapts to large increases or large decreases in food intake of several days' duration by means of a process called adaptive thermogenesis. Adaptive thermogenesis is one example of how the human body evolved to cope with feast-or-famine conditions.

Energy expenditure decreases during food restriction or starvation. Kilocalories are burned more efficiently. Adaptive thermogenesis causes an individual who is trying to lose weight either to lose at a slower rate or to stop losing weight. It makes weight loss difficult for many people but not impossible.

Overeating for several days will cause an increase in energy expenditure. Energy expenditure has been found to be higher than predicted during the refeeding of previously starved patients, especially within the first week (Hoffer, 1999).

Researchers do not yet understand why some people are unable to maintain energy balance. However, for about one-half the population the human body maintains energy balance.

Measurement of Energy

Both the energy (fuel) foods contain and the amount of energy the body uses can be measured. The methods used to measure energy are fairly universal.

Units of Measure

The energy content of food is measured in kilocalories, often abbreviated as kcalories or kcal. A kilocalorie is the amount of heat required to raise 1 kilogram of water 1°C. Kilocalories are what the media and people who are not health-care professionals incorrectly call "calories." In chemistry, a calorie is the amount of heat required to raise 1 gram of water 1°C. One kilocalorie contains 1000 times as much energy as one calorie. "Kilocalorie" is the term used throughout this text. Using kcalories for nutritional measurement eliminates the large numbers that use of the chemical term would necessitate.

The **joule** is another unit increasingly used to measure energy; you may encounter this term as you read scientific journals. One kilojoule is the amount of energy required to move a mass of 1 kilogram with an acceleration of 1 meter per second. The kilojoule is equal to 0.239 kilocalorie; a kilocalorie equals 4.184 kilojoules.

Energy Nutrient Values

The energy nutrients are carbohydrates, fat, and protein. Alcohol (ethanol) also yields energy. A food's kilocalorie value is determined by its content of protein, fat, carbohydrates, and alcohol. To review:

- 1 gram of carbohydrate equals 4 kilocalories (or 17 kilojoules)
- 1 gram of protein equals 4 kilocalories (or 17 kilojoules)
- 1 gram of fat equals 9 kilocalories (or 37.6 kilojoules)
- 1 gram of alcohol equals 7 kilocalories (or 29.3 kilojoules).

Water, fiber, vitamins, and minerals do not provide kilocalories. Clinical Calculation 6–1 demonstrates how to determine the energy content of a food item.

Determination of Energy Values

Foods

The energy content of individual foods is measured by a device called a bomb calorimeter, illustrated in Figure 6–1. A bomb calorimeter is an insulated container that has a chamber in which food is burned. The amount of heat (kilocalories) produced by the burning of the food is determined by the change in the temperature of a measured amount of water that surrounds the chamber. All energy in food is in the form of chemical energy. In a bomb calorimeter, the chemical energy stored in the food sample is transformed into heat energy. The following equation may facilitate understanding of this concept:

Protein + oxygen = heat energy + water + carbon dioxide

(Carbohydrate or fat may be substituted for protein in the equation.)

Human Body

A process similar to the combustion of food in the bomb calorimeter occurs in the body. The amount of energy the human body uses can be

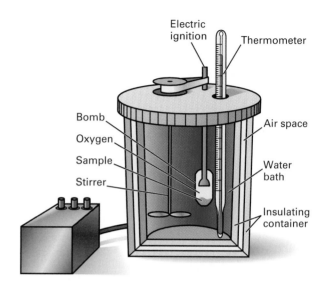

Figure 6–1:
Cross-section of a bomb calorimeter showing essential features. The food sample is completely burned in the inner section; heat produced is absorbed by the known volume of water in the surrounding section. Change in temperature provides the measure of heat produced (Reproduced by permission from Guthrie, HA: Introductory Nutrition, ed 7. Times Mirror/Mosby College Publishing, St. Louis, 1989)

measured directly or indirectly. Direct measurement of energy used by the human body requires expensive equipment that is used only in scientific research. Energy is measured directly by placing a person in an insulated heat-sensitive chamber and measuring the heat emitted by the body. Indirect measurement of energy is discussed in Clinical Application 6–1.

Components of Energy Expenditure

The human body requires energy (1) to meet its resting energy expenditure needs and (2) its physical activity requirements to digest, absorb, transport, and utilize nutrients. Physical activity includes the energy needed for voluntary activities, which are consciously controlled, such as running, walking, and swimming and involuntary activities.

Resting Energy Expenditure

Resting energy expenditure represents the energy expended or used by a person at rest. Resting energy expenditure (REE) requires more total kilocalories than physical activity in most people. Another term still in use in some scientific literature is basal metabolic rate (BMR). The major difference between resting energy and basal metabolic rate is that basal metabolic rate is always measured beginning at least 12 hours after the last meal and under certain conditions, such as controlled temperature and humidity.

Clinical Application 6–1 discusses the measurement of REE in hospitalized clients. The term REE is generally associated with the use of a respirometer. In practice, BMR and REE differ by less than 12 percent in

Clinical Calculation 6–1 Calculating the Energy Content of a Food Item

If you know the carbohydrate, fat, and protein content of a food item, you can readily calculate the food item's kilocalorie content. Two examples are shown below. One starch exchange contains 3 g of protein and 15 g of carbohydrate. Adding the protein and carbohydrate content in the starch exchange together equals 18.

	Carbohydrate (g)	Protein (g)	Fat (g)	Total (g)
One starch exchange	15	+ 3	+ 0	= 18

There are 4 kcal in 1 g each of carbohydrate and protein so all you need to do to obtain the kilocalorie content of the starch exchange is to multiply 4 by 18. Thus there are 72 kcal in one starch exchange.

One fat exchange contains 5 g of fat.

	Carbohydrate (g)	Protein (g)	Fat (g)	Total (g)
One fat exchange	0	+ 0	+ 5	= 5

There are 9 kcal in a gram of fat. To obtain the kilocaloric content of one fat exchange, multiply 5 by 9. Thus one fat exchange contains 45 kcal.

CLINICAL APPLICATION 6–1

Respiratory Gas Analyzer

The indirect method of measuring energy expenditure is done with a respiratory device called a respiratory gas analyzer or respirometer. The amount of carbon dioxide exhaled and the amount of oxygen consumed for a given period are recorded. From this data, the number of kilocalories expended by the client can be calculated. Kilocalorie expenditure, at rest, can be calculated from oxygen consumption and carbon dioxide production using the following equation (Cerra, 1984):

$$\text{Kilocalories per day}_2 = (3.8 \times \text{liter } O_2 \text{ used} + 1.2 \times \text{liter } CO2 \text{ produced}) \times 1.4$$

In clinical practice, the indirect measurement of energy expenditure is only done for clients who are at a high nutritional risk. A respirometer is an expensive piece of equipment. The health care worker is most likely to observe this procedure being performed in the intensive care unit of an acute care hospital.

healthy well-nourished clients, and the terms are used interchangeably (Subcommittee on the 10th Edition of the RDAs, 1989).

The kilocalories necessary to support the following contribute to resting energy expenditure:

1. Contraction of the heart
2. Maintenance of body temperature
3. Repair of the internal organs
4. Maintenance of cellular processes
5. Muscle and nerve coordination
6. Respiration (breathing)

REE accounts for approximately 66 percent of most people's total energy requirements.

Body composition influences resting energy expenditure. Individuals of similar age, sex, height, and weight with a higher percentage of muscle (lean body mass) have a higher REE than those with less muscle. It takes more energy, or kilocalories, to support lean body mass (protein) than to support body fat. Muscle tissue requires more kilocalories than does fat tissue, even when muscle tissue is resting. Therefore, the higher a person's body protein content, the more kilocalories he or she can eat and still maintain a stable body weight.

Estimating a person's resting energy expenditure is commonly done by using the equations found in Table 6–1. These equations take into account age, sex, and weight but ignore differences in body composition, climate, and genetic variability (discussed in the following sections). Although these equations are not completely accurate for all individuals, they can serve as a guide for menu planning and calculating tube and intravenous feedings. The ultimate test of how kilocalories eaten work in the body is to monitor body weight and kilocaloric intake over time—one reason nurses monitor clients' body weight and food intake and dietitians calculate clients' kcaloric intake.

AGE Resting energy expenditure varies with lean body mass, which varies with age. The highest rates of energy expenditure per pound of body weight occur during infancy and childhood. In adults, REE declines about 2 percent per decade because of a decline in lean body mass. The result is a reduced need for kilocalories. Individuals can slow the decline in lean body mass somewhat by increasing their exercise. An individual who fails either to decrease kilocaloric intake to compensate for this reduced need or to increase physical activity may experience a slow weight gain (see Wellness Tip 6–1).

SEX Differences in body composition between men and women occur as early as the first few months of life. The differences are relatively small until the child reaches age 10. During adolescence, body composition changes radically. Men develop proportionately greater muscle mass than women, who deposit fat as they mature. Consequently, REE differs by as much as 10 percent between men and women.

GROWTH Human growth is most pronounced during the growth spurts that take place before birth and during infancy and puberty. Kilocalories required per kilogram of body weight are highest during these growth

Wellness Tip 6–1

- To compensate for a decrease in resting energy expenditure as you grow older, increase exercise and decrease food intake.

Table 6–1 Equations for Calculating Resting Energy Expenditure

Sex Age Range (Years)	Equation to Obtain REE in Kilocalories per Day	
Men		
0-3	(60.9 × weight in kilograms)	−54
3-10	(22.7 × weight in kilograms)	495
10-18	(17.5 × weight in kilograms)	651
18-30	(15.3 × weight in kilograms)	679
30-60	(11.6 × weight in kilograms)	879
> 60	(13.5 × weight in kilograms)	487
Women		
0-3	(61.0 × weight in kilograms)	−51
3-10	(22.5 × weight in kilograms)	499
10- 18	(12.2 × weight ill kilogl ams)	746
18-30	(14.7 × weight in kilograms)	496
30-60	(8.7 × weight in kilograms)	829
> 60	(10.5 × weight in kilograms)	596

SOURCE: Adapted from the Subcommittee on the 10th Edition of the RDAs, 1989, p. 26.

spurts, because the kilocaloric cost of anabolism is greater than the kilocaloric cost of catabolism.

BODY SIZE People with large bodies require proportionately more energy than smaller ones. A tall individual uses more energy because he or she has a greater skin surface through which heat is lost than does a shorter person. A shorter person also has less muscle tissue or lean body mass than a taller person. In proportion to total body weight, the infant has a large surface area, loses more heat through the skin, and therefore has a proportionately high REE.

GENETICS REE is strongly influenced by individual genetic patterns. Each person, it appears, is programmed with a need to burn a certain number of kilocalories to maintain energy balance. This fact becomes apparent to health-care workers when counseling two very similar clients. Both clients may be of the same sex, of equal weight, perform similar types of physical activity, and have about the same body fat content. Yet each client may need to eat a different number of kilocalories to maintain a stable body weight. Many individuals have little control over the number of kilocalories required to meet the needs of REE.

CLIMATE Climate affects REE because kilocalories are needed to maintain body temperature. This fact pertains to extreme differences in external temperatures, whether cold or hot. In the United States, most people do not need to eat more kilocalories during colder months because the majority of living environments range from 68°F to 77°F. Outside, people usually protect themselves from extreme cold and shivering, which causes an increase in REE, by wearing warm clothes.

Clients with fevers also need extra kilocalories. Clinical Application 6–2 discusses this need.

Wellness Tips 6–2

- Choose sensible portion sizes: Fat-free and reduced-fat foods may not be low in kcalories.
- Kcalories count regardless of the source (fat, protein, or CHO).

Thermic Effect of Food

After a meal, the heat produced by the body is called the thermic effect of food (TEF). An older term for this energy cost is specific dynamic action (SDA). Energy is needed to chew, swallow, digest, absorb, and transport nutrients. Metabolism increases after eating. As metabolism increases, more kilocalories are used. Clinical Calculation 6–2 demonstrates the calculation of REE for a typical 18- to 30-year-old 154-pound man.

The consumption of protein and carbohydrates results in a much larger thermic effect than the consumption of fat. Fat in food is processed to body fat more efficiently than carbohydrate or protein. If an individual eats as many kilocalories from carbohydrate as from fat, he or she will store fewer of the carbohydrate kilocalories as body fat.

Kilocalories do count, however, regardless of the source. Consumers need to read food labels carefully. Sometimes a regular version of a food may actually contain fewer kcalories than the fat-free or reduced-fat version. For example, a regular fig cookie contains 50 kcalories, and one fat-free version contains 70 kcalories. One-half cup of regular ice cream contains 180 calories, and the same amount of one kind of reduced-fat ice cream contains 190 kcalories. Sometimes consumers are under the illusion that because the food they are eating is low-fat, they can eat unrestricted amounts (see Wellness Tip 6–2).

Physical Activity

For most of the U.S. population, the second cause of total energy expenditure is physical activity (see Wellness Tip 6–3). Some very active individuals may need more kilocalories as a result of physical activity than as a result of REE (Fig. 6–2). Professional athletes may burn a large number of kilocalories as a result of training and engaging in competition. Table 6–2 provides activity factors (energy needs per pound of body weight) associated with a range of pursuits. Multiply the activity factor by the REE to calculate a person's kilocaloric requirements. The energy cost of physical activity is frequently referred to as the thermic effect of exercise (TEE).

Energy needs can be calculated on the basis of body weight and adjusted for activity level as shown in Table 6–2. Clinical Calculation 6–3 demonstrates the calculation of daily energy allowance, which includes kilocalories needed for activity. Such calculations are approximations at best. The most accurate method to determine a client's kilocalorie requirement is to monitor both food intake and body weight over time.

Physical activity can greatly influence energy requirements (Box 6–1). For example, a 154-pound man (70 kilograms) may require only 2406 kilocalories on a very sedentary day and as many as 3938 kilocalo-

CLINICAL APPLICATION 6–2

Fever

Heat acts as a catalyst in most chemical reactions. A catalyst is a substance that speeds up a chemical reaction. Fever increases resting energy expenditure by about 7 percent for every 1°F increase in body temperature. Frequently, an individual with a fever is too ill to eat. Fruit juices with added glucose polymers or a nutritional supplement will give the client needed energy.

Clinical Calculation 6–2:
Calculating Resting Energy Expenditure

Sample calculations for a 154-lb, 18- to 30-year-old man's resting energy expenditure:

1. Convert weight in pounds to kilograms

$$\frac{\text{Weight in pounds}}{\text{Weight in pounds per kilogram}} = \text{Weight in kilograms}$$

$$\frac{154}{2.2} = 70 \text{ kg}$$

2. Locate equation from Table 6–1 and perform the calculation.

REE = (15.3 × weight in kilograms) + 679
REE = (15.3 × 70 kg) + 679
REE = 1071 + 679
REE = 1750 kcal per day

ries on a very active day. A 128-pound woman (58 kilograms) may require only 1856 kilocalories on a very sedentary day and as many as 3038 kilocalories on a very active day (Subcommittee of the 10th Edition of the RDAs, 1989).

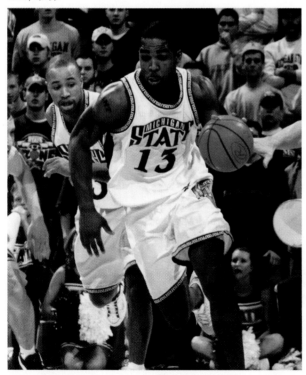

Figure 6–2:
A trained athlete may burn more kcalories as a result of physical activity than as a result of resting energy expenditure. (Courtesy of Kevin Fowler, Sports Information Michigan State University)

Wellness Tip 6–3

- Be active.

Thermic Effect of Exercise

Energy expended during exercise is only a portion of the total energy cost of physical activity. Exercise may also affect both REE and the TEF. Some clients' REE increases for up to 48 hours after exercise. Although the exact reason for this increase in REE is not known, the most plausible explanation is that the glycogen stores need to be refilled. Because exercise depletes glycogen stores, there is an energy cost to refill these stores during the postexercise period.

Adaptive Response to Exercise

An individual with well-developed muscles performs more efficiently—uses fewer kilocalories to perform a given amount of physical work—than an individual with less well developed muscles. As exercise is repeated, the body learns how to get the job done with the least effort (the body's adaptive response to exercise). If an individual has a weight loss due to increased exercise, he or she will eventually use fewer kilocalories to do a specific activity. Lighter people require fewer kilocalories for a given amount of exercise than heavier people do; it takes fewer kilocalories to move a smaller mass than a larger one.

Exercise and Appetite

Many exercise researchers think that exercise decreases appetite. **Appetite** is defined as a strong desire for food (or by extension for a pleasant sensation) based on previous experience that causes one to seek food for the purpose of tasting and enjoying. After exercise, a person's appetite may be less—that is, he or she may be satisfied with less food. Some types of exercise release a chemical in the brain called beta-endorphin. Beta-endorphin has an effect similar to that of natural morphine; it produces a state of relaxation. In effect, exercise can be a safe substitute for overeating in individuals who eat to decrease stress and tension.

Aerobic Exercise

Aerobic exercise is any activity during which the energy metabolism needed is supported by the amount of increase in oxygen inspired. Aerobic exercises increase physical fitness and involve large muscle groups. Vigorous workouts that last at least 30 minutes, such as fast walking, cycling, swimming, skating, rope jumping, aerobic dancing, hiking, jogging, and rowing require an increase in the amount of oxygen

Table 6–2 Energy Needs Based on Weight and Activity			
	Energy Needs in Kilocalories per Pound of Body Weight		
	Sedentary*	Moderately Active†	Active‡
Overweight	9–11	13	16
Normal weight	13	16	18
Underweight	13	18	18–23

*Patients with severly limited mobility
†Active students, sales clerks, many farm workers
‡Full-time athletes, unskilled laborers, Army recruits

Clinical Calculation 6–3: Calculating Daily Energy Allowance

Sample calculation for a moderately active person at his or her normal weight 5 of 150 lb.

1. Locate the kcal/lb needed from Table 6–2. Formula is:

   Number from table × weight in pounds.

2. Perform calculations:

   16 × 150 = 2400 kcal/day

Thus the estimated daily energy need for this person is 2400 kcal.

inspired. Any exercise that raises your pulse to target heart rate is an aerobic activity. To determine your target heart rate, see Clinical Application 6–3.

Aerobic exercise provides many health benefits, including:

- Decreased risk of cardiovascular disease
- Improved blood sugar control for people with diabetes
- Decreased risk of obesity
- Reversal or prevention of varicose veins
- Decreased risk of osteoporosis
- Improvement in the quality of sleep
- Improved hypertension control.

Anaerobic Exercise

Exercise during which energy needed is provided without an increase in the use of inspired oxygen is anaerobic exercise. Short bursts of vigorous activity, such as resistance or muscle strength training (weight lifting, for example), are forms of anaerobic exercise. Anaerobic exercise allows for muscle toning, the building of muscular strength and endurance, and the building of bone mass. This kind of training provides added strength and toughness, which help to reduce injury during aerobic exercise, prevents lower back problems, and allows for a more muscular appearance.

Diet and Activity

A healthy lifestyle depends on much more than diet alone. Physical activity makes a vital contribution to health, function, and performance. The

CLINICAL APPLICATION 6–3

Determining A Theoretical Target Heart Rate

The theoretical target heart rate is the rate you need to reach to achieve maximal aerobic effect. Determine your theoretical* target heart rate as follows:

l. Subtract your age from the number 220.

2. Multiply this number first by 65 percent and then by 80 percent. The two numbers should represent the range of heart beats per minute that you should try to maintain during aerobic exercise. Example of an 18-year-old woman:

$$220 - 18 = 202$$
$$202 \times 0.65 = 131$$
$$202 \times 0.80 = 161$$

This individual should exercise sufficiently to reach a heart rate of between 131 and 161 beats per minute.

*To monitor your heart rate during exercise, count the number of times your heart beats for 6 seconds and multiply by 10.

greatest benefit derived from physical activity is gained when a person moves from sedentary to moderate levels of activity. Current research indicates that the sedentary lifestyle of one in four Americans is extremely risky and to be avoided at all costs (Nieman, 1998).

Every American adult should engage in 30 minutes or more of moderate-intensity physical activity on most, preferably all, days of the week (Pale, et al., 1995)—that is, a total of 30 minutes per day of brisk walking, stair climbing, calisthenics, heavy gardening, or dancing. The activity need not be continuous but may be broken up into short sessions. For example, three brisk 10-minute walks would meet the minimum requirement. A person performing these activities for 30 minutes expends 200 total kilocalories. The President's Council on Physical Fitness and Activity has published an Activity Pyramid (Fig. 6–3).

Energy Intake

Two different surveys found that the average daily reported energy intakes for men were between 2359 and 2639 kilocalories per day. The average

Box 6–1 Kcalories expended in 30 minutes at various activities by 140 and 180 pound individuals

Activity	Kcalories expended by a 140-pound person	Kcalories expended by a 180-pound person
Sittng quietly	39	51
Walking	228	291
Running	396	5 10
Jogging	324	417
Cycling	192	246
Gardening	177	225
Golf (pull/carry clubs)	162	210
Golf (power cart)	75	96
Swimming (crawl, moderate pace)	270	348
Social dancing	192	246
Weight training	228	294

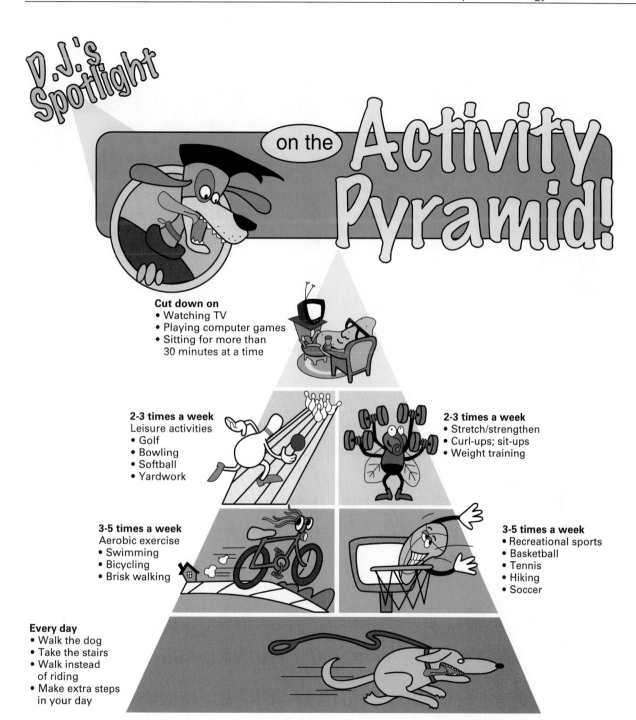

Cut down on
- Watching TV
- Playing computer games
- Sitting for more than 30 minutes at a time

2-3 times a week
Leisure activities
- Golf
- Bowling
- Softball
- Yardwork

2-3 times a week
- Stretch/strengthen
- Curl-ups; sit-ups
- Weight training

3-5 times a week
Aerobic exercise
- Swimming
- Bicycling
- Brisk walking

3-5 times a week
- Recreational sports
- Basketball
- Tennis
- Hiking
- Soccer

Every day
- Walk the dog
- Take the stairs
- Walk instead of riding
- Make extra steps in your day

Figure 6–3:
The President's Council Activity Pyramid for Children. Children should have some activity every day, vigorous activity 2 to 3 times a week, and minimal sedentary activity such as watching television and playing computer games.

daily reported intakes for women were between 1639 and 1793 kilocalories per day. The average reported intakes for women are of special concern because of the difficulty in incorporating all nutrients at recommended levels in a diet so low in kilocalories (National Research Council, 1989). The need for the average woman to increase energy output or physical activity is well documented.

Information from the Nationwide Food Consumption Survey has been used to compare energy intakes in 1965 with those in 1977. These data suggest that energy intake declined for both sexes by approximately 10 percent during those 10 to 20 years (National Research Council, 1989). The percentage of overweight men and women has been increasing in spite of the decrease in energy intake. Many experts attribute increased obesity to decreased energy expenditure. America is becoming an increasingly sedentary society. The current recommendation is that the typical person increase physical activity rather than decrease kilocalorie intake below the recommended energy allowance to achieve energy balance.

Kilocaloric Density of Foods

Some foods are more kilocalorically dense than other foods. Density is the quantity per unit volume of a substance. **Kilocaloric density** refers to the kilocalories contained in a given volume of a food. Foods with a high water and fiber content tend to have a lower kilocaloric density. Fruits and vegetables such as lettuce, watermelon, and celery are high in water content and low in kilocalories. A given volume of grapes has fewer kilocalories than an equal one of raisins because grapes contain more water than raisins.

Fats or foods high in fat have the highest kilocaloric density (Fig. 6–4). Whole-milk products, high-fat meat exchanges, fat exchanges, and foods made with these ingredients all contain appreciable amounts of fat. Table 6–3 lists several tips for decreasing the kilocaloric density of a diet.

Nutrient Density of Foods

Kilocaloric content alone should not be the criterion to decide whether to include a food in one's diet. The **nutrient density** of a food—the concentration of nutrients in a food compared with the food's kilocaloric content—is also an important consideration. If a food is high in kilocalories and low in nutrients, the nutrient density of the food is low. Empty kilocalories means that the food contains kilocalories and almost no nutri-

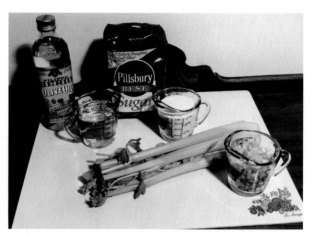

Figure 6–4:
One cup of celery contains 17 kcalories, 1 cup of sugar contains 770 calories, and 1 cup of oil contains 1925 kcalories. Celery is the least kcalorically dense (of the foods pictured), and oil is the most dense. Sugar is between celery and oil in kcaloric density.

ents; table sugar is an example of such a food. If a food is low in kilocalories and high in nutrients, the nutrient density of the food is high.

Cantaloupe is an example of a food with a high nutrient density—it is low in kilocalories, high in vitamin C, and contains a moderate amount of vitamin A. Skim milk and whole milk are similar in nutrient content; both types of milk contain about the same amounts of protein, calcium, and riboflavin. Eight ounces of skim milk provides about 90 kilocalories compared with 150 kilocalories in 8 ounces of whole milk. Skim milk thus has a higher nutrient density than whole milk.

Energy Allowances

The recommended dietary allowances for energy based on differences for age, sex, and body size are shown in Table 6–4. The kilocalories listed in the table are based on a reference man and woman. For example, the reference 15- to 18-year-old woman weighs 120 pounds and is 64 inches tall; actual energy requirements may vary widely within any given age group. Genetics may play a role in determining a person's actual energy requirement.

Note that the kilocaloric allowances for pregnant and lactating women are increased. A pregnant woman's energy allowance is 300 kilocalories beyond her nonpregnant allowance; a lactating woman's energy allowance is 500 kilocalories beyond her nonlactating allowance.

Dietary Recommendations

All the major national health organizations recommend that individuals maintain a healthy body weight. The American Heart Association recommends maintaining a healthy body weight to decrease the risk of heart and circulatory diseases. The American Cancer Society cites numerous studies suggesting that lower kilocaloric intake may lower an individual's risk of cancer. Most individuals would benefit by monitoring their weight and increasing their energy expenditure or decreasing their energy intake as necessary to maintain a healthy body weight.

TABLE 6–3 Tips for Decreasing the Kilocaloric Density of a Diet

- Use low-fat or nonfat dairy products including skim milk, cheese, and yogurt.
- Brown meats by broiling or cooking in nonstick pans with little or no fat. Avoid fried foods.
- Chill soups, stews, sauces, and broths. Lift off and discard hardened fat.
- Trim all visible fat from meat before cooking.
- Use water-packed, canned foods such as fruits and tuna.
- Use fresh fruits and vegetables often. Try to eat at least 2 1/2 cups of these foods each day.
- Use low-kilocalorie salad dressings.
- When you eat out, do not look at the menu. Instead, have an idea of what you would like to eat before you arrive at the restaurant. Explain to the waitress or waiter what you would like to eat.

TABLE 6–4 Recommended Dietary Allowances for Energy

Category	Age or Condition	Weight (kg)	Height (in)	REE† (kcal/day)	Average Energy Allowance (kcal/day)*	
					Per kg‡	Per day
Infants	0-0.5	6	24	320	108	650
	0.5-1	9	28	500	98	850
Children	1-3	13	35	740	102	1300
	4-6	20	44	950	90	1800
	7-10	28	52	1130	70	2000
Males	11-14	45	62	1440	55	2500
	15-18	66	69	1760	45	3000
	19-24	72	70	1780	40	2900
	25-50	79	70	1800	37	2900
	51+	77	68	1530	30	2300
Females	11-14	46	62	1310	47	2200
	15-18	55	64	1370	40	2200
	19-24	58	65	1350	38	2200
	25-50	63	64	1380	36	2200
	51+	65	63	1280	30	1900
Pregnant 1st trimester						+0
2nd trimester						+300
3rd trimester						+300
Lactating 1st 6 months						+500
2nd 6 months						+500

SOURCE: Adapted from the Subcommittee on the 10th Edition of the RDAs, 1989, p. 33. *Includes kilocalories needed for physical activity. ‡Does not include kilocalories needed for physical activity. †Based on a median age, weight, height, and light-to-moderate activity level.

Summary

Energy balance exists when energy intake equals energy output. A person whose body weight remains stable is usually in energy balance. In about one-half of the U.S. population, the capability of regulating energy intake and expenditure to accommodate daily variations is normal. When an individual is not in energy balance, he or she is gaining or losing body weight.

The human body needs energy for resting energy expenditure and voluntary physical activity. Energy allowances are calculated by multiplying an individual's resting energy expenditure by a factor for physical activity.

Foods high in water and fiber (fruits and vegetables) are low in kilocaloric density. Foods high in fat (fatty meats, oils, spreads, salad dressings,

and food made with these ingredients) are high in kilocaloric density. Foods that are low in kilocalories and contain substantial amounts of one or more nutrients are high in nutrient density. Individuals should try to consume nutritionally dense foods.

Americans have been decreasing both their food intake and activity for the past 30 years. The current recommendation is that individuals who gain weight while consuming their energy RDA should increase their activity to maintain energy balance rather than decrease intake.

Case Study 6–1

The Fairview Nursing Home holds a weekly client care conference. All the facility's residents have their nursing care plans reviewed on a rotating basis, with each client's nursing care plan being reviewed once every 3 months. All members of the health care team are often present at the conference. Team members may include the administrator, the physician, the director of nursing, the staff nurse, the nursing assistant, the activities director, the social worker, the dietitian, and the client or a family member representing the client.

Mr. G has been experiencing a slow weight gain. His weight history follows:

1/89	175 lb
3/89	177 lb
7/89	178 lb
9/89	180 lb
12/89	181 lb

Mr. G is 5 ft 8 in. tall and is 79 years old. He is alert, feeds himself, and has normal bowel and bladder function. Mr. G walks to the dining room three times a day. His favorite activity is watching television. He has good dentition and is on a regular diet. According to the appetite records kept by the nurse's aide, Mr. G's intake is good to excellent. He accepts all the major food groups. Mr G is concerned with his slow weight gain but claims he does not know what to do. To address the slow weight gain problem, the health care team and Mr. G developed the following nursing care plan.

Nursing Care Plan

Nursing Diagnosis   NANDA: Altered nutrition: More than body requirements (North American Nursing Diagnosis Association, 1999, with permission) Related to knowledge deficit as evidenced by admitted lack of understanding and a gain in weight of 3 percent over the past year

Desired Outcomes Evaluation Criteria	Nursing Actions/ Interventions	Rationale
NOC: Nutritional Status: (NOC) (Johnson, Maas, and Moorhead, 2000, with permission.)	NIC: Nutritional Counseling (McCloskey and Bulechek, 2000, with permission.)	
Client will select fresh fruits for desserts at 50 percent of all social activities.	Provide encouragement to the client to select fresh fruit at all social activites. Congratulate the client when he is able to retrain trom eating rich desserts. Remind the Dietary Department to serve fresh fruit at social functions.	Replacing kilocalorically dense cakes, pies, and cookies with fresh fruit will promote weight maintenance.
Client will keep a food diary and exercise log 1 day per week for the next 3 months.	Review the client's food record with him each week. Note all empty kilocalories consumed. Discuss the client's food selections and exercise log with him. Document results.	Self-monitoring of food intake and exercise will help the client focus on controlling his behaviors. Nurse's review of food records with the client while pointing out kilocalorically dense foods will educate the client about his negative behaviors.
Client will participate in the exercise program provided by the activities director at least seven times per week for the next 3 months.	Encourage the client to attend the exercise program or to walk ten minutes before each meal. Document the activity.	Exercise burns kilocalories and increases body protein content. A high body protein content is associated with increased energy expenditure.

Critical Thinking Questions

1. What would you do at the next client care conference if Mr. G changed his mind about weight control and said, "All I have left in life is food. I don't want to lose weight."

2. What would you do at the next client care conference if Mr. G had done everything asked but only managed to maintain his weight at 181 pounds?

 Study Aids

Subjects . . . .**Internet Sites**

Examples of moderate physical activity for adults . . . . .http://www./pmg.com/box

Activity Pyramid . . . . .http://www.schoolmenu.com/activity-pyramid.htm

NIH Consensus Statements: Physical activity . . . . .http://womenshealth.medscape.com/govmt/NIH

Activity calorie counter, body weight and activity
duration calculator . . . . .http://primusweb.com/cgi-bin/fpc/actcal.pl

Calories burned calculator http://128.95.122.195/nwcphp/features/calories.html

American College of Sports Medicine . . . . .www.acsm.org

President's Challenge . . . . .www.indiana.edu/~preschool

Nutrition Analysis Tool & Energy Calculator . . . . .www.einstein.wsd.wednet.edu/Sportsmed/fitness/fitorg.html

American Council on Exercise . . . . .www.acefitness.org

Chapter Review

1. The components of energy expenditure are _____ .
   a. Mental activity and physical activity
   b. Thermic effect of exercise and thermic effect of foods
   c. Resting energy expenditure, physical activity, and to a lesser extent the thermic effect of foods.
   d. Thermic effect of foods, physical activity, and thermic effect of exercise.

2. Energy homeostasis exists when:
   a. Kilocalories from food intake equal kilocalories used for energy expenditure.
   b. Kilocalories used for physical activity equal kilocalories used for energy expenditure.
   c. An individual is gaining weight.
   d. Kilocalories from food intake equal kilocalories used for resting energy expenditure.

Chapter Review (continued)

3. A kilocalorie is used to measure both
   a. Weight and percentage body fat
   b. Height and weight
   c. The units of energy used in the body and contained in foods
   d. Leanness and body-fat content
4. Kilocalories required per kilogram of body weight are highest during:
   a. Starvation
   b. Growth
   c. Weight loss
   d. Old age

5. Which of the following foods is the most kilocalorically dense?
   a. 1 cup of sugar
   b. 1 cup of celery
   c. 1 cup of skim milk
   d. 1 cup of margarine

Clinical Analysis

1. Monitoring a resident's weight is a government requirement in long-term care facilities. The goal is to prevent a slow weight loss, which, over time, can have health consequences. Mr. I, resident of Sunnybrook Nursing Home, has been experiencing an undesirable slow weight loss. His weight history is as follows:

   Feb   180 pounds
   June 175 pounds
   Oct   170 pounds

   As Mr. I's nurse, you should first:
   a. Encourage Mr. I to eat only twice a day.
   b. Call the doctor.
   c. Wait for the next client care conference to act on this problem.
   d. Monitor Mr. I's food intake to determine what he is eating.

2. A teacher noticed that many students in her fifth grade class were overweight. As a school project, the class kept food records for 3 days. A computer software program analyzed the records. Many students were eating less than their recommended dietary allowance for kilocalories but gaining weight nonetheless (a common problem among our nation's young). The teacher asked the class by a show of hands what they did after school and on weekends. Many of the same children who were overweight raised their hands when asked if they played mostly video games and watched television when not in school. The teacher shared this information with the school nurse and asked her to speak to the class. The school nurse correctly decided that:
   a. The teacher is overly concerned since the percent of overweight students approximates the percent of overweight adults in the community.
   b. The computer program must be in error.
   c. All the students need to increase their total intake, including foods from the major food groups.
   d. Many students would benefit from an increase in physical activity.

3. A client appears to be totally concerned with the kilocaloric density of foods and not at all concerned with the nutrient density of foods. You need to encourage the consumption of both types of foods. Which of the following behaviors do you need to discourage?
   a. The substitution of skim milk for 2% milk
   b. The avoidance of all meat, fish, and poultry
   c. The inclusion of dark green and yellow fruits and vegetables in the diet
   d. The inclusion of whole grains in the diet

Bibliography

Bennett, WI: Beyond overeating. N Engl J Med 332:10, 673, 1995.

Blair, SN: Diet and activity: The synergistic merger. Nutrition Today 30:3, 108, 1995.

Cerra, F: Pocket Manual of Surgical Nutrition. Mosby, St. Louis, 1984.

Groff, JL and Gropper, SS: Advanced Nutrition and Human Metabolism. 3rd edition. Wadsworth, St. Paul, MN, 1999.

Guthrie, HA: Introductory Nutrition, 7th ed. Times Mirror/Mosby College Publishing, St. Louis, 1989.

Hands, ES: Food Finder Food Sources of Vitamins and Minerals. ESHA Research, Salem, 1990.

Hoffer, LJ: Metabolic Consequences of Starvation. In Shils, ME (ed): Modern Nutrition in Health and Disease. 9th ed. Williams and Wilkins, Baltimore, 1999.

Johnson. M. Maas, M, and Moorhead, S: Nursing Outcomes Classification (NOC), ed 2. Mosby, Philadelphia, 2000.

Krahn DD, Rock C, Deckert MS, and Nairn DD, and Hasse SA: Changes in resting energy expenditure and body composition in anorexia nervosa during refeeding. J Am Diet Assoc 93:4, 1993.

McCloskey, JC and Bulechek, GM: Nursing Interventions Classification (NIC), 3rd ed. Mosby, Philadelphia, 2000.

National Research Council: Diet and Health: Implications for Reducing Chronic Disease Risk. Report of the Committee on Diet and Health, Food and Nutrition Board, Commission on Life Sciences. National Academy Press, Washington, DC, 1989, p. 110.

Nieman. DC: The Exercise-Health Connection. Human Kinetics Publishers. Champaign, Il, 1998.

North American Nursing Diagnosis Association: Nursing Diagnoses: Definitions and Classification 1999-2000, North American Diagnosis Association, Philadelphia, 1999.

Pale, RP: Physical activity and public health. JAMA 273:5, 402, 1995.

Pi-Sunyer, EX (ed.): Clinical Guidelines on the Identification, Evaluation, Treatment of Overweight and Obesity in Adults. NHLBI Obesity Education Initiative. US Dept. of Health and Human Services, June, 1998

Subcommittee on the 10th Edition of the RDAs. Food and Nutrition Board. Commission of Life Sciences. National Research Council: Recommended Dietary Allowances. National Academy Press, Washington, DC, 1989, pp. 24–38.

CHAPTER 7

Vitamins

LEARNING OBJECTIVES

After completing this chapter, the student should be able to:

1. Differentiate between fat-soluble and water-soluble vitamins.
2. State the functions of each of the vitamins discussed.
3. Name three good food sources for each of the vitamins discussed.
4. List diseases caused by specific vitamin deficiencies and identify associated signs and symptoms.
5. Describe the wise use of vitamin supplements.

The importance of vitamins was first recognized by the effects of their absence. Some deficiency diseases have been known for centuries, but it was not until the twentieth century that vitamins were isolated in the laboratory. This chapter considers the importance of vitamins in the body and in the diet, the general functions of vitamins, the classification of vitamins, and the use of vitamin supplements. Each of the vitamins is discussed from absorption through excretion, including functions, sources, recommended dietary allowances, dietary reference intakes, deficiencies, toxicities, and factors affecting stability.

The Nature of Vitamins

Vitamins are organic substances needed by the body in small amounts for normal metabolism, growth, and maintenance. Organic substances are derived from living matter and contain carbon. Vitamins themselves are not sources of energy, nor do they become part of the structure of the body. Vitamins act as regulators or adjusters of metabolic processes and as **coenzymes** (substances that activate enzymes) in enzymatic systems.

Specific Functions

Vitamin functions are specific; the bodily processes do not permit substitutes. Thus, vitamins are similar to keys in a lock. All the notches in a key have to fit the lock, or the key will not turn. One vitamin cannot perform the functions of another. If a person does not consume enough vitamin C, for instance, taking vitamin D will not correct the deficiency. Vitamin D is the wrong key for that lock.

Classification

A major distinguishing characteristic of vitamins is their solubility in either fat or water. This physical property is used to classify vitamins and is also significant for storage and processing of foods that contain vitamins and for the utilization of the vitamins in the body. Vitamins A, E, D, and K are fat soluble. The eight B-complex vitamins and vitamin C are water soluble. See Table 7–1 for a list of the 13 known vitamins. Choline, recently added to the DRI list, is discussed last.

Recommended Dietary Allowances

The amounts of vitamins recommended in the United States to meet the needs of almost all healthy individuals are listed by age and physiological status (Appendices F and H). Within this chapter examples are given for healthy adults, not pregnant or lactating women. Specified amounts vary in other countries.

Vitamins A, D, and E historically have been measured in International Units, a unit that appears on some labels. The RDAs, however, are listed in the metric system: micrograms and milligrams. There are no generic "units" that can be converted directly to the metric system. The amount designated by a unit is specific for each vitamin. The formulae to convert **International Units** to the metric system are given in Clinical Calculation 7–1.

Table 7–1 Classification of Vitamin

Fat Soluble	Fat Soluble
Vitamin A	B-Complex
Vitamin D	Thiamin
Vitamin E	Riboflavin
Vitamin K	Niacin
	Vitamin B_6
	Folic Acid
	Vitamin B_{12}
	Biotin
	Pantothenic acid
	Vitamin C

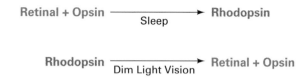

Figure 7–1:
Vitamin A and the protein opsin combine while we sleep to form rhodopsin. When we need to see in dim light, the rhodopsin breaks down into vitamin A and opsin.

Up to a year's supply of vitamin A is stored in the body, 90 percent of it in the liver. Excessive carotene is stored in adipose tissue, giving fat a yellowish tint, but it is harmless.

Functions of Vitamin A

Several crucial body functions depend on vitamin A, or retinol. It is necessary for vision, for healthy epithelial tissue, for proper bone growth, and for energy regulation.

CHEMICAL NECESSARY FOR VISION The eye is like a camera. It has a dark layer to keep out excess light, a lens to focus light, and a light-sensitive layer at the back of the eye, called the **retina**. In the retina, light rays are changed into electrical impulses that travel along the optic nerve to the back of the brain. The vitamin A metabolite retinol is part of the molecules of a chemical in the retina that is responsible for this conversion. The body can synthesize this chemical, called **rhodopsin**, or visual purple, only if it has a supply of vitamin A.

When the eye is functioning in dim light, rhodopsin is broken down into a protein, called **opsin**, and vitamin A. In darkness or during sleep, opsin and vitamin A are reunited to become rhodopsin. Figure 7–1 diagrams this reaction. The body can keep reusing the vitamin A, but some of it is depleted during each visual cycle. It is for this reason that a dietary deficiency produces **night blindness**. Clinical Application 7–1 discusses a practical method used to conserve a person's rhodopsin for night vision.

HEALTH OF EPITHELIAL TISSUE Epithelial **tissue** covers the body and lines the organs and passageways that open to the outside of the body. Skin is epithelial tissue, as are the surface of the eye and the lining of the alimentary canal. Epithelial tissue has a protective function, often producing mucus to wash out foreign materials. Vitamin A in the form of retinoic acid helps to keep epithelial tissue healthy by aiding the differentiation of specialty cells. This function, control of gene expression, has led some scientists to believe that vitamin A may play a role in cancer prevention. See Clinical Application 7–2 for more information on vitamin A and cancer.

Fat-Soluble Vitamins

More or less of the vitamin may be retained in the food, depending upon the methods of processing and storing. Compared with water-soluble vitamins, the fat-soluble vitamins A, D, E, and K are more stable and more resistant to the effects of oxidation, heat, light, and aging. Exposure to the sun and other kinds of dehydration, however, can adversely affect the fat-soluble vitamins.

Fat-soluble vitamins are absorbed from the intestine in the same way as fats, and, like fats, they can be stored in the body. Because the body can store fat-soluble vitamins, excessive intake can create health problems. Excessive intake of some forms of vitamins A and D can be fatal.

Vitamin A

Vitamin A comes in two forms: preformed vitamin A, **retinol**, and **provitamin A, carotene**. A preformed vitamin is already in a complete state in ingested foods. A **provitamin** requires conversion in the body to be in a complete state. Carotene (provitamin A) is converted to vitamin A in the intestine. The term "precursor" is often used interchangeably with the term "provitamin." A **precursor** is a substance from which another substance is derived.

Absorption, Metabolism, and Excretion

Of preformed vitamin A, 80 to 90 percent is absorbed, whereas of carotene, only 33 percent is absorbed. Too little dietary fat or lack of bile salts reduces its absorption. Vitamin A is transported bound to a retinol binding protein. This complex is too large for the kidney to filter, so it is retained in the body.

CLINICAL APPLICATION 7–1

Red Light Conserves Rhodopsin

Red light breaks down rhodopsin more slowly than do other wavelengths of light. for this reason aviators spend time in a red-lit room before flying at night. In the presence of red light, a buildup of rhodopsin occurs in the rods of the retina. Vision in dim light is thus enhanced. Red light is used on navigational instruments for the same reason.

NORMAL BONE GROWTH The mechanism by which vitamin A participates in bone growth and development is unclear. In children with vitamin A deficiency, some bones, such as those in the skull, stop growing, while other bones grow excessively.

ENERGY REGULATION Retinoic acid, a metabolite of vitamin A, has a role in heat production and the regulation of energy balance. The reason Arctic animals store large amounts of vitamin A may be related to these functions (see "Hypervitaminosis A" under "Vitamin A Toxicity"). Researchers are investigating this function of vitamin A and its implications for obesity control (Villarroya, 1998; Wolf, 1995).

Vitamin A Deficiency

Even though vitamin A is stored in the body, deficiencies can occur. In some parts of the world vitamin A deficiency is widespread. Cases are common in India, south and east Asia, Africa, and Latin America. The World Health Organization considers vitamin A deficiency to be a public health problem in over 60 countries, affecting an estimated 250 million preschool children (World Health Organization, 1995). Vitamin A deficiency is second only to protein-calorie malnutrition as a nutritional problem affecting young people.

Vitamin A deficiency in the United States is most often due to disease. For example, clients with long-lasting infectious disease, fat absorption problems, or liver disease are at risk of vitamin A deficiency. Vision loss attributed to hypovitaminosis A due to malabsorption following ileal-jejunal bypass 20 years earlier for morbid obesity was treated successfully with vitamin A supplementation (Purvin, 1999).

SIGNS AND SYMPTOMS Lack of vitamin A as retinol causes night blindness. In this condition the resynthesis of rhodopsin is too slow to allow quick adaptation to dim light.

Vitamin A is related to normal bone growth and development. In the person deficient in vitamin A, the cessation of bone growth produces brain and spinal cord injury. A deficiency can cause fetal malformations (Ross, 1999).

All epithelial tissue suffers because of vitamin A deficiency with consequent lack of retinoic acid. The person so affected may have sinus trouble, a sore throat, and abscesses in the ears, mouth, and salivary glands. The most serious effect is the thickening of the epithelial tissue covering the eye. **Xerophthalmia**, an abnormal thickening and drying of the outer surface of the eye, is a leading cause of blindness in some developing countries. An estimated 5 million children develop xerophthalmia each year, of whom 500,000 go blind (Sommer, 1995.) More than half of these blind children will die in childhood (Glasziou and Mackerras, 1993.)

TREATMENT AND PREVENTION Vitamin A supplements are used as adjunct treatment of infectious diseases. Cases of measles still cause 1.5 million deaths worldwide every year. Vitamin A supplementation to chil-dren hospitalized with measles reduced the risk of death about 60 percent overall and 90 percent in infants. The World Health Organization recommends vitamin A supplementation to all measles clients in developing countries (Fawzi, et a., 1993). In Japan, children with measles or respiratory syncytial virus infection given vitamin A had symptoms of shorter duration than children not supplemented, even in the absence of malnutrition (Kawasaki, et al., 1999).

Prevention of vitamin A deficiency involves three strategies: supplementation, fortification of foods, and diet diversification. The World Health Organization recommends vitamin A supplementation in conjunction with immunization clinics.

Significant improvement in vitamin A status has been obtained in Guatemala and Honduras through the fortification of sugar (Mora, Guere, and Mora, 1998).

A third approach is dietary diversification that is cheaper than supplementation or fortification, requires little or no foreign currency, promotes intakes of nutrients other than vitamin A, and does not "medicalize" food and nutrition. Thus, effective programs to eliminate vitamin A deficiency in poor countries will need a mix of supplementation, food fortification, and dietary diversification (Filteau and Tomkins, 1999).

Free educational materials (wall posters, books, videos) in English, French, and Spanish and vitamin A capsules may be obtained from Task Force "Sight and Life," P.O. Box 2116, CH 4002 Basel, Switzerland (Potter, 1997).

Recommended Dietary Allowances

The 1989 RDA for vitamin A is 800 **retinol equivalents** (RE) for women and 1000 RE for men. One RE corresponds to 1 **microgram** of retinol or 6 micrograms of beta carotene.

Food Sources and Preservation of Vitamin A

Preformed vitamin A (retinol) is found in animal foods such as liver, kidney, egg yolk, and fortified milk products. Two-thirds of the vitamin A in the American diet comes from carotene, a yellow pigment found mostly in fruits and vegetables. Its presence can be readily seen in foods such as carrots, sweet potatoes, squash, apricots, and cantaloupe. Although not as noticeable because chlorophyll masks the yellow color, carotene is also present in dark leafy green vegetables, including spinach, collards, broccoli, and cabbage. New evidence suggests that carotene is more readily absorbed from fruit than from vegetables because of the different structures surrounding the carotene (de Pee, West, et al., 1998).

Vitamin A is fairly stable to heat, but sunlight, ultraviolet light, air, and oxidation easily destroy it. Carrots that come packaged in plastic bags are better protected from light and air than the "bouquets" secured by a rubber band. Carotene content of a species of vegetable can vary with the vegetable's maturity, handling, and preparation (de Pee, Bloem, et al., 1998).

Vitamin A Toxicity

Whereas most other vitamin toxicities are a result of supplementation, hypervitaminosis A can be caused by foods. Fetal malformations can be caused by deficiency or excess of vitamin A. The hazard of excessive vitamin A to the fetus is discussed in Chapter 11.

CAROTENEMIA The condition resulting from ingesting too much carotene is called **carotenemia**. The person's skin becomes yellow, first on the palms of the hands and the soles of the feet. The whites of the eyes do not become yellow, however, as they do in people with jaundice caused by liver disease.

Carotenemia has occurred in infants fed too much squash and carrots. The skin returns to normal within 2 to 6 weeks after stopping the excessive intake. Carotenemia produces no other adverse effects.

HYPERVITAMINOSIS A   Vitamin A toxicity is called **hypervitaminosis A**. Symptoms of vitamin A toxicity are similar to those of a brain tumor causing increased intracranial pressure. Clients may complain of headaches and blurred vision and display signs of increased pressure within the skull. Other symptoms include pain in the bones and joints, dry skin, and poor appetite. Some clients have developed symptoms after consuming beef liver once or twice a week. Self-prescribed vitamin A supplements have produced liver failure. A client died after consuming 25,000 International Units (IU) daily for 6 years (Kowalski et al., 1994). The same intake was judged sufficient to cause cirrhosis in another study (Geubel et al., 1991).

One hazard of excessive vitamin A intake is unique to the Arctic. Polar bear liver has made both men and dogs sick. It contains 354,545 micrograms RE per 3-ounce serving—354 times the RDA for men. Other Arctic game poses similar hazards.

Vitamin D

Recently, vitamin D, which promotes bone growth, has come to be regarded as a hormone rather than a vitamin because of the way it works. Vitamin D receptors have been found in tissues not usually associated with bone metabolism such as adrenal glands, pancreas, prostate, and lymphocytes (Malloy and Feldman, 1999). Vitamin D has a role in immunity and can be protective against autoimmune processes (Boucher, 1998).

Absorption, Metabolism, and Excretion

Two forms of vitamin D are metabolically active. Vitamin D_2, **ergocalciferol**, is formed when ergosterol (provitamin) in plants is irradiated by sunlight. Vitamin D_3, **cholecalciferol**, is formed when 7-dehydrocholesterol (another provitamin) in the skin of animals or humans is irradiated by ultraviolet light or sunlight.

Both forms are absorbed into the blood. Like other fat-soluble vitamins, they are transported in the blood bound to protein. The liver alters the vitamin to **calcidiol**, an inactive form of vitamin D. By enzyme action, the kidney converts the calcidiol to **calcitriol**, the active form of vitamin D. Figure 7–2 diagrams the path of these processes.

Functions of Vitamin D

Vitamin D promotes normal bone mineralization in three ways. (1) Vitamin D stimulates DNA to produce transport proteins, which bind calcium and phosphorus, thus increasing intestinal absorption of these minerals. (2) Once these minerals have been absorbed into the blood, vitamin D stimulates bone cells to use them to build and maintain bone tissue. (3) Vitamin D stimulates the kidneys to return calcium to the bloodstream rather than to allow it to be lost in the urine.

Another control mechanism is also at work. **Parathyroid hormone** is secreted in response to a low serum calcium level. Parathyroid hormone causes the catabolism of bone to maintain a correct serum cal-

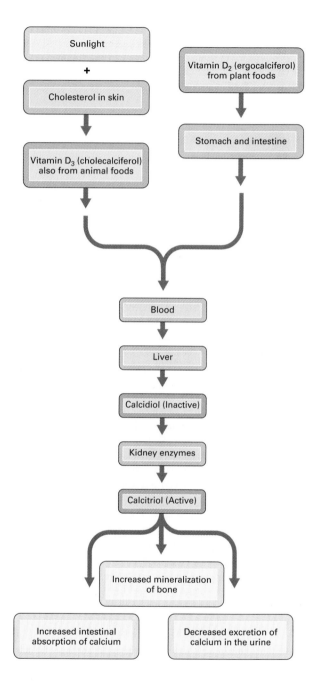

Figure 7–2:
Vitamin D, whether from food or synthesis in the skin, is metabolized by the liver and the kidneys to its active form.

cium level. The body's priority goal is maintenance of correct serum calcium for blood clotting, nerve function, and muscle contraction. Without this mechanism to sustain vital functions, a person would not live long enough to develop rickets, a disease of vitamin D deficiency.

Vitamin D Deficiency

Lack of sunshine or vitamin D, chronic liver or kidney disease, and rare genetic disorders are causes of vitamin D deficiency. Of particular concern are children whose bones are still growing.

RICKETS Vitamin D deficiency in children is called **rickets**. Twenty-four cases occurred in Philadelphia between 1974 and 1978 in children who belonged to a religious sect that wore long hooded robes (which blocked sunshine) and ate vegetarian diets (Brown, 1990). More recently, four cases were reported in New York, all children under 24 months who were breast-fed without formula supplements (Pugliese et al., 1998) and two cases in Philadelphia, children 14 and 15 months old breast-fed without supplements by mothers who eliminated dairy products from their own diets (Herman and Bulthuis, 1999). Additional cases of rickets in dark-skinned children being breast-fed but not receiving vitamin D supplements were reported in New England (Fitzpatrick et al., 2000), north Texas (Shah et al., 2000), and North Carolina (Kreiter et al., 2000). At greatest risk in the United States are dark-skinned children in northern, smoggy cities and breast-fed infants not exposed to sunlight. To prevent such deficiency diseases or to diagnose them early, healthcare providers should pay special attention to assessing the client's whole situation and not just concentrate on the immediate reason for the visit.

In Great Britain, evidence of subnormal serum levels of vitamin D without evidence of rickets was documented among Asian 2-year-old (Lawson and Thomas, 1999) and preschool children (Davies et al., 1999). In both studies, the lowest levels were predicted or found during the winter when exposure to sunshine and perhaps outdoor play are less common.

OSTEOMALACIA Vitamin D deficiency in adults is called **osteomalacia**. This deficiency disease occurs most often in women who have insufficient calcium intake and little sunlight exposure, and frequently among those who are pregnant or lactating. Women who immigrate to Europe and North America from Asia and the Middle East are particularly at risk (McLaren, 1999).

Environmental factors involved in osteomalacia are similar to those described for rickets. People whose skin is not exposed much to sunlight are at increased risk: cloistered nuns, office workers, residents of smoggy areas, and institutionalized elderly people. Low serum vitamin D levels, not frank osteomalacia, were found in free-living elderly Europeans (van der Wielen et al., 1995). A study of adults admitted to a medical service in a New England hospital determined that 22 percent had severe hypovitaminosis D and 34 percent had moderate deficiency (Thomas et al., 1998). Independent predictors of hypovitaminosis D in the Thomas research were inadequate vitamin D intake, winter season, and being housebound. Careful attention to a client's lifestyle and circumstances during assessment may uncover potential problems.

Because of the complex processes involved in vitamin D metabolism, liver or kidney disease can lead to bone deterioration. Chronic kidney failure has caused osteomalacia due to the inability of the kidneys to convert vitamin D to its active form. Dialysis unit protocols frequently call for pharmaceutical vitamin D supplementation.

SIGNS AND SYMPTOMS Children with rickets have soft, fragile bones. Classic deformities occur, such as bowlegs, knock knees, and misshapen skulls. **Tetany** in infants may be due to low levels of blood calcium.

Adults with osteomalacia also have increasing softness of the bones, causing deformities due to loss of calcium. The bones most commonly affected are those of the spine, pelvis, and lower extremities.

Dietary Reference Intakes

Vitamin D is measured in micrograms of cholecalciferol. Compared to the 1989 RDAs, the Dietary Reference Intakes call for decreased recommended levels for infants, children, and younger adults, and increased ones for older adults. One reason is that intestinal absorption of vitamin D decreases with age (Boucher, 1998) as does the capacity of the skin to synthesize cholecalciferol. The 1998 Adequate Intake for vitamin D is 5 micrograms for everyone through age 50, 10 micrograms from age 51 through 70, and 15 micrograms after age 70. Some authorities have suggested the new recommended levels are too low (Utiger, 1998; Vieth, 1999). The Tolerable Upper Intake Level (UL) is 50 micrograms for adults and children older than one year, and 25 micrograms for infants.

Sources of Vitamin D

Two sources of vitamin D are readily available to most people. Vitamin D is synthesized by the body, and it is added to most dairy products in the United States.

SUNLIGHT A major source of vitamin D is the body itself. Vitamin D is manufactured in the skin. Children with low dietary intakes may escape rickets if their exposure to sunlight is adequate.

Light-skinned adults can obtain the necessary 5 micrograms of cholecalciferol by exposing their hands, arms, and face to sunlight for 15 minutes twice a week. It is not possible to overdose on vitamin D from sunshine.

FOOD If a person is not exposed to sunshine, food sources of vitamin D become increasingly important. Few natural foods contain enough vitamin D to provide the recommended intakes. The major food source of vitamin D in the United States is fortified milk. Milk is the ideal food to link with vitamin D since it also contains calcium and phosphorus, which are necessary for bone anabolism. See Clinical Application 7–3 on the **fortification** of foods.

Historically, the means to obtain vitamin D was with cod liver oil. One teaspoonful contains 226 percent of children's Adequate Intake. Although it is a natural product, cod liver oil is a supplement, not a food.

Stability and Interfering Factors

Vitamin D is stable to heat and not easily oxidized. Little special handling of foods is necessary. A high-fiber diet interferes with the absorption of vitamin D. Abnormalities of absorption such as diarrhea, fat malabsorption, and biliary obstruction also may lead to vitamin D deficiency.

Vitamin D Toxicity

Since vitamin D is stored in the body, it is possible to ingest too much. Vitamin D from supplements or even foods can be hazardous to health.

MOST TOXIC OF VITAMINS Infants face increased risk from multiple fortified foods. Recent cases have been reported involving not dietary intake,

---

CLINICAL APPLICATION 7–3

Fortification of Foods: Use and Misuse

Fortification is the addition of nutrients to foods in amounts greater than normally present to prevent deficiencies. Many cereals are fortified with vitamins and minerals not normally found in grains. Fluid milk must be fortified with vitamin D in the United States, but there are no mandates for other dairy products.

Occasionally, intentions are better than practices. Between 1985 and 1991, 56 cases of hypervitaminosis D were identified in Massachusetts. Two individuals died as a result and nine were discharged from the hospital with residual effects. Although state law required an upper limit of 500 IU (12.5 micrograms) of vitamin D per quart, the implicated dairy's milk exceeded this by 70 to 600 times (Blank et al., 1995).

---

but errors of prescribing or dispensing supplemental vitamin D (Muhlendahl and Nawracala, 1999).

SIGNS AND SYMPTOMS Clinical manifestations of hypervitaminosis D include loss of appetite, nausea, vomiting, polyuria, muscular weakness, and constipation. The more serious consequences of vitamin D overdose result from calcium deposits in the heart, kidney, and brain.

Vitamin E

The third fat-soluble vitamin is vitamin E. Much less is known about vitamin E than about vitamins A and D. Observational studies have linked it to prevention of cardiovascular disease and of cancer (Meydani and Meisler, 1997), but intervention studies have not supported the finding. For example, a study of people at high risk for cardiovascular events found no difference in the occurrence of heart attacks, stroke, or death between those given supplemental vitamin E for 4.5 years and those given placebos (Yusuf et al., 2000).

Absorption, Metabolism, and Excretion

About 45 percent of vitamin E from ordinary foods is absorbed along with fat (Vitamin E, 1999). Most vitamin E is stored in adipose tissue. Maximum transfer of vitamin E across the placenta occurs just before term delivery. The significance of this phenomenon will become clearer in the discussion of premature infants in Chapter 12.

Functions of Vitamin E

The major function of vitamin E is as an **antioxidant**. The process by which a substance combines with oxygen is called **oxidation**. Several substances can be destroyed by oxidation, including vitamin E, vitamin A, and vitamin C. Some molecules become very unstable when they are oxidized. Their accelerated movements can damage nearby molecules. Vitamin E accepts oxygen instead of allowing other molecules to become unstable. In this role, vitamin E protects vitamin A and unsaturated fatty acids from oxidation. Vitamin E in lung cell membranes provides an important barrier against air pollution. It also protects the stability of the polyunsaturated fatty acids in the red blood cell membranes from oxidation in the lungs.

Oxidation is suspected of contributing to cataract formation and macular degeneration of the retina, although early research produced inconsistent findings. Clinical Application 7–4 describes some of the results of investigations into antioxidants and eye disease.

The role of vitamin E in immunity is under investigation. It is considered of possible benefit in improving immune responses in elderly people (Traber, 1999). Insufficient vitamin E has been found to cause immune cell membranes to become unstable (Meydani and Meisler, 1997).

Deficiency of Vitamin E

In animals, vitamin E deficiency produces sterility. In several species of animals, a deficiency of vitamin E suppresses the immune system, whereas supplementation stimulates it.

In humans, a progressive peripheral neuropathy occurs (Traber, 1999). In cases of chronic fat malabsorption, muscle weakness and forms of muscular dystrophy are seen. Premature infants with inadequate reserves of vitamin E develop anemia. Without sufficient vitamin E the membranes of the red blood cells break down easily when exposed to oxygen or an oxidizing agent. Severe vitamin E deficiency has profound effects on the central nervous system (Benomar et al., 1999). Even with adequate vitamin E intake, defects in the alpha-tocopherol transfer protein gene have produced ataxia and mental symptoms (Hoshino et al., 1999; Schuelke et al., 1999).

Dietary Reference Intakes

Vitamin E is measured in milligrams of **alpha-tocopherol equivalents (a-TE)**. Not all vitamin E is alpha-tocopherol. Another form, y–tocopherol, is assumed to substitute for alpha-tocopherol with an efficiency of just 10 percent and to provide much shorter antioxidant activity (Traber, 1999). The RDA is 15 milligrams for persons 14 years of age and older. The UI is 800 milligrams for 14- to 18-year-olds and 1000 milligrams for other adults. The need for vitamin E increases as the intake of polyunsaturated fatty acids increases. The recommended ratio of vitamin E/PUFA is 0.4 milligrams of d-a-alpha-tocopherol per gram of PUFA (Vitamin E, 1999).

Food Sources and Preservation of Vitamin E

The best source of vitamin E is vegetable oils, and the vegetable oils highest in alpha-tocopherol are the ones high in monounsaturated fatty acids such as olive and canola oils. In contrast, corn and soybean oils have a greater proportion of y–tocopherol, the less well retained form of vitamin E (Traber, 1999). Other sources are whole grains, wheat germ, milk, eggs, meats, fish, and leafy vegetables. Vitamin E is fairly stable on exposure to heat and acid. Normal cooking temperatures do not destroy it, but frying does. Vitamin E is unstable to light, alkalis, and oxygen.

Vitamin E Toxicity

Very large supplemental doses of more than 600 milligrams of alpha-tocopherol daily (40 times the RDA) for a year or longer may cause excessive bleeding, impaired wound healing, and depression. Clinical Application 7–5 describes a client with vitamin E toxicity.

Vitamin K

Nurses should understand the functions of vitamin K because it is often prescribed as a medication. Vitamin K also impacts the effectiveness of a commonly prescribed anticoagulant. Therefore, nurses must give clients who are taking vitamin K instructions regarding food intake.

CLINICAL APPLICATION 7–4

Antioxidants and Zinc in Eye Disease

In the western world, age-related macular degeneration is the most common cause of irreversible vision loss after the age of fifty. The center of the retina, or macula, deteriorates so that the person loses the ability to read, drive a car, or perform fine tasks, but still retains some peripheral vision. The cause is unknown, but risk factors include ultraviolet light and smoking. No cure has been discovered.

Researchers found that serum levels of vitamin E and zinc in people with age-related macular degeneration were significantly lower than those in people free of the disease (Belda et al., 1999). Zinc received weak support as protective against the development of some forms of early disease (Mares-Perlman et al., 1996). In contrast, no association between age-related macular degeneration and dietary intake was found for carotene, vitamins A and C, either from food or supplements, in one study (Smith et al., 1999) or for vitamins C and E in another (Mares-Perlman et al., 1996). Moreover, the use of supplements has not been shown to retard the disease process. A review of eight trials did not support a recommendation to use vitamin or mineral supplements to prevent progression of macular degeneration (Evans, 1999).

In the United States, the most common surgery performed on people over the age of 65 is to treat cataracts. A cataract is the clouding of the lens of the eye. Predisposing factors, in addition to age, are ultraviolet radiation, diabetes, smoking, and alcohol consumption (Cataract Management Guideline Panel, 1993).

Studies of nutrients and cataract formation also show uneven results. An analysis of women who used vitamin C supplements for ten years or more showed a 77 to 83 percent lower prevalence of lens opacities compared with women who did not use vitamin C supplements (Jacques et al., 1997). A check of blood levels, however, found the only serum carotenoid or tocopherol inversely related to cataracts was vitamin E, after adjusting for age, smoking, serum cholesterol, heavy drinking, and adiposity (Lyle et al., 1999b). When foods were studied instead of nutrients, individuals who consumed fewer than 3.5 servings of fruits or vegetables per day were found to be at increased risk of cataracts (Jacques and Chylack, 1991).

There are many antioxidants in addition to vitamins A, C, and E. Two carotenoids, lutein and zeaxanthin, found in spinach and collard greens, have been associated with a dose-dependent reduction in age-related macular degeneration (Hankinson and Stampfer, 1994) but only lutein was associated with a reduction in cataracts (Lyle et al., 1999a).

Many of the researchers concluded by recommending the "5 a day" Food Pyramid fruit and vegetable plan. They noted that health-conscious individuals who take vitamin supplements often consume nutrient-dense diets (Mares-Perlman, 1997).

Absorption, Metabolism, and Excretion

Two forms of vitamin K can meet the body's needs. Vitamin K_1, or **phylloquinone**, is the one found in plant foods. Vitamin K_2, or **menaquinone**, is synthesized by intestinal bacteria. A synthetic, water-soluble pharmaceutical form of vitamin K_1, **phytonadione**, can be administered orally or by injection.

Functions of Vitamin K

The role of vitamin K in blood clotting has been known and used clinically for a long time. More recently, a protein has been identified in bone that depends on vitamin K. Vitamin K participates with vitamin D in synthesizing this bone protein, which helps to regulate serum calcium levels. In addition, vitamin K-dependent proteins have been found in bone, cartilage, kidney, plaque in blood vessels, and numerous other soft tissues, although information on the mode of action remains to be discovered (Ferland, 1998).

BLOOD CLOTTING At least 13 different proteins plus the mineral calcium are involved in blood clotting. Vitamin K is necessary for the liver to make factors II (**prothrombin**), VII, IX, and X. Three additional coagulation proteins are vitamin K-dependent. These factors and proteins are key links in the chain of events producing a blood clot.

BONE METABOLISM Vitamin K influences bone metabolism by facilitating the synthesis of **osteocalcin**, a hormonally regulated calcium-binding protein made almost exclusively by the bone-building cells called **osteoblasts** (Collins and Gernacy, 1998; Xiao et al., 1997; Kanai et al., 1997). In animals, long-term vitamin K deficiency resulted

CLINICAL APPLICATION 7–5

Vitamin E Toxicity

A client was admitted to the hospital for **narcolepsy**, a disorder characterized by recurrent, uncontrollable, brief periods of sleep from which the individual is easily awakened. This client would fall asleep while driving his car.

Narcolepsy can be a sign of uremia, hypoglycemia, diabetes, hypothyroidism, increased intracranial pressure, tumor of the brainstem or hypothalamus, or absence epilepsy. If all of these causes are ruled out, the medical diagnosis is either classical or independent narcolepsy.

During her assessment, the dietitian discovered only one unusual nutritional practice. A clerk in a health foods store had recommended vitamin E. The patient had begun and continued this self-prescribed supplement.

The dietitian's investigation of vitamin E's adverse effects led her to suggest to the physician that the narcolepsy could be caused by excessive vitamin E. The client discontinued the vitamin E and the narcolepsy disappeared.

In this case, a thorough nutritional assessment and an inquiring attitude saved the client much discomfort (and his insurance company many dollars) by eliminating the need for extensive diagnostic tests. Often, clients do not regard dietary supplements as medications. The nurse should always ask specifically about what vitamin and mineral preparations the client is taking, and in what doses.

in stunted growth and bone crystallization problems (Groff, Gropper, and Hunt, 1995).

Deficiency of Vitamin K

The intestinal tract of the newborn infant is sterile. For this reason the baby is unable to produce vitamin K until the intestine is colonized with bacteria from the infant's environment, usually within 24 hours. To prevent bleeding problems, a dose of vitamin K may be administered to the mother late in labor or to the infant immediately after birth. In developing countries, vitamin K deficiency in the breast-fed newborn is a major cause of infant **morbidity** and **mortality** (Olson, 1999).

Deficiencies have been associated with disease and with drug therapy. Fat absorption problems may hinder vitamin K absorption, resulting in prolonged blood clotting time. Antibiotics kill the normal bacteria in the intestine along with the organisms causing an infection. In one study, 31 percent of clients with gastrointestinal disorders given antibiotics for prolonged periods developed vitamin K deficiencies (Krasinski and Russell, 1985).

Vitamin K may be useful for maintaining a positive balance of bone metabolism. One month of vitamin K supplementation of female athletes who showed low estrogen levels at baseline produced a 15 to 20 percent increase of bone formation markers and a 20 to 25 percent decrease of bone resorption markers (Craciun et al., 1998). The lack of vitamin K has also been linked to poor bone health. In hemodialysis clients, suboptimal plasma vitamin K levels were associated with increased risk of bone fracture (Kohlmeier et al., 1997).

The clinical decision-making path is not always clear. Priorities have to be set after weighing therapeutic and adverse effects of drugs. For example, vitamin K antagonist drugs are given after heart surgery to prevent clotting problems. In one set of these clients, one year of oral vitamin K antagonist therapy showed significantly lower osteocalcin (the calcium-binding protein made by the bone-building cells) levels than clients who were not receiving anticoagulants. although changes in bone mineral density were not detected in this period of time (Lafforgue et al., 1997).

Individuals at risk of vitamin K deficiency include newborn infants and adults who avoid green leafy vegetables and animal products, and clients with malabsorption syndromes. Careful assessment of dietary factors in these clients is warranted.

Recommended Dietary Allowances

The 1989 RDAs for adults 25 years of age and older for vitamin K are 65 micrograms for women and 80 for men. The typical U.S. diet supplies 300 to 500 micrograms.

Sources of Vitamin K

The body is capable of manufacturing some vitamin K. Many common foods also contain adequate amounts.

INTESTINAL SYNTHESIS Approximately half the body's needed vitamin K is manufactured by intestinal bacteria, a fact that has been best quantified in laboratory animals. It is uncertain whether the microorganisms manufacturing vitamin K live in the ileum or the colon. If in the colon, where

vitamin K is poorly absorbed, perhaps reflux of the vitamin into the ileum is a mechanism whereby absorption might be increased (Olson, 1999).

FOOD SOURCES Liver, green leafy vegetables, vegetables of the cabbage family, and milk are the best sources of vitamin K. Examples of the vegetables include lettuce, spinach, asparagus, kale, cabbage, cauliflower, broccoli, and Brussels sprouts.

Stability and Interfering Factors

Vitamin K resists heat but is unstable in the presence of oxygen, light, alkalis, and strong acids. Overconsumption of some vitamins can trigger a deficiency of others. In this case, megadoses of vitamins A and E have interfered with vitamin K. The anticoagulant **warfarin sodium** interferes with the liver's use of vitamin K—the desired effect of the medication.

Vitamin K Toxicity

The naturally occurring forms of vitamins K_1 and K_2 do not cause toxicity. Phytonadione, the pharmaceutical preparation of vitamin K_1, causes fewer adverse effects than earlier, stronger formulations. Nevertheless, special care must be taken when administering vitamin K to infants.

Table 7–2 summarizes the information on the fat-soluble vitamins. Table 7–3 summarizes the stability of vitamins to environmental conditions. See Clinical Application 7–6 for a description of two conditions that mimic deficiencies of fat-soluble vitamins.

Water-Soluble Vitamins

Vitamins that dissolve in water are vitamin C, or **ascorbic acid**, and the B vitamins. The B vitamins include **thiamin, riboflavin, niacin,** vitamin B_6, **folic acid,** vitamin B_{12}, **pantothenic acid,** and **biotin.** Another substance, choline, has sometimes been classified as a B vitamin or not a B vitamin. It has recently been given DRIs (see discussion toward the end of this chapter).

Cooking easily destroys water-soluble vitamins. For example, one-third to one-half of the vitamin content is lost in the cooking water of boiled vegetables.

Vitamin C

Most animals manufacture vitamin C in their livers. Humans, along with other primates, guinea pigs, some birds, some fish, and fruit-eating bats, cannot synthesize vitamin C.

Absorption, Metabolism, and Excretion

Vitamin C is absorbed from the small intestine. The adrenal and pituitary glands have the highest concentrations of vitamin C, but the greatest total amount is found in the liver and skeletal muscle.

As the amount of vitamin C consumed increases, the proportion of the vitamin that is absorbed decreases. In a study of healthy volunteers, 100 percent of a 200-milligram dose was absorbed. Seventy percent of a 500-milligram dose was absorbed, but 70 percent of the absorbed dose was excreted in the urine. Of the 1250-milligram dose, only 50 percent was absorbed, and nearly all of it was excreted in the urine (Levine et al., 1996).

Table 7–2 Fat-Soluble Vitamins

Vitamin	Adult RDA and Food Portion Containing RDA	Functions	Deficiency Disease	Signs and Symptoms of Deficiency	Best Sources
A	800 to 1000 RE 0.5 cup frzn. or canned carrots	Dim light vision Differentiation of epithelial cells Normal bone growth	Nightblindness Xerophthalmia	Nightblindness Sore throat, sinus trouble, ear and mouth abscesses Dry and thick outer covering of eye Blindness	Preformed: liver, kidney, egg yolk, fortified milk Provitamin: carrots, sweet potatoes, squash, apricots, cantaloupe, spinach, collards, broccoli, cabbage
D	5 µg	Increases intestinal absorption of calcium	Rickets	Bowlegs, knock-knees, misshapen skull Tetany in infants	Sunlight on skin Fortified milk Cod liver oil
	2 cups fortified milk	Stimulates bone production Decreases urinary excretion of calcium	Osteomalacia	Soft fragile bones, especially of spine, pelvis, lower extremities	
E	15 mg 5 tbsp corn oil	Antioxidant Protects polyunsaturated fatty acids in red blood cell membranes from oxidation in lungs	No specific term	Animals: sterility, suppression of immune system Humans: Muscle weakness; forms of muscular dystrophy Anemia in premature infants	Vegetable oils Whole grains, wheat germ
K	65 to 80 µg 0.75 cup raw cabbage	Used in manufacture of several clotting factors, including prothrombin Assists vitamin D to synthesize a regulatory bone protein	No specific term	Prolonged clotting time	Synthesis in large intestine Green leafy vegetables Liver

Functions of Vitamin C

Vitamin C has diverse functions in the body. It contributes to wound, burn, and fracture healing, serves as an antioxidant, and assists in the synthesis of neurotransmitters and steroid hormones. It enhances the absorption of iron and converts folic acid, a B vitamin, to an active form. It is necessary in the formation of **collagen**, the strong fibrous protein in connective tissue. Bone, skin, soft dental structures, and scar tissue all contain collagen.

ANTIOXIDANT Vitamin C is a powerful antioxidant. By preventing the uptake of oxygen by other molecules, it deters the destruction of tissue by unstable molecules. Vitamin C is more sensitive to oxidation than either vitamin E or vitamin A and will be oxidized before they are. Thus it is called the "antioxidants' antioxidant".

When combined with iron, the iron–ascorbate couple has demonstrated the opposite effect, pro-oxidant activity, in laboratory studies. Whether such actions occur in animals or humans is uncertain (Carr and

Frei, 1999) and lacking evidence (Levine et al., 1999) but warrants further study particularly in cases of iron overload or trauma that disperses free iron into the tissues (Jacob, 1999).

ADRENAL GLAND FUNCTION High concentrations of vitamin C are found in the **adrenal gland**s. These are the organs that secrete adrenalin, the "fight or flight" hormone, in times of stress. Vitamin C aids in the release of adrenalin from the adrenal glands. Emotional and physical stress increase the body's need for vitamin C by three to four times.

IRON ABSORPTION Vitamin C facilitates iron absorption. It acts with hydrochloric acid to keep iron in the more absorbable **ferrous** form. Four ounces of orange juice nearly quadruples the iron a person absorbs from plant foods he or she eats with it.

FOLIC ACID CONVERSION Vitamin C converts folic acid to an active form. For this reason deficiency of vitamin C can lead to **anemia** due to inefficient use of iron and folic acid.

Table 7–3 Factors Affecting Stability of Vitamins

Vitamin	Stable to				
	Oxygen	Heat	Light	Acids	Alkalies
Fat Soluble					
A	No	Yes	No	No	*
D	Yes	Yes	Yes	*	*
E	No	Yes	No	Yes	No
K	No	Yes	No	No	No
Water Soluble					
C	No	No	No	Yes	Yes
Thiamin	No	No	No	Yes/No†	No
Riboflavin	Yes	Yes	No	Yes	No
Niacin	Yes	Yes	Yes	Yes	Yes
B$_6$	*	Yes	No	Yes	No
Folic acid	No	No	No	No	Yes
B$_{12}$	No	Yes	No	No	No

*Data unavailable.
†Destroyed by tannic and caffeic acid; protected by ascorbic and citric acid.

Deficiency of Vitamin C

Until the 17th century, sailors on long voyages often died of **scurvy** due to lack of vitamin C. The disease develops within 3 months after vitamin C is eliminated from the diet.

SIGNS AND SYMPTOMS Early signs of scurvy are tender, sore gums that bleed easily and small skin hemorrhages due to weakened blood vessels. The late manifestations of scurvy relate to the breakdown of collagen. Wound healing is delayed; even healed scars may separate. The ends of long bones soften, become malformed and painful, and fractures appear. The teeth loosen in their sockets and fall out. Hemorrhages occur about the joints, stomach, and heart. Untreated, scurvy progresses to often sudden death, probably from internal bleeding.

TREATMENT Moderate doses of vitamin C will cure scurvy. A daily dose of 300 milligrams replenishes the body tissues in 5 days.

CURRENT PREVALENCE OF VITAMIN C DEFICIENCY As many as 25 percent of persons surveyed have a vitamin C intake well below the 1989 RDA of 60 milligrams. Intake may be less than half their 1989 RDA level for infants, teens, and elderly people. Low blood levels of vitamin C are more common in men than women and in people of lower socioeconomic status. The highest prevalance (20 percent) is reported in poor elderly men, who frequently live alone and consume a diet devoid of fresh fruits and vegetables (Jacob, 1999). People who avoid acidic foods and clients

---

CLINICAL APPLICATION 7–6

Conditions Mimicking Deficiencies of Fat-Soluble Vitamins

Protein Deficiency

Water and fat do not mix. To circulate fats in the water-based blood, the liver attaches fat-soluble vitamins to protein carriers. Sometimes a protein deficiency hinders the use of the fat-soluble vitamins.

Zinc Deficiency

Vitamin A is carried from storage in the liver to the tissues by a zinc-containing protein. For this reason zinc deficiency can mimic vitamin A deficiency.

---

receiving dialysis for kidney failure are also at increased risk of vitamin C deficiency. Case reports still appear in medical journals describing scurvy in people with alcoholism (Garg, Draganescu, and Albornoz, 1998).

Expanding the nursing assessment to include the social situation might uncover persons at increased risk of vitamin C deficiency.

Dietary Reference Intakes

The RDA of vitamin C for adults 19 years of age and older is 75 milligrams for women and 90 milligrams for men. An average intake of 46 milligrams per day should prevent scurvy (Carr and Frei, 1999). A daily intake of 200 milligrams completely saturates the tissues and will prevent deficiency for more than a month if intake is stopped (Levine et al., 1999). After major surgery or extensive burns, a client may need up to 1000 milligrams of vitamin C per day. The UL of vitamin C is 2000 milligrams for adults 19 years of age and older.

Food Sources of Vitamin C

Citrus fruits are excellent sources of vitamin C. Other good sources include peppers, tomatoes, white potatoes, cabbage, broccoli, chard, kale, turnip greens, asparagus, berries, melons, pineapple, and guavas. Three foods high in vitamins A and C are shown in Figure 7–3.

Stability and Preservation

Air, light, heat, and alkalis destroy vitamin C. Easily implemented food preparation procedures can minimize loss of vitamin C. Store orange juice in an opaque container that holds no more than an amount that can be consumed in a short time. Cook vegetables as quickly as possible; crisp-cooked is better than limp-cooked for retaining the vitamin C content. Boiling the cooking water for 1 minute before adding the food eliminates the dissolved oxygen that would otherwise oxidize the vitamin C.

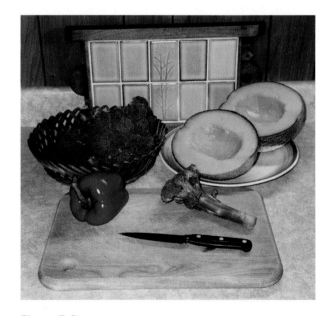

Figure 7–3:
Broccoli, cantaloupe, and red pepper are excellent sources of vitamins A and C.

Controlling the **pH** is also important. In years past many food establishments routinely added baking soda to vegetables to enhance their color, but the alkali also destroyed the vitamin C. Fortunately this practice is now illegal.

Interfering Factor

Smokers deplete vitamin C stores faster than nonsmokers do. Smokers need at least 100 milligrams per day to achieve the same tissue saturation that nonsmokers achieve with 60 milligrams (Levine et al., 1995). Plasma vitamin C concentrations increased significantly in smokers given a supplement of 500 milligrams of vitamin C daily for four weeks (Aghdassi, Royall, and Allard, 1999). Unfortunately, many smokers do not consume even the RDA.

Vitamin C Toxicity

Megadoses in amounts of 1000 to 2000 milligrams per day have produced nausea, abdominal cramps, and diarrhea. Because vitamin C increases the amount of iron absorbed, persons with diseases characterized by iron overload should avoid megadoses of ascorbic acid. Individuals prone to kidney stones are advised not to take megadoses of vitamin C because it is metabolized to oxalate, and kidney stones are often composed of calcium oxalate. By a different mechanism competing with uric acid for reabsorption by the kidney, megadoses of vitamin C theoretically could increase the risk of urate stones (Groff, Gropper, and Hunt, 1995).

Excessive vitamin C causes false readings in two common laboratory tests. Some urine glucose tests will read false-positive. Stool guaiac for occult blood will read false-negative.

An occasionally reported consequence of taking megadoses of vitamin C and then abruptly discontinuing them is **rebound scurvy.** The body cannot adjust quickly enough and continues to absorb a meager proportion of the now smaller dose (DePaola, Faine, and Palmer, 1999). A similar condition was reported in newborns whose mothers took supplemental vitamin C during pregnancy (Cochran, 1965). Even without megadose supplements, however, plasma vitamin C levels fall to deficiency levels within 1 to 3 weeks of removal of vitamin-rich fruits and vegetables from the diet (Johnston, 1999).

B-Complex Vitamins

Eight vitamins belong to the B-complex group: thiamin, riboflavin, niacin, vitamin B_6, folic acid, vitamin B_{12}, pantothenic acid, and biotin. They all function as coenzymes. A **coenzyme** joins with an enzyme to activate it. If a person lacks the coenzyme, the effect is the same as lacking the enzyme itself.

The fact that many of the actions of the B-complex vitamins are interrelated gives rise to a theory that combinations of low vitamin intakes may have a greater impact on health than the sum of their individual effects (Lowik et al., 1994). In 1992 to 1993 an epidemic of peripheral neuropathy in Cuba was attributed to deficiencies of thiamin, folate, vitamin B_{12}, and sulfur-containing amino acids. Increased risk was found among those who smoked, missed meals, drank alcohol, lost weight, or consumed excessive sugar (Roman, 1994). Some diseases, including beriberi and pellagra, are associated with deficiencies of a single B-vitamin.

Thiamin

Beriberi is the deficiency disease due to the lack of **thiamin**, a vitamin originally named B$_1$. The neurological symptoms of beriberi were recognized in China in 2600 BC, but it was not until 1937 that lack of thiamin was chemically identified as the causative agent. The enrichment of food products has almost eliminated this disease, but it is still seen in alcoholics and artificially nourished persons in the West and in persons in developing countries where enrichment may not be a standard practice.

ABSORPTION, METABOLISM, AND EXCRETION About one-half the body's thiamin is located in the skeletal muscles, but the heart, liver, kidneys, and brain also have high concentrations (Tanphaichitr, 1999). Thiamin is absorbed in the small intestine. The need for thiamin increases proportionately with carbohydrate intake. Excess thiamin is excreted in the urine.

FUNCTIONS OF THIAMIN Thiamin serves as a coenzyme in carbohydrate metabolism and may play a role in nerve conduction outside its contribution to energy metabolism (Tanphaichitr, 1999). It is involved in the production of energy from glucose and helps oxidize glucose to form a compound that stores energy. Thiamin is required to convert the essential amino acid **tryptophan** to niacin, another B vitamin.

DEFICIENCY People at increased risk of thiamin deficiency include breast-fed infants of thiamin deficient mothers, people whose carbohydrate intake is chiefly milled rice, and chronic alcoholics (Tanphaichitr, 1999). In the Orient, beriberi causes sudden death in young migrant workers who subsist on rice (McLaren, 1999). Individuals whose thiamin status is marginal may become deficient with an increased need for energy during strenuous activity, pregnancy, a growth spurt, or fever. Beriberi is characterized by neurological and cardiovascular abnormalities.

Initially, symptoms of beriberi such as anorexia, indigestion, and constipation occur because the digestive process is disrupted by impaired glucose metabolism. Without a continual supply of glucose for the central nervous system (CNS), apathy, fatigue, and muscle weakness set in. The **myelin sheaths** covering peripheral nerves eventually degenerate, resulting in paralysis and muscle atrophy. If the thiamin deficiency continues, cardiac failure and death are the result. In infantile beriberi, death may occur within a few hours if no thiamin is administered (Tanphaichitr, 1999).

Wernicke-Korsakoff syndrome is a neurological disorder caused by thiamin deficiency. Clients with **Wernicke's encephalopathy** display many motor and sensory deficits. Clients with **Korsakoff's psychosis** have short-term memory deficits. Wernicke-Korsakoff syndrome is often associated with chronic alcoholism because of chronic malnutrition and because thiamin is used to convert alcohol to energy. Wernicke's encephalopathy is most likely to be seen in alcoholic clients who receive carbohydrates without adequate thiamin replacement (McLaren, 1999). Thirty-two cases of Wernicke's encephalopathy were reported in Australia over a period of 33 months before 1991 when mandatory thiamin enrichment of bread-making flour began (Wood and Currie, 1995). In other cases, extraordinary losses of thiamin have occurred through vomiting (Ohkoshi, Ishii, and Shoji, 1994) or dialysis (Jagadha et al., 1987).

Artificial feeding with intravenous glucose without thiamin supplementation for more than a week produced cases of Wernicke's encephalopathy and lactic acidosis. One malnourished woman in the United Kingdom received a glucose-containing intravenous solution without the thiamin that had been suggested by the referring physician (Bamber, 1998). In the United States, six cases have been publicized by the Centers for Disease Control. Some clients demonstrated signs of Wernicke's encephalopathy whereas others developed acidosis from the accumulation of lactate due to the incomplete metabolism of glucose. Three clients died from lactic acidosis due to a shortage of multivitamins for total parenteral nutrition in 1989 (Centers for Disease Control, 1989), but although a similar shortage in 1996 produced three cases, it did not result in fatalities (Centers for Disease Control, 1997). The severe deficiencies developed in 7 to 34 days, highlighting the need to respect vitamin additives to intravenous solutions as essential, not just optional, therapy.

DIETARY REFERENCE INTAKES The RDAs for thiamin are 1.2 milligrams for adult males and 1.1 milligrams for adult females. The Adequate Intake (AI) level is 0.2 to 0.3 milligrams for infants. The need for thiamin increases as kilocaloric consumption increases. An athlete consuming 4000 kilocalories needs twice as much as an office worker consuming 1800 kilocalories. Fasting does not decrease the need for thiamin, however, because the need is proportional to energy expenditure, not simply food intake.

FOOD SOURCES Pork, wheat germ, yeast, black beans, black-eyed peas, sunflower seeds, and fortified cereals are the best sources. Many other commonly consumed foods contain lesser amounts. A person who chooses enriched grains and eats a balanced diet should have no problems with lack of thiamin.

STABILITY AND INTERFERING FACTORS Air and heat destroy thiamin. The destruction is especially pronounced in the presence of alkalis. For this reason, adding baking soda to green vegetables to retain their color or to dried beans to soften them inactivates the thiamin in the vegetables. An enzyme in raw fish, **thiaminase**, destroys up to 50 percent of thiamin. Tea also contains an **antagonist**.

TOXICITY Thiamin is rapidly excreted from the body by the kidneys. Thus no evidence of toxicity following oral administration of thiamin has been reported (Tanphaichitr, 1999). Excessive thiamin by injection, however, has been associated with adverse effects including convulsions, cardiac arrhythmias, and anaphylactic shock (Groff, Gropper, and Hunt, 1995).

Riboflavin

Riboflavin was encountered late in the 19th century when laboratory workers observed a yellow-green fluorescent pigment that formed crystals. The complex, originally named vitamin B_2, also contained niacin and vitamin B_6. Not until 1933 was riboflavin isolated and its identity as a vitamin established.

ABSORPTION, METABOLISM, AND EXCRETION Absorption of riboflavin occurs in the small intestine. Only small amounts are stored in the liver and kidneys, so daily needs must be met in the diet. In high doses, riboflavin imparts a bright yellow color to the urine (Yee, 1999).

FUNCTIONS Riboflavin is a coenzyme in the metabolism of protein and of other vitamins. Thyroid and adrenal hormones control the conversion of riboflavin to its active coenzymes, which are involved in many oxidative enzyme systems.

DEFICIENCY Riboflavin deficiency often occurs with thiamin and niacin deficiencies. A person who avoids all dairy products, however, may be deficient in riboflavin alone, a condition called **ariboflavinosis**. Signs of this deficiency include lesions on the lips and in the oral cavity, seborrheic dermatitis, scrotal or vulval skin changes, and normocytic anemia.

DIETARY REFERENCE INTAKES The RDAs for riboflavin are 1.3 milligrams for adult males and 1.1 milligrams for adult females. Infants' AI is 0.3 to 0.4 milligram.

Riboflavin needs increase as protein needs increase. Clients undergoing major healing processes, such as those with extensive burns, require more riboflavin than the average person.

FOOD SOURCES Good sources are organ meats, milk, whole or enriched grains, legumes, and vegetables.

STABILITY Riboflavin is relatively stable to heat but is sensitive to ultraviolet light. Cardboard milk cartons or opaque plastic bottles filter out more light than do clear glass bottles.

TOXICITY There is no known toxicitgy (Feinman and Lieber, 1999).

Niacin

Niacin, or nicotinic acid, is vitamin B_3. Lack of niacin causes a specific disease, pellagra.

ABSORPTION, METABOLISM, AND EXCRETION Not all nutrients present in a food are available to the body. Niacin is found in corn but in a bound form that cannot be absorbed. Treating the corn with lye, as is done in some Latin American cultures, frees the niacin for the body's use.

Not all the body's niacin has to come from preformed niacin in food. The liver can convert the amino acid tryptophan to niacin, but protein synthesis is given a higher priority than niacin formation (Cervantes-Laurean, McElvaney, and Moss, 1999). This is the only known vitamin with an amino acid for a provitamin.

FUNCTIONS OF NIACIN Niacin is a coenzyme in the production of energy from glucose. Niacin also participates in the synthesis of fatty acids.

DEFICIENCY **Pellagra** is the deficiency disease caused by the lack of niacin. It is endemic in India and parts of China and Africa (Cervantes-Laurean, McElvaney, and Moss, 1999). To have a deficiency, a person must have a diet lacking in both niacin and tryptophan. Adults can get up to 67 percent of their niacin from foods classified as complete proteins.

Pellagra has serious effects. The "three Ds" are its major symptoms: dermatitis, diarrhea, and dementia. The dermatitis is a red rash on the face, neck, hands, and feet. The rash is bilaterally symmetrical; on the hands and arms it sometimes resembles gloves. A recent case involved a 48-year-old man with alcoholism and a rash on his hands, forearms, and neck that he had had for two years. Treatment with nicotinamide cured his rash in two weeks (Isaac, 1998).

DIETARY REFERENCE INTAKES Niacin is measured in **niacin equivalents** (NE). One milligram of niacin equivalent is the same as 1 milligram of preformed niacin or 60 milligrams of tryptophan. The RDAs for niacin are 16 milligrams NE for adult males and 14 milligrams NE for adult females. The UL is 35 milligrams obtained from supplements or fortified foods.

FOOD SOURCES Preformed niacin occurs in significant amounts in meat, particularly red meat and liver. Other sources include peanuts and legumes. Coffee also contains niacin and prevents pellagra in cultures with low protein and high coffee intakes. The process of roasting coffee beans increases the niacin content by 30 times as nicotinic acid is formed from an alkaloid in the beans (Cervantes-Laurean, McElvaney, and Moss, 1999).

STABILITY Niacin is a water-soluble vitamin. Small amounts are lost in cooking water. Niacin is stable to heat, light, air, acid, and alkalis. It is the most environmentally stable vitamin.

TOXICITY Pharmacological doses of niacin cause flushing. Even reformulation of breakfast cereal to 100 percent of the RDA of vitamins, including niacin, has caused flushing and a rash in a person who consumed six cupsful for breakfast (Morse, Morse, and Patterson, 1999). The large doses prescribed to lower blood lipid levels over the long term can cause liver damage. A case of niacin toxicity from food is reported in Clinical Application 7–7. It explains how food poisoning epidemics are investigated and what the nurse's responsibilities are when assisting with the inquiry.

Vitamin B₆

Vitamin B_6 serves in many roles, but no deficiency disease is associated with a lack of it. The name for the pharmaceutical preparation of vitamin B_6 is **pyridoxine**.

ABSORPTION, METABOLISM, AND EXCRETION Vitamin B_6 is absorbed in the small intestine, mainly in the jejunum. It is found throughout the body, but 80 to 90 percent of it is in muscle tissue (Leklem, 1999). Riboflavin

---

CLINICAL APPLICATION 7–7

Niacin Toxicity

In late 1980, almost half the clients in a small nursing home in Illinois became ill after breakfast. Their faces became flushed, or they developed a rash 15 to 30 minutes after the meal. As in suspected food poisoning epidemics, the foods consumed were compared. Which food was eaten by all those who became ill, but by none of those who did not become ill? In this case, it was cornmeal mush.

Careful observation and documentation is important in food poisoning cases. The sequence of signs and symptoms may steer the investigators in the right direction. Often the signs and symptoms have disappeared by the time the physician arrives. In this nursing home, the signs and symptoms lasted only an average of 50 minutes.

If food poisoning is suspected, health authorities take samples of the food to examine in the laboratory. None of the leftover food should be discarded before health authorities arrive. The Food and Drug Administration tested the cornmeal from the nursing home's kitchen. It contained more than 1000 mg of niacin per pound. The recommended amount for cornmeal is 16 to 24 mg/lb.

Often a food poisoning epidemic has run its course by the time the source of the outbreak is known. In this case, the offending food was identified, but the method of contamination never was positively determined.

---

is needed to convert most naturally available vitamin B_6 to its functional coenzyme (Lowik et al., 1994).

FUNCTIONS Vitamin B_6 is a coenzyme in the synthesis and catabolism of amino acids. It is involved in the metabolism of more than 60 enzymes. Vitamin B_6 functions as a coenzyme in the conversion of tryptophan into niacin. It helps to manufacture antibodies. The hormone epinephrine and the neurotransmitters **dopamine** and **serotonin** all require vitamin B_6 as a coenzyme. It also participates in amino acid transport and the transfer of sulfur and nitrogen to form other compounds.

DEFICIENCY A deficiency of B_6 is unlikely because large amounts are present in the general diet. Nonetheless, factors such as drug interactions or errors in food processing may cause a deficiency. In the past, improperly processed commercial infant formula produced vitamin B_6 deficiencies.

Vitamin B_6 deficiency risk is increased by the use of oral contraceptives. Women who use oral contraceptives for more than 2 or 3 years require additional vitamin B_6 because of an abnormal tryptophan metabolism. Infants of mothers who took oral contraceptives for more than 30 months before pregnancy should also be monitored for deficiency.

Clinically, a person with a vitamin B_6 deficiency may present with anemia, neurological abnormalities, or impaired immune function. Infants usually display abnormal electroencephalogram tracings or convulsions. Adults more often suffer from various mouth lesions, depression, and confusion (Leklem, 1999).

DIETARY REFERENCE INTAKES The RDAs for vitamin B_6 are 1.3 milligrams for men and women through age 50, 1.7 milligrams for older men, and 1.5 milligrams for older women. An increase in protein metabolism increases the need for vitamin B_6. The UL is 100 milligrams for adults.

FOOD SOURCES Vitamin B_6 is widely distributed in foods. Pork and organ meats are the best animal sources. Whole grains and wheat germ are the best plant sources. Vitamin B_6 is not included in the enrichment process for breads; for this reason, whole wheat bread contains more vitamin B_6 than white bread. Other good sources include legumes, potatoes, oatmeal, and bananas.

STABILITY As with other water-soluble vitamins, vitamin B_6 is preserved when vegetables are cooked as quickly as possible. Vitamin B_6 is relatively stable to heat and acids, but very sensitive to light and easily destroyed by alkalis.

TOXICITY Pyridoxine toxicity has resulted from taking 2 to 6 grams per day for 2 to 40 months. These megadoses, 1100 to 3500 times the RDA, were self-prescribed. Signs and symptoms include sensory loss and numbness of the hands and feet, resulting in clumsiness and severe **ataxia**. Cessation of the drug permitted the return of some, but not all, functions. Even 200 milligrams per day has produced sensory neuropathy (Feinman and Lieber, 1999).

Folic Acid

Also known as its salt, folate, **folic acid** is involved in protein synthesis, including that of DNA and RNA, and in the maturation of red blood cells. The latter function explains its interrelationship with vitamin B_{12}, discussed next.

ABSORPTION, METABOLISM, AND EXCRETION The folic acid in food is usually bound to amino acids. The enzyme needed to separate the folic acid from the amino acids is folate conjugase. It is found in salivary, gastric, pancreatic, and jejunal secretions. The unbound folate is absorbed from the small intestine, primarily in its proximal third, and transported to the liver. In the liver some of the folate is processed for storage in the tissues and the liver, which holds about half the body's supply. Some folate is secreted into bile. When the gallbladder releases bile into the duodenum, the folate may again be split off and absorbed. This recycling process is important in making folate stores adequate for 2 to 4 months, compared with 1 to 4 weeks for thiamin stores. Excretion of folic acid occurs via bile and urine.

FUNCTIONS Folic acid is necessary for the formation of DNA. Thus, folate participates in the reproduction of every cell. Folic acid is active in cell renewal and is necessary for rapidly growing cells, including those in the gastrointestinal (GI) tract, blood, and fetal tissue.

DEFICIENCY Folic acid deficiency is probably the most common vitamin deficiency due to inadequate food intake. Only one fresh fruit or fresh vegetable daily is considered sufficient to eliminate this deficiency (Herbert, 1999). At risk are poorly nourished children and poverty-stricken people. Pregnant women, infants, and young children are also at risk because increased folic acid is needed during periods of rapid growth. An estimated one-third of the world's pregnant women are affected by folate deficiency (Herbert, 1999). The link between folic acid and neural tube defects in the developing fetus is discussed in Chapter 11. Causes of folic acid deficiency include inadequate intake, inadequate absorption, inadequate use, increased requirement, increased destruction, and increased excretion. In clients with chronic alcoholism, the fact that all six causes may coexist explains why about 80 percent of these individuals are folate deficient. A deficiency may also occur in conditions causing increased metabolic rates, such as infections and hyperthyroidism and those characterized by increased cell turnover such as severe burns and cancer (Herbert, 1999).

Folic acid deficiency results in impaired cell division and protein synthesis, including the faulty synthesis of red blood cells. Signs and symptoms include a red, smooth, and swollen tongue, heartburn, diarrhea, fainting, and fatigue. In addition, since folic acid functions in the production of heme, the person deficient in this vitamin develops **megaloblastic anemia**.

Although clients with folate deficiency do not develop the nerve damage seen in vitamin B_{12} deficiencies, they do manifest neurologic symptoms that include irritability, forgetfulness, and hostile and paranoid behavior. These symptoms improve markedly 24 hours after beginning treatment with folic acid (Herbert, 1999).

One positive result of folate deficiency occurs in tropical countries where it protects against malaria. The lack of folic acid stops the spread of the parasite by preventing its DNA from replicating (Herbert, 1999).

DIETARY REFERENCE INTAKES The RDA for folic acid is 400 micrograms for adults. Women capable of becoming pregnant should consume 400 micrograms of folic acid from fortified foods or supplements in addition to food folate. Pregnant women have an RDA of 600 micrograms. UL for synthetic folic acid obtained from supplements and/or fortified foods is 1000 micrograms for adults.

SOURCES OF FOLATE From the meat group, liver is a good source of folic acid. Green, leafy vegetables such as spinach, asparagus, and broccoli provide folic acid. Other vegetables containing appreciable folic acid are kidney and lima beans, beets, and vegetables of the cabbage family. Fruits providing folic acid are oranges and cantaloupe.

An alternate source of folate is thought to be synthesis by intestinal bacteria. An increase in serum folate concentration has been associated with an increase in dietary fiber intake. The rationale suggested was that the fiber enhanced the synthesis of folate by intestinal bacteria (Houghton et al., 1997).

STABILITY Folic acid is stable in the presence of alkalis but it is easily oxidized by light and acids. Some forms are easily destroyed by heat, so that cooking losses may be as high as 80 to 90 percent. To minimize losses, cook vegetables as quickly as possible.

INTERFERING FACTORS Alcohol, oral contraceptives, or zinc deficiency may interfere with the absorption of folic acid. Conjugase inhibitors in certain foods prevent the digestion of polyglutamate forms of folate and thus prevent its absorption. Some of the foods containing these conjugase inhibitors are legumes, lentils, cabbage, and oranges (Groff, Gropper, and Hunt, 1995).

Methotrexate, an anticancer drug, is a folic acid antagonist. Its purpose is to interfere with DNA in cancer cells, but it simultaneously affects normal cells. A more commonly used drug, aspirin, displaces folic acid from its carrier protein; the displaced folic acid is then excreted.

TOXICITY Folic acid toxicity is rare. Dose levels of over-the-counter vitamins have been limited to 400 micrograms to make it inconvenient to overdose. The limitation is not to prevent toxicity from folic acid but to avoid masking signs of pernicious anemia. The current opinion of the scientific community, however, is that intake of folate and folic acid up to 5,000 micrograms per day would have no adverse effects and that a more sophisticated blood test can be used to diagnose pernicious anemia (Workshop, 1999).

Recommended doses in healthy humans have not been reported to be toxic, but very large doses in laboratory animals have produced renal toxicity and convulsions. The interaction of folic acid with antiepileptic drugs is discussed in Chapter 17.

Vitamin B_{12}

Vitamin B_{12} is an essential coenzyme in fatty acid metabolism and nucleic acid synthesis. Vitamin B_{12} is stored to a greater extent than the other B vitamins, but diverse causes can precipitate vitamin B_{12} deficiency, leading to serious consequences and a specific disease condition.

ABSORPTION, METABOLISM, AND EXCRETION Efficient absorption of vitamin B_{12} requires a highly specific protein-binding factor called **intrinsic factor**, secreted by the gastric mucosal cells in the stomach. Vitamin B_{12}, also called **extrinsic factor**, combines with intrinsic factor in the proximal small intestine. In this way, intrinsic factor protects vitamin B_{12} from digestive enzymes and intestinal bacteria until the complex reaches the ileum where the vitamin is absorbed. About 1 percent of large pharmacological doses of vitamin B_{12} are absorbed by passive diffusion in the intestine (Weir and Scott, 1999).

Vitamin B_{12} is not freely absorbed. The amount absorbed depends upon the body's storage levels. Vitamin B_{12} has a long half-life, so that a person's stores last from 3 to 5 years. The principal storage site is the liver, which contains 50 percent of the body's supply.

FUNCTIONS Vitamin B_{12} is required in a series of reactions that precede the use of folic acid in DNA replication. In fact, without vitamin B_{12}, folic acid is unable to assist in the manufacture of red blood cells. Vitamin B_{12} is also essential for the synthesis and maintenance of myelin, the fatty insulation that permits speedy transmission of impulses along the nerves.

DEFICIENCY Persons may be at increased risk of vitamin B_{12} deficiency because of stomach pathology, intestinal disease, or diet. When a person lacks intrinsic factor, the result is a condition called **pernicious anemia**. The prevalence of the disease increases with age and is attributed to antibodies against gastric parietal cells and intrinsic factor. Pernicious anemia can also occur following the surgical removal of the stomach or a large portion of the stomach. In those cases vitamin B_{12} is not absorbed because intrinsic factor is missing.

People with **Crohn's disease** involving the ileum and those whose ileum has been removed do not absorb vitamin B_{12} efficiently. Dietary treatment is ineffective in such clients, to whom vitamin B_{12} traditionally is given by injection. The pharmaceutical names for vitamin B_{12} are **cyanocobalamin** or **hydroxocobalamin**. In several studies, large doses of cyanocobalamin administered orally have been reported to be effective in normalizing serum levels and blood pictures (Altay and Cetin, 1999; Hathcock and Troendle, 1991; Lederle, 1991) and neurologic abnormalities (Kuzminski et al., 1998). Nevertheless, a consensus has not been reached; oral administration is criticized as not preventing neurological damage (Freeman, 1999, 1992, and 1988).

Symptoms of vitamin B_{12} deficiency are, in usual order of appearance, numbness and tingling in the hands and feet, red blood cell changes, moodiness, confusion, depression, delusions, and overt **psychosis**. Eventually, irreparable nerve damage occurs, and finally, death. One study reported 28 percent of clients with neuropsychiatric disorders caused by vitamin B_{12} deficiency displayed no red blood cell pathology, suggesting cobalamin deficiency should be ruled out in clients with unexplained neuropsychiatric disorders (Lindenbaum et al., 1988).

Diagnosing vitamin B_{12} deficiency by examining red blood cells is difficult if the person consumes ample folic acid. The folic acid enables the body to continue manufacturing red blood cells in the correct size and number, but the neurological deterioration of pernicious anemia continues unabated. Other blood tests are more effective in diagnosing vitamin B_{12} deficiency.

Strict vegetarians are at risk of vitamin B_{12} deficiency because animal products are the best sources of vitamin B_{12}. In this case, additional vitamin B_{12}, from either food or supplements, is the treatment. A 33-year old-man who had been a strict vegetarian for many years without taking vitamin supplements became irreversibly blind as a result of to severe bilateral optic neuropathy. The condition was attributed to deficiencies of vitamin B_{12} and thiamin (Milea, Cassoux, and LeHoang, 2000).

DIETARY REFERENCE INTAKES The adult RDA for vitamin B_{12} is 2.4 micrograms. One ounce of beef liver contains 13 times this amount. Because 10 to 30 percent of older people may not absorb vitamin B_{12} from food well, the RDA table for men and women older than 50 suggests fortified foods or a vitamin supplement be used as the source for vitamin B_{12}.

FOOD SOURCES Vitamin B_{12} is synonymous with animal products that have derived their cobalamins from microorganisms. Healthy young adults who regularly eat meat, milk, cheese, or eggs are not at risk of vitamin B_{12} deficiency. Some plant foods may contain vitamin B_{12} from bacterial contamination or in the case of legumes, from the nitrogen-fixing bacteria on their roots. For strict vegetarians, nutritional yeast and vitamin B_{12}-fortified soymilk are more reliable food sources than relianceon bacterial contamination.

STABILITY AND INTERFERING FACTORS Vitamin B_{12} is stable to heat. However, light, acids, and alkalies inactivate it. Megadoses of vitamin C interfere with vitamin B_{12} absorption and utilization. The body's use of vitamin B_{12} is also impaired by a deficiency of vitamin B_6 and gastritis.

Recently Emphasized Vitamins

Two B vitamins are so widely distributed in foods that only special circumstances have produced deficiencies. Long-term total parenteral nutrition is one such situation.

PANTOTHENIC ACID The vitamin **pantothenic acid** plays a role in the metabolism of carbohydrates, fats, and proteins and in the synthesis of the neurotransmitter **acetylcholine**. No cases of deficiency of pantothenic acid have been documented in people who eat a variety of foods, but deficiencies have occurred in prisoner-of-war camps and have been produced experimentally (Plesofsky-Vig, 1999). There are no RDAs for pantothenic acid. Instead, an Adequate Intake (AI) of 5 milligrams has been set for adults. The average U.S. diet supplies 7 milligrams. Rich food sources include liver, yeast, egg yolk, milk, broccoli, Brussels sprouts, sweet potato, and dried beans. Bacteria in the colon are able to synthesize pantothenic acid (Said, 1999).

BIOTIN Closely related to folic acid and vitamin B_{12}, **biotin** is a coenzyme in the synthesis of fatty acids and amino acids. It is required to form **purines**, which are essential components of DNA and RNA. Oral biotin, even in pharmacological doses, is completely absorbed (Zempleni and Mock, 1999). Deficiencies have been seen in children displaying the chief sign of skin rash. Deficiencies may occur in clients fed intravenously who also receive antibiotics. Antibiotics kill the bacteria in the large intestine that synthesize biotin. Other clients who have developed biotin deficiency are those with alcoholism or gastrointestinal diseases and those on long-term anticonvulsant therapy or receiving long-term hemodialysis (Mock, 1999). The AI for biotin is 30 micrograms.

Avidin, a protein in raw egg white, binds with biotin. Humans given six raw egg whites per day developed dermatitis in 3 to 4 weeks. A week or two later they displayed mental changes, muscle pain, nausea, and loss of appetite. Five days of biotin therapy cured the symptoms. Good food sources of biotin include liver, kidney, meat, egg yolk, and tomatoes.

Choline

The organic compound **choline** is necessary for life. It occurs in the structure of membranes, modulates signaling within cells, and plays a vital role in brain development (Zeisel, 1999). Formerly classified as a B vitamin, this substance has been given an Adequate Intake under the Dietary Reference Intake system but is not listed as a vitamin. Choline is found in most animal tissues and is widely distributed in foods.

Choline facilitates movement of fat into the cells and decreases liver fat content by increasing phospholipid turnover. Deficiency of choline can result in fatty liver and hepatic cirrhosis. Choline is a primary component of acetylcholine, a neurotransmitter. It has produced memory improvement among healthy young people but its effect on elderly people has been disappointing (Groff, Gropper, and Hunt, 1995).

The AI for choline is 550 milligrams for men and 425 milligrams for women. The UL for choline is 3500 milligrams per day for adults. The best food sources of choline are eggs, liver, soybeans, wheat germ, and peanuts (Groff, Gropper, and Hunt, 1995)

People at increased risk of choline deficiency include growing infants, pregnant or lactating women, people with cirrhosis of the liver, and clients receiving **total parenteral nutrition (TPN)** (see Chapter 15). All of these individuals, especially those on limited diets or being artificially fed, may be at risk for deficiencies of other nutrients as well as choline.

Of the water-soluble vitamins, ascorbic acid is the most vulnerable to loss and niacin the most resistant. Table 7–4 summarizes information on vitamin C and six of the B-complex vitamins. In it and Table 7–2, although examples of food portions containing the RDA are given, it is for clarity only, not as a recommendation to use those specific foods to the exclusion of others. Table 7–5 and Figure 7– 4 summarize the sources of vitamins by food groups.

Vitamins as Medicine

Supplements

Vitamin supplements are not intended to be substitutes for a healthy diet. It should be clear from the discussion throughout the chapter that knowledge of vitamins is not complete. New functions and relationships are being discovered every year. The new Dietary Reference Intakes are designed to consider the effect of vitamin intake on chronic disease occurrence, rather than simply to prevent deficiency diseases. The single piece of advice that appears most frequently in the conclusions of researchers, however, is the admonition to eat five servings of fruits and vegetables every day. Figure 7– 5 is a reminder that fruit eaten out of hand is the original fast food.

If a person wishes to take supplements, it is best not to exceed 150 percent of the RDA for each vitamin (Omaye, 1998). This amount will pre-

vent deficiency in young, well individuals and toxicity is unlikely. Even so, people ought to consider vitamins as medications when their primary care providers ask what medications they are taking.

Evidence is accumulating that high levels of supplementation are associated with decreased risks of chronic diseases. Rather than self-medicate and risk overdosing or interfering with medications, individuals with special concerns should discuss their needs with their primary healthcare providers.

For the first time, the RDAs specify fortified foods or supplements for certain life-stage groups. It is recommended that people over 50 years of age obtain vitamin B_{12} from fortified foods or supplements. For all women who may become pregnant, the recommendation is to consume 400 micrograms of folic acid from fortified foods or supplements in addition to food folate to reduce the risk of neural tube defects in the fetus. This abnormality is discussed in Chapter 11, "Life Cycle Nutrition: Pregnancy and Lactation."

Pharmacological Uses

Vitamin supplements can be used to offset dietary deficiencies or to compensate for diseases causing malabsorption. They also have been given for some conditions unrelated to diet.

Treatment of Deficiencies

The obvious use of vitamins is to treat vitamin deficiencies. Vitamin C is the treatment for scurvy, vitamin D for rickets, niacin for pellagra, and vitamin B_{12} for pernicious anemia. Common uses in diseases causing malabsorption are discussed in Unit Three, "Clinical Nutrition."

Other Uses

MEGADOSES A dose ten times the RDA is called a **megadose**. Some individuals take huge doses of vitamin C in an attempt to prevent the common cold. Evidence of effectiveness has not been proven to the satisfaction of many scientists. A recent review of the literature, however, indicated a decrease of one-half day in the duration of symptoms of the cold in individuals taking vitamin C either daily or at the onset of a cold, but did not find long-term supplementation reduced the incidence of colds (Douglas, Chalker, and Treacy, 1999). Rebound scurvy has been reported when megadoses of vitamin C were discontinued abruptly.

TREATING NONNUTRITIONAL DISORDERS Many vitamins have uses unrelated to prevention or treatment of deficiencies. Vitamins A, E, C, riboflavin, and niacin are examples. Vitamin A derivatives are often prescribed to control acne and the wrinkles of aging. The hazards to the fetus are discussed in Chapter 11 on Pregnancy and Lactation. Clinical Application 7–8 discusses Vitamin C as a food additive intended to reduce the formation of cancer-causing compounds. A clinical trial of high doses of riboflavin to prevent migraine headaches has been reported (Schoenen, Jacquy, and Lenaerts, 1998). Topical application of niacin is being tested as an aid in identifying schizophrenia (Ward, et al., 1998). High doses of niacin, usually 3 to 6 grams per day, have been used to lower serum cholesterol but doses of 2 to 4.5 grams per day have caused macular edema and vision loss until the niacin was discontinued (Callanan, Blondi, and Martin, 1998).

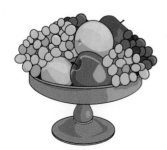

The Original Fast Food

Figure 7–5:
A reminder that fruits eaten out-of-hand are the original fast foods.

Table 7–4 Water Soluble Vitamins

Vitamin	Adult RDA and Food Portion Containing RDA	Functions	Deficiency Disease	Signs and Symptoms of Deficiency	Best Sources
C Ascorbic acid	60 mg 0.5 cup orange juice	Antioxidant Formation of collagen Function of adrenal glands Facilitates iron absorption Converts folic acid to active form	Scurvy	Bleeding mucous membranes Poor wound healing or reopening of scars Softened ends of long bones Teeth loosen, may fall out Death due to internal hemorrhage	Orange juice, grapefruit juice, cantaloupe, strawberries Peppers, Brussels sprouts, broccoli
B_1 Thiamin	1.1 to 1.2 mg 3.6 oz pork chop, lean only	Coenzyme in CHO metabolism Necessary to convert alcohol to energy	Beriberi	Anorexia, indigestion, constipation Apathy, fatigue, muscle weakness Deterioration of myelin sheaths—paralysis, muscle atrophy Wernicke-Korsakoff syndrome Death due to cardiac failure	Pork Black beans, black-eyed peas Sunflower seeds Fortified cereals
B2 Riboflavin	1.1 to 1.3 mg 1.1 oz beef liver, fried	Coenzyme in protein metabolism	Aribino-flavinosis	Lesions on lips and in mouth Seborrheic dermatitis Skin changes on scrotum or vulva Normocytic anemia	Beef liver Milk Fortified cereals Raw or cooked (not canned) mushrooms
B3 Niacin	14 to 16 mg niacin equivalents 3.6 oz water-packed tuna	Coenzyme in production of energy from glucose Assist in synthesis of fatty acids	Pellagra	Bilaterally symmetrical dermatitis on face, neck, hands, and feet Diarrhea Dementia	Tuna Chicken breast Beef liver
B6 Pyridoxine	1.3 to 1.7 mg 2.6 bananas	Coenzyme in synthesis and catabolism of amino acids	No specific term	Dermatitis Glossitis Convulsions	Beef liver Bananas Baked potatoes Baked chicken breast
Folate Folic acid	400 μg 6.3 oz beef liver	Essential to the formation of DNA Functions in formation of heme	No specific term	Red, smooth, swollen tongue Heartburn, diarrhea Fatigue, fainting Confusion, depression Macrocytic anemia	Beef liver Pinto beans Cooked asparagus Cooked spinach
B_{12} Cyanoco-balamin	2.4 μg 3.2 oz cooked lean beef	Necessary for folic acid use in DNA replication Synthesis and maintenance of myelin	Pernicious anemia (lack of intrinsic factor, not dietary)	Sore tongue Numbness and tingling of hands and feet Macrocytic anemia Moodiness, confusion Depression Delusions, psychosis	Meat Fish Shellfish Poultry Milk

Table 7–5 Sources of Vitamins by Food Groups

Vitamin	Synthesis/ Miscellaneous	Meats	Milk	Fruits/Vegetables	Grains
A		Liver	Fortified	Deep yellow, dark green leafy	
D	In skin	Liver, eggs, some fish	Fortified		
E				Vegetable oil	Wheat germ, whole grains
K	In intestine	Liver, eggs	Milk	Green leafy	
C				Fresh fruit, especially citrus Vegetables	
Thiamin		Pork		Green vegetables	Brewer's yeast
Riboflavin		Organ meats	Milk	Legumes	Brewer's yeast
Niacin	Coffee	Meat, tuna, eggs	Milk		Brewer's yeast, whole grains
B_6		Pork, organ meats, chicken, fish		Potatoes, bananas, legumes	Whole grains, wheat germ, oatmeal
Folic acid		Liver		Cabbage family, dark green leafy, beets, kidney beans, cantaloupe, oranges	Whole grains
B_{12}		Meat, eggs	Milk		
Pantothenic acid	In intestine	Liver, kidney, egg yolk	Milk	Dried beans, Brussels sprouts, sweet potato	
Biotin	In intestine	Meat, liver, kidney, egg yolk		Tomatoes	

CLINICAL APPLICATION 7–8

Vitamin C and Smoked Meat

Vitamin C blocks the formation of nitrosamines from nitrates. *Nitrates* are chemicals added to smoked and cured meats to preserve them and enhance their flavor. In the small intestine, however, nitrates combine with amino acids to form nitrosamines, which have been linked to some cancers. For this reason meat packers have begun adding vitamin C to protect against nitrosamine formation. Blocking the formation of nitrosamines in the intestinal tract is also suggested as support for a 200 milligram RDA (Levine et al., 1996).

Summary

Vitamins are organic substances required in minute quantities that are necessary for many bodily processes. They do not become part of the structure of the body.

Some deficiency diseases have been known and treated for centuries. It was not until the twentieth century, though, that each of the known vitamins was isolated in the laboratory.

Vitamins A, D, E, and K are fat-soluble and stable to heat. Sufficient dietary fat intake and adequate fat digestion and absorption are required for the proper utilization of these vitamins. Fat-soluble vitamins, especially A and D, can be stored in excess by the body, and for that reason can be sources of toxicity. Both vitamins A and D cause clear-cut deficiency diseases: xerophthalmia and night blindness for vitamin A and rickets for vitamin D.

The water-soluble vitamins, C and the B-complex vitamins, are not stored in the body in appreciable amounts. Vitamins C, B_{12}, thiamin, andniacin have specific diseases associated with deficiency: scurvy, pernicious anemia, beriberi, and pellagra, respectively.

Because of the interdependent functions of vitamins, people without special needs are advised to rely mainly on a varied, balanced, moderate diet for vitamins (Wellness Tips 7–1). Vitamin supplements will not compensate for a poor diet. People who take vitamins should limit their intake to 150 percent of the RDA, except individuals with special needs.

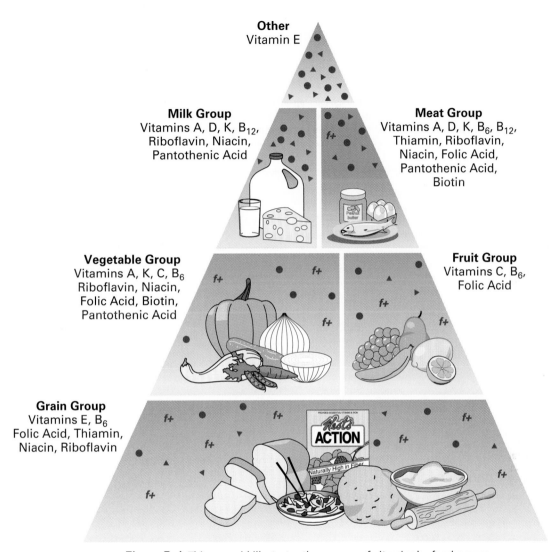

Other
Vitamin E

Milk Group
Vitamins A, D, K, B₁₂,
Riboflavin, Niacin,
Pantothenic Acid

Meat Group
Vitamins A, D, K, B₆, B₁₂,
Thiamin, Riboflavin,
Niacin, Folic Acid,
Pantothenic Acid,
Biotin

Vegetable Group
Vitamins A, K, C, B₆
Riboflavin, Niacin,
Folic Acid, Biotin,
Pantothenic Acid

Fruit Group
Vitamins C, B₆,
Folic Acid

Grain Group
Vitamins E, B₆
Folic Acid, Thiamin,
Niacin, Riboflavin

Figure 7–4: This pyramid illustrates the sources of vitamins by food groups.

Wellness Tips 7–1

- Eat 5 servings of fruits and vegetables each day. Whole foods contain nutrients and phytochemicals not found in vitamin tablets.
- Select whole grain products rather than refined ones to maximize vitamin content.
- Follow the Food Guide Pyramid. Limiting fat does not mean eliminating fat. Absorption of fat soluble vitamins requires fat intake.
- Seek advice from the healthcare provider if a whole category of food is excluded from the diet.
- If using a vitamin supplement, choose a multivitamin preparation instead of individual vitamins unless the health-care provider recommends them to treat particular conditions.
- Do not attempt to implement the findings of every new study on vitamins that is reported.
- When asked, be sure to include vitamin supplements on the list of medications you take.
- Avoid preformed vitamin A preparations. Beta-carotene is safer.
- Follow the recommended dosages, not to exceed 150 percent (one and one-half times) the RDA. In certain situations, vitamin supplementation has been associated with increases in infections or cancer. Bacteria and cancer cells need these nutrients, also. (Discussed in Chapter 12 on Infants, Children, and Adolescents and in Chapter 23 on Cancer.)

Case Study 7–1

Mr. J, a 79-year-old widowed man, prides himself on caring for himself in the past year since his wife died. His typical meal pattern is:

- Breakfast—egg, toast, jam, coffee
- Lunch—cheese or lunch meat sandwich, tea
- Dinner—canned stew or hash

Although Mr J has a refrigerator, he avoids buying fresh fruit or vegetables. He says he has difficulty consuming produce before it spoils. He seldom goes out to eat.
For the past few months Mr. J. has notices that his gums are tender. He stopped wearing his dentures when his gums began to bleed.
The visiting nurse confirmed the inflammation of the gums. When the nurse took Mr. J's blood pressure, she noted a red, flat rash where the blood pressure cuff had been.

Nursing Care Plan

Subjective Data	Sore gums
	Diet lacks fresh fruits and vegetables
Objective Data	Erythematous petechiae under blood pressure cuff
Nursing Diagnosis	NANDA: Altered Nutrition, less than body requirements, possible vitamin C deficiency (North American Nursing Diagnosis Association, 1999, with permission.) Related to lack of fresh fruit and vegetables as evidenced by sore bleeding gums and petechiae under blood pressure cuff.

Desired Outcomes Evaluation Criteria	Nursing Actions/ Interventions	Rationale
NOC: Nutritional Status (Johnson, Maas, and Moorhead, 2000, with permission.)	NIC: Nutritional Counseling (McCloskey and Bulechek, 2000, with permission.)	
Will consume foods containing 90 mg of vitamin C every day within 3 days	Teach importance of daily vitamin C	Little vitamin C is stored in the body; must be consumed every day.
	Explore acceptability of good sources of vitamin C; list amounts necessary to obtain 90 mg; recommend purchasing small quantities.	Foods would be better sources than vitamin supplements because other nutrients supplied also.
	If client selects frozen vegetables, teach to boil water 1 minute before adding vegetables and to cook quickly until crisp-tender.	Heat and oxygen destroy vitamin C.

Critical Thinking Question

1. What additional assessment data would be helpful as you work with Mr. J to increase his fruit and vegetable intake?
2. Speculate on the reasons the visiting nurse is calling on Mr. J. Can you think of medical conditions that would be directly affected by lack of vitamin C?
3. Mr. J wants to keep his present meal pattern and "take a vitamin pill" to correct his nutritional deficiencies. How would you respond?

 Study Aids

Subjects . . . . .Internet Sites
Fruits and vegetables http://www.5aday.com
http://www.dcpc.nci.gov/5aday/
Morbidity and mortality . . . . .http://www.cdc.gov/epo/mmwr
Nutrient information . . . . .http://nutrition.org
http://odp.od.nih.gov/ods/
http://www.fda.gov
http://www.healthfinder.gov
http://www.eyenet.org
Dietary supplements . . . . .http://www.nal.usda.gov/fnic/ibids.html
Pharmaceuticals . . . . .http://www.usp.org
http://www.rxlist.com

Chapter Review

1. Which of the following vitamins are water-soluble?
   a. A and C
   b. A, D, E, and K
   c. B and C
   d. B, D, E, and K

2. The vitamin that is essential to the synthesis of several blood clotting factors is:
   a. Vitamin A
   b. Vitamin B_6
   c. Vitamin C
   d. Vitamin K

3. Which of the following groups of foods would be the best sources of carotene?
   a. Apricots, cantaloupe, and squash
   b. Asparagus, beets, and sweet potatoes
   c. Broccoli, lettuce, and lima beans
   d. Lemons, oranges, and strawberries

4. Deficiency of vitamin A causes:
   a. Night blindness
   b. Pellagra
   c. Rickets
   d. Scurvy

5. In general, individuals who elect to take a vitamin supplement should:
   a. Buy the most economical product
   b. Limit the amounts to 150 percent of RDA levels
   c. Obtain a physician's prescription
   d. Select the most advertised product

Clinical Analysis

1. Ms. C is bringing her 3-month-old baby girl to the well-baby clinic. Ms. C states that the baby is taking 6 ounces of a commercial baby formula every 4 hours. Ms. C has not added solid foods to the baby's diet. She was told to wait until the baby is 4 months old before adding cereal. Ms. C is giving the baby the multivitamin preparation prescribed. She also has added cod liver oil to the infant's diet. "It's only a teaspoonful," she said. Ms. C's grandmother gave Ms. C cod liver oil as a child. Ms. C credits her grandmother's care during her own childhood for her strong bones and teeth. She admires her grandmother, who at age 75 still stands straight and tall. Which of the following pieces of information should the nurse gather first to focus on the situation presented?
   a. The amount of vitamin C in the multivitamin supplement
   b. The conditions under which the vitamins are stored
   c. Ms. C's technique for measuring the vitamins
   d. The total amount of vitamin D the infant receives each day

2. Mr. S has expressed interest in improving his diet. The nurse assessed Mr. S's usual intake, noting the absence of citrus fruit. He stated the acids upset his stomach. Which of the following suggestions to maximize vitamin C content in vegetables is appropriate?
   a. Adding baking soda to the cooking water
   b. Cooking thoroughly to kill any bacteria
   c. Eating good sources raw when possible
   d. Keeping food in a mesh bag to allow air to circulate

3. Ms. P has been taking oral contraceptives for three years. The nurse should assess her vitamin _____ intake and check for signs of deficiency.
   a. A
   b. B_6
   c. C
   d. D

Bibliography

Aghdassi, E, Royall, D, and Allard, JP: Oxidative stress in smokers supplemented with vitamin C. Int J Vitam Nutr Res 69:45, 1999.

Altay, C, and Cetin, M: Vitamin B_{12} absorption test and oral treatment in 14 children with selective vitamin B_{12} malabsorption. Pediatr Hematol Oncol 16:159-63, 1999.

Bamber, MG: Wernicke's encephalopathy [letter]. Lancet 352:655, 1998.

Belda, JI, et al.: Serum vitamin E levels negatively correlate with severity of age–related macular degeneration. Mech Ageing Dev 107:159, 1999.

Benomar, A et al.: Vitamin E deficiency ataxia associated with adenoma. J Neurol Sci 162:97, 1999.

Blank, S, et al.: An outbreak of hypervitaminosis D associated with the overfortification of milk from a home-delivery dairy. Am J Public Health 85:656, 1995.

Boucher, BJ: Inadequate vitamin D status: Does it contribute to the disorders comprising syndrome "X"? British Journal of Nutrition 79:315, 1998.

Brown, JE: The Science of Human Nutrition, Harcourt, Brace, Jovanovich, San Diego, 1990.

Callanan, D, Blodi, BA, and Martin, DF: Macular edema associated with nicotinic acid (niacin) [letter]. JAMA 279:1702, 1998.

Carr, AC, and Frei, B: Toward a new recommended dietary allowance for vitamin C based on antioxidant and health effects in humans. Am J Clin Nutr 69:1086, 1999.

Cataract Management Guideline Panel: Cataract in Adults: Management of Functional Impairment. U.S. Department of Health and Human Services, Rockville, MD, 1993.

Centers for Disease Control. Deaths associated with thiamine-deficient total parenteral nutrition. MMWR 38:43– 46, 1989. Accessed July 15, 1999 at http://www.cdc.gov/epo/mmwr/preview/mmwrhtml/00001339.htm

Centers for Disease Control. Lactic acidosis traced to thiamine deficiency related to nationwide shortage of multivitamins for total parenteral nutrition—United States, 1997. MMWR 38:43–46. Accessed July 15, 1999 at http://www.cdc.gov/epo/mmwr/preview/mmwrhtml/00001339.htm.

Cervantes-Laurean, D, McElvaney, NG, and Moss, J: Niacin. In Shils, ME, et al (eds): Modern Nutrition in Health and Disease ed 9. Lippincott Williams and Wilkins, Philadelphia, 1999.

Cochran, WA: Overnutrition in prenatal and neonatal life: A problem? Can Med Assoc J 93:893, 1965.

Collins, M, and Gernaey, A: Osteocalcin—the oldest surviving bone protein? Last updated May 1, 1998. Accessed August 5, 1999 at http://nrg.ncl.ac.uk/research/ancient-biomols/osteocalcin.html

Committee on Diet and Health. Food and Nutrition Board. Commission on Life Sciences. National Research Council: Diet and Health: Implications for Reducing Chronic Disease Risk. National Academy Press, Washington, DC, 1989.

Craciun, AM et al.: Improved bone metabolism in female elite athletes after vitamin K supplementation. Int J Sports Med 19:479, 1998.

Davies, PS, et al.: Vitamin D: Seasonal and regional differences in preschool children in Great Britain. Eur J Clin Nutr 53:195, 1999.

de Pee, S, Bloem, MW, et al.: Reappraisal of the role of vegetables in the vitamin A status of mothers in Central Java, Indonesia. Am J Clin Nutr 68:1068, 1998.

de Pee, S, West, CE et al.: Orange fruit is more effective than are dark green leafy vegetables in increasing serum concentrations of retinol and beta-carotene in school children in Indonesia. Am J Clin Nutr 68:1058, 1998.

DePaola, DP, Faine, MP, and Palmer, CA: Nutrition in relation to dental medicine. In Shils, ME, et al. (eds): Modern Nutrition in Health and Disease ed 9. Lippincott Williams and Wilkins, Philadelphia, 1999.

Douglas, RM, Chalker, EB, and Treacy, B: Vitamin C for the common cold. [Computer software]. The Cochrane Library, Oxford, 1999 issue 1. Abstract accessed through CINAHL, accession no. 1999023402.

Evans, JR: Antioxidant vitamin and mineral supplements for age-related macular degeneration. [Computer software]. The Cochrane Library, Oxford, 1999 issue 1. Abstract accessed through CINAHL, accession no. 1999022973.

Fawzi, WW, et al.: Vitamin A supplementation and child mortality. JAMA 269:898, 1993.

Ferland, G: The vitamin K-dependent proteins: An update. Nutr Rev 56:223, 1998.

Feinman, L, and Lieber, CS: Nutrition and diet in alcoholism. In Shils, ME, et al (eds): Modern Nutrition in Health and Disease ed 9. Lippincott Williams and Wilkins, Philadelphia, 1999.

Filteau, SM and Tomkins, AM: Promoting vitamin A status in low-income countries. Lancet 353: 1458, 1999.

Fitzpatrick S, et al.: Vitamin D-deficient rickets: A multifactorial disease. Nutr Rev 58:218, 2000.

Freeman, AG: Cyancobalamin—a case for withdrawal: Discussion paper. J R Soc Med 85:686, 1992.

Freeman, AG: Optic neuropathy and chronic cyanide intoxication: a review. J R Soc Med 18:103, 1988.

Freeman, AG: Oral or parenteral therapy for vitamin B_{12} deficiency. Lancet 353:410, 1999.

Garg, K, Draganescu, JM, and Albornoz, MA: A rash imposition from a lifestyle omission. Postgraduate Medicine 104:183, 1998.

Geubel, AP, et al.: Liver damage caused by therapeutic vitamin A administration: Estimate of dose-related toxicity in 41 cases. Gastroenterology 100:1710, 1991.

Glasziou, PP, and Mackerras, DEM: Vitamin A supplementation in infectious diseases: A meta-analysis. BMJ 306:366, 1993.

Groff, JL, Gropper, SS, and Hunt, SM: Advanced Nutrition and Human Metabolism, ed 2. West Publishing Co., Minneapolis, 1995.

Hankinson, SE, and Stampfer, MJ: All that glitters is not beta-carotene. JAMA272:1455, 1994.

Hathcock, JN, and Troendle, GJ: Oral cobalamin for treatment of pernicious anemia? JAMA 265:96, 1991.

Herbert, V: Folic acid. In Shils, ME, et al. (eds): Modern Nutrition in Health and Disease ed 9. Lippincott Williams and Wilkins, Philadelphia, 1999.

Herman, MJ, and Bulthuis, DB: Incidental diagnosis of nutritional rickets after clavicle fracture. Orthopedics. 22:254, 1999.

Hoshino, M, et al.: Ataxia with isolated vitamin E deficiency: A Japanese family carrying a novel mutation in the alpha-tocopherol transfer protein gene. Ann Neurol 45:809, 1999.

Houghton, LA, et al.: Association between dietary fiber intake and the folate status of a group of female adolescents. Am J Clin Nutr 66:1414, 1997.

Isaac, S: The "gauntlet" of pellagra. Int J Dermatol 37:599, 1998.

Jacob, RA: Vitamin C: In Shils, ME, et al. (eds): Modern Nutrition in Health and Disease ed 9. Lippincott Williams and Wilkins, Philadelphia, 1999.

Jacques, PF, and Chylack, LT: Epidemiologic evidence of a role for the antioxidant vitamins and carotenoids in cataract prevention. Am J Clin Nutr 53 (1 Suppl):352S, 1991.

Jacques, PF, et al.: Long-term vitamin C supplement use and prevalence of early age-related lens opacities. Am J Clin Nutr 66:911, 1997.

Jagadha, V, et al.: Wernicke's encephalopathy in patients on peritoneal dialysis or hemodialysis. Ann Neurol 21:78, 1987.

Johnson, M, Maas, M, and Moorhead, S: Nursing Outcomes Classification (NOC), ed 2. Mosby, Philadelphia, 2000.

Johnston, CS: Biomarkers for establishing a tolerable upper intake level for vitamin C. Nutr Rev 57:71, 1999.

Kanai, T, et al.: Serum vitamin K level and bone mineral density in postmenopausal women. Int J Gynecol Obstet 56:25, 1997.

Kawasaki, Y, et al.: The efficacy of oral vitamin A supplementation for measles and respiratory syncytial virus infection. Kansenshogaku Zasshi 73:104, 1999.

Kohlmeier, M, et al.: Bone health of adult hemodialysis patients is related to vitamin K status. Kidney Int 51:1218, 1997.

Kowalski, TE, Falestiny, M, Furth, E, et al.: Vitamin A hepatotoxicity: A cautionary note regarding 25,000 IU supplements. Am J Med 97:523, 1994.

Krasinski, SD, and Russell, RM: The prevalence of vitamin K deficiency in chronic gastrointestinal disorders. Am J Clin Nutr 41:639, 1985.

Kreiter, SR, et al: Nutritional rickets in African American breast-fed infants. J Pediatr 137:153, 2000.

Kuzminski, AM, et al.: Effective treatment of cobalamin deficiency with oral cobalamin. Blood 92:1191, 1998.

Lafforgue, P, et al.: Bone mineral density in patients given oral vitamin K antagonists. Rev Rhum Engl Ed 64:249, 1997.

Lawson, M, and Thomas, M: Vitamin D concentrations in Asian children aged 2 years living in England: Population survey. BMJ 318:28, 1999.

Lederle, FA: Oral cobalamin for pernicious anemia. JAMA 265:94, 1991.

Leklem, JE: Vitamin B_6. In Shils, ME, et al. (eds): Modern Nutrition in Health and Disease ed 9. Lippincott Williams and Wilkins, Philadelphia, 1999.

Levine, M, et al.: Criteria and recommendations for vitamin C intake. JAMA 281:1415, 1999.

Levine, M, et al.: Determination of optimal vitamin C requirements in humans. Am J Clin Nutr 62(suppl):1347S, 1995.

Levine, M, et al.: Vitamin C pharmacokinetics in healthy volunteers: Evidence for a recommended dietary allowance. Proc Nat Acad Sci USA 93:3704, 1996.

Lindebaum, J, et al.: Neuropsychiatric disorders caused by cobalamin deficiency in the absence of anemia or macrocytosis. N Engl J Med 318:1720, 1988.

Lowik, MRH, et al.: Interrelationships between riboflavin and vitamin B_6 among elderly people (Dutch Nutrition Surveillance System). Internat J Vit Nutr Res 64:198, 1994.

Lyle, BJ, et al.: Antioxidant intake and risk of incident age-related nuclear cataracts in the Beaver Dam Eye Study. Am J Epidemiol 149:801, 1999a.

Lyle, BJ, et al.: Serum carotenoids and tocopherols and incidence of age-related nuclear cataract. Am J Clin Nutr 69:272, 1999b.

Malloy, PJ, and Feldman, D: Vitamin D resistance. Am J Med 106:355, 1999.

Mares-Perlman, JA: Contribution of epidemiology to understanding relations of diet to age-related cataract. Am J Clin Nutr 66:739, 1997.

Mares-Perlman, JA, et al.: Association of zinc and antioxidant nutrients with age-related maculopathy. Arch Ophthalmol 114:991, 1996.

McCloskey, JC, and Bulechek, GM: Nursing Interventions Classification (NIC), ed 3. Mosby, Philadelphia, 2000.

McLaren, DS: Clinical manifestations of human vitamin and mineral disorders: A resume. In Shils, ME, et al. (eds): Modern Nutrition in Health and Disease ed 9. Lippincott Williams and Wilkins, Philadelphia, 1999.

Meydani, M, and Meisler, JG: A closer look at vitamin E. Postgraduate Medicine 102:199, 1997.

Milea, D, Cassoux, N, and LeHoang, P: Blindness in a strict vegan [letter]. N Engl J Med 342:897, 2000.

Mock, DM: Biotin. In Shils, ME, et al. (eds): Modern Nutrition in Health and Disease ed 9. Lippincott Williams and Wilkins, Philadelphia, 1999.

Mora, JO, Gueri, M, and Mora, OL: Vitamin A deficiency in Latin America and the Caribbean: An overview [Spanish]. Pan American Journal of Public Health 4:178, 1998.

Morse, JW, Morse, SJ, and Patterson, J: Niacin reaction: Common vitamin, uncommon ED diagnosis. Am J Emerg Med 17:320, 1999.

Muhlendahl, KE, and Nawracala, J: Vitamin D intoxication. European Journal of Pediatrics 158:266, 1999.

North American Nursing Diagnosis Association: Nursing Diagnoses: Definitions and Classification 1999–2000, North American Nursing Diagnosis Association, Philadelphia, 1999.

Ohkoshi, N, Ishii, A, and Shoji, S: Wernicke's encephalopathy induced by hyperemesis gravidarum, associated with bilateral caudate lesions on computed tomography and magnetic resonance imaging. Eur Neurol 34:177, 1994.

Olson, RE: Vitamin K. In Shils, ME, et al. (eds): Modern Nutrition in Health and Disease ed 9. Lippincott Williams and Wilkins, Philadelphia, 1999.

Omaye, ST: Safety facets of antioxidant supplements. Top Clin Nutr 14:26, 1998.

Plesofsky-Vig, N: Pantothenic acid. In Shils, ME, et al. (eds): Modern Nutrition in Health and Disease ed 9. Lippincott Williams and Wilkins, Philadelphia, 1999.

Potter, AR: Reducing vitamin A deficiency could save the eyesight and lives of countless children. BMJ 314:317, 1997.

Pugliese, MT, et al.: Nutritional rickets in suburbia. J Am Coll Nutr 17:637, 1998.

Purvin, V: Through a shade darkly. Surv Ophthalmol 43:335, 1999.

Roman, GC: An epidemic in Cuba of optic neuropathy, sensorineural deafness, peripheral sensory neuropathy and dorsolateral myeloneuropathy. J Neurol Sci 127:11, 1994.

Ross, AC: Vitamin A and retinoids. In Shils, ME, et al. (eds): Modern Nutrition in Health and Disease ed 9. Lippincott Williams and Wilkins, Philadelphia, 1999.

Said, HM: Cellular uptake of biotin: Mechanisms and regulation. J Nutr 129(2S Suppl):490S, 1999.

Schoenen, J, Jacquy, J, and Lenaerts, M: Effectiveness of high-dose riboflavin in migraine prophylaxis. Neurology 50:466, 1998.

Schuelke, M, et al.: Treatment of ataxia in isolated vitamin E deficiency caused by alpha-tocopherol transfer protein deficiency. J Pediatr 134:240, 1999.

Shah, M, et al.: Nutritional rickets still afflict children in north Texas. Tex Med 96:64, 2000.

Smith, W, et al.: Dietary antioxidants and age-related maculopathy: the Blue Mountains Eye Study. Ophthalmology 106:761, 1999.

Sommer, A: Vitamin A deficiency and its consequences: A field guide to detection and control ed 3. WHO, Geneva, 1995.

Tanphaichitr, V: Thiamin. In Shils, ME, et al. (eds): Modern Nutrition in Health and Disease ed 9. Lippincott Williams and Wilkins, Philadelphia, 1999.

Thomas, MK, et al.: Hypovitaminosis D in medical patients. N Engl J Med 338:777, 1998.

Traber, MG: Vitamin E. In Shils, ME, et al. (eds): Modern Nutrition in Health and Disease ed 9. Lippincott Williams and Wilkins, Philadelphia, 1999.

Utiger, RD: The need for more vitamin D. N Engl J Med 338:828, 1998.

van der Wielen, RPJ, et al.: Serum vitamin D concentrations among elderly people in Europe. Lancet 346:207, 1995.

Vieth, R: Vitamin D supplementation, 25-hydroxyvitamin D concentrations, and safety. Am J Clin Nutr 69:842, 1999.

Villarroya, F: Differential effects of retinoic acid on white and brown adipose tissues: An unexpected role for vitamin A derivatives on energy balance. Annals of the New York Academy of Sciences 839 (May 15), 1998.

Vitamin E. American Society for Nutritional Sciences. Accessed July 20, 1999 at http://www.nutrition.org/nutinfo/content/vie.shtml

Ward, PE, et al.: Niacin skin flush in schizophrenia: A preliminary report. Schizophrenia Research 29:269, 1998.

Weir, DG, and Scott, JM: Vitamin B12 "Cobalamin." In Shils, ME, et al. (eds): Modern Nutrition in Health and Disease ed 9. Lippincott Williams and Wilkins, Philadelphia, 1999.

Wolf, G: A regulatory pathway of thermogenesis in brown fat through retinoic acid. Nutrition Reviews 53:230, 1995.

Wood, B, and Currie, J: Presentation of acute Wernicke's encephalopathy and treatment with thiamin. Metab Brain Dis 10:57, 1995.

Workshop on Folate, B$_{12}$, and Choline. Nutrition 15:92, 1999.

World Health Organization: Global prevalence of vitamin A deficiency. WHO, Geneva, 1995.

Xiao, G, et al.: Ascorbic acid-dependent activation of the osteocalcin promoter in MC3T3-E1 proosteoblasts: Requirement for collagen matrix synthesis and the presence of an intact OSE2 sequence. Molecular Endocrinology 11:1103, 1997. Accessed August 5, 1999 at http://endo.edoc.com/mend/v11n8/1103-abs.html

Yee, AJ: Effectiveness of high-dose riboflavin in migraine prophylaxis. Neurology 52:431, 1999.

Yusuf, S, et al.: Vitamin E supplementation and cardiovascular events in high-risk patients. JAMA 342:154, 2000.

Zeisel, SH: Choline and phosphatidylcholine. In Shils, ME, et al. (eds): Modern Nutrition in Health and Disease, ed 9. Lippincott Williams and Wilkins, Philadelphia, 1999.

Zempleni, J, and Mock, DM: Bioavailability of biotin given orally to humans in pharmacologic doses. Am J Clin Nutr 69:504, 1999.

CHAPTER 8

Minerals

LEARNING OBJECTIVES

After completing this chapter, the student should be able to:

1. Compare and contrast minerals and vitamins.
2. Describe one or more functions of the main nutritive minerals.
3. List at least two food sources for each mineral and identify any nonfood sources.
4. Identify individuals at increased risk for mineral deficiencies.
5. Devise strategies to increase clients' calcium or iron intakes.

In a broad sense, minerals are obtained from the earth's crust. Through the effects of the weather, rocks that contain minerals are ground into smaller particles, which then become part of the soil. Growing plants absorb the minerals from the soil. Animals eat the plants, and humans eat both the plants and the animals. In this way, minerals become part of the food chain.

Minerals in Human Nutrition

Minerals make vital contributions to the growth and maintenance of health in the body. This chapter discusses the minerals important in human nutrition and the role each plays in the body. It describes some of the general functions of minerals and explains how minerals are classified in nutrition. It discusses the nutritional implications of the seven major and ten trace minerals; a note on the use of supplemental minerals concludes the chapter.

Functions of Minerals

Like vitamins, minerals help to regulate bodily functions without providing energy and are essential to good health. Minerals differ from vitamins in two ways: minerals are inorganic substances, and minerals become part of the structure of the body. Minerals represent 4 percent of total body weight.

Minerals become part of the body's structure and part of the body's enzymes. For instance, calcium and phosphorus combine to give bones and teeth their hardness. Iron becomes attached to the protein globin to form hemoglobin. Iodine becomes part of the thyroid hormones.

Most minerals serve a variety of functions in the body's regulatory and metabolic processes. Sodium is essential for maintaining fluid balance. Sodium, potassium, and calcium have critical functions in nerve and muscle activity. Potassium and phosphorus play significant roles in acid–base balance. A disruption of the body's balance of any one of these minerals, albeit not necessarily caused by diet, can be life-threatening.

Classification of Minerals

In nutrition, two groups of minerals exist: major and trace. Major minerals, also called macrominerals, are present in the body in quantities greater than 5 grams (approximately 1 teaspoonful). The body needs a daily intake of 100 milligrams (approximately 1/50 teaspoonful) or more of each of the major minerals.

Trace minerals, often called microminerals or trace elements, are present in the body in amounts less than 5 grams. Humans need a daily intake of less than 100 milligrams of each of the trace minerals. The term trace does not mean unimportant. Trace minerals make vital and often unique contributions to the body's functioning.

Major Minerals

The seven major minerals include calcium, sodium, and potassium, which are familiar to many people in a dietary context. The other four major minerals are phosphorus, magnesium, sulfur, and chloride.

Calcium

The body of a 150-pound adult contains approximately 3 pounds of calcium. Ninety-nine percent of this amount is in the bones and teeth. The remaining 1 percent of the calcium circulates in the body fluids. Of this 1 percent, one-quarter to one-half is bound to plasma proteins, while the rest travels as free particles that carry an electrical charge (ions). The ionized calcium moves freely from one fluid compartment to another and serves several important functions in the body.

Functions of Calcium

Calcium, with phosphorus, forms the hard substance of bones and teeth. Ample calcium and phosphorus alone will not guarantee strong bones and teeth, however. Vitamin D is necessary for calcium absorption. Exercise, particularly weight-bearing exercise, is also essential for strong bones. Very little calcium is deposited in fully formed teeth. Consequently, if calcium is lost from the teeth, it cannot be replaced. This is the reason dental cavities or caries cannot heal themselves.

Maximum accumulation of calcium in the bones occurs during the pubertal growth spurt, during which time bone mass increases 7 to 8 percent per year. The body's peak bone mass is achieved shortly after adult height is reached. Total body bone mass remains fairly constant through the reproductive years although various sites, such as the skull and the shaft of the femur, continue to add bone throughout life (Weaver and Heaney, 1999), but the balance is upset in the aging adult and with age, total body bone mass decreases. Age-related bone loss is most marked in postmenopausal women but also occurs in men.

Calcium also performs several vital metabolic functions in the nervous, muscular, and cardiovascular systems.

1. Calcium assists in manufacturing **acetylcholine**, a neurotransmitter (a chemical that enhances transmission of nerve impulses).
2. Calcium acts as a catalyst in initiating and controlling muscle contraction and relaxation. At the beginning of a muscle contraction, calcium is released from its storage area inside the muscle cell. At the end of a contraction, the calcium is again gathered into its storage area.
3. Calcium is a catalyst in the clotting process: it aids in the conversion of platelets to thromboplastin and in the conversion of **fibrinogen** to **fibrin**.
4. Calcium controls the passage of substances across cell membranes by affecting membrane permeability.
5. Calcium activates certain enzymes such as **pancreatic lipase** and is necessary for absorption of vitamin B_{12}.

Control Mechanisms for Calcium

Although it may seem to be a permanent substance, bone is 2 to 5 percent living cells that are constantly undergoing change. Bone is the body's bank account or storage area for calcium. As much as 700 milligrams of calcium is moved in and out of the bones each day. The bone calcium pool turns over every 10 to 12 years on average, but this turnover does not occur in the teeth (Weaver and Heaney, 1999). One reason for the changes in bone composition is to maintain the adult serum calcium concentration within the normal limits of 9 to 11 milligrams per 100 milliliters of serum. Another reason for the movement of calcium in and out of the bones is to renew the bone tissue. In this process bone cells called **osteoclasts** produce enzymes to destroy the protein matrix that holds the calcium phosphate in place. Other bone cells, called **osteoblasts** produce new matrix protein, which chemically attracts calcium and other nutrients to rebuild the bone.

Several hormones work together to accomplish these activities. Vitamin D is one of these hormones. Parathyroid hormone and calcitonin are the other two. Vitamin D is actually a hormone because it regulates tissue functions. It increases calcium absorption by the small intestine and increases calcium deposition in the bones and teeth.

Tiny glands behind the thyroid gland in the neck secrete **parathyroid hormone.** When the serum calcium level falls, the parathyroid glands secrete the hormone, which increases the withdrawal of calcium from the bone, thereby raising the serum calcium level. Additionally, parathyroid hormone increases the serum calcium level by stimulating the kidneys to return more calcium to the bloodstream instead of excreting it in the urine.

To balance the action of parathyroid hormone, the thyroid gland secretes another hormone, **calcitonin**, when the serum calcium level is high. It inhibits the release of calcium from bone. Figure 8–1 illustrates the complementary actions of parathyroid hormone and calcitonin.

Other hormones affect the body's use of calcium. One prominent one is estrogen. Its exact mechanism of action in bone metabolism is unknown, but research is continuing in efforts to explain the dramatic loss of bone structure following menopause. Evidence suggests that normal women's bone resorption increases when estradiol levels are low during the menstrual cycle so that fluctuating rates of bone resorption occur from menarche to menopause (Chiu et al., 1999). One mechanism proposed for the action of estrogen on bone metabolism is that estrogen suppresses inflammatory cytokines that promote production of osteoclasts. Thus when estrogen levels fall during menopause, the cytokines are more active permitting greater numbers of osteoclasts to be synthesized (Sunyer et al., 1999).

Dietary Reference Intakes of Calcium

The Adequate Intake (AI) for calcium for adults aged 19 to 50 years is 1000 milligrams. For those older than 50 the amount is 1200 milligrams.

Even with the bones as a reservoir, daily intake of calcium is important. Calcium can be obtained from animal or vegetable sources, but calcium from animal sources is more readily absorbed.

Sources of Calcium

ANIMAL SOURCES Milk and milk products are the best animal sources of calcium, followed by sardines, clams, oysters, and salmon. In milk, calcium is combined with lactose, which increases absorption. Even so, only 28 percent of the available calcium in milk is absorbed. Another advantageous component of milk is the protein the osteoblasts need to rebuild the bone matrix. In sum, milk is such an important source of calcium that it is virtually impossible to obtain adequate calcium without milk or dairy products. Figure 8–2 shows a child drinking milk with a "fast food" meal.

Table 8–1 lists the quantity of foods containing approximately 300 milligrams of calcium, the amount in 1 cup of milk. "Bargain" foods listed that are high in calcium but low in kilocalories include skim milk and plain yogurt. The "most expensive" sources of calcium, considering kilocalories, are hard and soft ice cream and large-curd, creamed cottage cheese. Table 8–1 reveals that not all dairy products are equally beneficial as sources of calcium, but this is not a call to abandon all fat intake. Consuming some fat with calcium increases the absorption of the mineral by slowing peristalsis.

Obtaining calcium from supplements is less desirable than obtaining it from foods. Milk products supply other nutrients, such as vitamin D and lactose, which assist in calcium absorption. Milk is also a major source of

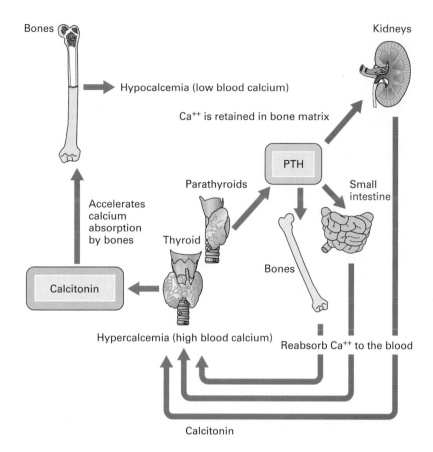

Figure 8–1:
Parathyroid hormone raises serum calcium levels when they are too low. Calcitonin from the thyroid gland lowers serum calcium levels when they are too high. (Reprinted from Thomas, 1997, page 286, with permission.)

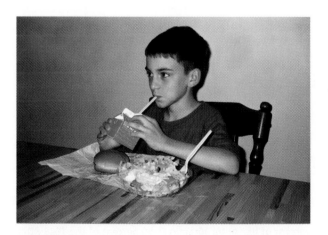

Figure 8–2:
This child has a balanced meal from a fast food restaurant: a small hamburger, a salad, and milk. Growing bones and teeth need calcium from milk products.

riboflavin and protein. Figure 8–3 shows the percentages of the AIs or RDAs for vitamins A and D, protein, thiamin, and riboflavin an adult woman could obtain from 3 cups of skim milk. Clinical Application 8–1 describes some of the contaminants in "natural" calcium supplements.

PLANT SOURCES Good plant sources of calcium include rhubarb, spinach, greens (turnip, beet), broccoli, kale, tofu, and legumes. In all cases vegetables yield more calcium when cooked. Some experts question how much the body is actually able to absorb owing to multiple interfering factors.

Another good plant source is calcium-fortified orange juice. An unusual source of calcium for Navajo Americans is the ash derived from the branches and needles of the juniper tree. The ash is used to flavor various foods, such as cornmeal mush and pancakes and Navajo tea. One teaspoon of the ash supplies roughly the calcium in one glass of milk (Christensen, et al., 1998). This is an example of the contribution of traditional food selection and processing to health.

Absorption and Excretion

In general, the percentage of available calcium absorbed from vegetables is considerably less than that absorbed from milk. For example,

TABLE 8–1 Quantities of Food Containing Approximately 300 Milligrams of Calcium, Equal to One Cup of Milk, in Order of Energy Content

Food	Amount	Kilocalories
Skim milk	1.0 cup	86
Grated Parmesan cheese	4.3 tbsp	99
Plain low-fat yogurt	0.7 cup	101
Swiss cheese	1.1 oz	118
2 percent milk	1.0 cup	121
Whole milk	1.0 cup	150
Cheddar cheese	1.5 oz	171
Processed American cheese	1.7 oz	180
Low-fat yogurt with fruit	0.9 cup	199
Blue cheese	2.0 oz	200
Vanilla milkshake	0.9 cup	273
2 percent low-fat cottage cheese	2.0 cups	410
Hard ice cream, vanilla	1.7 cups	459
Soft ice cream	1.3 cups	479
Cottage cheese, creamed, large curd	2.25 cups	529
Sherbet	2.9 cups	786

only 5 percent of the total calcium found in spinach is absorbed. Several factors can interfere with the absorption and retention of calcium: oxalates, phytic acid, and excessive intakes of protein or dietary fiber (see Table 8–2).

Some vegetables contain salts of oxalic acid called oxalates. **Oxalates** bind with the calcium present in the vegetable to produce calcium oxalate, an insoluble form of calcium that is excreted in the feces. The calcium content not bound to oxalates is available for absorption, however, and oxalates do not interfere with the absorption of calcium from other foods. Chard, spinach, beet leaves, rhubarb, cranberries, and gooseberries all contain oxalic acid. Unusually high intake of these foods may cause oxalic acid poisoning (see Clinical Application 8–2).

Cereals contain a substance that forms an insoluble complex with calcium. This interfering substance is **phytic acid**, the storage form of phosphorus in seeds. Foods with heavy concentrations of phytate, such as wheat bran cereal and dried beans, reduce calcium absorption significantly. For other plants rich in calcium such as broccoli and cabbage, the

TABLE 8–2 Factors Affecting Calcium Absorption and Excretion

Increase Absorption	Decrease Absorption	Increase Excretion
Acidity	Alkalinity	Excessive animal protein
Estrogen	Insoluble dietary fiber	Excessive sodium
Lactose or sucrose	Oxalic acid	Caffeine
Protein	Phytic acid	
Vitamin D	Vitamin D deficiency	

CLINICAL APPLICATION 8–1

Contents of Natural Calcium Supplements

Shells, bones and dolomite are natural sources of calcium that are used as dietary supplements. Much of the calcium found in shells and bones is in the form of calcium phosphate, one of the most difficult calcium compounds to absorb. In addition, shells and bones often contain excessive amounts of mercury and lead (Ross, Szabow, and Tebbett, 2000; Scelfo and Flegal, 2000).

Dolomite is a limestone that is rich in both calcium and magnesium. It also may contain lead, mercury, arsenic and aluminum. Because of the possibility of contamination, it is best to obtain calcium from food sources whenever possible. When this is not possible, pharmaceutical products are preferable to natural supplements.

calcium is as easily absorbed as that in milk. The difficulty becomes the volume necessary to absorb the quantity of calcium in a glass of milk: 2.3 servings of cabbage or 4.5 servings of broccoli (Weaver and Heaney, 1999).

The overall effect of oxalic and phytic acids on calcium availability in most diets usually is not significant. People who avoid dairy products, however, may need careful attention to meal planning. Ovovegetarian and vegan clients should be instructed to seek calcium fortified products, such as orange juice and calcium-set tofu, to bolster their intake of the mineral.

Adequate protein intake facilitates calcium absorption, but excessive intake of protein increases urinary loss of calcium. Eating 100 grams or more of protein a day, not unusual for many Americans, increases urinary excretion of calcium. Over a wide range of protein intake, for each additional gram of dietary protein consumed, one additional milligram of calcium was shown to be spilled in the urine (Krall and Dawson-Hughes, 1999a). When protein is accompanied by a high phosphorus intake, the calcium loss is lessened considerably. Fortunately, in the American diet, foods high in protein usually are high in phosphorus as well.

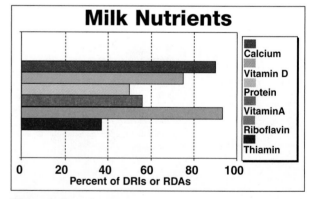

Figure 8–3:
Milk supplies many nutrients in addition to calcium. Three cups of skim milk provide a woman between 25 and 50 years of age with 90 percent of her AI for calcium, 75 percent of her AI for Vitamin D, 50 percent of the 1989 RDA for protein, 56 percent of the 1989 RDA for Vitamin A, 93 percent of her 1998 RDA for riboflavin and 37 percent of her 1998 RDA for thiamin. The kilocaloric cost for all these nutrients is a miniscule 258 kilocalories.

CLINICAL APPLICATION 8–2

Oxalic Acid Poisoning

It is possible to be poisoned by ingesting too much of one or more foods that contain oxalic acid. Cranberries, gooseberries, chard, spinach, beet leaves, and rhubarb are high in oxalic acid. For example, one normal serving of rhubarb contains one-fifth the toxic dose. Rhubarb leaves contain three or four times as much as the stalks. Ingesting a fairly small amount of leaf then, can poison a child.

One way to minimize the chance of oxalic acid poisoning is to consume foods that contain calcium with foods high in oxalic acid. The calcium combines with the oxalate, which then passes through the intestine harmlessly. Calcium absorption will be decreased, however.

Calcium absorption is hindered by excessive intake of insoluble dietary fiber. It passes through the alimentary canal undigested. Any calcium that binds with dietary fiber is also excreted.

Two substances interfering with calcium retention in the body are sodium and caffeine. For every 500 milligram increase in sodium intake, an additional 10 milligrams of calcium is spilled in the urine (Krall and Dawson-Hughes, 1999a). A direct effect of high sodium intake on bone loss at the hip has been demonstrated (Lau and Woo, 1998). Caffeine is thought to reduce reabsorption of calcium by the kidney, thus increasing urinary losses. The caffeine equal to 2 to 3 cups of coffee accelerated bone loss from the spine and total body in postmenopausal women who consumed less than 744 milligrams of calcium per day. It is uncertain if the effect was due to lessened absorption of calcium or to replacement of milk in the diet with caffeinated beverages (Weaver and Heaney, 1999). Regardless, it seems clear that if a person's calcium intake is low or marginal, drinking many caffeinated beverages could make a difference in bone health.

Gastric acidity increases the solubility of calcium salts. Calcium supplements taken with a meal are better absorbed than when taken without food, possibly due to delayed emptying time of the stomach (Weaver and Heaney, 1999).

Calcium Deficiencies

Calcium deficiency in children can contribute to poor bone and tooth development. Rickets is more directly related to vitamin D deficiency than calcium deficiency except in premature infants, whose skeletons still need much added mineral. Two other conditions related to calcium balance are osteoporosis and tetany.

OSTEOPOROSIS According to the World Health Organization, **osteopenia** is bone mineral density 1 to 2.5 standard deviations below the mean of healthy young adults, whereas **osteoporosis** is bone mineral density more than 2.5 standard deviations below the mean (Greenspan, 1999). Osteoporosis permits fractures to occur following minimal trauma. Bones commonly affected are the hip, wrist, and vertebrae.

Osteoporosis is most common in postmenopausal, fair-complected white women. A woman loses 2 to 5 percent of bone tissue per year immediately before and for about 8 years after menopause. The most rapid loss of bone occurs in the first five years after menopause. Men and black women lose bone mass also, but because their skeletons

are generally heavier, they are at lower risk of osteoporosis. Blacks have higher bone mineral density than whites and Asians, a difference that is noted beginning in early childhood (Krall and Dawson-Hughes, 1999a). Figure 8–4 shows an X-ray of a normal bone and one of an osteoporotic bone.

The exact cause of osteoporosis is unknown. It is presumed to have many causes, but it is more closely associated with a deficiency of calcium than with a deficiency of vitamin D. Furthermore, population studies have not demonstrated a relationship between calcium intake and osteoporosis in all countries. Researchers are investigating genetic variations in vitamin D receptors that might help to explain population differences in bone density and rates of bone loss (Krall et al., 1995). Clinical Application 8–3 discusses some of the research on osteoporosis.

Treatments may be tailored to the individual client's situation. In cases marked by high bone turnover (increased osteoclastic resorption), hormone replacement therapy, calcitonin, or bisphosphonates (to suppress osteoclast formation or activity) may be helpful. In cases with low bone turnover (decreased osteoblastic activity), fluoride or parathyroid hormone may be prescribed (Lane, 1997).

TETANY Despite the hormonal control of serum calcium and the large reservoir in the bones, serum calcium sometimes falls below normal. An actual lack of calcium or a lack of ionized calcium may cause tetany. A serum calcium level that is too low is called **hypocalcemia**. If the signs and symptoms described below appear, the condition is called **tetany**. Causes include parathyroid deficiency, vitamin D deficiency, and alkalosis.

Parathyroid deficiency has been caused by accidental removal of the parathyroid glands during thyroidectomy but more often is caused by

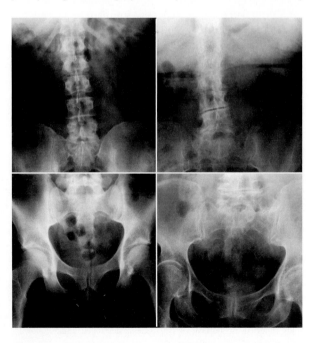

Figure 8–4:
X-rays of a normal bone on the left with an osteoporotic bone on the right. (Courtesy of Dr. Russell Tobe.)

CLINICAL APPLICATION 8–3

RESEARCH ON OSTEOPOROSIS

More than 25 million people in the United States have osteoporosis, the major factor in fractures in the elderly. Annually in the United States, osteoporotic fractures occur at the hip (250,000), at the spine (500,000), or at the forearm (250,000) totaling approximately $14 billion in direct costs (Greenspan, 1999).

Two major factors in the development of osteoporosis are the bone mass developed from birth to age 30 and rate of loss of bone mass in later life. Contributing to both of these factors are genetics, estrogen levels, calcium intake, vitamin D supply, and exercise. Researchers have investigated all of these topics.

Bone Mass Development. Children given calcium supplements increased their bone mass faster than their identical twins (Johnston et al., 1992). The effect was lost when supplementation stopped, however. Recollection of milk consumption before age 25 was a significant independent predictor of bone mineral density (Murphy et al., 1994).

Rate of Bone Loss. The rate of bone loss in women is greatest in the five years immediately after menopause. Until 30 to 40 percent of bone mass is lost, it is not detectable on x-ray, but **dual-energy x-ray absorptiometry (DEXA)** permits earlier diagnosis.

In a study of female twins, the one who smoked more had less bone mass than the one who smoked less. Women who smoke one pack of cigarettes daily through adulthood will reach menopause with an average deficit of 5 to 10 percent in bone density, sufficient to increase the risk of fracture (Hopper and Seeman, 1994). In a three-year study of elderly men and women, smoking accelerated bone loss from the femoral neck and total body, possibly related to less efficient calcium absorption (Krall and Dawson-Hughes, 1999b).

Alcohol also contributes to bone loss because it is toxic to osteoblasts and suppresses bone formation. Higher alcohol intake was significantly related to osteoporosis (Blaauw et al., 1994).

Hormone Therapy. Healthy white women, 3 to 6 years post menopause, who received estrogen and progesterone with calcium and vitamin D lost less bone mineral than women who received only calcium and vitamin D. The latter group lost less than the placebo group receiving just vitamin D (Aloia et al., 1994).

Calcium Intake. Four years of calcium supplementation of post menopausal women, with an average age of 58 years, reduced the rate of loss of bone mineral density and the number of fractures compared to a control group (Reid et al., 1995). Clients diagnosed with osteoporosis

who were given cyclical slow-release fluoride and calcium for four years suffered significantly fewer new vertebral fractures than the control group receiving just calcium (Pak et al., 1995).

Vitamin D Supply. Individuals with an intake less than 2.5 micrograms in Norway had a significant increase in the risk of hip fracture (Meyer et al., 1995). In a study in the Netherlands, compared to age-matched healthy people, hip fracture patients had lower serum vitamin D concentrations mainly due to low exposure to sunshine (Lips et al., 1987). Healthy postmenopausal women supplemented to 20 micrograms of vitamin D showed less bone loss from the femoral neck than women supplemented to 5 micrograms. All the women received equal amounts of calcium (Dawson-Hughes et al., 1995).

Both Calcium and Vitamin D. Postmenopausal women supplemented with 10 micrograms of vitamin D and calcium showed a modest increase in spinal bone mineral density compared to women receiving only equal amounts of calcium (Dawson-Hughes et al., 1991). Healthy ambulatory women, with an average age of 84 years, who received vitamin D and calcium supplements suffered 43 percent fewer hip fractures than women receiving placebo (Chapuy et al., 1992). Men and women 65 years of age or older showed moderately reduced bone loss in the femoral neck, spine, and total body when given calcium and vitamin D supplements for three years. The supplemented group also suffered fewer nonvertebral fractures than the placebo group (Dawson-Hughes et al., 1997).

Exercise. Weight-bearing exercise stimulates osteoblastic activity. Loss of bone mass in immobile patients is well known. Postmenopausal women in a 1-year walking program maintained spinal bone mineral density, whereas the control group did not (Nelson et al., 1991). Women coached in two 45-minute high-intensity strength training sessions per week for 1 year showed some improvement in bone density, muscle mass and strength, and balance compared to control group (Nelson et al., 1994). Increased muscle mass, strength, and balance lessen the risk of falling, bone density aside.

Recommendations. Because osteoporosis develops in response to multiple factors, including a genetic component, no "one size fits all" plan to stave off the disease is advocated. Lifetime adequate intakes of calcium and vitamin D, along with sufficient exercise, will increase bone mass. If calcium supplementation is chosen, the bioavailability of various products should be considered. Estrogen supplementation at menopause is appropriate for some women. A total program should be discussed with the physician.

edema following thyroid surgery or by disease of the gland. One recent study reported 4.6 percent of 109 patients developed tetany following subtotal thyroidectomy, all on the first postoperative day (Yamashita et al., 1999). Tetany related to vitamin D deficiency can result from inadequate sunlight, malnutrition, or impaired kidney function.

In **alkalosis**, because of the excessive alkalinity of body fluids, a greater number of calcium ions are bound to serum proteins, effectively inactivating the calcium. Therefore, nerve and muscle function is impaired. Alkalosis may be caused by the loss of acid (due to vomiting or gastric suction) or by the ingestion of alkalis (for example, sodium bicar-

Phosphorus Intake and Calcium Balance

In the past, the ratio of calcium to phosphorus was considered to be crucial to proper calcium balance. Now authorities believe that the calcium-to-phosphorus ratio is less important that the adequacy of calcium intake. Results of research indicate that a high phosphorous intake has little or no effect on calcium balance in humans; intake of 2 g of phosphorus (two and one-half times the RDA) per day did not affect calcium balance in adult men regardless of calcium intake (National Research Council 1989).

bonate). Alkalosis can even be caused by breathing too rapidly, either in response to fear or through mechanical ventilation. The result is excessive loss of carbon dioxide. In the blood, carbon dioxide is transported as carbonic acid. Thus, when too much carbon dioxide is exhaled, the alkalinity of the blood increases and produces tetany.

Early symptoms of tetany are nervousness, irritability, numbness, and tingling of the extremities and around the mouth, and muscle cramps. Diagnostic signs are Trousseau's sign and Chvostek's sign. In **Trousseau's sign**, inflation of the blood pressure cuff above systolic pressure for 3 minutes causes ischemia of the peripheral nerves, increasing their excitability. What the examiner sees is muscle spasms of the forearm and hand. In **Chvostek's sign**, a tap over the facial nerve in front of the ear causes a twitch of the facial muscles on that side. Figure 8–5 depicts these diagnostic signs.

Because of the many functions of calcium, tetany is a medical emergency. Untreated, it can progress to respiratory paralysis, seizures or coma, heart dilatation, and blood clotting problems.

Calcium Toxicity

A serum calcium level that is too high, above 11 milligrams per 100 milliliters of serum in adults, is called **hypercalcemia**. It can be caused by **hyperparathyroidism** and other diseases, by vitamin D poisoning, by

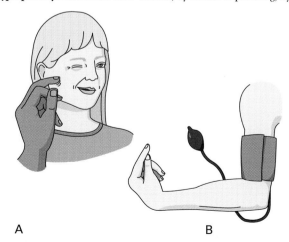

A **B**

Figure 8–5:
Indications of hypocalcemia: (a) a positive Chvostek's sign and (b) positive Trousseau's sign

antacids, but almost never by ingestion of foods. Idiopathic hypercalcemia associated with vitamin D toxicity is seen most frequently in infants. Kidney stones are not usually caused by dietary calcium but by malfunctioning kidneys that permit too much calcium to be spilled into the urine (Weaver and Heaney, 1999).

In a series of 100 clients with hypercalcemia, the most common causes were malignancy and hyperparathyroidism. The third most common cause was milk-alkali syndrome, including three people who underwent surgery for parathyroid disease before the diagnosis was established (Beall and Scofield, 1995).

Milk-alkali syndrome, a condition caused by ingestion of excessive absorbable alkali and milk, is characterized by high blood calcium and a more alkaline urine that predisposes to the formation of calcium deposits in the kidney. It was associated with the milk and cream and antacid treatment of peptic ulcers that was common years ago. Recent cases, in which some clients required hemodialysis for renal failure, resulted from self-prescribed calcium carbonate tablets (Abreo et al., 1993; Beall and Scofield, 1995). Individuals reported taking 2 to 18 grams daily, usually for indigestion. (Package instructions caution not to take more than 8 grams per day and not to use that dose for more than 2 weeks without consulting a physician.) Some concern is raised about the use of calcium carbonate to prevent osteoporosis. These cases emphasize the importance of a careful dietary and medication history and of client teaching regarding over-the-counter as well as prescription medications.

Phosphorus

Phosphorus occurs in bones and teeth as calcium phosphate. The body of a 154-pound man contains about 700 grams of phosphorus, 80 percent in bone and 9 percent in skeletal muscle (Knochel, 1999). Phosphorus is closely associated with calcium both in foods and in interrelated metabolic functions in the body. See Clinical Application 8–4 for information on phosphorus intake and calcium balance.

Phosphorus is a component of DNA and RNA. The storage forms of energy **adenosine diphosphate (ADP) and adenosine triphosphate (ATP)** contain phosphorus. Phosphorus is an essential mineral in **phospholipids**, which are structural components of cells. Phospholipids contain glycerol, fatty acids, and phosphorus. Lecithin, a part of cell membranes, and myelin, the insulating covering of many nerves are phospholipids. Phosphorus is contained in almost all enzymes, and phosphorus compounds are used as a buffer system to maintain the pH of the blood between 7.35 and 7.45.

Control Mechanism for Phosphorus

A higher proportion of phosphorus is absorbed from the diet than calcium. Seventy percent of dietary phosphorus is absorbed, and the remaining 30 percent is excreted in the feces. Absorption occurs in the jejunum, the middle portion of the small intestine. The same factors that affect calcium absorption are at work for phosphorus.

Low levels of serum phosphorus stimulate the kidney to produce more active vitamin D. The vitamin D then increases the absorption of phosphorus from the intestinal tract. Excess phosphorus is excreted by the kidney in response to parathyroid hormone.

Dietary Reference Intakes and Sources of Phosphorus

The 1998 RDAs for phosphorus are 700 milligrams for men and women aged 19 and older. Phosphorus, essential in plant and animal cells, is widespread in foods. Animal protein is the best source of phosphorus, especially lean meat. Good plant sources include nuts and legumes.

Deficiency of Phosphorus

Phosphorus deficiency is unlikely to be a function of diet. Certain diseases or medications, however, produce **hypophosphatemia**. A condition called **refeeding syndrome**, related to imbalances in phosphorus, occurs when wasted or starved clients are given nutrients in excess of what their bodies can handle (Chapter 24). In addition, hypophosphatemia has occurred in persons who ingested a diet low in phosphorus while also taking a phosphate-binding drug, such as the antacid, aluminum hydroxide. In the client with alcoholism, the clinical picture of severe hypophosphatemia could be mistaken for delirium tremens because the client may suffer from hallucinations (Knochel, 1999).

Hyperparathyroidism is a disease that causes excess excretion of phosphorus. In this disease, parathyroid hormone causes withdrawal of calcium from the bones. Since the two are combined in the bones, phosphorus is lost along with calcium. Chronic kidney disease often produces the same result.

Phosphorus Toxicity

Hyperphosphatemia caused by dietary overload is unusual. Cases have occurred in infants given only cow's milk, which has twice the phosphorus content of human milk and infant formula during the first few weeks of life. The cow's milk diet, too much for an infant's immature kidneys, overtaxes the infant's ability to maintain homeostasis. Other cases of hyperphosphatemia have occurred following excessive or chronic administration of sodium phosphates used as a saline laxative or as an enema. Clients with conditions that would increase the permeability of the intestine are at special risk when using these ordinarily harmless products.

Sodium

The adult body contains about 90 grams of sodium, approximately 3 ounces. Two-thirds of the sodium in the body is in the blood and other extracellular fluids. The other one-third is in the bones.

Sodium, which has a major role in maintaining fluid balance in the body, is also necessary for the transmission of electrochemical impulses along nerve and muscle membranes and is a component of two phosphate buffers.

The intestine readily absorbs sodium. Only about 5 percent of dietary sodium travels within the intestine to remain in the feces. To maintain a normal level of sodium in the blood, the kidney either reabsorbs sodium and returns it to the bloodstream or allows it to be spilled in the urine. A hormone from the adrenal cortex, **aldosterone**, stimulates the kidney to return sodium to the bloodstream.

Recommended Intake and Sources of Sodium

The average American intake is 4 to 6 grams of sodium per day. The maximum daily intake recommended is 2400 milligrams (National Research Council, 1989). A safe minimum intake for infants and young children is considered to be 23 milligrams per kilogram of body weight. For adults, a safe minimum is 500 milligrams per day. Pregnancy and lactation needs are estimated to be 69 milligrams and 139 milligrams, respectively, over the adult minimum (Subcommittee on the 10th Edition of the RDAs, 1989).

Table salt, the major dietary source of sodium, is 40 percent sodium and 60 percent chloride. One teaspoonful (5 grams) of salt contains about 2 grams of sodium, nearly the maximum recommended daily intake. Many foods, such as milk, milk products, and several vegetables, are naturally high in sodium. Most of the sodium we consume is from the salt or sodium-containing additives in processed foods, although salt is not so necessary to maintaining year-round food stocks as it was years ago when, for instance, meat was salted to preserve it. Table 8–3 compares the sodium content of relatively unprocessed foods with processed versions.

Deficiency of Sodium

Deficiency of sodium is associated primarily with increased sodium loss. Conditions such as diarrhea, vomiting, heavy sweating, or kidney disease may cause low serum sodium. The technical name for low serum sodium, less than 135 milliequivalents per liter in adults, is **hyponatremia**. A serum sodium that is low, not because of an absolute lack of sodium, but because of an excess of water is called **dilutional hyponatremia**. One condition producing this effect, the syndrome of inappropriate secretion of antidiuretic hormone (SIADH), is discussed in Chapter 9.

Sodium Toxicity

The reported 4 to 6 grams of sodium in the average American diet is probably an underestimate. Frequently such surveys do not account for all sources of sodium. Healthy people excrete excess sodium without immediate adverse effects. Because of the previously discussed loss of calcium with high sodium intake, long-range adverse effects may accrue for individuals at risk for osteoporosis. For people with hypertension, heart disease, or kidney disease, the control of sodium balance becomes an important issue. An excess of sodium in the blood, greater than 145 milliequivalents per liter in adults, is called **hypernatremia**.

TABLE 8–3 Comparison of Sodium Content in Fresh and Processed Foods

Fresh Food	Sodium (mg)	Processed Food	Sodium (mg)
Natural Swiss cheese, 1 oz.	74	Pasteurized, processed Swiss cheese, 1 oz.	388
Lean roast pork, 3 oz.	65	Lean ham, 3 oz.	930
Whole raw carrot, 1	25	Canned carrots, 1/2 cup	176
Tomato juice, canned without salt, 1 cup	24	Tomato juice, canned with salt, 1 cup	881

Potassium

The adult body contains about 270 grams of potassium, approximately 9 ounces. Ninety-eight percent of this potassium is inside the cells, where it helps to control fluid balance.

In addition to fluid balance, potassium is essential for the conduction of nerve impulses and the contraction of muscles, including one vital muscle, the heart. Potassium helps to maintain acid–base balance and is required for the conversion of glucose to glycogen.

The kidney responds to systemic alkalosis by excreting potassium to conserve hydrogen. Retaining the hydrogen will make the blood more acidic and help to correct the alkalosis. Conversely, in acidosis, the body responds by excreting hydrogen and retaining potassium.

Estimated Minimum Intake of Potassium

There are no RDAs established for potassium. The estimated minimum amount for healthy adults is 2000 milligrams per day. The average American diet contains 2000 to 4000 milligrams of potassium.

Sources of Potassium

Potassium is present in all plant and animal cells. Only fats, oils, and white sugar have negligible amounts of potassium. One cup of cooked, dry lima beans contains 1163 milligrams. Foods that supply almost half the minimum amount include 1 cup of winter squash, 1 cup of cooked pinto beans, or 1 baked potato with skin. Fruits are good sources of potassium. Over 500 milligrams are contained in 1 cup of sliced banana, 1/3 cup of dried apricots or peaches, 1/3 cantaloupe, or 3/4 cup of prune juice.

Deficiency of Potassium

A potassium deficiency is related to diet only in cases of severe protein calorie malnutrition. **Hypokalemia**, a serum potassium less than 3.5 **milliequivalents** per liter, can be fatal if prolonged or severe. Hypokalemia may be caused by diarrhea, vomiting, laxative abuse, alkalosis, and protein–calorie malnutrition. Deficiency symptoms include fatigue, muscle weakness, irregular heart rhythm, nausea, vomiting, and decreased reflexes.

Potassium Toxicity

A potassium level greater than 5.0 milliequivalents per liter is **hyperkalemia**. The normal kidney excretes potassium effectively so that excessive dietary intake rarely causes hyperkalemia. Intravenous intake is a different matter, so that a client's urine output should be verified before administering an infusion containing potassium. Serum levels of 10 to 12 milliequivalents per liter usually produce cardiac arrest (Brensilver and Goldberger, 1996).

Potassium toxicity is most often the result of diabetic acidosis, kidney failure, adrenal insufficiency, or severe dehydration. Hyperkalemia may also be caused by excessive destruction of cells in burns, crushing injuries, or severe infections. Vague muscle weakness usually appears first, followed by flaccid paralysis beginning in the legs and moving up the body. The heart's rhythm is affected, and characteristic changes appear on the electrocardiogram. The muscles supplied by the cranial nerves are usually spared. The client remains alert and apprehensive (Brensilver and Goldberger, 1996).

Magnesium

The body contains about 1 ounce of magnesium, about 53 percent of which is combined with calcium and phosphorus in the bones and 27 percent is located in muscle tissue (Shils, 1999). The rest is found in other tissues and body fluids.

Magnesium is involved in more than 300 essential metabolic reactions (Shils, 1999). Magnesium is necessary for the transmission of nerve impulses and the relaxation of skeletal muscles after contraction. It activates enzymes for the metabolism of carbohydrates, fats, and proteins, including protein synthesis. Magnesium activates the enzymes that add the third phosphate group to ADP to form ATP. It also aids in the release of energy from muscle glycogen. As a cofactor in calcium utilization, magnesium not only aids bone formation but also helps to hold calcium in tooth enamel, thus preventing tooth decay.

Magnesium competes with calcium for absorption in the upper small intestine but evidence suggests magnesium is also absorbed in the large intestine (Shils, 1999). As magnesium intake increases, the percentage absorbed decreases. The kidney selectively excretes excess magnesium.

Dietary Reference Intakes and Sources of Magnesium

The 1998 RDAs for magnesium are 400 to 420 milligrams for adult males and 310 to 320 milligrams for adult females. Focusing on magnesium status by assessing dietary intake may mislead the healthcare provider. Questions have been raised about the accuracy of the tables of food composition in relation to magnesium. The data are inadequate or missing for some foods (Shils, 1999).

Magnesium is widely distributed in foods, especially plant foods, because it is part of the chlorophyll molecule. Green vegetables are good sources of magnesium. One cup of cooked spinach contains 150 milligrams; other good sources are seeds, legumes, shrimp, and some bran cereals.

Interfering Factors and Deficiency of Magnesium

High intakes of some nutrients may interfere with the absorption of magnesium. Phosphorus, calcium, fat, and protein are four such nutrients.

Inadequate diets do not generally cause magnesium deficiency. Deficiency may accompany protein–calorie malnutrition, but it is usually the result of increased magnesium excretion or decreased magnesium absorption. Excessive excretion of magnesium can result from major surgery, vomiting, diarrhea, or diuretic therapy. Magnesium absorption is decreased in malabsorption syndromes and chronic alcoholism.

Magnesium deficiency may exacerbate the increased neuroirritability in cases of acute alcohol withdrawal. The association of magnesium with the nervous system is also being studied in regard to migraine headaches. Half of the clients suffering from migraine headaches have shown low levels of ionized magnesium and obtained relief from magnesium infusions. Other trials of oral supplements showed decreased frequency of migraine headaches (Mauskop and Altura, 1998).

Magnesium deficiency is a common occurrence, especially in older people on poor diets, clients with chronic alcoholicism, and those who use diuretics (Santinelli et al., 1999). In one study, 20 percent of the clients admitted to a medical intensive care unit had a deficiency of magnesium (Reinhart and Desbiens, 1985). Insufficient magnesium impairs central nervous system activity and increases muscular excitability. Because magnesium metabolism is intricately linked to calcium metabolism, magnesium-deficient clients display the signs of tetany. Other signs include disorientation, convulsions, and psychosis. Relief of signs and symptoms may take 60 to 80 hours after treatment begins (Brensilver and Goldberger, 1996).

Magnesium Toxicity

Ordinarily, magnesium levels do not build up in the blood except as a result of kidney disease. A person with magnesium toxicity has the following signs: lethargy, sedation, hypotension, slow pulse, and depressed respirations. Respiratory or cardiac arrest may ensue. Because of magnesium's close link to calcium, the effects of magnesium toxicity can be blocked by administering calcium.

Sulfur

Sulfur is a component of the cytoplasm of every cell. It is especially notable in hair, skin, and nails, where the **disulfide linkages** help to hold the amino acids in their distinct shapes. Sulfur is a component of thiamin, biotin, insulin, and heparin. A protective function of sulfur is that of combining with toxins to neutralize them.

Important sources of sulfur are cheese, eggs, poultry, and fish. Cases of deficiency of sulfur are unknown. Only people with a severe protein deficiency lack this mineral.

Chloride

Whenever an industrial accident involving chlorine occurs, such as the derailment of a chlorine tanker car, the surrounding area is quickly evacuated because of the chemical's toxic effects. A harmless form of chlorine, chloride, far from being poisonous, is a required nutrient. The body contains about 90 grams of chloride. Chloride is found in hydrochloric acid in the stomach and in fluid outside of the cells. Chloride is involved in the maintenance of normal fluid balance and proper acid–base balance. The estimated minimum recommended intake for chloride ranges from 180 to 300 milligrams for infants and is 750 milligrams for adults. Table salt, which is 60 percent chloride, contains about 3 grams of chloride per teaspoon (5 grams).

Loss of gastrointestinal fluids through severe vomiting, nasogastric suctioning, or diarrhea is a common cause of chloride deficiency. Chloride deficiency occurred in infants because chloride was omitted from the formula they received. Long-term sequelae in some of these children included cognitive impairments, visual-motor difficulties, and attention deficit disorder (Kaleita, Kinsbourne, and Menkes, 1991).

See Table 8–4 for a summary of the major minerals.

Trace Minerals

Trace minerals are present in the body in amounts less than 5 grams and have a recommended intake of less than 100 milligrams per day. Many trace minerals occur in such small amounts that they are difficult to measure and analyze; thus their physiological functions and possible roles in nutrition are not completely understood. For example, lead, gold, and mercury are found in body tissue but only, as far

as is known, as the result of environmental contamination; see Clinical Application 8–5.

Eight trace minerals have probable, but as yet not clearly delineated, functions in human nutrition. This group includes aluminum, arsenic, boron, cadmium, nickel, tin, silicon, and vanadium. Arsenic is a notorious poison often employed in detective stories. Cadmium is one of the most dangerous occupational and environmental poisons, but a high calcium intake is protective against toxicity (Brzoska and Moniuszko-Jakoniuk, 1998).

Aluminum is a toxic metal frequently found in the environment. Concern has been raised about aluminum toxicity through ingestion in pharmaceuticals, food, and water, through injections of contaminated intravenous or total parenteral nutrition solutions or kidney dialysis solutions, and through inhalation in the workplace (Greger and Sutherland, 1997). Boron has been related to bone, mineral, and lipid metabolism, energy utilization, and immune function (Penland, 1998). It has been researched as a supplement to enhance athletic performance but further investigation is recommended (Naghii, 1999). Vanadium has been found to have insulin-mimetic effects and is the subject of ongoing research (Verma, Cam, and McNeill, 1998).

Ten trace minerals have well known bodily functions and nine have been assigned RDAs, Adequate Intakes (AI), or Estimated Safe and Adequate Daily Dietary Intakes (ESADDIs). Four of them are commonly recognized for their relationship with health: iron, iodine, fluoride, and zinc. The other six are selenium, chromium, copper, manganese, cobalt, and molybdenum. These ten minerals are discussed individually in the sections below, starting with iron.

Iron

For a nutrient with functions as vital as those of iron, the amount in the male body is very slight—about 3.8 grams, approximately the weight of a penny. Women's bodies average 2.3 grams. The body conserves its supply of iron by recycling the mineral released from the catabolism of worn-out red blood cells. In adult men, about 95 percent of the iron needed for RBC production comes from this source and only 5 percent from the diet. Infants who are rapidly growing, however, derive 70 percent of their need from recycled iron and 30 percent from the diet (Centers for Disease Control, 1998b).

Functions of Iron

Iron is essential to hemoglobin formation. **Hemoglobin**, the oxygen-carrying component of the red blood cell, is composed of heme, the non-protein portion that contains iron, and globin, a simple protein. Iron is also a component of **myoglobin**, a protein located in muscle tissue. Myoglobin stores oxygen within the muscle cells. When the body needs an immediate supply of oxygen, as during strenuous exercise, myoglobin releases its stored oxygen. Iron is also present in enzymes that permit the oxidation of glucose to produce energy.

Because the brain has the highest metabolic rate of any organ, it requires high levels of iron and oxygen. Iron is required for the synthesis of myelin and of the neurotransmitters serotonin and dopamine. Areas of the brain related to movement contain relatively high amounts of iron. The

TABLE 8–4 Major Minerals

Mineral	Adult RDA and Food Portion Containing RDA	Functions	Signs and Symptoms of Deficiency	Signs and Symptoms of Excess	Best Sources
Calcium	1000-1200 3.3–4 cups milk	Structure of bones and teeth Nerve conduction Muscle contraction Blood clotting	Tetany Osteoporosis Rickets	Renal calculi Calcification of soft tissue	Milk Sardines, oysters, clams, salmon
Phosphorus	700 mg 2.2 cups chili with beans	Structure of bones and teeth Component of DNA and RNA Component of ADP and ATP Component of phospholipids (i.e., myelin) Buffer	Increased calcium excretion Bone loss Muscle weakness	Tetany Convulsions Renal insufficiency	Lean meat Milk
Sodium	None*	Fluid balance Transmission of electrochemical impulses along nerve and muscle membranes	Hyponatremia	Hypernatremia	Table salt Processed foods Milk and milk products
Potassium	None*	Conduction of nerve impulses Muscle contraction	Hypokalemia (not usually dietary)	Hyperkalemia (not usually dietary)	Cooked dry lima beans Pinto beans Winter squash Baked potato Banana Dried apricots or peaches Cantaloupe Prune juice
Magnesium	310-320 (female) 400-420 mg (male) 0.6 to 0.75 cup sunflower seeds	Transmission of nerve impulses Relaxation of skeletal muscle Aids bone formation Helps hold calcium in teeth	Impaired CNS function Tetany	Weakness Depressed respirations Cardiac arrest	Sunflower seeds Sesame seeds Cashews Spinach Wheat germ
Sulfur	None	Component of some amino acids Gives shape to hair, skin, and nails	None known	None known	Protein foods
Chloride	None*	Component of hydrochloric acid Maintains fluid and acid base balance	In infants: failure to thrive, lethargy, muscle weakness	None known	Table salt Seafood Milk Meat Eggs

*See Table of Estimated Sodium, Chloride, and Potassium Minimum Requirements of Healthy Persons (Appendix J).

concentrations in the **basal ganglia** are similar to that in the liver (Connor and Beard, 1997).

About 80 percent of the iron in a healthy body is available for carrying oxygen: hemoglobin contains 65 percent, myoglobin 10 percent, and iron-containing enzymes 3 percent. The remainder is stored. The main storage form of iron in the body is a protein–iron compound called **ferritin**. It is kept in the liver, spleen, and bone marrow for future use. When surplus iron accumulates in the blood because of the rapid destruction of red blood cells, the excess is stored in the liver in another compound, **hemosiderin**.

Absorption of Iron

The body tightly conserves its supply of iron. Most dietary iron is absorbed in the duodenum. When red blood cells are destroyed after their usual life span of 120 days, their iron is stored for reuse. Once iron is absorbed, there is no effective mechanism for excreting the excess. Fortunately, under normal conditions, the body is selective about absorbing iron.

FACTORS AFFECTING AMOUNTS As the body's need for iron increases, so does the proportion absorbed. In a healthy person, 5 to 15 percent of the iron in foods is absorbed. An anemic person, however, absorbs as

CLINICAL APPLICATION 8–5

LEAD POISONING (PLUMBISM)

Lead is a contaminant in the human body. The effects of lead toxicity, such as neurological damage and retardation, can be devastating and permanent. Over the past 25 years in the United States, mean blood lead levels of children declined by 80 percent and the number of children with elevated blood lead levels decreased by 90 percent (Ryan et al., 1999). Specifically, the prevalence of a blood lead level of 10 micrograms per 100 milliliters of blood in 1 to 5 year old children fell from 88.2 percent in the late 1970s to 8.9 percent in 1991.

Even so, nearly 900,000 children less than 6 years old in the United States still have elevated blood lead levels (Matte, 1999). A small local study revealed incomplete implementation of screening mandates and less-than-recommended follow-up of elevated results (Markowitz, Rosen, and Clement, 1999). Low-income children and black children are at 8 times and 5 times higher risk for lead poisoning, respectively, than other U.S. children (Ryan et al., 1999). A California study identified Mexican-born children at higher risk than Hispanic children born in the United States (Snyder et al., 1995).

Food is not the chief source of lead. Years ago, "painters' colic" or chronic lead poisoning was a fairly common occupational hazard. Today, sweet-tasting lead-based paint in older homes is the primary source of poisoning in inner-city children. Approximately 57,000 pre-1978 houses are estimated to have some leaded paint, and approximately 11 percent of pre-1980 homes are estimated to have soil lead concentrations exceeding 1000 parts per million (Matte, 1999). A paint chip the size of a penny may contain from 50 to 100 micrograms of lead. This amount, ingested daily for 3 months, could accumulate to 100 times the tolerable level for adults.

Some childhood cases have been discovered after the family pets were affected. In both situations the source of lead was exterior renovation in the neighborhood (Dowsett and Shannon, 1994). The child may not actually be eating paint chips. A principal mode of ingestion is that of lead dust on hands, toys, and household objects (Ryan et al., 1999).

Other sources of lead are automobile emissions from leaded gasoline, lead in or lead glazes on serving utensils, solder in metal cans, contaminated food products (Kakosy, Hudak, and Naray, 1996). Decreasing blood levels of lead in children have been correlated with diminishing amounts of lead in gasoline (Stromberg, Schutz, and Skerfring, 1995). Removing lead from gasoline in the 150 countries still permitting its use would prevent a large number cases of lead poisoning (Ryan et al., 1999). Small outbreaks of lead poisoning were traced to items brought into the United States by international travelers. Ten members of an extended family in California were poisoned by candy packaged in ceramic jars from Mexico. Thirteen members of an extended family in Michigan had elevated blood lead levels traced to a spice purchased in Iraq (Centers for Disease Control, 1998a). More uncommon sources of lead poisoning are ingested curtain weights or fishing sinkers (Mowad, Haddad, and Gemmel,

1998) and retained shrapnel from gunshot wounds (Farrell et al., 1999). Two cases of plumbism in toddlers were traced to pool cue chalk (Miller et al., 1996).

Hyperactivity has been linked to both lead poisoning and iron deficiency. There is evidence that suggests that these two conditions, not additives, allergens, or sugar, are the causes of hyperactivity. Lead poisoning and iron deficiency have risk factors in common and both cause neurological effects.

Early diagnosis and treatment of lead poisoning are essential. Foremost is the avoidance of further exposure through environmental control. Several nutritional tactics can be used in addition. Iron and calcium supplementation can be started so these minerals will compete with lead for absorption. A reduced fat diet and frequent meals also decrease gastrointestinal absorption of lead. Use of chelating agents that will bind with lead are recommended if the blood lead level is greater than 45 micrograms per 100 milliliters (Committee on Environmental Health, 1998). Even children successfully treated and kept away from further intake showed lasting brain damage in 25 percent of the cases.

Concern about the lead content in aging municipal water pipes prompted the Environmental Protection Agency (EPA) to lower the permissible lead level from 50 parts per billion to 15 parts per billion. Older homes also may have plumbing that could possibly contaminate the drinking water. Ten infants were poisoned from formula reconstituted with lead-contaminated water (Shannon and Graef, 1992). Since boiling increases the concentration of lead in water, the need to boil water for infant formula needs individual evaluation. To decrease the chance of lead leaching into drinking or cooking water, (1) flush the system for two minutes in the morning before drawing water and (2) use cold water. Local health departments should be able to direct people to appropriate laboratories if they wish to have their water tested.

Universal screening is recommended in communities with inadequate local data on blood lead levels and in communities with 27 percent or more of housing units built before 1950. Targeted screening is recommended in communities where 12 percent or fewer children have blood lead levels of 10 micrograms per 100 milliliters or higher or where fewer than 27 percent of the houses were built before 1950. Selecting children to screen focuses on such risk factors as the housing or day care facilities, family history of lead poisoning, birth country's prevalence of lead poisoning, likelihood of folk remedies being used, and the family's financial resources (Committee on Environmental Health, 1998).

One California county found that reported ingestion of dirt, dust or paint, use of foods canned in foreign countries, birth outside the United States, living within one block of a freeway, treatment with a lead-based home remedy, use of pottery or ceramic vessels for cooking, eating, or drinking, and having ever been to Latin America predicted elevated blood lead levels (Snyder et al., 1995)

much as 50 percent. Even though the proportion decreases with increased supply, the absolute amount absorbed increases. The entire process of iron absorption and its regulation are incompletely understood (Beutler, 1997).

The amount of dietary iron that is absorbed is determined by the amount of ferritin already present in the intestinal mucosa (where ferritin is formed). The iron obtained from ingested food is bound to a protein called **apoferritin** to form ferritin. When the total supply of apoferritin has been bound to iron, any additional iron in the gut is rejected and eliminated in the feces. Absorbed iron combines with a protein in the blood, **transferrin**, which transports iron to the bone marrow for hemoglobin synthesis, to the liver for storage, or to the body cells. Hemoglobin synthesis requires adequate protein and traces of copper, in addition to iron.

FACTORS AFFECTING RATES OF ABSORPTION Two types of iron are found naturally in food: heme iron and nonheme iron. **Heme iron** is bound to the hemoglobin and myoglobin in meat, fish, and poultry. Forty percent of the total iron in these animal sources is heme iron. Because heme iron is composed of ferrous iron, (Fe^{2+}), it is rapidly transported and absorbed intact. The other 60 percent of the total iron in meat, fish, and poultry, and all the iron in plant sources, is **nonheme** iron. Heme iron is two to three times more absorbable than nonheme iron (Centers for Disease Control, 1998b).

The absorption of nonheme iron is slow because it is closely bound to organic molecules in foods as **ferric iron** (Fe^{3+}). In the acidic medium of the stomach, the oxygen is removed from ferric iron during a chemical reaction called reduction. The end product is **ferrous iron**, which is more soluble and bioavailable. See Figure 8–6 for an overview of the steps involved in the process of iron absorption.

FACTORS ENHANCING ABSORPTION Several factors increase the absorption of iron through very different mechanisms. Consumption of large amounts of alcohol damages the intestine, which then permits absorption of increased amounts of iron. A high calcium intake increases iron absorption because the calcium combines with phosphates and phytates so that they are not available to inhibit iron absorption. Vitamin C forms a soluble compound with iron, negating the effect of phytates (see below) and increasing the absorption of iron. Finallly, an MFP (meat, fish, poultry) factor increases the absorption of iron. Nonheme iron absorption is increased when meat, fish, or poultry is consumed at the same time.

FACTORS INTERFERING WITH ABSORPTION When less gastric acid is present, whether because of antacids or gastric resection, less iron is absorbed. Phytic acid from cereals (wheat, rice, and maize) and nuts (walnuts, peanuts, hazelnuts) and oxalic acid from certain vegetables both combine with iron, reducing its availability. Other minerals compete with iron for binding sites. Excesses of copper, zinc, or manganese decrease absorption of each other and of iron.

Nonheme iron can be locked out of the absorption process by substances called **tannates**, which are found in tea and coffee. Tea may reduce iron absorption by 60 percent; coffee by 40 percent, Table 8–5 summarizes the factors that affect iron absorption. People who consume vegetarian diets should be especially careful to construct optimal menus. Practical suggestions to enhance iron and zinc nutrition in vegetarian diets are given in Table 8–6.

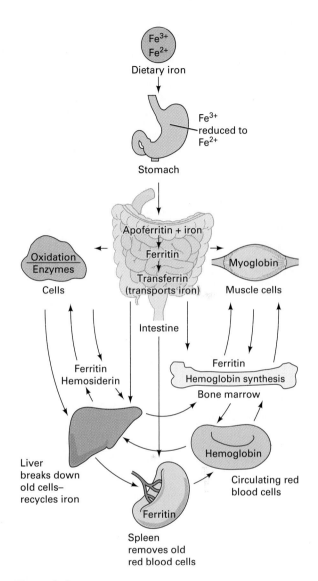

Figure 8–6:
In the process of dietary iron absorption, iron is absorbed primarily in the small intestine and may be transported or stored to meet the body's needs.

Excretion of Iron

No known mechanism exists to regulate the excretion of iron. Small amounts of iron are lost daily in sweat, hair, shed skin cells, and urine.

TABLE 8–5 Factors Affecting Iron Absorption

Increase	Decrease
Large alcohol intake	Less gastric acid
High calcium intake	Coffee or tea (tannates)
Vitamin C	Phytic or oxalic acids
Meat, fish, or poultry	Excessive copper, manganese, or zinc intake

TABLE 8–6 IMPROVING IRON AND ZINC NUTRITION WITH VEGETARIAN DIETS

Goal	Strategy	Rationale
Increase the total amount of iron and zinc consumed.	Select foods rich in iron and zinc at all meals. Consume cereals and pasta fortified with these nutrients.	Obtaining sufficient iron and zinc without animal products requires careful planning.
Make use of contamination iron.	Use cast iron cookware or steel woks for vegetable casseroles or curries, spaghetti sauces, or stewed fruits.	Moist, acidic foods have increased iron content when thus cooked for a long period. Even 20 minutes has shown an effect (Fairweather-Tait, Fox, and Mallilin, 1995).
Expand the intake of absorption enhancers.	Consume fermented foods such as yogurt and oriental soy products (tempeh, miso, natto, and soy sauce). Include a good source of vitamin C at every meal.	Certain organic acids (citric, lactic, malic, and tartaric) prevent the formation of insoluble iron and zinc phytates. Ascorbic acid is the most effective enhancer of nonheme iron absorption when consumed with the nonheme iron. It reduces ferric to ferrous iron that is more soluble at the pH of the duodenum and small intestine. Vitamin C also forms a stable complex with iron thus preventing iron from complexing with phytates and tannins (Lubin et al., 1997).
Reduce the intake of absorption antagonists.	Consumption of both sprouted whole grain cereals and legumes and yeast-leavened baked products can potentially reduce the phytic acid content of a meal.	Microbial fermentation can enhance bioavailability of iron and zinc via hydrolysis induced by microbial phytase enzymes derived from microflora on the surface of cereal grains or from yeast.
	Soak legumes before cooking.	Soaking reduces the phytic acid of most legumes since it is relatively water-soluble.
	Delay drinking tea and coffee until at least two hours after meals.	These beverages reduce nonheme iron absorption 35 to 64 percent.
Avoid taking high doses of mineral supplements.	Dietary sources alone are unlikely to compromise iron and zinc status.	Antagonistic interactions between copper and zinc and between nonheme iron and zinc are most likely when high doses of supplemental zinc and nonheme iron are ingested without food.

Adapted from Gibson, Donovan, and Heath, 1997.

Recommended Dietary Allowances of Iron

The values set for the 1989 RDA are based on the assumption that only 10 to 15 percent of the iron in ingested foods is absorbed. The RDAs for iron are: 10 milligrams for men, children aged 6 months to 10 years, and women over the age of 51 years, 15 milligrams for women of reproductive age and lactating women, and 30 milligrams for pregnant women.

Sources of Iron

The western diet contains an estimated 5 to 7 milligrams of iron per 1000 kilocalories. In the United States, one-third of dietary iron is supplied by grains, one-third by meats, and one-third by other sources. Absorption varies among the sources of iron also. Ten to 30 percent of iron is absorbed from liver and other meats; less than 10 percent is absorbed from eggs; and less than 5 percent is absorbed from grains and most vegetables.

Many foods are fortified with iron but its bioavailability depends upon the compounds used. If the added iron is metallic iron, very little can be absorbed (Fairbanks, 1999). Spinach, iron supplements, and contamination iron are absorbed at a 2 percent rate. Clinical Application 8–6 describes one way iron becomes available from nonfood sources. To show that all foods are not equal in nutrient content, the labeled percentages of iron and calcium in ready-to-eat cereals popular with children are compared in Figure 8–7. Manufacturers sometimes change these amounts. People who are trying to maximize their nutritional intake must read labels.

Deficiency of Iron

Anemia is a condition of insufficient hemoglobin to provide oxygen to the cells of the body. The features of the red blood cells are characteristic of various anemias. In iron deficiency anemia, the red blood cells are **microcytic** (smaller than normal) and **hypochromic** (contain less hemoglobin, giving the cell less color than normal).

Although iron deficiency is the most common nutritional cause of anemia worldwide, iron is not the only nutrient required for adequate blood formation. Some of the other nutrients needed include protein, the vitamins C, E, B_{12}, riboflavin, pyridoxine, folic acid, and the mineral copper.

Insufficient intake of iron, excessive blood loss, malabsorption, or lack of gastric hydrochloric acid can lead to **iron deficiency anemia**. The most common nutrient deficiency in the United States is that of iron. Even before the person becomes anemic, his cognitive performance can be impaired (Scrimshaw, 1991). Investigation of central nervous system development in infants in Chile showed marked differences in auditory conduction time in anemic infants compared with nonanemic ones at follow-up despite effective iron therapy, suggesting altered myelination as a possible explanation (Roncagliolo et al., 1998).

CLINICAL APPLICATION 8–6

CONTAMINATION IRON

Cooking in iron pots can increase the iron content of foods. This source of dietary iron is called contamination iron. Significant transfer occurs during simmering of acidic foods, especially tomatoes. For instance, 3-1/2 oz of spaghetti sauce cooked for 3 hours in a cast iron pot contains almost 90 mg of iron, compared to less than 5 mg of iron when cooked in a glass container (Zhou and Brittin, 1994). An East Indian practice of cooking curries in cast iron woks also was shown to increase iron content 4- to 12-fold (Fairweather-Tait, Fox, and Mallillin, 1995). The absorption rate of contamination iron is the same as that of supplements, 2 percent.

OCCURRENCE Iron deficiency is the most common single-nutrient-deficiency disease in the world. In tropical countries where intestinal **helminthiasis** is common, prevalence of iron deficiency is especially high. In India, where hookworm disease is prevalent and vegetarianism is mandated by religion, iron deficiency is nearly universal (Fairbanks, 1999). Iron deficiency also affects an estimated 94 million people in the Americas (Darnton-Hill et al., 1999).

At particular risk are African-Americans, Hispanic Americans, Native Americans, and poor people of all ethnic groups. In the United States, iron deficiency was found in 9 percent of toddlers aged 1 to 2 years and in 9 to 11 percent of adolescent girls and women in their reproductive years. Iron deficiency anemia was found in 3 percent and 2 to 5 percent of those groups respectively. These percentages represent approximately 700,000 toddlers and 7.8 million women with iron deficiency and 240,000 toddlers and 3.3 million women with iron deficiency anemia (Looker et al., 1997). Even so, the number of children in the United States with iron deficiency is decreasing, an outcome due largely to fortification of cereals and infant formulas.

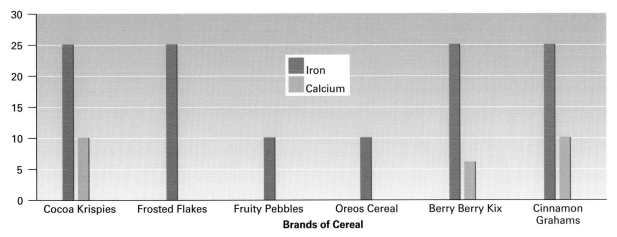

Percent of Iron and Calcium of a 2000 kcal diet contained in certain brands of cereal

Figure 8–7:
Three-fourths of a cup of each of these cereals supplies the indicated percentage of iron and calcium, assuming a 2000 kilocalorie diet. The tallest bars represent 25 percent. Other values are 10, 6, and 0 percent. Serving the usual way with milk would increase the percentage of calcium obtained.

RISK OF IRON DEFICIENCY Individuals at greatest risk of iron deficiency are young children and women of childbearing age, especially low-income minority women, who have 12 or fewer years of education or have had four or more children (Looker et al., 1997). Children 4 months to 3 years old, adolescents, and pregnant women should be monitored carefully for signs of iron deficiency because of their increased needs. All women in their menstrual years are at risk, a risk that increases with use of an intrauterine contraceptive device, which increases blood loss.

ASSESSMENT DATA Although no single test is diagnostic for iron deficiency, a common test to determine the hemoglobin level of the blood delivers valuable assessment data. The normal level for men is 14 to 18 grams per 100 milliliters of blood; for women it is 12 to 16 grams. A second common laboratory test is the **hematocrit**. This test measures the percentage of red blood cells in a volume of blood. Normal hematocrit levels are 40 to 54 percent for men and 36 to 46 percent for women. Hemoglobin and hematocrit levels are late indicators of iron deficiency.

In early iron deficiency, before hemoglobin and hematocrit readings drop, **serum transferrin** levels rise. The person with early iron deficiency will, providing the body is attempting to compensate, manufacture more transferrin to increase iron-carrying capacity. A new measure of iron status is **plasma transferrin receptor**. It increases even in mild deficiency and is unaffected by inflammation, making it a useful diagnostic aid for clients with inflammatory diseases (Connor and Beard, 1997).

TREATMENT PRECAUTIONS After a person has been treated for iron deficiency, iron therapy should be continued for several months after hemoglobin and hematocrit levels return to normal. This prolonged therapy will enable the body to rebuild iron stores.

Although oral iron supplements can cause side effects such as nausea and constipation and have been blamed for noncompliance with therapy, those factors have not been found to be the main reasons for discontinuing treatment. Rather, worldwide, the failure to complete therapy was most often caused by lack of availability of the supplements due to inadequate program support or insufficient service delivery (Galloway and McGuire, 1994).

In developing countries with high levels of infectious diseases, iron administration for anemia has been followed by increased morbidity from infections. Bacteria also require iron, and when the body's supply increases they thrive. Improved vitamin A status may protect against this potentially harmful effect of iron supplementation. The precise interaction between iron and vitamin A is uncertain (Ribaya-Mercado, 1997).

Iron Toxicity

For most people, there is little risk of developing iron overload from the diet. Iron absorption is effectively controlled in healthy people even when meat intake is high and foods are fortified (Hallberg, Hulthen, and Garby, 1998). Nevertheless, iron toxicity is seen in iron metabolism disorders, chronic alcoholism, or iron poisoning.

Surplus iron is stored in the liver as hemosiderin. When large amounts of hemosiderin are deposited in the liver and spleen, a condition called **hemosiderosis** results.

If prolonged, it can lead to **hemochromatosis**, a disease of iron metabolism in which iron accumulates in the tissues. A person with this relatively common, autosomal-recessive disease suffers from impaired liver function, blood sugar disturbances, joint pain, and skin discoloration. Cardiac failure and death may follow. The incidence of iron overload in parts of Africa is the highest in the world where some postmortem studies reported hepatic iron sufficient to cause cirrhosis at a prevalence of more than 10 percent (Gordeuk, 1992). An estimated 10 to 15 percent of Caucasians of northern European descent may be carriers of the gene that was identified in 1996.

Clients with alcoholism, although often lacking many other nutrients, sometime suffer from iron overload. Some alcoholic beverages themselves contain a significant amount of iron. For example, inexpensive red wines contain 10 to 350 milligrams of iron per liter. The problem may be more complex than just oversupply. Most alcoholic cirrhosis clients with iron overload have hereditary hemochromatosis whereby alcohol abuse increases the risk of cirrhosis but does not cause the iron overload (Fairbanks, 1999).

Toxicity from supplemental iron tablets is a major threat to children. The absorptive controls for dietary iron are circumvented by the large amounts of soluble iron in pharmaceutical preparations. Iron is the most common cause of pediatric poisoning deaths reported to poison control centers in the United States. As few as five or six tablets of a high-potency product could prove fatal for a 22-pound child. During 1991, of 5144 ingestions of iron supplements reported to poison control centers in the United States, 11 were fatal. An additional 2 deaths were caused by prenatal multivitamin preparations with iron. Between June 1992 and January 1993, five toddlers in the Los Angeles area died from ingesting iron supplements (Centers for Disease Control, 1993).

Since mid-1997, all iron-containing drugs and dietary supplements have carried a warning notice regarding children's risk of poisoning. In addition, most products containing 30 milligrams or more of iron per dosage unit must be packaged as individual doses to make it more time-consuming or troublesome for a small child to consume many tablets.

Health-care providers should impress upon parents the enormous threat medications and supplements pose for small children. The products should be stored out of reach, out of sight, with child-resistant caps intact. If a child ingests any medication or supplement, a poison control center should be consulted immediately without waiting for signs and symptoms to appear.

Iodine

Iodine can be found in the muscles, thyroid gland, skin, and skeleton. The body of the average adult contains 20 to 50 milligrams of iodine, 70 to 80 percent of it in the thyroid gland in the neck.

Function of Iodine and Control of the Thyroid Gland

The thyroid gland secretes **thyroxine (T_4)** and **triiodothyronine (T_3)** in response to the **thyroid stimulating hormone (TSH)** from the anterior pituitary gland. Both T_3 and T_4 increase the rate of oxidation in cells, thereby increasing the rate of metabolism. The only known function of iodine is its participation in the synthesis of T_4 and T_3. When serum levels of T_3 and T_4 are adequate, secretion of TSH ceases.

Absorption and Excretion of Iodine

Iodine is easily absorbed from all portions of the intestinal tract. Of the absorbed iodine, 33 percent is used by the thyroid cells for the synthesis of T_4 and T_3, and the remaining 67 percent is excreted in the urine. After performing their functions, T_4 and T_3 are degraded by the liver, and the iodine content is excreted in bile.

Recommended Dietary Allowance and Sources of Iodine

The 1989 RDA for iodine is 150 micrograms for adult men and women. Iodine can come from foods, either naturally present or fortified, or from incidental sources.

IODINE IN FOODS Foods that are naturally high in iodine include saltwater fish, shellfish, and seaweed. The iodine content in plants varies with the mineral content of the soil in which they are grown. The amount of iodine present in eggs and dairy products depends on the animals' diets. Using food tables to calculate iodine intakes has resulted in erroneous estimates of intake since the regions producing the food analyzed would vary significantly regarding the iodine content of the soil. Table salt fortified with iodine (1 milligram of iodine in 10 grams of salt) has been available in the United States since 1924.

INCIDENTAL IODINE Sometimes iodine is present as a side effect of processing. For example, iodine solutions are used to sterilize milk pasteurization vats; some iodine may remain on the vat and be mixed into the next batch of milk to be processed. Iodine is also used to improve the texture of bread dough. A third source of incidental iodine is FDA Red Dye #3.

Deficiency of Iodine

Because the normal function of the thyroid gland depends on an adequate supply of iodine, a deficiency may result in goiter, cretinism, or myxedema. Since the introduction of iodized salt, these deficiency diseases are rarely encountered in North America. Between 1922 and 1927, with the implementation of a statewide prevention program, the goiter rate in Michigan declined from 38.6 percent to 9.0 percent (Centers for Disease Control, 1999a). At particular risk of iodine deficiency are vegans who consume sea salt, which contains virtually no iodine, rather than iodized salt. In a group of North American strict vegetarians, 12 percent developed hypothyroidism (Remer, Neubert, and Manz, 1999). Diagnosis of thyroid malfunction can be readily evaluated by measuring protein-bound iodine and the serum levels of T_4 and T_3.

LOCAL EFFECTS When the thyroid gland does not receive sufficient iodine, it increases in size, attempting to increase production. The gland may reach 1 to 1.5 pounds (about 500 to 700 grams). This enlargement of the thyroid is called **goiter**. Sometimes the gland may attain sufficient size to impede breathing (Tsukada et al., 1999). Unfortunately, replacement of iodine does not always reduce the goiter after the thyroid has enlarged. In some cases, prolonged deficiency results in thyroid tissue which produces T_3 and T_4 in response to dietary iodine rather than TSH. Iodine given to these people may cause hyperthyroidism (Medeiros-Neto, 1995; Pennington, 1990).

Goiter has been known as a disease entity since 3000 BC. Because of iodine-poor soil, the Great Lakes states and the Rocky Mountain states once were considered the "goiter belt." Now that food supplies are obtained nationwide and iodized salt is readily available, goiter is less common in this country. In contrast, worldwide, 211 million people have goiter, and 1.6 billion people are at risk for iodine deficiency, particularly in mountainous areas or those with eroded soil.

SYSTEMIC EFFECTS Iodine deficiency is the most common cause of preventable mental defect in the world (Hetzel and Clugston, 1999). Severe **hypothyroidism** during pregnancy results in **cretinism** in the newborn. As a consequence of the mother's thyroid deficiency, the infant exhibits mental and physical retardation. Cretinism is a congenital condition (present at birth). About 20 million people in developing countries are at risk for overt cretinism due to iodine deficiency. **Endemic** cretinism affects up to 10 percent of the people living in severely iodine-deficient areas of India, Indonesia, and China (Hetzel and Clugston, 1999).

Prevention must focus on treating the iodine deficiency in the mother. Hypothroidism due to iodine deficiency occurring in older children and adults is called **myxedema**. In areas where food fortification is difficult to implement, treatment may consist of iodized oil administered by injection, which can suffice for 3 to 4 years, or oral iodized walnut, soybean, or peanut oils that have a duration of 1 to 2 years (Hetzel and Clugston, 1999).

Factors Interfering with Iodine

Substances called **goitrogens** may block the body's absorption or utilization of iodine. Goitrogens are found in vegetables belonging to the cabbage family, including cauliflower, broccoli, Brussels sprouts, rutabaga, and turnips. The only food linked to goiter is cassava, a starchy root eaten in developing countries. The persistence of goiter in Greece despite correction of iodine deficiency suggests a possible role for a naturally occurring goitrogen (Doufas et al, 1999).

Iodine Toxicity

Toxicity has been reported with intakes of 2000 to 3200 micrograms, but normal diets of natural foods are likely to supply just 1000 micrograms per day (Hetzel and Clugston, 1999). The exception would be a diet containing large quantities of marine fish, seaweed, or contamination iodine. Toxicity from iodine has occurred in parts of Japan from the ingestion of large amounts of seaweed. Too much iodine can cause either hypo- or hyperthyroidism. In autoimmune thyroid disease, high dietary iron may induce hypothyroidism or "iodine goiter" and may also cause skin lesions similar to acne. The opposite effect, iodine-induced hyperthyroidism, results from the thyroid gland becoming autonomous and ignoring the controlling attempts by thyroid stimulating hormone.

Fluoride

In body fluids fluorine exists as fluoride, a salt of hydrofluoric acid or as an ion. About 99 percent of the body fluoride accumulates as fluorapatite in the bones and teeth. It seems to make bone mineral less soluble and hence less likely to be reabsorbed. Soluble fluoride such as sodium fluoride is rapidly absorbed from the stomach and small intestine. Increased gastric secretion increases its rate of absorption, and aluminum hydroxide (the antacid) inhibits absorption (Nielsen, 1999).

Function of Fluoride

In addition, low levels of fluoride in saliva can decrease the rate of demineralization and enhance remineralization of early carious lesions (DePaola, Faine, and Palmer, 1999). The incorporation of fluoride into teeth strengthens them and renders them better able to resist the bacterial acids that cause dental caries. For this reason, fluoride is often added to water supplies, mouthwashes, and toothpastes, or taken as a prescription supplement. The use of fluoridated water and fluoride supplements has resulted in a 30 to 50 percent decrease in children's caries. In addition, fluoridated mouth rinses and toothpastes have reduced the incidence of caries in children by about 40 percent. A study in Louisiana showed that Medicaid-eligible children 1 to 5 years old in communities without fluoridated water were three times more likely to require dental treatment in a hospital operating room than Medicaid-eligible children in communities with fluoridated water. The resulting costs of dental treatment were approximately twice as much for the first group as for the second (Centers for Disease Control, 1999b).

Dietary Reference Intakes and Sources of Fluoride

The AI for fluoride has been set at 4 milligrams for men and 3 milligrams for women.

One of the main sources of fluoride is drinking water that has been fluoridated at a cost of approximately 30 cents per person per year. About 50 percent of the community water supply in the United States serving about 52 percent of the population is fluoridated, to a concentration of one part per million. This amount equals 1 milligram per liter of water. In England and Wales, less than 10 percent of the population receives fluoridated water. The issue still evokes controversy (Coggon and Cooper, 1999). Food sources of fluoride include fish, fish products, and tea. Also, foods prepared in fluoridated water have increased levels of fluoride. Additional sources of fluoride are supplements and fluoride-containing dental products.

Fluoride Toxicity

Excessive, prolonged ingestion of fluoride results in **fluorosis**, a condition that can cause mottled discoloration of the teeth in children (from birth to 8 or 10 years old). Fluorosis has been observed when the concentration of fluoride has reached 2 parts per million. The fluorosis produced by this dose may be cosmetically unacceptable, but the teeth are sound. Just as an excess of iodine can cause the same symptoms as deficiency (i.e., goiter), a fluoride concentration of 4 parts per million is associated with increased dental caries.

Zinc

Estimated content of zinc in adult humans is 1.5 to 2.5 grams, over 95 percent of it within the cells. Zinc is a component of all body tissues. As much as 20 percent of total body zinc is found in the skin (Andrews and Gallagher-Allred, 1999). Greater concentrations are found in the eyes, hair, bone, and male reproductive organs than in other tissues. Zinc is essential for the growth and repair of tissues because it is involved in the synthesis of DNA and RNA. Zinc is incorporated into the structure of more than 200 enzymes for protein and DNA synthesis, and it is associated with the hormone insulin. It is also necessary for the metabolism of all the energy nutrients. The production of active vitamin A for the visual pigment rhodopsin requires zinc. It is necessary for the formation of collagen, which is necessary for wound healing. Zinc also protects against disease through its role in providing immunity and is the subject of research with the common cold.

The form of the compound and the vehicle carrying it makes a difference in the zinc's effectiveness. Some researchers report that zinc gluconate lozenges started within 24 to 48 hours of the onset of symptoms

and taken every 2 hours while awake reduced the duration and severity of colds (Marshall, 1998), others that zinc acetate lozenges can be judged to be beneficial (Eby, 1997). In 1999, however, in answer to charges by the Federal Trade Commission, two companies agreed not to make unsubstantiated claims for their zinc products (Federal Trade Commission, 1999).

Absorption and Control of Zinc

Zinc is released from foods in the acid environment of the stomach and absorbed from the small intestine through the same absorption sites as iron. Control of zinc levels is achieved through limitations on absorption and excretion into intestinal waste. As the concentration of zinc in the intestinal lumen increases, the percentage absorbed decreases, but the total amount absorbed increases. Up to 40 percent of zinc in animal products is absorbed, compared with 15 percent in high-phytate diets (Sandstrom, 1995). Absorption is increased during lactation, but citric acid and picolinic acid do not appear to increase absorption (King and Keen, 1999). The body does not store zinc.

Unabsorbed zinc and the zinc in pancreatic secretions are excreted through intestinal wastes. The liver removes excessive zinc effectively. An abnormal zinc metabolism has been observed in people with diabetes, but zinc's role in the etiology of diabetes is as yet unknown. Healthy people excrete no zinc in the urine, but in catabolic conditions, zinc (as well as potassium, creatinine, and nitrogen) appears in the urine from the breakdown of muscle tissue.

Recommended Dietary Allowances and Sources of Zinc

The 1989 RDAs for zinc are 12 milligrams for females ages 11 to 50 and 15 milligrams for those 51 years of age and older. For males ages 11 and older, the RDA in 1989 was set at 15 milligrams.

The best dietary sources of zinc are shellfish and red meat; the source of the food is significant. Three ounces of shucked Eastern oysters contain 121 milligrams, but Western oysters only 17 milligrams. More popular foods high in zinc are canned pork and beans (7.45 milligrams in half cup), canned chili with beans (5.13 milligrams in 1 cup), wheat germ (4.73 milligrams in quarter cup), and beef sirloin steak or rump roast (4.45 and 4.21 milligrams, respectively, in 3 ounces).

Interfering Factors for Zinc

Iron and zinc compete for the same absorption sites. Thus, if a person's intake of iron is two to three times that of zinc, the absorption of zinc is reduced. Decreased absorption of zinc has been noted when a 30-milligram supplement of iron is taken. Pregnant women taking 60 milligrams of iron daily should also take supplemental zinc (King and Keen, 1999).

Vitamin and mineral supplements with a ratio greater than 3 to1of iron to zinc inhibit zinc absorption. Calcium, excess folate, fiber, phytates, and **chelating agents** all reduce the absorption of zinc. Zinc itself is a chelating agent protecting the body from poisoning from lead and cadmium. If a person has marginal zinc status, high intakes of coffee, cocoa, tea, or whole grain products (especially if unleavened) may lower zinc levels because of their phytate content.

Deficiency of Zinc

Clinical zinc deficiency is not commonly diagnosed in the United States. In other parts of the world, zinc deficiency is widespread, especially where the population subsists on cereal grains. The possibility of subclinical zinc deficiency in the United States exists since the U.S. food supply provides only 12.3 milligrams per person per day. Zinc intake correlates directly with protein consumption. Groups at risk because of limited meat intake include the poor, the elderly, and vegetarians. A reliable, sensitive laboratory index is needed to identify people at risk of zinc deficiency (King and Keen, 1999).

In Colorado, a group of healthy children, short for their ages, were supplemented with 5 milligrams of zinc daily and gained more height than an unsupplemented control group of comparable children. In contrast, zinc supplementation in children who had normal height for age did not increase their growth (King and Keen, 1999).

Zinc deficiency in adults can also occur as a result of diseases that either hinder zinc absorption or cause excessive amounts of zinc to be excreted in the urine. Most types of stress or inflammatory processes, such as sepsis, burns, head injury, or multiple trauma, cause increased urinary losses of zinc (Boosalis, Stuart, and McClain, 1995). Some of the clinical conditions that may precipitate zinc deficiency include acute myocardial infarction, alcoholic cirrhosis, celiac disease, Crohn's disease, and lymphoma. A rare autosomal recessive disease, **acrodermatitis enteropathica**, causes zinc deficiency through an unknown defect in absorption and is fatal if untreated.

Less severe deficiency of zinc produces the symptoms of abnormal fatigue, decreased alertness, impaired night vision, anorexia, and diminished sense of taste and smell. Signs of severe zinc deficiency include skin lesions, hypopigmentation of the hair (giving it a reddish cast), patchy **alopecia**, diarrhea, and corneal edema. Other signs are retarded growth (dwarfism), delayed sexual maturation (if deficiency occurs during critical growth periods), low sperm counts, and delayed healing of wounds and burns.

Zinc deficiency impairs wound healing as the result of decreased collagen synthesis. Oral zinc supplementation has not been shown to be generally beneficial in the healing of chronic venous or arterial leg ulcers, but limited evidence was found of benefit in individuals with low serum zinc levels (Wilkinson and Hawke, 1998). Because serum zinc levels greater than 400 milligrams per deciliter may inhibit wound repair, supplemental zinc should not be given to clients who are not deficient. Supplementation speeds the healing process only in the truly deficient client.

Zinc Toxicity

Because zinc can be toxic if consumed in excessive amounts, it should be obtained from foods in the diet and not from routine or long-term supplementation. Supplemental doses only two to three times the RDA can interfere with copper absorption and lead to copper deficiency. Supplementation at the RDA level blocks the exercise effect of increasing serum levels of high-density lipoproteins (HDLs), the "good cholesterol." Amounts ten times the RDA—150 milligrams per day—have been shown to impair white blood cells and decrease HDLs (Subcommittee on 10th edition of RDAs, 1989).

Copper

The healthy adult body contains 50 to 120 milligrams of copper. Absorption of copper occurs in the stomach and upper intestine and varies inversely with intake. It is stored in the liver and excreted in feces as a component of bile salts.

Copper is a cofactor for enzymes involved in hemoglobin and collagen formation. It helps to incorporate iron into hemoglobin and to transport iron to the bone marrow. As a component of Factor V, copper is necessary for blood clotting. It also is required for normal development and function of cells of the immune system. Copper helps to oxidize glucose and release energy. It is required for skeletal mineralization and cardiac function. Copper is necessary for melanin pigment formation and for maintaining myelin sheaths.

Copper is believed to be readily absorbed from the stomach, duodenum, and jejunum. Although the uptake and metabolism of copper in humans are not well understood, the main route of excretion is thought to be the biliary tract (Spiegel and Willenbucher, 1999).

Estimated Safe and Adequate Daily Dietary Intake and Sources of Copper

The ESADDI for copper is 1.5 to 3 milligrams for adults. In the United States, adult intake averages 1 to 2 milligrams. The World Health Organization has proposed a limit of 2 milligrams per liter for drinking water (Olivares et al., 1998). Unfortunately, data are missing on the copper content of many foods listed in or programmed into databases for nutritional analysis. Also, a food's copper content depends upon its handling. The best sources of copper are organ meats, shellfish, nuts, legumes, chocolate, and whole cereals. A 3-ounce serving of liver contains 3 milligrams of copper.

Interfering Factors and Deficiency of Copper

High intakes of zinc, iron, calcium, and manganese interfere with copper absorption. The recommended iron-to-copper ratio is 10 to 17:1, but 80 percent of infant formulas examined were found to have ratios exceeding 20:1 (Johnson, Smith, and Edmonds, 1998). As little as 18.5 milligrams of zinc per day was shown to impair copper absorption. Overt signs of copper deficiency developed in people taking 150 milligrams (10 times the RDA) of zinc daily for two years (King and Keen, 1999). Some studies have expressed concern over fortifying foods and formulating supplements with iron and zinc but not copper or manganese. Even in supplements containing copper, the compound selected by the manufacturer more often than not was a poorly absorbed form of copper (Johnson, Smith, and Edmonds, 1998).

Phytates hinder absorption by forming more stable complexes with copper than with calcium or iron. An alkaline medium inhibits copper absorption. A dose of 15 antacid tablets per day may precipitate copper and induce deficiency.

Copper deficiency is not known to occur in adults under normal conditions, but it has occurred as a result of the administration of **total parenteral** nutrition (TPN) solutions deficient in copper. Total parenteral nutrition is an intravenous feeding designed to meet all of a person's nutritional needs. Copper deficiency has also occurred in premature infants exclusively fed cow's milk; the result is an anemia that does not respond to iron supplementation.

Because of its link with iron utilization, copper deficiency produces a hypochromic, microcytic anemia. Other manifestations of copper deficiency are skeletal demineralization, impaired immune function, and depigmentation of the skin and hair. A hereditary abnormality that blocks the absorption of copper from the gastrointestinal tract causes **Menkes' disease**. It is an X-linked recessive trait occurring 1 in 50,000 to 100,000 live births. The natural history of the disease involves cerebral degeneration, retarded growth, and death by the age of 3 years. Intravenous administration of copper corrects the blood levels but does not improve brain function or slow the progressive deterioration (Turnlund, 1999).

Copper Toxicity

Clients treated with an artificial kidney that used copper tubing, some who consumed acidic foods stored in copper vessels, and infants fed water high in copper have experienced toxicity. A defect in the excretion of copper into the bile causes **Wilson's disease**. It is inherited as an autosomal recessive trait, occurring in 1 of 200,000 people in the United States (Turnlund, 1999). As a result, copper accumulates in various organs, particularly the liver, kidneys, and brain. Chelation therapy may be augmented by a dietary prescription to avoid foods high in copper.

Selenium

Most selenium occurs in proteins as a component of amino acids. The mineral selenium is part of an enzyme that works with vitamin E to protect cellular compounds from oxidation. In this role, selenium functions as an antioxidant. Selenium and vitamin E have a reciprocal sparing relationship (each spares the other). Selenium forms part of the protein matrix of the teeth, appears necessary for iodine metabolism, and helps to protect the liver from cirrhosis. It contributes to the work of drug-metabolizing enzymes and plays a role in preventing heavy metal poisoning from mercury, cadmium, and silver (Burk and Levander, 1999). In addition, a possibly unique selenoprotein occurring in the sperm mitochondrial capsule is vital to the integrity of sperm flagella (Holben and Smith, 1999).

The highest concentrations of this mineral occur in the liver, kidneys, and heart. About 50 to 100 percent of selenium is absorbed without regard to nutritional status. Rather, urinary excretion maintains homeostasis of the nutrient. Currently, no suitable methods of determining clinical selenium status are available (Burk and Levander, 1999).

The 2000 RDA for selenium for adults is 55 micrograms. The Tolerable Upper Intake Level (UL) is 400 micrograms. Adolescence, pregnancy, and lactation increase the need for selenium, whereas a high intake of vitamin E reduces it. The amount of selenium present in plant foods depends on the selenium content of the soil and water where the foods are grown. In Finland, selenium is added to the soil. The selenium in the British diet fell from 65 to 31 micrograms per day after switching from North American wheat to European wheat (Burk and Levander, 1999). Seafood, meats, eggs, and grains are the best dietary sources of selenium.

Selenium deficiencies have been produced in animals but are unlikely in humans who eat meat on a regular basis. Nevertheless, there are some exceptions. Clients being maintained long-term on special formulas, such as that used to treat phenylketonuria, should have the formula checked for adequacy of trace nutrients. Several clients being maintained

on TPN have developed heart disease that responded to selenium treatment. A deterioration of the heart due to selenium deficiency has occurred in residents of the province of Keshan, China. The fatality rate of **Keshan disease** is as high as 80 percent, and once heart failure occurs, supplementation does not reverse it. Researchers have linked selenium deficiency in mice to a mutation of an avirulent virus to a virulent one producing myocardial disease. Significantly, the virulent strain then caused heart disease in non-selenium-deficient mice, an unusual situation in which a host's nutritional status affected the genetic composition of a microorganism (Burk and Levander, 1999).

Toxicity from selenium occurs in animals grazing on selenium-rich land. In humans, selenium toxicity occurred when the amount in a supplement was 125 times the correct dose. Signs and symptoms of selenium toxicity include fatigue, nausea and vomiting, garlic or sour-milk breath odor, and nail and hair loss. Animals that consume excessive selenium exhibit nervous-system impairment and die of respiratory failure.

Chromium

The adult body contains 4 to 6 milligrams of chromium. High concentrations are found in the bone, kidneys, liver, muscle, spleen, and pancreas. Only about 0.5 to 2 percent of dietary chromium is absorbed. The chief organ of excretion is the kidney.

Chromium is associated with RNA and DNA and is a cofactor in the activation of enzymes involved in fat and cholesterol metabolism. It potentiates insulin action. Chromium is thought by some researchers to increase the cellular uptake of glucose by helping to bind insulin to its receptor sites on the cell membranes. The complex achieving this transfer was called **glucose tolerance factor (GTF)**, but attempts to isolate or synthesize GTF have been unsuccessful, leaving the precise mechanism in doubt (Nielsen, 1996). Four different chromium compartments in the body have been identified with different half-lives of chromium displayed by clients with and without diabetes (Stoecker, 1999).

The ESADDI for chromium for adults ranges from 50 to 200 micrograms. The World Health Organization rated the minimum mean population daily intake likely to meet normal needs at approximately 33 micrograms (Nielsen, 1996). Stressors that increase the need for chromium or increase its loss include an elevated intake of simple sugars, strenuous exercise or physical work, infection, and physical trauma. Vitamin C and aspirin increase absorption, but antacids decrease it.

Brewer's yeast, whole grains, some cereals, and broccoli are good sources of chromium. Other sources are meats, especially organ meats, cheese, mushrooms, prunes, nuts, asparagus, beer, wine, and seasonings such as thyme and black pepper. Chromium is leached from stainless steel, particularly with acid foods.

Chromium deficiency impairs the effectiveness of insulin and usually results in an elevated blood glucose or glucose intolerance. In some clients receiving TPN, chromium, not insulin, successfully lowered blood sugar levels. Lack of sufficient chromium intake is also associated with coronary artery disease. Supplementation with chromium has improved blood lipid levels.

Dietary chromium toxicity usually occurs as a result of eating contaminated foods; the characteristic symptom is a disagreeable metallic taste in the mouth. A more common cause is absorption of a different form of chromium through the skin or lungs in an industrial setting. Stainless steel welding may be the most common source of this contamination (Stoecker, 1999).

Manganese

The body contains only 10 to 20 milligrams of manganese, which is found in highest concentrations in the bones and glands. Manganese is a cofactor of enzymes involved in energy metabolism and is required for bone formation. The metabolism of manganese is not completely known. About 40 percent of the manganese ingested is absorbed. Its concentration seemingly is regulated by absorption in the small bowel and excretion, 90 percent of which occurs through the bile (Alves et al., 1997) often within minutes of absorption (Greger and Malecki, 1997). Unlike nutrients that fulfill unique functions, other minerals can sometimes substitute for manganese. One such mineral is magnesium.

The ESADDI for manganese is 2 to 5 milligrams for adults. The best sources of manganese are wheat bran, legumes, nuts, and leafy green vegetables. Other good sources are cereal grains, coffee, and tea. Excessive intakes of iron, zinc, or copper cause decreased manganese absorption.

Low serum manganese levels have been reported in people with diabetes, pancreatic insufficiency, protein–calorie malnutrition, and some types of epilepsy. The client displays weight loss, hypocholesterolemia, nausea, vomiting, dermatitis, and changes in hair color. The best-documented case involved a child on total parenteral nutrition whose bone demineralization was cured by manganese supplements (Nielsen, 1999).

Toxicity due to dietary intake has not been reported in healthy people, but miners exposed to manganese dust over prolonged periods have suffered liver and central nervous system damage (including severe psychiatric symptoms), muscle spasms, and monotone voice. Those at risk for manganese toxicity are clients receiving parenteral nutrition and those with decreased liver function or **cholestasis**. A case of manganese toxicity resulted from long-term parenteral nutrition following small intestine resection; the study demonstrated that serum manganese levels can be normal while cerebral levels remain elevated (Alves et al., 1997).

The clinical picture of manganese toxicity resembles that of Parkinson's disease. Two children receiving long-term parenteral nutrition at home showed manganese in the basal ganglia on magnetic resonance imaging (MRI) without overt clinical signs. Over time the deposited manganese was removed by the body, indicating a good prognosis in the absence of neurological signs and liver disease (Kafritsa et al., 1998). Six other cases involving total parenteral nutrition were reported (Komaki et al., 1999; Nagatomo et al., 1999; and Reynolds et al., 1998).

Cobalt

As an essential component of the vitamin B_{12} molecule, cobalt is necessary for red blood cell formation, but a role for the ionic form of cobalt has not been demonstrated (Groff, Gropper, and Hunt, 1995). An RDA for cobalt has not been established. Foods that provide vitamin B_{12} are good sources of cobalt; these foods are meats, poultry, fish, shellfish, and milk.

Cobalt deficiency has not been reported in humans or animals. Very large pharmaceutical doses have produced an excess of red blood cells (polycythemia) in humans, and chronic high doses over time can produce goiter (Lindeman, 1987).

Molybdenum

Molybdenum, a cofactor for enzymes involved in protein synthesis, is found primarily in the liver, kidneys, bone, and adrenal glands. It is absorbed in the stomach and small intestine and is mainly excreted in urine, but also in bile to some extent (Nielsen, 1999).

The ESADDI for adults is 75 to 250 micrograms. Daily intake from the average diet provides 200 to 500 micrograms. Sources of molybdenum are milk, organ meats, legumes, and grains. Because molybdenum is a copper antagonist, high levels of copper decrease the absorption of molybdenum.

One client on TPN was treated as molybdenum deficient. His signs and symptoms were caused by an inability to process sulfur-containing amino acids. His clinical picture was of increased pulse rate and respiratory rate, visual defects, night blindness, irritability, and coma. After discontinuation of his intake of sulfur-containing amino acids and supplementation with molybdenum, the symptoms disappeared (National Research Council, 1989).

No definite molybdenum toxicity has been documented in humans. In Russia, intakes of 10 to 15 milligrams of molybdenum per day (40 times the U.S. ESADDI) have been associated with hyperuricemia and gout.

A summary of the main food sources of each of the trace minerals discussed in this chapter appears in Table 8–7. The food groups contributing to the intake of major and trace minerals is illustrated in Figure 8–8.

Supplementation

Excessive intake of nutrients can be as harmful as insufficient intake. For healthy people, foods are the preferred source of minerals rather than medicinal supplementation (Wellness Tips 8-1). People who take supplements should not take more than the RDAs, the AIs, or the ESADDIs for each mineral. In the case of some minerals, toxicity is possible at levels slightly above the recommended or estimated intake amounts. In addition, an excess of one mineral may cause a deficiency of another.

Wellness Tips 8–1

- Implement the Daily Food Guide Pyramid. Keep score to identify goals to emphasize.
- Attempt to restrain your taste for salt. It is a learned preference and can be unlearned.
- If you choose to use a mineral supplement, select a balanced one, not individual minerals unless under your professional health-care provider's direction.
- If you choose to use a mineral supplement, select a pharmaceutical one, not one of raw materials.
- Be extremely cautious and skeptical of remedies or foods privately imported into the United States.
- Consult your health-care provider if it has been necessary to make daily use of over-the-counter medicines such as antacids for 2 weeks.
- Treat dietary supplements as medicine. Lock them in childproof cupboards. Do not take medicines in front of children lest they imitate you.

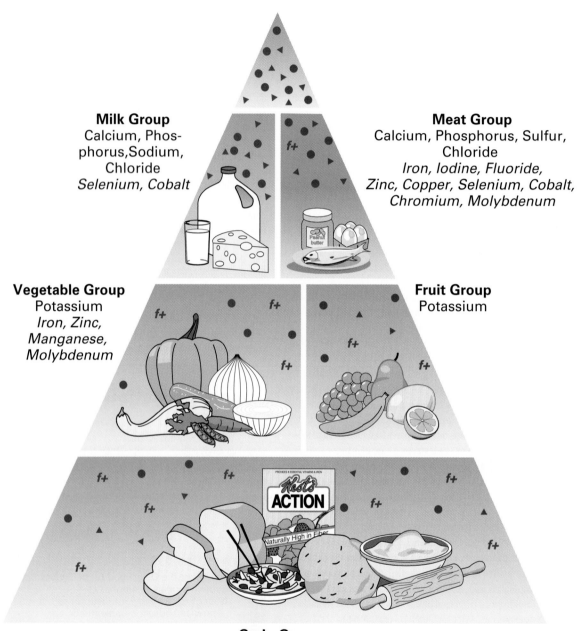

Milk Group
Calcium, Phos-
phorus,Sodium,
Chloride
Selenium, Cobalt

Meat Group
Calcium, Phosphorus, Sulfur,
Chloride
*Iron, Iodine, Fluoride,
Zinc, Copper, Selenium, Cobalt,
Chromium, Molybdenum*

Vegetable Group
Potassium
*Iron, Zinc,
Manganese,
Molybdenum*

Fruit Group
Potassium

Grain Group
Magnesium
*Zinc, Copper, Chromium,
Manganese, Molybdenum*

Figure 8–8:
This pyramid illustrates the food groups supplying the various minerals. Italics indicate trace minerals.

Table 8–7 Trace Minerals

Mineral	Adult RDA or AI and Food Portion Containing RDA	Function	Signs and Symptoms of Deficiency	Signs and Symptoms of Excess	Best Sources
Iron	15 mg (female) 10 mg (male) 2–3 tbsp Blackstrap molasses	Component of hemoglobin	Fatigue, listlessness Impaired cognition Hypochromic, microcytic anemia	Hemosiderosis Hemochromatosis	Liver, other organ meats Blackstrap molasses Oysters Red meat
Iodine	150 mcg 0.3 tsp iodized salt	Components of thyroid hormones	Goiter Cretinism Myedema	Acne-like lesions Goiter	Iodized salt Saltwater seafood
Fluoride	3–4 mg 3–4 L fluorinated water	Hardens teeth	Dental caries	Mottled teeth Increased caries	Fluoridated water Seafood
Zinc	12 mg (female) 15 mg (male) 0.8 to 1 cup canned pork and beans	Involved in DNA and RNA synthesis Component of >200 enzymes Associated with insulin Required for production of active vitamin A Necessary for formation of collagen Serves role in immunity Essential role in sexual maturation Integral role in energy metabolism, including alcohol detoxification	Growth failure Hypogonadism Poor would healing Impaired night vision Abnormal taste and smell	Copper deficiency Cancellation of effect of exercise on HDLs Impaired white blood cells	Oysters Canned pork and beans Canned chili with beans Wheat germ Beef sirloin steak or rump roast
Copper	None*	Cofactor for enzymes involved in hemoglobin and collagen formation Component of Factor V in clotting sequence Necessary for melanin formation Required to maintain myelin	Anemia Demineralization of skeleton Depigmentation of skin and hair Impaired immune function	Copper deposits in liver, kidneys, and brain	Oysters Liver Fortified cereal
Selenium	55 mcg Amount in food varies with region	Antioxidant Interchangeable with vitamin E for some functions	Keshan cardiomyopathy	Nail and hair loss Nervous system impairment	Seafood Liver Meats Dairy products
Chromium	None*	Cofactor in enzymes used in fat and cholesterol metabolism Component of glucose tolerance factor	Glucose intolerance Elevated blood lipids	Rare related to food Metallic taste	Brewer's yeast Whole grains Meats

Continued on next page

Table 8–7 Trace Minerals (continued)

Mineral	Adult RDA and Food Portion Containing RDA	Function	Signs and Symptoms of Deficiency	Signs and Symptoms of Excess	Best Sources
Manganese	None*	Cofactor of enzymes involved in energy metabolism Required for bone formation Essential for normal brain function Magnesium may substitute for manganese in some functions	Weight Loss Hypercholesterolemia Nausea Vomiting Dermatitis Changes in hair color	Not reported due to diet Miners: liver damage Parkinson-like syndrome—monotone voice, CNS impairment	Wheat bran Legumes Nuts Leafy vegetables
Cobalt	None	Component of vitamin B_{12}	Not reported	Polycythemia Goiter	Meat, poultry Fish, shellfish Milk
Molybdenum	None*	Cofactor for enzymes involved in protein synthesis	TPN patient: Inability to process sulfur-containing amino acids	Hyperuricemia Gout	Organ meats Legumes Grains

*See Table of Estimated Safe and Adequate Daily Intakes (ESADDI) of Selected Vitamins and Minerals (Appendix I).

Summary

Minerals are inorganic substances that are necessary for good health. Like vitamins, they help to regulate body functions without providing energy. Unlike vitamins, minerals become part of the body's structure and enzymes.

In human nutrition, minerals are classified as major or trace. Major minerals are present in the body in amounts of 5 grams (1 teaspoonful) or more; the daily recommended intake is 100 milligrams or more.

Trace minerals are those present in amounts smaller than 5 grams; the daily recommended intake is less than 100 milligrams.

People can be adversely affected by either insufficient or excessive intakes of minerals, as is true of vitamins. Strangely, some minerals pro-duce the same symptoms in both cases. When a client is nourished only by a very restrictive diet or by intravenous feedings for a long time, deficiencies of trace minerals may become apparent. In the United States, increasing the intake of two minerals, iron and calcium, has the potential to improve the health of millions of people.

Food is the safest source of nutrients. To prevent possible toxicity, people who take supplements should limit intake to RDA, AI, or ESADDI levels. Pharmaceutical preparations are preferred to "natural" supplements, whose strengths may be uncertain and that may contain possible contaminants.

Case Study 8–1

Mrs. B is a 34-year-old woman who has related her fear of osteoporosis to the nurse. A recent visit to a 75-year-old aunt crystallized this fear. The aunt has become stooped and recently broke her hip. Mrs. B is especially concerned because she has often been told she resembles this aunt. Mrs. B asks, "Is there anything I can do to prevent this from happening to me?"

A 24-hour recall of dietary intake revealed a total of 1 cup of milk and no other dairy products. Mrs. B did consume two 3 oz. servings of meat. Mrs. B has three small children and stated that they are exercise enough for her. She sits outside and watches them play on every nice day.

Mrs. B is 5 ft. 3 in. tall and weighs 110 lb. She is Caucasian with fair skin.

Nursing Care Plan

Subjective Data	Fear of osteoporosis
	Family history positive for osteoporosis
	Less than AI for calcium previous 24 hours
	Meeting Food Pyramid guideline for meat group
	No planned exercise program
Objective Data	Height: 5 ft, 3 in.
	Weight: 110 lb
	Caucasian, fair, slight build
Nursing Diagnosis	NANDA: Health seeking behavior (North American Nursing Diagnosis Association, 1999, with permission.)
	Regarding preventive measures for osteoporosis related to fear of repeating aunt's experience as evidenced by request for information

Desired Outcomes Evaluation Criteria	Nursing Actions/ Interventions	Rationale
NOC: Health seeking behavior (Johnson, Maas, and Moorhead, 2000, with permission.)	NIC: Self-modification assistance (McCloskey and Bulechek, 2000, with permission.)	
Client will list appropriate actions to maintain a strong skeleton after teaching session.	Teach client how to consume 1000 mg of calcium daily: 3 cups of milk or equivalent.	One cup of milk contains approximately 300 mg of calcium + 100 mg from other sources
	Teach client factors favoring calcium absorption: moderate protein intake.	High protein intake causes increased calcium excretion by the kidneys.
	Teach client role of exercise in making bones strong.	Weight-bearing exercise stimulates the osteoblasts to build bone.

Critical Thinking Question

1. What additional dietary information would you need before recommending good sources of calcium for Mrs. B?
2. Suppose Mrs. B implements the suggested interventions. What other assessment data would be helpful to broaden the scope of preventing osteoporosis?
3. Is the problem described in the Case Study a significant one for a 34-year-old woman? Why or why not?

Study Aids

Subjects	Internet Sites
Dairy Products	http://www.nationaldairycouncil.org
	http://www.milk.co.uk/
	http://www.whymilk.com
Fluoride	http://www.ada.org/consumer/fluoride/fl-menu.html
	http://www.iupui.edu/it/iuortho/fluoride.html
	http://cda.org/public/pubhsrvc.html
Iodine and Goiter	http://encarta.msn.com/find/search.asp?tr=122&search=goiter
	http://www.idrc.ca/mi/idddocs/idd293.htm
	http://endocrineweb.com/goiter/html
Iron	http://www.ironpanel.org.au
	http://www.hemochromatosis.org
	http://text.nlm.nih.gov/cps/www/cps.28.html
	http://www.ama-assn.org/scipubs/journals/archive/jama/vol_277/no_12/oc6c11a.htm
	http://cpmcnet.columbia.edu/texts/gcps/gcps0032.html
Osteoporosis	http://www.nof.org
	http://www.osteo.org
Plumbism	www.hud.gov/lea
	www.leadlisting.org
	www.ama-assn.org/consumer.htm
Poison Control	http://www.fda.gov/fdac/features/296_kid.html
	http://vm.cfsan.fda.gov/~dms/bgiron.html
Sodium	http://www.nalusda.gov/fnic/dga95/sodium.html

Chapter Review

1. Like vitamins, minerals give no energy to the body. Unlike vitamins, minerals:
   a. Are completely absorbed from the intestinal tract
   b. Become part of the structure of the body
   c. Cause few clinical problems because of their great abundance in foods
   d. Cannot accumulate to the extent that they cause problems
2. Calcium is necessary for strong bones and teeth. It is also necessary for:
   a. Maintaining stomach acidity
   b. Enabling muscle contraction
   c. Preventing blood clots
   d. Assisting with the production of insulin
3. From which of the following sources of iron is the greatest percentage of iron absorbed by the average person?
   a. Eggs
   b. Ferrous sulfate tablets
   c. Meat
   d. Vegetables
4. Which of the following individuals would be at greatest risk for a mineral deficiency?
   a. Someone who consumes no dairy products.
   b. Someone who consumes no shellfish.
   c. Someone who consumes no red meat.
   d. Someone who drinks tea or coffee with every meal.
5. The most common nutrient deficiency in the United States is that of:
   a. Calcium
   b. Iodine
   c. Iron
   d. Zinc

Clinical Analysis

Mrs. H is a 30-year-old mother of three children all under 5 years of age. On her 6-week postpartum visit, her hemoglobin level was 10 grams per 100 milliliters of blood. She is given a prescription for ferrous sulfate and referred to the office nurse for nutrition counseling regarding her iron intake.

Mrs. H tells the nurse that she eats what the children eat; cold cereal and milk for breakfast, peanut butter and jelly sandwiches and maybe a banana for lunch, and casseroles of tuna or hamburger for dinner. Mrs. H is a heavy coffee drinker, consuming 10 cups per day, two with each meal and a total of four others during "coffee breaks."

The H family is lower middle-class. Mr. H is a long-distance truck driver and is away from home for long intervals. Mrs. H has some knowledge of iron needs and sources because of her three pregnancies. She is reluctant to continue the ferrous sulfate she has been taking throughout her pregnancy. "It binds me up," she tells the nurse. Also, Mrs. H maintains she cannot eat liver: "It gags me."

1. To maximize Mrs. H's iron intake with as little change in her habits as possible, the nurse would want to know:
   a. Whether Mrs. H drinks regular or decaffeinated coffee
   b. What kinds of cereal Mrs. H consumes
   c. At what time of day the H family eats
   d. Whether or not Mrs. H has tried veal liver
2. Which of the following statements by Mrs. H would indicate she understood the nurse's instructions correctly?
   a. "I should eat a little meat, fish, or poultry with every meal containing grain and fruit and vegetable sources of iron."
   b. "I should increase the fiber in my diet because it will increase the absorption of iron."
   c. "If I want an alcoholic beverage, beer contains the most iron in a readily absorbable form."
   d. "Since I am taking an iron supplement, it is not important how I eat."
3. To meet the safety needs of the H children, the nurse instructs Mrs. H to keep her ferrous sulfate in a locked cupboard. The reason for this is:
   a. Interactions of iron tablets with vitamin supplements intended for children can cause deficiencies of water soluble vitamins.
   b. The human body has no effective means of excreting an overload of iron.
   c. Iron poisoning, although rare, can occur if a child ingests more than 30 tablets of ferrous sulfate.
   d. Because iron binds with calcium, an overdose of iron would cause rickets.

Bibliography

Abreo, K, Adlakha, A, and Kilpatrick, S, et al.: The milk-alkali syndrome. Arch Intern Med 153:1005, 1993.

Aloia, JF, et al.: Calcium supplementation with and without hormone replacement therapy to prevent postmenopausal bone loss. Ann Inter Med 120:97, 1994.

Alves, G, et al.: Neurologic disorders due to brain manganese deposition in a jaundiced patient receiving long-term parenteral nutrition. J Parenter Enteral Nutr 21:41, 1997.

Andrews, M, and Gallagher-Allred, C: The role of zinc in wound healing. Adv Wound Care 12:137, 1999.

Beall, DP, and Scofield, RH: Milk-alkali syndrome associated with calcium carbonate consumption. Medicine 74:89, 1995.

Beutler, E: How little we know about the absorption of iron. Am J Clin Nutr 66:419, 1997.

Blaauw, R, et al.: Risk factors for the development of osteoporosis in a South African population. South African Med J 84:328, 1994.

Boosalis, MG, Stuart, MA, and McClain, CJ: Zinc metabolism in the elderly. In Morley, JE, Glick, Z, and Rubenstein (eds): Geriatric Nutrition ed 2. Raven Press, Ltd, New York, 1995.

Brensilver, JM, and Goldberger, E: A Primer of Water, Electrolyte, and Acid–Base Syndromes, ed 8. FA Davis, Philadelphia 1996.

Brzoska, MM, and Moniuszko-Jakoniuk, J: The influence of calcium content in the diet on cumulation and toxicity of cadmium in the organism. Arch Toxicol 72:63, 1998.

Burk, RF, and Levander, OA: Selenium. In Shils, ME, et al., (eds): Modern Nutrition in Health and Disease ed 9. Lippincott Williams and Wilkins, Philadelphia, 1999.

Centers for Disease Control: Achievements in public health, 1900–1999. MMWR 48:905, 1999a. Accessed 3/23/2000 at http://www.cdc.gov/epo/mmwr/preview/mmwrhtml/mm4840a1.htm

Centers for Disease Control: Lead poisoning associated with imported candy and powdered food coloring—California and Michigan. MMWR 47:1041, 1998a. Accessed 3/23/2000 at http://www.cdc.gov/epo/mmwr/preview/mmwrhtml/00055939.htm

Centers for Disease Control: Recommendations to Prevent and Control Iron Deficiency in the United States. MMWR 47:1, 1998b. Accessed 3/26/2000 at http://www.cdc.gov/epo/mmwr/preview/mmwrhtml/00051880.htm

Centers for Disease Control: Toddler deaths resulting from ingestion of iron supplements—Los Angeles, 1992–1993. MMWR 42:111, 1993. Accessed 11/27/1999 at http://www.cdc.gov/epo/mmwr/preview/mmwrhtml/00019593.htm

Centers for Disease Control: Water fluoridation and costs of Medicaid treatment for dental decay—Louisiana, 1995–1996, MMWR 48:753, 1999b. Accessed 9/6/99 at http://www.cdc.gov/epo/mmwr/preview/mmwrhtml/mm4834a2.htm

Chapuy, MC, et al.: Vitamin D_3 and calcium to prevent hip fractures in elderly women. N Engl J Med 327:1637, 1992.

Chiu, KM et al.: Changes in bone resorption during the menstrual cycle. J Bone Miner Res 14:609, 1999.

Christensen, NK, et al.: Juniper ash as a source of calcium in the Navajo diet. J Am Diet Assoc 98:333, 1998.

Coggon, D, and Cooper, C: Fluoridation of water supplies. Brit Med J 319:269, 1999. Accessed 3/27/2000 at http://www.bmj.com/cgi/content/full/319/7205/269

Committee on Environmental Health, American Academy of Pediatrics: Screening for elevated blood lead levels. Pediatrics 101:1072, 1998.

Connor, JR, and Beard, JL: Dietary iron supplements in the elderly: To use or not to use? Nutrition Today 32:102, 1997.

Darnton-Hill, I, et al.: Iron and folate fortification in the Americas to prevent and control micronutrient malnutrition: An analysis. Nutr Rev 57:25, 1999.

Dawson-Hughes, B, et al.: Effect of calcium and vitamin D supplementation on bone density in men and women 65 years of age or older. N Engl J Med 337:670, 1997.

Dawson-Hughes, B, et al.: Effect of vitamin D supplementation on wintertime and overall bone loss in healthy postmenopausal women. Ann Intern Med 115:505, 1991.

Dawson-Hughes, B, et al.: Rates of bone loss in postmenopausal women randomly assigned to one of two dosages of vitamin D. Am J Clin Nutr 61:1140, 1995.

DePaola, DP, Faine, MP, and Palmer, CA: Nutrition in relation to dental medicine. In Shils, ME, et al., (eds): Modern Nutrition in Health and Disease ed 9. Lippincott Williams and Wilkins, Philadelphia, 1999.

Doufas, AG, et al.: The predominant form of non-toxic goiter in Greece is now autoimmune thyroiditis. Eur J Endocrinol 140:505, 1999.

Dowsett, R, and Shannon, M: Letter to the Editor. N Engl J Med 331:1661, 1994.

Eby, GA: Zinc ion availability—the determinant of efficacy in zinc lozenge treatment of common colds. J Antimicrob Chemother 40:483, 1997.

Fairbanks, VF: Iron in medicine and nutrition. In Shils, ME, et al. (eds): Modern Nutrition in Health and Disease ed 9. Lippincott Williams and Wilkins, Philadelphia, 1999.

Fairweather-Tait, SJ, Fox, TE, and Mallilin A: Balti curries and iron. Br Med J 310:1368, 1995.

Farrell, SE, et al.: Blood lead levels in emergency department patients with retained lead bullets and shrapnel. Acad Emerg Med 6:208, 1999.

Federal Trade Commission: QVC Cable Network and maker of Cold-eeze zinc lozenges agree to settle FTC charges. 11/23/99. Accessed 3/4/2000 at http://www.ftc.gov/opa/1999/9911/qvcquig.htm

Galloway, R, and McGuire, J: Determinants of compliance with iron supplementation: Supplies, side effects, or psychology? Soc Sci Med 39:381, 1994.

Gibson, RS, Donovan, UM, and Heath, A-LM: Dietary strategies to improve the iron and zinc nutriture of young women following a vegetarian diet. Plant Foods Hum Nutr 51:1, 1997.

Gordeuk, VR: Dietary iron overload [reply to letter]. N Engl J Med 326:1705, 1992.

Greenspan, SL: A 73-year old woman with osteoporosis. JAMA 281:1531, 1999.

Greger, JL, and Malecki, EA: Manganese: How do we know our limits? Nutrition Today 32:116, 1997.

Gregor, JL and Sutherland, JE: Aluminum exposure and metabolism. Crit Rev Clin Lab Sci 34:439, 1997.

Groff, JL, Gropper, SS, and Hunt, SM: Advanced Nutrition and Human Metabolism, ed 2. West, Minneapolis, 1995.

Hallberg, L, Hulthen, L, and Garby, I: Iron stores in man in relation to diet and iron requirements. Eur J Clin Nutr 52:623, 1998.

Hetzel, BS, and Clugston, GA: Iodine. In Shils, ME, et al. (eds): Modern Nutrition in Health and Disease ed 9. Lippincott Williams and Wilkins, Philadelphia, 1999.

Holben, DH, and Smith, AM: The diverse role of selenium within selenoproteins: A review. J Am Diet Assoc 99:836, 1999.

Hopper, JL, and Seeman, E: The bone density of female twins discordant for tobacco use. N Engl J Med 330:387, 1994.

Johnson, M, Maas, M, and Moorhead, S: Nursing Outcomes Classification (NOC), ed 2. Mosby, Philadelphia, 2000.

Johnson, MA, Smith, MM, and Edmonds, JT: Copper, iron, zinc, and manganese in dietary supplements, infant formulas, and ready-to-eat breakfast cereals. Am J Clin Nutr 67:1035S, 1998.

Johnston, CO, et al.: Calcium supplementation and increases in bone mineral density in children. N Engl J Med 327:82, 1992.

Kafritsa, Y, et al.: Long-term outcome of brain manganese deposition in patients on home parenteral nutrition. Arch Dis Child 79:262, 1998.

Kakosy, T, Hudak, A, and Naray, M: Lead intoxication epidemic caused by ingestion of contaminated ground paprika. Clinical Toxicology 34:507, 1996.

Kaleita, TA, Kinsbourne, M, and Menkes, JH: A neurobahavioral syndrome after failure to thrive on chloride-deficient formula. Dev Med Child Neurol 33:626, 1991.

King, JC, and Keen, CL: Zinc. In Shils, ME, et al. (eds): Modern Nutrition in Health and Disease ed 9. Lippincott Williams and Wilkins, Philadelphia, 1999.

Knochel, JP: Phosphorus. In Shils, ME, et al. (eds): Modern Nutrition in Health and Disease ed 9. Lippincott Williams and Wilkins, Philadelphia, 1999.

Komaki, H, et al.: Tremor and seizures associated with chronic manganese intoxication. Brain Dev 21:122, 1999.

Krall, EA, et al.: Vitamin D receptor alleles and rates of bone loss: Influences of years since menopause and calcium intake. J Bone Miner Res 10:978, 1995.

Krall, EA, and Dawson-Hughes, B: Osteoporosis. In Shils, ME, et al. (eds): Modern Nutrition in Health and Disease ed 9. Lippincott Williams and Wilkins, Philadelphia, 1999a.

Krall, EA, and Dawson-Hughes, B: Smoking increases bone loss and decreases intestinal calcium absorption. J Bone Miner Res 14:215, 1999b.

Lane, JM: Osteoporosis: medical prevention and treatment. Spine 22:32S, 1997.

Lau, EM, and Woo, J: Nutrition and osteoporosis. Curr Opin Rheumatol 10:368, 1998.

Lindeman, RD: Minerals in medical practice. In Halpern, SL (ed): Quick Reference to Clinical Nutrition ed 2.JB Lippincott, Philadelphia, 1987.

Lips, P, et al.: Determinants of vitamin D status in patients with hip fracture and in elderly control subjects. Am J Clin Nutr 46:1005, 1987.

Looker, AC, et al.: Prevalence of iron deficiency in the United States. JAMA 277:973, 1997.

Lubin, BH, et al.: Nutritional anemias. In Walker, WA, and Watkins, JB (eds): Nutrition in Pediatrics, ed 2. BC Decker, Hamilton, Ontario, 1997.

Markowitz, M, Rosen, JF, and Clemente, I: Clinician follow-up of children screened for lead poisoning. Am J Public Health 89:1088, 1999.

Marshall, S: Zinc gluconate and the common cold. Review of randomized controlled trials. Can Fam Physician 44:1037, 1998.

Matte, TD: Reducing blood lead levels. JAMA 281:2340, 1999.

Mauskop, A, and Altura, BM: Role of magnesium in the pathogenesis and treatment of migraines. Clin Neurosci 5:24, 1998.

McCloskey, JC, and Bulechek, GM: Nursing Interventions Classification (NIC), 3 ed. Mosby, Philadelphia, 2000.

Medeiros-Neto, G: Iodide deficiency disorders. In DeGroot, LJ (ed): Endocrinology ed 3 vol I. WB Saunders, Philadelphia, 1995.

Meyer, HE, et al.: Risk factors for hip fracture in a high incidence area: A case-control study from Oslo, Norway. Osteoporosis Int 5:239, 1995.

Miller, MB, et al.: Pool cue chalk: A source of environmental lead. Pediatrics 97:916, 1996.

Mowad, E, Haddad, I, and Gemmel, DJ: Management of lead poisoning from ingested fishing sinkers. Arch Pediatr Adolesc Med 152:485, 1998.

Murphy, S, et al.: Milk consumption and bone mineral density in middle aged and elderly women. Br Med J 308:939, 1994.

Nagatomo, S, et al.: Manganese intoxication during total parenteral nutrition: Report of two cases and review of the literature. J Neurol Sci 162:102, 1999.

Naghii, MR: The significance of dietary boron, with particular reference to athletes. Nutr Health 13:31, 1999.

National Research Council: Diet and Health: Implications for Reducing Chronic Disease Risk. Report of the Committee on Diet and Health, Food and Nutrition Board, Commission on Life Sciences. National Academy Press, Washington, DC, 1989.

Nelson, M, et al.: A 1 year walking program and increased dietary calcium in postmenopausal women: Effects on bone. Am J Clin Nutr 53:1304, 1991.

Nelson, ME, et al.: Effects of high-intensity strength training on multiple risk factors for osteoporotic fractures. JAMA 272:1909, 1994.

Nielsen, FH: Controversial chromium: Does the superstar mineral of the Mountebanks receive appropriate attention from clinicians and nutritionists? Nutrition Today 31:226, 1996.

Nielsen, FH: Ultratrace minerals. In Shils, ME, et al. (eds): Modern Nutrition in Health and Disease ed 9. Lippincott Williams and Wilkins, Philadelphia, 1999.

North American Nursing Diagnosis Association: Nursing Diagnoses: Definitions and Classification 1999–2000, North American Nursing Diagnosis Association, Philadelphia, 1999.

Olivares, M, et al.: Copper in infant nutrition: Safety of World Health Organization provisional guideline value for copper content of drinking water. J Pediatr Gastroenterol Nutr 26:251, 1998.

Pak, CYC, et al.: Treatment of postmenopausal osteoporosis with slow-release sodium fluoride. Ann Intern Med 123:401, 1995.

Penland, JG: The importance of boron nutrition for brain and psychological function. Biol Trace Elem Res 66:299, 1998.

Pennington, JAT: A review of iodine toxicity reports. J Am Diet Assoc 90:1571, 1990.

Reid, IR, et al.: Long-term effects of calcium supplementation on bone loss and fractures in postmenopausal women: A randomized controlled trial. Am J Med 98:331, 1995.

Reinhart, RA, and Desbiens, NA: Hypomagnesemia in patients entering the ICU. Crit Care Med 13:506, 1985.

Remer, T, Neubert, A, and Manz, F: Increased risk of iodine deficiency with vegetarian nutrition. Brit J Nutr 81:45, 1999.

Reynolds, N, et al.: Manganese requirement and toxicity in patients on home parenteral nutrition. Clin Nutr 17:227, 1998.

Ribaya-Mercado, JD: Importance of adequate vitamin A status during iron supplementation. Nutr Rev 55:306, 1997.

Roncagliolo, M, et al.: Evidence of altered central nervous system development in infants with iron deficiency anemia at 6 month: Delayed maturation of auditory brainstem responses. Am J Clin Nutr 68:683, 1998.

Ross, EA, Szabo, NJ, and Tebbett, IR: Lead Content of Calcium Supplements. JAMA 284:1425, 2000.

Ryan, D, et al.: Protecting children from lead poisoning and building healthy communities. Am J Public Health 89:822, 1999.

Sandstrom, B: Considerations in estimates of requirements and critical intake of zinc: Adaption, availability and interactions. Analyst 120:913, 1995.

Santinelli, et al.: Magnesium deficiency and dizziness: A case of electrolyte imbalance. Geriatrics 54:67, 1999.

Scelfo, GM, and Flegal, AR: Lead in calcium supplements. Environ Health Perspect 108:309, 2000.

Scrimshaw, NS: Iron deficiency. Scientific Am 265:46, 1991.

Shannon, M, and Graef, J: Hazard of lead in infant formula [letter]. N Engl J Med 326:137, 1992.

Shils, ME: Magnesium. In Shils, ME, et al. (eds): Modern Nutrition in Health and Disease ed 9. Lippincott Williams and Wilkins, Philadelphia, 1999.

Snyder, DC, et al.: Development of a population-specific risk assessment to predict elevated blood lead levels in Santa Clara County, California. Pediatrics 96:643, 1995.

Spiegel, JE, and Willenbucher, RF: Rapid development of severe copper deficiency in a patient with Crohn's Disease receiving parenteral nutrition. J Parenter Enteral Nutr 23:169, 1999.

Stoecker, BJ: Chromium. In Shils, ME, et al. (eds): Modern Nutrition in Health and Disease ed 9. Lippincott Williams and Wilkins, Philadelphia, 1999.

Stromberg, U, Schutz, A, and Skerfring, S: Substantial decrease in blood lead in Swedish children, 1978–94, associated with petrol lead. Occup Environ Med 52:764, 1995.

Subcommittee on the 10th Edition of the RDAs. Food and Nutrition Board. Commission on Life Sciences. National Research Council: Recommended Dietary Allowances, ed 10. National Academy Press, Washington, DC, 1989.

Sunyer, T, et al.: Estrogen's bone-protective effects may involve differential IL-1 receptor regulation in human osteoclast-like cells. J Clin Invest 103:1409, 1999.

Thomas, CL (ed): Tabor's Cyclopedic Medical Dictionary ed 18. FA Davis, Philadelphia, 1997.

Tsukada, H, et al.: Intrathoracic retroesophageal goiter causing tracheal stenosis. Jpn J Thorac Cardiovasc Surg 47:174, 1999.

Turnlund, JR: Copper. In Shils, ME, et al. (eds): Modern Nutrition in Health and Disease ed 9. Lippincott Williams and Wilkins, Philadelphia, 1999.

Verma, S, Cam, MC, and McNeill, JH: Nutritional factors that can favorably influence the glucose/insulin system: Vanadium. J Am Coll Nutr 17:11, 1998.

Weaver, CM, and Heaney, RP: Calcium. In Shils, ME, et al. (eds): Modern Nutrition in Health and Disease ed 9. Lippincott Williams and Wilkins, Philadelphia, 1999.

Wilkinson, EAJ, and Hawke, CI: Does oral zinc aid the healing of chronic leg ulcers? Arch Dermatol 134:1556, 1998.

Yamashita, H, et al.: Postoperative tetany in Graves Disease: Important role for vitamin D metabolites. Ann Surg 229:237, 1999.

Zhou, Y, and Brittin, HC: Increased iron content of some Chinese foods due to cooking in steel woks. J Am Diet Assoc 94:1153, 1994

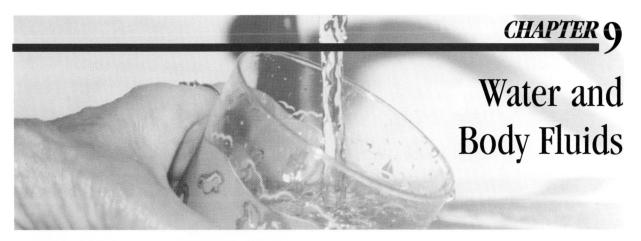

CHAPTER 9

Water and Body Fluids

LEARNING OBJECTIVES
After completing this chapter, the student should be able to:
1. Describe the locations and functions of water in the body.
2. Discuss the body's control mechanisms for maintaining fluid and electrolyte balance.
3. Recognize how buffer systems maintain acid–base balance.
4. List amounts of water usually gained and lost by adults in a day.
5. Differentiate insensible from sensible water loss.
6. Identify methods of assessing water balance in the body.
7. Distinguish between heat exhaustion and heat stroke with respect to cause and first-aid treatment.

The need for water is more urgent than the need for any other nutrient in the body. Human beings can live a month without food but only 6 days without water. This chapter explains why water is so important in the body and discusses ways in which water balance is achieved. The assessment and treatment of fluid volume deficit and fluid volume excess are also discussed.

The distribution and movement of water in the body are intricately bound to certain elements. Understanding this relationship requires knowledge of the essentials of atomic structure. This chapter begins, then, with a discussion of how atoms interact with one another.

Interactions between Atoms

An element is a primary, simple substance that cannot be broken down by ordinary chemical methods into any other substance. There are more than 105 known elements. Oxygen is an element, as are sodium, chlorine, and the other minerals discussed in the previous chapter.

Atoms

Elements are composed of smaller parts called **atoms**. In the center of an atom is the nucleus, which contains protons and neutrons and gives an atom its weight and mass. Circling around the nucleus like satellites are electrons. These electrons are arranged in a consistent manner: a maximum of two in the orbit or shell closest to the nucleus, and a maximum of eight in each of the outer shells. The ability of an atom to react chemically depends on the number of "empty slots" in the outermost electron shell.

Chemical Bonding

A **compound** is a substance created by the chemical bonding (joining) of two or more different kinds of atoms (elements). A chemical bond is the force that binds atoms together. A compound is formed when atoms share electrons or when one atom donates one or more electrons to another atom. For example, water (a liquid) is formed when two atoms of hydrogen (a colorless, odorless gas) are joined with one atom of oxygen (another colorless, odorless gas).

Similarly, sodium chloride (table salt) is a compound of sodium (an unstable, silvery white, waxy, soft metal) and chlorine (a greenish yellow poisonous gas). Sodium and chlorine are so chemically active that in nature they are always found bound to each other or to other elements (Fig. 9–1).

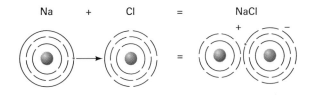

Figure 9–1:
Formation of an ionic bond. An atom of sodium loses an electron to an atom of chlorine. The two ions formed have unlike charges, are attracted to one another and form a molecule of sodium chloride. (From Scanlon and Sanders, 1995, p. 25, with permission.)

A sodium atom has only one electron in its outer shell; a chlorine atom has seven. In close proximity, the sodium atom donates the electron in its outer shell to the outer shell of the chlorine atom. With the loss of its electron, the sodium now has an electrical charge of +1 and is called a sodium **ion** (Na+). Ions with positive charges are referred to as cations. The chlorine atom, which gained an electron, now has a charge of -1 and is called a chloride ion (Cl–). Ions with negative charges are referred to as **anions**.

Because these ions have opposite charges (+ and -) they are attracted to one another and unite, forming sodium chloride (NaCl). The chemical bond that holds the sodium and chloride ions together is called an **ionic bond**. There are other types of chemical bonds (not discussed here). Sodium can donate its single electron to other elements beside chlorine, and other elements can form ionic bonds as well.

An **electrolyte** is an element or compound that, when dissolved in water, separates (dissociates) into ions capable of conducting an electrical current. These electrically charged particles are then available to take part in other chemical reactions. Clinical Application 9–1 discusses examples of uses and hazards related to electrolytes in the body.

Distribution of Water in the Body

More than half of body weight is water, which is found in and around the cells, within the blood and lymph vessels, and in various body cavities. Some tissues have significantly more water than others: muscle tissue is 70 percent water, fat tissue is 30 percent water, and bone tissue is 10 percent water. A man's body is 60 to 65 percent water and a woman's body is 50 to 54 percent water. Men have a higher water content because of their greater muscle mass.

Age affects the proportion of water in a body. Compared with the 50 to 65 percent for women and men, an infant's body is 75 percent water. Premature infants may be 80 percent water by weight. Infants, especially premature infants, are at high risk of fluid imbalances because of the proportion and distribution of water in their bodies. The adult proportion of water to body weight is reached at about 9 to 12 months of age.

Aging also affects adult proportions of water in the body. Women experience a 17 percent decrease in total body water from the third to the eighth decade, compared with an 11 percent decrease for men in the same time period. This change is a reflection of the decline in lean body mass and occurs chiefly with the cell compartments (Pfeil, Katz, and Davis, 1995).

Fluid Compartments

Body fluids are contained in intracellular and extracellular compartments (see Fig. 9–2). These compartments are separated by semipermeable membranes, which allow some substances to pass through and prevent the passage of other substances. Water passes freely through the membranes. Ten recently identified water transport proteins, called **aquaporins**, explain the speed at which water moves across cell membranes. Aquaporins are membrane proteins that function as water-selective channels in the plasma membranes of many cells (Dibas, Mia, and Yorio, 1998; Knoers and Deen, 1998). Research indicates that aquaporins may be involved in conditions such as cataract formation, hypertension, edema, heart failure, and hydrocephalus (Connolly, Shanahan, and Weissberg, 1996). As more is learned about aquaporins in health, it may be possible to develop new drug treatments to target specific areas of malfunction in disease.

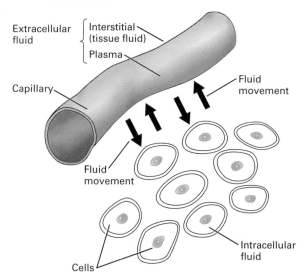

Figure 9–2:
Three fluid compartments of the body. In distributing nutrients and disposing of waste, fluid moves from capillaries to interstitial fluid, to the cell, and vice versa. (From Scanlon and Sanders, 1995, p. 438, with permission.)

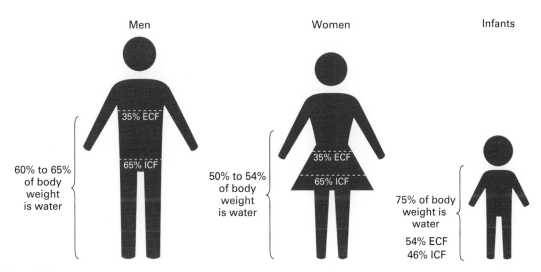

Figure 9–3:
The relative amounts of body weight that are intracellular and extracellular water in men, women, and infants.

Intracellular Fluid

The fluid inside the cells is called intracellular. In adults, intracellular water constitutes 65 percent of body water. In infants, 46 percent of the body water is intracellular.

Extracellular Fluid

All fluid outside the cells is extracellular. In adults, 40 percent of the body's water is extracellular; in infants, 54 percent is extracellular. Figure 9–3 illustrates the proportions of intracellular to extracellular fluid in men, women, and infants. The difference is important, because extracellular fluid is more easily and rapidly lost to the outside of the body than is intracellular fluid. Extracellular fluid includes interstitial, intravascular, lymph, and transcellular fluids.

INTERSTITIAL FLUID Located between the cells or surrounding the cells, **interstitial fluid** assists in transporting substances between the cells and the blood and lymph vessels.

INTRAVASCULAR FLUID **Intravascular fluid** is found within the blood vessels, arteries, arterioles, capillaries, venules, and veins. The liquid part of the blood is called **plasma;** minus the clotting elements the liquid part of the blood is called **serum.** As is illustrated in Figure 9–4, 91.5 percent of the plasma is water.

LYMPHATIC FLUID The venous system cannot collect and return all the fluid from the tissues to the heart. The **lymph,** via the lymphatic vessels, assists in returning the fluid part of the blood to the heart.

TRANSCELLULAR FLUID The **transcellular fluids** include cerebrospinal fluid, pericardial fluid, pleural fluid, synovial fluid, intraocular fluids, and gastrointestinal secretions. The transcellular fluids are constantly being secreted into their spaces and reabsorbed into the vascular system.

Functions of Water

Water has important functions in the body. As a component of cells, water helps give the body shape and form. It is a constituent of the structure of many of the body's large molecules such as protein and glycogen. Some body water also serves as a lubricant, as in mucus secretions and joint fluid.

Water helps to regulate body temperature. It absorbs the heat produced by fever and the heat resulting from metabolic processes. On average, tissue metabolism generates 100 kilocalories per hour. The blood carries excess heat to the skin where it is dissipated by sweating or radiation. (The later Clinical Calculation 9–4 gives an example involving evaporative water loss in fever.)

Water is a **solvent** for minerals, vitamins, glucose, and other small molecules. (The substance that is dissolved in a solvent is called a **solute.**) As a solvent, water is able to transport nutrients to the cells and carry waste products away from the cells. In addition, it becomes a medium for chemical reactions and participates in chemical reactions, as may be seen in many of the digestive processes, such as the breakdown of proteins to amino acids. See Table 9–1 for a summary of the functions of water.

Absorption, Metabolism, and Storage of Water

No storage tanks for water exist in the body. Water continually moves from one body compartment to another and is often reused by the body to perform different tasks. A small amount of water can be absorbed into the bloodstream from the stomach. A liter of water can be absorbed from the small intestine in an hour.

Table 9–1 Functions of Water
• Gives shape and form to cells
• Helps form the structure of large molecules
• Serves as a lubricant
• Helps to regulate body temperature
• Serves as a solvent
• Transports nutrients to cells
• Carries waste products away from cells
• Is a medium for chemical reactions
• Participates in chemical reactions

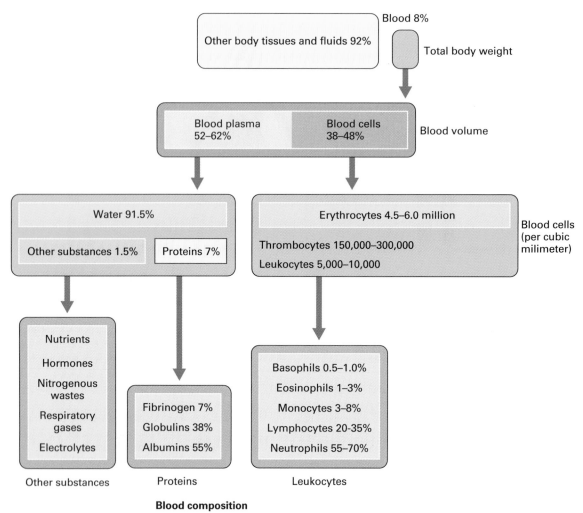

Blood composition

Components of blood and relationship of blood to other body tissues

Figure 9–4:
The blood comprises 8 percent of the body weight. The largest single component of the blood is water. (Reprinted from Thomas, 1997, p. 235, with permission.)

The metabolism of the energy nutrients produces water. Each energy nutrient produces a different amount of metabolic water: 1 gram of carbohydrate produces 0.60 gram, 1 gram of fat produces 1.07 grams, and 1 gram of protein produces 0.41 gram. One ounce of pure alcohol requires 8 ounces of water for its metabolism. Alcohol, rather than quenching thirst, can cause dehydration and increased thirst.

Under conditions that have disrupted the individual's automatic adaptive mechanisms, water may be retained. The accumulation of excessive amounts of fluid between the cells (in the interstitial compartments) is called **edema**. Hypothyroidism, congestive heart failure, severe protein deficiency, and some kidney conditions may cause such water retention. Excessive water can be dispersed throughout the body, also. This condition is called **water intoxication**. It can be caused by excessive water intake (either by the intravenous or gastrointestinal route), cerebral concussion,

or hormonal disorders. Many of the symptoms are caused by diluting the concentration of the electrolytes in the body's fluid compartments.

Water Balance

For optimum health, the water lost through the kidneys, skin, lungs, and large intestine must be continually replaced. The electrolyte content of all body fluids must also be maintained within narrow limits. The body has automatic monitoring and regulating mechanisms to achieve this balance or homeostasis.

The Effect of Electrolytes on Water Balance

Each fluid compartment has an electrolyte composition that best serves its needs. Each of the fluid compartments has automatic mechanisms that are designed to keep it electrically neutral or balanced. The positive ions within a compartment must equal the negative ones. When shifts and losses occur, compensating shifts and gains take place to reestablish electroneutrality.

Regulation of Fluid Balance

Fluid balance is regulated by electrolytes because cells have no mechanism for holding onto water molecules, which pass freely through all membranes. However, cells can control the movement of electrolytes, and water tends to remain wherever the concentration of electrolytes is highest. In practical terms, water will follow high concentrations of electrolytes such as sodium, the ion most closely associated with water balance.

Important Body Electrolytes

Major mineral ions strongly influence not only water balance but also osmotic pressure, blood pressure, and acid–base balance, which will be discussed later in the chapter. Cations of importance in body fluids are sodium, potassium, calcium, and magnesium. Anions of importance include chloride, bicarbonate, phosphate, and sulfate. Sodium (Na^+) is the main electrolyte in extracellular fluid (ECF). Potassium (K^+) is the main electrolyte in intracellular fluid (ICF). Ionized sodium, potassium, and chloride are the solutes that maintain the balance between the intracellular and extracellular compartments. See Table 9–2 for a summary of the major body electrolytes.

Measurement of Electrolytes

Electrolytes are measured by the total number of particles in solution rather than their total weight, because chemical activity is determined by the concentration of electrolytes in any given solution. The unit of measure used in the United States is the **milliequivalent** expressed as milliequivalents per liter. The concentration of a pharmaceutical electrolyte in solution is also measured in milliequivalents per liter. Clinical Calculation 9–1 shows the conversion of milligrams of sodium chloride to milliequivalents.

Osmotic Pressure

Osmosis is the movement of water (or another solvent) across a semipermeable membrane from an area with fewer particles to one with more particles. The result, as long as the difference is reasonable, is an equalization of concentration on either side of the membrane. Clinical Application 9–2 describes an experiment to demonstrate osmosis.

Osmosis is a passive process. The movement of some substances, however, is active. Some substances require active transport mechanisms to push them through a membrane. Two such transport mechanisms are the sodium pump and the potassium pump. Located in cell membranes, these pumps are actually proteins that can move ions. **Sodium pumps** move sodium ions out of the cells (and the water follows). **Potassium pumps** move potassium ions into the cells. In this manner, the electrolyte concentrations of the intracellular and extracellular fluid compartments are maintained. Active transport requires energy.

DETERMINATION OF OSMOTIC PRESSURE When two solutions on either side of a semipermeable membrane have different concentrations, pressure develops. This pressure, which is exerted on the semipermeable membrane, is called **osmotic pressure**. Osmotic pressure causes a solvent such as water to cross the membrane, while the solutes (particles) that are outside the membrane cannot go through.

The size of the molecule and its ability to ionize determines the number of particles in a given concentration. Electrolytes readily ionize in solution. Disaccharides and monosaccharides do not ionize. Without the appropriate enzymes to split the disaccharide into its component monosaccharides, the disaccharide molecule remains intact. Just as there are more tacks in a pound than there are spikes in a pound, there are more particles in a given volume containing 100 kilocalories of a monosaccharide such as glucose compared with 100 kilocalories of a disaccharide such as lactose. The larger number of particles per unit volume exerts more osmotic pressure.

OSMOLARITY OF BODY FLUIDS The measure of the osmotic pressure exerted by the number of particles per volume of liquid is referred to as

Table 9–2 Major Body Electrolytes

Electrolyte	Fluid Compartment*	Functions
Cations		
Sodium (Na^+)	Extracellular	Major cation in ECF. Na^+ concentration in fluids determines the distribution of H_2O by osmosis. With Cl^- and HCO_3^-, Na^+ regulates acid-base balance.
Potassium (K^+)	Intracellular	Major cation in ICF. K^+ with Na^+ maintains water balance. With Na^+ and H^+, K^+ regulates acid-base balance.
Calcium	Extracellular†	Participates in permeability of cell membranes, transmission of nerve impulses, muscle action.
Magnesium (Mg^{2+})	Intracellular	Regulates nerve simulation and normal muscle action.
Anions		
Chloride (Cl^-)	Extracellular	Major anion in ECF. Helps maintain water balance and acid-base balance.
Bicarbonate (HCO_3^-)	Extracellular	Most important ECF buffer.
Phosphate (HPO_4^{2-})	Intracellular	Within the ICF, phosphates and proteins buffer 95 percent of the body's carbonic acid and 50 percent of other acids.

*ECP and ICF both contain all the cations and anions listed in this table but are labeled as either ECP or ICF according to the concentration. For example, sodium ions make up 142 of the total 155 milliequivalents per liter (of the cations) in the ECF.
†Of the cations, 3 percent in ECF and 1 percent in ICF.

Clinical Calculation 9–1 Converting Milligrams to Milliequivalents

Milligram is a measure of weight. Milliequivalent is a measure of the concentration of electrolytes (number of particles) per volume of solution. The usual amount of solution on which electrolytes are reported is 1 L.

To convert milligrams to milliequivalents, it is necessary to know the number of milligrams per liter, the molecular weight of the substance, and its valence. Valence, a number indicating the combining power of an atom, is found in many dictionaries.

A teaspoonful of table salt in 1 L of water will produce a 0.5 percent solution. (Isotonic sodium chloride is 0.9 percent.) How would the electrolytes be reported in milliequivalents? A teaspoonful is roughly 5 g. Since table salt is 40 percent sodium and 60 percent chloride, the liter of 0.5 percent salt water would contain 2 g (2000 mg) of sodium and 3 g (3000 mg) of chloride.

Two other values are needed: atomic or molecular weights, and valences. The atomic weight for sodium is 22,9898. Sodium has a valence of 1. The formula for converting milligrams to milliequivalents is:

$$mEq/L = \frac{(mg/L) \times valence}{molecular\ weight}$$

Filling in the sodium values we know for this case, we have:

$$mEq/L = \frac{2000\ (mg/L) \times 1}{22.9898} = 85\ mEq/L\ of\ sodium$$

Continuing, we can use the same formula with different values to calculate the milliequivalents of chloride. The atomic weight for chlorine is 35.453. Chlorine has a valence of 1.

Filling in the values for chloride, we have:

$$mEq/L = \frac{3000\ (mg/L) \times 1}{35.453} = 85\ mEq/L\ of\ chloride$$

Then, adding the sodium and chloride, we have:

$$87 + 85 = 172\ mEq/L\ in\ the\ 0.5\ percent\ solution.$$

its **osmolarity**. The unit of measure for osmotic activity is the **milliosmole**. Clinically, osmolarity is usually reported in milliosmoles per liter.

Osmolality, in contrast, is the measure of the osmotic pressure exerted by the number of particles per weight of solvent. Clinically, osmolality is usually reported in milliosmoles per kilogram.

The osmolality of human blood serum is about 300 milliosmoles per kilogram. (Laboratory texts list various ranges between 280 and 310 milliosmoles per kilogram.) Values above 350 milliosmoles per kilogram indicate a grave prognosis (Brensilver and Goldberger, 1996).

Most serum osmolarity is a function of sodium, potassium, and chloride. In the extracellular fluid, sodium is the primary determinant of osmolality.

OSMOLALITY AND NUTRITION Fluids are designated isotonic if they approximate the osmolality of the blood plasma. Fluids exerting less

osmotic pressure than plasma are labeled **hypotonic**. Those exerting greater osmotic pressure than plasma are called **hypertonic**.

Achieving the correct osmolality of fluids administered intravenously (by needle or tube into the vein) is very important. A solution that is too concentrated pulls water out of the red blood cells, and the cells shrivel and die. A solution that is too weak allows water to be pulled into the red blood cells until the cells burst.

Examples of isotonic fluids are 5 percent glucose in water and 0.9 percent sodium chloride. Only isotonic sodium chloride is given with red-blood cell products to avoid shrinking or bursting the red blood cells.

Less concentrated solutions of glucose and sodium chloride and plain water are hypotonic. Stronger solutions are hypertonic. Solutions containing sufficient nutrients to provide all a person's known needs are so strong that they must be infused into a large vein in the chest so that they are diluted quickly by the liberal volume of blood flowing past the infusion port or catheter. This procedure is discussed in Chapter 15.

Oral fluids also can be categorized by osmotic pressure. Plain water is hypotonic. Whole milk at 275 milliosmoles per liter is close to isotonic. Ginger ale with 510 milliosmoles per liter and 7-Up with 640 are both hypertonic. The significance of these differences will become apparent in the later section on treatment of fluid volume deficit.

SERUM ELECTROLYTES The electrolyte content of blood can also be reported in milliequivalents per liter. Normal serum sodium is 135 to 145 milliequivalents per liter. In most cases, because sodium is the most influential extracellular ion, osmolarity of the extracellular fluid can be estimated clinically by doubling the serum sodium value. Normal serum sodium doubled would be 270 to 296 milliosmoles per liter. Normal osmolality of the serum is about 300 milliosmoles per kilogram. This simple method gives a close approximation.

The other ion that health-care providers monitor carefully in clients with potential fluid and electrolyte imbalances is potassium. Most of the potassium in the body is inside the cells, at a concentration of 150 milliequivalents per liter. By contrast, potassium concentration in the blood is only 3.5 to 5.0 milliequivalents per liter. Even slight variations above or below these values can produce severe consequences. The heart muscle is particularly sensitive to high or low levels of potassium; abnormal levels can produce cardiac arrest.

Electrolyte Imbalances

Table 9–3 lists the normal values for serum sodium and serum potassium, along with the technical names and some of the signs and symptoms for deviations from the normal. Many other signs, including the direct meas-

CLINICAL APPLICATION 9–2

Osmosis in the Kitchen

To make sauerkraut, the cabbage is sliced very fine and placed in the bottom of a crock. Salt is then added to the dry cabbage. This is repeated, layer after layer, until the crock is full. At this point, much liquid will already have gathered, pulled from the cabbage pieces by the concentrated salt. After the cabbage ferments for 5 or 6 weeks, the crock is really full of "extra" juice.

To try a tiny batch of sauerkraut use 2 tsp of canning salt per pound of cabbage.

urement of serum electrolytes and the results of electrocardiograms, assist in the diagnosis. Dire consequences can result from any of these four imbalances. If the nurse recognizes and reports early signs and symptoms, the need for drastic treatment measures may be averted. Unfortunately, older clients may display fewer signs and symptoms than younger ones do (Pfeil, Katz, and Davis, 1995). The clinical chapters present more information about electrolyte imbalances commonly accompanying various disease conditions.

The Effect of Plasma Proteins on Water Balance

The body has highly developed mechanisms that maintain the constant flow of water and nutrients to the cells and the flow of water and waste materials from the cells. Adequate blood pressure is necessary for this transport system to function. Blood pressure is the force exerted against the walls of the arteries by the beating heart. It is reported in two numbers, 120/80, for example (measured in millimeters of mercury). The top number is the pressure when the heart beats, called **systolic pressure**. The bottom number is the pressure between beats, called the **diastolic pressure**. One of the factors necessary to maintain blood pressure is a sufficient volume of blood in the arteries and veins.

Water and nutrients in the blood are pushed out through the thin walls of the capillaries into the interstitial fluid by **hydrostatic pressure** (blood pressure) supplied by the heart. From the interstitial compartment, the water and nutrients cross cell membranes to bathe and nourish the cell. Plasma proteins, including albumin, remain in the capillaries because they are too large to squeeze through the capillary wall. Inside the blood vessels, the plasma proteins exert **colloidal osmotic pressure** (COP). The COP, now greater than the hydrostatic pressure, pulls water and waste materials from the interstitial fluid back into the blood capillaries. Thus, the volume of fluid within the blood vessels is maintained and the venous blood is returned to the lungs to take up oxygen, then to the heart to be recirculated. However, osmotic pressure within the cell is still being maintained by the balance of fluid and electrolytes as described above. Clinical Application 9–3 describes a condition in which a low serum protein is the cause of water imbalance.

CLINICAL APPLICATION 9-3

Protein-Energy Malnutrition and Water Balance

Starving children often look plump. They are not fat but edematous. These children are victims of kwashiorkor, a disease of protein-energy malnutrition. It occurs most often in children just after weaning when there is not enough protein in their diets to replace their mothers' milk.

Protein plays a crucial role in maintaining the volume of fluid in the blood vessels. These children develop edema because they do not have enough plasma proteins remaining in the capillaries to pull water back into the circulatory system. Thus, it accumulates in the interstitial spaces. Once treatment begins the plasma proteins will pull the retained water into the blood and the children will appear emaciated. This is a reminder that appearances can be deceiving. Malnutrition occurs in this country also. A thorough assessment may identify problem areas that on first glance are not apparent.

Body Regulation of Water Intake and Excretion

The body has mechanisms that regulate both the intake and the excretion of water. Normally, thirst governs water intake. The excretion of water is controlled mainly by two hormones: Antidiuretic hormone causes the body to reabsorb (retain) water; aldosterone causes the body to retain sodium.

Thirst Mechanism

Thirst is the desire for fluids, especially water. Thirst normally occurs when 10 percent of the intravascular volume is lost or when cellular volume is reduced by 1 to 2 percent. When there is too little water in the blood (or, put another way, when the solutes are too concentrated), there is an increase in the osmotic pressure of the blood. Special sensors in the **hypothalamus** monitor the osmotic pressure of the blood as it circulates in the brain. When the hypothalamus detects an increase in the osmotic pressure, it triggers the desire to drink. Sometimes the thirst mechanism

---

Table 9–3 Signs and Symptoms of Abnormal Serum Sodium and Potassium Levels

	Low	Normal	High
Sodium			
Lab value	Less than 135 mEq/L	135-148 mEq/L	Greater than 148 mEq/L
Condition	Hyponatremia		Hypernatremia
Symptoms	Irritability		Thirst
	Anxiety		Fatigue
Signs	Muscle twitching		Flushed skin
	Fingerprinting over the sternum		Sticky mucous membranes
	Seizures		Agitation
	Coma		Coma
Potassium			
Lab value	Less than 3.5 mEq/L	3.5-5.0 mEq/L	Greater than 5.0 mEq/L
Condition	Hypokalemia		Hyperkalemia
Symptoms	Nausea and/or vomiting		Irritability
	Paresthesias, esp. lower extremities		Abdominal cramps
			Weakness, esp. lower extremities
Signs	Decreased bowel sounds		Irregular pulse
	Weak, irregular pulse		Cardiac arrest if greater than
	Coma		8.5 mEq/L

goes awry. In such cases, because the precise neural control of thirst is unknown, conscious control of fluid intake is the mode of treatment (McKenna and Thompson, 1998).

Antidiuretic Hormone

If thirst is not alleviated, the sensors in the hypothalamus increase the secretion of **antidiuretic hormone (ADH)** from the posterior pituitary gland. ADH, also named **vasopressin**, causes the kidneys to return more water to the bloodstream rather than spill it into the urine. This effect is accomplished through the action of Aquaporin 2, the only water channel currently known to be activated by vasopressin.

Antidiuretic hormone has an additional effect of arterial vasoconstriction. By constricting blood vessels, it increases blood pressure. (When someone places a finger over the end of a garden hose and partly blocks the opening, the amount of water flowing is the same as before, but the smaller outlet increases the pressure.)

Sometimes the ADH mechanism goes awry. In **diabetes insipidus** the hypothalamus does not secrete ADH or the kidneys do not respond appropriately. Diabetes insipidus can be caused by brain tumor, surgery, trauma, infection, radiation injury, or congenital conditions. If the hypothalamus is not secreting ADH, a pharmaceutical preparation can be given. Clinical Application 9–4 tells about a condition called syndrome of inappropriate secretion of antidiuretic hormone (SIADH).

Aldosterone

The release of **aldosterone**, a hormone secreted by the adrenal glands, is another water-balancing mechanism in the body. It causes sodium ions to be returned to the bloodstream by the kidneys rather than to be spilled into the urine. Sodium, the most influential extracellular ion, pulls water along with it.

The trigger for the release of aldosterone is decrease in pressure of the blood supplying kidney tissue. In response, the kidneys produce **renin**. Renin acts as an enzyme to split angiotensinogen, a serum globulin secreted by the liver, to form angiotensin I. Enzymes in the lungs convert angiotensin I to **angiotensin II**. Angiotensin II constricts the body's blood vessels which increases blood pressure and also stimulates the secretion of aldosterone and ADH. Aldosterone then increases sodium retention, which retains water along with it. ADH also increases water retention and thus the blood volume is increased (Figure 9–5).

Another side of sodium retention is potassium loss. Within fluid compartments, positively charged particles must equal negatively charged ones. When sodium is retained, to maintain electroneutrality the kidney excretes more potassium, also under the influence of aldosterone.

Acid–Base Balance

The body is well equipped to digest and metabolize acidic and basic foods without jeopardizing its acid–base balance. The use of substances such as baking soda to treat an upset stomach should be discouraged, however, since the baking soda can be absorbed into the blood, thereby affecting the total body systems. Antacids designed to treat stomach upsets, used according to directions, are a better choice than baking soda.

Electrolytes play an important role in maintaining the correct acidity or alkalinity of various body fluids. Acids are compounds that yield

---

CLINICAL APPLICATION 9–4

Syndrome of Inappropriate Secretion of Antidiuretic Hormone (SIADH)

Normally, increased osmolality of the blood stimulates the posterior pituitary gland to release ADH. When enough water is returned to the bloodstream by the kidney, the ADH secretion stops.

Several situations cause ADH to be released inappropriately. Certain lung tumors produce an ADH-like substance. Other lung conditions such as pneumonia, tuberculosis, and asthma have caused SIADH. Other cancers, stress, surgery, some anesthetics, pain and morphine have been implicated in increased release of ADH. Medications such as chlorpropamide and oxytocin as well as various antidepressants, anticonvulsants, and cancer chemotherapeutic agents have precipitated SIADH. Even paradoxical reactions to thiazide diuretics have been reported (van Assen and Mudde, 1999; Wierzbicki, Ball, and Singh, 1998). Conditions directly affecting the brain (including the hypothalamus and the pituitary gland) such as meningitis, brain tumors, and subarachnoid hemorrhage have been liked to SIADH.

The signs and symptoms of SIADH are those of hyponatremia. In this case it is dilutional hyponatremia. The client has enough sodium, but it is diluted in too much retained water. Initially, the client becomes apprehensive. When the serum sodium drops to 120 to 125 mEq per liter, neurological signs appear, owing to edema of the brain cells. The client becomes irritable, apathetic, and displays personality changes. Other signs of hyponatremia include tremors, hyperactive reflexes, muscle spasms, and convulsions. Fingerprints remain over the sternum due to the excess intracellular fluid. Urine osmolality (Brensilver and Goldberger, 1996). When the serum sodium drops to less than 115 mEq per liter, seizures, coma, and permanent neurological damage can occur.

Effective treatment of SIADH is based upon discovering and removing the cause of the condition. Beyond that, or in the instance of a postoperative or stress reaction, treatment involves diuretic therapy and fluid restriction. The client is given precisely prescribed amounts of fluids throughout the day. Over a period of several days, through obligatory excretion, the client's body will excrete the extra water

---

hydrogen ions when dissociated in solution. The more hydrogen ions a solution contains, the more concentrated the acid. Bases, or alkalis, are substances that accept hydrogen ions. The acidity or alkalinity of a substance is measured according to a scale called **pH**. The pH scale ranges from 0 to 14: Acids are rated 0 to 6.999; 7 is neutral; bases are above 7. One on the scale would indicate a strong acid and 14 a strong base. Figure 9–6 illustrates the pH scale showing placement of acid, neutral, and alkaline fluids.

The balance between too much and too little acid in body fluids is maintained by the action of the lungs, the kidneys, and the buffer systems of the body. The purpose of buffer systems is to minimize significant changes in the pH of the body fluids by controlling the hydrogen ion (H^+)

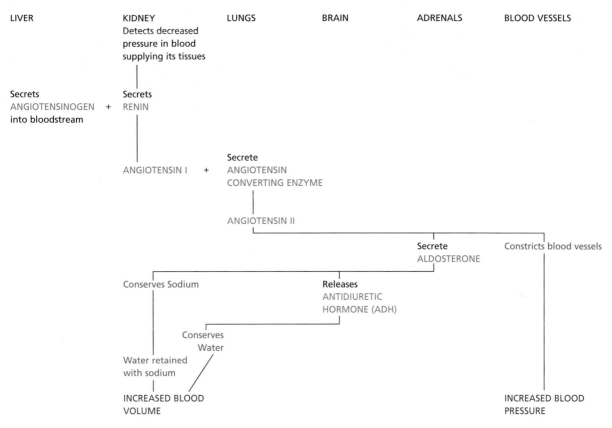

Figure 9–5:
Hormonal control of water balance. Although the kidneys do most of the work, the complex process also involves the liver, lungs, brain, adrenal glands, and blood vessels.

concentration. Buffers are substances that can neutralize both acids and bases. Bicarbonate (HCO_3^-) is the most important buffer in the extracellular fluid. Phosphate (HPO_4^{2-}) and proteins are two important buffers in the intracellular fluid.

Extracellular Fluid

The normal pH of the extracellular fluid (including the blood and interstitial fluid) is 7.35 to 7.45. It is slightly alkaline, despite the acidity of the body's waste products. The body is continually working to maintain correct pH within this narrow range. If the serum pH drops below 6.8 or rises above 7.8, death usually results.

Extracellular fluid contains both positive sodium ions (Na^+) and negative bicarbonate ions (HCO_3^-). When a strong acid is introduced to the fluid, a chemical reaction takes place. The end products of this reaction are sodium chloride (a salt), which is neutral, and carbonic acid (a weak acid). The **carbonic acid** breaks down to carbon dioxide and water. The carbon dioxide is excreted by the lungs (exhaled) and the water is excreted by the kidneys.

Another chemical reaction takes place when a strong base (alkali) is introduced into the fluid system. When a strong base enters the system, carbon dioxide and water (the two main waste products of cellular metabolism) react to form carbonic acid to counteract the alkaline effect of the

base. The end products of this reaction are water and a weak base that does not drastically affect the pH.

Respiratory System

The lungs help maintain pH by varying the amount of carbon dioxide (CO_2) exhaled. Excess carbon dioxide makes the body fluids more acidic because it reacts to form **carbonic acid**, a source of hydrogen ions. Too much carbonic acid, or too much of any acid, results in **acidosis**, a condition that causes the lungs to automatically increase the rate and depth of breathing, eliminating more carbon dioxide and water.

This respiratory response to acidosis begins within minutes of an increase in acidity. Respiratory compensation for acidosis is 50 to 75 percent effective and is an extremely important component in the regulation of pH. Normally, the respiratory system has one or two times the buffering power of all chemical buffers in the body.

Renal System

The respiratory system acts quickly but can eliminate only carbonic acid. Other acids, as well as excess carbonic acid, must be eliminated in the urine. The kidney spills or retains hydrogen, sodium, and bicarbonate ions as necessary to maintain an acceptable pH in the blood. For example, in response to acidosis, the kidneys excrete hydrogen ions and reabsorb sodium and bicarbonate ions. Conversely, in response to alkalosis, the kidneys conserve hydrogen ions and excrete sodium and bicarbonate ions. The kidneys initiate these actions within 24 hours but require 3 to 4 days to compensate for changes in blood pH.

Intracellular Fluid

The normal pH of the intracellular fluid is 6.8 to 7.0, slightly acid to neutral. Within the intracellular fluid, organic phosphates and proteins are the most important buffers. These substances buffer 95 percent of the body's carbonic acid and 50 percent of other acids. Protein is the most powerful and plentiful buffer system in the body. Of the body's proteins, hemoglobin has the largest buffering capacity. Thus the red blood cells have 70 percent of the buffering power of the blood. This buffering capacity allows large quantities of carbon dioxide to be transported from the tissues to the lungs with only a small change in venous pH compared with arterial pH.

When the blood contains excessive hydrogen ions, they move into the cells to be buffered. Then, to maintain electroneutrality, potassium moves from the intracellular compartment to the extracellular (intravascular), raising serum potassium levels.

Recommended Dietary Allowance

There is no RDA for water. Unless they are on a high-salt or high-protein diet, adults need one milliliter per kilocalorie per day. A person on a 1500-kilocalorie diet should take in 1.5 liters of liquid. Adults require 2 to 4 percent of their body weight as water daily. The 154-pound person would need 3 to 6 pounds of water. A pint is approximately a pound, so 3 to 6 pounds would be 1 1/2 to 3 quarts of liquid. Of this amount, at least

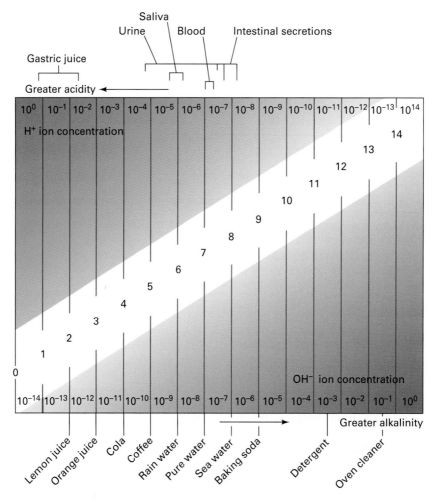

Figure 9–6:
Representation of the pH scale with usual readings for body fluids, beverages, and household products. (Reprinted from Thomas, 1997, p. 1458, with permission.)

60 percent should be consumed as water and the remainder obtained from foods and metabolic water.

Infants have a greater need for water than adults. Their basal heat production per kilogram is twice that of adults. To rid their bodies of the heat and waste products, they need 1.5 milliliters of water per kilocalorie ingested (compared with the 1 milliliter per kcalorie adults require). Infants must drink 10 to 15 percent of their body weight to maintain health, compared with the 2 to 4 percent that adults need. As discussed in Chapter 12, breast milk alone can supply the infant's needed water.

Sources of Water

Much of our water is consumed in other beverages. Adults consume 6 cups of water per day in beverages.

Water may contain other nutrients. Hard water has calcium, magnesium, and often iron. Water conditioners used to soften water replace the calcium, magnesium, and iron with sodium. Drinking softened water increases some people's sodium intake excessively. In fact most experts recommend that the cold water at the kitchen sink be unsoftened.

We obtain about 4 cups of water per day in foods. Skim milk is 91 percent water, and whole milk is 88 percent water. Some foods that are solids also have a high water content: head lettuce is 96 percent water, celery is 95 percent water, and raw carrots are 88 percent water. Other foods that contain a large percentage of water include apples (84 percent), grapes (81 percent), bananas (74 percent), hard-cooked eggs (75 percent), drained tuna (61 percent), and chicken breast or thigh (52 percent). Whole wheat bread is 38 percent water; its water content drops to 29 percent when the bread is toasted.

Water is also a product of metabolism. The average person acquires 1 cup of water per day from this process.

Losses of Water

We lose water in obvious ways, such as in perspiration and urine. These means are called **sensible water losses**. We also lose water in less obvious ways, such as through breathing, which are called **insensible water losses**.

Sensible Water Losses

Sensible water losses include losses of the major extracellular ions, sodium and chloride. Three important routes commonly account for sensible water losses: through the skin as perspiration, through the kidney as urine, and through the gastrointestinal tract in the feces.

Perspiration

Evaporation of sweat from the skin is the main means of dissipating the heat produced in the body by exercise. To produce 1 liter of perspiration requires 600 kilocalories. In extreme cases, a person may perspire at the rate of 2 liters per hour. For example, during a marathon race, runners may lose 6 to 7 percent of their body weight, primarily as perspiration. A 150-pound person would lose 10 1/2 pounds, or 4.8 liters of fluid. To the extent that sweat drops from the body, it is not useful for evaporative cooling (Gisolfi, 1996).

Sweat is not pure water. It is salty to the taste and is hypotonic. One liter of perspiration contains 45 milliequivalents of sodium, 5 milliequivalents of potassium, and 58 milliequivalents of chlorine. In this instance, the milliosmole value is the same as the milliequivalent value (because all the ions are monovalent) so the milliequivalents can be added to obtain an osmolarity of 108 milliequivalents per liter of perspiration.

For a sweat loss of less than 5 or 6 liters, rehydration with water suffices. Intense work in a very hot environment (a foundry or mine) may result in "miner's cramps" believed to be caused by sodium depletion. In this case, sports drinks or salt tablets may be indicated (Groff, Gropper, and Hunt, 1995).

Urine

In the normal, healthy person, with average exertion throughout the day, urine output is roughly equal to liquid intake, usually 1200 to 1500 milliliters per day. A well-hydrated individual produces light yellow or straw-colored urine.

Two commonly consumed substances increase urine output without a compensatory contribution to the water balance of the body. They are alcohol and caffeine. Alcohol blocks ADH activity, thus permitting more water to be spilled in the urine (Klotz, 1998). A study of healthy adults found that caffeine led to negative fluid balance. These individuals normally drank coffee but abstained from caffeine-containing substances for 5 days before the study. The first day of the study, their water requirements were met with mineral water. The second day, 6 cups of coffee containing 642 milligrams of caffeine replaced part of the mineral water. As a result, urine output increased significantly and body weight and total body water decreased significantly. Despite these losses, only 2 of the 12 subjects experienced thirst (Neuhauser-Berthold et al., 1997).

A minimum amount of urine must be excreted each day to carry away the waste products resulting from metabolic processes. This function, called **obligatory excretion**, eliminates 400 to 600 milliliters per day.

The hourly urine output of seriously ill clients must be monitored. The amounts must be interpreted in relation to the client's whole situation. Even if a person is losing massive amounts of fluid through the gastrointestinal tract, such losses do not rid the body of metabolic wastes as efficiently as the kidney does. Adults should excrete 1 to 2 liters of urine in 24 hours—an average of 40 to 80 milliliters per hour—although the amount varies throughout the day and night. Clinical Calculation 9–2 shows a method of determining a desirable hourly urine output for children.

Gastrointestinal Secretions

Abnormal gastrointestinal function can cause extensive fluid loss. When the secretion occurs from a point high in the gastrointestinal tract, the resulting symptoms differ from those that occur when the secretion is from a point lower in the tract. Gastric juice is acid, while intestinal juices are alkaline. Therefore, conceptually, gastrointestinal losses are divided into those lost above the outlet of the stomach, the pylorus, and those lost below it.

ABOVE THE PYLORUS The common causes of losses above the pylorus are vomiting or stomach suctioning. Two organs secrete digestive juices

Clinical Calculation 9–2 Hourly Urine Output in Children

Children should excrete between 0.5 and 2 milliliters of urine per kilogram of body weight per hour. What would be a normal hourly urine output for a child who weighs 50 pounds?

First convert pounds to kilograms. There are 2.2 pounds per kilogram.

$$\frac{50 \text{ lb}}{2.2 \text{ lb/kg}} = 22.7 \text{ kg}$$

To find the desirable range of output, multiply the child's weight in kilograms by the desired factors of 0.5 to 2 mL per kilogram.

$$22.7 \times 0.5 = 11.4 \text{ mL/h}$$
$$22.7 \times 2 = 45.4 \text{ mL/h}$$

Thus the 50-lb child normally should excrete between 11 and 45 mL/h of urine.

Clinical Calculation 9–3 Insensible Water Loss Through the Skin

The rule of thumb for insensible water loss through the skin is 6 mL/kg per 24 hours. Let us look at a 154-lb client to see what his or her amount of water loss would be in a 24-hour period. First, convert pounds to kilograms:

$$\frac{154 \text{ lb}}{2.2 \text{ lb/kg}} = 70 \text{ kg}$$

Then multiply the client's weight (in kilograms) by the amount of water loss per kilogram:

$$70 \text{ kg} \times 6 \text{ mL/kg} = 420 \text{ mL}$$

Thus, this client's insensible water loss is a 24-hour period is expected to be 420 mL

humidity (Kleiner, 1999). Clinical Calculation 9–3 gives a client example of insensible water loss. Burns, phototherapy, radiant warmers, or fever will increase the amount of insensible water loss. Fever increases evaporative losses by about 12 percent per Celsius degree of temperature elevation. Clinical Calculation 9–4 shows how **evaporative water losses** are calculated. Table 9–4 lists average fluid gains and losses for 24 hours.

Assessment of Water Losses

Gathering data on water losses is quite straightforward. Because water is more than 50 percent of body weight, with few exceptions a loss of water shows up in the client's weight. Recording the liquid a client takes in and puts out is a second means of tracking water balance.

Clinical Calculation 9–4 Evaporative Water Loss in Fever

Fever increases the amount of evaporative loss by 12 percent for every degree Celsius of fever. If the 154-lb client in Clinical Calculation 9–3 had a fever of 102.2°F, how much additional evaporative loss would he or she sustain?

Temperatures can be reported in Fahrenheit or Celsius degrees and the conversion formulas account for the fact that the Celsius scale sets freezing at zero and the Fahrenheit sets it at 32 degrees.

To convert Fahrenheit to Celsius, subtract 32 and multiply by 5/9.

$$102.2 - 32 = 70.2 \times 5/9 = 39 \text{ degrees C}$$

The client had insensible losses of 420 mL. Normal body temperature on the Celsius scale is 37°.

To convert Celsius to Fahrenheit, multiply by 9/5 and add 32.

$$37 \times 9/5 = 66.6 + 32 = 98.6 \text{ degrees F}$$

The client has an elevation of 2 degrees C, which would increase evaporative loss by 24 percent.

$$420 \text{ mL} \times .24 = 100.8 \text{ mL additional evaporative water loss.}$$

$$420 \text{ mL} + 100.8 \text{ mL} =$$
$$520.8 \text{ total insensible water loss through the skin.}$$

above the pylorus, the salivary glands in the mouth and the gastric glands in the stomach. Both of these secretions are isotonic, so their loss threatens electrolyte balance to a greater extent than loss of an equal amount of perspiration would. The ions lost in secretions above the pylorus are sodium, potassium, chloride, and hydrogen.

About 1 liter of saliva per day is mixed with food or just swallowed. The stomach secretes about 1.5 to 2.5 liters of gastric juice per day. If gastric juices are lost, hydrogen ions in the hydrochloric acid are also lost, putting the person at risk for alkalosis.

BELOW THE PYLORUS The usual causes of losses below the pylorus are diarrhea or intestinal suctioning. Gastrointestinal secretions below the pylorus also are isotonic. They contain sodium, potassium, and bicarbonate. About 2 to 3 liters of intestinal secretions per day flow into the bowel to digest food. Normally, bile is released from the gallbladder into the small intestine at the rate of 1 liter per day. The total gastrointestinal secretions amount to 6.5 to 8.5 liters per day. Yet, because water is absorbed back into the blood from the large intestine, normal feces from an adult contain only 100 to 200 milliliters of water.

See Clinical Application 9–5 for a discussion of conditions resulting from exposure to extreme heat.

Insensible Water Losses

An invisible amount of water is lost through the lungs and the skin. These are insensible losses. An amount between 800 and 1000 milliliters of water is lost each day via the lungs and skin. Breath is visible only in very cold weather. Even in warmer weather and indoors, people lose 400 milliliters of water per day in exhaled air. Deep respirations or a dry climate increase the amount of water lost.

The insensible loss of water through the skin is evaporative. It is almost pure water and nearly electrolyte-free. This insensible water loss amounts to 6 milliliters per kilogram of body weight in 24 hours, which is a baseline amount.

Environmental conditions influence the amount of water lost. Greater losses occur at high temperatures, at high altitudes, and in low

CLINICAL APPLICATION 9–5

HEAT-RELATED ILLNESSES

Exposure to extreme heat may overtax the body's adaptive capabilities. Between 1979 and 1996, high temperatures caused an average of 381 deaths annually in the United States (Centers for Disease Control, 1999). Approximately half of these deaths occurred in people older than 65 years. Figure 9–7 depicts the average annual rate of heat-related deaths by age group. The annual death rate from hyperthermia is higher for men than for women aged 35 or more and for black people than for white people, although the reasons underlying these differences are unknown. Persons at risk of hyperthermia when exposed to excessive heat for prolonged periods include those of advanced age, those who live alone, and those with cardiovascular or respiratory diseases or with mental illnesses. Drugs such as alcohol, antipsychotic medications, major tranquilizers, and anticholinergic agents increase risk.

Loss of more than 3 percent of body weight due to dehydration is an important risk factor for heat-related illnesses (Barrow and Clark, 1998). Depending upon the extent of the stressor and the body's ability to adapt, the person may experience heat edema, heat cramps, heat syncope, heat exhaustion, or heat stroke.

A particularly difficult situation occurs in a crowd. Individuals in the center of a mass of bodies are unable to cool themselves through normal physiological mechanisms. This phenomenon is called the "Penguin Effect" after the practice of penguins to huddle together, ostensibly to conserve heat (Blows, 1998). In certain crowds, moreover, heat production is increased, as in pop concerts where the audience cheers and dances. If the people are shoulder-to-shoulder as in an audience or on a commuter train, a person may faint but remain upright, thwarting the normal mechanism of restoring circulation to the brain.

Heat Edema

In heat edema, unacclimatized people experience swelling in the feet and ankles and other dependent areas of the body during hot summer months, caused by transient peripheral vasodilation and orthostatic pooling when they sit or stand for a long time. Elevating the legs and exercising periodically may improve the condition until the person becomes acclimatized (Barrow and Clark, 1998).

Heat Cramps

Heat cramps are painful spasms of the muscles of the arms, legs, or abdomen caused by exertion and loss of sodium. Treatment involves stretching the muscle and replacing fluid and salt. An oral rehydration solution using 1 teaspoon of salt to 1 quart of water can be helpful (Barrow and Clark, 1998). Caution is necessary because overhydrating with hypotonic intravenous fluids has led to hyponatremia (Herfel et al., 1998).

Heat Syncope

Heat syncope is an episode of heat-related fainting that usually follows rising from a sitting or lying position. The skin blood vessels have dilated to promote cooling, leaving insufficient blood circulating to the brain. Once the person falls down, his or her brain is re-perfused, and the person recovers consciousness.

To treat heat syncope, have the client lie down in a cooler location and replace the water deficit (Barrow and Clark, 1998).

Heat Exhaustion

In heat exhaustion, the client suffers the loss of water and sodium chloride in sweat. The client's temperature is usually less than 102.2°F (39°C). He or she suffers from dizziness, weakness, and fatigue, but remains coherent. The pulse is weak, thready, and rapid. Respirations are shallow and quiet. The skin is cool, clammy, and sweaty. First-aid treatment consists of moving the client to a cooler environment. The client should lie down with the feet elevated, and clothing should be loosened. If the person can drink it, 1/2 teaspoon of salt in 1/2 glass of water will begin to replace the water and sodium chloride lost. The salt-in-water treatment should be repeated every 15 minutes, and the client's temperature should be monitored until the emergency team arrives.

Heat Stroke

Heat stroke is a life-threatening medical emergency. The death rate averages 25 percent (Hett and Brechtelsbaluer, 1998), but medical studies have shown that cooling the client to a temperature of less than 39.9°C (103.8°F) within 30 minutes improves survival (Dematte et al,. 1998).

The client with heat stroke fails to perspire because the body can no longer regulate body temperature. The client has an extremely elevated temperature, 105°F (40.6°C) or above. With this level of hyperthermia, many body enzymes become denatured so that chemical reactions cannot occur (Curtis, 1997). The client's mental state goes from lethargy to disorientation, delirium, and coma. The skin is flushed, hot, and typically dry but could be wet if the client's condition has just progressed to heat stroke from heat exhaustion (Curtis, 1997). The pulse is full and bounding. Breathing is difficult and respirations are loud. The first aid treatment of heat stroke includes complete quiet with the head elevated, removal of clothing, and bathing the extremities with cool water. Fanning the person increases the evaporation rate until the medical team arrives.

Heat stroke ranks third behind head and neck trauma and cardiac disorders as a cause of death among United States high school athletes (Barrow and Clark, 1998). Hyperthermia and dehydration caused the deaths of three collegiate wrestlers within 33 days in 1997. Those young men were attempting to dehydrate themselves before the official weigh-in in order to compete in desired weight classes (Centers for Disease Control, 1998).

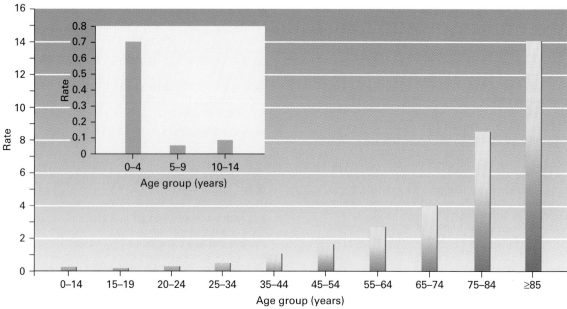

*Per million population.

†Underlying cause of death attributed to excess heat exposure classified according to the International Classification of Diseases, Ninth Revision, as code E900.0, "due to weather conditions"; code E900.1, "of manmade origin"; or E900.9, "at unspecified origin."

Figure 9–7:
Average annual rate per 1 million population) of heat–related deaths, by age group—United States, 1979– 1996. (From Centers for Disease Control, 1999.)

Weight

Rapid weight changes usually are a reflection of fluid balance. Daily weight is the single most important indicator of fluid status. An easy way to relate volume to weight is to remember "A pint is a pound the world around." One liter is 1 kilogram or 2.2 pounds. Individuals who have lost only one percent of body weight in water have experienced impaired temperature regulation and decreased capacity for physical work (Gisolfi, 1996). Acute weight loss in adults is rated as follows: mild volume deficit—2 to 5 percent loss; moderate volume deficit—5 to 10 percent loss; severe volume deficit—10 to 15 percent loss. A loss greater than 15 percent can be fatal (Horne, Heitz, and Swearingen, 1991).

Fluid balance in the infant is much more precarious. Because a greater proportion of their body water is in the extracellular space, infants can lose it more rapidly than can adults. Therefore, a loss of 5 percent of body weight in an infant merits medical attention.

Sudden weight changes are not always due to fluid shifts. If a client receives no oral, enteral, or parenteral nutrition, the loss of body tissue may amount to 0.3 to 0.5 kilogram per day.

Intake and Output

In addition to monitoring weight, recording liquid intake and output is a common nursing action. In the healthy person, liquid intake and output should be approximately equal. Measuring intake is easier than measuring output, but still is frequently inaccurate. Most institutions post the amounts that food and beverage containers hold. Amounts remaining should be measured and subtracted from the total liquid served.

Rather than assume that clients have consumed everything missing from the pitcher or tray, the nurse should ask if they drank the fluid (as opposed, say, to giving it to a visitor). Updating the intake form throughout the day rather than at the end of a shift is likely to produce a more

TABLE 9–4 Average Fluid Gains and Losses in Adults in 24 Hours			
Fluid Gains		**Fluid Losses***	
Energy metabolism	300 mL	Kidneys	1200–1500 mL
		Skin	500–600 mL
Oral fluids	1100–1400 mL	Lungs	400 mL
Solid foods	800–1000 mL	Intestines	100–200 mL
Total	2200–2700 mL	Total	2200–2700 mL
*Includes sensible and insensible losses.			

Charting Tips 9–1

Be Specific and Document
- Be specific when teaching clients.
- Record both the content and the client's response to the material.
- One client was told to "drink a lot of fluid" when he was discharged from the hospital. He interpreted this to be 3 to 4 gallons per day! His kidneys did their best, but kidneys cannot produce plain water. In a few days, the client was back in the hospital for correction of electrolyte imbalance. This outcome could have been prevented if the client had been taught to drink a specific amount of fluid rather than "a lot."

complete record. Record the amount of water from ice chips as one-half of their volume. One cup of ice chips yields only 1/2 cup of water.

Fluid that is lost into a dressing or a diaper can be estimated by weighing it. Subtract the dry material's weight from the total. One gram of weight equals 1 milliliter of water. **Specific gravity** is the weight of a substance compared with that of distilled water. Normal specific gravity of urine is 1.010 to 1.025. A lower value is common in newborns. So, although the weight of a diaper wet with urine is not exactly the same as if it were wet with water, this method of recording incontinent urine is adequate in most situations.

In a sick person, intake and output totals may not balance every day. The client's intake and output should be analyzed over a period of several days because a one-day evaluation could prove misleading. Of utmost importance is the ability to see the big picture. See Charting Tips 9–1 for teaching and documentation tips.

Water Imbalances

Two common imbalances are fluid volume deficit and fluid volume excess.

Fluid Volume Deficit

In fluid volume deficit, the individual experiences vascular, interstitial, or cellular dehydration. For every liter of fluid lost, core temperature rises 0.3 degree Celsius, cardiac output decreases one liter per minute, and heart rate increases eight beats per minute (Coyle and Montain, 1992). In the body's effort to compensate, fluid moves from one compartment to another; the client's situation is constantly changing.

Losses of Fluid

Fluid losses can be external or internal. Treatments may differ, but the signs and symptoms of fluid volume deficit are similar, whatever the cause.

EXTERNAL LOSSES Fluids lost to the outside of the body are called **external fluid losses**; gastrointestinal losses are the most common. Vomiting or diarrhea are just two of the ways in which gastrointestinal fluids are lost. But medical treatments such as gastrointestinal suctioning or surgical rerouting of intestinal contents also produce fluid deficit. Hemorrhage causes not only fluid loss but also the loss of blood cells.

INTERNAL LOSSES It may be hard to imagine, but fluids can be "lost" inside the body. Edema is excessive fluid accumulation in the interstitial fluid compartment. Although the fluid remains inside the body, it is outside the blood vessels and lost to the circulation.

As a result of injury or trauma, capillary permeability increases so that more fluid and cells can travel to the site of the injury to begin repairs or healing. This process also causes the swelling, or edema, at the site of an injury—blisters at the site of burns, for example. Fluid leaves the vessels and accumulates in the skin. Correct fluid replacement is a high priority for severely burned clients.

There are also several places in the body where vast amounts of fluid can accumulate. These losses are called **third-space losses**. Several liters of fluid can accumulate in the bowel when a person has a bowel obstruction. Certain diseases can cause **ascites**, the accumulation of fluid (often amounting to several liters), not within the bowel but around it in the abdominal cavity. Other third-space losses involve internal bleeding or the collection of fluid in the chest cavity. An alert nurse can spot an early clue to third-space losses. Decreasing urine output in spite of seemingly adequate fluid intake demands further assessment.

Assessment of Fluid Volume Deficit

Loss of fluid may be mild and corrected easily if the client has and obeys the body's thirst command to drink. On the other hand, the client's life may be threatened if the fluid loss is severe or sudden.

SYMPTOMS The thirst response is triggered when 10 percent of intravascular volume is lost or when cellular volume is reduced by 1 to 2 percent. Thus, thirst is a symptom of fluid volume deficit. The client may also suffer a loss of appetite or be nauseated because of decreased blood flow to the intestines. Other symptoms of fluid deficit are headache, light-headedness, and fatigue (Kleiner, 1999).

SIGNS Clients who have a fluid volume deficit are less able to maintain their blood pressure immediately after rising from a lying or sitting position. This sign is called **orthostatic hypotension**. The nurse measures the blood pressure with the client lying or sitting, asks the client to stand, and immediately retakes the blood pressure. A drop of 15 millimeters or mercury in either systolic or diastolic blood pressure upon standing suggests fluid volume deficit. A narrowing of **pulse pressure** (the difference between systolic and diastolic readings) also occurs with fluid volume deficit.

In an effort to maintain perfusion of the tissues, the body compensates for a lowered blood pressure by an increase in pulse rate. Taking a pulse when lying or sitting and immediately after rising is another method of assessing fluid volume deficit. An increase of 20 beats per minute upon standing merits further assessment.

Decreased skin **turgor** or elasticity is a sign of fluid volume deficit associated with sodium loss. To assess skin turgor, pinch the skin on the forearm, over the sternum, or on the back of the hand. If the skin stays pinched, suspect fluid volume deficit. This is a less reliable sign in the elderly, whose skin has lost much of its elasticity.

Another sign of fluid volume deficit can be found in the client's mouth. Besides dry mouth, many longitudinal furrows of the tongue are visible instead of the single one in the well-hydrated adult.

Delayed filling of hand veins is a sign of fluid volume deficit. To assess vein filling, raise the hand above the heart. Normally, the veins will collapse in 3 to 5 seconds. Then lower the hand below the heart. The veins should refill in 3 to 5 seconds. The veins of a person with fluid volume deficit require more than 5 seconds to refill.

The symptoms of loss of appetite and nausea attributable to fluid deficit may progress to the sign of vomiting; the cause is decreased blood flow to the intestines.

Fluid volume deficit produces changes in certain laboratory readings. Urine color is easily observed, and urine's specific gravity can be measured at the bedside. Clients also show increases in hemoglobin and hematocrit levels unless they have lost red blood cells through hemorrhage.

Special attention must be given to the assessment of infants. Because 75 percent of the infant's body weight is water and 54 percent of the water is extracellular, dehydration from fluid loss can occur rapidly. Signs to assess in the infant, in addition to poor skin turgor and dry mucous membranes, are depressed fontanel ("soft spot" in skull), sunken eyes, and lack of tears when crying.

SHOCK If fluid volume deficit continues, the client goes into shock. The loss of 20 to 25 percent of intravascular volume produces shock. **Shock** is an acute peripheral circulatory failure due to loss of circulatory fluid or derangement of circulatory control. Signs of shock are decreased blood pressure and increased pulse. The person's skin is pale, cool, and clammy from perspiration. Urine output may be less than 15 milliliters per hour.

Treatment of Fluid Volume Deficit

In the treatment of fluid volume deficit, it is essential to correct the cause of the fluid depletion. Hypotonic fluids are given in order to replace fluid volume and correct electrolyte imbalances (Clinical Application 9–6). If possible, use the oral route. Be aware that oral electrolyte solutions, although effective in maintaining hydration, do not necessarily reduce stool volume or the duration of diarrhea.

Because lack of a visible therapeutic effect sometimes discourages use of the electrolyte solutions, alternate formulations are being investigated (Thillainayagam, Hunt, and Farthing, 1998). Thickened hydration solutions are also available for clients who have difficulty swallowing thin liquids. A dietitian should be consulted before using food thickeners, inasmuch as some of them bind with water making it less available for absorption.

An alternative to intravenous rehydration in selected clients is the use of hypodermoclysis. In this technique, fluid is introduced into the subcutaneous tissue, in the thighs or abdomen, for instance, usually by means of a pair of needles. A drug may be used to aid in dispersal of the solution. Hypodermoclysis may be appropriate if the client has an adequate blood pressure and requires hypotonic or isotonic solutions of 2 or 3 liters per day (Abdulla and Keast, 1997).

If hypertonic solutions are given orally to correct fluid loss, the concentrated solution would remain in the stomach longer than water, providing satiety and restraining water intake (Brensilver and Goldberger, 1996). Additionally, hypertonic solutions draw fluid from the bowel wall into the lumen; the result would be osmotic diarrhea. Some commercial laxatives and enemas are hypertonic solutions that work in this way.

Maximal sodium and water absorption is thought to occur with a glucose concentration of 10 to 25 grams per liter. Higher concentrations allow less sodium and water to be absorbed, in addition to causing osmotic diarrhea. Cola beverages, ginger ale, and apple juice are poor choices for rehydration in prolonged diarrhea, owing to their high glucose

and low electrolyte concentrations. In contrast, attempts to rehydrate with large volumes of plain water inhibit thirst and produce a diuretic response (Maughan, Leiper, and Shirreffs, 1997).

Another situation that causes electrolyte imbalance can occur if a client in shock requires blood transfusions. Clinical Application 9–7 discusses hyperkalemia following blood transfusion.

Fluid Volume Excess

The opposite of fluid volume deficit is fluid volume excess. The individual is retaining fluid intracellularly or extracellularly. Fluid compartments do not operate in isolation: if one is out of balance, the other compartments eventually will be affected as the body attempts to equalize osmotic pressure across the compartments.

Gains of Fluid

If the kidney and the hormones from the adrenal and pituitary glands are functioning normally, excess water is excreted from the body in the urine. When a person becomes ill and these control mechanisms stop working, fluids shift from the intravascular and interstitial spaces to the intracellular space so as to equalize osmotic pressure.

CLINICAL APPLICATION 9–6

Oral Electrolyte Solutions

Originally, oral electrolyte solutions were designed to combat diarrheal diseases in developing countries. They proved so useful that they have since been modified for use in Western nations.

One commonly used oral electrolyte solution is Pedialyte. It is available over the counter without a prescription. One liter of Pedialyte contains:

Electrolytes
45 mEq sodium
20 mEq potassium
35 mEq chloride
30 mEq citrate, a base

The total osmolarity of Pedialyte is mildly hypotonic, about 269 milliosmoles per liter. Pedialyte also illustrates electroneutrality. The sodium and potassium are cations carrying positive charges. The chloride and citrate are anions carrying negative charges.

45 mEq Na$^+$	35 mEq Cl$^-$
+20 mEq K$^+$	+30 mEq citrate$^-$
65 cations	65 anions

Pedialyte is designed for maintenance of an infant or child experiencing vomiting or diarrhea. If the client becomes dehydrated, medical attention is needed. Intravenous fluids or an oral rehydration solution of different composition from Pedialyte may be prescribed for the dehydrated client. Loss of 5 percent of body weight indicates dehydration.

Pedialyte also has the ideal concentration of glucose to promote sodium and water absorption, 25 g/L. In contrast, athletic beverages contain concentrated sweeteners to mask the bitter taste of the electrolytes (Brensilver and Goldberger, 1996).

CLINICAL APPLICATION 9–7

Hyperkalemia following Blood Transfusion

A person who has hemorrhaged may need blood replacement. Red blood cells do not live as long in the blood bank as they do in the human body. Potassium is the major cation in red blood cell (intracellular). When the red blood cells die and their cell walls rupture, potassium is spilled into the serum.

Blood that has been stored for a prolonged period may contain up to 30 mEq per liter of potassium due to the destruction of the red blood cells. This may not sound like a lot, but potassium is usually administered intravenously at a concentration of 40 mEq per liter to a person who is potassium depleted. The person receiving a blood transfusion may have a serum potassium level that is nearly normal, and the old blood containing a higher concentration of potassium may push him or her into hyperkalemia. The nurse should be aware of the age of fresh blood products to be given and identify clients at risk of hyperkalemia.

Inflammation increases the fluid in interstitial space, causing edema. In most cases, localized edema is not life threatening. The accumulation of fluid in the brain (cerebral edema) or in lung tissue (pulmonary edema), however, is a life-threatening condition. Cerebral edema may result from tumors, toxic chemicals, or infection. Pulmonary edema can be a consequence of a failing heart or irritation of the lung, as when a client inhales toxic gases.

Assessment of Fluid Volume Excess

Many of the presenting signs and symptoms of fluid volume excess are opposite those of fluid volume deficit. One symptom common to both is loss of appetite.

SYMPTOMS   The client with fluid volume excess complains of loss of appetite and nausea. In this case the symptoms are due to edema of the gastrointestinal tract, rather than decreased blood flow as in fluid volume deficit.

SIGNS   The same edema of the gastrointestinal tract causing the anorexia and nausea causes the sign of vomiting. Because the brain cells are extremely sensitive to changes in the internal environment, a person with fluid volume excess exhibits deteriorating consciousness.

Increased fluid in the blood decreases the proportion of red blood cells to total volume. Consequently, the hematocrit reading is decreased. The increase in blood volume causes an increased pulse pressure. The same technique described under fluid volume deficit is used to assess hand veins. With fluid volume excess the veins will not empty 3 to 5 seconds after raising the hand above the heart.

Increased blood flow to the kidneys causes increased urine output if the kidneys are functioning. The increased systolic blood pressure due to the excessive fluid pushes more fluid into the interstitial space, causing edema. Firm pressure over a bone, the ankle, or the top of the foot, forces some of the fluid aside. If the indentation remains visible for 5 seconds, it is called pitting edema. Table 9–5 lists signs and symptoms for fluid volume deficit and fluid volume excess.

Treatment of Fluid Volume Excess

As with fluid volume deficit, the remedy for fluid volume excess is to treat the cause. Osmotic diuretic drugs such as mannitol remain in the plasma. By increasing the osmotic pressure there, these drugs pull excess fluid from the cells to be excreted by the kidney.

Nutritionally, the client may be on a restricted fluid regimen. The physician may prescribe an intake of no more than 1000 milliliters in 24 hours. This amount compensates for insensible losses through the skin and lungs. It is essential for the nurse to supply fluid as prescribed and to teach the client the reason for the restriction. Over a period of several days, the obligatory urine output and any diuretic therapy will help the client's body to excrete the excess fluid.

TABLE 9-5 Signs and Symptoms of Abnormal Fluid Volume

	Fluid Volume Deficit	Fluid Volume Excess
Symptoms		
Gastrointestinal	Thirst	Loss of appetite (edema of the bowel)
	Loss of appetite (decreased blood to intestines)	Nausea
Signs		
General	Weight loss	Weight gain
	Depressed fontanel (infant)	Edema
	Sunken eyes (infant)	
	Lack of tears when crying (infant)	
Skin and mucous membranes	Dry mucous membranes	Skin stretched and shiney
	Decreased skin turgor	
Cardiovascular system	Orthostatic hypotension (pressure decrease of 15 mmHg in systolic or diastolic)	Increased hematocrit values
		Increasing pulse pressure
	Increased pulse rate upon standing	Emptying of hand veins takes longer than 5 seconds
	Increased hematocrit values (unless red blood cells also lost)	
	Narrowing pulse pressure	
	Filling of hand veins takes longer than 5 seconds	
Urinary	Decreased urine output	Polyuria
	Concentrated urine	Dilute urine
Gastrointestinal	Vomiting (decreased blood to intestines)	Vomiting (edema of intestines)
	Longitudinal furrows on tongue	
Central nermous system	Confusion, disorientation	Deteriorating consciousness

Summary

Water is our most essential nutrient. It constitutes at least half of everyone's body weight. The amount of water varies with the type of tissue, with gender, and with age. Body fluids are held in two compartments: intracellular fluid is the water within the cells; extracellular fluid is the water outside the cells. The latter includes intravascular fluid, lymph, interstitial, and transcellular fluid.

Water has many vital functions in the body. It gives shape and form to the cells, helps form the structure of large molecules, serves as a lubricant, and helps regulate body temperature. As a solvent, water transports solutes to and from the cells, is a medium for chemical reactions, and participates in chemical reactions. Because of its vital importance, everyone should take care to stay well hydrated (Wellness Tips 9-1).

The human body has no storage tanks for water. When necessary, the body can absorb water rapidly. Although some water can be absorbed from the stomach, 1 liter per hour can be absorbed from the small intestine.

The movement, distribution, and composition of body fluids are influenced and controlled by electrolyte and plasma protein concentrations. In the extracellular fluid, sodium is the major cation and chloride is the major anion. The major cation in the intracellular fluid is potassium. Ionized sodium, potassium, and chloride are the solutes that maintain the balance between the extracellular and intracellular compartments.

A complex system regulates the amount of water retained or excreted by the kidney. Aldosterone and ADH are hormones that cause retention of sodium and water, respectively. The hypothalamus stimulates the thirst mechanism when fluids inside the cells become too concentrated (with solutes).

Acid–base balance is maintained in the body by the action of the lungs, the kidneys, and chemical buffers. Bicarbonate is the most important buffer in the extracellular fluid. Phosphate and protein are two important buffers in the intracellular fluid.

Wellness Tip 9–1

- Tally your intake of fluids for a day. If it is less than optimum, consciously decide to drink fluids at specified intervals. Select trigger events (before meals, after a bathroom break) to consume a healthful beverage.
- Tally your intake of caffeinated and alcoholic beverages for a day. Subtract that amount from the total for the day when analyzing your intake. Analysis may reveal the potential for chronic underhydration and stimulate a change of habits.
- Establish modest goals to be achieved. When those are met, increase the amount of fluids you will try to consume.
- Enter any exercise period well hydrated.
- If you know you have lost electrolytes in sweat, consume a sports drink or fruit or vegetable juice with a salty snack food along with plain water

The body's sources of water include beverages, foods, and water from the metabolism of the energy nutrients (except alcohol). Water can be lost through the skin, lungs, kidneys, and intestinal tract. Although still present in the body, fluid can be lost to circulation through third spacing. The single most important measure of fluid balance is daily weight.

Since most fluid losses are hypotonic, the fluids usually used to correct fluid volume deficits and electrolyte imbalances are hypotonic. The use of hypertonic fluids would have the opposite effect, pulling more water out of the tissues and into the bowel or bloodstream.

Fluid volume excess can be local or generalized. The most dangerous sites for local edema are the brain and the lungs. Generalized fluid volume excess can make exorbitant demands on the heart. Common treatments for fluid volume excess are diuretics and fluid restriction.

Case Study 9–1

Mr. N, a 75-year-old retired office worker, recently arrived from his summer home in the North to his winter home in Florida. He had anticipated enjoying the 85°F weather. He left temperatures in the forties. Although Mr. N had hired someone to care for his small yard while he was away from Florida, there were still a number of chores to be done, which he tackled with a vengeance.

After 1-1/2 hours, Mr. N began to get a headache. He felt a bit weak and dizzy, but continued his work. He was nearly finished with the outside tasks.

Half an hour later, Ms. N found her husband lying on the ground and called to their neighbor, a retired nurse, who was reading in her lanai.

The nurse noted that Mr. N's skin was pale and cool but that he was perspiring profusely. He was conscious and coherent but said he felt weak. The nurse took Mr. N's pulse. It was 90 beats per minute, regular but weak. His respirations were 12 per minute and shallow.

The nurse provided the emergency care described in the following nursing care plan. (Of course, she did not write it all out before helping Mr. N.)

Nursing Care Plan

Subjective Data	Has worked outside in 85°F heat 2 hours
	Headache, weakness, dizziness
	Recently arrived from colder climate
Objective Data	Conscious, coherent
	Skin pale, cool, wet with perspiration
	Pulse 90, regular and weak
	Respirations 12 and shallow
Nursing Diagnosis	NANDA: Fluid volume deficit (North American Nursing Diagnosis Association, 1999, with permission.)
	Related to excessive loss of hypotonic fluid (sweat) as evidenced by wet, pale skin and weak, rapid pulse.

Desired Outcomes Evaluation Criteria	Nursing Actions/ Interventions	Rationale
NOC: Thermoregulation (Johnson, Maas, and Moorhead, 2000, with permission.)	NIC: Fluid/Electrolyte Management (McCloskey and Bulechek, 2000, with permission)	
Client will remain conscious and oriented, with a pulse no greater than 90, until the emergency team arrives.	Instruct Ms N to call emergency medical services and return to help.	In an emergency situation, the nurse stays with the client. Potential electrolyte imbalance requires medical care.
	Loosen Mr. N's clothing.	Mr. N. is already in a state of shock. Loosening the clothing will allow maximum air exchange and permit relaxation.
	With Ms. N, move client to shade or provide shade where he lies.	Mr. N must get out of the sun. Depending on the situation, he might be moved indoors, but perhaps the two women could not manage to move him.
	Keep client lying down with legs elevated slightly.	Lying down permits maximum blood circulation to the brain. Raising the legs increases the return of blood to the heart. The head should not be lowered because this causes venous congestion in the brain.
	Send Ms. N to kitchen for 1/2 glass water with 1/2 teaspoonful of salt in it. Administer salty water to Mr. N.	Although this is a hypertonic solution, sodium is readily absorbed by the intestine, so it is unlikely to cause osmotic diarrhea. Only 5 percent of consumed sodium remains in the feces. Sodium levels in the blood are controlled by the kidneys. This client has lost water and sodium chloride in perspiration.

Critical Thinking Question

1. What would you include in a presentation on preventing heat-related illnesses for an audience of elderly residents such as Mr. N, who follow the sun for the winter?
2. Reread the narrative. At what points in the narrative or in your expansion of the story could you envision Mr. N avoiding this incident?
3. The case study narrative does not discuss Mr. N's usual dietary intake. What dietary modifications can you think of that would make Mr. N's situation of overworking in the heat more critical?

Study Aids

Subjects . . . .**Internet Sites**

Heat-related Illness . . . . .http://www.methodisthealth.com/health/nutrition/WATER.HTML
http://www.pp.okstate.edu/ehs/training/heat.htm
http://www.pp.okstate.edu/ehs/chapters/heat.htm
http://www.princeton.edu/~oa/safety/heatill.html
http://www.redcross.org/tips/august/augtip98.html
http://www.aafp.org/patientinfo/heatill.html
http://travelhealth.com/heat.htm

Multilingual Patient Information http://mhcs.health.nsw.gov.au/health-public-affairs/mhcs/publications/healthgen/HTS-496.html
http://mhcs.health.nsw.gov.au/health-public-affairs/mhcs/publications/nutrition/bhc-3055.html

Water Needs http://mayohealth.org/mayo/9706/htm/thirst.htm

Chapter Review

1. Which of the following people has the greatest percentage of body weight as water?
   a. A 154-pound man
   b. A 120-pound woman
   c. An 8-pound girl, 4 days old
   d. An 18-pound boy, 14 months old
2. Which of the following represents the approximate amount of water contained in oral fluids consumed by the average adult?
   a. 100–200 milliliters
   b. 500–600 milliliters
   c. 800–1000 milliliters
   d. 1100–1400 milliliters
3. Heat exhaustion is caused by:
   a. Insufficient secretion of ADH
   b. Loss of water and salt in sweat
   c. Inability to perspire
   d. Retention of excessive water
4. When aldosterone secretion is increased, _____ is retained by the kidney and _____ is excreted to maintain electroneutrality.
   a. Sodium, potassium
   b. Potassium, sodium
   c. Calcium, hydrogen
   d. Hydrogen, potassium
5. If a person's body is too acid, the automatic response of the body is to:
   a. Increase sweat production
   b. Retain water
   c. Decrease rate and depth of breathing
   d. Increase rate and depth of breathing

Clinical Analysis

Baby I, a 4-month-old boy, has developed diarrheal stools within the past 2 days. At birth he weighed 7 pounds 8 ounces. Since then he has gained steadily. Three days ago he weighed 12 pounds 8 ounces. Baby I's present weight is 12 pounds 2 ounces.

Mrs. I has been feeding the baby his usual formula. He drinks eagerly but then has an explosive bowel movement with loud crying. Baby I has had six bowel movements per day instead of his usual two.

1. With this history, what physical assessment measures would the nurse include initially?
   a. Skin turgor, fontanel fullness, moisture of mucous membranes
   b. Condition of hair, strength of grasp, presence of sucking reflex
   c. Heart sounds, lung sounds, blood pressure
   d. Urine specific gravity, observation of diaper rash
2. Which of the following recommendations by the nurse would show understanding of supportive care of this client?
   a. Give Baby I whole milk to maintain nutrition.
   b. Continue, as Mrs. I has been doing, to allow the bowel to empty itself.
   c. Substitute orange juice for the formula for 3 days.
   d. Start Baby I on an oral electrolyte solution.
3. The nurse instructs Mrs. I to return for additional care for Baby I if one of the following events takes place. Which one would indicate the need for reassessment of Baby I?
   a. The baby sleeps soundly and has to be awakened for a night feeding.
   b. The baby has three loose bowel movements the day after beginning treatment.
   c. The baby continues to lose weight or passes blood in the stool.
   d. The baby gains more than 2 ounces per day.

Bibliography

Abdulla, A, and Keast, J: Hypodermoclysis as a means of rehydration. Nurs Times 93:54, 1997.

Barrow, MW, and Clark, KA: Heat-related illnesses. Am Fam Physician. 58:749, 1998.

Blows, WT: Crowd physiology: the 'penguin effect.' Accid Emerg Nurs 6:129, 1998.

Brensilver, JM, and Goldberger, E: A Primer of Water, Electrolyte, and Acid Base Syndromes, ed 8. FA Davis, Philadelphia, 1996.

Centers for Disease Control: Heat-related illnesses and deaths— Missouri, 1998, and United States, 1979– 1996. Morbidity and Mortality Weekly Report. 48:469, 1999. Accessed 8/11/99 at http://www.cdc.gov/epo/mmwr/preview/mmwrhtml/mm4822a2.htm

Centers for Disease Control: Hyperthermia and dehydration-related deaths associated with intentional rapid weight loss in three collegiate wrestlers—North Carolina, Wisconsin, and Michigan, November–December 1997. Morbidity and Mortality Weekly Report. 47:105, 1998. Accessed 8/24/99 at http://www.cdc.gov/epo/mmwr/preview/mmwrhtml/00051388.htm

Connolly, DL, Shanahan, CM, and Weissberg, PL: Water channels in health and disease. Lancet 347:210, 1996.

Coyle, EF, and Montain, SJ: Benefits of fluid replacement with carbohy-drate during exercise. Med Sci Sports Exerc 24:S324, 1992.

Curtis, R: OA guide to heat related illnesses and fluid balance. Accessed 9/6/99 at http://www.princeton.edu/~oa/safety/heatill.html

Dematte, JE, et al.: Near-fatal heat stroke during the 1995 heat wave in Chicago. Ann Intern Med 129:173, 1998.

Dibas, AI, Mia, AJ, and Yorio, T: Aquaporins (water channels): Role in vasopressin-activated water transport. Proc Soc Exp Biol Med. 219:183, 1998.

Gisolfi, CV: Fluid balance for optimal performance. Nutr Rev 54:S159, 1996.

Groff, JL, Gropper, SS, and Hunt, SM: Advanced Nutrition and Human Metabolism, ed 2. West, Minneapolis, 1995.

Herfel, R, et al.: Iatrogenic acute hyponatraemia in a college athlete. Br J Sports Med 32:257, 1998.

Hett, HA, and Brechtelsbaluer, DA: Heat-related illness. Postgraduate Med 103:107, 1998.

Horne, MM, Heitz, UE, and Swearingen, PL: Fluid, Electrolyte, and Acid–Base Balance. Mosby Year Book, St Louis, 1991.

Johnson, M, Maas, M, and Moorhead, S: Nursing Outcomes Classification (NOC), ed 2. Mosby, Philadelphia, 2000.

Kleiner, SM: Water: An essential but overlooked nutrient. J Am Diet Assoc 99:200, 1999.

Klotz, RS: The effects of intravenous solutions on fluid and electrolyte balance. Journal of Intravenous Nursing 21:20, 1998.

Knoers, NV, and Deen, PM: Aquaporin molecular biology and clinical abnormalities of the water transport channels. Curr Opin Pediatr 10:428, 1998.

Maughan, RJ, Leiper, JB, and Shirreffs, SM: Factors influencing the restoration of fluid and electrolyte balance after exercise in the heat. Br J Sports Med 31:175, 1997.

McCloskey, JC, and Bulechek, GM: Nursing Interventions Classification (NIC), 3 ed. Mosby, Philadelphia, 2000.

McKenna, K, and Thompson, C: Osmoregulation in clinical disorders of thirst appreciation. Clin Endocrinol 49:139, 1998.

Neuhauser-Berthold, M, et al.: Coffee consumption and total body water homeostasis as measured by fluid balance and bioelectrical impedance analysis. Ann Nutr Metab 41:29, 1997.

North American Nursing Diagnosis Association: Nursing Diagnoses: Definitions and Classification 1999–2000, North American Nursing Diagnosis Association, Philadelphia, 1999.

Pfeil, LA, Katz, PR, and Davis, PJ: Water Metabolism. In Morley, JE, Glick, Z, and Rubenstein, LZ (eds): Geriatric Nutrition ed 2. Raven, New York, 1995.

Scanlon, VC, and Sanders, T: Essentials of Anatomy and Physiology, ed 2. FA Davis, Philadelphia, 1995.

Thillainayagam, AV, Hunt, JB, and Farthing, MJG: Enhancing clinical efficacy of oral rehydration therapy: Is low osmolality the key? Gastroenterology 114:197, 1998.

Thomas, CL (ed): Tabor's Cyclopedic Medical Dictionary ed 18. FA Davis, Philadelphia, 1997.

van Assen, S, and Mudde, AH. Severe hyponatremia in an amiloride/hydrochlorthiazide-treated patient. Neth J Med 54:108, 1999.

Wierzbicki, AS, Ball, SG, and Singh, NK: Profound hyponatraemia following an idiosyncratic reaction to diuretics. Int J Clin Pract 52:278, 1998.

CHAPTER 10

Digestion, Absorption, Metabolism, and Excretion

LEARNING OBJECTIVES

After completing this chapter, the student should be able to:

1. List the anatomic structures that make up the gastrointestinal tract.
2. Describe the processes of digestion, absorption, metabolism, and excretion.
3. Discuss how cells use nutrients.
4. Describe appropriate dietary treatments for lactose intolerance, lipid malabsorption, food allergies, and gluten-sensitive enteropathy.
5. List the ways the body eliminates waste.

Every part of the human body requires nutrients for energy, maintenance, and growth. Food supplies the necessary nutrients. Food is composed of complex substances that must be broken down to simpler forms that the cells can use.

The cell is the ultimate destination for the nutrients found in food. Digestion, absorption, and metabolism are the three interrelated processes that act on food to prepare it for use by the body. A fourth process, excretion, is the elimination of undigestible or unusable substances. This chapter discusses all the bodily activities, organs, and systems involved in these major processes.

The Major Processes

The first step in preparing food for use by the cells is digestion. Digestion is the process by which food is broken down mechanically and chemically in the gastrointestinal tract into forms small enough for absorption to occur. The end products of digestion move from the gastrointestinal tract into the blood or lymphatic system in a process called absorption.

After absorption, the nutrients usually are transported to the liver, where they may be adjusted to suit the needs of the body. Metabolism, the sum of all physical and chemical changes that take place in the body, determines the final use of the individual nutrients as well as medications. What the cells have no use for becomes waste that is eliminated through excretion.

Digestion

Digestion takes place in the alimentary canal and the accessory organs.

Alimentary Canal

The alimentary canal is a long, muscular tube that extends through the body from the mouth to the anus. It includes the oral cavity, pharynx, esophagus, stomach, small intestine, and large intestine. Muscle rings, called sphincters, separate segments of the alimentary canal. They act as valves to control the passage of food. When the muscles contract, the passageway closes; when the muscles relax, the passageway opens. Mucosa lines the alimentary canal. It secretes mucus, which lubricates the canal and helps facilitate the smooth passage of food. The mucosa secretes the digestive enzymes of the stomach and small intestine.

Accessory Organs

Three organs located outside of the alimentary canal are considered part of the digestive system—the liver, gallbladder, and pancreas. They make important contributions to the digestive process.

Liver

The liver is the second largest single organ in the body (skin is the largest). The liver performs many functions, but its primary digestive function is the production of bile. Bile is important in breaking down dietary fats. Bile exits the liver by the hepatic duct (a duct is a narrow tube that permits the movement of fluid from one organ to another). A later section in this chapter discusses some of the tasks the liver performs after the absorption of nutrients.

Gallbladder

The gallbladder is a 3- to 4-inch sac that concentrates and stores bile until it is needed in the small intestine. Bile is delivered to the small intestine through the common bile duct. About 2 to 3 cups of bile are secreted each day into the alimentary canal.

Pancreas

The pancreas secretes enzymes that are involved in the digestion of all the energy nutrients. These secretions are collectively known as pancreatic juice. Pancreatic juice is carried to the small intestine via the pancreatic and common bile ducts.

Digestive Action

Mechanical and chemical digestion occur simultaneously throughout the alimentary canal. Mechanical digestion is the physical breaking down of food into smaller pieces. Chemical digestion involves the splitting of complex molecules into simpler forms.

Mechanical Digestion

Examples of mechanical digestion include chewing or mastication, swallowing, peristalsis, and emulsification. Peristalsis is a wavelike movement that propels food through the entire length of the alimentary canal. This one-way movement is caused by the alternate contraction and relaxation of the circular and longitudinal muscles that make up the external muscle layer of the alimentary canal. Other muscular activity churns the food, reducing it to successively smaller particles and mixing it with digestive secretions. All of these muscular actions are regulated by a network of nerves within the wall of the alimentary canal. Emulsification is discussed later in this chapter.

Chemical Digestion

Many chemical reactions are involved in digestion. For example, the conversion of starch to maltose, of fat to glycerol and fatty acids, and of protein to amino acids all involve the process of hydrolysis. The hydrolysis of nutrients is achieved mostly through the action of digestive enzymes, which are present in saliva, gastric juice, pancreatic juice, and intestinal juice.

Each enzyme is specific in its action; it acts only upon a particular substance and no other. Enzymes sometimes require the presence of additional substances such as activators, coenzymes, or hormones to make them active. More than 500 are enzymes involved in the digestive process; this chapter discusses a few of the major ones.

In addition to enzymes, other secretions and chemicals are used in the chemical digestion of food, including mucus, electrolytes, and water. Mucus lubricates passages and facilitates the movement of food. It also protects the inside walls of the alimentary canal from acidic solutions. Electrolytes are substances that conduct an electric current in solution (see previous chapter). One example of an electrolyte is the hydrochloric acid (HCl) the stomach secretes. HCl performs many functions necessary to the digestive process, discussed later in this chapter.

CONTROL OF SECRETIONS The amount of mucus, electrolytes, water, and enzymes released during the digestive process depends on several factors. Hormones frequently initiate a given secretion. For example, the acid content of the food mixture in the stomach causes the release of a hormone called secretin. The release of secretin in the small intestine causes the pancreas to send pancreatic juices into the small intestine.

Emotions and conditioned responses can affect the amount of a secretion released. For example, the smell of a roasting turkey on Thanksgiving Day causes the release of hydrochloric acid in the stomach.

Stress and tension can also produce this effect, sometimes with deleterious results.

The presence of food in the gastrointestinal tract can influence the release of alimentary canal secretions. Coffee drinking, for instance, causes a hormone to be released into the stomach that in turn causes the secretion of hydrochloric acid. Another trigger for the release of bile from the gallbladder is the presence of fat in the small intestine. A chain of reactions whereby one event causes another and then another is very common in all biological systems.

END PRODUCTS OF DIGESTION Four to six hours after a meal, the body has broken down the food into some trillion molecules. Each of the energy nutrients is broken down into simpler molecules. Carbohydrates are digested into monosaccharides. Fats are broken down into molecules of glycerol, fatty acids, and monoglycerides. The end products of protein digestion are amino acids and small peptides. It is thought that as much as one-third of dietary protein is absorbed into mucosal cells as dipeptides and tripeptides. Vitamins, minerals, and water are also released during digestion.

The Food Pathway

Food passes through the mouth into the oral cavity, where it is chewed and exposed to chemicals in the saliva. The tongue voluntarily forces the mass of food, called a bolus, into the pharynx, which is responsible for the reflex action of swallowing. When swallowed, the bolus enters the esophagus, a muscular, mucus-lined tube, and is propelled downward by peristalsis to the stomach. Both mechanical and chemical digestion occur in the stomach, reducing the food to a semifluid mass that is then released into the small intestine. Further digestion takes place in the small intestine, and most of the absorption of nutrients occurs there as well. Any food remaining after digestion and absorption passes into the large intestine and is excreted as fecal matter.

Oral Cavity

The oral cavity, the hollow space in the skull directly behind the mouth, includes the roof of the mouth, the cheeks, and the floor of the mouth. Within the oral cavity are the teeth, tongue, and the openings of the ducts of the salivary glands.

DIGESTIVE ACTION Food entering the oral cavity is chewed and thus broken into smaller particles. This mechanical action increases the surface area of the food for exposure to saliva, a digestive secretion produced by the salivary glands. Saliva moistens and softens the food for swallowing and contains the digestive enzyme known as salivary amylase. Salivary amylase converts starch to maltose (a disaccharide) or to shorter chains of glucose. Because simple sugars (monosaccharides) require no digestion, some absorption of them may occur in the mouth. A few medications such as nitroglycerin are absorbed in the mouth. The chemical digestion of carbohydrates (starch) continues until the hydrochloric acid in the stomach halts the action of the salivary amylase. After being chewed, the bolus (food mass) is maneuvered backward by the tongue into the pharynx. Box 10–1 introduces the dietary treatment of dysphagia.

Box 10–1 Dietary Treatment for Dysphagia

Approximately 15 million people in the United States have a swallowing disorder called dysphagia, literally meaning difficulty swallowing. Many swallowing disorders go undiagnosed. Although a swallowing disorder may prompt a cough, this does not always occur. Food particles may pass unnoticed into the lungs (aspiration) allowing bacteria to multiply. Such "silent" aspiration, which has been observed in people in the aftermath of a stroke, carries with it the serious risk of pneumonia and death (Cataldo, 1999).

Diets for dysphagia that safely meet nutrient needs range from nothing by mouth (NPO) to total oral feedings. Candidates for oral feedings should demonstrate the ability to perform a safe swallow by a bedside evaluation or a modified barium swallow; be alert and able to follow directions; and be oriented to self and the task of eating. Dysphagia diets provide graduated steps from the most easily managed food to the ones most difficult to manage (Lewis and Redder, 1996):

- Liquids range from thick to thin.
- Solids range from pureed to regular.
- The most conservative starting point is thickened liquids and pureed textures.
- Liquids and solids may be progressed independently.

The most precise diet orders specify both the texture of solid foods and the consistency of liquids as well as other therapeutic modifications.

The use of thickening agents to modify the consistency of beverages, soups, and pureed foods is both an art and a science. Commercial thickening agents, instant potato flakes, unflavored gelatin, and dehydrated baby foods and cereals can all be used to thicken foods. The nurse should recognize that thickening agents may:

- Become thicker with time
- Add significant carbohydrate kcalories to clients' diets
- React differently in various foods
- Affect palatability of the thickened item (Lewis and Redder, 1999)

Staff need to be trained to follow recipes and mix complementary flavors. For example, tomato juice can be used to thin spaghetti sauce.

Some foods change their consistency at body temperature, such as ice cream and gelatin. Foods with mixed consistency such as vegetable soups with "chunks" and cereal with milk may not be appropriate for a given individual because he or she may not be able to swallow a food of mixed consistency. For individuals who have problems forming a food bolus, foods such as rice, scrambled eggs, corn, peas, and legumes may cause a problem. These foods do not form a cohesive bolus. For other patients, foods that crumble, such as crackers, cornbread, and unmoistened ground meats may not be appropriate. Thus, each patient needs his or her diet highly individualized.

A preprinted sheet of dos and don'ts is of limited usefulness for many of these clients. A nurse, speech therapist, occupational therapist, and a registered dietitian may collectively devote many sessions to the development of an individualized diet plan and to determine the best position for the client during feeding times. Usually the patient should be sitting upright with hips at a 90 degree angle, shoulder slightly forward, and feet flat on the floor or firmly supported (The American Dietetic Association, 1996). Poorly functioning institutional systems may lack the resources and sometimes delay evaluation and treatment for these clients. The nurse can do much to help these clients by referring them to healthcare providers who can spend the time to work with them.

Signs and symptoms that indicate dysphagia include:

- "Gurgly" voice
- Coughing or choking with food and fluid intake
- Nasal regurgitation
- Pocketing of food in cheeks
- Drooling
- Difficulty in initiating a swallow
- Excessive chewing
- Poor tongue control
- Poor lip closure
- Lack of body position control
- Slurred speech
- Refusal to eat
- Absence of gag reflux
- Excessive time spent eating
- Multiple swallows required to clear a single bolus of food
- Pain upon swallowing
- Verbal complaints of food stuck in the throat
- Lack of attention to eating

Upon observation, these patients may have a documented weight loss, edema, poor skin turgor, and open wounds. These are all signs of poor nutrition.

Tips for safe swallowing include:

- Eat slowly
- Avoid distractions while eating
- Do not talk while eating
- Remove loose dentures
- Sit up while eating
- Position head correctly
- Use a teaspoon and take only one-half teaspoon of food or liquids at a time
- Swallow completely between bites or sips
- Select foods and fluids of appropriate consistency

Pharynx

The pharynx is a muscular passage between the oral cavity and the esophagus. No digestive action occurs there. The pharynx continues the movement of the bolus by the reflexive action of swallowing. The bolus then enters the esophagus.

Esophagus

The esophagus is a muscular tube about 10 inches long that takes food from the pharynx to the stomach. No digestive action occurs there. Peristalsis forces the bolus into the stomach with the help of mucous secretions. Between the esophagus and the stomach is the cardiac sphincter (the first portion of the stomach is called the cardia), which opens to permit passage of the food. The sphincter closes after the passage of food to prevent the backup of stomach contents.

Stomach

The stomach is a J-shaped sac that extends from the esophagus to the small intestine. Folds in the mucous membrane, called rugae, smooth out when the stomach is full. They allow the stomach to expand. There is no need to eat constantly, partly because the stomach serves as a reservoir for food—it takes 4 to 6 hours for food to pass completely through to the small intestine. Gastric juice, the collective secretions of the stomach, consists of hydrochloric acid, mucus, and the enzymes pepsin, rennin, and gastric lipase.

DIGESTIVE ACTION In the stomach, the chemical digestion of protein begins and further mechanical digestion takes place. Some water and minerals, certain drugs, and alcohol are absorbed in the stomach. Even before food enters the mouth, the sight or smell of food can cause the gastric mucosa to excrete the hormone gastrin. This hormone stimulates the secretion of gastric juice so that there is some present in the stomach when the food arrives. The stomach's lining is partially protected from the corrosive effects of gastric juice by mucus.

The hydrolysis of protein is initiated when hydrochloric acid activates and then converts pepsinogen to its active form, pepsin. A protein molecule consists of as many as hundreds of amino acids joined together by peptide bonds. Such chains of amino acids linked by peptide bonds are called polypeptides. Pepsin breaks down large polypeptides into smaller polypeptides. In infants, the milk protein casein is broken down by the enzyme rennin. The action of rennin coagulates (curdles) the milk. In addition to activating pepsin, hydrochloric acid destroys harmful bacteria, makes certain minerals such as iron and calcium more absorbable, and maintains the pH (1 to 2) of the gastric juice.

Some butterfat molecules of milk are also broken down into smaller molecules in the stomach. The enzyme that accomplishes this breakdown is gastric lipase. This enzyme is most active in infants; the more alkaline environment of the infant's stomach enables gastric lipase to work more effectively than in adults.

The mechanical digestion that occurs in the stomach is a result of the churning action of the muscular walls. This muscular activity agitates the contents of the stomach, thoroughly mixing the food with gastric juice. In this way, the food is reduced to a semifluid mass of partially digested material called chyme. Peristaltic waves push the chyme toward the pyloric sphincter, the valve separating the stomach from the small intes-

tine. With each peristaltic wave, a small amount of chyme is forced through the pyloric sphincter into the small intestine.

Small Intestine

The small intestine is the longest portion of the alimentary canal, approximately 20 feet (610 cm) in length. It extends from the pyloric sphincter of the stomach to the large intestine. The small intestine is looped and coiled in the central part of the abdominal cavity, surrounded by the large intestine. It consists of three parts: the duodenum is the first 10 inches, the jejunum is the middle 8 feet, and the ileum is the last 11 feet. Ninety percent of the digestive action in the alimentary canal and nearly all absorption of the end products of digestion occur in the small intestine. Its anatomy is discussed further in the section on absorption.

The entry of chyme into the duodenum stimulates the secretion of two hormones, secretin and cholecystokinin. Collectively, these hormones are responsible for the secretion and release of bile and the secretion of pancreatic juice. Secretin stimulates the production of bile by the liver and the secretion of sodium bicarbonate juice by the pancreas. The bile salts in bile emulsify fats, and sodium bicarbonate juice (which is alkaline) neutralizes the gastric juice that enters the duodenum. This neutralization is necessary to prevent damage to the lining of the duodenum. Mucus secreted by intestinal glands also provides some measure of protection against such damage.

Cholecystokinin stimulates the contraction of the gallbladder, an action that forces stored bile into the duodenum. It also stimulates the secretion of pancreatic enzymes, which are essential for the breakdown of carbohydrates, fats, and proteins. Intestinal juice is also secreted in response to the presence of chyme in the duodenum. Peristaltic action of the small intestine mixes together the bile, the pancreatic juice, and the intestinal juice with the chyme as it moves toward the colon. The collective action of these juices yields the final end products of the digestive process.

DIGESTION OF CARBOHYDRATES Carbohydrate digestion is completed through the action of pancreatic and intestinal enzymes. Pancreatic amylase breaks down any remaining starch into maltose. The disaccharides maltose, sucrose, and lactose are reduced to monosaccharides by the action of three enzymes located in the walls of the small intestine. Each of these enzymes is specific for a given disaccharide: maltase breaks down maltose to glucose and glucose, sucrase breaks down sucrose to glucose and fructose, and lactase breaks down lactose to glucose and galactose. Often, low levels of these enzymes can lead to intolerances for the respective disaccharides.

In fact, approximately 70 percent of the world's population has some degree of lactose intolerance. This intolerance is the result of a lack of the intestinal enzyme lactase. Clinical Application 10–1 discusses carbohydrate intolerances, including lactose intolerance. Table 10–1 lists food items that are lactose-free, low in lactose, and high in lactose. Table 10–2 contains a lactose-restricted diet with a sample menu.

DIGESTION OF FATS Fats are emulsified by bile salts in the small intestine before they are digested further. Emulsification is the physical breaking up of fats into tiny droplets. In this way, more surface area of the fat is exposed to the chemical action of the enzyme pancreatic lipase. Pancreatic lipase completes the digestion of fats by reducing triglycerides

CLINICAL APPLICATION 10–1

Carbohydrate Intolerances

Some individuals are deficient in one or more of the enzymes lactase, maltase, or sucrase. They are unable to digest these disaccharides into monosaccharides. The resulting disease is called a lactose intolerance, maltose intolerance, or sucrose intolerance.

Lactose intolerance, the most common of these diseases, may occur in 60 percent to 100 percent of Hispanics, blacks, and southeast Asians. The condition can be hereditary or can be secondary to other disease processes involving the small intestine. Symptoms of a lactose intolerance include abdominal cramping and pain, loose stools, and flatulence (gas) after eating or drinking milk products.

Dietary treatment of a lactose intolerance involves three steps: (1) identifying food items that contain lactose; (2) eliminating all sources of lactose from the diet; and (3) establishing an individual tolerance level for the client on a trial-and-error basis. The tolerance levels for lactose vary widely among individuals.

The lactose content of cheeses varies. One gallon of milk is required to produce 1 lb of cheese. During cheese making, the whey is separated from the curd. The whey is the liquid and the curd is the solid material (similar to the curd in cottage cheese). Most of the lactose in cheese is contained in the whey. In ripened cheese, the small amount of lactose entrapped in the curd is transformed into lactic acid, which does not require lactase for absorption.

Generally, cheese must age for more than 90 days to be lactose free. The following cheeses are considered hard ripened (low in lactose): blue, brick, Brie, Camembert, Cheddar, Colby, Edam, Gouda, Monterey, Muenster, Parmesan, Provolone, and Swiss. The following cheeses are considered "soft cheeses" and thus contain more lactose: cream cheese, Neufchatel, ricotta, mozzarella, and cottage cheese.

Clients on a lactose-free diet should read all labels carefully to see if milk or milk solids, lactose, or whey have been added to the products. Many toothpastes or over-the-counter medications contain a small amount of lactose. Generally, the amount is very small and is tolerated well.

Lactaid is an over-the-counter product specially designed for individuals with a lactose intolerance. Lactaid is a natural enzyme that is available in liquid or tablet form. The liquid form is typically added to milk, whereas the tablet form is chewed before consumption of a food product containing lactose. Some grocery stores also sell milk that has been pretreated with Lactaid. This product will digest 70 percent of the lactose in a product into glucose galactose. As a result, most lactose-intolerant persons can drink Lactaid-treated milk or eat foods that contain lactose and digest it comfortably. Milk treated with Lactaid is slightly sweeter than regular milk. The sweeter taste results naturally when lactose is broken down into glucose and galactose.

A lactose-restricted diet may be low in calcium, riboflavin, and vitamin D. Clients should be instructed in alternative sources of these nutrients or advised to take supplements.

Table 10–1 Lactose Content of Foods

Lactose-Free Foods		Low-Lactose Foods (0–2 g/serving)	
Broth-based soups		1/2 cup	Milk treated with lactase enzyme
Plain meat, fish, poultry, peanut butter		1/2 cup	Sherbet
Breads that do not contain milk, dry milk solids, or whey		1–2 oz	Aged cheese
		1 oz	Processed cheese
Cereal, crackers		Butter or margarine	
Fruit, plain vegetables		Commercially prepared foods containing dry milk solids or whey	
Desserts made without milk, dry milk solids or whey		Some medications and vitamin preparations may contain a small amount of lactose. Generally, the amount is very small and is tolerated well.	
Tofu and tofu products, such as tofu-based ice cream substitute			
Nondairy creamers			
High-Lactose Foods (5 to 8 g/serving)			
1/2 cup	Milk (whole, skim, 1 percent, 2 percent, buttermilk, sweet acidophilus)	1/2 cup	White sauce
		1/2 cup	Party chip dip or potato topping
1/8 cup	Powdered dry milk (whole, nonfat, buttermilk—before reconstituting)	3/4 cup	Creamed or low-fat cottage cheese
		1 cup	Dry cottage cheese
1/4 cup	Evaporated milk	3/4 cup	Ricotta cheese
3 tbsp	Sweetened condensed milk	2 oz	Cheese food or cheese spread*
3/4	Heavy cream	3/4 cup	Ice cream or ice milk
1/2 cup	Half and half	1/2 cup	Yogurt†
1/2 cup	Sour cream		

*Lactose content is higher than that of aged cheese and of processed cheese because of the addition of whey powder and dry milk solids.
†Yogurt may be tolerated better than foods with similar lactose content because of hydrolysis of lactose by bacterial lactase found in the culture. Tolerance may vary with the brand and processing method.
Source: Mayo Clinic Diet Manual, with permission.

Table 10–2 Lactose-Restricted Diet

Description: This diet restricts foods which contain lactose. Soy milk substitutes are used as a milk replacement. Individual tolerances should be taken into consideration as some clients may tolerate foods low in lactose. (See Table 10–1)

Note: All labels should be read carefully for the addition of milk, lactose, or whey.

Indications: This diet is used for the management of patients exhibiting the signs and symptoms of lactose intolerance, Crohn's disease, short bowel syndrome, or colitis. Persistent diarrhea and excessive amounts of gas may be lessened by decreasing lactose intake.

Nutritional adequacy: This diet is low in calcium, riboflavin, and vitamin D. Supplementation is recommended

Food Group	Allowed	Avoided
Milk	Hard, ripened cheese Ensure Sustacal Ensure Plus Soy milk Lactaid-treated milk Coffee Rich	Unripened cheese Fluid milk Powdered milk Milk chocolate Cream Most chocolate drink mixes Most coffee creamers

Breads and Cereals	Most water-based bread (French
	   Italian, Jewish)
	Graham crackers
	Ritz crackers without cheese
		Bread to which milk or lactose
		   has been added (Check label)

Fruits	Any	None
Vegetables	Fresh, frozen, or canned without milk	Creamed, buttered, or breaded vegetables
Meats	Those not listed under avoided Kosher prepared meat or milk products	Breaded or creamed meat, fish, poultry Most luncheon meats Sausage Frankfurters

Desserts and
  Miscellaneous
  Items
	Angel food cake
	Gelatin desserts
	Milk-free cookies
	Popcorn (with milk-free margarine)
	Pretzels
	Mustard, catsup
	Pickles
		Most commercially made desserts
		Sherbet
		Ice cream
		Cream candies
		Toffee
		Caramels
		Most chewing gums

SAMPLE MENU

Breakfast	Lunch/Dinner
1/2 cup orange juice 1/2 cup cream of wheat 2 slices whole grain milk-free bread 2 tsp milk-free margarine Jelly Coffee 1/2 cup nondairy "creamer"	3 oz baked chicken Baked potato 1/2 cup carrots Sliced tomato 1 slice milk-free bread 2 tsp milk-free margarine Angel food cake with fresh fruit topping Coffee

to diglycerides and monoglycerides, fatty acids, and glycerol. Lingual lipase is an important enzyme in infants, although not in adults.

DIGESTION OF PROTEIN Although hundreds of enzymes are involved in protein digestion, this text reviews only a few of the major ones. The shorter polypeptides resulting from the digestive action in the stomach are broken down even further by the action of pancreatic and intestinal enzymes. Two of the major pancreatic enzymes that are responsible for this additional protein-splitting are trypsin and chymotrypsin. Both trypsin

and chymotrypsin have inactive precursors that are activated by other enzymes.

The intestinal wall also secretes a group of enzymes known as peptidases. The peptidases act on the smaller molecules produced by the pancreatic enzymes, reducing them to single amino acids and small peptides, the final end products of protein digestion.

Table 10–3 summarizes the digestion of carbohydrates, fats, and proteins by body organ (mouth, stomach, and small intestine). The Table

Table 10–3 Summary of Digestion

Nutrient	Mouth and Esophagus	Stomach	Small Intestine
Carbohydrates	*Mechanical* Mastication Swallowing Peristalsis Mucus	*Mechanical* Peristalsis Mucus	*Mechanical* Peristalsis Mucus
	Chemical Salivary amylase	*Chemical* None	*Chemical* Pancreatic enzymes: 　Pancreatic amylase Intestinal enzymes: 　Maltase 　Sucrase 　Lactase
Monosaccharides			
Fats yield	*Mechanical* Mastication Swallowing Peristalsis Mucus	*Mechanical* Peristalsis Mucus	*Mechanical* Peristalsis Mucus Gallbladder: 　Bile*
	Chemical None Lingual lipase in infants	*Chemical* Gastric lipase†	*Chemical* Pancreatic enzymes: 　Pancreatic 　lipase
Glycerol, fatty acids, 　and monoglycerides			
Proteins yield	*Mechanical* Mastication Swallowing Peristalsis Mucus	*Mechanical* Peristalsis Mucus	*Mechanical* Peristalsis Mucus
	Chemical None	*Chemical* Rennin Pepsin Hydrochloric acid	*Chemical* Pancreatic enzymes: 　Trypsin 　Chymotrypsin Intestinal enzymes: 　Peptidases
Amino acids and 　small peptides			

*Emulsifies fat.
†Digests butterfat only.

10–3 subcategories identify whether the digestive action is mechanical or chemical.

Absorption

The end products of digestion move from the gastrointestinal tract into the blood or lymphatic system in a process called absorption. The lymphatic system transports lymph from the tissues to the bloodstream. This system is technically part of the circulatory or cardiovascular system. Eventually, all fluid in the lymphatic system enters the blood. It is only after nutrients have been absorbed into either the blood or lymphatic system that the cells of the body can use them.

The end products of digestion include the monosaccharides from carbohydrate digestion, the fatty acids and glycerol (and often monoglycerides) from fats, and small peptides and amino acids from protein digestion. Absorption occurs primarily in the small intestine.

Small Intestine

The inner surface of the small intestine has mucosal folds, villi, and microvilli to increase the surface area for maximum absorption (Fig.

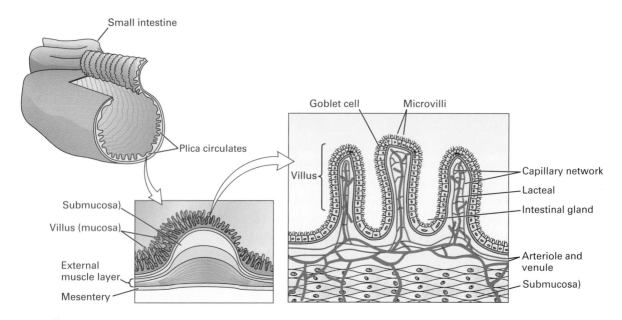

Figure 10–1:
Cross-section of the small intestine. The multiple folds greatly increase the furface area of the small intestine. (With permission, Scalon and Sanders, *Essentials of Anatomy and Physiology*, FA Davis.)

10–1). The mucosal folds are like pleats in fabric. On each fold ("pleat") are millions of finger-like projections, called villi. Each villus has hundreds of microscopic, hairlike projections (resembling bristles on a brush), called microvilli, on its surface. The large surface area resulting from this arrangement fosters the movement of nutrients into the blood or lymphatic system. The structure of the mucosa serves as a unit that accomplishes the absorption of nutrients.

Within each villus is a network of blood capillaries and a central lymph vessel called a lacteal. The villi absorb nutrients from the chyme by way of these blood and lymph vessels. Monosaccharides, amino acids, glycerol (which is water soluble), minerals, and water-soluble vitamins are absorbed into the blood in the capillary network. Because short- and medium-chain fatty acids have fewer carbons in their chain length, they are more water soluble than long-chain fatty acids. Thus, they are absorbed directly into the blood as well.

These water-soluble nutrients, including short- and medium-chain fatty acids, eventually enter into hepatic portal circulation (via the portal vein) and travel to the liver. Hepatic portal circulation is a subdivision of the vascular system by which blood from the digestive organs and spleen circulates through the liver before returning to the heart. In the liver, the nutrients are modified according to the needs of the body.

Because long-chain fats are not soluble in water and the blood is chiefly water, the fat-soluble nutrients cannot be absorbed directly into the blood. Instead, fat-soluble nutrients—including long-chain fatty acids, any monoglycerides remaining from fat digestion, and fat-soluble vitamins—are first combined with bile salts as a carrier. Then, this complex of fat-soluble materials is absorbed into the cells lining the intestinal wall.

Once the fat is absorbed, the bile separates from it and returns to recirculate. Within the intestinal cells, any remaining monoglycerides are reduced to fatty acids and glycerol by an enzyme. Glycerol, fatty acids, and absorbed long-chain fatty acids are recombined (within the intestinal cells) to form human triglycerides in a process called triglyceride synthesis.

The newly formed triglycerides and any other fat materials present (such as cholesterol) are covered with special proteins, forming lipoproteins called chylomicrons. The chylomicrons are released into the lymphatic system via the lacteals. Remember that the lymphatic system is connected to the blood system. The protein "wrapping" these packages of fat enables the chylomicrons to move into the blood via the thoracic lymphatic duct (and hence into portal blood). In the liver, lipids are also modified to suit the needs of the body before distribution to body cells. Table 10–4 describes some of the nutrient modifications that are made in the liver.

Table 10–4 Metabolic Modifications in the Liver	
Energy Nutrient	**Modification**
Carbohydrates	Fructose and galactose changed to glucose, excess glucose converted to glycogen
Lipids	Lipoproteins formed, cholesterol synthesized, triglycerides broken down and built
Amino acids	Nonessential amino acids manufactured, excess amino acids deaminated and then changed to carbohydrates or fats, ammonia removed from the blood, plasma proteins made
Other	Alcohol, drugs, and poisons detoxified

Table 10–5 Factors Decreasing Absorption

Medications	Antacids
	Laxatives
	Birth control pills
	Anticonvulsants
	Antibiotics
Parasites	Tapeworm
	Hookworm
Surgical procedures	Gastric resections
	Any surgery on the small intestine
	Some surgical procedures on the large intestine
Disease states	Infection
	Tropical sprue
	Gluten-sensitive enteropathy
	Hepatic disease
	Pancreatic insufficiency
	Lactase deficiency
	Sucrase deficiency
	Maltase deficiency
	Circulatory disorders
	Cancers involving the alimentary canal
Medical complications	Effects of radiation therapy
	Chemotherapy

Note: Most of these conditions will be discussed in later chapters.

Further passage of undigested food is controlled by the ileocecal valve, which relaxes and then closes with each peristaltic wave. This valve prevents backflow and ensures that chyme remains in the small intestine long enough for sufficient digestion and absorption.

Large Intestine

The large intestine, also called the colon, extends from the ileum (last part of the small intestine) to the anus. When the chyme leaves the small intestine, it enters the first portion of the large intestine, the cecum (the appendix, an organ with no known function, is attached to the cecum). Chyme leaves the cecum and travels slowly through the remaining parts of the large intestine: the ascending colon, the transverse colon, the descending colon, the sigmoid colon, the rectum, and the anal canal.

Water is the main substance absorbed by the large intestine. However, the absorption of some minerals and vitamins also occurs in the colon. Most of the water, up to 80 percent, is extracted in the cecum and the ascending colon and returned to the bloodstream. Vitamins synthesized by intestinal bacteria, including vitamin K and some of the B-complexes, are absorbed from the colon. After absorption and digestion have taken place, the remaining waste products are eliminated in the feces through the rectum.

Elimination of Unabsorbed Materials

Absorption of water into the bloodstream slowly reduces the water content of the material left inside the large intestine, and the waste product has a solid consistency. This solid material is the feces. Mucus, the only secretion of the large intestine, provides lubrication for the smooth passage of the feces. By the time feces reaches the rectum, it consists of 75 percent water and 25 percent solids. The solids include cellular wastes, undigested dietary fiber, undigested food, bile salts, cholesterol, mucus, and bacteria.

CLINICAL APPLICATION 10–2

Surgical Removal of All or Part of the Alimentary Canal

Clients may need to have a portion of the small intestine surgically removed for a variety of reasons. These clients are frequently at a nutritional risk because they are either permanently or temporarily unable to absorb essential nutrients. In such cases, a nutritional assessment is indicated. In the past, some clients elected to have a portion of the alimentary canal removed to lose weight. This procedure is discussed in the weight control chapter.

Indigestible Carbohydrates

The body cannot digest some forms of carbohydrates because it lacks the necessary enzyme to split the appropriate molecule. Some vegetables and legumes contain these indigestible sugars and fibers. Intestinal gas is formed in the colon by the decomposition of undigested materials. Examples of gas-forming foods are beans, onions, radishes, and vegetables of the cabbage family.

Factors Interfering with Absorption

Malabsorption is the inadequate movement of digested food from the small intestine into the blood or lymphatic system. Malnutrition can be caused by malabsorption. Table 10–5 lists factors that interfere with the absorption of nutrients. Note in the table that many diseases, medications, and some medical treatments have a negative impact on the absorption of nutrients. Clinical Application 10–2 discusses surgical removal of all or part of the alimentary canal and the effect on absorption. Clinical Application 10–3 discusses inadequate absorption.

CLINICAL APPLICATION 10–3

Inadequate Absorption

Visually inspecting a client's feces can confirm a suspicion of poor digestion or poor absorption. Large chunks of food indicate a problem with digestion. A large amount of liquid or near-liquid stools suggests poor absorption. A simple question directed to the client, such as "Are your stools formed?" can provide some information. Sometimes, however, client's concept of normal may be different from the health-care providers

The cells lining the inside layer of the small intestine have a very short life. The smallest structures are replaced every 2 to 3 days. Although this rapid cell turnover helps to promote healing after injury, it also allows vulnerability to any nutritional deficiency or process that might interfere with cell reproduction.

"Gut failure" is a term used to describe a situation in which the small intestine fails to absorb nutrients properly. Symptoms include diarrhea, malabsorption, and a poor response to oral feedings. A vicious cycle starts when the cells lining the small intestine fail to reproduce because they do not have the necessary nutrients for cell replacement. The result is chronic diarrhea caused by malabsorption. In turn, the malabsorption leads to malnutrition which prevents cell reproduction. Fig. 10–2 diagrams this cycle.

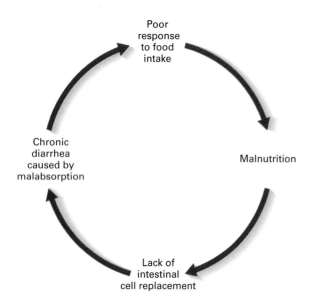

Figure 10–2:
"Gut failure." Gut failure is a self-perpetuating cycle. Poor response to food intake leads to poor intestinal cell regeneration, which leads to chronic diarrhea caused by malabsorption.

Steatorrhea

Some diseases and medications result in the malabsorption of fat. In these conditions, clients have steatorrhea, or fat in the stools. Frequently the condition is caused by the inhibition of pancreatic lipase, an enzyme necessary for the digestion of fats. Clinical Application 10–4 discusses lipid malabsorption and dietary treatment.

Nontropical Sprue

Nontropical sprue is a disorder of the small intestine. This disease is commonly referred to as celiac disease or gluten-sensitive enteropathy. Gluten-sensitive enteropathy results from the toxic effects that occur from the ingestion of gluten, a protein present in the following grains: wheat, rye, oats, and barley. Individuals with this disease suffer from a wide variety of nutritional problems.

The result of the toxic effect of gluten is the direct destruction of intestinal cells. This may be related to an allergic reaction and can be either severe or mild. In the severe form, the loss of the intestinal mucosa causes lactose intolerance.

Treatment in this situation would involve the use of medium-chain triglycerides to increase the kilocaloric content of the diet and a lactose-free, gluten-free diet. This is a complex diet for the healthcare professional to plan and for the client to follow. Usually, frequent consultations with the physician regarding the status of the client's intestinal cells are necessary. These clients are often malnourished. As such, the client benefits from being kept on this severe a diet only until intestinal cell regeneration is

---

Lipid Malabsorption

Some clients for a variety of reasons are unable to digest and absorb long-chain fatty acids. For these clients, the use of MCT (medium-chain triglyceride) oil is indicated. MCT oil can provide a kilocalorie source for patients with a fat malabsorption problem.

Any food that contains fat must be fitted into the diet of any client who suffers from a lipid malabsorption. The American Dietetic and Diabetes Associations' Exchange Lists for Menu Planning can be used as a guide in planning this type of diet. Usually the physician will order a specified number of grams of fat high in long-chain fatty acids. A typical low-fat diet order may read: 40-g fat diet. Such a diet may be planned as follows:

Exchange	Number of Exchanges/ Day	Grams of Fat
Skim milk	Unlimited	0
Starches	8	4 (0.5 g of fat/exchange
Fruits	Unlimited	0
Vegetables	Unlimited	0
Meat, lean	7	21 (7 x 3 g/exchange)
Fat	3	15 (3 x 5 g/exchange) 40 g fat/day

The MCT oil is then added to the diet as necessary to bring the kilocalories up to meet the client's kilocalorie requirement.

Some physicians prefer to treat a lipid disorder with medication. Pancrease is one of the medications indicated for steatorrhea secondary to pancreatic insufficiency, as in cystic fibrosis or chronic alcoholic pancreatitis (discussed in Gastrointestinal chapter). Pancrease is an enzyme that digests nutrients.

---

completed. Once the client is able to tolerate both lactose and long-chain triglycerides, these should be included in the diet. This will increase the client's compliance in maintaining a high kilocalorie intake and assist in treating the malnutrition.

In milder forms, only a gluten-restricted diet is indicated (Table 10–6). Gluten is present in a number of prepared foods that contain thickened sauces. Extensive client teaching is necessary for a positive client outcome. Removal of all forms of wheat, rye, oats, and barley from the diet frequently results in remission or improvement within weeks. Table 10–7 lists products that can be substituted for flour in many recipes.

Food Allergies

A food allergy is a sensitivity to a food that does not cause a negative reaction in most people. Individuals may be genetically predisposed to a food allergy. Almost any food can cause an allergic reaction, but more than 90 percent of food allergies in the U.S. are attributed to cow's milk, eggs, fish, crustaceans, peanuts, soybean, tree nuts, and wheat (Taylor, Hefle, and Munoz-Furlong, 1999). Some food allergies may be due to an alteration in absorption. The susceptible person absorbs a part of a food before it

Table 10–6 Gluten-restricted Diet

Description: The diet is free of cereals that contain gluten: wheat, oats, rye, and barley.

Indications: This diet is used to treat the primary intestinal malabsorption found in celiac disease.

Adequacy: Unless an effort is made to increase kilocalories, the energy intake may be inadequate to replace previous weight loss. This diet may not meet the RDA for B-complex vitamins, especially thiamin. Iron intake may be inadequate for the premenopausal woman.

Food Groups	Foods That Contain Gluten	Foods That May Contain Gluten	Foods That Do Not Contain Gluten
Beverage	Cereal beverages (e.g., Postum), malt, Ovaltine, beer and ale	Commercial* chocolate milk; cocoa mixes; other beverage mixes; dietary supplements	Coffee; tea; decaffeinated coffee; carbonated beverages; chocolate drinks made with pure cocoa powder; wine; distilled liquor
Meat and meat substitutes		Meat loaf and patties, cold cuts and prepared meats, stuffing, breaded meats, cheese foods and spreads; commercial souffles, omelets, and fondue; soy protein meat substitutes	Pure meat, fish, fowl, egg, cottage cheese, and peanut butter
Fat and oil		Commercial salad dressing and mayo, gravy, white and cream sauces, nondairy creamer	Butter, margarine, vegetable oil
Milk	Milk beverages that contain malt	Commercial chocolate milk	Whole, low-fat, and skim milk; buttermilk
Grains and grain products	Bread, crackers, cereal, and pasta that contain wheat, oats, rye, malt, malt flavoring, graham flour, durham flour, pastry flour, bran, or wheat germ; barley; millet; pretzels; communion wafers	Commercial seasoned rice and potato mixes	Specially prepared breads made with wheat starch† rice, potato, or soybean flour or cornmeal; pure corn or rice cereals; hominy grits; white, brown, and wild rice; popcorn; low protein pasta made from wheat starch
Vegetable		Commercially seasoned vegetable mixes; commercial vegetables with cream or cheese sauce; canned baked beans	All fresh vegetables; plain, commercially frozen or canned vegetables

*The terms "commercially prepared" and "commercial" are used to refer to partially prepared foods purchased from a grocery or food market and to prepared foods purchased from a restaurant.

†Wheat starch may contain trace amounts of gluten. Avoid if not tolerated.

(continued)

Table 10–6 Gluten-restricted Diet (Continued)

Food Groups	Foods That Contain Gluten	Foods That May Contain Gluten	Foods That Do Not Contain Gluten
Fruit		Commercial pie fillings	All plain or sweetened fruits; fruit thickened with tapioca or cornstarch
Soup	Soup that contains wheat pasta; soup thickened with wheat flour or other gluten-containing grains	Commercial soup, broth, and soup mixes	Soup thickened with cornstarch potato rice or soybean flour; pure broth
Desserts	Commercial cakes, cookies and pastries	Commercial ice cream and sherbet	Gelatin; custard; fruit ice; specially prepared cakes, cookies, and pastries made with gluten-free flour or starch; pudding and fruit filling thickened with tapioca, cornstarch, or arrowroot flour
Sweets		Commercial candies, especially chocolates	
Miscellaneous		Ketchup; prepared mustard; soy sauce; commercially prepared meat sauces and pickles; vinegar; flavoring syrups (syrups for pancakes or ice cream)	Monosodium glutamate; salt; pepper; pure spices and herbs; yeast; pure baking chocolate or cocoa powder; carob; flavoring extracts; artificial flavoring

SAMPLE MENU

Breakfast	Lunch/Dinner
1/2 cup orange juice	Chicken breast
Cocoa Puffs, Sugar Pops, puffed rice	Baked potato
2 slices gluten-free bread	1/2 cup broccoli
1 poached egg	Lettuce/tomato salad
1 cup milk	French dressing
2 tsp margarine	Sour cream
Jelly	1/2 cup milk
	Cornstarch pudding

Note: Medications may contain trace amounts of gluten. A pharmacist may be able to provide informatin on the gluten content of medications.

Mayo Clinic Diet Manual, 1988, with permission.

Table 10–7 Substitutions for 2 Tablespoons of Wheat Flour
3 tsp cornstarch
3 tsp potato starch
3 tsp arrowroot starch
3 tsp quick-cooking tapioca
3 tbsp white or brown rice flour

has been completely digested. The incomplete digestion of protein in particular is responsible for many allergic reactions.

The body does not recognize the sequence of amino acids (because the protein was absorbed partly undigested) and therefore treats the protein as a foreign substance and tries to destroy it. This attempt produces the symptoms of food allergy, including skin rash, nausea, vomiting, diarrhea, intestinal cramps, swelling in various parts of the body, and spasm of the small intestine. An allergen may also be inhaled into the body. For example, the smell of peanuts may cause an allergic reaction in susceptible people.

Once diagnosed, the treatment for a food allergy is to avoid the offending food. This is difficult even with the current U.S. labeling laws and especially challenging when eating away from home or in foreign countries.

Food allergies are frequently diagnosed in children. One approach used to treat these clients is the Allergy I and Allergy II diets. The Allergy I diet is limited to rice, lamb, and a few fruits and vegetables, and therefore eliminates most common food allergens, including wheat, eggs, and milk. The Allergy II diet includes a few meats, potatoes, and a few more fruits and vegetables. This second diet is completely free of cereal, milk, and eggs. These diets are typically used for one to two weeks. If symptoms are relieved, selected foods are gradually added back into the diet one at a time. Chewing gum, vitamin pills, and certain medications such as antibiotics and antihistamines should be discontinued during the test period. These diets are often prescribed for any apparent allergic response with a multitude of varying and individual symptoms including rash, sinus congestion, headache, wheezing, cough, etc.

The Allergy I and II diets are not nutritionally adequate. Both diets are deficient in calcium, riboflavin, thiamin, folic acid, vitamin B_6, magnesium, and possibly Vitamin C for all ages. In addition, iron is inadequate for teenagers and premenopausal women. For this reason, these diets are not recommended for long-term use. Allergy I and II diets are presented in Table 10–8.

Metabolism

After digestion and absorption, nutrients are carried by the blood (usually after being modified in the liver cells) to all cells of the body. After entry into the cells, the nutrients from food undergo many chemical changes, which result in either the release of energy or the use of energy. Metabolism is the sum of all chemical and physical processes continuously going on in living organisms, comprising both anabolism and catabolism. Catabolic reactions usually result in the release of energy. Anabolic reactions require energy. The next section describes how cells utilize the end products of digestion to meet the energy needs of the body.

Catabolic Reactions

Glucose, glycerol, fatty acids, and amino acids can be broken down even further. These nutrients are held together by bonds that require energy to

form and that, when broken, release energy. The breakdown of the fuel-producing nutrients yields carbon dioxide, water, heat, and other forms of energy. The carbon dioxide is eventually exhaled, and the water becomes part of the body fluids or is eliminated in the urine. Fifty percent or more of the total potential energy usually is lost as heat. The remaining available energy is temporarily stored in the cells as ATP, adenosine triphosphate.

ATP, a high-energy compound that has three phosphate groups in its structure, is thus available in all cells. Practically speaking, ATP is the storage form of energy for the cells since each cell has enzymes that can initiate the hydrolysis (breakdown through the addition of water) of ATP. In this reaction, one or more phosphate groups split off and subsequently release energy. If one phosphate group is removed, the result is ADP (adenosine diphosphate) plus phosphate.

Many steps are involved in the catabolic process responsible for the release of this energy. These steps require one or more of the following agents: enzymes, coenzymes, and/or hormones. Some vitamins and minerals act as coenzymes. Oxygen is also necessary for the full release of any potential energy. This addition of oxygen to the reaction is called oxidation. During the many steps that occur, the energy is released little by little and stored as ATP. The breakdown process includes the formation of intermediate chemical compounds such as pyruvate (pyruvic acid) and acetyl CoA. Acetyl CoA can be broken down further by entering a series of chemical reactions known as the Krebs cycle or the TCA (tricarboxylic acid) cycle. Figure 10–3 is a simplified schematic of the steps involved in the release of energy by the cells.

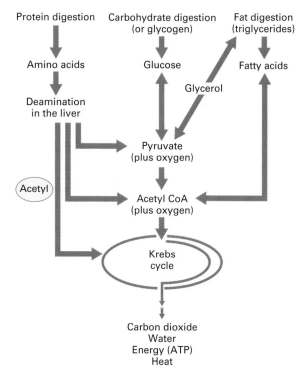

Figure 10–3:
Energy production in the cells. Energy is released bit by bit during the further breakdown of amino acids, glucose, glycerol, and fatty acids.

Table 10–8 Allergy I and II Diets

Allergy I

Food Group	Allowed Foods
Bread, cereal, rice, and pasta group	Rice, rice wafers, rice biscuits, Rice Chex, puffed rice, rice flakes, cream of rice, tapioca, white rice
Vegetable group	Beets, carrots, chard, lettuce, sweet potatoes, yams
Fruit group	Apricots, cranberries, peaches, pears, juice of allowed fruit; unsweetened or sweetened with sucrose
Meat, poultry, fish, dry beans, eggs, and nut group	Lamb
Milk, yogurt, and cheese group	None
Fats, oils, and sweets group	Any vegetable oil or shortening, margarine without milk solids Cane or beet sugar Salt White vinegar, and tapioca

SAMPLE MENU

Breakfast	Lunch/Dinner
Hot cream of rice cereal 2 Rice biscuits 1/2 cup peaches 2 tsp. apricot preserves 1/2 cup peach juice (drained from canned peaches	Lamb chop or ground lamb patty 1/2 cup cooked white rice Baked sweet potato 1/2 cup canned pears Cranberry juice

Allergy II

Food Group	Allowed Foods
Bread, cereal, rice and pasta group	Tapioca, soy flour, potato flour, white and sweet potatoes
Vegetable group	Soybean sprouts, lettuce, spinach, chard, carrots, beets, artichoke, squash, asparagus, peas, string beans, and lima beans
Fruit group	Sucrose-sweetened and unsweetened apricots, cranberries, peaches, pears, pineapple, and prunes and the juices of these fruits
Meat, poultry, fish, dry beans, eggs, and nuts group	Lamb, beef, chicken, bacon, veal, and soybeans
Milk, yogurt, and cheese group	None
Fats, oils, and sweets	Any vegetable oil and shortening, margarine without milk solids Cane or beet sugar (sucrose) Salt, white vinegar, tapioca

SAMPLE MENU

Breakfast	Lunch/Dinner
1/2 cup pineapple chunks 2 slices of bacon 1/2 cup fried potatoes fried in oil 1 cup pineapple juice	4 oz. lamb, beef, chicken, veal or 1/2 cup soybeans Boiled potatoes 2 tsp. milk free margarine 1/2 cup of cooked carrots Lettuce wedge with oil and vinegar Stewed prunes 1 cup cranberry juice

Storage of Excess Nutrients

If the cells do not have immediate energy needs, the excess nutrients are stored. Glucose is stored as glycogen in liver and muscle tissue; surplus amounts are converted to fat. Glycerol and fatty acids are reassembled into triglycerides and stored in adipose tissue. Amino acids are used to make body proteins; any excess is deaminated (stripped of nitrogen) and ultimately used for glucose formation or stored as fat. If energy is not available from food, the cells will seek energy in body stores.

Anabolic Reactions

Once immediate energy needs have been met, the cells utilize the nutrients as needed for growth and repair of body tissue. The cellular supply of ATP is used first. When this instant energy source is exhausted, glycogen and fat stores are used. In addition to building up body protein, other anabolic reactions include the recombination of glycerol and fatty acids to form triglycerides and the formation of glycogen from glucose.

Excretion of Waste Products

Materials of no use to the cells become waste that is eliminated through excretion. Solid waste and some liquid is disposed of in the feces. The digestive system needs assistance from other body systems in the disposal of nonsolid waste. The lungs dispose of gaseous waste. Most liquid waste is sent first to the kidneys and then to the bladder to be eliminated in the urine. Some liquid waste is disposed of by the skin through perspiration.

Carbon dioxide (CO_2) is a gas that is eliminated through the lungs each time one exhales. The amount of carbon dioxide exhaled depends on the type of fuel (lipid, protein, or carbohydrate) and/or the source of fuel that the body is currently burning for energy. For example, more CO_2 is produced when carbohydrates are being utilized than with protein or fat.

The skin removes some of the liquid waste in the form of perspiration or water, and some is excreted in the feces. The kidneys eliminate most of the excess water, sodium, hydrogen, and urea. Urea is synthesized in the liver from the nitrogen resulting from the breakdown of amino acids. Some water is also removed from the body each time one exhales.

Summary

The cell is the ultimate destination for the nutrients in food. For food to be of use to the cells, it must first be broken down into many tiny particles and then absorbed into the body. Digestion is the process whereby food is broken down into a form usable by the cell: carbohydrates are broken down to monosaccharides, fats are reduced to glycerol and fatty acids, and proteins are split to yield amino acids. This is accomplished by both mechanical and chemical means. Secretions from the salivary glands, stomach, small intestine, liver, and pancreas assist in chemical digestion. Absorption refers to the movement of food from the gastrointestinal tract into the blood and lymphatic system. Metabolism involves the two processes of anabolism and catabolism. The liver plays a major role in metabolism.

After absorption, water-soluble nutrients go directly to the liver for further processing. The liver releases the nutrients into the bloodstream

for delivery to the cells. Most of the fat-soluble nutrients are absorbed into the lymphatic system before entering the bloodstream. Short- and medium-chain triglycerides are absorbed differently than long-chain triglycerides. The cells remove the nutrients from the bloodstream as needed for energy and growth. Energy is released little by little from the end products of digestion in a series of chemical reactions. Energy nutrients not needed immediately by the cells are placed in storage as glycogen and adipose tissue.

The metabolism of food produces waste. Waste products are released from the body in the feces, urine, perspiration, and exhaled air.

Many ailments and diseases are related to the structure and function of the gastrointestinal system. Many forms of malabsorption, including disaccharide intolerances and gluten-sensitive enteropathy, are related to structural damage of the small intestine.

Case Study 3-1

Mr. H is a 25-year-old man, 6 ft tall and weighing 170 lb (dressed without shoes). He has a medium frame, as determined by measuring his wrist circumference. Mr. H has just been admitted to the hospital on your service for an elective arthroscopic (surgical procedure) on his right knee. During the nursing admission process, Mr. H complained of gas pains and frequent loose stools. He stated that he does not avoid any particular foods and has a healthy appetite. He claims to

drink about three cups of milk each day. The client complains of a loss of 5 lb during the prior month. Mr. H needs to use the restroom twice during the interview to "move his bowels." The second time you inspect the stool. The client's stool is loose, and unformed.

The next day you note that a diagnosis of lactose intolerance has been made. A lactose-restricted diet is ordered.

The following nursing care plan originates on the day the client is admitted. The physician uses the information collected from the nurse in making his or her diagnosis. Please note that the client has already met the first desired outcome and part of the second; they have been charted. The client has not met the third desired outcome.

Nursing Care Plan

Subjective Data	Client complains of gas pains and loose stools. Client states that he does not avoid any particular foods. He drinks milk.
Objective Data	Client observed to use the restroom twice in 10 minutes to defecate. Visual inspection shows stool to be loose and unformed
Nursing Diagnosis	Nursing Diagnosis NANDA: Diarrhea (North American Nursing Diagnosis Association, 1999) related to client's complaints of loose stools as evidenced by the client's need to use the restroom twice in a 10-mitlute period and by direct observation of one loose and unformed stool.

Desired Outcomes Evaluation Criteria	Nursing Actions/ Interventions	Rationale
Treatment Behavior: Illness (NOC) (Johnson, Maas, and Moorhead, 2000)	Diarrhea Management (NIC) (McCloskey and Bulechek, 2000)	
The client will assist in ruling out causes for his loose stools and report his signs and symptoms to the nurse.	Teach the client to observe and record the pattern, onset, frequency, characteristics, amount, time of day, and precipitating events related to occurrence of diarrhea. Refer client to the dietitian to determine usual food intake and nutritional status. Determine exposure to recent environmental contaminants, that is, drinking water; food handling practices; and proximity to others who are ill. Review drug intake for medications affecting absorption (see Table 10–5, Factors Decreasing Absorption).	Observation and documentation of the client's response to these factors will assist in determining the cause of his loose stools.
The client will eliminate causative factors at once after these factors have been determined	Follow through with the elimination of causative factors, restrict intake if necessary, note change in drug therapy, if any.	Elimination of the causative factors should decrease the frequency of loose, unformed stools. The client needs to be instructed on the relationship of his diarrhea to causative factors.
The client will have formed stools within 24 hours after the causative factors have been eliminated.	Document stool consistency.	Whenever possible an objective measure should be used to evaluate the success of any client intervention. Stool consistency is an objective measure for treatment response to diarrhea and malabsorption.

Critical Thinking Questions

1. The client asks you how long he will need to follow this diet and will he ever be able to reintroduce milk into his diet. What do you tell him?
2. What would you tell the client if the diet were only partially effective in controlling the diarrhea?

 Study Aids

Subjects	.Internet Sites
Dysphasia	.http://www.dysphagia-diet.com/index.html
Food allergies	.http://www.foodallergy.org
Gluten-free diet	.http://www.gluten-free.com
Digestion, absorption, and metabolism American College of Gastroenterology	.http://www.acg.gi.org
Links to sites that focus on gluten intolerance	.http://www.gluten-free.org

Chapter Review

1. An appropriate snack for a child on a gluten-free diet would be:
   a. crackers and peanut butter
   b. 1/2 cheese sandwich
   c. potato chips and an oatmeal cookie
   d. rice cakes and a banana
2. Solid body waste is stored in the _____.
   a. large intestine
   b. gallbladder
   c. small intestine
   d. stomach
3. Gaseous waste is expelled _____.
   a. in the urine
   b. in the feces
   c. through the lungs
   d. through the skin
4. The end products of protein digestion are _____.
   a. glycerol and fatty acids
   b. amino acids
   c. fatty acids
   d. monosaccharides
5. A food commonly responsible for an allergic reaction
   is_____.
   a. chicken
   b. peanuts
   c. rice
   d. carrots

Clinical Analysis

1. The nurse is visiting Mr. D, who is receiving home health care. His caregiver is concerned that Mr. D. chokes on liquids but swallows semi-solid food well. Which of the following actions by the nurse would be the most appropriate?
   a. Observe Mr. D's efforts to swallow liquids.
   b. Recommend a fluid restriction
   c. Refer Mr. D to a speech therapist
   d. Contact Mr. D's physician
2. Brenda, a 3-year-old, has been admitted to the pediatric unit with a diagnosis of celiac disease. She has a gluten-free diet ordered. Which of the following meals would be compatible with the diet order?
   a. Goulash, green beans, and milk
   b. Hamburger on bun, French fries, and a chocolate shake
   c. Tomato soup, grilled cheese, applesauce, and a cookie
   d. Baked chicken, baked potato, sour cream, green beans, peaches, and milk
3. Mr. P is on a low-fat diet (20 grams) to control his steatorrhea. An appropriate snack would be _____.
   a. fruit
   b. nuts
   c. cheese
   d. cookies

Bibliography

American Dietetic Association: Manual of Clinical Dietetics, ed 5, ADA, Chicago, 1996.

Caltaldo, CW, DeBruyne, LK, and Whitney, EN: Nutrition and Diet Therapy, ed 5. Wadsworth, Belmont, CA, 1999.

Feldman, M, et al.: Gastrointestinal and Liver Disease, ed 6. WB Saunders, Philadelphia, 1998.

Johnson, M, Maas, M, and Moorhead, S: Nursing Outcomes Classification (NOC), ed 2. Mosby, Philadelphia, 2000.

Lewis, MM, and Kidder, JA: Nutrition Practice Guidelines for Dysphagia. The American Dietetic Association, Chicago, Il.1996.

McCloskey, JC, and Bulechek, GM: Nursing Interventions Classification (NIC), ed 3. Mosby, Philadelphia, 2000.

North American Nursing Diagnosis Association: Nursing Diagnoses: Definitions and Classification 1999–2000, North American Nursing Diagnosis Association, Philadelphia, 1999.

Pecora, AA: Lactose Intolerance. Osteopathic Medical News 7:7, 1990.

Pemberton, CM, et al.: Mayo Clinic Diet Manual: A Handbook of Dietary Practice, ed 6. BC Decker, Philadelphia, 1988.

Scalon, VC, and Sanders, T: Essentials of Anatomy and Physiology, ed 2., FA Davis, Philadelphia, 1995.

Skipper, A: Dietitians Handbook of Enteral and Parenteral Nutrition, ed. 2. Aspen Publishers, Inc. Gaithersburg, Maryland, 1998.

Taylor, SL, Hefle, SL, and Munoz-Furlong, A: Food allergies and avoidance diets. Nutr Today 34:15, 1999.

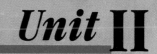

Unit II

Family and Community Nutrition

CHAPTER 11

Life Cycle Nutrition: Pregnancy and Lactation

LEARNING OBJECTIVES
After completing this chapter, the student should be able to:

1. Compare the nutritional needs of a pregnant woman with those of a nonpregnant woman of the same age.
2. Contrast the nutritional needs of a pregnant adolescent with those of a pregnant adult.
3. Explain why folic acid intake is critical in pregnancy.
4. Discuss the dietary treatment of common problems of pregnancy.
5. List three advantages that breast-feeding confers on the mother

The needs for many nutrients change at different stages of life. Social, economic, and psychological circumstances also influence nutritional status. Human beings are most vulnerable to the impact of poor nutrition during periods of rapid growth. If the essential nutrients are not present to support growth, permanent damage to tissues and organs can occur. This chapter focuses on the period of most rapid growth, that of the unborn child.

Nutrition during Pregnancy

An expectant mother's nutritional status can affect the outcome of pregnancy. For example, during the first month of **gestation**, it is crucial that the mother be well nourished so that the **placenta** that forms will be healthy. As well, within 2 to 3 months of conception all the major body organs are formed in the **embryo**. From the beginning of the third month until birth, the developing child is called a **fetus**. Because the fetus obtains nutrients from the mother's diet or body stores, its health depends on her nutritional intake.

The placenta is not just a passive conduit for nutrients, however. It can selectively extract nutrients of the appropriate form, for instance long-chain essential fatty acids and alpha-tocopherol (vitamin E), suited to the needs of the fetus (James, 1997).

After the birth and weaning of the child, the mother needs time to rebuild her nutrient stores. Occurrence of a second pregnancy within 6 months of delivery is associated with adverse outcome (Kitzman, 2000).

Poor outcomes of pregnancy include spontaneous abortion (miscarriage), premature delivery, a **low-birth-weight (LBW) infant,** a **small-for-gestational-age (SGA) infant**, and mental and physical abnormalities in the newborn. These complications are not evenly distributed throughout the population. Analysis of over one-half million birth records in New York City showed that overall, black women had a substantially higher risk of LBW infants than did white women; the risk for black women, however, varied with birthplace and census-tract economic classification. Caribbean and African-born women had birth outcomes similar to those of white women and even better than those of white women in communities in the lowest third of income classification (Fang, Madhavan, and Alderman, 1999).

The best action an expectant mother can take for her unborn child is to enter the pregnancy with good nutrient stores and to consume a well-balanced diet while pregnant. She must also avoid harmful substances, such as alcohol and contraindicated drugs, including over-the-counter and prescription preparations.

From **implantation** to birth, the fertilized **ovum** (which weighs less than 100 micrograms) develops into an infant who weighs about 3.4 kilograms (7.5 pounds) on the average. During this period of rapid growth and development the mother needs additional nutrients, including kilocalories, protein, and certain vitamins and minerals.

Energy Needs

Increased energy is needed to sustain the mother and for the development of the fetus and the placenta. From the third through the sixth month, much of this energy supports the growth of the uterus (womb) and other maternal tissues. During the seventh through ninth months, the third trimester, much of the energy supports the fetus and the placenta. To meet this increased metabolic workload and to spare protein for tissue building, the pregnant woman needs an additional 300 kilocalories per day throughout the pregnancy. Maintaining blood glucose levels in the mother is vital because the fetus's blood glucose level is always lower than the mother's (McGanity, Dawson, and Van Hook, 1999).

Protein Needs

Protein is required to build fetal **tissue**. The mother also needs adequate protein for growth of her tissues. Her blood volume increases in anticipation of blood loss at delivery. Her breasts develop in preparation for lactation. Her uterus enlarges and fills with a sac containing **amniotic fluid**. For these reasons, an additional 10 grams of protein per day are needed. Translating this need to the exchange system, 1 extra cup of milk (8 grams of protein) and 1 additional ounce of meat (7 grams of protein) would more than meet the increased protein requirement.

A complication arises if a woman with phenylketonuria (PKU) consumes a regular diet during pregnancy. The high level of phenylalanine in such a woman's bloodstream can cross the placenta and cause fetal malformations and defects. Careful monitoring of blood levels of phenylalanine and provision of a special medical food (see Clinical Application 5–3 in Chapter 5) are begun before conception and continued throughout the pregnancy. Strict control of phenylalanine blood levels is likely to reduce the risk of congenital defects from 80 percent to near zero (McGanity, Dawson, and Van Hook, 1999).

All women should be asked directly if they have ever had a special diet prescription. It may be difficult to convince even known clients with PKU to change their diets, but even harder if the person's medical history is vague. Because women of childbearing age with PKU may have been taken off the special diet after age 4 to 6, they may have little memory of this part of their medical history. The health-care worker should investigate further when a woman cites a history of troubled pregnancies: congenital abnormalities, a mentally retarded infant, spontaneous abortion, or stillbirth. Women needing careful screening for PKU include those born prior to 1967, those who immigrated to the United States, those with a history of seizures, and those who have low IQs (Acosta and Wright, 1992).

Vitamin Needs

Pregnant women have an increased need for some vitamins. They must avoid taking excessive amounts of others because of potential hazard to the fetus.

Water-Soluble Vitamins

Increased amounts of certain B vitamins, especially folic acid, and vitamin C are needed during pregnancy. Vitamin C is needed to (1) convert folic acid to an active form, (2) enhance the absorption of iron, and (3) help to form connective tissues. Women who have been using oral contraceptives have been found to have lower blood levels of folate, vitamin C, vitamins B_6 and B_{12}, and beta-carotene that may take four months to return to normal after the drugs have been discontinued (Hally, 1998). Increased metabolic demands make intake of some of the other B vitamins necessary in additional amounts; they include thiamin, riboflavin, niacin, and vitamin B_6. These B vitamins are all coenzymes involved in the metabolism of the energy nutrients.

A CDC guideline recommends that a woman who has previously borne a child with a neural tube defect (NTD) take 4 milligrams of folic acid per day from one month before conception through the first trimester (Centers for Disease Control, 1992). As part of the revision of the RDAs, the National Academy of Sciences has recommended that all women of childbearing potential consume 400 micrograms of synthetic folic acid daily from fortified foods or a supplement in addition to food folate from a varied diet (1998).

Box 11–1 contains a review of research pertinent to implementing these recommendations. None of the studies suggests that folic acid supplementation will prevent all cases of NTD; evidence also supports genetic and environmental influences. A higher incidence of NTD in Newfoundland, Quebec, northern China, parts of India, Scotland, and Ireland stimulated a search for a genetic cause. Women with histories of NTD pregnancies attained lower serum folate levels than control subjects following oral doses of folate (Schoral et al., 1993).

The identification of a gene producing an abnormality in an enzyme necessary to folate metabolism bolsters the argument for genetic susceptibility, but it is estimated to be responsible for only 13 percent of NTDs (Whitehead et al., 1995). The fact that the abnormal **allele** is thermolabile may help explain the increased occurrence of NTD associated with a history of fever or the use of a hot tub or sauna in the first trimester (Milunsky et al, 1992). Almost half the Irish population is either **heterozygous** or **homozygous** for the affected thermolabile gene, but its low rate of detectable effects has led researchers to search for additional mechanisms producing NTDs (James, 1997).

Assembling these pieces of the research puzzle to devise a comprehensive, cost-effective, and harmless public policy is a daunting task. For the first time since 1943, the U. S. Food and Drug Administration issued a fortification order. Since January 1, 1998, 43 to 140 micrograms of folic acid per pound have been added to all enriched foods in an attempt to reduce the occurrence of NTDs. Breakfast cereals can be fortified with up to 400 micrograms per serving, and the FDA permits the labels of foods containing sufficient amounts of folate to claim that the products may reduce the risk of having a pregnancy affected with NTD (Centers for Disease Control, 1996).

Fat-Soluble Vitamins

For pregnant women older than 25 years of age, an adequate diet usually provides the needed additional vitamins D, E, and K. Because of the risk of fetal deformities, vitamin A consumption beyond the RDA is contraindicated during the first trimester. Risk to the fetus was increased if the mother took 10,000 IU or more of supplemental vitamin A daily, especially before the seventh week of pregnancy. This risk specifically involves preformed vitamin A, not carotene (Rothman et al., 1995). Avoidance of vitamin A in excess of the RDA is recommended, although a dose-response relationship to major malformations was not demonstrated (Mastroiacovo, 1999). See the RDA tables (Appendices F and H) for the specific amounts recommended for each vitamin during pregnancy.

Vitamin A, sometimes used to treat acne, could pose a risk to the fetus of a teenager who unintentionally becomes pregnant. The risk of a major congenital abnormality in a child exposed to isotretinoin, a vitamin A metabolite, in utero during the first trimester appears to be increased about 25 times (Futoryan and Gilchrest, 1994). Pastuszak, Koren, and Rieder (1994) found that although 77 percent of women taking isotretinoin knew it to be teratogenic, 38.5 percent used no contraception, 23.1 percent experienced contraceptive failure, and 8 percent discontinued contraception during therapy.

Despite a pregnancy prevention program started by the manufacturer of isotretinoin in 1988, approximately 900 pregnancies occurred

Box 11–1 Implementing the Research on Folic Acid and Neural Tube Defects

The neural tube is embryonic tissue that develops into the brain and spinal cord. A critical time in the development of this structure is from conception through the fourth week of pregnancy. Interference with normal development produces major congenital defects including **anencephaly, meningoencephalocele, spina bifida,** and **meningocele.**

In the United States, approximately 4,000 pregnancies are affected by neural tube defects (NTDs) each year; 50 to 70 percent of them could be prevented with daily intake of 400 micrograms of folic acid throughout the period before and after conception (Centers for Disease Control, 1999a). Overall, focusing on known cases would not be an effective population strategy since about 95 percent of women who deliver infants with NTDs have not previously delivered infants with these defects (Czeizel and Dudas, 1992). The lifetime cost of one case of spina bifida is estimated to be $349,133 (Romano et al., 1995).

The effectiveness of folic acid was demonstrated in a large randomized trial conducted in seven countries. Women with a history of NTD pregnancy were given 4 mg of folic acid per day. Control groups received placebos or other vitamins. The study was stopped early to permit treatment of all participants because the folic acid reduced the risk of a subsequent child with NTD by 70 percent (MRC Vitamin Study Research Group, 1991).

The dose of folic acid just sufficient to prevent NTD in women without a positive history has not been determined. A dose of 0.8 mg of folic acid reduced NTD to zero in 2104 women without prior occurrences. By comparison, 6 NTD cases were noted among 2050 control subjects (Czeizel and Dudas, 1992).

How to use this research to prevent NTD has provoked much discussion. Unfortunately, the neural tube develops when many women are unaware they are pregnant. In addition, more than half of all pregnancies in the United States are unplanned, and 13.2 million sexually active women of child-bearing age are not using effective contraception (Romano et al., 1995). Pre-conception health counseling is the ideal but not the norm.

Several approaches to NTD prevention have been considered: dietary, pharmaceutical, and food fortification. Dietary intake of folic acid is desirable but difficult to implement. First, folates obtained from foods are not as well absorbed as folic acid (Centers for Disease Control, 1992). Bioavailability of dietary folate is about 50 percent (Pérez-Escamilla, 1995). Second, only 8 percent of adult women obtained 400 micrograms of dietary folate from 1976 through 1980 (Romano et al., 1995). Third, two registered dietitians required 30 hours to develop a one-week menu that included 400 micrograms of folic acid daily (Bendich, 1994).

Supplementation by pharmaceutical folic acid would be less cumbersome and less time-consuming than dietary counseling but would miss a large proportion of women at risk. In addition, some women resist taking folate supplements when pregnant or in general (Bower et al., 1997). Nevertheless, counsel congruent with that of the U.S. Public Health Service and the Centers for Disease Control has been strongly advised lest healthcare providers be held liable for its omission (Rush, 1994). Using supplements, consumers would spend an estimated $132,000 to prevent each case of NTD (Romano et al., 1995).

Fortification of food is another method. It would cost an estimated $65,000 to $92,000 per case of NTD prevented, much less expensive than pharmaceutical supplementation (Romano et al., 1995). One hazard of fortification is the masking of vitamin B_{12} deficiency. Although pernicious anemia is more common in older people than younger ones, adding folic acid to everyone's food supply theoretically would increase the risk of neurologic damage due to undiagnosed pernicious anemia (Rush, 1994). No reports of delayed diagnosis have been published since 1973 (Oakley, Adams, and Dickinson, 1996), however, and neurological signs and symptoms of pernicious anemia do occur without anemia (Dickinson, 1995). An additional concern is that of folic acid interfering with anticonvulsant medications, but numerous controlled trials have demonstrated no effect by oral folic acid at doses up to 20 mg daily (Romano, et al., 1995).

Women are slowly becoming aware of the need for sufficient folic acid and even more slowly implementing the recommendations. A comparison of the findings of national surveys of 18- to 45-year-old women in 1995 and 1998 (Centers for Disease Control, 1999a) follows:

Reported Knowledge and Behavior	1995 (percent)	1998 (percent)
Had heard of folic acid	52	68
Knew folic acid helps prevent birth defects	5	13
Knew folic acid should be taken before pregnancy	2	7
Currently taking a vitamin supplement containing folic acid	28	32

Food fortification may help but is not designed to completely meet the preconception and first trimester needs of fertile women, hence the revised RDA for folate, specifying synthetic sources. Opportunities to educate clients abound. Pediatric nurses should counsel adolescent girls as well as mothers of younger children. Nurses caring for women of reproductive age in any setting can help to decrease their clients' risks of NTDs by making this subject a priority for teaching.

In addition to general education, areas with high rates of NTD can be targeted for specific interventions. A project in the Texas counties bordering Mexico recruited women who had given birth to an infant with NTD. In 14 border counties, the rate of NTD-affected pregnancies was 13.8 per 10,000 live births for Hispanic women compared with 8.8 per 10,000 live births for Caucasian women. Counseling and folic acid supplements were provided, the dose dependent upon whether or not contraception was practiced. Women who used no contraception were given 4 milligrams compared to 400 micrograms for women using contraception. Early results indicate the folic acid to be effective in reducing the risk for NTD among Hispanic women. Even this carefully aimed intervention was not perfectly received by the 36 percent of the women eligible for the program who refused enrollment, quit, or were lost to follow-up (Centers for Disease Control, 2000b).

between 1989 and 1998 in women enrolled in the Boston University Accutane Survey. CDC follow-up of isotretinoin-exposed pregnancies in California revealed that all the respondents knew the drug should not be used during pregnancy, but only 7 percent followed the contraceptive protocol and 57 percent reported having intercourse without contraception at the time of the exposed pregnancy. None of the respondents reported being referred for the free contraceptive counseling that is part of the prevention program (Centers for Disease Control, 2000a). Both of these studies illustrate the need for more effective teaching of clients receiving prescriptions for isotretinoin. Women of childbearing age taking isotretinoin should adhere to strict contraceptive protocols, including simultaneous use of two methods. No one should donate blood during or for 30 days after therapy (Nursing 2000, 2000).

By contrast, vitamin A deficiency is a greater problem than toxicity in developing countries. Either preformed vitamin A or provitamin A (beta carotene) was shown to reduce mortality related to pregnancy by 40 to 49 percent in Nepal (West et al., 1999), a country in which night blindness is considered an annoyance of pregnancy reportedly affecting 16 percent of women (Christian et al., 1998).

Mineral Needs

Minerals become part of the structure of the body whereas vitamins do not. Both the mother and the fetus require minerals to build new tissues.

Iron

During pregnancy the mother's blood volume increases about 35 percent, and her volume of red blood cells increases by 21 to 26 percent. Additional iron is needed for the red blood cells in the fetus, placenta, and umbilical cord. Iron is transported to the fetus regardless of the mother's iron status. The total iron need for a single-fetus pregnancy is estimated to be 0.8 to 1 gram. During the third trimester, 3 to 4 milligrams of iron per day is transferred to the fetus (Fairbanks, 1999).

Iron deficiency anemia during the first two trimesters of pregnancy is associated with twice the risk for preterm delivery and three times the risk for producing a LBW infant. Since 1979, anemia prevalence among low-income pregnant women in the United States has been fairly stable. In 1993, it was 9 percent, 14 percent, and 37 percent for the first, second, and third trimesters (Centers for Disease Control, 1998b).

Fortunately, the body adjusts to limited or abundant sources of iron. Absorption of iron is enhanced in the second and third trimesters of pregnancy. In women who are not taking an iron supplement, iron absorption increases from 6.5 percent early in pregnancy to 14.3 percent at term. This rate drops to 8.6 percent with an iron supplement.

The Centers for Disease Control recommend educating clients about iron-rich foods and those that enhance iron absorption as well as prescribing a daily 30-milligram supplement beginning when clients enter prenatal care (1998b). One common preparation is ferrous sulfate. A 150-milligram dose of ferrous sulfate contains 30 milligrams of iron, the 1989 RDA for pregnancy. If iron needs are not met, a pregnant woman may develop **iron-deficiency anemia**. Even when she takes supplements, the woman's hemoglobin and hematocrit should be monitored every 2 to 3 months. Lower values are expected during the first and second trimesters because of expanding blood volume. Among women who do not take iron supplements, the hemoglobin and hematocrit levels remain low during the third trimester, but in women with adequate iron intake, the values gradually rise toward prepregnancy levels (Centers for Disease Control, 1998b).

Prescribing an iron supplement does not necessarily mean the woman will take it. Side effects or economic factors may influence the extent to which a woman takes her supplements. Clinical Application 11–1 illustrates the principles of knowing the client as well as the subject matter and seeking feedback on one's teaching.

Calcium

Calcium is the chief mineral in the adult body, with the bones serving as a storage depot. When serum calcium is low, the bones demineralize to restore the serum level. For most well-nourished women, the demand for calcium by the fetus does not appear to negatively affect their bones (Ritchie et al, 1998). As with iron, intestinal absorption of calcium increases during pregnancy. In a longitudinal study, the average proportion of calcium absorbed increased from 32.9 percent at prepregnancy to 49.9 percent during the second trimester and to 53.8 percent during the third trimester (Ritchie et al., 1998). One reason for this increased absorption is the ability of the placenta to convert inactive vitamin D to the active form. Chapters 7 and 8 describe the effects and interactions of calcium and vitamin D.

Pregnancy-associated osteoporosis, a rare complication, has been recognized for 40 years but is still not well understood. In one case, a 23-year old woman suffered compression fractures of 5 vertebrae and then recovered bone mineral density rapidly in the six months following delivery, although not to normal levels. The literature shows that, mysteriously, most women are not affected in their subsequent pregnancies (Liel, Atar, and Ohana, 1998).

CLINICAL APPLICATION 11–1

Effective Teaching

Often the facts presented by a healthcare provider who is educating a client are misunderstood by the client or perceived as counter to the client's goals. The following incidents illustrate the point (Galloway and McGuire, 1996).

1. When anemic pregnant women were give iron tablets, they took the supplement until they felt better and then stopped, thinking they were cured. Prevention is a new concept to people in many countries.

2. Anemic pregnant women accepted the notion of iron supplements to correct "too little blood" but were fearful that too much iron would give them too much blood so that they would bleed more extensively at delivery.

3. Presenting the idea that iron would produce bigger babies was a disincentive for anemic pregnant women who thought they then would face a more difficult labor.

Teaching is more than just presenting facts, especially when the goal is changed behavior. Local knowledge and perspective are essential to the healthcare provider who is promoting a new health practice.

The Adequate Intake (AI) for calcium for pregnant and lactating women 19 years of age and older is 1000 milligrams. For women 18 years of age and younger, the amount is 1300 milligrams. These amounts can be obtained from 3.3 to 4.3 servings of milk or milk products equivalent in calcium. (Lactose intolerance is discussed in Chapter 10.)

Phosphorus and Magnesium

In addition to calcium, two other minerals involved in skeletal formation are also in great demand during pregnancy: phosphorus and magnesium. For pregnant women 25 years of age and older, the allowance recommended for phosphorus is 1.5 times the amount allowed for nonpregnant women. The 1998 RDA for magnesium is slightly increased over that of nonpregnant women.

Iodine

As part of thyroid hormones, iodine is essential to the control of metabolism. During the second half of pregnancy, resting energy expenditure increases by as much as 23 percent. In the United States, a pregnant woman's usual need for iodine is met, like that of other adults, by the use of iodized salt. In parts of the world with endemic cretinism, supplementation is beneficial (Mahomed and Gulmezoglu, 1999).

Fluoride

The fetus begins to develop teeth at the 10th to 12th week of pregnancy. Fewer dental caries were found in infants of mothers whose diets were supplemented with 1 milligram of fluoride daily than in those of unsupplemented mothers (Glenn, Glenn, and Duncan, 1982). In a later study, however, Leverett et al. (1997) did not find a strong caries-preventive effect after following children to 5 years of age.

Zinc

Zinc is not mobilized from the mother's tissues. To provide for the fetus, the mother needs constant intake. Zinc deficiency has been associated with abnormally long labors and delivery of small and malformed infants. Zinc supplementation was associated with fewer preterm deliveries and less perinatal mortality (McGanity, Dawson, and Van Hook, 1999). African-American women with low plasma zinc levels who took a zinc supplement delivered heavier infants than did the control group. The greatest increase occurred in women with prepregnant body mass indices (BMIs) of less than 26 (Goldenberg et al., 1995). Three servings of meat or meat substitute per day will provide adequate zinc for the pregnant woman. See the RDA tables (Appendices F and H) for the specific amount recommended for each mineral during pregnancy.

Water and Weight Gain

The average increase in plasma volume during pregnancy is 49 percent (O'Connor, 1994). The increase in total body water is about 7 liters or approximately 15 pounds (Van Loan et al., 1995). The pregnant woman needs about 6 to 8 cups of water per day. Because some women fear excessive weight gain, the nurse should reinforce the need for adequate fluid intake.

The amount of weight a woman is expected to gain during pregnancy has varied over the years. The current recommendation is based on a BMI, which incorporates the woman's height and weight before pregnancy. Clinical Calculation 11–1 shows the procedure to determine a goal for

---

Clinical Calculation 11–1 Determining Recommended Weight Gain During Pregnancy

$$\text{Body mass index (BMI)} = \frac{\text{Weight in kilograms}}{\text{Height in meters}^2}$$

Suppose a woman is 5 ft, 4 in tall and weighs 125 lb.

$$5 \text{ ft, } 4 \text{ in} = 64 \text{ in}$$
$$1 \text{ m} = 39.371 \text{ in}$$

$$\frac{64}{39.371} = 1.6 \text{ m}$$

$$\frac{125 \text{ lb}}{2.2 \text{ lb/kg}} = 56.8 \text{ kg}$$

$$\text{BMI} = \frac{56.8}{(1.6)^2} = \frac{56.8}{2.56} = 22.2$$

Looking at the table below, we see that 22.2 is in the normal category. Recommended weight gain for this woman is 25 to 35 lb.

BMI Category	Recommended Weight Gain for Pregnancy	
	Kilograms	Pounds
<19.8 = Low	12.5–18	28–40
19.8–26 = Normal	11.5–16	25–35
26–29 = High	7–11.5	15–25
>29 = Obese	6	15

Young adolescents and black women should strive for gains at the upper end of the recommended range. Women whose height is less than 157 cm (62 in) should strive for gains at the lower end of the range.

---

weight gain in pregnancy. A woman of normal weight should gain 2 to 4 pounds during the first trimester, followed by a pound a week for the remainder of the pregnancy. Figure 11–1 is a graph on which the woman can plot her weight gain.

Obese women (a BMI > 29 before pregnancy) have increased risk of complications such as hypertension and diabetes and of surgical delivery by Caesarian section. Those with a prepregnancy BMI over 28 run twice the risk of NTD-affected fetuses, independent of folate status and supplement use (McGanity, Dawson, and Van Hook, 1999).

Weight gain during pregnancy is not perfectly correlated with birth weight but it is inversely related to perinatal mortality (McGanity, Dawson, and Van Hook, 1999). Only among pregnant women who smoked did the amount of weight gain predict small-for-gestational-age infants. To have delivered infants equal in size to those of nonsmokers, the smokers would have had to gain 44 pounds rather than the 26 cited as a standard (Muscati, Gray-Donald, and Newson, 1994).

Meal Pattern

Relatively few modifications in the Food Pyramid recommendations for adults are needed for mature women who become pregnant. They can meet their needs and those of the fetus by consuming one additional serv-

The Weighting Game Weight Graph

Your Beginning Weight _ _ _ _ _ _ lbs.

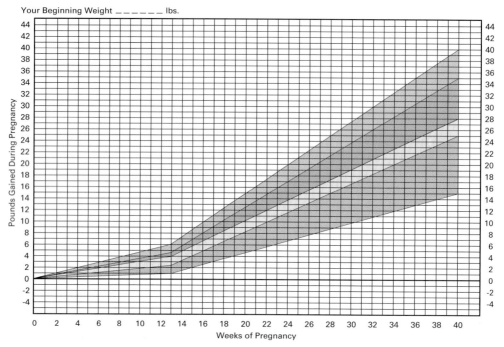

Weeks of Pregnancy

Adapted from the National Academy of Science's **Nutrition during Pregnancy**, 1990.

If your weight was normal before you became pregnant, try to keep your weight in the yellow/orange range.

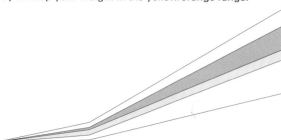

If your weight was much higher than ideal, your weight gain should be in the blue range.

This is not the time to lose weight. Try to gain weight at a steady pace. Report any sudden and/or unexplained weight changes to your health care provider.

If you were underweight before you became pregnant, your weight gain should be in the orange/pink area.

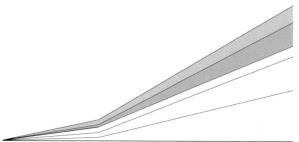

Here's How It All Adds Up	
Baby	7-8½ pounds
Amniotic fluid	2 pounds
Placenta	2-2½ pounds
Increased blood volume	4–5 pounds
Tissue fluid	3–5 pounds
Increased weight of uterus	2 pounds
Body changes for breast feeding	1–4 pounds
Mother's stores*	4–6 pounds
	25–35 pounds

*Mother's stores are reserves of extra fat and probably a little protein. These serve as a source of energy to support the work of pregnancy. These stores also supply energy for labor and delivery and for milk production after birth.

TABLE 11–1 Daily Food Guide in Pregnancy and Lactation

	Pregnant Adult	Pregnant Adolescent*	Lactation
Milk, cups	3–4	4–5	3–4
Meat, oz	6	6	6
Fruit, servings			
High vitamin C	2	2	2
Other	2	2	3
Vegetable, servings			
High vitamin A	1	1	1–2
Starch/Bread, servings	10	11	10
Other	2–4	2–4	2–4
Other foods	To meet kilocaloric needs	To meet kilocaloric needs	To meet kilocaloric needs

*Meets adolescent RDA except for iron and folic acid.

ing of milk, an additional ounce of meat, and one additional source of vitamin C each day.

Pregnant teenagers need nutrients to provide for their own growth as well as that of the fetus. They should have an additional serving from each of the milk and starch/bread groups over and above the number of servings recommended for mature pregnant women. Clinical Application 11–2 relates the particular hazards of teenage pregnancy.

Moderation is suggested in implementing the meal pattern. For instance, overfeeding of protein to pregnant women may be counterproductive. Giving high-protein supplements to pregnant women, many of whom were adolescents, seems to have reduced birth weight. Similar effects have been seen by animal breeders (James, 1997). Table 11–1 can be used as a food guide for pregnant adult women and adolescents during pregnancy and lactation.

Careful food selection is critical for pregnant vegetarian women. Strict vegetarians, particularly, may be prescribed a vitamin and mineral supplement that at a minimum provides folate, vitamin B_{12}, iron, and zinc (McGanity, Dawson, and Van Hook, 1999).

Food Assistance

Supplemental food assistance is available for families in the Food Stamp Program and for women and children in the Supplemental Feeding Program for Women, Infants, and Children (WIC). The latter program serves 7 million people each month, about one-fourth of them pregnant and lactating women (McGanity, Dawson, and Van Hook, 1999).

Substances to Avoid

Women are urged to eliminate certain substances from their diets while they are pregnant. Alcohol, caffeine, and soft cheeses are three such substances that merit special mention. Tobacco and cocaine use also affect fetal nutrition.

Alcohol

First recognized in 1973, fetal alcohol syndrome (FAS) is the major cause of mental retardation in the Western world (Murphy-Brennan and Oei,

1999). FAS occurs in 30 to 50 percent of alcoholic mothers' offspring. The fetus is most vulnerable to FAS during the first trimester when basic structural development occurs. Often, the woman does not know that she is pregnant until late in the first trimester.

Children with FAS, a completely preventable condition, are malformed and suffer from mental retardation (Fig. 11–2). Because researchers have not been able to determine how much alcohol is safe to ingest during pregnancy, women who are planning a pregnancy should be encouraged to abstain from alcohol for the good of the fetus. Unfortunately, prevention projects have been shown to raise awareness of FAS but have not evoked behavior change (Murphy-Brennan and Oei, 1999; Kaskutas et al, 1998).

The task of protecting the unborn is formidable. As many as 12.5 percent women of childbearing age reported consuming an average of seven or more drinks per week or five or more drinks on at least one occasion during the previous month (Centers for Disease Control, 1997). Unfortunately, women who consumed the most alcohol also saw the least

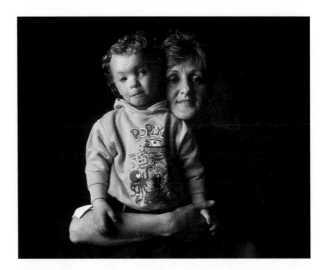

Figure 11–1:
GREAT BEGINNINGS: The Weighting Game Weigh Graph. This is an example of a chart on which a woman can plot her weight gain during pregnancy. (From the Great Beginnings Calendar, ed 2, 1991. Courtesy of NATIONAL DAIRY COUNCIL, with permission

Figure 11–2:
Specific facial signs of fetal alcohol syndrome include microcephaly or small head size, small eyes and or short eye openings, and an underdeveloped upper lip with flat upper lip ridges. (Photo by George Steinmetz, reproduced with permission.)

CLINICAL APPLICATION 11–2

Teenage Pregnancy

The United States has the highest rate of teenage pregnancy in the industrialized world (McGanity, Dawson, and Van Hook, 1999). In 1997 in the United States, 500,000 teenagers gave birth to infants. About 90,000 of these infants were the teenage mother's second child. Of mothers aged 15 to 17, 87 percent were unmarried, compared with 72 percent of mothers aged 18 to 19 (Ventura, Mathews, and Curtin, 1998). Not surprisingly, 80 to 85 percent of teenage pregnancies are unplanned (Rhinehart and Gabel, 1998).

Birth rates for teenagers vary by ethnic background. Black teenagers have the highest rate, followed by Hispanic teenagers. As the graph in Figure 11–3 illustrates, birth rates (number of live births per 1,000 women) for teenagers have declined by 15 percent since 1991. Risk factors for early sexual activity, which predicts early fertility, include lower socioeconomic status, less education, substance and alcohol abuse, single-parent households, and a history of abuse (Rhinehart and Gabel, 1998; Wellings et al., 1999).

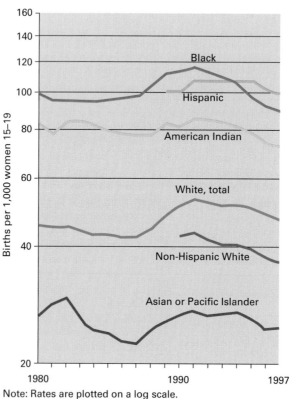

Note: Rates are plotted on a log scale.

Figure 11–3:
Birth rate for teenagers 15 to 19 by race and Hispanic origin: United States, 1980–97. (From Ventura, Mathews, and Curtin, 1998.)

The average girl does not reach her full height or attain gynecologic maturity until age 17. When pregnant before that age, she herself is still growing and has a fetus to nourish as well.

Nutrients most often lacking in the pregnant teenager's diet are folate, vitamins A, E, and B_6, calcium, iron, zinc, and fiber. In addition, kilocaloric intake is usually insufficient to meet daily needs. The 11- to 14-year-old expectant mother requires 2700 kcal per day, the 15- to 18-year old, 2400 kcal.

Teenage mothers are at increased risk of complications of pregnancy, such as preeclampsia and premature delivery. Infants born to mothers under the age of 16 are twice as likely to be of low birth weight as infants born to mothers age 20 and older, and three times more likely to die in the first month of life as infants of older mothers (Story, 1997).

The cause is not solely age-related, however. Complications of pregnancies are more strongly associated with poor nutrition than with maternal age. Because teenage pregnant girls tend to enter prenatal care later than older pregnant women, improving access to prenatal care and focusing on nutritional needs when providing that care are important steps toward reducing the poor outcomes of teenage pregnancy (Story, 1997).

---

risk-associated drinking during pregnancy (Stutts, Patterson, and Hunnicutt, 1997).

Caffeine

The effects of caffeine consumption during pregnancy have been studied with inconsistent results. In some studies, caffeine consumption during pregnancy has been associated with spontaneous abortion (Fernandes et al., 1998; Klebanoff et al., 1999; Parazzini et al., 1998), low-birth-weight babies (Eskenazi et al., 1999; Fernandes et al., 1998; Santos et al., 1998b), and sudden infant deaths (Ford et al., 1998). Caffeine intake has also been associated with delays in achieving pregnancy (Boluman et al., 1997; Jensen et al., 1998). In other studies, however, no relation to caffeine was found with spontaneous abortion (Fenster et al., 1997), low birth weight, preterm delivery, intrauterine growth retardation (Santos et

al., 1998a), or sudden infant deaths (Alm et al., 1999). Vlajinac et al (1997) found a reduction in infant birth weight associated with caffeine among nonsmoking mothers only, perhaps because smoking shortens the half-life of caffeine (Eskenazi, 1999). Changes in fetal heart rate and breathing patterns have been observed even with moderate caffeine intake that apparently gave the mother no noticeable signs. Moreover, caffeine is secreted in breast milk and has a half-life of up to 100 hours in infants (Eskenazi, 1999). Therefore, limiting caffeine intake is prudent advice for pregnant or lactating women and for women desiring to become pregnant.

Soft Cheeses and Ready-to-Eat Meats

Listeriosis is a bacterial infection that is particularly virulent for fetuses, with a case-fatality rate of 30 percent in newborns and almost 50 percent if the onset occurs in the first four days of life (Chin, 2000). The causative organism, *Listeria monocytogenes*, is transmitted from the mother (who may be asymptomatic) to the fetus in utero or through the birth canal. The infection may result in abortion or septicemia or meningitis in the newborn. Other individuals at risk are the elderly, those with impaired immune systems, and farm workers.

Outbreaks of listeriosis have been associated with raw or contaminated milk, soft cheeses, contaminated vegetables, and ready-to-eat meats. The reservoir of the organism is soil, forage, water, mud, and silage (Chin, 2000). An outbreak from August 1998 through January 6, 1999 sickened at least 50 people in 11 states resulting in six adult deaths and two spontaneous abortions (Centers for Disease Control, 1999b). The mode of transmission in this case was hot dogs traced to a single packing plant. The FDA also issued a health warning after finding *Listeria monocytogenes* in cold-smoked fish products (U.S. Department of Health and Human Services, 2000).

Listeria infections during pregnancy can cause influenza-like symptoms, with fever and chills. Illness may not appear until 2 to 8 weeks after a person has eaten the contaminated food (Centers for Disease Control, 1999b). If the infection is diagnosed, antimicrobial therapy may prevent fetal infection and the associated high mortality (Yonekura and Mead, 1999).

In addition to the general rules for safe food handling, pregnant women and immunocompromised individuals should

1. Avoid soft cheeses (feta, Brie, Camembert, blue-veined, and Mexican-style cheese). Hard cheeses, processed cheeses, cream cheese, cottage cheese, and yogurt may be eaten safely.
2. Cook leftover foods or ready-to-eat foods (hot dogs) until steaming hot (165°F).
3. Although the risk for listeriosis associated with foods from deli counters is low, pregnant women and immunocompromised individuals may avoid these foods altogether or thoroughly reheat cold cuts before eating (Centers for Disease Control, 1998a).

Tobacco

Pregnant women who smoke one or more packs of cigarettes per day deliver infants weighing about one-half pound less than those delivered by nonsmoking women. The infants also have an increased risk of perinatal mortality. Increases in the number of abortions and preterm deliveries are also related to smoking. Physiologically, smoking causes a decrease in the oxygen-carrying capacity of the blood of up to 10 percent and vasoconstriction of the blood vessels of the placenta. To maintain normal blood levels, smokers need three times the intake of folic acid and twice the intake of vitamin C as nonsmokers. Lower vitamin C levels are associated with weakened amniotic membranes containing less collagen leading to premature rupture of the membranes and early delivery. Limiting cigarette use to fewer than 5 per day reduces the ill effects on the fetus to a statistically insignificant level (McGanity, Dawson, and Van Hook, 1999).

Cocaine

Cocaine crosses the placenta and can be detected in the infant's intestinal waste for up to eight weeks. Chronic cocaine addiction causes a weight deficit in the fetus of as much as 500 grams (1.1 pounds). In addition, the infant usually suffers from immature mental development that may be related

directly to the drug or to malnutrition of the mother, which has been likened to wartime intrauterine starvation (McCanity, Dawson, and Van Hook, 1999).

Common Problems and Complications of Pregnancy

The physiological changes that take place in a woman's body during pregnancy may cause a variety of possible medical conditions. Some of the more common problems such as morning sickness and leg cramps are usually annoying but only occasionally require medical intervention. Other conditions, such as pregnancy-induced hypertension and gestational diabetes, are more complicated and hazardous and require medical treatment.

Common Problems

Four of the most common problems of pregnancy are morning sickness, leg cramps, constipation, and heartburn. Pica (discussed later) is a regional complaint that is mainly influenced by culture.

MORNING SICKNESS Hormonal changes cause the nausea and vomiting of pregnancy. The occurrence and duration of these symptoms vary widely, and their occurrence is not confined to mornings. Control of the problem without medication is the goal. Eating dry crackers before getting out of bed is the classic preventive. Other suggestions include (1) avoid fatty foods in favor of fruits and complex carbohydrates taken in small, frequent meals; (2) consume cold foods rather than hot foods; (3) drinking liquids between rather than with meals; and (4) eat a high-protein snack at bedtime. In most cases, morning sickness subsides after the first trimester. A review of randomized controlled trials concluded that, aside from antiemetic medication (which was effective but produced side effects—and there is little information on fetal effects), pyridoxine (vitamin B_6) was effective in reducing the severity of nausea. Ginger may be of benefit, but the evidence is weak (Jewell and Young, 1999).

LEG CRAMPS Pregnant women often complain of leg cramps. One possible cause may be neuromuscular irritability due to low serum calcium. Increasing calcium intake is the prescribed treatment, following this reasoning. Another theory postulates a high serum phosphorus level in relation to calcium as the cause. The treatment is for the woman to substitute a calcium supplement for some of her milk intake, thus decreasing serum phosphorus level. Because of its close link to calcium metabolism, magnesium deficiency has been postulated to cause leg cramps. In a small study, magnesium supplementation was helpful (Dahle et al., 1995). Advice directed to athletes may also be applicable to pregnant women suffering from leg cramps. Staying well hydrated is of prime importance, followed by maintaining adequate intakes of potassium, sodium, calcium, and magnesium. A noninvasive procedure to prevent muscle cramps is to stretch the muscles before exercise and, for nighttime cramps, before bedtime (Stamford, 1993).

CONSTIPATION The growing uterus presses on the intestines, causing constipation. Adequate fluid intake, regular exercise, and a high-fiber diet should relieve this condition. The suggested amount of fiber intake, 30 grams per day, should be achieved with food rather than pharmaceutical preparations. Foods high in fiber but relatively low in kilocalories are listed in Table 11–2.

HEARTBURN A burning sensation beneath the breastbone is called heartburn. Hormonal changes cause relaxation of the cardiac sphincter,

TABLE 11-2 Nutrient-Dense Foods High in Fiber

Food	Quantity	Grams of Dietary Fiber	Kilocalories
Grains			
All bran	1/3 cup	10	70
Bran buds	1/2 cup	11.5	109
100% Bran	1/2 cup	10	89
Fruits			
Applesauce, unsweetened	1 cup	4	106
Orange sections, raw	1 cup	4	85
Pear, d'Anjou raw with skin	one	6	120
Prunes, ckd. unsweetened	1/2 cup	4.5	114
Strawberries, fresh	1 cup	4	45
Vegetables			
Baked beans, in tomato sauce with pork	1/2 cup	7	129
Lima beans, ckd. from frozen	1/2 cup	8	94
Broccoli, raw	one spear	6	42
Brussels sprouts, ckd. from raw	1 cup	6	60
Kidney beans, canned	1/2 cup	8.5	108
Navy beans, ckd. from dry	1/2 cup	8	130
Black-eyes peas, ckd. from dry	1/2 cup	10.5	99

located between the esophagus and the stomach. That and the upward pressure on the diaphragm from the enlarging uterus cause reflux of gastric contents into the esophagus and the burning sensation.

Heartburn can be controlled by avoiding spicy or acidic foods and taking small, frequent meals. Sitting up for an hour after a meal may help. Pregnant women should not self-medicate with sodium bicarbonate or antacids. The bicarbonate can be absorbed, producing alkalosis. Antacids decrease iron absorption by decreasing gastric acids, thus increasing the risk of anemia.

PICA The compulsive ingestion of nonfood items, usually dirt, clay, laundry starch, or ice is called **pica**. It is an ancient behavior. Most notable in some regions of the southern United States, pica occurs in conjunction with inadequate diets due to poverty, but it also occurs in women at other socioeconomic levels. Many women with pica have it only during pregnancy, believing it cures the annoyances of pregnancy or ensures a beautiful baby. Others contend that the substances they ingest taste good to them.

Health concerns about pica include inadequate nutrition due to substitution of nonfood items for nutritious foods, iron deficiency anemia, constipation, and lead poisoning. Laundry starch interferes with iron absorption. A study in Texas showed significantly lower hemoglobin levels at delivery for women who admitted to having pica than for women who did not (Rainville, 1998). Ingestion of clay may lead to fecal impaction. If the substance ingested includes paint chips, lead poisoning may result.

Women who have migrated to an area where pica is uncommon may continue the custom. A caring, nonjudgmental assessment on the nurse's part may encourage a woman to reveal that she has a craving for and is eating strange things; it could open the door to a teaching opportunity.

Complications of Pregnancy

Three complications of pregnancy with nutritional ramifications are hyperemesis gravidarum, pregnancy-induced hypertension, and gestational diabetes.

HYPEREMESIS GRAVIDARUM Severe nausea and vomiting persisting after the fourteenth week of pregnancy is called **hyperemesis gravidarum**. Estimated to occur in 2 percent of pregnancies, it can be life threatening, causing dehydration, electrolyte imbalance, and weight loss. It develops most often in Western countries and in first pregnancies. Many approaches have been used to treat it: rehydration, antiemetics without teratogenic effects, bedrest, and psychiatric intervention. Treatments are used that will not harm the fetus.

In a one-year study, for all 20 women admitted to the hospital with hyperemesis gravidarum, intravenous saline with multivitamins was an effective treatment. The clients received nothing by mouth until the vomiting subsided, which occurred in all the patients within 24 hours. The intravenous treatment lasted for ten days. Two women suffered relapses 3 to 4 weeks later. The treatment was repeated and the vomiting stopped. All clients gave birth to healthy babies weighing at least 5.5 pounds with no congenital abnormalities (van Stuijvenberg et al., 1995).

PREGNANCY-INDUCED HYPERTENSION A clear cause for pregnancy-induced hypertension has not been determined. It occurs in 5 to 7 percent of pregnancies and causes edema and proteinuria, as well as elevated blood pressure. The signs and symptoms appear after the 20th week of pregnancy, usually in the 2 months before term. **Pregnancy-induced hypertension (PIH)**, also called preeclampsia-eclampsia syndrome, is potentially life threatening for both the mother and the fetus; its cause is unknown. Excesses or deficiencies of magnesium, calcium, polyunsaturated fatty acids, zinc, cadmium, and sodium have been investigated as contributing factors. The syndrome occurs most frequently in women under 20 or over 35 years of age who are pregnant for the first time, and in women who have had five or more pregnancies. Risk of this syndrome is heightened by personal or family histories of diabetes, hypertension, or vascular or renal disease.

Pregnancy-induced hypertension may progress from mild preeclampsia to severe preeclampsia to eclampsia. The signs of **preeclampsia** are hypertension, edema, and proteinuria (protein in the urine). When the client becomes eclamptic, edema of the brain can cause convulsions and coma.

Mild preeclampsia is characterized by a systolic blood pressure increase of 30 millimeters of mercury or a diastolic increase of 15 millimeters of mercury over prepregnancy levels. It is treated with bed rest and possibly a high-protein diet to replace that lost in the urine. Diuretics are not used because they would aggravate the condition by increasing the permeability of the kidney's filtering system, causing greater losses of protein.

Severe preeclampsia is characterized by a systolic blood pressure greater than 160 millimeters of mercury or a diastolic pressure greater than 110 millimeters of mercury. Clients with severe preeclampsia are hospitalized to provide rest and to monitor the mother and the fetus. Sedative drugs may be prescribed to lessen the irritability of the brain.

Eclampsia is an obstetrical emergency that occurs in 1 of 200 cases of preeclampsia. The mother is in immediate danger of convulsing. She requires intensive nursing care because she is at high risk of cerebral hemorrhage, circulatory collapse, and kidney failure. The fetus, too, is in grave danger. Eclampsia is a major cause of maternal morbidity and mortality, especially in underdeveloped nations (Belfort, Anthony, and Saade, 1999).

Good prenatal care, including weight and blood pressure monitoring and urine testing, and early intervention are the keys to minimizing the hazard of pregnancy-induced hypertension. Calcium supplementation has been shown to reduce the risk of preeclampsia and of preterm birth (Crowther et al., 1999) and to benefit women who have increased risk of PIH or who have low calcium intake (Atallah, Hofmeyr, and Duley, 1999; Kulier et al., 1998).

GESTATIONAL DIABETES Pregnancy, a natural "stress test" of a woman's physiological adaptation, may precipitate the onset of diabetes in some women (McGanity, Dawson, and Van Hook, 1999). This condition, known as **gestational diabetes**, is detected by glucose tolerance tests, which are recommended as a routine part of prenatal care. Gestational diabetes, so called even if insulin is used or if the hyperglycemia persists after delivery (Gabbe, 1998), is discussed in detail in the chapter on diabetes mellitus.

The Breast-Feeding Mother

One of the goals of Healthy People 2010 is to increase to 75 percent the proportion of mothers who breast-feed in the early postpartum period, to 50 percent those who breast-feed until the infant is 6 months old, and to 25 percent of mothers who breast-feed until the infant is 1 year old. In 1998, 64 percent of mothers were breast-feeding in the early postpartum period, but only 29 percent were nursing at 6 months, and 16 percent at one year (U.S. Department of Health and Human Services, 2000). Breast-feeding was most common in the Western states (where 75 percent of infants were initially breast-fed) and among women who were older, college educated, **multiparous**, not employed outside the home, and those who had infants of normal birth weight (Ryan, 1997). Figure 11–4 shows breast-feeding rates in the United States from 1965 through 1995. The following chapter discusses the advantages of breast milk for the infant. In the next section, we consider nutritional implications of breast-feeding for the mother.

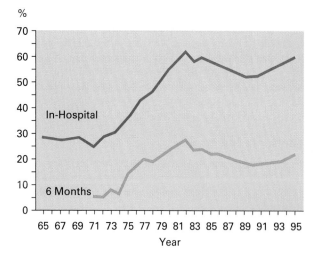

Figure 11–4:
U.S. breast-feeding rates: 1965 through 1995. (Reproduced with permission from Pediatrics, Vol 99, Page 12, 1997.)

Nutritional Needs

Recommended additional foods for a breast-feeding woman are two milk exchanges, one meat exchange, and one fruit or vegetable high in vitamin C. An increase in fluid intake of 1 liter per day is also advised. While exclusively breast-feeding their infants for 6 months, lactating women preserved their lean body mass by consuming 55 percent more protein than the nonlactating control group (Motil et al., 1998).

To produce milk, the breast-feeding mother requires 160 to 300 milligrams of calcium per day (Council on Scientific Affairs, 1997). To meet this need, the mother's skeleton is depleted of calcium at the rate of 1 percent per month regardless of calcium and vitamin D supplementation (Weaver and Heaney, 1999). Breast-feeding mothers, compared with formula-feeding mothers and nonpregnant, nonlactating women, had significant decreases in bone mineral content at the spine, femoral neck, total hip, and whole body. The reason for the differences is unclear, but these changes were not related to calcium intake, breast-milk calcium concentration, vitamin D-receptor genotype, postpartum weight change, or use of the progesterone-only contraceptive pill (Laskey et al., 1998). What is becoming clear is that human lactation is associated with alterations in calcium metabolism that are independent of dietary calcium intake and unresponsive to increases in calcium intake. Little evidence exists that indicates breast-feeding has a detrimental effect on long-term bone health (Prentice, 1997).

Energy

A breast-feeding mother requires an additional 500 kilocalories per day from food. Although 750 kilocalories are required, the remainder should be derived from fat stores. The calculation is as follows. Thirty ounces of breast milk a day at 20 kilocalories per ounce equals to 600 kilocalories total. Another 150 kilocalories are needed to make the milk. The RDA allows for 500 of these 750 kilocalories from food. The other 250 kilocalories are expected to be taken from fat stores laid down for this purpose during pregnancy.

Effect of Maternal Deficiencies

Even if a mother lacks some nutrients in her current diet, her milk contains the correct level of nutrients. The lack of nutrients in the mother's diet ultimately affects her nutrient stores, but while she nurses, she usually produces good-quality milk, but in less quantity. If the mother's diet is low in vitamin C, however, her milk also will be deficient in the vitamin. In an otherwise well-nourished mother, the use of a vitamin supplement does not increase the vitamin content of her milk.

Benefits to the Mother

Several advantages to the mother are associated with breast-feeding. It helps the uterus return to its nonpregnant state more quickly. Breast-feeding is convenient and less costly than bottle feeding, and may be protective against later premenopausal breast cancer and postmenopausal hip fractures.

Aids Uterine Involution

During breast-feeding, the sucking of the infant stimulates the release of **oxytocin** from the posterior pituitary gland in the brain. Oxytocin causes the uterine muscles to contract and helps return the uterus to its nonpregnant size.

Convenience at Less Cost

Breast milk is always ready at the correct temperature. There is no formula to make or contamination to worry about. The additional foods the mother consumes are less expensive than infant formula.

Lessens Risk of Breast Cancer

Over the long term, breast-feeding has been associated with a decreased risk of breast cancer later in life. In a Japanese study, the risk was lowest among premenopausal women who had ever lactated for 7 to 9 months (Yoo et al., 1992). Other researchers have found lactation associated with slight reductions in the risk of premenopausal and some postmenopausal breast cancer (Fruedenheim et al., 1997; Gilliland et al., 1998), of premenopausal and postmenopausal breast cancer (Furberg et al., 1999), and of postmenopausal breast cancer (Newcomb et al., 1999). These are statistical proportions for the group, not an individual guarantee

Techniques of Breast-Feeding

The medical and nursing staff will assist the mother to start breast-feeding her infant. Mothers nursing twins or premature babies will need additional education and support (Ellings, Newman, and Bowers, 1998). Some general principles to aid in breast-feeding have been established.

The mother and infant should be permitted to spend as much time together as possible during the first 24 hours after birth. This practice permits bonding of infant and mother. Some areas encourage fathers to "room in," also, to bond with the baby.

One correct position for breast-feeding is shown in Figure 11–5. It is tummy to tummy. The infant should face the breast squarely. If the breast is very large, the mother must take care to prevent it from blocking the infant's nose lest it impede infant's breathing. When nursing, the infant should grasp the entire areola (the colored portion around the nipple) to prevent the nipples from becoming sore.

Most infants will take 80 to 90 percent of the milk from each breast in the first 4 minutes of nursing. Because nursing stimulates further milk production, the mother should alternate which breast is first offered to the infant. This method allows the infant to empty the first breast offered and to finish feeding on the other breast if it is still hungry or is just enjoying the experience. At the next feeding, the mother should start with the breast the infant finished on the time before.

Encouraging Breast-Feeding

Although the American Academy of Pediatrics states the ultimate decision on feeding method is the mother's, pediatricians are encouraged to provide information on the benefits and methods of breast-feeding so that the mother can make an informed choice (American Academy of Pediatrics, 1997). A meta-analysis indicated that providing formula or coupons for formula upon discharge negatively affected the mothers choice to breast-feed (Perez-Escamilla 1994), but other evidence suggests the choice of feeding method is based on prenatal advice (Perez-Escamilla, 1998). Motivational videotapes played in prenatal clinic waiting rooms were associated with increased duration of breast-feeding (Gross et al., 1998).

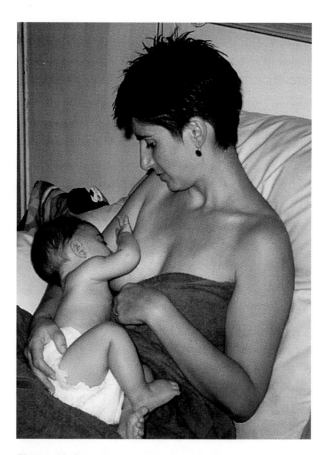

Figure 11–5:
One correct breast-feeding position, tummy-to-tummy. The infant takes the entire areola in its mouth. Notice how focused the mother is on the baby.

Use of peer counselors was effective in increasing breast-feeding rates (Long et al., 1995) and duration (Morrow et al., 1999; Schafer et al., 1998). Women who attended a single breast-feeding support meeting before 6 weeks postpartum were three times as likely as to breast-feed beyond 6 months as were nonattenders (Chezem and Friesen, 1999). Other breast-feeding support resources include the La Leche League and Internet Web sites.

Adoptive mothers have successfully breast-fed their infants by stimulating the breasts for several weeks before the baby arrived in the home. Additional bank breast milk or formula can be given through a narrow tube that lies next to the nipple (Elia, 1994). Even a child adopted at 5 months of age was breastfed until 8-1/2 months of age (Lambert, 1996). An adoptive mother who breast-fed two children maintains an adoptive breast-feeding resource website. It is listed under FourFriends.com with the other Internet Sites in the Study Aids section at the end of the chapter.

Maternal Contraindications to Breast-Feeding

Most women can feed their infants at breast. There are a few contraindications to breast-feeding including the mother's exposure to toxic chemicals, the mother's use of illegal drugs and certain medications, and certain illnesses in the mother. Untreated active tuberculosis is one of those illnesses. In the United States, maternal infection with human immunodeficiency virus (HIV) is a contraindication (Committee on Pediatric AIDS, 1995). The physician is the best source of guidance in a particular case. Galactosemia, a contraindication due to a metabolic defect in the infant, is discussed in Chapter 12.

In developing countries, the risks of malnutrition and other infectious diseases may be more immediate than the risk of HIV. A glimpse of the difficulty in coping with the AIDS epidemic in Africa is shown by a clinical trial in Kenya. It involved HIV seropositive pregnant women who were randomized to breast-feeding or formula feeding.

The conditions of the formula-fed group were far superior to the average family's situation. Free formula was provided that would have cost 300 U.S. dollars for a 6-month supply. Only women with access to municipally treated water were eligible for the study, and staff taught correct formula preparation. Infants were fed by cup rather than with artificial nipples to minimize contamination. Nurses followed-up clients at home within 2 weeks of the birth and then as needed. At the end of 2 years, significantly fewer of the formula-fed infants were infected with HIV compared with the breast-fed infants (32 to 50 percent); however, the overall infant mortality at 2 years was not significantly different (Nduati et al., 2000).

Exposure to Toxic Chemicals

Certain chemicals, such as DDT and PCB, have been shown to be **teratogenic**, causing congenital defects. Concern has been raised about the transmission of toxic chemicals to the infant through breast milk. Once ingested, if the body has no means of excreting the chemicals; the contaminants are stored in adipose tissue. When the lactating mother's fat stores are mobilized to produce milk, it, too contains the chemicals.

Some experts believe that the risk to the infant is minimal unless the mobilization of the mother's fat is due to inadequate intake. Others say that there is no hazard unless the woman has had occupational exposure to the chemicals or has consumed a large amount of fish from contaminated waters. Recently in Britain, high levels of dioxins and PCBs were found in breast milk. While the matter is still under study, and efforts continue to reduce environmental contamination, health-care providers in Britain believe the benefits of breast-feeding outweigh the risks posed by the chemicals (Wise, 1997). Women with concerns about the issue should discuss them with their health-care providers.

Medication Use

Many medications are secreted in breast milk. The physician should be consulted about both prescription and nonprescription drugs the mother takes.

Substances that are often not thought of as drugs may also affect the breast-fed infant. These include alcohol and caffeine. Here again, experts offer opposite advice to the breast-feeding mother. While some recommend abstinence, others think that the moderate use of alcohol and caffeine is acceptable. The primary-care provider is the best source of advice for the individual client.

Altered Physiology or Pathology

In the United States, absolute contraindications to breast-feeding include AIDS and active tuberculosis. Acute or chronic diseases in the mother also may preclude breast-feeding. Some are heart disease, severe anemia, and nephritis. If the woman becomes pregnant again, she will have to stop breast-feeding.

The use of breast-feeding as a method of birth spacing has been shown to be 98 percent successful for 4 to 6 months under certain conditions: if the infant feeds frequently, if no supplementary feedings are given, and so long as the woman remains amenorrheic (Bhler, 1997; Treffers, 1999; van Unnik and van Roosmalen, 1998; World Health Organization, 1999). Because estrogen inhibits lactation, the WHO advises against its use as an oral contraceptive during lactation. Alternative methods of contraception should be instituted once the woman gives up breast-feeding.

Wellness Tips 11–1

- Women of reproductive age should maximize their nutritional status before pregnancy, including optimizing their weight and nutrient stores.
- Obtaining prepregnancy counseling and seeking prenatal care early in the pregnancy are means to focus on wellness and prevention of complications.
- Those who have been using oral contraceptives should delay 4 months before attempting pregnancy to permit blood levels of folate, vitamins B_6 and B_{12}, and beta-carotene to return to normal after discontinuing the oral contraceptive. An alternative method of contraception should be used in the interim.
- All women capable of becoming pregnant should consume 400 micrograms of synthetic folic acid daily. This amount is in addition to food folate. Although synthetic folic acid is used to fortify grains, the surest means to obtain this amount of folic acid is with a multi-vitamin supplement.
- It is best to avoid consuming large amounts (>10,000 IU/day) of preformed vitamin A during the first trimester because of its teratogenic potential. The medication isotretinoin, a vitamin A metabolite, is prescribed for intractable acne and bears specific warnings pertaining to contraception that must be heeded.
- Substances to avoid for 8 weeks before and during pregnancy include alcohol and foods related to the transmission of Listeria monocytogenes—soft cheeses and ready-to-eat meats—as well as tobacco, and cocaine.

Nursing Makes a Difference

In a replication of an earlier study, home visits by nurses to pregnant women and to the mother and child after hospital discharge improved the subsequent life choices made by the woman. The nursing visits focused not only on immediate needs but also on clarifying goals, identifying barriers, and planning the women's futures related to education, employment, and child-bearing. Compared with a control group, the women visited by the nurses had fewer subsequent pregnancies, fewer closely spaced pregnancies, and longer intervals between the births of first and second children. The visits continued over two years, but the improvements in lifestyles were maintained for five years (Kitzman, et al., 2000). Nursing does make a difference in clients' lives. Wellness Tips 11–1 summarizes key information nurses can use in client education.

Summary

To support her own and the fetus's growth, a pregnant woman requires increased intake of kilocalories, protein, B and C vitamins, iron, iodine, and zinc. Recent efforts to prevent neural tube defects in the embryo have included revision of the RDA for folic acid and fortification of grains with folic acid. Substances for the pregnant woman to avoid are alcohol, caffeine, certain soft cheeses, and immoderate or supplemental intake of preformed vitamin A, along with tobacco and cocaine.

A pregnant teenage client is at especially high nutritional risk. Her own body still needs adequate nutrients for growth, and she also has a fetus to nourish.

Nutritional interventions are sometimes helpful for common complaints of pregnancy: morning sickness, leg cramps, constipation, and heartburn. Tact and diplomacy may be required to counsel women who have pica. Medical intervention and nutritional support are indicated for clients with hyperemesis gravidarum, pregnancy-induced hypertension (preeclampsia and eclampsia), or gestational diabetes.

Breast-feeding offers benefits to the mother. It aids uterine involution and offers convenience since the milk is constantly ready-to-feed. Some maternal contraindications to breast-feeding are exposure to toxic chemicals, ingestion of certain medications and drugs, and some illnesses, including AIDS and tuberculosis.

Case Study 11–1

Ms. T is a 21-year-old sexually active woman who has been followed in a family planning clinic for three years. She has been faithful about keeping appointments and taking her oral contraceptives and the pyridoxine that was prescribed. She is taking no other medications or vitamin supplements. Now she relates that she is seriously considering becoming pregnant. Her boyfriend proposed at her 21st birthday celebration. She denies knowledge of means to minimize fetal risk and states she drinks "a beer" or a glass of wine on Saturdays and Sundays. She does not smoke. She received the standard measles, mumps, and rubella (MMR) vaccination as a child.

Ms. T is a 5 ft. 3 in. woman and weighs 136 lb. Her wrist measures 5.5 in. Her hemoglobin was 14 g/dL and hematocrit was 42 percent last month.

Nursing Care Plan

Subjective Data	Expressed interest in becoming pregnant
	Regular moderate alcohol intake
	History of compliance with medical regimen
	Immunized against measles, mumps, and rubella
Objective Data	115 percent of healthy body weight
	Hemoglobin 14 g/dL, within normal limits (WNL)
	Hematocrit 42 percent, within normal limits (WNL)
Nursing Diagnosis	NANDA: Risk for injury, fetal (North American Nursing Diagnosis Association, 1999, with permission.)
	Related to lack of knowledge of measures to decrease risk to embryo

Desired Outcomes Evaluation Criteria	Nursing Actions/ Interventions	Rationale
NOC: Risk Control (Johnson, Maas, and Moorhead, 2000, with permission.)	NIC: Health Education (McCloskey and Bulechek, 2000, with permission.)	
Will affirm intention to abstain from alcohol when attempting to achieve a pregnancy and throughout gestation.	Teach Ms. T about fetal alcohol syndrome.	No amount of alcohol is presumed to be safe in pregnancy.
	Use photographs of affected children.	"A picture is worth 1,000 words." Photographs introduce visual learning and impact feelings.
Will begin taking a daily multi-vitamin, multi-mineral supplement within a week.	Instruct Ms. T to select a vitamin preparation containing 400 micrograms of folic acid.	This is the 1998 RDA for all women capable of becoming pregnant.
	Review the value of a varied diet and good sources of food folate.	The 1998 RDA also emphasizes the importance of food folate. *(Continued)*

Nursing Care Plan (Continued)

Desired Outcomes / Evaluation Criteria	Nursing Actions / Interventions	Rationale
Will recount the limits to vitamin A intake during pregnancy.	Inform Ms. T of RDA for vitamin A in pregnancy. Alert Ms. T to the large amounts of preformed vitamin A in liver and liver products. Caution against supplements of vitamin A in addition to the multi-vitamin, multi-mineral tablet.	Teratogenic effects usually occur during the 1st trimester.
	Discuss the safety of beta-carotene (provitamin A) in pregnancy.	Beta-carotene has not been associated with birth defects. Supplements containing provitamin A are considered safe for pregnant women at the RDA level.
Will list actions to take to minimize exposure to Listeria infection.	Provide Ms. T with a list of cheeses to avoid and those that are considered safe. Review rules for safe handling of ready-to-eat meats.	Because the incubation period of Listeria is up to 8 weeks, avoidance of possibly contaminated food should begin well before conception.
	Alert her to report flu-like symptoms to her primary healthcare provider.	
Will discuss the discontinuation of oral contraceptive therapy and attempting conception with the primary healthcare provider before changing her regimen.	Advise Ms. T about the possibility of birth defects with some oral contraceptives.	Progestins may cause birth defects if taken early in pregnancy (Nursing 2000, 2000).

Critical Thinking Question

1. If Ms. T were to achieve a pregnancy, what would her month-by-month recommended weight gain be?
2. What additional assessment data would you obtain to design a comprehensive, personalized nursing care plan with her?
3. Are there other issues you believe ought to be raised with Ms. T before she attempts to become pregnant? Are they more or less important than the ones addressed in the Nursing Care Plan? Why?

 ## Study Aids

Subjects	Internet Sites
Pregnancy	http://www.nal.usda.gov/fnic/pubs/bibs/topics/pregnancy/preghp/html
	http://www.noah.cuny.edu/pregnancy/pregnancy.html
Breast-feeding	http://lalecheleague.org
	http://www.nursingmother.com
	http://www.prairiernet.org/laleche/otherInternet.html
	http://www.fourfreinds.com/abrw/
Fetal Alcohol Syndrome	http://www.nofas.org
	http://depts.washington.edu/fadu/
	http://www.jdmc.org/fase.htm
	http://azstarnet.com/~tjk/fashome.htm
	http://thearc.org/misc/faslist.html
	http://www.accessone.com/~delindam/
	http://www.arbi.org
Listeriosis	http://vm.cfsan.fda/gov/~dms/listeren.html
	http://www.healthfinder.gov/text/docs/Doc0205.htm
	http://health.state.ny.us/nysdoh/consumer/lister.htm
	http://www.ci.nyc.ny.us/html/doh/html/cd/cdis.html
	http://nevdgp.org.au/Travel/dis/lister.htm
Neural tube defects	http://text.nlm.nih.gov/cps/www/cps.48.html
	http://www.modimes.org/Programs2/FolicAcid/Default.htm
	http://cpmcnet.columbia.edu/texts/gcps/gcps0052.html
	http://www.cps.ca/english/statements/DT/dt95-01.htm
	http://www.asbah.demon.co.uk/folicacid.html

Chapter Review

1. A pregnant woman should consume one more serving of milk than she consumed when not pregnant and
   a. Two additional servings of deep green leafy or yellow vegetables
   b. One additional ounce of meat and an extra serving of a good source of vitamin C
   c. Three additional whole grain bread servings
   d. Two extra servings of fresh fruit and at least four total servings of "free" vegetables from the ADA Exchange Lists
2. Which of the following substances is contraindicated during pregnancy
   a. Alcohol
   b. Cocoa
   c. Coffee
   d. Tea
3. Compared to a pregnant adult, the pregnant teenager should consume 1 additional serving of both:
   a. Fruit and meat
   b. Milk and meat
   c. Milk and starch/ bread
   d. Vegetable and fruit
4. The 1998 RDA for folic acid specifies 400 micrograms of synthetic folic acid from fortified foods or supplements for
   a. All women capable of becoming pregnant
   b. Women taking oral contraceptive medications
   c. Women of northern European descent
   d. Breast-feeding mothers
5. If a pregnant woman complains of heartburn, she should be instructed to:
   a. Increase her intake of milk products
   b. Decrease her overall food intake
   c. Rest in bed after eating
   d. Avoid spicy or acidic foods

Clinical Analysis

Ms. T is a 15-year-old girl who thinks that she is 2 months pregnant. She confides to the school nurse that she is not sure if she should have an abortion. She has not told anyone else of the pregnancy. Her purpose in disclosing the information to the school nurse is to obtain assistance with weight control so she has more time to make up her mind.

1. Based on the above information, which one of the following interventions would be of highest priority at this time?
   a. Designing a weight control program that is high in calcium
   b. Giving information on the desirability of breast-feeding the infant
   c. Instructing the girl regarding substances that are likely to harm the fetus
   d. Scheduling a visit with a social worker to help the girl decide on a course of action
2. Knowing that adolescents are often lacking in certain nutrients, the nurse would want to assess the girl's intake of:
   a. Cola, coffee, and tea
   b. Fruits, vegetables, milk, and red meat
   c. Fried foods and pastries
   d. Poultry, seafood, and white bread
3. Ms. T complains of morning sickness. The nurse instructs her to:
   a. Eat breakfast later in the morning.
   b. Drink at least two glasses of liquid with every meal.
   c. Increase her intake of whole-grain breads and cereals to two servings per meal.
   d. Drink a large glass of skim milk at bedtime.

Bibliography

Acosta, RB, and Wright, L: Nurses' role in preventing birth defects in off-spring of women with phenylketonuria. JOGNN 21:270, 1992.
Alm, B, et al.: Caffeine and alcohol as risk factors for sudden infant death. Arch Dis Child 81:107, 1999.
Anderson, AS: Folic acid: The message we're failing to get across. Prof Care Mother Child 5:64, 66, 1995.
American Academy of Pediatrics Work Group on Breastfeeding. Breastfeeding and the use of human milk. Pediatrics 100:1035, 1997.
Atallah, AN, Hofmeyr, GJ, and Duley, L: Calcium supplementation during pregnancy for preventing hypertensive disorders and related problems. [Computer software]. The Cochrane Library, Oxford, 1999 issue 2. Abstract accessed through CINAHL, accession no. 1999040187.
Barrett, JFR, et al.: Absorption of nonhaeme iron from food during normal pregnancy. Br Med J 309:79, 1994.
Belfort, MA, Anthony, J, and Saade, GR: Prevention of eclampsia. Semin Perinatol 23:65, 1999
Bendich, A: Folic acid and prevention of neural tube defects: Critical assessment of FDA proposals to increase folic acid intakes. J Nutr Educ 26:294, 1994.
Bhler, E: [Breast feeding as family planning in a global perspective]—Norwegian. Tidsskr Nor Laegeforen 117:704, 1997.

Bolumar, F, et al.: Caffeine intake and delayed conception: A European multicenter study on infertility and subfecundity. European Study Group on Infertility Subfecundity. Am J Epidemiol 145:324, 1997.
Bower, C, et al.: Promotion of folate for the prevention of neural tube defects: Knowledge and use of periconceptional folic acid supplements in Western Australia, 1992 to 1995. Aust N Z J Public Health 21:716, 1997.
Centers for Disease Control: Accutane-exposed pregnancies—California, 1999. MMWR 49:28, 2000a. Accessed 4/12/2000 at http://www.cdc.gov/epo/mmwr/preview/mmwrhtml/mm4902a.htm
Centers for Disease Control: Alcohol consumption among pregnant and childbearing-aged women—United States, 1991 and 1995. MMWR 46:346, 1997. Accessed 9/19/99 at http://www.cdc.gov/epo/mmwr/preview/mmwrhtml/00047306.htm
Centers for Disease Control: Knowledge about folic acid and use of multivitamins containing folic acid among reproductive-aged women—Georgia. MMWR 45:793, 1996. Accessed 9/13/99 at http://www.cdc.gov/epo/mmwr/preview/mmwrhtml/00043735.htm
Centers for Disease Control: Knowledge and use of folic acid by women of childbearing age—United States, 1995 and 1998. MMWR 48:325, 1999a. Accessed 9/13/99 at http://www.cdc.gov/epo/mmwr/preview/mmwrhtml/00056982.htm

Centers for Disease Control: Neural tube defect surveillance and folic acid intervention—Texas–Mexico border, 1993–1998. MMWR 49:1, 2000b. Accessed 4/12/2000 at http://www.cdc.gov/epo/mmwr/preview/mmwrhtml/mm4901a1.htm

Centers for Disease Control: Multistate outbreak of listeriosis—United States, 1998. MMWR 47:1085, 1998a. Accessed 9/19/99 at http://www.cdc.gov/epo/mmwr/preview/mmwrhtml/00056024.htm

Centers for Disease Control: Recommendations for the use of folic acid to reduce the number of cases of spina bifida and other neural tube defects. MMWR 41 (No. RR-14):1, 1992.

Centers for Disease Control: Recommendations to prevent and control iron deficiency in the United States. MMWR 47:1, 1998b. Accessed 9/13/99 at http://www.cdc.gov/epo/mmwr/preview/mmwrhtml/00051880.htm

Centers for Disease Control: Update: multistate outbreak of listeriosis—United States, 1998–1999. MMWR 47:1117, 1999b. Accessed 9/19/99 at http://www.cdc.gov/epo/mmwr/preview/mmwrhtml/00056169.htm

Chezem, J, and Friesen, C: Attendance at breast-feeding support meetings: relationship to demographic characteristics and duration of lactation in women planning postpartum employment. J Am Diet Assoc 99:83, 1999.

Chin, J (ed): Control of Communicable Diseases Manual ed 17. American Public Health Association, Washington, DC , 2000.

Christian, P, et al.: An ethnographic study of night blindness "ratauni" among women in the Terai of Nepal. Soc Sci Med 46:879, 1998.

Committee on Pediatric AIDS. Human breast milk, breastfeeding, and transmission of human immunodeficiency virus in the United States. Pediatrics 96:977, 1995.

Council on Scientific Affairs, American Medical Association: Intake of dietary calcium to reduce the incidence of osteoporosis. Arch Fam Med 6:495, 1997.

Crowther, CA, et al.: Calcium supplementation in nulliparous women for the prevention of pregnancy-induced hypertension, preeclampsia and preterm birth: An Australian randomized trial. Aust N Z J Obstet Gynaecol 39:12, 1999.

Czeizel, AE, and Dudas, I: Prevention of the first occurrence of neural-tube defects by periconceptual vitamin supplementation. N Engl J Med 327:1832, 1992.

Dahle, LO, et al.: The effect of oral magnesium substitution on pregnancy-induced leg cramps. Am J Obstet Gynecol 173:176, 1995.

Dickinson, CJ: Does folic acid harm people with vitamin B_{12} deficiency? Q J Med 88:357, 1995.

Elia, I: Adoptive breastfeeding. Nursing Standard 8:20, 1994.

Ellings, JM, Newman, RB, and Bowers, NA: Prenatal care and multiple pregnancy. JOGNN 27:457, 1998.

Eskenazi, B et al.: Associations between maternal decaffeinated and caffeinated coffee consumption and fetal growth and gestational duration. Epidemiology 10:242, 1999.

Eskenazi, B, Caffeine—filtering the facts. N Engl J Med 341:1688, 1999.

Fairbanks, VF: Iron in medicine and nutrition. In Shils, ME, et al. (eds): Modern Nutrition in Health and Disease ed 9. Lippincott Williams and Wilkins, Philadelphia, 1999.

Fang, J, Madhavan, S, and Alderman, MH: Low birth weight: Race and maternal nativity—impact of community income. Pediatrics 103:e5, 1999. Accessed 10/29/1999 through http://www.pediatrics.org

Fenster, L, et al.: Caffeinated beverages, decaffeinated coffee, and spontaneous abortion. Epidemiology 8:515, 1997.

Fernandes, O, et al.: Moderate to heavy caffeine consumption during pregnancy and relationship to spontaneous abortion and abnormal fetal growth: a meta-analysis. Repro Toxicol 12:435, 1998.

Food and Drug Administration: Food standards: Amendment of standards of identity for enriched grain products require addition of folic acid. Federal Register 61:8781, 1996.

Ford, RP, et al.: Heavy caffeine intake in pregnancy and sudden infant death syndrome. Arch Dis Child 78:9, 1998.

Freudenheim, JL, et al.: Lactation history and breast cancer risk. Am J Epidemiol 146:932, 1997.

Furberg, H, et al.: Lactation and breast cancer risk. Int J Epidemiol 28:396, 1999.

Futoryan, T, and Gilchrest, BA: Retinoids and the skin. Nutrition Reviews 52:299, 1994.

Gabbe, SG: The gestational diabetes mellitus conferences. Diabetes Care 21, Suppl 2, B1, 1998.

Galloway, R, and McGuire, J: Daily versus weekly: How many iron pills do pregnant women need? Nutr Rev 54:318, 1996.

Gilliland, FD, et al.: Reproductive risk factors for breast cancer in Hispanic and non-Hispanic white women: The New Mexico Women's Health Study. Am J Epidemiol 148:683, 1998.

Glenn, FB, Glenn, WD, and Duncan, RC: Fluoride tablet supplementation during pregnancy for caries immunity: A study of the offspring produced. Am J Obstet Gynecol 143:560, 1982.

Goldenberg, RL, et al.: The effect of zinc supplementation on pregnancy outcome. JAMA 274:463, 1995.

Gross, SM, et al.: Counseling and motivational videotapes increase duration of breast-feeding in African-American WIC participants who initiate breast-feeding. J Am Diet Assoc 98:143, 1998.

Hally, SS: Nutrition in reproductive health. Journal of Nurse-Midwifery 43:459, 1998.

James, WPT: Long-term fetal programming of body composition and longevity. Nutr Rev 55:S31, 1997.

Jensen, TK, et al.: Caffeine intake and fecundability: A follow-up study among 430 Danish couples planning their first pregnancy. Reprod Toxicol 12:289, 1998.

Jewell, D, and Young, G: Treatments for nausea and vomiting in early pregnancy. [Computer Software]. The Cochrane Library, Oxford, 1999 issue 1. Abstract accessed through CINAHL, accession no. 1999023380.

Johnson, M, Maas, M, and Moorhead, S: Nursing Outcomes Classification (NOC), ed 2. Mosby, Philadelphia, 2000.

Kaskutas, LA, et al.: Reach and effects of health messages on drinking during pregnancy. Journal of Health Education 29:11, 1998.

Kitzman, H, et al.: Enduring effects of nurse home visitation on maternal life course. JAMA 283:1983, 2000.

Klebanoff, MA, et al.: Maternal serum paraxanthine, a caffeine metabolite, and the risk of spontaneous abortion. N Engl J Med 341, 1639, 1999.

Kulier, R, et al.: Nutritional interventions for the prevention of maternal morbidity. Int J Gynaecol Obstet 63:231, 1998.

Lambert, J: Adoptive breastfeeding: A personal experience. Breastfeeding Review 4:85, 1996.

Laskey, MA, et al.: Bone changes after 3 months of lactation: Influence of calcium intake, breast-milk output, and vitamin D-receptor genotype. Am J Clin Nutr 67:685, 1998.

Leverett, DH, et al.: Randomized clinical trial of the effect of prenatal fluoride supplements in preventing dental caries. Caries Research 31:174, 1997.

Liel, Y, Atar, D, and Ohana, N: Pregnancy-associated osteoporosis: Preliminary densitometric evidence of extremely rapid recovery of bone mineral density. Southern Medical Journal 91:33, 1998.

Long, DG, et al.: Peer counselor program increases breastfeeding rates in Utah Native American WIC population. J Human Lact 11:279, 1995.

Mahomed, K, and Gulmezoglu, AM: Maternal iodine supplements in areas of deficiency. [Computer software]. The Cochrane Library, Oxford, 1999 issue 2. Abstract accessed through CINAHL, accession no. 1999040422.

Mastroiacovo, P, et al.: High vitamin A intake in early pregnancy and major malformations: A multicenter prospective controlled study. Teratology 59:7, 1999.

McCloskey, JC, and Bulechek, GM: Nursing Interventions Classification (NIC), 3 ed. Mosby, Philadelphia, 2000.

McGanity, WJ, Dawson EB, and Van Hook, JW: Maternal nutrition. In Shils, ME, et al. (eds): Modern Nutrition in Health and Disease ed 9. Lippincott Williams and Wilkins, Philadelphia, 1999.

Milunsky, A, et al.: Maternal heat exposure and neural tube defects. JAMA 268:882, 1992.

Morrow, AL, et al.: Efficacy of home-based peer counseling to promote exclusive breast-feeding: A randomized controlled trial. Lancet 353:1226, 1999.

Morrow, JD, and Kelsey, K: Folic acid for prevention of neural tube defects: Pediatric anticipatory guidance. Journal of Pediatric Health Care 12:55, 1998.

Motil, KJ, et al.: Lean body mass of well-nourished women is preserved during lactation. Am J Clin Nutr 67:292, 1998.

MRC Vitamin Study Research Group: Prevention of neural tube defects: Results of the Medical Research Council Vitamin Study. Lancet 338:131, 1991.

Murphy-Brennan, MG, and Oei, TP: Is there evidence to show that fetal alcohol syndrome can be prevented? J Drug Educ 29:5, 1999.

Muscati, SK, Gray-Donald, K, and Newson, EE: Interaction of smoking and maternal weight status in influencing infant size. Can J Public Health 85:407, 1994.

Nduati, R, et al.: Effect of breastfeeding and formula feeding on transmission of HIV-1. JAMA 283:1167, 2000.

Newcomb, PA: Lactation in relation to postmenopausal breast cancer. Am J Epidemiol 150:174, 1999.

North American Nursing Diagnosis Association: Nursing Diagnoses: Definitions and Classification 1999–2000, North American Nursing Diagnosis Association, Philadelphia, 1999.

Nursing 2000 Drug Handbook. Springhouse Corporation, Springhouse, PA, 2000.

Oakley, GP, Adams, MJ, and Dickinson, CM: More folic acid for everyone, now. J Nutr (Suppl)126:251 S, 1996.

Oakley, GP, and Erickson, JD: Vitamin A and birth defects. N Engl J Med 333:1414, 1995.

O'Connor, DL: Folate status during pregnancy and lactation. Adv Exp Med Biol 352:157, 1994.

Parazzini, F, et al.: Coffee consumption and risk of hospitalized miscarriage before 12 weeks of gestation. Hum Reprod 13:2286, 1998.

Pastuszak, A, Koren, G, and Rieder, MJ: Use of the Retinoid Pregnancy Prevention Program in Canada: Patterns of contraception use in women treated with isotretinoin and etreinate. Reprod Toxicol 8:63, 1994.

Pérez-Escamilla, R, et al.: Infant feeding policies in maternity wards and their effect on breast-feeding success: an analytical overview. Am J Public Health 84:89, 1994.

Pérez-Escamilla, R: Periconceptual folic acid and neural tube defects: Public health issues. Bull Pan Am Health Organ 29:250, 1995.

Pérez-Escamilla, R: Prenatal and perinatal factors associated with breast-feeding initiation among inner-city Puerto Rican women. J Am Diet Assoc 98:657, 1998.

Prentice, A: Calcium supplementation during breast-feeding. N Engl J Med 337:558, 1997.

Rainville, AJ: Pica practices of pregnant women are associated with lower maternal hemoglobin level at delivery. J Am Diet Assoc 98:293, 1998.

Rhinehart, SN, and Gabel, LL: Teenage pregnancy: an update on impact and preventive measures. Family Practice Recertification 20, 61, 1998.

Ritchie, LD, et al.: A longitudinal study of calcium homeostasis during human pregnancy and lactation and after resumption of menses. Am J Clin Nutr 67:693, 1998.

Romano, PS, et al.: Folic acid fortification of grain: An economic analysis. Am J Public Health 85:667, 1995.

Rothman, KJ, et al.: Teratogenicity of high vitamin A intake. N Engl J Med 333:1369, 1995.

Rush, D: Periconceptional folate and neural tube defect. Am J Clin Nutr (suppl) 59:511S, 1994.

Ryan, AS. The resurgence of breastfeeding in the United States. Pediatrics 99(4), 1997. Accessed 9/15/99 at http://www.pediatrics.org/cgi /content/full/99/4/e12

Santos, IS, et al.: Caffeine intake and low birth weight: a Population-based case-control study. Am J Epidemiol 147:620, 1998a.

Santos, IS, et al.: Caffeine intake and pregnancy outcomes: a meta-analytic review. Cad Saude Publica 14:523, 1998b.

Schafer, E, et al.: Volunteer peer counselors increase breastfeeding duration among rural low-income women. Birth: Issues in Perinatal Care and Education 25:101, 1998.

Schoral, CJ, et al.: Possible abnormalities of folate and vitamin B_{12} metabolism associated with neural tube defects. Ann NY Acad Sci 678:81, 1993.

Stamford, B: Muscle cramps. Physician and Sportsmedicine 21:115, 1993.

Steinmetz, G: Fetal alcohol syndrome. National Geographic 181:36, 1992.

Story, M: Promoting healthy eating and ensuring adequate weight gain in pregnant adolescents: Issues and strategies. Ann N Y Acad Sci 817:321, 1997.

Stutts, MA, Patterson, LT, and Hunnicutt, GG: Females' perception of risks associated with alcohol consumption during pregnancy. American Journal of Health Behavior 21:137, 1997.

Treffers, PE: [Breastfeeding and contraception]-Dutch. Ned Tijdschr Geneeskd 143:1900, 1999.

United States Department of Health and Human Services. Healthy People 2010. Accessed 4/14/00 at http://web.health.gov/healthypeople/document/html/volume2/16mich.htm#_TOC471971365

U.S. Department of Health and Human Services: FDA issues nationwide health warning about Royal Baltic cold-smoked fish products. HHS News March 10, 2000. Accessed 3/12/2000 at http://www.fda.gov/bbs/topics/NEWS/NEW00719.html

Van Loan, MD, et al.: Fluid changes during pregnancy: Use of bioimpedance spectroscopy. J Appl Physiol 78:1037, 1995.

van Stuijvenberg, ME, et al.: The nutritional status and treatment of patients with hyperemesis gravidarum. Am J Obstet Gynecol 172:1585, 1995.

van Unnik, GA, and van Roosmalen, J: [Lactation-induced amenorrhea as birth control method] – Dutch. Ned Tijdschr Geneeskd 142:60, 1998.

Ventura, SJ, Mathews, TJ, and Curtin, SC: Declines in teenage birth rates, 1991–97: National and state patterns. National Vital Statistics Reports 47 number 12. National Center for Health Statistics, Hyattsville, MD, 1998. Accessed 9/20/99 at http://www.cdc.gov/nchswww/data /nvs47_12pdf

Vlajinac, HD, et al.: Effect of caffeine intake during pregnancy on birth weight. Am J Epidemiol 145:335, 1997.

Weaver, CM, and Heaney, RP: Calcium. In Shils, ME, et al. (eds): Modern Nutrition in Health and Disease ed 9. Lippincott Williams and Wilkins, Philadelphia, 1999.

Wellings, K, et al.: Teenage fertility and life chances. Rev Reprod 4:184, 1999.

West, KP, Jr, et al.: Double blind, cluster randomized trial of low dose supplementation with vitamin A or beta carotene on mortality related to pregnancy in Nepal. Brit Med J 318:570, 1999.

Whitehead, AS, et al.: A genetic defect in 5,10 methylenetetrahydrofolate reductase in neural tube defects. Q J Med 88:763, 1995.

Wise, J: High amounts of chemicals found in breast milk. Brit Med J 314:1501, 1997. Accessed 4/16/2000 at http://www.bmj.com/cgi/content/full/314/7093/1501/j

World Health Organization Task Force on Methods for the Natural Regulation of Fertility: World Health Organization multinational study of breast-feeding and lactational amenorrhea. III Pregnancy during breast-feeding. Fertil Steril 72:431, 1999.

Yonekura, ML, and Mead, PB: Protocols: OB/GYN infection. Listeria infection in pregnancy. Contemporary OB/GYN 44:16, 1999.

Yoo, K-Y, et al.: Independent protective effect of lactation against breast cancer: A case–control study in Japan. Am J Epidemiol 135:726, 1992.

CHAPTER 12

Life Cycle Nutrition: Infancy, Childhood, Adolescence

LEARNING OBJECTIVES

After completing this chapter, the student should be able to:

1. Describe normal growth patterns and corresponding nutritional needs for a full-term infant, a toddler, a school-age child, and an adolescent.
2. Explain why breast milk is uniquely suited to the human infant's capabilities.
3. Compare the advantages and disadvantages of breast-feeding and formula-feeding.
4. Discuss the rationale for the sequence in which semisolid foods are introduced into an infant's diet.
5. List causes and treatments of five common nutritional problems of infancy.
6. Summarize common nutritional problems of the preschool child.
7. Relate ways in which a child can be encouraged to establish good nutritional habits.
8. Identify areas of concern regarding an adolescent's diet.

Good nutrition is of paramount importance for both infants and children. Because of public health efforts, U.S. infant mortality rates decreased significantly between 1915 and 1997. Of every 1000 infants born alive in 1915, approximately 100 died before the age of 1 year, compared with a mortality rate of 7.2 in 1997 (Centers for Disease Control, 1999a).

That is a significant achievement, yet in 1999 the United States ranked 17th of 50 countries in infant mortality rate (Infant mortality, 1999). Certain ethnic groups bear a greater risk than others. Black infants are more than twice as likely to die as white infants. American Indian/Alaska Native infants and Hispanics of Puerto Rican origin also have higher death rates than white infants (Centers for Disease Control, 1999a), although infant mortality rates for American Indians have fallen

from 62.7 infant deaths per 1000 live births in 1955 to 9.4 in 1991 (Story et al., 1998). An undetermined portion of these decreases can be attributed to improved nutrition and sanitation, including pure drinking water.

This chapter focuses on periods of rapid growth during infancy, childhood, and adolescence. In addition to nutritional needs for all periods of growth, the stages of physical and **psychosocial development** are discussed for these ages, noting ways in which food relates to psychosocial development.

Psychosocial Development

American psychoanalyst **Erik Erikson** formulated a theory of psychological development based on an individual's interactions with other people. Erikson divided life into eight stages, each of which involves a psychosocial developmental task to be mastered and an opposite negative trait that emerges if the task is not mastered. Even if a developmental task is successfully mastered, a new situation may arise, challenging the person to reaffirm his or her mastery.

Erikson's developmental tasks through adolescence are outlined in Table 12–1. This chapter and the next discuss the ways that nutrition and food can influence psychosocial development.

Nutrition in Infancy

Growth, the progressive maturation and increase in size of a living thing, entails the synthesis of new protoplasm and multiplication of cells. Infancy, the first year of life, is a critical period for the growth of essential organs. Health-care workers use certain milestones to judge the adequacy of a baby's growth.

Table 12–1 Erikson's Theory of Psychosocial Development

Stage of Life	Developmental Task	Opposing Negative Trait
Infancy	Trust	Distrust
Toddler	Autonomy	Doubt
Preschooler	Initiative	Guilt
School-age child	Industry	Inferiority
Adolescent	Identity	Role confusion

Growth

The only time human beings grow faster than in infancy is the 9 months before they are born. A baby's birth weight should double by age 4 to 6 months and triple by 1 year. An infant who weighs 7 pounds at birth, for example, should weigh 14 pounds at 6 months and 21 pounds at 1 year. From a birth length of about 20 inches, a baby grows to about 30 inches by age 1.

The infant's *rate of growth* is more significant than absolute values. Is the infant progressing at a reasonable pace? A gain of 5 to 8 ounces per week is expected during the first 4 or 5 months. Thereafter, a gain of 4 to 5 ounces per week until the first birthday is reasonable.

Evidence suggests that breast-fed and formula-fed infants have different growth rates after 3 months of age. A study found that formula-fed boys were significantly heavier than breast-fed boys at each month between the ages of 7 to 18 months. For girls the differences occurred between 6 and 18 months of age. Dewey and coworkers recommend the use of separate growth charts for breast-fed infants (Dewey, et al., 1992).

During the first few days after birth, a baby loses weight as it adjusts to its new environment and food supply. The amount of weight lost should not exceed 10 percent of the birth weight. The newborn (or neonate, as a baby is called during its first 28 days after birth) usually returns to its birth weight within 14 days.

The period most critical to brain development extends from conception into the second year of life. Brain cells increase most rapidly before birth and during the first 5 or 6 months after birth. To attain maximum brain growth, the baby needs optimal nutrition. Severe protein-calorie malnutrition in the last trimester of pregnancy or the first 6 months of life may decrease the number of brain cells by as much as 20 percent.

Development

Development is the gradual process of changing from a simple to a more complex organism. Becoming a mature individual involves psychosocial and physical changes, not only an increase in size.

Psychosocial Development

The psychosocial developmental task of the infant is to learn to **trust** (Table 12-1). The parent who responds promptly and lovingly to the infant's cries is teaching the baby to trust, laying the foundation for future human relationships. If the caregiver handles the infant inconsistently gently one time and roughly the next—however, the baby learns to mistrust. If the psychosocial task of trust is not accomplished, it lays a groundwork of mistrust and suspicion in the individual's personality.

In situations where physical care is provided but a tender relationship does not develop, infants may actually suffer stunted physical growth. **Failure to thrive** (FTT) has become a medical diagnosis for severely underweight infants; some authorities suggest that the term is used as a euphemism for undernutrition (Duggan, 1997).

An infant can explore the world through feeding and foods. New foods encourage experimentation. Babies like to poke their fingers into the food. When attempting to feed themselves they may turn the spoon upside down on the way to their mouths. Consistent acceptance from parents teaches the infant to trust his or her world. Parents should not, for example, laugh at a particular behavior of their child one time and scold the next.

Physical Development

Development proceeds at a different pace in various tissues and organs. Proper feeding practices are based on the maturation rate of body organs.

GASTROINTESTINAL SYSTEM The infant's gastrointestinal system is very different from the adult's. For several months, an infant's salivary and pancreatic amylases are inadequate to easily digest complex carbohydrates. Infants have lingual lipase for the digestion of fat, an enzyme that adults lack.

An infant's intestinal tract is also immature. It resembles a chain-link fence rather than a sieve, allowing whole proteins to be absorbed into the bloodstream. The more mature intestine permits absorption of amino acids but not whole proteins. This is one reason many foods that often cause allergies are not offered to the infant under one year of age.

Infants have to be fed often. A newborn's stomach holds about an ounce. By 1 year of age, the stomach holds about 8 ounces. An adult's stomach, by comparison, can hold about 2 quarts.

NERVOUS SYSTEM Development of nervous tissue, bile, and hormones requires fat and cholesterol. Because of the rapid growth of the brain and the nervous system, the infant requires adequate fat and cholesterol in its diet.

A **term infant** does have some well-developed reflexes. One of these is the **rooting reflex**. When the infant's cheek is stroked, the head turns toward that side to nurse. For the first 3 or 4 months, the infant suckles by using an up-and-down motion of the tongue. If semisolid food is offered at this time, the natural motion of the tongue tends to spit it out.

After 4 months, the infant can suck using orofacial muscles. The tongue moves back and forth instead of up and down. At this point, semisolid food is more likely to be swallowed than spit out. By 6 months of age, the infant has enough hand-to-eye coordination to put food and other objects into its mouth. A 7-month-old infant can chew appropriate foods.

URINARY SYSTEM An infant's kidneys are immature and have limited capacity to filter solutes. Not until the end of the second month can the infant's kidneys excrete the waste of semisolid foods (as discussed later, feeding of semisolids often is delayed another 2 months, however). By the infant's first birthday, the kidneys have reached full functional capacity.

Nutritional Needs of the Term Infant

A normal pregnancy is 38 to 42 weeks. Breast milk is the natural food for human infants. Its characteristics are the standard for infant formulas, which replicate many of the components of breast milk but which cannot supply all of its desirable qualities.

Protein

Because of the extensive tissue building that occurs, an infant's 1989 RDA for protein is 13 grams per day for the first 6 months and 14 grams for the second 6 months of life. By comparison, the RDA for protein is 63 grams for adult males and 50 grams for adult females.

The protein in breast milk is easy for the infant to digest. Human milk contains 70 percent whey and 30 percent casein compared to 18 percent whey and 82 percent casein in cow's milk. The whey portion of milk consists of soluble proteins that are easily digested. The major whey protein in breast milk is alpha-lactalbumin, with an amino acid pattern much like that of the body tissues. The infant's body can absorb it easily and, without much processing, can use it for building tissue. Gastric emptying is faster with human milk than cow's milk formula. In contrast, the major whey protein in cow's milk is beta-lactoglobulin, the protein often blamed for cow's milk allergy and colic (Schanler, 1997).

Energy

Infants need much higher relative energy intakes than do adults, primarily because the resting metabolic rates of infants and their needs for growth and development are so high. Normal pulse rate is 120 to 150 beats per minute; normal respiratory rate is 30 to 50 breaths per minute. Because of the large proportion of skin surface to body size, temperature regulation takes significant energy. An activity such as crying may double the infant's energy expenditure.

A newborn requires 100 to 120 kilocalories per kilogram of body weight per day. If a 154-pound (70-kilogram) man consumed energy at the rate of a newborn, he would take in 7000 to 8400 kilocalories per day. By the end of the first year of life, the infant requires only 80 to 100 kilocalories per kilogram of body weight.

CARBOHYDRATE The carbohydrate in breast milk is easily digested by the infant. Breast milk contains amylase that is 40 to 60 times more active than that of cow's milk (Lo, 1997). The lactose in milk provides galactose, which is necessary for brain cell formation.

One source of carbohydrate an infant must not be given is honey (see Clinical Application 12–1).

FAT An infant needs 30 to 55 percent of kilocalories from fat as a concentrated source of energy because of the small capacity of the infantile stomach. The developing nervous system also requires fat because approximately 60 percent of the structural material of the brain consists of lipids, mainly arachidonic and docosahexaenoic (very-long-chain) fatty acids (Phylactos, et al., 1994). These latter two fatty acids are essential for retinal and neural development (Lo, 1997). They are found in red cell membranes and human milk, but not in cow's milk (Schanler, 1997). Since breast milk contains the necessary lipase to begin digestion for the infant, about 95 to 98 percent of the fat in human milk is

---

CLINICAL APPLICATION 12–1

Honey is a Danger to Infants

No honey should be given to an infant until after the first birthday because it frequently contains organisms that the infant cannot fight off. After the age of one, the infant's intestinal flora have matured sufficiently to prevent colonization by the botulism spores (David, 1996).

Bees may contaminate honey with botulism spores acquired from plants or the soil. Processing the honey does not destroy these spores. If ingested by the infant, the spores become active in its intestinal tract and produce a toxin. This is a serious, even potentially fatal, situation because the toxin affects the nervous system.

Botulism spores occur in many places. Honey is not the only source. Other foods and even dust contain botulism spores. In fact, in only 20 percent of the reported cases of infant botulism had the infant been fed honey, but feeding the infant honey increases the risk 8 times (David, 1996).

Box 12–1 Research Links Cognitive Abilities to Breast-Feeding

Preterm breast-fed infants showed significantly higher IQ scores at age 8 than formula-fed infants even after controlling for social class and education (Lucas, et al., 1992).   One possible explanation is that until recently infant formula did not contain arachidonic and docosahexaenoic (DHA) fatty acids, the main components of brain tissue (Phylactos, et al., 1994). Supplementing formula for preterm infants with DHA suggested a link with improved visual acuity and cognitive ability (Carlson, et al., 1994).

Long-term follow-up also showed the importance of breast-feeding to cognitive development. Adolescents who as full-term infants were breast-fed longer than 12 weeks tested significantly better in verbal and reasoning IQ than those breast-fed less than 12 weeks (Greene, et al., 1995). Duration of breast-feeding was a significant predictor of later cognitive or educational outcomes even after adjusting for maternal age and education, family socioeconomic status, family income, living standards, infant birth weight, birth order, and gender (Horwood and Fergusson, 1998).

---

absorbed. Box 12–1 identifies research linking cognitive development to breast-feeding.

EVALUATION The best indicator of adequate kilocaloric intake is a normal growth rate according to standard growth charts. Measurements should be made every 3 months; they can be graphed on growth charts such as those that appear in Appendix D.

Vitamins

The RDA tables (see Appendices F and H) specify vitamin intake for infants aged 0 to 6 months and 6 to 12 months. Infants need all the vitamins that other humans need, but in different amounts.

Cow's milk contains nine times the vitamin B_{12} of breast milk from Caucasian women consuming a mixed diet. Research indicated that vegan women produced milk containing only one-fourth to one-third as much vitamin B_{12} as women on a mixed diet (Weir and Scott, 1999). Even cow's milk is not a good source of the vitamin compared with meat. Studies have described severe vitamin B_{12} deficiencies with grave neurological deterioration in 4- to 8-month-old infants. Half the breast-feeding mothers were vegetarians, but half were not (Graham, Arvela, and Wise, 1992).

Human breast milk contains more vitamin C, but less vitamin D, than cow's milk. The cholesterol in breast milk functions as a precursor of vitamin D that is produced in the skin, a benefit to infants who receive some exposure to sunlight. Because of other hazards of exposure to sun, however, a vitamin D supplement may be a wiser choice. Parents should consult their primary health-care providers for advice.

In adults, intestinal bacteria produce vitamin K to meet an individual's needs. Until the infant's intestine becomes colonized with *Escherichia coli*, he or she is at risk for bleeding problems. In this regard, formula-fed infants have an advantage over breast-fed babies, because breast milk supports proliferation of lactobacilli rather than *E. coli* (Lo, 1997). This fact contributes to the infant morbidity and mortality caused by vitamin K deficiency seen worldwide in breast-fed infants (Olson, 1999). The usual method of prevention of hemorrhagic disorders is an intramuscular dose of vitamin K within 1 hour after birth (Zipursky, 1999).

Special situations that warrant vitamin supplementation are discussed later in this chapter.

Minerals

Infants need the same minerals as other human beings. Breast milk contains only one-third the sodium, potassium, and chloride, and one-eighth the phosphorus of cow's milk, an amount that accommodates the limited function of the infant's kidneys. Breast milk also contains less iron than cow's milk, but the infant absorbs 49 percent of it compared with 10 percent from cow's milk. Several factors in breast milk promote iron absorption: less protein and phosphorus, more lactose and ascorbate (Lo, 1997).

Breast milk contains about one-sixth to one-quarter of the calcium of cow's milk. The infant is able to absorb 67 percent of the calcium in breast milk, compared with 25 percent of the calcium in cow's milk, possibly because the high phosphorus content of cow's milk produces decreased absorption and increased excretion of calcium (Lo, 1997). The bioavailability of zinc in breast milk is 60 percent, compared with 43 to 50 percent in cow's milk and 27 to 32 percent in infant formulas (Lo, 1997).

These differences in mineral content affect the osmolality of the milk. See Clinical Application 12–2 for additional information on the extra minerals' effect on the workload of the kidneys. The data show why unmodified cow's milk is inappropriate for young infants.

Fluoride should not be administered to infants until after 6 months of age. Even then, supplementation is necessary only if the water supply is severely deficient (less than 0.3 ppm), whether the infant is breast-fed or formula-fed (American Academy of Pediatrics, 1997).

Water

The infant's body is about 75 percent water. By the age of 1, the body has developed so it has the adult proportion of about 60 percent water. The daily turnover of water in the infant is approximately 15 percent of body weight.

Breast milk contains more water than cow's milk. Even in desert climates, an infant can be adequately hydrated on breast milk alone. An infant will regulate its intake of formula to obtain sufficient energy. If the formula is dilute, the baby will take more of it; if concentrated, less. This self-regulating mechanism is not perfect, however, since the infant may consume excess formula to quench its thirst.

The Breast-Fed Infant

Breast-feeding is known to be a superior source of nutrition for the infant yet breast-feeding rates in the United States are only 50 and 60 percent. Between 1984 and 1989 the proportion of newborn infants initially breast-fed declined from 60 to 52 percent, but then reverted to 60 percent in 1995. By 6 months of age 22 percent of all infants were still receiving some breast milk, compared with 24 percent in 1984 and 18 percent in 1995 (Freed, 1993; Ryan, 1997).

CLINICAL APPLICATION 12–2

Renal Solute Loads

When selecting a formula it is important to distinguish two measures of osmotic pressure. One is the osmotic pressure the formula presents to the gut. The other examines what remains to be excreted by the kidney after digestion, absorption, and metabolism have taken place. These leftovers are excess electrolytes and by-products of protein metabolism. The osmotic pressure of these leftovers presented to the kidney for disposal is called the renal solute load. It varies considerably from one formula to another. When dealing with an infant's immature digestive and urinary systems, selecting an appropriate formula may be crucial to health. Below is a comparison of several infant feedings with the intestinal osmolality and the renal solute load listed. Because infant formulas are often changed in response to new scientific information, the following chart is offered as an example only. The agency's dietitian or pharmacist should be consulted for the latest information. As always, the standard of comparison is human breast milk. Unmodified cow's milk would place the greatest burden on the infant's immature renal system.

Milk Formula	Intestinal Osmolality (mOsm/kg)	Renal Solute Load (mOsm/L)
Human breast milk	300	101
Milk-based Formulas		
Enfamil	300	132*
Similac	290	105
Milk-based Reduced Electrolyte		
SMA	300	128
Similac 60/40	260	96
Soy-based Formula		
Isomil	250	122
Nursoy	296	172
3.3 percent cow's milk	275	275

Sources: Klish and Montandon, 1987; Thorp, Pierce, and Deedwanea, 1987; and *Enfamil, 1999.

In Scandinavia, the belief that it is unethical to feed infants synthetic formulas necessitates a system of human milk banks (Sturman and Chesney, 1995). One of the goals of Healthy People 2010 is to increase to 75 percent the proportion of mothers who breast-feed in the early postpartum period, to 50 percent those who breast-feed until the infants are 6 months old, and to 25 percent of mothers who breast-feed until the infants are 1 year old (U.S. Department of Health and Human Services, 2000).

Practices conducive to breast-feeding and lactation include initiation of breast-feeding in the delivery or birthing room, frequent feedings, unlimited suckling time, and no supplementation (Janken et al., 1999.) Breast-feeding immediately after delivery is contraindicated if the mother is heavily medicated or if the newborn has a gestational age of less than 36 weeks or an **Apgar score** of less than 6 (Bear and Tigges, 1993.) Pediatricians are encouraged to work actively to deter hospital practices that discourage breast-feeding such as postpartum separation of mother and baby and distribution of formula discharge packs (American Academy of Pediatrics, 1997).

The need for increased follow-up by health-care providers was shown in a study in Cincinnati. Mothers who called someone about breast-feeding problems turned to family or friends 34.7 percent of the time, to the lactation consultant 16.5 percent, to the pediatrician 8.8 percent, to the obstetrician or midwife 8.2 percent, to a breast-feeding support group 5.9 percent, and to the birth hospital 2.5 percent of the time (Kuan et al., 1999). Of the 522 women in that study, 29 percent had stopped breast-feeding by 8 weeks postpartum.

The American Academy of Pediatrics recommends that breast-feeding continue for at least 12 months and that supplements (water, glucose water, or formula) and pacifiers be avoided or, if used at all, only after breast-feeding is well established (1997). Among mothers planning postpartum employment, the use of supplementary bottle feeding in the hospital was significantly related to a shorter period of breast-feeding, as was receipt of formula samples by mail (Chezem et al., 1998). To keep the infant interested in breast-feeding, nurses in Toronto and Kansas City have learned to cup-feed infants who temporarily could not be put to breast. This is a procedure in common use in Africa (Mulford, 1995). As with many child-care procedures, cup-feeding an infant should not be attempted casually or without adequate training. Clinical Application 12–3 discusses the storage of human milk.

Composition of Breast Milk

All breast milk is not alike; its composition adjusts to the infant's needs during the weeks an infant is nursing, even during the course of a single feeding. Breast milk varies from mother to mother and even in one mother with the time of day. It also varies with the lactation cycle as discussed below.

COLOSTRUM The milk secreted for the first 2 to 4 days after the birth of the baby is called *colostrum*. It is a thin, yellow, cloudy fluid. Colostrum is high in proteins such as immunoglobulins, in fat-soluble vitamins, in minerals, and is low in fat.

CLINICAL APPLICATION 12–3

Storage of Human Milk

Care must be taken when breast milk is expressed and stored for later feeding. Contamination by skin bacteria is a major problem. If breast milk is to be stored for more than 48 hours, it should be frozen or autoclaved. Refrigeration, freezing, and autoclaving all decrease the milk's immune factors such as IgA and may destroy lipases. One small study, however, showed IgA concentration to be unaffected by refrigerating samples for 72 hours (Jocson, Mason, and Schanler, 1997). Nutrients such as vitamin A, nitrogen, calcium, phosphorus, sodium, zinc, iron, and copper are not markedly affected. Heat treatment may negatively affect several vitamins or their binding proteins (Lo, 1997).

Because transmission of HIV to infants by breast milk has been documented, the American Academy of Pediatrics recommended that milk banks screen donors for HIV infection and predisposing risk factors and pasteurize all specimens. In addition, workers exposed to frequent or prolonged exposure to breast milk should wear gloves (American Academy of Pediatrics, 1995).

TRANSITIONAL MILK Transitional milk follows colostrum and continues through the second week after delivery. Transitional milk contains lactose, fat, and water-soluble vitamins at the level of mature milk. It is produced in larger quantities than is colostrum.

MATURE MILK As breast-feeding becomes established, the mother produces mature milk, which varies in composition. At 3 months, for instance, immunoglobulins make up a smaller portion of the proteins than when the baby is younger.

During a feeding, the constituents of the milk change. The milk contains more fat at the end of a feeding than in the beginning. Mature breast milk generally is 2 percent fat at the beginning of a feeding and up to 7 percent at the end (Borowitz, 1988). Fat provides satiety, or a feeling of fullness or satisfaction. If the infant received high-fat milk at the beginning of a feeding, it might become contented and stop nursing. The variation in content also offers the infant a variety of taste experiences. Despite the fact that some of their milk contains 7 percent fat, breast-fed infants at 1 year have serum cholesterol levels equal to those of formula-fed infants.

Effects of exercising by the mother on the composition of breast milk have been investigated. A case was reported of a baby nursing as usual and then crying apparently from abdominal pain after breast-feeding following his mother's five-mile run. This occurred three times. Testing the breast milk for lactic acid before and after running revealed no differences. The mother was a competitive runner who solved the dilemma by pumping her breasts and discarding the milk after running and feeding the baby formula for this feeding only (Duffy, 1997).

Another study showed lactic acid levels in breast milk were significantly elevated for 90 minutes after strenuous exercise (Carey, Quinn, and Goodwin, 1997) but not after moderate intensity exercise (Carey, Quinn, and Goodwin, 1997; Quinn and Carey, 1999). Breast milk contained significantly lower amounts of IgA for 10 to 30 minutes after exhaustive exercise but recovered in 1 hour (Gregory et al., 1997), but concentrations of calcium, phosphorus, magnesium, potassium, and sodium were not altered by maximal exercise (Fly, Uhlin, and Wallace, 1998).

Unique Advantages of Breast-Feeding

Two well-documented advantages to breast-feeding have not been duplicated by formulas. The first is the protection against disease that a mother's milk provides. The second is a lowered risk of allergies in the infant. Even a few weeks of breast-feeding benefits the infant. Additional advantages beginning to be reported are a negative association with obesity and an enhancement of performance on IQ tests (see Box 12–1).

PROTECTION AGAINST DISEASE Breast-fed infants have been shown to be sick less frequently than formula-fed babies. This benefit is most important in developing countries where sanitation, hygiene, and immunization are major public health issues. Gastrointestinal infections are the leading cause of infant mortality worldwide. In fact, fluid and electrolyte imbalances caused by infection kill more children than any other disease or disaster. Even in the United States in 1993 and 1994, infants who received formula only showed an 80 percent increase in risk of diarrhea and a 70 percent increase in risk of ear infection compared with infants who were breast-fed exclusively (Scariati, Grummer-Strawn, and Fein, 1997).

Breast milk, through bifidus growth factors, promotes a particular kind of bacteria, *Lactobacillus bifidus*, in the baby's intestine rather than *E. coli*. Although the normal adult intestine harbors *E. coli*, it can cause diarrhea in children. The *L. bifidus* produces acids that retard the growth of organisms such as staphylococci, shigella, protozoa, and yeast, which can cause disease. Another component of breast milk, lactoferrin, an iron-binding protein, competes with any bacteria for iron and kills some organisms such as *Streptococcus mutans* and *Vibrio cholerae* (Goldman, Goldblum, and Schmalstieg, 1997).

Among the infection-fighting agents in breast milk are leukocytes or white blood cells (WBCs). The highest concentration of WBCs in human milk occurs in the first few days of lactation, 1 to 3 million per milliliter. About 35 to 55 percent of the WBCs are macrophages that kill microorganisms (Goldman, Goldblum, and Schmalstieg, 1997).

Much remains to be learned about the protective properties of human milk. Because certain immune factors appear in infants in amounts that could not be merely transferred through breast milk, it is thought that breast-feeding stimulates the activity of the infant's own immune system. Breast-feeding primes the infant to produce higher blood levels of interferon-a in response to respiratory syncytial virus infection (Goldman, Goldblum, and Schmalstieg, 1997).

Breast milk also contains the protein immunoglobulin A (IgA), an antibody against viruses and bacteria. Many proteins, if taken orally, would be digested. IgA, however, is resistant to acidity and enzymes that break down protein, so it is effectively transferred to the infant in the mother's milk. Moreover, IgA is supplied in the greatest amount during the first 3 months of lactation, when an infant's immune system is the weakest. Many of the immunologic components of human milk decline in concentration as the infant matures, presumably better able to take over his or her own defenses against infection (Goldman, Goldblum, and Schmalstieg, 1997).

Attempts to replicate human milk include addition of nucleotides to formula to assist the infant's immune response. Nucleotides are the structural units of nucleic acids, such as DNA and RNA. Such supplementation of formula has led to higher concentrations of some antibodies and a significant decrease in the incidence of diarrhea, an advantage conferred by unknown mechanisms (Pickering et al., 1998).

PREVENTION OF ALLERGIES The young infant's gastrointestinal tract can permit the passage of whole proteins into the bloodstream. These proteins can stimulate an allergic response in susceptible infants. Contrary to earlier opinion, infants can be allergic to their own mother's milk. The successful treatment of infant allergy by having the mother avoid cow's milk protein and several other items suggests that food allergy during breast-feeding may be due to multiple foods (de Boissieu, Matarazzo, and Dupont, 1997).

Breast-fed infants whose mothers avoided dairy products, eggs, fish, peanuts, and soybeans had fewer and milder cases of eczema than breast-fed infants of mothers consuming unrestricted diets (Chandra, Puri, and Hamed, 1989). Some improvement of infant eczema followed the implementation of a strict diet for the mother, but significant improvement followed discontinuing breast-feeding (Isolauri et al., 1999).

Even diet during pregnancy seems to influence the development of allergy. Pregnant women who consumed peanuts more often than once a week were more likely to have a peanut-allergic child than mothers who consumed peanuts less frequently. In this study, exclusive breast-feeding did not prevent peanut sensitization (Frank et al., 1999). Dietary modification before week 22 of the pregnancy and throughout lactation has been recommended to prevent allergies in the infant born to a family with a history of allergies (Hampton, 1999).

Other researchers are less certain of the value of dietary modification during lactation in preventing allergy in infants. One reason is described as the multifactorial nature of **atopic** disease (Vandenplas, 1997). Many factors contribute to the development of allergies. Other investigators found no relation between a maternal avoidance diet (in which eggs, cow's milk, and fish were avoided) during the first 3 months of lactation and allergy in the children at 10 years of age (Hattevig, Sigurs, and Kjellman, 1999).

Either gross or occult gastrointestinal bleeding may result from cow's milk allergy (Lo, 1997). Once an infant becomes allergic to cow's milk, the risk of other allergies developing increases. Fortunately, most infants outgrow food allergies by age 2. Exclusive breast-feeding for more than 1 month after birth has offered significant prevention of food allergies to children at 3 years of age and of respiratory allergies at 17 years of age, whereas 6 months of breast-feeding was required to prevent eczema until age 3 (Saarinen, and Kajosaari, 1995).

NEGATIVE ASSOCIATION WITH OBESITY In a population study of Bavarian 5- and 6-year-old children, the prevalence of obesity in children who had never been breast-fed was 4.5 percent compared with 2.8 percent in breast-fed children. These differences were unrelated to social class or lifestyle (von Kries et al., 1999).

Specific Genetic Abnormalities and Breast-Feeding

The infant's lack of an enzyme to metabolize galactose is an absolute contraindication to breast-feeding. This condition of **galactosemia** is inherited as an autosomal recessive trait and occurs once in every 40,000 to 50,000 live births. The infant is fed a substitute formula containing no lactose or galactose.

The mother of an infant with phenylketonuria (discussed in Clinical Application 5–4) often chooses to feed the child only the special formula. Breast-feeding the baby requires both limited amounts of breast milk and the special formula. To determine the amount of breast milk the child may consume to keep its blood levels within the therapeutic limits requires constant monitoring and consultations, but it has been done successfully. Every state has at least one medical center for treating metabolic defects. The maternal and child health division of the state health department can assist with locating such a facility (Duncan and Elder, 1997).

The Formula-Fed Infant

As good as it is, exclusive breast-feeding is not possible for all mothers. Infants can be well nourished with commercial formulas, which are made to nearly duplicate human milk.

The processing of infant formulas in the United States has been regulated by law since 1980. These products have been so well received that

CLINICAL APPLICATION 12–4

Soy Protein Formulas

The isolated soy protein formulas being marketed today are all free of cow's milk protein and lactose and are iron-fortified. Prospective studies of high-risk infants suggest that soy protein-based formula is no better than cow's milk formula in preventing allergies. Nor have controlled trials shown soy protein-based formulas to be better than cow's milk formulas for treating colic. A side effect of the manufacturing process is an aluminum content of 600 to 1300 ng/mL compared to the 4 to 65 ng/mL of human milk. The high aluminum content, for which no function is known in humans, may contribute to the reduced skeletal mineralization seen in preterm infants.

The American Academy of Pediatrics recommended the following appropriate uses for soy protein-based formulas:

- For term infants whose nutritional needs are not being met from breast milk or cow's milk formulas

- For infants with galactosemia and hereditary lactase deficiency

- For term infants for whom the parents desire a vegetarian diet

- For documented cases of lactose intolerance following acute gastroenteritis

- For infants with documented IgE-mediated allergy to cow's milk protein

In contrast, the Academy *does not* recommend soy protein-based formula under the following circumstances:

- For routine treatment of colic

- For healthy or high-risk infants to prevent atopic disease

- For infants with documented cow's milk protein-induced enteropathy or enterocolitis because such infants are often sensitive to soy protein

- For preterm infants weighing <1800 grams (4 lbs)

(Summarized from American Academy of Pediatrics, 1998b).

---

95 percent of formula-fed infants receive commercial products rather than a homemade formula. Commercial formulas for full-term infants must contain 20 kilocalories per ounce. The formula osmolality may be no more than 400 milliosmoles per kilogram. Commercial formulas are designed to imitate human breast milk but differ from it in protein, fat, and mineral content.

Formulas contain more protein than breast milk. The cow's milk proteins do not contain the optimal amino acids for human infants, so enough protein is included in the formula to provide a sufficient distribution of amino acids.

The saturated fats of cow's milk are poorly digested by the infant. In infant formulas, the saturated fats are removed and replaced by vegetable oils.

Formulas are treated to lower the sodium content of cow's milk, but most formulas nonetheless contain more sodium than breast milk, which has 7 milliequivalents per liter. Formulas can be purchased with or without added iron, but the American Academy of Pediatrics strongly advo-

cates iron-fortified formulas, and recommends that the manufacture of infant formulas containing less than 4 milligrams of iron per liter be discontinued (American Academy of Pediatrics, 1999).

Formula Preparations

Commercial formulas come in three forms: powder (to mix with water), liquid concentrate, and ready-to-feed. Less waste occurs with the powdered formula. A smaller amount can be mixed for the young infant. Opened cans of liquid formula may be stored covered in the refrigerator but must be used within 48 hours. Prepared bottles of formula should be discarded once they have been out of the refrigerator for 1 hour or have been offered to the infant.

In Western countries with safe drinking-water supplies, the use of clean rather than sterile technique often is sufficient. Parents will receive specific instructions from their health-care providers. Nevertheless, separate utensils should be kept for formula preparation. Parents should be cautioned that equipment cannot be adequately sanitized in a microwave oven. Extreme caution is required if a microwave oven is used for infant foods because heat may be unevenly distributed and continues to build up in the food even after it is removed from the oven.

The importance of feeding the correct-strength formula must be impressed upon the parents. Either too concentrated or too dilute a formula can cause severe electrolyte imbalances. Some cases have been fatal.

Feeding Techniques

Contrary to the rigid feeding practices of some years ago, the current practice is to feed the infant when it is hungry. Most of the time the infant evolves a schedule whereby it demands a feeding approximately every 4 hours. By the age of 2 to 3 months, the baby probably will have eliminated one feeding so the schedule is five times a day. By 6 months, most infants are feeding four times a day.

The baby is positioned in the crook of the arm almost as if breast-feeding. The parent's or caregiver's touch is important to the infant's development. The nipple hole should be large enough for milk to drip out on its own, without the parent shaking the bottle. The bottle should be tipped so that the nipple is kept full of milk at all times to prevent the infant from swallowing air while feeding. "Propping" an infant with a bottle is never acceptable because (1) choking is a real hazard and (2) the infant needs to be held to develop a closeness with the parent or caregiver.

The daily formula intake for an infant should be 1.5 to 2 ounces per pound of body weight. At this rate, a 7-pound baby would take 10.5 to 14 ounces a day. An infant of this size would be feeding six times a day, so it would take 1.75 to 2.3 ounces per feeding. A 14-pound baby would be taking 21 to 28 ounces in four feedings of 5.25 to 7 ounces. A single feeding should never exceed 8 ounces.

Ongoing observation of the infant's urinary output is used to confirm the adequacy of intake. The infant's urine should be light yellow and voided several times per day. Major changes in output merit medical attention.

Special Formulas

Manufacturers have devised formulas for special needs. Infants who are allergic to cow's milk, those with galactosemia or lactose intolerance, and those with fat-absorption problems all need special formulas. See Clinical Application 12–4 for a brief description of such formulas, which are often

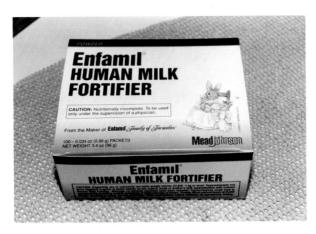

Figure 12–1:
Human Milk Fortifier, when added to human milk, increases the amount of protein, carbohydrates, and selected vitamins and minerals available to meet the needs of rapidly growing low-birth-weight infants.

soy-based. Unfortunately, soy proteins may also cause allergies in as many as 35 percent of infants allergic to cow's milk (Moon and Kleinman, 1995). Studies found that soymilk formula did not protect high-risk infants from eczema (Chandra, Puri, and Hamed, 1989) or from atopic disease and food allergy (Chandra, 1997). Goat's milk is not an acceptable option for an infant allergic to cow's milk. Bellioni-Businco et al. (1999), recommended a warning to that effect be placed on goat's milk formulas.

Other special formulas can be prescribed for infants with multiple allergies. One technique is to break down whole proteins into smaller components that may not stimulate an allergic response. Consumption of a whey hydrolysate formula by mothers (beginning in late pregnancy and continuing for 6 months postpartum) and their infants was determined to help prevent allergy development in 4-month-old infants (Fukushima et al., 1997). An amino acid formula improved the weight gain and decreased symptoms in infants allergic to extensively hydrolyzed cow milk protein formulas (de Boissieu, Matarazzo, and Dupont, 1997). Extensively hydrolyzed formula, along with abstinence from cow's milk until 9 months of age and of egg and fish until 12 months of age, prevented development of allergy during the first 18 months of life, whereas partially hydrolyzed formula did not (Oldacus et al., 1997).

The full-term infant's digestive, nervous, and urinary systems are immature—even a greater issue for premature infants. Clinical Application 12–5 summarizes some of the nutritional problems and appropriate interventions used for premature infants.

Hazards of Formula-Feeding

On a few occasions, improperly manufactured formulas have been responsible for vitamin and mineral deficiencies in infants. This is an unacceptable, but fortunately rare, occurrence. A more common hazard, and one an individual nurse can monitor, is the improper preparation and use of formulas by the parent. Formulas can be (1) the wrong dilution, (2) prepared with contaminated water, or (3) kept at feeding temperature too long. Body temperature is "just right" for bacteria to multiply, whether in the body or in a formula bottle.

Choice of Breast or Bottle

In the United States, infants can be well nourished whether breast- or formula-fed. To raise a child successfully takes more than simply supplying the correct ratio of nutrients. Mothers should not be coerced into breast-feeding because breast-feeding meets the physician or nurse's needs; their informed decision should be respected and supported.

Semisolid Foods

No proof exists of the folk wisdom that the early feeding of solid food to infants promotes their sleeping through the night. At 3 months, 75 percent of infants sleep all night, regardless of diet.

If solid foods are introduced too early, the infant may develop allergies because of the permeability of the intestine. Infants given four or more types of solid food before 4 months of age had 2.35 times the risk of childhood eczema as infants not so fed. The number of foods, not specific foods, increased the risk (Fergusson, Horwood, and Shannon, 1990). Additionally, solid foods, especially high-protein items, add to the renal solute load (Wharton, 1997). Most physicians recommend starting semisolid foods at about 4 to 6 months of age.

The infant should achieve voluntary control of swallowing at about 3 to 4 months. Before being offered solid food, the infant should be able to control his or her head and trunk. With this ability the baby can turn away when satisfied. By this time the infant has doubled its birth weight, is drinking 8 ounces of formula or a similar estimated amount of breast milk, and yet becomes hungry in less than 4 hours.

In introducing solid food it is important to follow the infant's lead. To avoid later feeding problems, solid foods should be started when the baby is interested. Babies ready for solid food are hungry and not fussy about tastes (Figure 12–2). Children learn from adults; parents should avoid showing distaste for particular foods.

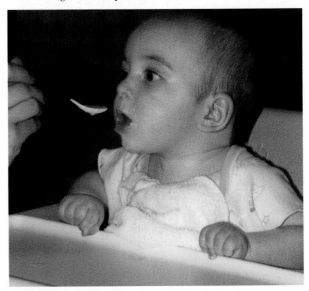

Figure 12–2:
This 5-month-old baby is experiencing semisolid food for the first time. His readiness is clear. Notice how eager he is, how focused on the spoon.

CLINICAL APPLICATION 12–5

Premature Infants

Premature infants are born before 37 weeks' gestation. A low-birth-weight (LBW) infant weighs less than 2500 g (5.5 lb) at birth. A very low-birth-weight (VLBW) infant has been defined as weighing less than 1500 g (3.3 lb) (Cheung, Peliowski, and Robertson, 1998; Rogowski, 1998) and an extremely low birth weight (ELBW) infant as weighing less than 1000 g (2.2 lb) (Piecuch et al., 1997; Yaseen, 1996). An infant can be both premature and LBW or VLBW.

Not all premature infants weigh less than 2500 g. Nor are all LBW infants premature, but birth weight is the most potent single predictor of an infant's future health status. LBW infants are 20 times more likely to die as normal-weight infants. Although LBW infants make up just 7 percent of the births in the United States, they comprise almost 66 percent of deaths in the first year of life. There is a substantial association between intellectual function and LBW, even greater with VLBW.

Compared with full-term infants, premature infants have an even larger proportion of their bodies as water. The antidiuretic hormone and aldosterone mechanisms develop in the last weeks of gestation so VLBW infants have virtually no response to these hormones designed to conserve water (Yaseen, 1996). They have less protein and fat than babies born at term. Their bones are poorly calcified and their muscles are poorly developed. There is almost no glycogen. The sucking reflex is not developed prior to the 32nd or 34th week of gestation. As a result, premature infants often require tube feeding through the gastrointestinal tract or intravenous feeding.

Tube feeding will conserve energy even in an infant who is able to suck. Tube feedings at body temperature (37°C, 98.6°F) produced fewer gastric residuals than formula administered at room temperature (24°C, 75.2°F) or at a cool temperature (10°C, 50°F). No difference was noted between the last two (Gonzales et al., 1995). Esophageal peristalsis is absent and the esophageal sphincter is weak, leading to increased danger of aspiration. The liver is immature in enzyme systems and in iron stores.

Fat digestion is limited by decreased activity of pancreatic lipase. Fat absorption is limited by a deficiency of bile salts. Despite this, preterm infants fed formula supplemented with the omega-3 fatty acid docosahexaenoic acid (DHA) showed improved visual acuity in the first half of infancy in one trial and improved performance on tests of mental development in another trial (Carlson et al., 1994). In a trial of term infants, those fed formula supplemented with DHA and or DHA and arachidonic acid (AA) showed visual acuity development equal to the breast-fed infants used as the "gold standard" group (Birch et al., 1998). Those two fatty acids are permitted in infant formula in 60 countries, but as of early 2000, not in the United States.

Protein digestion and absorption functions are relatively intact. Carbohydrate absorption also is intact, but digestion is limited by decreased pancreatic and salivary amylase activity and delayed development of lactase. Of particular concern in premature infants with immature lungs, is the proportion of carbohydrate and fat in the feedings. Carbohydrate metabolism produces more carbon dioxide than fat metabolism does. Consequently, constant monitoring and adjusting of intake may be necessary.

Special formulas for premature infants are designed to provide for the infant's growth needs despite the immature digestive system. Glucose polymers and medium-chain triglycerides are used to construct a formula that will take advantage of the infant's digestive capabilities. The premature infant has high energy needs. If given 120 kcal/kg of body weight enterally, the infant will grow at about the same rate as if still in the uterus. Special growth grids for premature infants are available. These are based on conceptual age or the expected due date. Premature infants should have their chronological age corrected by gestational age until age 18 months for head circumference, 24 months for weight, and 40 months for length (Duggan, 1997).

Vitamin supplements are needed because the infant's intake is so small. Maximal transfer of vitamin E across the placenta occurs just before full-term delivery, but assessment of its status clinically is problematic (vanZoeren-Grobben et al., 1998). Vitamin E stabilizes red blood cell membranes. If deficient, the infant suffers from hemolytic anemia. Vitamin E also delays the onset of retinopathy in infants receiving oxygen (Bohles, 1997). Vitamin A is paramount for fetal lung development because retinoic acid selectively regulates surfactant proteins and riboflavin deficiency has been caused by phototherapy for hyperbilirubinemia of newborns (Bohles, 1997). Once adequate intakes of fortified human milk or preterm formulas are taken by the premature infant, vitamin supplementation may be discontinued until weaning to regular formula (Schanler, 1997).

Premature infants may need to have their diets supplemented with the minerals calcium, phosphorus, and sodium. Rickets of prematurity can occur in the second postnatal month due not to the lack of vitamin D but to the lack of calcium and phosphorus. Prematurity is associated with increased dental caries, but fluoride intake recommendations have been established only for full-term infants (Zlotkin, Atkinson, and Lockitch, 1995). Sodium needs will increase as the infant grows. Monitoring serum and urine sodium levels will alert the physician to the infant's changing needs.

Not all mothers of premature infants can begin lactation. The milk of those who do differs significantly from the milk of mothers who deliver at term: the breast milk of the mother of a premature baby has more protein, sodium, and host defense factors but insufficient calcium, phosphorus, and magnesium. The incidence of any infection and sepsis/meningitis are significantly reduced in human milk-fed VLBW infants compared with exclusively formula-fed VLBW infants (Hylander, Strobino, and Dhanireddy, 1998). In one case, a mother did not decide to breast-feed her premature infant until it was 2 days old, but with an intensive day and night program of expressing her milk using much assistance and support from the staff, lactation was established (Turnbull, 1999).

To better meet the premature infant's needs, human milk fortifiers have been developed. Enfamil Human Milk Fortifier is a powdered supplement that can be added to human milk for premature infants older than 2 weeks who are rapidly growing (Mead Johnson, 1999). The fortifier adds protein, carbohydrate, vitamins, and minerals to the breast milk, and the mother's antibodies are still available to the baby. See Figure 12–1. A liquid human milk fortifier, Similac Natural Care, is produced by Ross Products Division of Abbott Laboratories (Anderson and Pittard, 1997).

When infants are fed by stomach tube, the milk remaining in the stomach from the previous feeding is drawn out and measured. This is called a gastric residual. Depending upon the amount of the gastric residual, the scheduled feeding may be withheld to allow the stomach to empty. In a study of 108 infants fed either fortified human milk or preterm formula, those receiving the human milk had fewer gastric residuals for which feedings were withheld, fewer major complications, and were discharged approximately 2 weeks earlier that those fed the preterm formula. The authors recommended that increased use of fortified human milk feeding should be endorsed in all neonatal nurseries (Schanler, Shulman, and Lau, 1999).

Waiting too long to introduce solid foods may delay the infant's acquiring the skill to manipulate the tongue appropriately. Some infants who have not started spoon-feeding by 6 months of age show considerable delay in adapting from the milking action of the mouth to the chewing and tongue-rolling action needed to handle solid foods (Wharton, 1997).

How to Feed

New foods should be introduced one at a time, so if a problem develops, it can be readily identified. A food should be tried for 3 to 5 days before the infant is permitted to reject it. Only a taste or two is sufficient for the first try. Even if the baby takes the food eagerly, small amounts should be given to keep a sufficient appetite for milk.

The parent should heat a small amount to serve the infant. Food that has been heated and not consumed should be discarded because of possible contamination with salivary enzymes and bacteria. Food that has been opened but not heated can be stored in the covered jar in the refrigerator if it will be used in 2 to 3 days. A commonly used schedule for introducing new foods appears in Table 12–2. The baby's physician may modify it to meet individual needs. Care must be taken to offer only food that the infant can chew and swallow safely (Clinical Application 12–6).

This is a critical time in the infant's life. Eating adult foods is a skill that the babies must learn, but their culture affects the food choices they will be offered. They may have had a preview of various flavors in utero or through breast milk. Amniotic fluid has been shown to acquire a garlic odor after capsules containing its essential oil were ingested by pregnant women (Mennella, Johnson, and Beauchamp, 1995). The mother's diet influences the taste of her breast milk as well as the reaction of the infant to particular foods (discussed under "Colic"). Infants offered a vegetable 10 times significantly increased their intakes of the vegetable, but those fed breast milk had a greater intake of the vegetable than did formula-fed infants (Sullivan and Birch, 1994).

Weaning the Infant

Teaching the infant to use a cup is a gradual process. Often the baby will show an interest in the cup at 4 to 6 months. For these early experiments water can be offered. For many of the reasons already discussed, the American Academy of Pediatrics recommends breast-feeding for at least 12 months (1997). If the mother decides to wean the child before then,

---

CLINICAL APPLICATION 12–6

Avoiding Choking Accidents

Each year several hundred infants are asphyxiated by food. This is a hazard for older children as well. On average, one death every 5 days is reported in children from infancy to 9 years of age.

Hot dogs, or frankfurters, are involved most often. Hot dogs, apples, cookies, and biscuits cause choking most often in infants. Peanuts and grapes are the most dangerous for 2-year-old children, while 3-year-olds still face a risk from hot dogs.

Other foods that are often implicated in choking accidents are listed below. Because there are many other foods the child can eat safely, the prudent course is to avoid all of the foods listed. If a choking incident occurs, any caregiver needs to be able to administer cardiopulmonary resuscitation (CPR) should it become necessary. Training in CPR should be sought by all parents or parents-to-be. Small children should always be supervised while they are eating.

Hard Foods	Stringy Foods	Sticky Foods	Plug shaped Foods
Apples	Beans	Bread	Grapes
Carrots	Celery	Chewing gum	Hot dogs
Cookies		Peanut butter	
Corn			
Hard candy			
Nuts			
Peanuts			
Popcorn			
Raisins			
Raw vegetables			
Seedy items (e.g., watermelon)			

---

the replacement for breast milk should be formula, not unmodified cow's milk. The bottle-fed infant may not be ready to give up the bottle until 12 to 14 months of age. If bedtime bottles have not been used, weaning will proceed more rapidly. It is best to substitute the cup for the bottle for one feeding period at a time. Use the new schedule for 5 days or so, and then substitute the new method for a second feeding. Allowing the infant to set the pace will make the task easier.

Table 12–2 Suggested Schedule for Infant Foods

Age of Infant	Food	Ratinale/Precautions
4 months	Infant cereal mixed with formula	Because of risk of allergies, rice offered first; wheat after age 12 months. Read labels: some mixed infant cereals contain wheat.
5 to 6 months	Strained vegetables	Less sweet than fruits; less likely to be rejected if offered before fruit.
6 to 7 months	Strained fruits	Will be well accepted; humans have strong preference for sweets.
6 to 8 months	Finger foods (bananas, crackers)	Encourages self-feeding. Different textures may aid speech development.
7 to 8 months	Strained meats	Offer variety. See Clinical Application 12–6)
10 months	Strained or mashed egg yolk	Start with 1/2 tsp. Due to possible allergy, delay egg white till 1 year old.
1 0 months	Bite-sized cooked foods	Select appropriate foods. See Clinical Application 12–6.
12 months	Foods from adult table	Select suitable foods, prepared according to baby's abilities.

Table 12–3 Nutritional Problems in Infancy

Problem	Intervention	Comments
Regurgitation	Handle baby gently. Burp well; sit up after feeding.	Very common for first 6 months; not serious unless vomiting is projectile or bile-tinged.
Hiccoughs	Offer water to drink. Continue regular feedings.	May be caused by swallowed air.
Constipation	1/2 oz prune juice with 1/2 oz water; or 1/2 tsp dark corn syrup per feeding	Rare in breast-fed infants.
Burns to mouth	Shake formula after heating; test well.	Formula warmed in microwave oven continues to increase in temperature after removal.
Nursing-bottle syndrome	Do not use milk or juice as bedtime bottle. Do not put sweetener on pacifier.	See Clinical Application 3–1 .

Health-care providers face special challenges attempting to teach Western child-care methods to immigrants. Appropriate strategies include learning the mothers' beliefs, carefully monitoring the infants' progress, and adapting advice to balance culturally mandated practices (Thomas and de Santis, 1995).

Nutritional Problems in Infancy

Iron-deficiency anemia is the most prevalent nutritional deficiency in children in the United States. Other problems related to nutrition are allergies, intestinal injury induced by cow's milk protein, colic, and diarrhea. Additional problems of nutrition in infancy are summarized in Table 12–3. The table includes some home remedies, but if an infant does not improve rapidly from a nutrition-related problem, medical attention should be sought.

Iron-Deficiency Anemia

Exclusive breast-feeding for 4 to 6 months, without supplementary liquid, formula, or food, is a method of primary prevention of iron deficiency anemia. When exclusive breast-feeding ceases, iron-fortified formula should be given (Centers for Disease Control, 1998).

Sometimes a child drinks so much milk that he or she does not take in enough iron-rich foods. The result is iron-deficiency anemia. The type of milk is significant. In Great Britain, 33 percent of 18-month-old children receiving unmodified cow's milk were anemic, compared with 2 percent of those receiving an iron-supplemented formula (Williams et al., 1999). In the United States, 87.9 percent of formula-fed infants were reported to be meeting the 1989 RDA for iron in their diets between 1994 and 1996 (Centers for Disease Control, 1998).

In Spain, pre-school children showed better iron status if meat had been included in their diets during their eighth month or earlier, compared with those who were given meat later (Requejo et al., 1999). Cultural practices affect even the youngest members of a family. East Indian mothers living in Great Britain did not feed their children beef if they were Hindu, or pork or meats not "halal" if they were Moslem, and often did not replace the nutrients in those items with equivalent foods (Wharton, 1997).

OCCURRENCE In the United States, children between the ages of 9 and 18 months are at the highest risk of any age group for iron deficiency caused by inadequate intake of iron. Children from low-income families and black or Mexican-American children are at higher risk for iron deficiency than children from middle- or high-income families or white children (Centers for Disease Control, 1998).

Other risk factors for iron-deficiency include premature birth, low birth weight, malnutrition, adolescent parents, single mothers, absent fathers, maternal depression, low parental educational level, and parental psychiatric problems. Often many of these risk factors occur in a given family.

Mild levels of anemia delay motor development, but more severe deficiency is related to impaired cognition, possibly related to cerebral iron during this period of rapid brain growth (de Andraca, Castillo, and Walter, 1997). A population-based study showed an increased likelihood of mild or moderate mental retardation associated with anemia, independent of birth weight, maternal education, sex, race-ethnicity, the mother's age, or the child's age at entry into the Supplemental Feeding Program for Women, Infants, and Children (WIC) (Hurtado, Claussen, and Scott, 1999). In Great Britain, Asian children seem to have a higher prevalence of iron deficiency than white children, possibly because the luxury status of milk in some tropical countries leads parents to overvalue its benefit to children (Duggan, 1993).

EARLY DIAGNOSIS To be sure that iron deficiency anemia is diagnosed promptly in infants and toddlers, monitoring of the hemoglobin level is recommended through the infant's second birthday. Normal hemoglobin levels are 14 to 24 grams per 100 milliliters in the newborn, 10 to 15 grams per 100 milliliters in the infant. Tests of early iron deficiency (serum ferritin and iron-binding capacity) are not routinely performed, however, one reason the American Academy of Pediatrics recommends universal use of iron-fortified formula (1999).

TREATMENT OF IRON-DEFICIENCY ANEMIA Treatment of iron-deficiency anemia may include medication and ingestion of iron-fortified foods or foods naturally high in iron. Treatment should produce a normal hemoglobin level in 1 to 2 months (Deglin and Vallerand, 1999). Red meats, especially liver, are high in iron. The parent should offer the iron-rich foods at the beginning of the meal, when the infant is hungry. After the baby has eaten the strained or pureed foods, breast milk or formula may be given.

To help prevent iron-deficiency anemia, tea should only be offered to a child after the first birthday, if at all. As little as 1 cup of tea per day decreases the absorption of iron from both plant sources and milk in 6- to 12-month-old infants. (Merhav et al., 1985). Although unmodified cow's milk is not a good source of iron, fortified formula is a good source and breast milk is relatively so.

A number of special circumstances make vitamin or mineral supplementation desirable. Some of these situations appear in Table 12–4.

Allergies

Introducing certain foods too early increases the likelihood that the child will develop allergies. Special caution is needed for infants with a family history of allergies. If a parent or sibling has allergies, the infant's risk of developing allergies doubles (Wharton, 1997), but the specific allergens affecting the individuals in the family may differ (Taylor, Hefle, and Munoz-Furlong, 1999).

COMMON FOOD ALLERGENS IN INFANCY An **allergen** is a substance that provokes an abnormal individual hypersensitivity. Allergies develop, for the most part, when a person is exposed to an allergen, usually a protein, which sensitizes the individual to that item, causing the immune system to produce IgE antibodies. True food allergies affect 1 to 2 percent of the total population, but as many as 5 to 8 percent of children under 3 years of age (Taylor, Hefle, and Munoz-Furlong, 1999). Cases have been reported of infants displaying hypersensitivity reactions upon the first known exposure to foods (in these cases, milk, egg, or peanut) leading to the conclusion that the sensitizing dose was delivered in utero, through breast milk, or through inadvertent administration of the offending food (Van Asperen, Kemp, and Mellis, 1983).

An area of technology that bears watching is genetically engineered foods. A project designed to improve the nutritional quality of soybeans by introducing a Brazil nut gene was stopped when a majority of volunteers allergic to Brazil nuts reacted to the modified soybean (Seeds of Change, 1999). Cow's milk protein is an allergen that affects only 1 to 3 percent of children.

The identification of allergies to orange juice inspired an important change in infant feeding. Formerly, infants were given orange juice as the first food to complement evaporated milk formulas. However, there is enough vitamin C in both breast milk and commercial formulas to prevent scurvy. Currently, if additional vitamin C is needed, a synthetic product is usually prescribed to avoid the allergens in orange juice.

Wheat protein and egg-white protein can also be allergens to infants. Other foods that have caused allergies in infants are peanut butter, nuts, and chocolate. Peanuts and peanut products are probably the leading cause of fatal and near fatal **anaphylaxis** caused by food (Sampson, 1996). Clinical Application 12–7 summarizes a report on six fatal and seven near-fatal cases of anaphylaxis following ingestion of an allergen in which multiple errors of judgment are evident. Food allergies should never be underestimated. The Food Allergy Network provides educational materials to assist in analyzing labels for ingredients with allergenic potential. Its Web site can be accessed at http://www.foodallergy.org (Taylor, Hefle, and Munoz-Furlong, 1999).

The British government has advised women with close family members with allergic reactions, asthma, hay fever, or **eczema**, to avoid eating peanuts when pregnant or breast-feeding (Kmietowicz, 1998). Other authors conclude that the development of food allergies in high-risk infants (those with two parents with allergies) can be delayed but not prevented (Taylor, Hefle, and Munoz-Furlong, 1999).

SIGNS AND SYMPTOMS Food allergies may produce signs and symptoms in the gastrointestinal tract and other systems. They can cause skin and respiratory problems as well. An infant may have **hives**, eczema, or other rashes; asthma, bronchitis, wheezing; or a runny nose, called "allergic rhinitis."

The signs and symptoms of food allergies may appear as long as 5 days after exposure to the allergen. Thus, if 5 days are allowed to elapse between the introduction of each new food, chances are better that any allergens will be readily identified.

In some cases involving older children or adults, the allergen may be inhaled. Cooking vapors from legumes caused asthma in one report (Garcia-Ortiz et al., 1995). Other researchers in Spain identified weak associations between asthma and unloading of soybeans from ships (Ballester et al., 1999). Allergens from dissimilar sources also can evoke an allergic response. Cautions pertaining to cross-sensitivity to latex among persons allergic to various foods appear in Clinical Application 12–8.

TREATMENT OF ALLERGIES Soy formula has been used to treat children allergic to cow's milk protein, but soy also can cause allergies. Other special formulas contain hydrolyzed protein in an attempt to break up the protein into small pieces so that the body does not recognize the antigen.

Table 12-4 Vitamin-Mineral Supplementation for Infants

Supplement	Prescribed for	Situation or Rationale
Vitamin		
D	Breast-fed infants	If sunlight exposure to head, arms, hands is less than 1 hour per week
E	Premature infants	See Clinical Application 12–5.
K	All infants	Given immediately after birth
C	2-week-old formula-fed infants, if vitamin is not in formula	Synthetic preferable to juices. Orange juice especially, may be allergen.
Folic acid	Evaporated milk formula-fed infant	Sterilizing heat destroys folic acid.
B_{12}	Breast-fed infant, if mother is strict vegetarian	
Mineral		
Calcium	Premature infants	See Clinical Application 12–5
Phosphorus	Premature infants	See Clinical Application 12–5.
Iron	Term infant, when birth weight has doubled	Iron-fortified formula is available
	Formula-fed premature, from onset	
	Fortified human milk-fed premature, when full enteral feeding established (Schanler, 1997)	
Fluoride	All > 6 months of age	If water contains < 0.3 ppm

CLINICAL APPLICATION 12–7

Anaphylactic Reactions to Food

Allergy to food can be fatal. An analysis of 13 anaphylactic reactions to food identifies points along the critical path that had the potential to alter the outcome. Of 13 cases identified, 6 were fatal. In all cases, the client was known to be asthmatic and to be allergic to some food. None of the clients was aware that the allergen was present in the foods consumed. The items were candy, cookies, and pastry. Symptoms began soon after ingestion, but in some cases abated before becoming severe.

Of particular significance is the fact that fewer than half the children had self-injectable epinephrine prescribed and only one of the six children used a dose. The average delay between ingestion of the allergenic food and receipt of a dose of epinephrine was two and one-half times as long in the fatal cases as in the nonfatal cases. Also, more of the

fatal cases occurred in public places rather than a private home. These and other similarities and differences are tabulated below, followed by recommendations for the management of potential for anaphylaxis.

Several recommendations came from this study:

- Epinephrine should be prescribed, kept available, and used for clients with IgE mediated food allergies.

- Children and adolescents who have an allergic reaction to food should be observed for 3 to 4 hours after the reaction at a center capable of dealing with anaphylaxis.

- Parents of such children should be taught to ensure a rapid response by schools and other institutions.

(Summarized from Sampson, Mendelson, and Rosen, 1992.)

SITUATIONAL FACTOR	FATAL CASES		NEAR-FATAL CASES	
Age of client (average and range)	11.5 years 2 to 16 years		12.4 years 9 to 17 years	
Gender	1 male 5 females		2 males 5 females	
Known to have asthma	6		7	
Cause of anaphylactic reaction	Peanuts Cashews Eggs	3 2 1	Filberts Milk Peanuts Brazil nuts Walnuts	2 2 1 1 1
Average number of foods identified as allergenic for each client	1.7		2	
Onset of symptoms	3 to 30 minutes		1 to 5 minutes	
Location	School Fair Home	4 1 1	Home Relative's home Friend's home Vacation home	2 2 2 1
Parent present at site	3		4	
Had a prescription for self-injectable epinephrine	3		3	
Used the self-injectable dose	0		1	
Number of minutes after ingestion that any epinephrine was given (average and range)	93.3 15 to 180		36.4 10 to 130	

The normal gastrointestinal microorganisms contribute to the gut mucosal defense barrier. A strain of *Lactobacillus* promotes local antigen-specific immune responses, prevents permeability defects, and confers controlled antigen absorption. *Lactobacillus* GG, added to extensively hydrolyzed whey formula, given to formula-fed infants with atopic eczema significantly improved their dermatitis in the one-month study, compared with infants receiving the same formula without *Lactobacillus* (Majamaa and Isolauri, 1997).

Many infants outgrow food sensitivities by age 1 or 2. It is important not to permanently exclude foods from the diet on the basis of the first year's experience. The physician should be reminded of diet limitations so

that an appropriate time can be chosen to reintroduce the offending foods. An exception is allergy to peanuts and other nuts, which is rarely outgrown (Sampson, 1996).

Cow's Milk Protein-Induced Intestinal Injury

Approximately 1 percent of infants incur intestinal injury from cow's milk protein. The signs include failure to thrive, fever, vomiting, diarrhea that may test positive for blood, and anemia resulting from the blood loss. Treatment consists of removing cow's milk protein from the diet, possibly until age 2. Gluten-containing foods should also be removed from the diet if the intestinal injury is severe. Other foods that often cause allergic symp-

CLINICAL APPLICATION 12–8

LATEX ALLERGIES AND FOOD HYPERSENSITIVITY

Individuals allergic to latex have demonstrated hypersensitivity to foods botanically unrelated to latex. Among the fruits and nuts identified as allergens are avocado, banana, chestnut, fig, kiwi, mango, melon, papaya, passion fruit, peach, peanut, pineapple, and tomato (Brehler et al., 1997; SaraOclar et al., 1998). Anaphylaxis occurred in many of those cases (Blanco et al., 1994; Cinquetti et al., 1995; Llatser, Zambrano, and Guillaumet, 1994). Researchers have identified components common to latex and some of the fruits (Delbourg et al., 1996; Latasa et al., 1995). Latex allergy should be ruled out in individuals allergic to any of those foods before performing clinical procedures utilizing latex gloves (Rodriquez et al., 1993).

toms in children, citrus fruits, chocolate, eggs, nuts, peas, and fish, are best avoided until age 2 (Savilahti, 1981).

Colic

An estimated 10 to 20 percent of infants have colic (Jacobson and Melvin, 1995). The infant with colic is unhappy and fussy. He or she may cry for hours, starting late in the afternoon, just when caregivers are also tired and cranky.

POSSIBLE CAUSES Any time multiple, diverse treatments are proposed, it is likely that the basic cause of a condition is unknown, as is the case with colic. Spasms of the muscles of the colon are blamed, hence the name colic. The abdomen is tense and the infant draws its legs up to its belly. Distention may result from swallowing air. The pain seems to be relieved by the passage of gas or flatus.

If the baby is bottle-fed, it may be that the nipple holes are too big or too small, increasing the amount of air swallowed. If the infant is overfed, bacteria will ferment the excess milk in the intestine, forming gas.

The breast-fed infant might be swallowing air because of incorrect nursing position. Breast-fed infants seem to get gas from some of the same foods that give adults gas. Maternal intake of cruciferous vegetables, onion, chocolate, or cow's milk was shown to be associated with colic in exclusively breast-fed infants (Lust, Brown, and Thomas, 1996). It is also possible that the baby may be allergic to antigens in the mother's milk. In two studies, a majority of breast-fed infants with colic were cured when the breast-feeding mother stopped drinking cow's milk (Jakobsson and Lindberg, 1978, 1983). The authors of these studies suggest that nursing mothers abstain from cow's milk as a first treatment for infantile colic.

Other contributing factors may include fatigue or chilliness in the baby or tensions or emotional upsets in the mother. Compared to mothers of noncolicky infants, mothers of infants with colic were more bothered by the infants' temperament and were more likely to characterize the infants as difficult (Jacobson and Melvin, 1995). Allergies and lactose intolerance should be ruled out first.

TREATMENT OF COLIC Holding the baby upright, burping, or giving it some warm water sometimes helps. Diluting the formula or offering cold formula has been successful with some babies. Other interventions

reported to soothe colicky infants are swaddling, carrying the infant, using a pacifier, rocking, and soft repetitive sounds (Jacobson and Melvin, 1995).

Even though their baby's condition is stressful for them, the parents should try not to be overly concerned. Most infants grow and gain weight despite colic. Infantile colic generally resolves by the time the baby is 4 to 6 months old (American Academy of Pediatrics, 1998b).

Diarrhea

Seventy-five percent of an infant's body weight is water, 54 percent of it extracellular. For this reason, an infant is at special risk of rapid dehydration from diarrhea.

CAUSES Infants are subject to osmotic diarrhea. Overfeeding and food intolerances are common causes of diarrhea. Apple juice may produce diarrhea in infants because of carbohydrate malabsorption.

The most common cause of infectious **enteritis** in human infants is rotavirus. Worldwide, rotavirus is associated with about one-third of the cases of diarrhea requiring hospitalization in children younger than 5 years old (Chin, 2000). Rotavirus is the most important cause of mortality (estimated at 600,000 deaths yearly) due to dehydrating diarrhea in infants and children throughout the world (Bernstein et al., 1999). In developing countries, rotavirus causes an estimated 870,000 cases of enteritis per year. Severe vomiting may accompany the diarrhea.

Children between 6 months and 2 years of age are most susceptible; by age 3 most individuals have antibodies against the virus. The fecal-oral route is its probable mode of transmission but the virus survives for long periods on hard surfaces, in contaminated water, and on hands. Because the rate of illness is comparable in industrialized and developing countries, improved sanitation is unlikely to decrease the incidence of the disease (American Academy of Pediatrics, 1998a). Breast-feeding does not affect infection rates but may reduce the severity of the gastroenteritis (Chin, 2000). Human milk mucin has protected mice from rotavirus infection and presumably serves the same function in infants (Goldman, Goldblum, and Schmalstieg, 1997).

PATHOPHYSIOLOGY As a result of diarrhea, the wall of the intestine may become inflamed. The inflammation diminishes the amount of lactase produced, so the infant exhibits temporary lactose intolerance. Distension, cramps, and osmotic diarrhea ensue.

TREATMENT Electrolyte solutions (discussed in Chapter 9) are life-saving not only in developing countries but also in North America. Ceralyte, Pedialyte, or Oralyte are available at nearly all drug stores and grocery stores. The Centers for Disease Control (1999b) advises parents to keep two bottles or packages of these products on hand to use when the child develops diarrhea, following the package instructions according to the child's age. Sports drinks are not adequate substitutes for these solutions. Liquids at room temperature are often better tolerated than warm or cold beverages.

Children who are breast-feeding, taking formula or eating solids should continue to follow their usual diet (Centers for Disease Control, 1999b). Breast-feeding should be continued during diarrheal episodes because withholding of breast milk has been associated with progression of dehydration as has failing to give oral rehydration solution (Bhattacharya et al., 1995).

Box 12–2 Healthy Eating Index

The Healthy Eating Index (HEI) is a measure of diet quality devised by the United States Department of Agriculture Center for Nutrition Policy and Promotion. It has 10 components scored with up to 10 points each for a possible perfect score of 100. The first five components are based upon the Food Guide Pyramid (grains, vegetables, fruits, milk, and meat), numbers 6 through 8 on fat consumption (total, saturated, cholesterol), number 9 on sodium, and number 10 on variety. A Healthy Eating Index score above 80 implies a good diet, one between 51 and 80 a diet that needs improvement, and one less than 51 a poor diet.

As is readily visible in Figure 12–4, diet quality goes steadily downhill from ages 2 to 16. The decline is most closely linked to reductions in scores for fruit and milk consumption (Lino et al., 1998). The data were gathered by a nationally representative survey of about 5000 children conducted between 1994 and 1996. Specific findings of this report are discussed in the sections devoted to the various age groups.

Assessment of parents' knowledge and sources of information on home care is advised. Often information obtained from Internet web sites is erroneous and out of date. For instance, only 20 percent of traditional medical sources identified by web searches offered advice congruent with the guidelines by the American Academy of Pediatrics on treatment of diarrhea. The source of the information, even if a major academic medical center, did not guarantee correct advice, and various departments within an institution sometimes offered conflicting recommendations (McClung, Murray, and Heitlinger, 1998).

In developing countries, zinc supplementation has reduced the prevalence (Lira, Ashworth, and Morris, 1998) and duration of diarrhea (Faruque et al., 1999; Penny et al., 1999), with pronounced effects among those who were underweight or malnourished (Roy et al., 1998; Roy et al., 1997). It is unclear whether zinc supplementation corrects a deficiency to promote the clinical improvement or exerts its action in another manner (Folwaczny, 1997); the extent to which zinc supplementation interacts with copper absorption is also unclear (Bhutta, Nizami, and Isani, 1999; Fuchs, 1998).

WHEN TO CALL THE PHYSICIAN Diarrhea is common in infants and can sometimes be life threatening. A parent should seek medical treatment immediately if the child loses 5 percent of his or her body weight, has prolonged vomiting that prevents retaining of liquids, or shows blood in the stool. Other signs requiring immediate medical attention are a fever equiv-

alent to 101.5°F, orally, or signs of dehydration (decreased urination, sunken eyes, tearless crying, extreme thirst, dry or sticky mouth, or unusual drowsiness or fussiness (Centers for Disease Control, 1999b). A lack of improvement after 24 hours following these recommendations also deserves professional consultation. Among the treatments shown to be effective are special elemental formulas (Eliason and Lewan, 1998) and oral treatment with Lactobacillus GG along with oral rehydration. The latter reportedly resulted in the shortest duration of diarrhea (Rautanen et al., 1998).

Nutrition in Childhood

Childhood covers the growth periods of the toddler (1 to 3 years), the preschool child (3 to 6 years), and the school-age child (6 to 12 years). The child's nutritional needs become more like those of adults after the first birthday. A Food Guide Pyramid from the U. S. Department of Agriculture for 2- to 6-year-old children is illustrated in Figure 12–3. Suggestions for implementing the Food Pyramid for 2- to 6-year old children are described in Table 12–5. A measure of diet quality devised by the U. S. Department of Agriculture, the Healthy Eating Index (HEI), is explained in Box 12–2. It covers children and adolescents ages 2 to 16. The data gathered on 5,000 children using the HEI is graphed in Figure 12–4.

Nutrition of the Toddler

During the toddler years growth is slower than during infancy and, although activity increases, the proportional need for kilocalories decreases compared with infancy. So the child's appetite slackens.

Nevertheless, the child has to eat. How and what the family eats will influence the child's habits and tastes for many years. How family members treat one another and the toddler at mealtimes and at other times is more important than the precise amount of food the toddler swallows at each meal. Being forced to eat a distasteful food because "it's good for you" has imprinted permanent avoidance behaviors on some individuals. Conversely, some parents expand their repertory of menu choices to set good examples for their children (Devine et al., 1998).

Psychosocial Development

According to Erikson, the psychosocial developmental task of the toddler is to build **autonomy,** or independence. Every 2-year-old knows the word "No." One way parents can assist the toddler to achieve autonomy is to encourage choices from acceptable alternatives (Fig. 12–5). If the parents

Table 12–5 Food Pyramid for 2- to 6-year-olds		
Food Group	**Number of Servings**	**Serving Suggestions**
Bread/Cereal	Six or more	Select whole-grain breads and iron-fortified cereals.
Fruit	Two or more	Include 4 oz of orange juice or other food high in vitamin C
Vegetable	Three or more	Include one vegetable high in vitamin A. Crisp-cooked, warm rather than hot vegetable preferred
Meat	Two servings	Child-size servings of red meat are essential for RBC synthesis.
Milk	Two servings	Not to be overdone at expense of blood-forming nutrients. Low-fat milks are now permissible.

insist that the child eat certain items or amounts, he or she may learn to use food rejection as a means of gaining attention. Later, more serious eating problems may result from such interactions.

Physical Growth and Development

During the toddler years, growth slows. The expected weight gain in the second year may be just 4 to 6 pounds. Height may increase by about 4 inches. By age 2, though, head circumference reaches two-thirds of its adult size.

The toddler is aptly named. One of the skills being acquired during this time is walking upright. As this skill is being perfected, the child's muscles of the back, buttocks, and thighs are enlarging. The bones are becoming more mineralized and baby fat is disappearing. Along with the gross motor skill of walking, the toddler's fine motor control improves. He or she is able to use eating utensils with more finesse. The spoon is likely to reach the mouth still filled with food. The toddler's mouth is more sensitive than an adult's mouth. Foods are eaten better at lukewarm temperatures rather than hot. Thus, dawdling at the table may have a physiological basis.

Food Guide Pyramid for Young Children: A Daily Guide for 2- to 6- Year Olds

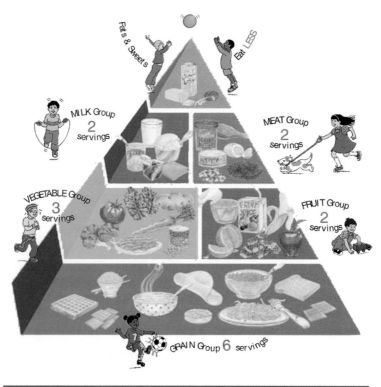

WHAT COUNTS AS ONE SERVING?

GRAIN GROUP
1 slice of bread
$\frac{1}{2}$ cup of cooked rice or pasta
$\frac{1}{2}$ cup of cooked cereal
1 ounce of ready-to-eat cereal

VEGETABLE GROUP
$\frac{1}{2}$ cup of chopped raw
or cooked vegetables
1 cup of raw leafy vegetables

FRUIT GROUP
1 piece of fruit or melon wedge
$\frac{3}{4}$ cup of juice
$\frac{1}{2}$ cup of canned fruit
$\frac{1}{4}$ cup of dried fruit

MILK GROUP
1 cup of milk or yogurt
2 ounces of cheese

MEAT GROUP
2 to 3 ounces of cooked lean meat, poultry, or fish
$\frac{1}{2}$ cup of cooked dry beans, or
1 egg counts as 1 ounce of lean meat
2 tablespoons of peanut butter count as 1 ounce of meat

FATS AND SWEETS
Limit calories from these.

Four- to six-year-olds can eat these serving sizes. Offer 2- to 3-year-olds less, except for milk.
Two-to six-year-olds need a total of 2 servings from the milk group each day.

Figure 12–3:
Food Guide Pyramid for Young Children and Planning Chart. This adaptation of the Food Guide Pyramid is designed to assist caregivers to provide healthful meals for children from 2 to 6 years of age. An accompanying tally sheet to identify areas for improvement and to instruct the preschool child in the cardinal principles of nutrition: balance, moderation, and variety can also be downloaded (United States Department of Agriculture, March 25, 1999).

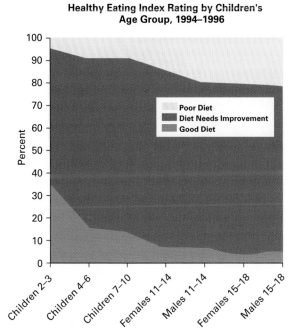

Healthy Eating Index Rating by Children's Age Group, 1994–1996

Legend:
- Poor Diet
- Diet Needs Improvement
- Good Diet

(Y-axis: Percent, 0 to 100. X-axis categories: Children 2–3, Children 4–6, Children 7–10, Females 11–14, Males 11–14, Females 15–18, Males 15–18)

Figure 12–4:
This Healthy Eating Index graph illustrates the steady downward slope of diet quality from that of 2- and 3-year olds to that of 15- to 18-year olds. (From Nutrition Insights, Center for Nutrition Policy and Promotion, United States Department of Agriculture, October 1998. Accessed 09/16/1999 at http://www.usda.gov/cnpp)

Nutrition Fundamentals

The toddler needs all the essential nutrients. The need for many nutrients increases proportionately with body size throughout the growth years. These needs, coupled with the toddler's poorer appetite, stretch the parents' ingenuity and patience.

FOOD LIKES Toddlers like finger foods. From a variety of finger foods, the child learns about texture. Toddlers prefer plain foods to most mixtures such as casseroles. Familiar combinations, though, may be relished. Some popular dishes are macaroni and cheese, spaghetti, and pizza.

MEALTIMES Toddlers are learning social skills as well as good nutritional habits. Eating is a social experience for adults most of the time; toddlers appreciate company also. Visiting other homes might introduce food items and experiences not encountered at home.

Keeping to a regular schedule will help maintain the child's food intake. A 1-year-old's stomach holds just 1 cup. Eating regular meals and nutritious snacks helps to prevent fatigue and control the appetite. However, if high-sugar snacks are used to assuage hunger before a meal, the more nutritious foods at the meal may be taken poorly.

NEW FOODS After the pureed foods of infancy, parents will be pleased to offer more attractive plates of food to the toddler. Brightly colored foods are appealing. Nevertheless, chewing may not be well developed. Tough meat or very fibrous vegetables are not for the toddler.

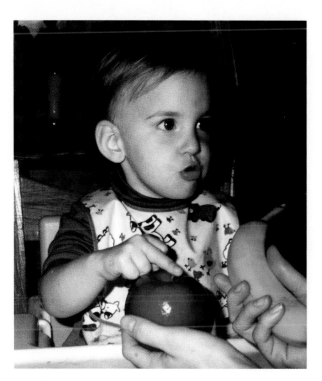

Figure 12–5:
Autonomy is achieved in small steps. This 19-month-old girl is choosing her dessert.

All of the foods that were not recommended until after the first birthday can be gradually introduced. These include unmodified cow's milk, egg white, wheat, citrus fruits, seafood, chocolate, and nut butters. The careful parent will continue to introduce foods one at a time and watch for reactions.

Because of the toddler's small stomach capacity, small servings are all that can be tolerated. A serving is one-fourth to one-fifth the size of an adult serving. A good rule of thumb is to serve 1 tablespoonful for each year of age. Even very young children make their wishes known through body movements, pushing food away, closing their mouths, and turning away from the feeder. The astute parent will respond to these cues before the child resorts to crying to communicate distress. Even at 8 to 12 months, 65 to 72 percent of children exhibited strong likes and dislikes and by 24 months, 91 percent did so (Skinner et al., 1998).

Daily intake should include one serving of a vitamin C-rich fruit or vegetable and one serving of a green leafy or yellow vegetable. Difficult as it may be, the parent should limit sugar and encourage consumption of fiber in cereals as well as in other foods. Beginning at age 2, an amount of fiber in grams equal to the child's "age + 5" is recommended. Thus, a 2-year-old should consume foods containing 7 grams of fiber with sufficient fluid to permit optimal passage through the intestinal tract. Iron-fortified cereals with at least 5 grams of fiber and no more than 3 grams of fat per serving are the best choices. In addition, cereals made from at least 51 percent whole grain can carry a health claim that in a low-fat diet, the cereals may reduce the risk of heart disease (Separating, 1999).

Offering three meals and three nutritious snacks daily will increase the likelihood that the toddler will obtain sufficient nourishment. The wise parent will avoid hazardous foods (review Clinical Application 12–6). Sometimes chopping the food into very tiny pieces eliminates a choking hazard. Nevertheless, a toddler should not be left alone while eating.

Because the kidneys become mature about age 1, the toddler can tolerate salt in moderation. The liking for salty foods is an acquired taste. Because of the association between salt and high blood pressure later in life, the prudent parent will discourage the consumption of heavily salted foods.

MILK AND FAT INTAKE Since iron-deficiency anemia is common in toddlers, the Centers for Disease Control (1998) recommends that milk intake be limited to 24 ounces per day to maintain the appetite for iron-enriched cereals, meats, and iron-rich fruits and vegetables. The term "milk anemia" refers to iron deficiency anemia caused by overconsumption of milk and underconsumption of iron-rich foods. Whether due to excessive milk (or juice) consumption or to lack of iron-rich foods, iron deficiency is found in 9 percent (700,000) of 1- to 2-year-old children and iron deficiency anemia in 3 percent. This prevalence probably reflects the fact that only 43.9 percent of 1- to 2-year-olds' diets contain 100 percent of the 1989 RDA for iron (Centers for Disease Control, 1998).

Although anemia is a risk to vegetarian children, it is also a risk for omnivores. Vegan diets are not adequate for young growing children, and are likely to be associated with malnutrition, especially if the diets result from authoritarian dogma (Hackett, Nathan, and Burgess, 1998). A key factor appears to be the exclusion of dairy products.

The American Academy of Pediatrics (1998c) recommends that between ages 2 and 5, the proportion of energy from fat be reduced to 30 percent of a child's intake, but not less than 20 percent. In contrast, the Canadian Pediatric Society recommended tapering fat intake from 50 percent of kilocalories at age 2 to 30 percent by the end of adolescence (Olson, 1995). Under either set of guidelines, 1- to 2-year-old children should drink whole milk to provide adequate fat for the still-growing brain.

The Quality of Toddlers' Diets

In one study, toddlers' HEI scores averaged 73.8, which, although it is the highest children's score, is still below the level of 80 used to define a good diet. The children's diets were scored above 8.0 in grains, cholesterol, sodium, and variety. None of the components were scored below the 5.1 that signifies a poor diet. The lowest scores were 5.4 for saturated fat and 5.9 for vegetables. More than 50 percent of the children met the dietary recommendations for grains, fruits, cholesterol, sodium, and variety.

A smaller study illustrates some of the variety in toddlers' meals. From a list of 196 foods, toddlers' and family preferences were tallied. The average number of foods that had been offered to 2-year-old children was 152.6, with a range of 96 to 190. Corn, mashed potatoes, and French fries were the only vegetables that more than 85 percent of the children liked and ate, with French fries the clear favorite because they were the only items liked and eaten by all the children. Only 11.2 percent of the 196 foods were disliked and no specific food was disliked by even half the children (Skinner et al., 1998).

Nutrition of the Preschool Child

The preschool child requires all the nutrients necessary for other human beings. This is a delightful time of enthusiastic learning, including food

preferences. Because food is consumed every day, opportunities to teach good nutritional practices abound.

Psychosocial Development

Erikson's theory postulates **initiative** as the psychosocial task to be mastered by the preschool child. Within their capabilities, children should be encouraged to set and achieve some goals of their own. This is a delightful time of enthusiastic learning, including food preferences. Children can participate in planning and preparation of meals. They should be prompted to help in the kitchen, not just with the cleanup. Preschool children love to make fancy cookies and showy relishes. Making even simple things like gelatin desserts gives the child a sense of accomplishment.

By making the meal a social time and eating slowly themselves, parents can encourage the same behavior in the child. Exemplifying good manners will be more productive than criticizing the child's manners. It is helpful for children to have company their own age. Children have been observed to stay at the table longer and to eat more in the company of their peers. Exchanging visits with a friend's child will begin to broaden the child's horizons.

Physical Growth and Development

From the third to the sixth year, a child continues to gain 4 to 5 pounds per year. A gain in height of about 2 inches per year is average. Adequacy of growth should be assessed every 6 to 12 months. Growth charts remain the standard against which a given assessment is judged.

Nutrition Fundamentals

Preschool children are very active. A 3-year-old may need 1300 to 1500 kilocalories per day. But the child may have little appetite. Serving sizes for 4- to 6-year-old children are the same as those for adults.

DEVELOPING GOOD HABITS The preschool child responds best to regular mealtimes. When the adult meal will be served late, the parents have to decide if it would be better to allow the child to socialize with adults at a late meal or to feed the child early.

Preschoolers, like toddlers, cannot eat enough in only three meals to meet their needs. By age 3, a child is able to verbalize hunger. A good supply of wholesome snacks will serve the conscientious parent well. Such items as cottage cheese, low-fat yogurt, fresh fruit, raw vegetables, milk, fruit juices, graham crackers, or fig bars all are nutrient dense and low in fat. So long as the parent still has control over the child's world, concentrated sweets such as candy and soda pop should be strictly limited.

Tableware appropriate for the preschool child will ease tensions during mealtimes. Unbreakable dishes that are designed for stability, with deep sides to permit scooping the food onto a spoon or fork, are practical choices. Small glasses and cups, also unbreakable, with a squat design and low center of gravity, will serve the child's and the parents' needs well.

It is not too early to emphasize the importance of cleanliness. Regularly washing hands before meals and brushing teeth after meals will cultivate good health habits.

NEW FOODS Parents should offer new foods one at a time in small amounts. Trying something new is most acceptable at the beginning of the meal when the child is hungriest. A taste or two is sufficient if new foods are offered at regular intervals. As many as 10 exposures to new foods are required before the child readily accepts the new taste (Birch, 1996).

Parents have the advantage over their children of being able to select the food offered. Items the parents dislike will not regularly grace the family table. Children, too, should be permitted their preferences. This advice is not permissive, just practical. If an argument over food develops into a power struggle, as sometimes happens, the child will never admit to liking the food, even when it turns out to be quite tasty.

Nutritional Problems

IRON-DEFICIENCY ANEMIA Between 1988 and 1994, 3 percent of 3- to 5-year-old children were found to be iron deficient and less than 1 percent were anemic (Centers for Disease Control, 1998). Children in low-income families are particularly susceptible to iron-deficiency anemia. Fortunately, the situation is improving. In 1985, only 3 percent of the 6-month to 6-year-old children in low-income households were anemic compared with 8 percent in 1975. This advance is attributed to the WIC program.

DENTAL HEALTH The destruction of tooth enamel by dental caries, discussed in Chapter 3, is a problem for all economic groups. The "baby" teeth, as well as the permanent teeth, deserve care and professional attention. In order for teeth to be correctly brushed, the parent may have to do it. Regular dental checkups should be a part of the preschool child's routine. Adequate dentition supports good nutrition. In contrast, fluorosis has occurred as a result of the overuse of supplements and the ingestion of toothpaste. Children younger than 6 years are likely to swallow rather than to expectorate toothpaste. A pea-sized portion of toothpaste is sufficient (DePaola, Faine, and Palmer, 1999).

CHILD-CARE PROGRAMS In 1999, 60 percent of the nation's children (13 million preschoolers, including 6 million babies and toddlers) were regularly receiving care from people other than their parents or guardians. The American Dietetic Association has addressed the means of meeting children's nutrition and nutrition education needs in a safe, sanitary, supportive environment (American Dietetic Association, 1999). Some of the specific recommendations follow.

- If the child is in the program 4 to 7 hours per day, the child-care program should be responsible for meeting one-third of the child's daily nutrition needs; if the child is in the program 8 or more hours per day, it should be responsible for meeting half to two thirds of the child's daily nutrition needs.

- The program should offer food at least every 3 hours, but not force it on the child or withhold it when the child fails to consume other food.

- Caregivers should not add extra salt or sugar to food.

- Good institutional food management practices should be implemented including good handwashing, service with plates and utensils (rather than foam cups and plates, which pose a choking hazard), adequate refrigeration, and proper storage of supplies.

- Nutrition education can include food preparation, identification of colors and shapes, counting, field trips, and keeping parents informed.

SPECIAL ASSESSMENT TECHNIQUES nutrition screening tool for use with children up to 6 years old appears as Box 12–3. The questionnaire is filled out by the primary caregiver to help identify potential nutrition problems. Each "yes" answer is awarded the number of points to the right on that line. The child's score is the point total, and a score of 4 or more indicates a probable problem that should be assessed further.

The Quality of Preschool Children's Diets

As an overall score, preschool children received a mean of 67.8 on the HEI. The only areas in which they averaged more than 8 points were in cholesterol and sodium. More than 50 percent of these preschool children met the dietary recommendations for cholesterol, sodium, and variety (Lino et al., 1998). Of 3- to 5-year-olds, 61.7 percent met the 1989 RDA for iron (Centers for Disease Control, 1998).

Another government report grouped children aged 2 to 5 years together. Data gathered on these children indicate areas of dietary intake that need improvement. For instance, approximately half of the 2- to 5-year-old boys and girls consumed at least 2 servings of fruits and 6 servings of grains per day. About 40 percent of the children received at least 2 servings of milk per day. Only one-quarter of them ate at least 3 servings of vegetables. As for meat or alternates, only 10 percent of the boys and 7 percent of the girls consumed 5 ounces per day, and 12 percent of the children consumed less than 1 ounce per day.

All of the children in the sample reported only 15 percent of the grains eaten were whole grains and only 57 percent of the vegetables eaten were other than white potatoes (U.S. Department of Agriculture, February 1999). Only 45 percent of 4- to 6-year-olds consumed enough fiber to meet the "age + 5" recommendation. For this age group, vegetables and low-fiber breads provided more fiber than other food categories. Substituting high-fiber breads and cereals for low-fiber ones is a suggested strategy (Hampl, Betts, and Benes, 1998).

Basically, a health educator could concentrate on any Food Pyramid category with good probability of improving children's diets. For preschool children, most of the messages will have to be designed for the parent, the babysitter, the day-care provider, and the preschool teacher. The lessons could be explicit instruction about nutrition or implicit teaching by example and by providing healthful food in the particular setting. Some preschool programs specify acceptable foods for parents to provide as snacks for the class.

The American Academy of Pediatrics recommends supplements only for children at nutritional risk. Such children include those from deprived families, those who are neglected or abused, those suffering from eating disorders or implementing fad diets, those on reduction diets for obesity, those diagnosed with chronic diseases (for instance, cystic fibrosis and inflammatory bowel disease), and children on vegetarian diets. Despite this authoritative advice, 54.4 percent of 3-year-olds were regularly receiving dietary supplements, most often combination vitamin and mineral preparations. The mothers of these children were more likely to be non-Hispanic white, married, affluent, better-educated, and receiving care from a private health-care provider than mothers of children not receiving supplements.

Only for iron supplements was the pattern reversed. The mothers of children receiving only iron supplements were more likely to be black and less-educated and have lower household income than the rest of the mothers sampled. (Yu, Kogan, and Gergen, 1997).

Box 12–3 A Nutrition Screening Tool for Young Children

The PEACH Survey consists of 17 "yes" or "no" questions carrying weights from 1 to 4. It is designed to be self-administered by a child's primary caregiver. The tool was validated on children from birth to age 5 against a pediatric dietitian's assessment. A score of 4 or more indicates a probable nutrition problem.

PEACH* Survey

Agency: _____   Date: _____
Child's Name: _____   Date of Birth: _____
Address: _____   Phone #: _____

Please circle YES or NO for each question as it applies to your child.

Does your child have a health problem (do not include colds or flu). If yes, what is it?	YES	NO	1
Is your child: Small for age: ___ Too thin? ___ Too heavy? ___ (If you check any of the above, please circle YES)	YES	NO	3
Does your child have feeding problems? If yes, what are they?	YES	NO	3
Is your child's appetite a problem? If yes, describe:	YES	NO	1
Is your child on a special diet? If yes, what type of diet?	YES	NO	2
Does your child take medicine for a health problem (Do not include vitamins, iron, or fluoride)? Name of medicine(s):	YES	NO	1
Does your child have food allergies? If yes, to what foods?	YES	NO	1
Does your child use a feeding tube or other special feeding method? If yes, explain:	YES	NO	4
Circle YES if your child does not eat any of these foods: Milk ___ Meats ___ Vegetables ___ Fruits ___ (Check all that apply)	YES	NO	1
Circle YES if your child has problems with: Sucking ___ Swallowing ___ Chewing ___ Gagging ___ (Check all that apply)	YES	NO	3
Circle YES if your child has problems with: Loose stools ___ Hard stools ___ Throwing up ___ Spitting up ___ (Check all that apply)	YES	NO	3
Does your child eat clay, paint chips, dirt, or any other things that are not food? If yes, what?	YES	NO	2
Does your child refuse to eat, throw food, or do other things that upset you at mealtime? If yes, explain:	YES	NO	2
For infants **under 12 months** who are bottle fed: Does your child drink less than 3 (8-ounce) bottles of milk per day?	YES	NO	1
For children **over 12 months**: (Check if applies and circle the YES) Is your child **not** using a cup? ___ Is your child not finger feeding ___	YES	NO	1
For children **over 18 months**: Does your child still take most liquids from a bottle?	YES	NO	2
Circle YES if your child is not using a spoon.	YES	NO	2

*Parent Eating and Nutrition Assessment for Children with Special Health Needs

Total = ☐

The Parent Eating and Nutrition Assessment for Children with Special Health Needs (PEACH) survey

---

In sum, with the possible exception of iron, vitamin-mineral supplements in the United States seem to be given to children who are at least rather than most nutritional risk. As with other individuals taking vitamin-mineral supplements, supplementation should not be perceived as an excuse for consuming an inadequate diet, but rather an enhancement of the diet. Foods in a balanced, varied diet provide nutrients and other substances for which RDAs or AIs have not been set because of lack of adequate data.

Nutrition of the School-Age Child

Few modifications in foodstuffs are necessary to accommodate the school-age child. A balanced diet suitable for healthy adults, emphasizing intake of protein, vitamins, and minerals will also be good for a school-age child. Overemphasis on limiting foods is not advised. Diets should not be restricted because of the energy, fat, or sugar content of any one food, nor should foods be labeled "good" or "bad." In the first case, food may be regarded as medicine, and in the second, as "forbidden fruit." Neither viewpoint fosters positive attitudes.

The total diet is key: does it provide variety, balance, and moderation? Severely curbing intake of meat and milk may result in undersupplying energy, iron, zinc, and calcium. After the age of 5 years, the child's fat intake should amount to no more than 30 percent and no less than 20 percent of energy (American Academy of Pediatrics, 1998c). Some fat is needed to supply essential fatty acids and to aid in absorption of fat-soluble vitamins. When 4- to 10-year-old children reduced their fat intake by 8.5 percent, effective strategies included replacing higher-fat foods with lower-fat ones, especially with milk, and eating more servings of fruits, vegetables, and very low-fat desserts. Their overall energy and nutrient intakes remained adequate (Dixon et al., 1997).

Psychosocial Development

According to Erikson, the developmental task of the school-age child is **industry.** The school years are the years to build competence in many different skills. School work, sports, hobbies, and chores at home permit the child to recognize the worth of work. Making and keeping commitments is part of developing industry.

School-age children can participate in planning menus, shopping for food, preparing the meals, as well as cleaning up afterwards (Fig. 12–6). As with younger children, limiting the child to washing the dishes or taking out the garbage will be more likely to foster a sense of inferiority than habits of industry. In addition, working with the parents or siblings on food preparation and clean-up can foster teamwork and togetherness.

Nutrition education continues in school. Interactions with other children and school experiences expose a child to different foods and different cultures. Increased knowledge following educational projects is fairly easily verified, but procuring and demonstrating changed attitudes and behavior is more difficult. Approximately 60 percent of school children in the United States participate in school lunch programs. Comprehensive demonstration projects were successful in reducing fat content of lunches from 40 to 30 percent of kilocalories, assisting teachers with nutrition education projects, and increasing opportunities for the children to be physically active (Harris et al., 1997). Educational messages directed at children should be focused on foods, not nutrients.

Growth and Health

By age 6, a child should weigh twice as much as at age 1. Suppose that a 7-pound infant who weighed 21 pounds at 1 year gained 5 pounds in the second year and 4 pounds per year through age 6. At age 6, the child would weigh 42 pounds, or twice the 1-year weight.

By school age, the effects of good or poor nutrition will begin to be apparent. The well-nourished child will display most of the qualities listed in Table 12–6. The poorly nourished child will be lacking in a significant number of these qualities.

Nutrition Fundamentals

School-age children, especially those 8 to 10 years old, generally have good appetites and like almost all foods. Vegetables are the least liked of the food groups. Sixty-five percent of 6- to 11-year-old children consume less than the recommended amount of fiber (Williams, Bollela, and Wynder, 1995).

Breakfast is very important. The child needs energy and other nutrients to last until lunch. Breakfast should contain one-fourth to one-third of the day's nutrients. In New Jersey, 25 percent of African-American elementary school children who skipped breakfast were found to consume less than 50 percent of the RDAs for energy, vitamin C, calcium, and iron (Sampson et al., 1995). Research has demonstrated a positive effect of breakfast on thinking, especially in children at nutritional risk (Pollitt, 1995).

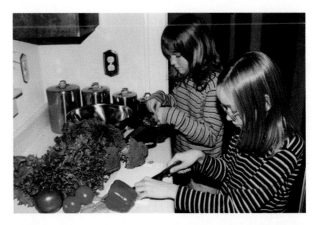

Figure 12–6:
A dinner invitation to a friend can involve culinary practice.

The School Breakfast Program, subsidized by the U. S. Department of Agriculture, serves over 6 million children a meal that provides one fourth to one third of the children's RDAs for energy and selected nutrients. It is available even in schools without kitchen facilities. Participation is higher in rural areas and among boys, children in the lower grades, African-American and Hispanic children, and those in low-income households (Kennedy and Davis, 1998).

The school-age child needs adequate protein intake for developing muscle and laying down bone matrix. Calcium is necessary to build dense bones. The body anticipates the adolescent growth spurt; the greatest retention of calcium and phosphorus precedes the rapid growth of adolescence by 2 years or more. Therefore, a liberal intake of milk and milk products

TABLE 12–6 Indications of Good Nutrition in the School-Age Child

General appearance	Alert, energetic
	Normal height and weight
Skin and mucous membranes	Skin smooth, slightly moist; Mucous membranes pink, no bleeding
Hair	Shiny, evenly distributed
Scalp	No sores
Eyes	Bright, clear, no fatigue circles
Teeth	Straight, clean, no discoloration or caries
Tongue	Pink, papillae present, no sores
Gastrointestinal system	Good appetite, regular elimination
Musculoskeletal system	Well-developed, firm muscles; erect posture, bones straight without deformities
Neurological system	Good attention span for age; not restless, irritable, or weepy

before the age of 10 gives a child a great advantage. Calcium supplementation increased bone density 3 to 5 percent over 3 years in prepubertal twins compared with their identical twins receiving placebos (Johnston et al., 1992). Moderation in sodium intake is indicated, because sodium intake negatively influenced increases in trabecular bone mineral density in girls younger than 11 years of age (Gunnes and Lehmann, 1996).

Exercise

Exercise can help the school-age child achieve growth and development in several areas. Weight-bearing exercise stimulates the osteoblasts, the bone-building cells. In girls younger than 11 years of age, changes in bone mineral density were most related to weight-bearing physical activity but also were dependent upon calcium intake (Gunnes and Lehmann, 1996). Exercise and activity balance energy intake to achieve weight control. Exercise, especially team sports, fosters interactions with peers. Activities that are likely to become lifetime interests should be especially encouraged. Unlike sports such as football that are played by few adults, skill at tennis or similar sports may provide an outlet for a lifetime.

Problem Areas

School-age children are generally so active that they may have trouble sitting still. Requiring them to spend 15 to 20 minutes at the table for meals will increase the likelihood that they will eat a complete meal.

Between 1977 and 1994, milk consumption by 6- to 11-year-olds declined by 24 percent among boys and 32 percent among girls while consumption of non-citrus fruit juices increased by 308 percent, of fruit drinks by 36 percent, and of carbonated beverages by 23 percent. In one study, however, children without a source of milk at the noon meal failed to consume the 1989 RDA for calcium (Johnson, Panely, and Wang, 1998). The RDA for calcium was increased in 1998; it is unlikely that the situation has improved.

Only 32 percent of 7- to 10-year-olds were found to consume enough fiber to meet the "age + 5" recommendation. For this age group vegetables and low-fiber breads provided more fiber than other food categories. Substituting high-fiber breads and cereals for low-fiber ones is a suggested strategy (Hampl, Betts, and Benes, 1998).

Some children are bothered by caffeine. Eight ounces of hot chocolate or 12 ounces of cola contain 50 milligrams of caffeine. Two such beverages in a 60-pound child are the equivalent of 8 cups of coffee in a 175-pound man. If the child has difficulty sleeping or has an irregular pulse, the first factor to investigate is caffeine intake.

In contrast, little scientific evidence exists to link sugar consumption to hyperactivity (Kinsbourne, 1994; Wolraich et al, 1994; Wolraich, Wilson, and White, 1995). A few children might be adversely affected, but a widespread association has been disproved.

The Quality of School-Age Children's Diets

The mean overall score of 7- to 10-year-old children on the HEI was 66.6. The only areas that would have rated "good" were on the cholesterol component at 8.7 and the variety component at 8.1. The same two areas were the only ones in which more than 50 percent of the children met dietary recommendations (Lino et al., 1998).

Of 6- to 11-year old boys, 60 percent consumed at least 6 servings of grains per day but of girls, only 46 percent. Approximately one-fourth of this age group consumed the recommended number of servings of vegetables and fruits. Food consumption diverged by gender for dairy products and meat with boys likely to consume more servings of dairy foods than girls (52 to 40 percent) and 5 ounces of meat or alternatives (23 to 11 percent). These children showed the same preference for refined grains and white potatoes as the preschoolers did (U.S. Department of Agriculture, February 1999). Of 6- to 11-year-old children, 79.8 percent of the boys and 60.9 percent of the girls met the 1989 RDA for iron intake (Centers for Disease Control, 1998).

The use of nutritional supplements for children was not included in those reports. In England and Scotland, a survey of 15,275 children between the ages of 4 and 12 years revealed that 15.9 percent used nutritional supplements, mainly multivitamins. Those most likely to receive supplements were younger children, of non-English, non-Scottish descent, those from smaller families, whose parents did not smoke, whose mothers were more educated, and whose fathers were in non-manual occupations (Bristow et al., 1997). Whether a comparable situation regarding school-age children exists in the United States is unknown, but some similar characteristics were associated with vitamin-mineral supplementation for 3-year-old children in this country. The advice of the American Academy of Pediatrics is to supplement only children at nutritional risk (Yu, Kogan, and Gergen, 1997).

Eating dinner with the family was associated with improved diet quality for 9- to 14-year-old children. A survey of 16,202 children revealed that those eating family dinner oftener consumed more fruits and vegetables and less fried food and soda than those who ate dinner with the family less often. More than half the 9-year-olds dined with the family every day, compared with about one-third of the 14-year-olds (Gillman et al., 2000).

Nutrition in Adolescence

Adolescence is the period that extends from the onset of **puberty** until full growth is reached. For most individuals, adolescence occurs between the ages of 12 and 20. Adolescence is second only to infancy in the nutritional requirements necessary for growth and development.

Psychosocial Development

Achieving their own **identity** is the developmental task Erikson identified for adolescents, including accepting their capabilities. In this process, teenagers "try on" various identities. Peers exert a major influence on a teenager's decisions. Adolescents pick up fads instantly and drop them just as suddenly. Food fads are part of the same pattern.

Opportunities abound for teaching adolescents about nutrition, but only 38 percent of 1,117 ninth-graders reported that their health-care providers had discussed the health benefits of calcium with them. Students in one study who knew about the link between calcium intake and osteoporosis consumed significantly more calcium than those without that knowledge (Harel et al., 1998).

Overcoming barriers is the challenge. Only 26 percent of college students surveyed were motivated by health concerns and reported dietary intakes to match their beliefs. The researchers characterized the remainder of the students as likely to be "turned off" by nutrition-oriented messages (Horacek and Betts, 1998). In New Orleans, high school students averaged 39 percent on a test of knowledge about fruits and vegetables prepared by the National Cancer Institute, with white students scoring significantly higher than African-American students (Beech et al., 1999). Targeting knowledge and behavior were goals of an intervention project featuring a media campaign, classroom workshops, school meal modification, and parental support.

Students at the intervention high schools showed a significant difference in knowledge scores and demonstrated a significant 14 percent increase in consumption of fruits and vegetables in the first 3 years. At follow-up, however, consumption of fruits and vegetables by students in the high schools used as a control group also increased to the point that the groups were equal (Nicklas et al., 1998), illustrating the difficulty of isolating influences on behavior in free-living people over a long period of time. The students at the control-group high schools no doubt received some of the same messages about healthy diets from other sources than those prepared for students at the intervention schools.

Oftentimes, modifying systems or communities offers the best chance of improving nutritional outcomes. A first step is understanding the client's perspective.

A program in California aimed to improve nutrition and physical fitness in 10- to 14-year-old minority youth in low-income communities. Assessment indicated that adolescents in the target communities spent about 40 percent of the family food dollar and prepared about 13 meals per week for themselves or their families without the necessary knowledge or skills to plan, buy, or prepare food. Further, they avoided outdoor exercise for fear of crime, and many of them believed they would not live long enough to reap the benefits of reduced chronic disease should they even try to modify their lifestyles. Consequently, their leisure activities focused on television and eating or meeting their friends at a fast food restaurant, one of the few clean, brightly lit, safe places in the neighborhood (Hinkle, 1997).

Physical Growth and Development

The term *growth spurt* is accurate. A teenager who may seem not to grow as much as others the same age will suddenly sprout like a weed, seemingly overnight. Boys and girls differ in the timing and completion of the growth spurt. Table 12–7 summarizes the ages of typical adolescent growth spurts. Growth is not completed at ages 15 to 19, only the growth spurt. Growth of the skeleton during adolescence contributes to about 45 percent of the adult skeletal mass (Heald and Gong, 1999).

Nutrient Needs of the Adolescent

Because of their growing and developing bodies, adolescents need more energy, vitamins, and protein than school-age children or adults.

Energy

The adolescent may require 60 to 80 kilocalories per kilogram of body weight per day, that is, 2700 to 3600 kilocalories for a 100-pound teenager. Boys need more kilocalories than girls. A 15-year-old girl requires 2100

kilocalories, whereas a 15-year-old boy requires 3000 kilocalories. The boy may be in a growth spurt, whereas the girl has probably completed hers. In addition, the gender differences in body composition become apparent. Boys' bodies develop more metabolically active muscle tissue while girls' bodies naturally increase fat stores that use less energy to maintain.

Vitamins and Minerals

The adolescent athlete may need up to 6000 kilocalories per day. Thiamin and niacin are related to energy expenditure, and riboflavin is needed for protein utilization; the need for these B-vitamins is increased in the athlete. A training table laden with extra whole-grain or enriched bread and milk should meet these vitamin needs.

Emotional or physical stress can increase the utilization of vitamin C by three or four times so fruits and vegetables are important components of the diet in adolescents undergoing multiple changes in their lives and their bodies. As discussed in Chapter 8, zinc is necessary for DNA and protein synthesis, and overt deficiency produces retarded growth and delayed sexual maturation. Before an adolescent eliminates red meat from the diet he or she should consider the best sources of zinc—shellfish and red meat. High-school athletes do seem more likely to use vitamin and mineral supplements than other teenagers (Sobal and Marquart, 1994), but teaching or counseling may be indicated to help young athletes make informed decisions. Some common substances thought to enhance athletic performance are discussed in Chapter 16.

Fiber

Adolescents 12 to 18 years old are the least likely age group to meet the "age plus 5" level of fiber intake. Seventy-seven percent of boys and 89 percent of girls consumed less than this amount (Williams, Bollela, and Wynder, 1995).

Food Pyramid Modification

The adolescent diet should consist of the adult distribution of foods, except that three servings of milk or milk products should be ingested. Since one-fourth of the adolescent's kilocalories come from snacks, these "between-meal meals" should be nutritionally dense and chosen to balance the diet.

Problem Areas

Two common nutritional problems of teenagers are overenthusiastic weight control and poor choices of foods.

Weight Control

Adolescents with BMIs greater than 30 should be referred for medical diagnosis and follow-up. Many dieting teens, however, are not overweight. Self-prescribed weight reduction diets are common among American women and girls. Of the psychosocial factors investigated in 2,536 normal-weight and underweight female adolescents, the strongest contributing factor differentiating dieters from nondieters was low self-esteem (Pesa, 1999). To prevent unhealthy dieting, nutritional education programs should incorporate activities to build self-esteem.

Unfortunately, Americans are lured by the "quick fix," promising instant results. Most often the diet consultants who promise quick results do so with an unbalanced diet. Of 30,000 adolescents surveyed in Minnesota, 12 percent reported dieting within the prior year, 30 percent reported binge eating, 12 percent reported self-induced vomiting, and 2

Table 12–7 Adolescent Growth Spurts		
	Age in Years	
Status	**Boys**	**Girls**
Begins	12 to 13	10 to 11
Peaks	14	12
Completed	19	15

percent reported using diuretics or laxatives for weight control. In this group, vegetarians were twice as likely to report dieting more than 5 times a year than nonvegetarians, 4 times as likely to report intentional vomiting, and 8 times as likely to use laxatives for weight control (Neumark-Sztainer et al., 1998).

As is discussed below, some adolescents may adopt vegetarianism as a means to control weight and body shape rather than for ecological or spiritual reasons. Regardless of the reason they have become vegetarians, these adolescents need special assessment of their nutritional status and dietary intakes.

Athletes who compete in events in which lower body weight is an advantage may adopt unhealthy dieting practices. Female athletes, especially, may eliminate meat from their diets in efforts to control their weight and body shapes at the risk of protein, iron, and zinc deficiencies. A female athlete who consumes a meatless diet should be assessed for those nutritional deficiencies as well as an eating disorder. Loosli and Ruud (1998) reported that **amenorrhea** in athletes has been strongly associated with meatless diets (87 percent) and eating disorders (62 percent). On the positive side, implementation of a minimal weight program for Wisconsin high school wrestlers resulted in significantly fewer weight-cutting practices and bulimic behaviors (Opplinger et al., 1998). The danger of weight cutting though dehydration is discussed in Chapter 9, and principles of safe weight reduction as well as **bulimia** and **anorexia nervosa** are covered in Chapter 18.

Poor Food Choices

Some fast-food restaurant chains offer salads, light salad dressings, and reduced-fat milks. There are some healthy choices possible. However, the old standbys on the fast-food menus are generally higher in kilocalories, fat, sugar, and sodium than are similar items prepared at home. Carbonated beverage consumption is associated with bone fractures in ninth and tenth grade girls. Among physically active girls, cola beverages, in particular, are highly associated with bone fractures (Wyshak, 2000).

As undesirable as a steady diet of fast food might be, it cannot be blamed for causing acne. About 80 percent of adolescents suffer from acne, starting about age 12 to 13 in girls and 14 to 15 in boys. Acne is caused by sex hormones stimulating the sebaceous glands. The skin becomes oilier and the ducts to the glands sometimes plug up, permitting the accumulation of harmful bacteria. There is as yet no convincing evidence that dietary indiscretions cause acne.

The Quality of Adolescents' Diets

The quality of adolescent diet continues its downward spiral. The overall HEI scores for 11- to 14-year-olds are 62.2 for males and 63.5 for females. For those 15 to 18 years of age, the scores are 60.7 for males and 60.9 for females. The only component scores above 8.0 were recorded for cholesterol by girls and for variety by 11- to 14-year-old boys. All of these groups had 50 percent of their members meeting the dietary recommendations for cholesterol and variety (except that only 37 percent of 15- to 18-year old females met the standard for variety). These adolescents' scores for the fruit component of the HEI were the worst tallied for any of the children: 3.5 for

11- to 14-year-old boys, 3.9 for girls; 2.8 for 15- to 18-year-old boys, 3.1 for girls (Lino et al., 1998).

Three-quarters of 12- to 19-year-old boys consumed the recommended servings of grains. Over half of them ate the recommended servings of vegetables, dairy products, and meat. Less than one-fourth consumed the recommended fruit servings. By contrast, in none of the categories did even 50 percent of the 12- to 19-year-old girls report eating the recommended number of servings. They came close in the grain category, with 49 percent. Eating 3 vegetables a day was recorded for 38 percent, but only about one-quarter met the recommended servings of fruit, dairy, and meat (U.S. Department of Agriculture, February 1999).

Only 24 percent of 12- to 19-year-old females in the USDA study reported consuming 5 ounces of meat or alternatives (for this tabulation, eggs, nuts, seeds, and soybean products). Given that low intake, the fact that 9 percent of 12- to 15-year-old nonpregnant girls and 11 percent of 16- to 19-year-old nonpregnant girls are iron deficient is not surprising. The corresponding percentages for iron-deficiency anemia are 2 and 3 percent. The boys of this age group have much better iron stores than girls. Only 1 percent or fewer of 12- to 19-year-old boys were iron deficient or anemic. No doubt these results relate to the 83.1 percent of the boys whose diets met the RDA for iron, compared with 27.7 percent of the girls (Centers for Disease Control, 1998).

Assessments of ninth-graders' dietary intakes of calcium were equally dismal. Only 11 percent consumed the RDA for calcium, with boys consuming 57 percent and girls 45 percent of the 1998 RDA for calcium, which has since been increased. Students not consuming dairy products at all amounted to 21 percent of the respondents (Harel et al., 1998). Substituting soft drinks for milk may contribute to the low intake of calcium. In 1994, about three fourths of adolescent boys drank an average of 34 ounces of soft drinks per day, and two thirds of the girls drank 23 ounces per day (Johnson, Panely, and Wang, 1998).

An association of inadequate food intake with socioeconomic status has been reported. In the Minnesota survey, 40 percent of the students from low socioeconomic backgrounds reported eating fruits and vegetables less than once a day.

Overweight Children and Adolescents

A widespread problem is the increasing prevalence of overweight children older than 3 years. Box 12–4 provides the data, including the variations associated with gender and ethnicity. As is explained in the later chapter on weight control, the solution to overweight and obesity involves not only diet.

Many factors have been investigated as contributing to obesity in children and adolescents, including too little activity and excessive or misguided parental control. Television viewing has been examined as a marker of inactivity. The amount of television viewing has been correlated with ethnicity and obesity. Adolescent non-Hispanic blacks reported a mean of 20.4 hours of television or video viewing per week compared with that for non-Hispanic whites of 13.1 hours (Gordon-Larson, McMurray, and Popkin, 1999). A 2-year randomized, controlled field trial found that

---

Box 12–4 Overweight in Childhood and Adolescence

Overweight has a significant prevalence in young people, as well as in adults. Because a separate chapter is devoted to the subject of weight control, the problem is only briefly described here.

There are no generally accepted definitions of overweight and obesity for youths. Either term is used to define children and adolescents above the 85th or above the 95th percentiles of a reference group for their age and sex. Thus, comparison of prevalence figures becomes difficult.

A clearer distinction relates overweight to measures of body mass index (BMI) and obesity to measures of skinfold thickness that reflect fatness or adiposity. It follows that when the criterion is the BMI, the correct term would be overweight, not obese. Using the 95th percentile as a cutoff is more likely to be specific for obesity than if the 85th percentile were used (Troiano and Flegal, 1998), and the following percentages are based on the 95th percentile. Thus defined, between 1988 and 1994 (Centers for Disease Control, 1997), 13.7 percent of children and 11.5 percent of adolescents were overweight. As depicted in Table 12–8, the prevalence varies by ethnicity, gender, and age.

Comparing prevalence figures for those years to ones collected from 1976 to 1980, prevalence of overweight increased in both sexes and in all age groups except preschool children. There was increased prevalence in 4- and 5-year-old girls, but no significant trend of increasing prevalence of overweight for 2- and 3-year-old children. The increases in mean BMIs for males ranged from 0.6 in 7-year olds to 2.1 in 14-year olds. For females, the average increases in BMIs ranged from 0.5 in 15-year olds to 1.9 in 13-year olds (Troiano and Flegal, 1998).

---

for girls in grades 6 and 7, each hour less of television viewing led to a lowered prevalence of obesity (Gortmaker et al., 1999).

In addition to excessive television viewing, the lack of physical education in schools contributes to children's sedentary lifestyle. Only about 36 percent of youth participate in physical activity in school every day. To address childhood obesity at the community level requires school administrators to reconsider and revise their physical activity policies and programs (Hill and Trowbridge, 1998). Our culture's emphasis on competitive sports often excludes those students most in need of physical activity.

Parents often encourage their children to overeat. Studies have shown that infants are able to regulate the amount of energy they consume when formulas of varying kilocaloric density are fed. Later on, overly restrictive and rigid parental control tends to impede children's ability to self-regulate food intake (Birch, 1996). Children who are least able to adjust their intake of energy in response to the energy content of the diet generally have parents who exert greater control over their children's eating. Moreover, many parents who are authoritarian in their control of child feeding demonstrate uncontrolled eating themselves (Picciano, McBean, and Stallings, 1999). Formula-feeding is also suggested as contributing to lack of self-control in children's eating behavior. Mothers who formula-feed are able to overfeed the infant, insisting that a certain amount be swallowed, whereas breast-feeding mothers do not know how much the infant has consumed so the baby is permitted to stop nursing when it has had enough (Birch and Fisher, 1998).

The conditions permitting or encouraging overweight among youth have evolved over a period of years. No single change is going to reverse the trend. Multiple interventions and strategies are needed for individuals, families, communities, and the nation. The gravity of the situation is evident as pediatricians are seeing more hypertension, dyslipidemia, and non-insulin-dependent diabetes mellitus in obese children. If these trends continue, more efforts and resources will be required to treat these adult diseases in children (Hill and Trowbridge, 1998).

Summary

During periods of rapid growth the need for nutrients is critical. The lack of nutrients or the excessive intake of certain substances during such periods may cause serious, permanent damage in the individual. Both infancy and adolescence are characterized by rapid growth.

While infants require the same nutrients as adults, they need them in different amounts. Breast milk is especially suited to the human infant because the protein, fat, and carbohydrate in breast milk are tailored to the infant's digestive capabilities. After the age of 4 months, semisolid and then solid foods are added to the diet gradually. Nutritional problems in infancy include iron-deficiency anemia, allergies, colic, and diarrhea.

Childhood includes the growth periods of the toddler, the preschool child, and the school-age child. Growth and development during childhood are not as rapid as during infancy. However, the total amounts of nutrients recommended continue to increase with age to meet body needs. Toddlers and preschoolers should be assessed for iron-deficiency anemia.

During adolescence, the final growth spurt of childhood occurs. Physical growth and development are rapid and sexual maturity is attained. Energy, protein, vitamins, and minerals are needed in increasing amounts. Adolescent girls often lack enough calcium in their diets. Major problems in adolescents are self-prescribed reduction diets and poor choices of food. Wellness Tips 12-1 summarizes healthy practices for the nutrition of infants, children, and adolescents.

Table 12–8 Percentages of Overweight Children above the 95th Percentile for Their Age and Sex

ETHNIC GROUP	OVERWEIGHT MALES		OVERWEIGHT FEMALES	
	6 to 11 years old	12 to 17 years old	6 to 11 years old	12 to 17 years old
Mexican American	18.8%	15.0%	15.8%	14.0%
Non-Hispanic black	14.7%	12.5%	17.9%	16.3%
Non-Hispanic white	13.2%	11.6%	11.9%	09.6%

Data from Centers for Disease Control, 1997.

Wellness Tips 12–1

- Habits and attitudes formed in children and youths may last a lifetime. Healthy practices are worth pursuing and may prevent obesity and its attendant disease risks.
- Eating should be pleasurable but portions may need to be limited to achieve moderation, balance, and variety.
- For infants, resist proceeding too fast with new foods. Watching the baby's response to new foods may be entertaining, but long-range effects may be less desirable, such as allergies.
- Ensure the toddler's safety by avoiding any food that might cause choking. Provide sufficient iron-rich foods to prevent anemia.
- Pre-schoolers need frequent healthy snacks to complement the usual 3-meals-a-day pattern.
- Drinking milk with meals would improve the nutrition of many 6- to 12-year-old children. Carbonated beverages or fruit drinks should not displace milk in a healthy diet.
- School-age and adolescent individuals should have enough exercise to permit them the pleasures of eating a healthy diet without incurring overweight or obesity.
- Adolescents need individualized assessment for eating disorders or inappropriate dieting and obesity, both of which are more prevalent in females than in males. Females, particularly, should consume the recommended servings of milk.
- For most children, increasing their intakes of fruit and milk would greatly improve their nutritional state.

Case Study 12–1

Ms. S is a public health nurse whose assignment includes an inner city high school. The principal asked for Ms. S's assistance in improving the students' nutritional and fitness states. A committee was formed that included students, teachers (classroom, home economics, and physical education), cafeteria and kitchen staff, parents, a dietitian from a nearby hospital, YMCA staff, neighborhood business owners, and city officials. The following nursing care plan reflects the program they devised after many meetings.

Nursing Care Plan

Subjective Data	Focus groups with students revealed their opinions of food and physical activity
	A school-wide survey solicited suggestions for classroom content, menu items, and physical activities
Objective Data	Analysis of school lunch menus revealed an average fat content of 38 percent of kilocalories
	Vending machines in and around school offered only high-fat snacks or those with empty kilocalories
	Inspection of building usage identified two days after school when the gym was empty but other parts of the building were in use.
Nursing Diagnosis	NANDA: Potential for Enhanced Community Coping (North American Nursing Diagnosis Association, 1999, with permission.)

Desired Outcomes Evaluation Criteria	Nursing Actions/ Interventions	Rationale
NOC: Community Health Status (Johnson, Maas, and Moorhead, 2000, with permission.)	NIC: Environmental Management: Community (McCloskey and Bulechek, 2000, with permission)	
Students will have increased opportunities to choose healthful foods in and around school	Analyze lunch menus periodically to select areas to improve and to note progress.	Prioritizing changes is important to budget resources. Feedback to cafeteria staff will help maintain their interest and effort to improve.
	Include fresh fruit and vegetables on every lunch menu	Fresh fruits and vegetables can offer vitamins, minerals, and fiber as well as decrease the dominance of high-fat items on the menu.
	Use student tasters to develop low-fat versions of popular dishes	Palatability is critical in devising dishes the students will eat.
	Diversify contents of vending machines to include dairy products, fruit juices, cereal-and-dried-fruit snacks.	Items must be available to give students the opportunity to choose.
Students will demonstrate higher goals for their physical fitness	Evaluate the place of physical education in the curriculum and campaign for needed changes.	To effectively prepare students for life requires offering skill development for an active life.
	Institute fitness testing in physical education classes.	Feedback to students allows them to track their progress.
	Insure that 75 percent of time in physical education class is active.	Inactivity is a major contributor to overweight. PE class should not add to the problem.
	Institute activities students suggest, such as ethnic dances and games other than major sports in the U.S.	Capitalizing on students' interests will recognize the value of their ideas. Later activities might broaden the scope to activities from other cultures.
	Arrange for supervised activities in the gym after school on the days the building would be open for other events. Vary the activities.	If community or volunteer leaders could be recruited, the cost would be minimized for the school and the students. A variety of activities would attract students other than the usual athletes who are active anyway.

Nursing Care Plan (Continued)

Desired Outcomes Evaluation Criteria	Nursing Actions/ Interventions	Rationale
Students will increase knowledge of healthful eating practices within time and budgetary constraints	Design and promote a practical course in skills of modern life for both genders.	Practical courses will attract a different student than strictly academic courses do.
	Devise short instructional units on planning, purchasing, and preparing healthful food for classroom or after school activity sessions.	Short units would give immediate feedback on the value of the information. Consuming the day's lesson is a bonus.
	Incorporate field trips to grocery stores as appropriate.	Expanding the students' perception of the choices open to them would offer the opportunity to increase variety in their diets.

Critical Thinking Questions

1. What additional interventions might be used to improve nutritional intake and increase physical activity in these students?
2. Identify possible barriers to implementing the outlined program. Suggest strategies to overcome them.
3. It is possible the committee's goals are not compatible with those of many of the students in this high school. How could the students be persuaded to value a more healthful lifestyle?

 Study Aids

Subjects	.Internet Sites
Information for Parents	.http://www.ianr.unl.edu/pubs/foods/g1249.htm
	http://nutrition.ucdavis.edu/briefs.html
	http://ificinfo.health.org/index3.htm
	http://www.dole5aday.com
	http://www.gerber.com/health/honey.html
	http://www.gerber.com/health/veg_diets.html
	http://www.gerber.com/health/flavor.html
	http://www.gerber.com/health/oral.html
	http://www.gerber.com/health/eggfree.html
	http://www.gerber.com/health/milk-free.html
	http://www.gerber.com/health/wheatfree.html
	http://www.kidshealth.org/parent/index.html
Activities for Children	.http://www.nppc.org/foodfun.html
	http://www.asfsa.org/kidzone
	http://www.kidshealth.org/kid/index.html
	http://www.kidshealth.org/teen/index.html
	http://www.dole5aday.com/menu/kids/menu.htm
Infant Formula Manufacturers	.http://www.meadjohnson.com/product/hcp-infant
	http://abbott.com/health/pediatricnutrition.htm
	http://carnationbaby.com
Client Information in Many Languages	.http://mhcs.health.nsw.gov.au/health-public-affairs/ mhcs/publications/BHC_3415.html
	http://mhcs.health.nsw.gov.au/health-public-affairs/mhcs/publications/BHC_5070.html
	http://mhcs.health.nsw.gov.au/health-public-affairs/mhcs/publications/BHC_4985.html
Allergies	.http://www.medicalert.org
	http://www.aaaai.org
	http://www.aaaai.org/aadmc
	http://www.foodallergy.org
	http://allergy.mcg.edu
	http://aafa.org
	http://ificinfo.health.org/index11.htm

Chapter Review

1. A nurse in a clinic would identify which of the following infants as needing additional assessment of growth?
   a. Baby girl A, 4 months old, birth weight 7 pounds 6 ounces, present weight 14 pounds 14 ounces
   b. Baby boy B, 2 weeks old, birth weight 6 pounds 10 ounces, present weight 6 pounds 11 ounces
   c. Baby boy C, 6 months old, birth weight 8 pounds 8 ounces, present weight 14 pounds 8 ounces
   d. Baby girl D, 2 months old, birth weight 7 pounds 2 ounces, present weight 9 pounds 10 ounces

2. Which of the following are advantages of breast milk that formula does not provide?
   a. Less fat and cholesterol
   b. More antibodies and less risk of allergy
   c. More fluoride and iron
   d. More vitamin C and vitamin D

3. Which of the following combinations of foods is appropriate for a 6-month-old infant?
   a. Cocoa-flavored wheat cereal, orange juice, and strained chicken
   b. Graham crackers, strained prunes, and stewed tomatoes
   c. Infant cereal, mashed banana, and strained squash
   d. Mashed potatoes, strained beets, and chopped hard-cooked egg

4. If a family is following the dietary guidelines of the American Academy of Pediatrics, which of the following is it important not to eliminate from the school-age child's diet?
   a. Caffeine
   b. Fat
   c. Salt
   d. Sugar

5. Which of the following individuals is at greatest nutritional risk?
   a. 3-month-old infant being fed commercial formula
   b. 3-year-old child who drinks 3 cups of milk a day
   c. 8-year-old child who eats four chocolate chip cookies and drinks 2 glasses of milk after school
   d. 16-year-old girl who is pregnant and attempting weight loss

Clinical Analysis

1. Mrs. T is having her 2-month-old son checked in the well-baby clinic. She tells the nurse that the baby is not sleeping through the night yet. Mrs. T's mother advised her to start the infant on cereal to "fill him up" at bedtime. Despite the nurse's instructions, Mrs. T says she is going to try her mother's idea. Which of the following would be most important if Mrs. T chooses to start the cereal?
   a. Following the cereal with a bedtime bottle to wash it down
   b. Making cream of wheat very thin and feeding the baby with an eyedropper
   c. Putting infant cereal into a bottle and enlarging the nipple hole
   d. Using infant rice cereal mixed with formula

2. Ms. C has given a 24-hour dietary recall for her 18-month-old son. The nurse is alert to identify common causes of choking. To avoid choking accidents, which of the following groups of foods would be considered safest for a toddler?
   a. Apple quarters, green beans, and chicken noodle casserole
   b. Grapes, carrot strips, and macaroni and cheese
   c. Diced peaches, mashed potatoes, and spaghetti
   d. Watermelon chunks, cheese-stuffed celery, and sliced frankfurters

3. Ms. K has delivered a 3-pound 8-ounce premature infant. She had planned to breast-feed. Upon which of the following statements should the nurse base her teaching?
   a. Fortified human breast milk for premature infants is strongly recommended by some experts.
   b. Because of their larger proportion of body weight as water, premature infants need supplemental water after every feeding.
   c. Formula feeding is advisable because room temperature feedings are better absorbed than those at body temperature.
   d. Breast feeding a premature offers no advantage to the infant and is difficult for the mother because of the necessary supplements.

Bibliography

American Academy of Pediatrics Committee on Infectious Diseases: Prevention of rotavirus disease: Guidelines for use of rotavirus vaccine. Pediatrics 102:1483, 1998a.

American Academy of Pediatrics Committee on Nutrition: Iron fortification of infant formulas. Pediatrics 104:119, 1999.

American Academy of Pediatrics Committee on Nutrition: Cholesterol in childhood. Pediatrics 101:141, 1998c.

American Academy of Pediatrics Committee on Nutrition: Soy protein-based formulas: Recommendations for use in infant feeding. Pediatrics 101:148, 1998b.

American Academy of Pediatrics Committee on Pediatric AIDS: Human milk, breastfeeding, and transmission of human immunodeficiency virus in the United States. Pediatrics 96:977, 1995.

American Academy of Pediatrics Work Group on Breastfeeding: Breastfeeding and the use of human milk. Pediatrics 100:1035, 1997.

American Dietetic Association: Position of the American Dietetic Association: Nutrition standards for child-care programs. J Am Diet Assoc 99:981, 1999.

Anderson, DM, and Pittard, WB: Update on neonatal nutrition therapy. Top Clin Nutr 13:8, 1997.

Ballester, F, et al.: Asthma visits to emergency rooms and soybean unloading in the harbors of Valencia and A Coruna, Spain. Am J Epidemiol 149:315, 1999.

Bear, K, and Tigges, BB: Management strategies for promoting successful breast-feeding. Nurse Practitioner 18:50, 1993.

Beech, BM, et al.: Knowledge, attitudes, and practices related to fruit and vegetable consumption of high school students. J Adolesc Health 24;244, 1999.

Bellioni-Businco, B, et al.: Allergenicity of goat's milk in children with cow's milk allergy. J Allergy Clin Immunol 103:1191, 1999.

Bernstein, DI, et al.: Efficacy of live, attenuated, human rotavirus vaccine 89-12 in infants: A randomized placebo-controlled trial. Lancet 354:287, 1999.

Bhattacharya, SK, et al.: Risk factors for the development of dehydration in young children with acute watery diarrhea: A case-control study. Acta Paediatr 84:160, 1995.

Bhutta, SA, Nizami, SQ, and Isani, Z: Zinc supplementation in malnourished children with persistent diarrhea in Pakistan. Pediatrics 103:e42, 1999.

Birch, LL: Children's food acceptance patterns. Nutr Today 31:234, 1996.

Birch, LL, and Fisher, JO: Development of eating behaviors among children and adolescents. Pediatrics 101:539, 1998.

Birch, EE, et al.: Visual acuity and the essentiality of docosahexaenoic acid and arachidonic acid in the diet of term infants. Pediatr Res 44:201, 1998.

Blanco, C, et al.: Latex allergy: Clinical features and cross-reactivity with fruits. Ann Allergy 73:309, 1994.

Bohles, H: Antioxidative vitamins in prematurely and maturely born infants. Int J Vitam Nutr Res 67:321, 1997.

Borowitz, D: Pediatric nutrition. In Feldman, EB: Essentials of Clinical Nutrition. FA Davis Company, Philadelphia, 1988.

Brehler, R, et al.: "Latex-fruit syndrome": Frequency of cross-reacting IgE antibodies. Allergy 52:404-10, 1997.

Bristow, A, et al.: The use of nutritional supplements by 4-12 year olds in England and Scotland. Eur J Clin Nutr 51:366, 1997.

Campbell, MK, and Kelsey, KS: The PEACH survey: A nutrition screening tool for use in early intervention programs. J Am Diet Assoc 94:1156, 1994.

Carey, GB, Quinn, TJ, and Goodwin, SE: Breast milk composition after exercise of different intensities. J Hum Lact 13:115, 1997.

Carlson, SE, et al.: Long-chain fatty acids and early visual and cognitive development of preterm infants. Eur J Clin Nutr 48:S27, 1994.

Centers for Disease Control. Achievements in public health, 1900–1999: Healthier mothers and babies. MMWR 48:849, 1999a. Accessed 10/1/1999 at http://www.cdc.gov/epo/mmwr/preview/mmwrhtml/mm4838a2.htm

Centers for Disease Control. Childhood diarrhea: Messages for parents. 1999b. Accessed 10/29/1999 at http://www.cdc.gov/od/oc/parents/

Centers for Disease Control: Prevalence of overweight among children, adolescents, and adults–United States, 1988–1994. MMWR 46:199, 1997. Accessed at http://www.cdc.gov/ejpo/mmwr/preview/mmwrhtml/00046647.htm

Centers for Disease Control: Recommendations to prevent and control iron deficiency in the United States. MMWR 47:1, 1998. Accessed 09/13/1999 at http://www.cdc.gov/epo/mmwr/preview/mmwrhtml/00051880.htm

Chandra, RK: Five-year follow-up of high-risk infants with family history of allergy who were exclusively breast-fed or fed partial whey hydrolysate, soy, and conventional cow's milk formulas. J Pediatr Gastroenterol Nutr 24:380, 1997.

Chandra, RK, Puri, S, and Hamed, A: Influence of maternal diet during lactation and use of formula feeds on development of atopic eczema in high risk infants. Br Med J 299:228, 1989.

Cheung, PY, Peliowski, A, and Robertson, CM: The outcome of very low birthweight neonates (</=1500 g) rescued by inhaled nitric oxide: Neurodevelopment in early childhood. J Pediatr 1998:735, 1998.

Chezem, J, et al.: Lactation duration: Influences of human milk replacements and formula samples on women planning postpartum employment. JOGNN 27:646, 1998.

Chin, J (ed): Control of Communicable Diseases Manual 17 ed. American Public Health Association, Washington, DC, 2000.

Cinquetti, M, et al.: Latex allergy in a child with banana anaphylaxis. Acta Paediatr 84:709, 1995.

David, J: Honey: An avoidable risk factor for infant botulism. Pediatric Basics #76, 1996. Accessed 09/27/1999 at http://www.gerber.com/health/honey.html

de Andraca, I, Castillo, M, and Walter, T: Psychomotor development and behavior in iron-deficient anemic infants. Nutr Rev 55:125, 1997.

de Boissieu, D: Multiple food allergy: A possible diagnosis in breastfed infants. Acta Paediatr 86:1042, 1997.

de Boissieu, D, Matarazzo, P, and Dupont, C: Allergy to extensively hydrolyzed cow milk proteins in infants: Identification and treatment with an amino acid-based formula. J Pediatr 131:744, 1997.

Deglin, JH, and Vallerand, AH: Davis's Drug Guide for Nurses, ed 6. FA Davis Company, Philadelphia, 1999.

Delbourg, MF, et al.: Hypersensitivity to banana in latex-allergens of 33 and 37 kD. Ann Allergy Asthma Immunol 76:321, 1996.

DePaola, DP, Faine, MP, and Palmer, CA: Nutrition in relation to dental medicine. In Shils, ME, et al. (eds): Modern Nutrition in Health and Disease ed 9. Lippincott Williams and Wilkins, Philadelphia, 1999.

Devine, CM, et al.: Life-course influences on fruit and vegetable trajectories: Qualitative analysis of food choices. JNE 30:361, 1998.

Dewey, KG, et al.: Growth of breast-fed and formula-fed infants from 0 to 18 months: The DARLING study. Pediatrics 89:1035, 1992.

Dixon, LB, et al.: The effect of changes in dietary fat on the food group and nutrient intake of 4- to 10-year old children. Pediatrics 100:863, 1997.

Duffy, L: Breastfeeding after strenuous aerobic exercise: A case report. J Hum Lact 13:145, 1997.

Duggan, C: Failure to thrive: Malnutrition in the pediatric outpatient setting. In Walker, WA, and Watkins, JB: Nutrition in Pediatrics, 2 ed. BC Decker, Hamilton, Ontario, 1997.

Duggan, MB: Cause and cure for iron deficiency in toddlers. Health Visitor 66:250, 1993.

Duncan, LL, and Elder, SB: Breastfeeding the infant with PKU. J Hum Lact 13:231, 1997.

Eliason, BC, and Lewan, RB: Gastroenteritis in children: Principles of diagnosis and treatment. Am Fam Physician 58:1769, 1998.

Enfamil/Enfamil with Iron. Mead Johnson Web page. Accessed 10/02/1999 at http://www.meadjohnson.com/products/hcp-infant/penfaml1.html

Faruque, AS, et al.: Double-blind, randomized, controlled trial of zinc or vitamin A supplementation in young children with acute diarrhea. Acta Paediatr 88:154, 1999.

Fergusson, DM, Horwood, IJ, and Shannon, FT: Early solid feeding and recurrent childhood eczema: A 10-year longitudinal study. Pediatrics 86:541, 1990.

Fly, AD, Uhlin, KL, and Wallace, JP: Major mineral concentrations in human milk do not change after maximal exercise testing. Am J Clin Nutr 68:345, 1998.

Folwaczny, C: Zinc and diarrhea in infants. J Trace Elem Med Biol 11:116, 1997.

Frank, L, et al.: Exposure to peanuts in utero and in infancy and the development of sensitization to peanut allergens in young children. Pediatr Allergy Immunol 10:27, 1999.

Freed, GL: Breast-feeding, time to teach what we preach. JAMA 269:243, 1993.

Fuchs, GJ: Possibilities for zinc in the treatment of acute diarrhea. Am J Clin Nutr 68 (2 Suppl):480S, 1998.

Fukushima, Y, et al.: Preventive effect of whey hydrolysate formulas for mothers and infants against allergy development in infants for the first 2 years. J Nutr Sci Vitaminol 43:397, 1997.

Garcia-Ortiz, JC, et al.: Bronchial asthma induced by hypersensitivity to legumes. Allergol Immunopathol Madr 23:38, 1995.

Gillman, MW, et al.: Family dinner and diet quality among older children and adolescents. Arch Fam Med 9:235, 2000.

Goldman, AS, Goldblum, RM, and Schmalstieg, FC: Protective properties of human milk. In Walker, WA, and Watkins, JB: Nutrition in Pediatrics, 2 ed. BC Decker, Hamilton, Ontario, 1997.

Gonzales, I, et al.: Effect of enteral feeding temperature on feeding tolerance of premature infants. Neonatal Network 14:39, 1995.

Gordon-Larsen, P, McMurray, RG, and Popkin, RM: Adolescent physical activity and inactivity vary by ethnicity: The National Longitudinal Study of Adolescent Health. J Pediatr 135:301, 1999.

Gortmaker, SL, et al.: Reducing obesity via a school-based interdisciplinary intervention among youth: Planet Health. Arch Pediatr Adolesc Med 153:409, 1999.

Graham, SM, Arvela, OM, and Wise, GA: Long-term neurologic consequences of nutritional vitamin B_{12} deficiency in infants. J Pediatr 121:710, 1992.

Greene, LC, et al.: Relationship between early diet and subsequent cognitive performance during adolescence. Biochemical Society Transactions 23:376S, 1995.

Gregory, RL, et al.: Effect of exercise on milk immunoglobulin A. Med Sci Sports Exerc 29:1596, 1997.

Gunnes, M, and Lehmann, EH: Physical activity and dietary constituents as predictors of forearm cortical and trabecular bone gain in health children and adolescents: a prospective study. Acta Paediatr 85:19, 1996.

Hackett, A, Nathan, I, and Burgess, L: Is a vegetarian diet adequate for children? Nutr Health 12:189, 1998.

Hampl, JS, Betts, NM, and Benes, BA: The "age + 5" rule: Comparisons of dietary fiber intake among 4- to 10-year-old children. J Am Diet Assoc 98:1418, 1998.

Hampton, SM: Prematurity, immune function and infant feeding practices. Proc Nutr Soc 58:75, 1999.

Harel, A, et al.: Adolescents and calcium: What they do and do not know and how much they consume. J Adolesc Health 22:225, 1998.

Harris, KJ, et al.: Reducing elementary school children's risks for chronic diseases through school lunch modifications, nutrition education, and physical activity interventions. JNE 29:196, 1997.

Hattevig, G, Sigurs, N, and Kjellman, B: Effects of maternal dietary avoidance during lactation on allergy in children at 10 years of age. Acta Paediatr 88:7, 1999.

Heald, FP, and Gong, EJ: Diet, nutrition, and adolescence. In Shils, ME, et al. (eds): Modern Nutrition in Health and Disease ed 9. Lippincott Williams and Wilkins, Philadelphia, 1999.

Hill, JO, and Trowbridge, FL: Childhood obesity: Future directions and research priorities. Pediatrics 101:570, 1998.

Hinkle, AJ: Community-based nutrition interventions: Reaching adolescents from low-income communities. Ann NY Acad Sci 817:83, 1997.

Horacek, TM, and Betts, NM: Students cluster into 4 groups according to the factors influencing their dietary intake. J Am Diet Assoc 98:1464, 1998.

Horwood, LJ, and Fergusson, DM: Breastfeeding and later cognitive and academic outcomes. Pediatrics 101:e9, 1998. Accessed 9/15/1999 at http://www.pediatrics.org/cgi/content/full/101/1/e9

Hurtado, EK, Claussen, AH, and Scott, KG: Early childhood anemia and mild or moderate mental retardation. Am J Clin Nutr 69:115, 1999.

Hylander, MA, Strobino, DM, and Dhanireddy, R: Human milk feedings and infection among very low birth weight infants. Pediatrics 102:E38, 1998.

Infant mortality and life expectancy for selected countries, 1999. Accessed 12/31/2000 at http://www.infoplease.com/ipa/A0004393.html

Isolauri, E, et al.: Breast-feeding of allergic infants. J Pediatr 134:27, 1999.

Jacobson, D, and Melvin, N: A comparison of temperament and maternal bother in infants with and without colic. Pediatr Nurs 10:181, 1995.

Jakobsson, I, and Lindberg, T: Cow's milk as a cause of infantile colic in breast-fed infants. Lancet 2:437, 1978.

Jakobsson, I, and Lindberg, T: Cow's milk proteins cause infantile colic in breast-fed infants: A double-blind crossover study. Pediatrics 71:268, 1983.

Janken, JK, et al.: Changing nursing practice through research utilization: Consistent support for breast-feeding mothers. Applied Nursing Research 12:22, 1999.

Jocson, MAL, Mason, EO, and Schanler, RJ: The effects of nutrient fortification and varying storage conditions on host defense properties of human milk. Pediatrics 100:240, 1997. Accessed 10/02/1999 through http://www.pediatrics.org/all.shtml

Johnson, M, Maas, M, and Moorhead, S: Nursing Outcomes Classification (NOC), ed 2. Mosby, Philadelphia, 2000.

Johnson, RK, Panely, C, and Wang, MQ: The association between noon beverage consumption and diet quality of school-age children. Journal of Child Nutrition and Management 22:95, 1998.

Johnston, CC, et al.: Calcium supplementation and increases in bone mineral density in children. N Engl J Med 327:82, 1992.

Kennedy, E, and Davis, C: US Department of Agriculture School Breakfast Program. Am J Clin Nutr 67 (suppl):798S, 1998.

Kinsbourne, M: Sugar and the hyperactive child. N Engl J Med 330:355, 1994.

Klish, WJ, and Montandon, CM: Nutrition and upper gastrointestinal disorders. In Halpern, SL (ed): Quick Reference to Clinical Nutrition, ed 2. JB Lippincott Company, Philadelphia, 1987.

Kmietowicz, Z: Women warned to avoid peanuts during pregnancy and lactation. Brit Med J 316:1926, 1998.

Kuan, LW, et al.: Health system factors contributing to breastfeeding success. Pediatrics 104:e28, 1999. Accessed 10/24/1999 through http://www.pediatrics.org

Latasa, M, et al.: Fruit sensitization in patients with allergy to latex. J Investig Allergol Clin Immunol 5:97, 1995.

Lino, M, et al.: Report card on the diet quality of children. Nutrition Insights 9: October 1998. Accessed 9/26/1999 through http://www.usda.gov/cnpp

Lira, RI, Ashworth, A, and Morris, SS: Effect of zinc supplementation on the morbidity, immune function, and growth of low-birth-weight, full-term infants in northeast Brazil. Am J Clin Nutr 68 (2Suppl):418S, 1998.

Llatser, R, Zambrano, C, and Guillaumet, B: Anaphylaxis to natural rubber latex in a girl with food allergy: Pediatrics 94:736, 1994.

Lo, CW: Human milk: Nutritional properties. In Walker, WA, and Watkins, JB: Nutrition in Pediatrics, 2 ed. BC Decker, Hamilton, Ontario, 1997.

Loosli, AR, and Ruud, JS: Meatless diets in female athletes: A red flag. Phys Sportsmed 26:45, 1998.

Lucas, A, et al.: Breast milk and subsequent intelligence quotient in children born preterm. Lancet 339:261, 1992.

Lust, KD, Brown, JE, and Thomas, W: Maternal intake of cruciferous vegetables and other foods and colic symptoms in exclusively breast-fed infants. J Am Diet Assoc 96:46, 1996.

Majamaa, H, and Isolauri, E: Probiotics: A novel approach in the management of food allergy. J Allergy Clin Immunol 99:179, 1997.

McCloskey, JC, and Bulechek, GM: Nursing Interventions Classification (NIC), 3 ed. Mosby, Philadelphia, 2000.

McClung, HJ, Murray, RD, and Heitlinger, LA: The Internet as a source for current patient information. Pediatrics 101:e2, 1998. Accessed 5-3-00 at http://www.pediatrics.org/cgi/content/full/101/6/e2

Mead Johnson Nutritionals. Enfamil human milk fortifier literature. Received by FAX 10/27/1999.

Mennella, JA, Johnson, A, and Beauchamp, GK: Garlic ingestion by pregnant women alters the odor of amniotic fluid. Chemical Senses 20:207, 1995.

Merhav, H, et al.: Tea drinking and microcytic anemia in infants. Am J Clin Nutr 41:1210, 1985.

Moon, A, and Kleinman, RE: Allergic gastroenteropathy in children. Annals of Allergy, Asthma, and Immunology 74:5, 1995.

Mulford, C: Swimming upstream: Breastfeeding care in a nonbreastfeeding culture. JOGNN 24:464, 1995.

Neumark-Sztainer, D, et al.: Lessons learned about adolescent nutrition from the Minnesota Adolescent Health Survey. J Am Diet Assoc 98:1449, 1998.

Nicklas, TA, et al.: Outcomes of a high school program to increase fruit and vegetable consumption: Gimme 5—a fresh nutrition concept for students. J Sch Health 68:348, 1998.

North American Nursing Diagnosis Association: Nursing Diagnoses: Definitions and Classification 1999-2000, North American Nursing Diagnosis Association, Philadelphia, 1999.

Nursing 2000 Drug Handbook. Springhouse Corporation, Springhouse, PA, 2000.

Oldacus, G, et al.: Extensively and partially hydrolyzed infant formula for allergy prophylaxis. Arch Dis Child 77:4, 1997.

Olson, RE: The dietary recommendations of the American Academy of Pediatrics. Am J Clin Nutr 61:271, 1995.

Olson, RE: Vitamin K. In Shils, ME, et al. (eds): Modern Nutrition in Health and Disease ed 9. Lippincott Williams and Wilkins, Philadelphia, 1999.

Opplinger, RA, et al.: Wisconsin minimum weight program reduces weight-cutting practices of high school wrestlers. Clin J Sport Med 8:26, 1998.

Penny, ME, et al.: Randomized, community-based trial of the effect of zinc supplementation, with and without other micronutrients, on the duration of persistent childhood diarrhea in Lima, Peru. J Pediatr 135(2 Pt 1):208, 1999.

Pesa, J: Psychological factors associated with dieting behaviors among female adolescents. J Sch Health 69:196, 1999.

Phylactos, AC, et al.: Polyunsaturated fatty acids and antioxidants in early development. Possible prevention of oxygen-induced disorders. Eur J Clin Nutr (suppl 2) 48:S17, 1994.

Picciano, MF, McBean, LD, and Stallings, VA: How to grow a healthy child: A conference report. Nutr Today 34:6, 1999.

Pickering, LK, et al.: Modulation of the immune system by human milk and infant formula containing nucleotides. Pediatrics 101:242, 1998.

Piecuch, RE, et al.: Outcome of extremely low birth weight infants (500 to 999 grams) over a 12-year period. Pediatrics 100:633, 1997. Accessed 10/29/1999 through http://www.pediatrics.org

Pollitt, E: Does breakfast make a difference in school? J Am Diet Assoc 95:1134, 1995.

Quinn, TJ, and Carey, GB: Does exercise intensity or diet influence lactic acid accumulation in breast milk? Med Sci Sports Exerc 31:105, 1999.

Rautanen, T, et al.: Management of acute diarrhea with low osmolarity oral rehydration solutions and Lactobacillus strain FF. Arch Dis Child 79:157, 1998.

Requejo, AM, et al.: The age at which meat in first included in the diet affects the incidence of iron deficiency and ferropenic anaemia in a group of pre-school children from Madrid. Int J Vitam Nutr Res 69:127, 1999.

Rodriquez, M, et al.: Hypersensitivity to latex, chestnut and banana. Ann Allergy 70:31, 1993.

Rogowski, J: Cost-effectiveness of care for very low birth weight infants. Pediatrics 102:35, 1998.

Roy, SK, et al.: Impact of zinc supplementation on persistent diarrhea in malnourished Bangladeshi children. Acta Paediatr 87:1235, 1998.

Roy, SK, et al.: Randomized controlled trial of zinc supplementation in malnourished Bangladeshi children with acute diarrhea. Arch Dis Child 77:196, 1997.

Ryan, AS: The resurgence of breastfeeding in the United States. Pediatrics 99:e12, 1997. Accessed 9/15/1999 at http://www.pediatrics.org/cgi/content/full/99/4/e12

Saarinen, UM, and Kajosaari, M: Breastfeeding as prophylaxis against atopic disease: Prospective follow-up study until 17 years old. Lancet 346:1065, 1995.

Sampson, AE, et al.: The nutritional impact of breakfast consumption on the diets of inner-city African-American elementary school children. J Natl Med Assoc 87:195, 1995.

Sampson, HA: Managing peanut allergy. Br Med J 312:1050, 1996.

Sampson, HA, Mendelson, L, and Rosen, JP: Fatal and near-fatal anaphylactic reactions to food in children and adolescents. N Engl J Med 327:380, 1992.

SaraOclar, Y, et al.: Latex sensitivity among hospital employees and atopic children. Turk J Pediatr 40:61, 1998.

Savilahti, E: Cow's milk allergy. Allergy 36:73, 1981.

Scariati, PD, Grummer-Strawn, LM, and Fein, SB: A longitudinal analysis of infant morbidity and the extent of breastfeeding in the United States. Pediatrics 99:e5, 1977. Accessed 9/16/1999 at http://www.pediatrics.org/all.shtml

Schanler, RJ: The low-birth-weight infant. In Walker, WA, and Watkins, JB: Nutrition in Pediatrics, 2 ed. BC Decker, Hamilton, Ontario, 1997.

Schanler, RJ, Shulman, RJ, and Lau, C: Feeding strategies for premature infants: Beneficial outcomes of feeding fortified human milk versus preterm formula. Pediatrics 103:1150, 1999.

Seeds of change. Consumer Reports 64: 41, 1999.

Separating the wheat from the chaff. Consumer Reports 64:30, 1999.

Skinner, JD, Carruth, BR, Houck, K, et al.: Mealtime communication patterns of infants from 2 to 24 months of age. JNE 30:8, 1998.

Skinner, JD, et al.: Toddlers' food preferences: Concordance with family members' preferences. JNE 30:17, 1998.

Sobal, J, and Marquart, LF: Vitamin/mineral supplement use among high school athletes. Adolescence 29:835, 1994.

Story, M, et al.: Nutritional concerns in American Indian and Alaska native children: Transitions and future directions. J Am Diet Assoc 98:170, 1998.

Sturman, JA, and Chesney, RW: Taurine in pediatric nutrition. Pediatr Clin North Am 42:879, 1995.

Sullivan, SA, and Birch LL: Infant dietary experience and acceptance of solid foods. Pediatrics 93:271, 1994.

Taylor, SL, Hefle, SL, and Munoz-Furlong, A: Food allergies and avoidance diets. Nutr Today 34:15, 1999.

Thomas, JT, and de Santis, L: Feeding and weaning practices of Cuban and Haitian immigrant mothers. J Transcult Nurs 6:34, 1995.

Thorp, FK, Pierce, P, and Deedwania, C: Nutrition in the infant and young child. In Halpern, SL (ed): Quick Reference to Clinical Nutrition, ed 2. JB Lippincott Company, Philadelphia, 1987.

Troiano, RP, and Flegal, KM: Overweight children and adolescents: Description, epidemiology, and demographics. Pediatrics 101(3 Suppl):497, 1998. Accessed through http://www.Pediatrics.org

Turnbull, F: Promoting health: breastfeeding in PICU. Paediatric Nursing 11:39, 1999.

United States Department of Agriculture. The Food Guide Pyramid for Young Children. March 25, 1999. Accessed 9/26/1999 at http://www.usda.gov/cnpp/KidsPyra/index.htm

United States Department of Agriculture. Pyramid Servings Data. 1994-96 Continuing Survey of Food Intakes by Individuals. February 1999. Accessed 10/05/1999 at http://www.barc.usda.gov

United States Department of Health and Human Services. Healthy People 2010. Accessed 4/14/00 at http://web.health.gov/healthypeople /document/html/volume2/16mich.htm#_TOC471971365

Van Asperen, PP, Kemp, AS, and Mellis, CM: Immediate food hypersensitivity reactions on the first known exposure to the food. Arch Dis Child 58:253, 1983.

Vandenplas, Y: Myths and facts about breastfeeding: Does it prevent later atopic disease? Acta Paediatr 86:1283, 1997.

vanZoeren-Grobbin, D, et al.: Vitamin E status in preterm infants: Assessment by plasma and erythrocyte vitamin E-lipid ratios and hemolysis tests. J Pediatr Gastroenterol Nutr 26:73, 1998.

von Kries, R, et al.: Breast feeding and obesity: Cross sectional study. Brit Med J 319:147, 1999. Accessed 09/15/1999 at http://www.bmj.com/cgi/content/short/319/7203/147

Weir, DG, and Scott, JM: Vitamin B_{12} "Cobalamin." In Shils, ME, et al. (eds): Modern Nutrition in Health and Disease ed 9. Lippincott Williams and Wilkins, Philadelphia, 1999.

Wharton, B: Weaning: Pathophysiology, practice, and policy. In Walker, WA, and Watkins, JB: Nutrition in Pediatrics, 2 ed. BC Decker, Hamilton, Ontario, 1997.

Williams, CL: Importance of dietary fiber in childhood. J Am Diet Assoc 95:1140, 1149, 1995.

Williams, CL, Bollela, M, and Wynder, EL: A new recommendation for dietary fiber in childhood. Pediatrics 96:985, 1995.

Williams, J, et al.: Iron supplemented formula milk related to reduction in psychomotor decline in infants from inner city areas: Randomized study. Brit Med J 318:693, 1999.

Wolraich, ML, et al.: Effects of diets high in sucrose or aspartame on the behavior and cognitive performance of children. N Engl J Med 330:301, 1994.

Wolraich, ML, Wilson, DB, and White, JW: The effect of sugar on behavior or cognition in children. JAMA 274:1617, 1995.

Wyshak, G: Teenaged girls, carbonated beverage consumption, and bone fractures. Arch Pediatr Adolesc Med 154:610, 2000.

Yaseen, H: Fluid, electrolyte and nutritional requirements of extremely premature infants during the first days of life: Pathophysiology and guidelines. Neonatal Intensive Care 9:39, 1996.

Yu, SM, Kogan, MD, and Gergen, P: Vitamin-mineral supplement use among preschool children in the United States. Pediatrics 100:e4, 1997. Accessed 4/23/2000 at http://www.pediatrics.org/cgi/content/full/100/5/e4

Zipursky, A: Prevention of vitamin K deficiency bleeding in newborns. Br J Haematol 104:430, 1999.

Zlotkin, SH, Atkinson, S, and Lockitch, G: Trace elements in nutrition for premature infants. Clin Perinatol 22:223, 1995.

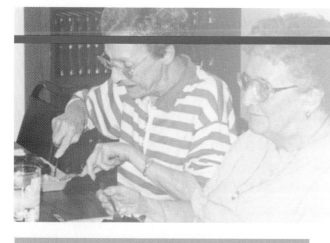

CHAPTER **13**

Life Cycle Nutrition: The Mature Adult

LEARNING OBJECTIVES

After completing this chapter, the student should be able to:

1. Identify the foods and food groups most likely to be lacking or excessive in the diets of adults.
2. Describe the changes in the older adult's body that affect nutritional status.
3. Explain how a nutritional assessment of an older adult differs from that of a younger one.
4. Illustrate ways in which food can be used to aid in the developmental tasks of adulthood.
5. List several suggestions to improve food intake for older people in a variety of living situations.

The life cycle of human growth and development continues throughout the adult years. Both psychosocial and physical developments continue as a person matures. This chapter discusses the impact on nutrition of the physiological and psychosocial changes that occur during young, middle, and older adult years. Because much of this book emphasizes the nutritional needs of the average adult, the main focus of this chapter is the older adult.

Overall food consumption of American adults poorly matches the Food Guide Pyramid recommendations, as Figure 13–1 illustrates. Whites of high socioeconomic status have reduced their consumption of high-fat foods (1989–1991 compared with 1965) and followed other dietary guidelines to a greater extent than have either whites or blacks of middle or low socioeconomic status (Popkin, Siega-Riz, and Haines, 1996). Even so, a major threat to health in adulthood is being overweight (Box 13–1). Weight control is discussed in detail in Chapter 18.

Young Adulthood

Young adulthood spans ages 18 through 39. Not all 18-year-olds are adults, developmentally speaking, nor are all 40-year-olds middle-aged in

thought or behavior. Chronological age is a convenient means of grouping people but may have limited applicability to a given individual.

Psychosocial Development

For identifying the patient's stage of psychosocial development, chronological age is not as important as a person's life situation. During the early years of young adulthood, the individual may be completing the adolescent task of identity. According to Erik Erikson, the developmental task of young adulthood is **intimacy** (Table 13–1). For example, people who delay commitment to a life partner until their 30s and 40s will probably be working at achieving intimacy; other 40-year-olds may be tackling the next task of generativity.

To achieve intimacy, the individual strives to build reciprocal, caring relationships. The word "intimacy" may suggest sexuality, but intimate relationships are not necessarily sexual. Solid friendships are based on intimacy, the revealing of oneself to another, at a special, quiet dinner perhaps. Failure at the task of intimacy could result in isolation. At this stage, perhaps more than with other developmental tasks, it is apparent that a person chooses what he or she is to become.

Nutrition in the Young Adult

Throughout this book, the RDAs and AIs for individual nutrients, as well as dietary guidelines, have been specified. Often the age categories in the literature differ from source to source. Any division into young, middle, and older adulthood is somewhat arbitrary.

The nutritional gender differences noted in children and adolescents continue to be shown in young men and women between the ages of 20 and 39 (Table 13–2). Women, according to the U.S. Department of Agriculture in 1999 were a little closer to achieving the goal of less than 30 percent of kilocalories derived from fat, 32 percent, compared with men's 34 percent. They tied men for fruit consumption but otherwise had poorer diets than men. More than half the men consumed the numbers of servings recommended in the Food Guide Pyramid for the grain, vegetable, and meat groups. By contrast, not even half the women did so for a single food group. Whole-grain consumption constituted only 13 percent of men's grain intake and 15 percent of women's. Choices in vegetables were heavily slanted toward white potatoes. Of the vegetables reported, about 38 percent of men's servings and 31 percent

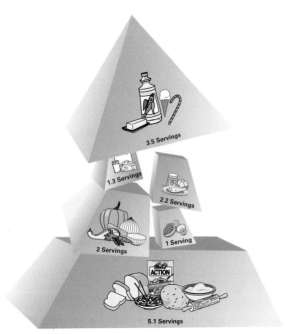

Figure 13–1:
The Tumbling Pyramid. Actual consumption of foods in the United States shows the meat group as the only food group for which intake corresponds with recommendations. (From Eating in America Today, ed 2, National Live Stock and Meat Board, courtesy of National Cattlemen's Beef Association, with permission.)

of women's were white potatoes (United States Department of Agriculture, February 1999).

Although 24-hour recall data are insufficient to evaluate an individual's nutritional status, recall data from large groups can serve to identify problem areas. An analysis of cereal consumption in women of childbearing age revealed that those who ate ready-to-eat breakfast foods twice in a two-week period had a mean daily folate intake of 220 micrograms, compared with 137 micrograms for women who consumed cereal less frequently. Neither group approached the recommended 400-microgram RDA, however (Albertson, Tobelmann, and Marquart, 1997). In Louisiana, 37 percent of young adults skipped breakfast and thereby increased by two to five times their risk of having an inadequate diet. Two-thirds of those who skipped breakfast had a snack before lunch (Nicklas, et al, 1998). If those snacks consisted of nourishing food, fortified ready-to-eat cereal instead of doughnuts, for example, the day's overall nutrient intake would improve.

> **Box 13–1** The Prevalance of Overweight and Inactivity in Adults
>
> In 1960–1962 the prevalence of overweight in persons 20 to 74 years of age was 24.3%. By 1988–1994 the prevalence of overweight in persons 20 years of age and older was 33.3% in men and 36.4% in women (Kuczmarski et al., 1994). Over half of black, non-Hispanic Americans (52.3%) and Mexican Americans (50.1%) were overweight, compared with 33.5% of white, non-Hispanic Americans (Centers for Disease Control, 1997).
>
> No doubt contributing to the increased prevalence of overweight is inactivity. Between 1988 and 1991, 17 percent of men and 27 percent of women 20 years of age and older reported no leisuretime physical activity. The groups with the greatest percentage of individuals reporting no leisuretime physical activity were Mexican American women (46%), non-Hispanic black women (40%), and Mexican American men (33%). For almost all subgroups that reported leisuretime physical activity, the most popular pursuits were walking and gardening/yard work (Crespo et al., 1996).

Middle Adulthood

The middle adult years are those between ages 40 and 65. Mandatory retirement rules in the past designated age 65 as the beginning of old age. Now the age range for middle age is more flexible.

Psychosocial Development

Erikson's task of **generativity** involves guiding the next generation to adopt one's values and serving as a mentor. In this way, middle-aged adults can attain a measure of immortality, by influencing not only their own children, but also their students or protégés at work.

Teaching family members to prepare traditional foods, for example, may help a person achieve generativity.

Nutrition in Middle Adulthood

In 1999, the U.S.D.A. indicated that more than half the 40- to 59-year-old men consumed the number of servings recommended by the Food Guide Pyramid for grain, vegetables, and meat. The 40- to 59-year-old women reported marginally better intakes than did the 20- to 39-year-olds. Exactly 50 percent of the 50- to 59-year-old women consumed at least 3 servings of vegetables on the days surveyed. See Table 13–3. These middle-aged adults chose only 14 to 17 percent of their grains as whole grains. They were slightly more inclined than the 20- to 39-year-olds to choose vegetables other than white potatoes, which for 40- to 59-year-old men comprised 29 percent of their vegetables and for women 27 percent. The men

Table 13–1 Erikson's Theory of Psychosocial Development in Maturity

Stage of Life	Developmental Task	Opposing Negative Trait	Use of Food to Achieve Task
Young Adult	Intimacy	Isolation	Arranging candlelight dinner
Middle Adult	Generativity	Stagnation	Teaching someone to prepare family favorite or ethnic dishes
Older Adult	Integrity	Despair	Using food fragrances or memories of food to reminisce

TABLE 13–2 Reported Compliance with Food Guide Pyramid Recommendations by Men and Women 20 to 39 Years of Age

	20 to 29 Year Old Men	30 to 39 Year Old Men	20 to 29 Year Old Women	30 to 39 Year Old Women
At least 6 Servings of Grains	71 percent	70 percent	41 percent	41 percent
At least 3 Servings of Vegetables	67 percent	69 percent	43 percent	44 percent
At least 2 Servings of Fruit	23 percent	23 percent	20 percent	23 percent
At least 5 ounces of Meat Equivalents*	63 percent	66 percent	25 percent	27 percent
At least 2 Servings of Dairy Products	30 percent	30 percent	17 percent	19 percent

*For this tabulation includes meat, poultry, fish, simulated meat products, eggs, tofu, peanut butter, nuts and seeds, but excludes dry beans and peas that were included with vegetables.
United States Department of Agriculture, February 1999

and the 40- to 49-year-old women consumed 34 percent of their kilocalories as fat, compared with 33 percent by the 50- to 59-year-old women (United States Department of Agriculture, February 1999).

The U.S.D.A. report does not indicate the rationale for selecting certain menu items. The knowledge that, for example, middle-aged women avoided dairy products for fear of gaining weight or because of lactose intolerance could affect educational efforts. Analysis of data from 1989 to 1991 revealed that six food categories accounted for 47.8 percent of adults' fiber intake. Yeast bread contributed 14.6 percent, ready-to-eat cereal 8 percent, dried beans and lentils 7.9 percent, white potatoes 7.3 percent, tomatoes 5.7 percent, and pasta 4.3 percent (Subar et al., 1998). Given their inclinations to select refined grains and the already large contribution of yeast bread to fiber intake, inspiring middle-aged adults to select whole grains more frequently should help boost fiber intake.

Older Adulthood

The older population in the United States is changing demographically. Life expectancy in 1900 was 45 years. Current life expectancy for women is 78 years and for men 71 years. In 1900, 4 percent of the population was over age 65; now the percentage is at 12 percent (25 million people) and growing. Barring major calamities, by early in this century 20 percent of the population will be over 65 years of age, and 11 percent will be over 75 years of age. The fastest-growing segment of the population is people older than 85.

This aging of the population is attributed to improved sanitation, an increased concern for safety, and control of communicable diseases. In 1900, 1 in 10 infants died; now the figure is 1 in 100. In the days of the "Wild West," a woman usually died before her youngest child left home. A man would have one horse his entire adult life (the average life span of horses is 25 years). The work world was harsh. Children worked in heavy industry. The death of one miner a week in a relatively small mining operation was commonplace. Today, by contrast, the major causes of death in adults are heart disease, cancer, and stroke. All of them are linked to lifestyle, including a dietary component.

Distinctions Among Older Adults

As a group, older adults display a wide range of interests and abilities. Some are content to stay at home and work in the garden. Others travel extensively. Only 10 percent are confined in any serious way. In a roomful of 3-year-old children, individuals are more like each other than in a roomful of 70-year-old adults. In old age, people become "more like themselves," accentuating traits they have had all along. Many older people have difficulty changing their behavior patterns, including those related to food.

The stereotype of old folks in a nursing home is just that, a stereotype. Only 5 percent of older adults live in nursing homes. That 5 percent, however, represents more than 1 million clients. This subgroup of the older population has special nutrient needs. Up to 50 percent cannot feed themselves. Often they have very low calcium intakes and low intakes of vitamin A, vitamin C, thiamin, riboflavin, and iron. If they do not receive sufficient sun exposure or do not consume fortified dairy products, they are at increased risk for vitamin D deficiency.

Psychosocial Development

Erikson's developmental task for older adults to achieve is **integrity,** in the sense of being whole or complete. Those who accomplish this task will look back on their lives as worthwhile. Although they

TABLE 13–3 Reported Compliance with Food Guide Pyramid Recommendations by Men and Women 40 to 59 Years of Age

	40 to 49 Year Old Men	50 to 59 Year Old Men	40 to 49 Year Old Women	50 to 59 Year Old Women
At least 6 Servings of Grains	68 percent	59 percent	39 percent	37 percent
At least 3 Servings of Vegetables	62 percent	67 percent	49 percent	50 percent
At least 2 Servings of Fruit	27 percent	30 percent	23 percent	31 percent
At least 5 ounces of Meat Equivalents*	65 percent	61 percent	27 percent	25 percent
At least 2 Servings of Dairy Products	29 percent	20 percent	16 percent	14 percent

*For this tabulation includes meat, poultry, fish, simulated meat products, eggs, tofu, peanut butter, nuts and seeds, but excludes dry beans and peas that were included with vegetables.
United States Department of Agriculture, February 1999

may have suffered some failures and have some regrets, they are able to see their lives in perspective. They can forgive themselves for their faults because they know they did the best they could with what they had.

A technique to help the older person achieve integrity is reminiscence. Asking an older person to recall special foods can stimulate reminiscence. Familiar food odors oftentimes will evoke memories.

Socially, older adults often must adapt to the loss of friends and relatives. The death of a spouse demands a tremendous adjustment. The accompanying depression and new responsibility for tasks the spouse performed may significantly affect an older person's food intake.

Physical Changes of Aging

Just as adolescents have a changing body image, so do older adults. Even without frank disease, the physical abilities of older adults diminish. "Middle-age spread" gives way to dwindling bulk and waning strength. Among the body systems significantly changed in the aging process are the integumentary, sensory, gastrointestinal, urinary, musculoskeletal, nervous, endocrine, and cardiovascular systems.

Integumentary System

Many changes take place in the skin as a person ages. As subcutaneous fat is lost, the skin becomes dry and wrinkled. Less elasticity is present to spring back after a pinch to the forearm, the usual site assessed for hydration status (the skin of the forehead or over the breastbone is a more reliable site in the elderly client than the forearm). The older adult also loses some of the ability to synthesize vitamin D from sunshine. An 80-year-old person requires almost twice as much time in the sun to produce a given amount of vitamin D as a 20-year-old (Ryan, Eleazer, and Egbert, 1995).

Sensory System

Four senses become markedly less acute as a person ages: vision, hearing, taste, and smell. Because the sense receptors do not deteriorate equally, some of the sense loss is attributed to changes in the central nervous system. Extensive variation exists among individuals.

EYES Vision is reduced. The older person sees reds, oranges, and yellows better than blues and violets. Clouding of the lens of the eye—cataract formation—decreases overall vision. The fine print labels on food items may be illegible to the elderly. Older eyes do not adjust well to glare.

Vision changes may make grocery shopping burdensome. Food preparation may become not only difficult but also hazardous if the person cannot see adequately. Poor vision was shown to be associated with lower protein and energy intakes in home health-care clients, independent of other medical conditions (Payette et al, 1995).

EARS The sound receptors in the inner ear deteriorate. First to be lost is the ability to perceive high tones. The older person with poor hearing usually hears men's voices better than women's. Hearing aids do not fully compensate for the hearing loss. In fact, they often magnify sideline noise to the point of distracting the wearer. The result may be social isolation when it becomes too laborious to interact with others. Socializing at meals may become embarrassing or frustrating and older people may avoid such interaction.

NOSE AND TONGUE For the sense of taste to function well, the sense of smell must also be intact. Food tastes bland when a person has a head cold. Many, but not all, older adults have dulled senses of smell and taste that they begin to notice about age 60. The sense of smell is frequently more impaired by aging than is the sense of taste, but both faculties are important to help protect the person from noxious elements in the environment. Blindfolded older subjects showed only half the ability of younger ones to recognize blended tastes, a loss attributed mainly to declining olfactory senses (Morley, 1997).

Taste receptors are concentrated on the tongue's surface but also are located at the base of the tongue, on the soft palate, and other areas of the nasopharynx. The traditional taste receptors permit recognition of sweet, sour, salty, and bitter sensations, but functions of taste nerves have been shown to transmit qualities of metallic and chalky (Schiffman, 1997). The sense of taste declines in most but not all aging clients. Usually salt receptors are most affected and sweet receptors least affected (Morley, 1997). Increasing the amounts of seasonings and condiments may be the older person's solution to diminishing taste sensations.

Gastrointestinal System

Particularly crucial to nutrition is gastrointestinal function. Hundreds of processes are required for the proper digestion, absorption, and metabolism of foods. Many functions of the gastrointestinal system decline significantly in older people.

By the age of 65, approximately 40 percent of Americans are edentulous or toothless and another 20 percent have lost half of their teeth (Martin, 1995). Missing teeth or those in poor repair and the general condition of the mouth can affect the amounts and textures of foods consumed. The major cause of tooth loss in the older adult is not dental caries but **periodontal** disease, which affects the gums.

Dentures, like hearing aids, only partially compensate. Dentures are only 20 percent as efficient as natural teeth (Martin, 1995). Furthermore, a denture cannot be effective if the underlying tissue is in poor condition. Box 13–2 illustrates a self-administered dental screening form designed to alert older people to their need for dental care. It was validated with a clinical dental examination on 165 people 65 to 94 years old, correctly identifying 82 percent of those with dental disease. Notice that not all the items are weighted equally.

The production of saliva decreases sharply in older adults. This condition is called **xerostomia**. Chewing and swallowing become more difficult, and food intake may be affected. Also with age, less mucus and smaller quantities of enzymes are secreted.

Atrophic gastritis, a chronic inflammation of the stomach lining, with decreases in size of the glands and mucous membranes, occurs in 10 to 30 percent of the U.S. population over the age of 60 (Russell, Rasmussen, and Lichtenstein, 1999). An extreme case is **achlorhydria**, the absence of hydrochloric acid in the stomach. Either of these conditions may interfere with protein digestion and with vitamin and mineral absorption. Vitamin B_{12} may remain locked to the food protein, and less iron will be absorbed in the more alkaline environment.

Intestinal motility decreases because of lessened muscle tone. Medications may interfere with electrolyte balance, also diminishing muscle tone. By the age of 70, the liver loses 18 percent of its weight and has reduced capabilities.

Box 13–2 The D-E-N-T-A-L Screening Survey Form

Certain dental conditions have been known to interfere with proper nutritional intake and possibly disposing a person to involuntary weight loss. Please answer the following questions regarding your dental health by placing a check before the conditions that apply to you.

		Point Value
___	Dry mouth	(2)
___	Eating difficulty	(1)
___	No recent dental care (within 2 years)	(1)
___	Tooth or mouth pain	(2)
___	Alteration or change in food selection	(1)
___	Lesions, sores, or lumps in the mouth	(2)

If you have scored more than 2 points on this survey you may have a dental problem that could be affecting your overall health and general well-being. We urge you to seek dental care as soon as possible for a check-up.

(Bush et al., 1996, with permission.)

Urinary System

The kidneys lose about 10 percent of their weight by the time an adult reaches the age of 70. At age 80, the blood flow to the kidneys is half of what it was at age 35. This compromised kidney function makes urine samples less reliable for nutrient analyses in the elderly. Two laboratory tests frequently are used to assess renal function: a blood urea nitrogen (BUN) test and a serum creatinine test. An increase in the BUN level usually indicates a decrease in kidney function. It may also be elevated in dehydration or if a excessive protein is presented to the liver for breakdown, as with a high-protein diet or with gastrointestinal bleeding.

Conversely, the BUN may be decreased in liver disease. Patients with even slightly elevated BUNs may not be able to excrete the waste products from protein metabolism. Caregivers must be judicious about giving high-protein nutritional supplements to older people with elevated BUNs. Creatinine, an end product of creatine metabolism, is excreted very efficiently by the healthy kidney. The amount of creatinine produced is proportional to the individual's skeletal muscle mass and remains fairly constant in the absence of extensive muscle damage. The serum creatinine test has the advantage over the BUN of being little affected by dehydration, malnutrition, or liver function. Creatinine levels may not detect decreased kidney function, however, if a slow decline in renal function occurs simultaneously with a slow decrease in muscle mass, as happens in the aging process (Watson and Jaffe, 1995). Consequently both tests may be performed to obtain a more complete diagnostic picture.

Musculoskeletal System

The major loss of body mass in the older adult involves muscle mass. This decreased lean body mass may be due in part to lessened physical activity and to alterations in protein metabolism possibly related to diminished anabolic hormone concentrations (Groff, Gropper, and Hunt, 1995). By age 70, a person's skeletal muscle diminishes by 40 percent. Because muscle is a more metabolically active tissue than fat, energy needs decline with the diminished muscle mass.

Nutritional deprivation and catabolic states can affect the muscles of respiration in the chest and diaphragm. Because the older person relies more on the diaphragm than the chest muscles to breathe, a full stomach may impede breathing to a greater extent than in a younger person (Quinn, 1997). The effect of respiratory disease on nutrition is discussed in greater detail in Chapter 24.

Perhaps more noticeable than the overall loss of muscle is the loss of height in older people. The average lifetime loss of height amounts to 2.9 centimeters (1.16 inches) in men and 4.9 centimeters (1.96 inches) in women. A major cause of this loss of height is osteoporosis. The bone loss amounts to about 8 percent per decade after age 35, so that by the age of 70, 25 percent of the bone structure is gone.

Joint surfaces are roughened by arthritis. By age 50, half of all adults have degenerative joint disease. Arthritis impairs the use of the hands for opening jars, chopping raw foods, and cutting cooked foods at the table. Arthritis also impairs the operation of the mandibular joint of the jaw for chewing.

Nervous System

By the time a person reaches old age, the brain has endured a lifetime of stressors. Blood flow to the brain decreases because of narrowing of the arteries. Thirst sensation becomes less operative, increasing the risk of uncompensated dehydration. One theory for the decrease in brain volume is a decrease in brain water content other than cerebrospinal fluid (Pfefferbaum et al., 1999). Adaptation to stress is less effective as people age. For instance, mortality from heat stroke rises sharply in people older than 60 years.

Various nutrients have been tested in relation to cognitive performance. For instance, glucose is the brain's preferred fuel. Performance by elderly individuals on memory tests was better following glucose ingestion than after saccharin ingestion (Gold, 1995). In a group of individuals of age 65 and older, higher ascorbic acid and beta-carotene plasma levels were associated with better memory performance in one study (Perrig, Perrig, and Stahlin, 1997) but not in another that found vitamin E effective (Perkins et al., 1999).

Special concerns of nourishing clients with dementia are discussed in Clinical Application 13–1. One type of dementia, Alzheimer's disease, affects approximately 4 million adults in the United States (Tully et al., 1997).

Endocrine System

The average older person is slowing down. Resting energy expenditure (REE) decreases, especially in the brain, skeletal muscle, and heart. The older adult's REE may be 10 to 12 percent less than a younger person's. Lost muscle mass is replaced, if at all, by adipose tissue that is less active metabolically than muscle.

The pancreas often secretes inadequate amounts of insulin, leading to diabetes mellitus (Chapter 19). Receptors in the kidney for antidiuretic hormone (ADH) may function poorly to produce a less effective response. Levels of aldosterone also decrease with age. Both of these changes make maintaining fluid volume more difficult for an older person than a younger one (Morrisson, 1997).

The immune system is less effective in the older person than in the younger one. The thymus gland, essential to the maturation of the thymic lymphoid cells (T cells), reaches maximum size at puberty and then

CLINICAL APPLICATION 13–1

Nutrition and Dementia

Care of clients with dementia challenges family and health-care providers. Clients progressively lose the ability for self-care, including feeding. A simple tool to assess the client's level of functioning is the Eating Behavior Scale, reproduced below. The six items assessed direct the caregivers to an appropriate strategy to assist the client without taking over a task the client still can perform.

Managing the client's environment is a major part of the care of the client with dementia. Dining rooms should be quiet and have adequate lighting. Having the same seat gives the client a familiar experience each meal. Offering one course at a time and providing appropriate but limited utensils, large-handled if necessary, are strategies that have been effective. Dishes with high sides to enable the client to scoop up the food onto a spoon or fork may prove useful. Offering finger foods that are within the client's capabilities to manage also may increase nutritional intake with minimal staff assistance.

Clients with dementia must be reminded of the steps involved in self-feeding: putting the food on the spoon,

directing it to the mouth, swallowing. Verbal cues or guiding the client's hand can get him or her started or keep the process going. Despite the surroundings, common courtesies can be effective in reminding clients of social expectations. Introducing the client to the other people at the table, providing a cup rather than a carton for milk, and offering foods separately rather than mixing them all together can contribute to maintaining a person's dignity (Kayser-Jones and Schell, 1997; Tully et al., 1997).

The effect of quiet music in the dining room on client behavior has been researched in various settings. Selections with a slow tempo—at or below the human heart rate—have usually been used to dampen environmental noises that might otherwise startle clients. Fewer incidents of agitated behaviors occurred during the weeks that music was played compared with weeks without music (Denney, 1997). Since staff members also heard the music, perhaps some of the effect was obtained by relaxing them also. Creating a pleasant environment at mealtime is an attempt at normalcy for demented clients.

National Institutes of Health Warren G. Magnuson Clinical Center
Nursing Department
Eating Behavior Scale (EBS)

Patient # _____   Admit Date _____   Observation Date _____

Observer initials_____   Meal Start _____   Finished _____

Patient room _____   Day room _____   Time–minutes_____

Circle only one answer: Maximum Score = 18   Total = _____

Observed Behavior	I.*	V.**	P.***	D.****
Was the patient:				
1. Able to initiate eating?	3	2	1	0
2. Able to maintain attention to meal?	3	2	1	0
3. Able to locate all food?	3	2	1	0
4. Appropriately using utensils?	3	2	1	0
5. Able to bite, chew and swallow without choking?	3	2	1	0
6. Able to terminate meal?	3	2	1	0
Comments				

   *I. = Independent
  **V. = Verbal prompts
 ***P. = Physical assistance
****D. = Dependent

begins involution. T cells are important to the body's cellular immune response to viruses, fungi, malignant cells, and foreign tissue grafts.

Cardiovascular System

As the older adult continues to age, there is (1) a decrease in cardiac output and (2) a slower heart rate. In response to exercise, the heart rate does not increase as effectively as in youth, nor does it return to normal as rapidly. Because of these diminishments, the elderly are at risk for diseases of the heart. Dietary modifications for heart disease are discussed in Chapter 20 on cardiovascular disease.

Nutrition in the Older Adult

The Food Guide Pyramid or one modified for adults older than 70 years can be used for assessment and counseling. Information has been gathered on the nutrition of older Americans regarding energy, vitamins, minerals, and water.

Food Pyramids

The Food Guide Pyramid serves the older adult well up to the age of 70. It is the standard against which the following survey results are measured.

In 1994 to 1996, none of the groups 60 years and older reported an intake of fat at 30 percent of kilocalories or less. Men reported a fat intake of 33 percent of total kilocalories and women 32 percent. Individuals aged 60 to 69 consumed grains, vegetables, and meat products at a better rate than did people over 70 years of age. In both age groups in every category a higher percentage of men than of women consumed the recommended number of servings.

Table 13–4 lists the percentages of older men and women reporting consumption of food groups as recommended by the Food Guide Pyramid. It shows that in only four of the twenty categories did more than half the respondents consume the recommended servings and those respondents were all men. Whole grains were given short shrift. Men selected whole grains for 17 percent of their grains, and women consumed 19 percent of their grains as whole. As with younger adults, the mainstay vegetable was the white potato, consisting of about 27 percent of the vegetables consumed by men and 24 percent of those chosen by women (U.S. Department of Agriculture, February 1999).

The approximate percentages of adult men and women, aged 20 to 60 and older, who consumed recommended servings from the major food groups are shown in Figure 13–2. In virtually every category, more men than women ate the recommended number of servings. With the exception of fruit and one slight reversal by the two younger groups of women in reporting vegetable intake, a greater proportion of younger people than older ones consumed the recommended number of servings.

A special Modified Food Guide Pyramid for People Over 70 Years of Age has been published (Figure 13–3). Eight servings of water provides a new foundation of the pyramid. The grain, vegetable, fruit, and meat minimum recommendations are the same as the Food Guide Pyramid with the addition of symbols for fiber in each of them to emphasize the food groups that are good sources of fiber. The milk group minimum is 3 servings instead of 2. Fat recommendation is unchanged, but a pennant is added at the top of the pyramid signifying calcium, vitamin D, and vitamin B_{12} supplementation (Russell, Rasmussen, and Lichtenstein, 1999).

Available evidence suggests that older people need almost the same intake from all nutrients as do other adults, with the exception of kilocalories. Energy needs decrease with age. Thus, there is less leeway for indiscretions and empty kilocalories in the diet.

Energy

It is estimated that older adults need about 5 percent fewer kilocalories per decade after the age of 40. Small changes have been recommended in intakes from carbohydrates, fats, and protein. As with younger people, the simplest criterion for the suitability of intake is the maintenance of a healthy body weight. There is much variation in energy expenditure within the elder population.

Older adults should have at least 30 minutes a day of moderate activity. It can be 30 minutes at one time or two 15-minute sessions or three 10-minute sessions. A one-year, twice weekly weight training program for white women, ages 50 to 70 years, resulted in significant increases in strength, balance, and estimated total body muscle mass compared to a control group (Nelson, 1994). An exercise routine should be introduced gradually. On average, physically active people live longer than inactive people do, even if exercise is started late in life. Exercise reduces the risk of chronic diseases and makes individuals feel healthier and look younger.

The proportion of energy to be obtained from carbohydrate, fat, and protein is changed slightly for older adults. Older people should derive 50 to 60 percent of their kilocalories from carbohydrates. Fats should contribute 20 to 30 percent of the kilocalories. Limiting fats should also increase comfort because fat absorption is delayed in older people leading to a feeling of fullness. Particularly among the elderly, rigid application

TABLE 13–4 Reported Compliance with Food Guide Pyramid Recommendations by Men and Women 60+ Years of Age

	60 to 69 Year Old Men	Men Older than 70 Years	60 to 69 Year Old Women	Women Older than 70 Years
At least 6 Servings of Grains	58 percent	49 percent	28 percent	28 percent
At least 3 Servings of Vegetables	61 percent	53 percent	46 percent	40 percent
At least 2 Servings of Fruit	36 percent	42 percent	34 percent	36 percent
At least 5 ounces of Meat Equivalents*	55 percent	37 percent	27 percent	17 percent
At least 2 Servings of Dairy Products	23 percent	24 percent	12 percent	15 percent

*For this tabulation includes meat, poultry, fish, simulated meat products, eggs, tofu, peanut butter, nuts and seeds, but excludes dry beans and peas that were included with vegetables.
United States Department of Agriculture, February 1999

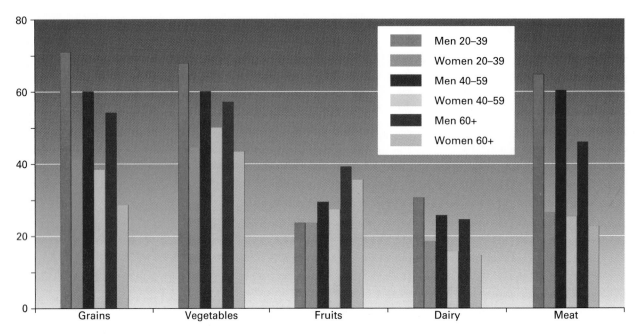

Figure 13–2:
Approximate percentages of individuals, sorted by age and gender, who reported consuming the recommended servings from the major food groups. (Interpreted from U.S. Department of Agriculture, February 1999.)

of diet rules may be inappropriate. Restricting fat so as to eliminate whole milk and eggs, which are easily eaten and relatively inexpensive, could endanger nutrition in the short term for uncertain long-term benefits.

An intake of protein at the level of 0.8 gram per kilogram of ideal body weight is recommended for healthy people. Some authorities suggest increasing the protein allotment for the elderly, but no consistent relationship between protein intake and serum albumin level has been found in elderly people (Freedman and Ahronheim, 1986). One reason for this may be related to liver function. A normally functioning liver is necessary to construct albumin molecules from the ingested protein and resulting amino acids. If liver function is impaired, no amount of protein intake will produce normal blood albumin levels.

Mortality rates from all causes were found to be highest in people over 71 years of age with the lowest serum albumin levels; mortality decreased as albumin levels increased. It is uncertain if serum albumin reflects nutritional status or disease presence and severity (Corti et al, 1994). For a given individual, serum albumin levels can indicate nutritional status, pathology, or both. An additional reason for moderate protein intake concerns calcium use. A high protein intake also increases calcium loss in the urine.

Vitamins

Vitamin intake and usage are potential problems for the elderly. Deficiencies of vitamins A, D, and C, niacin, and B_{12} are most frequently a concern. Excesses are possible, also, especially in people who self-medicate on megadoses of vitamins.

FAT-SOLUBLE VITAMINS Because fat-soluble vitamins are stored in the body, it may take a long time for a deficiency to present clinical signs.

Assessment of the individual's long-standing food habits might help to pinpoint a person's risks.

Vitamin A plays a role in bone metabolism, but more is not necessarily better. In the elderly, excessive levels of vitamin A are associated with increased bone loss. With dietary intake of retinol greater than 1.5 milligrams per day, compared with intake of less than 0.5 milligrams of retinol per day, bone mineral density was reduced 14 percent at the lumbar spine, 10 percent in the femoral neck, and risk of hip fracture was doubled (Melhus et al., 1998).

As discussed in the Chapter 7 on vitamins, the older person's intestinal absorption of vitamin D and synthesis of it in the skin is diminished compared with that of younger adults. The 1998 RDAs reflect those physiological changes by increasing the RDAs to 10 micrograms for 51- to 70-year-old people and to 15 micrograms for those older than 70. Milk is an excellent source of vitamin D because it is fortified. The elderly person who is most likely to be deficient in vitamin D is one who stays indoors, does not consume enough milk or milk products, and does not take a vitamin supplement.

New roles have been discovered for vitamin E. Besides its function as a scavenger of free radicals, it has been linked to improved immune function. A deficiency of vitamin E causes immune cell membranes to become unstable (Meydani and Meisler, 1997). High plasma vitamin E concentrations have been associated with lower incidences of infectious disease, and supplementation for 4 months has improved certain measures of cell-mediated immune responses (Meydani et al., 1997).

Vitamin K can be depleted relatively more quickly than the other fat-soluble vitamins. Besides its role in the clotting of blood, vitamin K contributes to bone metabolism. It is not surprising, therefore, that low serum

Modified Food Pyramid for 70+ Adults

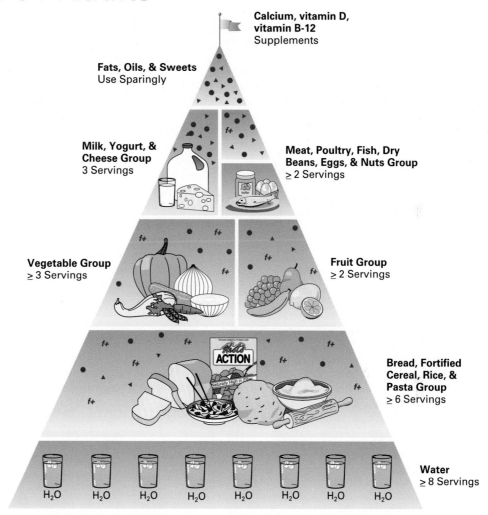

Calcium, vitamin D, vitamin B-12
Supplements

Fats, Oils, & Sweets
Use Sparingly

Milk, Yogurt, & Cheese Group
3 Servings

Meat, Poultry, Fish, Dry Beans, Eggs, & Nuts Group
≥ 2 Servings

Vegetable Group
≥ 3 Servings

Fruit Group
≥ 2 Servings

Bread, Fortified Cereal, Rice, & Pasta Group
≥ 6 Servings

Water
≥ 8 Servings

H_2O H_2O H_2O H_2O H_2O H_2O H_2O H_2O

● Fat (naturally occurring and added)
▲ Sugars (added)
f+ Fiber (should be present)
    These symbols show fat, added sugars, & fiber in foods.

Figure 13–3:
The Modified Food Guide Pyramid for People Over Seventy Years of Age
(From Russell, Rasmussen, and Lichtenstein, 1999. Reprinted with permission of J Nutr 129:752, American Society for Nutritional Sciences.)

levels of vitamin K have been found in clients with hip fractures. A daily intake of lettuce, the food that contributed the most dietary vitamin K to a group of women followed for 10 years, compared to one or fewer servings per week, was associated with 45 percent decrease in the risk for hip fracture (Feskanich et al., 1999). As a corollary, clients receiving warfarin have been observed to have lower bone mineral density than others (Bonjour, Schurch, and Rizzoli, 1996).

WATER-SOLUBLE VITAMINS The 2000 RDA for older adults is the same amount of vitamin C, 90 milligrams for men and 75 milligrams for women, as for younger adults. Older adults living at home generally have a better vitamin C status than those living in institutions. The independent elderly may spend more money on fruits and vegetables than institutions do, or poor cooking and serving practices in institutions may destroy the vitamin C in foods. "Widower's scurvy" refers to the condition developing in a man following the death of his wife and subsequent poor dietary intake of vitamin C (Morrisson, 1997).

Eating patterns affect the intake of B vitamins. Older adults who eat little meat and consume little milk or milk products containing tryptophan are at risk for niacin deficiency.

Older adults have decreased gastric juice, which contains intrinsic factor. Because of this, senior adults may develop a vitamin B_{12} deficiency, especially those with limited meat consumption. The meat group supplies 66 percent of the total dietary vitamin B_{12} (National Live Stock and Meat Board, 1995).

Minerals

Minerals of particular concern in the elderly are iron and calcium. In Chapter 8, see Table 8–1 for alternate recommendations for calcium intake and Clinical Application 8–3 to review research on osteoporosis.

Iron absorption is impaired by decreased gastric acidity, whether due to aging or to antacid use. Anemia is not always the result of aging or nutritional deficits. Hidden blood losses should be suspected and their sources sought in the anemic elderly person, just as in younger clients.

Water

Many older people have problems maintaining fluid balance. Sometimes the difficulty is self-inflicted. Loss of sphincter muscle tone in women and difficulty urinating in men may prompt older people to limit their fluid intake. Healthy older adults need 6 to 8 glasses of water per day, enough to produce about 1.5 liters of light yellow urine. Another standard for daily water intake, barring pathology, is 30 mL/kg body weight. For a 154-pound (70 kg) individual this amounts to 70 ounces or 8.75 cups of water.

Dehydration in the elderly can result in abnormal organ functioning. One of the signs of dehydration in the elderly is confusion. If no one is alert to these mental changes, the person may compound his or her difficulties by forgetting to take medications or eat meals. Signs of dehydration in the elderly are listed in Table 13–5. The increase in pulse rate upon standing is a valid assessment technique for fluid volume status in the elderly except when heart disease, cardiac medications, or artificial pacing would block the response (Weinberg, Minaker, and the Council on Scientific Affairs, 1995).

Patients who are immobilized may need as many as 12 to 14 glasses of water per day. Immobility increases the calcium loss from bones which then circulates in the blood until the kidney excretes the excess. A large fluid intake dilutes the urine so that the calcium does not form stones.

Common Problems Related to Nutrition

Although constipation, osteoporosis, and protein-energy malnutrition are problems for all age groups, they represent special concerns for geriatric clients.

Constipation

A person may complain of acute constipation (lack of stool) or of chronic constipation (general difficulty passing bowel movements). Recommended methods to achieve bowel regularity include increasing fluid intake, consuming high-fiber foods, taking time for elimination, and exercising.

Doubling the person's water intake, medical conditions permitting, is the first step. Increasing fresh fruit and vegetable intake is the second. Helping the client determine his or her normal bowel evacuation pattern (after each meal, once a day, every other day, etc.) is the third step. Time should be set aside to have a bowel movement according to that pattern. Drinking a warm beverage often stimulates evacuation. In addition, exercise promotes regular bowel movements.

Many older individuals have the idea that they must have a bowel movement every day when that may not be their pattern. Sometimes older adults adopt the routine use of laxatives to correct bowel habits. For such people, the program mentioned above will not provide instant resolution. If they adhere to the regimen, however, it is possible to overcome even long-standing constipation.

Arthritis

Arthritis refers to a group of diseases characterized by inflammation of various joints. Osteoarthritis, also called degenerative joint disease (DJD), by conservative estimate affects an estimated 21 million people in the United States (Lawrence et al., 1998). Risk factors include aging, obesity, and overuse or abuse of joints as with athletic or occupational stress. An additional risk factor, estrogen replacement therapy, was recently reported (Sahyoun et al., 1999b). Weight control is the prime nutritional factor in the prevention and treatment of osteoarthritis. Women with BMIs greater than 32 at initial interview had significantly higher risks of developing arthritis than women with BMIs between 19 and 21.9 (Sahyoun et al., 1999a).

In contrast to osteoarthritis, which is a local disease, rheumatoid arthritis is a systemic disease generally thought to be of autoimmune origin. Conservative estimates place the number of people affected at 2.1 million, 70 percent of them women (Lawrence et al., 1998). Because it is a systemic disease, efforts have been directed toward influencing the course of the disease through dietary or supplemental means. Among the suggested interventions are the following. A vegan diet is purported to improve symptoms by eliminating sources of arachidonic acid from which

Table 13–5 Signs of Dehydration in the Elderly	
Body System	**Sign**
Skin and mucous membranes	Skin warm and dry
	Decreased turgor; pinch test may be inaccurate due to loss of elasticity
	Furrowed tongue
	Elevated temperature
Cardiovascular	Elevated pulse
Urinary	Increased specific gravity
	Increased urinary sodium
Musculoskeletal	Weakness
Neurological	Confusion

eicosanoids are formed and which mediate inflammatory rheumatic diseases (Adam, 1995).

The effect of omega-3 and omega-6 fatty acids is under investigation (Alexander, 1998; de Deckere, et al., 1998; Kremer, 1996). Other nutrients being studied in relation to rheumatoid arthritis are vitamin E, selenium, beta-carotene, and zinc (Adam, 1995). Until the results of these studies are reported, Martin (1998) recommends consuming a varied diet and supplements as necessary, but avoiding megadosing and self-imposed elimination diets along with testing of suspected food intolerances under clinical supervision.

Osteoporosis and Fractures

The pathophysiology and prevention of osteoporosis is discussed in Chapter 8 in Clinical Application 8–3. This section examines only the risks of and results of hip fracture, which although half as common as reported vertebral fractures, is much more likely to be diagnosed and treated. It is estimated that only one third of vertebral fractures are clinically diagnosed.

Each year in the United States, hip fractures result in approximately 300,000 hospital admissions and $9 billion in direct medical costs (Centers for Disease Control, 1998). Of these hip fractures, 92 percent occur in clients at least 65 years old (Cooper, 1997). The best tool available to assess risk of osteoporotic fracture in postmenopausal women is the measurement of bone mineral density (BMD). A decrease of one standard deviation (SD) in femoral BMD is comparable to a 14-year increase in age on the risk of hip fracture. Yet many women are unaware that they have osteoporosis, a situation that may change following implementation of standardized coverage by Medicare for bone density tests for high-risk people, which began July 1, 1998 (Centers for Disease Control, 1998).

The lifetime risk of incidence of hip fracture is 25 percent for women and 5 percent for men. By the age of 85, 35 percent of women and 4 percent of men sustain a hip fracture (Rousseau, 1997) a figure that coincides almost perfectly with the 35 percent of 80-year-old women who meet the World Health Organization definition of osteoporosis, two SDs below the mean of young adults' BMD (Slemenda, 1997).

Other risk factors for hip fractures are white race, decreased visual acuity, impaired neuromuscular function, cognitive impairment, residence in a nursing home, inactivity, use of sedative or anticonvulsant medications, and being tall. All these factors have been discussed earlier or are self-explanatory, except height. Engineering analysis of the hip indicates greater resistance to fracture in shorter femoral necks, which occur in shorter people (Slemenda, 1997). It can be readily seen that many clients have more than one of these risk factors. In the case of hip fractures, obesity is protective (Grisso et al., 1994; Paganini-Hill et al., 1991). Suggested mechanisms include padding of the bone by adipose tissue, increased BMD from increased loading in ambulation, and production of estrogenic steroids by adipose tissue (Vellas et al., 1995).

Hip fracture often initiates a downward spiral in health. Only 50 percent of clients regain their mobility and independence (Johnell, 1997), 40 percent are unable to walk independently one year after the fracture, and 27 percent enter a nursing home for the first time (Cooper, 1997). About 8 percent of men and 3 percent of women older than 50 die while hospitalized for their hip fractures. Mortality one year after hip fracture is 36 percent for men and 21 percent for women and is much higher in older men (Cooper, 1997).

Weight Loss and Protein–Energy Malnutrition

Some people in the United States simply do not get enough food to eat (Box 13–3). The main reason individuals do not consume enough protein or enough kilocalories is lack of money. To rectify the situation for older adults, the federal government, with an amendment to the Older Americans Act, established meal programs for senior citizens. Low-cost meals are offered at central gathering places and/or delivered to the homebound. Senior citizens participate in some 2200 such local meal programs (Figure 13–4).

Lower nutritional status has been shown to be associated with older age, female sex, and living alone (Ranieri et al., 1996). A syndrome called **anorexia of aging** is described in Box 13–4. One of the most treatable psychologic causes of weight loss in the older person is depression. Ninety percent of older depressed clients experience weight loss, compared with 60 percent of younger depressed people. SCALES, a rapid office practice screen for risk of protein-energy malnutrition, is shown in Table 13–6. Two components of the screen are serum albumin and cholesterol. A serum albumin level less than 3.2 g/dL is highly predictive of mortality in hospitals, and a cholesterol level of less than 156 mg/dL is the best predictor of mortality in nursing homes (Morley, 1997).

Nonterminally ill hospitalized elderly who consumed less than 50 percent of their calculated energy requirements had average serum albumin levels of 2.9 g/dL and/or serum cholesterol levels of 154 mg/dL. They also had 8 times the risk of in-hospital death and 2.9 times the risk of death within 90 days as those whose nutrient intake was better than 50 percent of requirements (Sullivan, Sun, and Walls, 1999). Malnutrition contributes to many complications of illness, such as pressure ulcers (Clinical Application 13–2). Inadequate kilocaloric intake has been correlated with increased mortality in the elderly (Elmstahl et al., 1997; Incalzi et al., 1998).

Individual assessment is the key to planning nutritional care. For example, milk-based supplements that are both nutrient-dense and easy to consume might be a dietary recommendation for a person who is losing weight or one who cannot chew. To accommodate dentures, the per-

---

Box 13–3 Food Insufficiency

Between 1988 and 1994, 4.1 percent of the people surveyed were designated "food insufficient" if the family respondent reported that the family sometimes or often did not get enough food to eat. Food insufficiency was primarily related to poverty but not the region of the country, with a prevalence of 15.2 percent in Mexican Americans, 7.7 percent in non-Hispanic black Americans, and 2.5 percent in non-Hispanic white Americans. Food insufficiency was significantly related to the head of the family having less than a high school education (Alaimo et al., 1998).

In a study of preschool children, adult women, and the elderly, the strongest association between food insufficiency and decreased nutrient intakes was found with the elderly. In food-insufficient households, the mean energy intake of the elderly was only 58 percent of the recommended amounts, and intake of calcium, vitamin E, vitamin B_6, magnesium, and zinc was less than 66 percent of their recommended amounts (Rose and Oliveira, 1997).

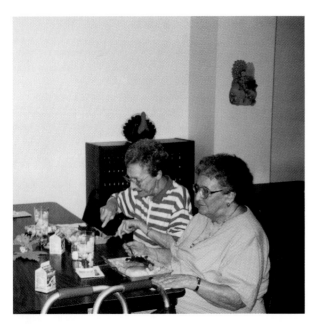

Figure 13–4:
These women partake of an evening meal served at their place of residence under the auspices of the Older Americans Act and managed by a county agency.

son may reduce his or her intake of meats, fresh fruits, and vegetables and may need assistance selecting appropriate substitute items. One study showed dietary intake in home healthcare clients was not related to chewing ability, however (Payette et al., 1995). A recommended procedure for learning to eat and drink with dentures is discussed in Clinical Application 13–3.

The Nursing Process and the Elderly

Although elderly people are not all alike, often they do have some common problems (Table 13–7).

Assessment

Special care is necessary when assessing the elderly to ensure marginal deficiencies are detected before major problems occur. Nutritional assessment tools for use with older adults were developed by the Nutrition Screening Initiative, a joint project of the American Academy of Family Physicians, the American Dietetic Association, and the National Council on Aging, Inc. "Determine Your Nutritional Health" is a self-administered

---

Table 13–6 SCALES, A Rapid Office Practice Screen for Protein-Energy Malnutrition

S: sadness
C: cholesterol < 4.14 mmol/L (160 mg/dL)
A: albumin < 40 g/L (4 g/dL)
L: loss of weight
E: eating problems (cognitive or physical)
S: shopping problems or inability to prepare a meal

(Morley, 1997. Reprinted with permission)

Box 13–4 The Anorexia of Aging

Humans (and other animals) of advanced age have reduced food intake. Older humans become sated earlier than younger ones, the result of decreased enjoyment of food and of altered hormonal and neurotransmitter regulation of food intake (Morley, 1997).

Changes in the physiology of the aging body explain this phenomenon in the otherwise healthy individual. Diminished ability to smell and taste may make eating less enjoyable. Because gastric emptying is slowed, an older person feels full longer after a meal. Increased levels of circulating cholecystokinin, a hormone credited with satiating activity, occur in aged individuals. Other physiologic causes are under investigation as a result of animal studies.

In addition to physiologic causes of anorexia, social, psychological, and medical conditions impact the older person's appetite. Social causes include isolation, poverty, lack of transportation to obtain food, and unappealing environment or food selection, particularly for institutionalized clients. Psychological causes include bereavement and depression. Preparing solitary meals and eating alone discourages balance and variety. Depression affected over 33 percent of outpatients and nursing home residents with weight loss (Morley, 1995). Medical causes include drug side effects, Parkinson's disease (increased muscular movement), stroke (swallowing disorders, self-care deficit for feeding). Given the incidence of multiple chronic diseases in the elderly, treated with multiple medications that may affect food intake, the high rate of anorexia is understandable.

Unfortunately protein–energy undernutrition is seldom recognized and, even if diagnosed, frequently goes untreated. Early identification and appropriate interventions can interrupt the downward spiral. Compared with clients not receiving supplements, clients with hip fractures receiving protein-rich nutritional supplements manifested lower rates of complications and death not only in the immediate postoperative period but also for 6 months afterward (Krall and Dawson-Hughes, 1999).

---

checklist with scoring directions to evaluate risk. The Level I Screening Tool is designed to be administered by professionals in health or social service programs and includes directions for appropriate referrals. The Nutrition Screening Initiative also devised a Level II Screening Tool for use in physicians' offices and health-care institutions that includes a clinical examination, skinfold measurements, and laboratory tests (Quinn, 1997). These two instruments are reproduced in Appendix C.

Implementation

Suggestions to increase the nourishment of elderly clients appear in Table 13–8. Keep in mind that there is no single answer suitable for every problem. Nutritional supplements may help maintain weight in individuals with poor appetites or eating problems, but a more economical choice may be

CLINICAL APPLICATION 13–2

Nutrition and Pressure Ulcers

The basic cause of pressure ulcers is impaired circulation from the weight of the body on a bony prominence or by shearing forces from pulling on the skin that damages the underlying tissue. Risk factors include immobility, inactivity, incontinence, impaired consciousness, and malnutrition. Progression of the ulcer from intact skin to an open, sometimes very deep sore increases the challenge to control infection, to replenish nutrient losses from the wound, and to promote healing.

People of any age experiencing the risk factors may develop pressure ulcers, but 50 percent occur in clients over the age of 70. Some 90 percent tend to form below the waist. Prevalences have been reported of 3.0 to 4.6 percent in general hospitals, 14.9 percent in intermediate care facilities, and 35 percent in skilled nursing facilities (Osterweil, Wendt, and Ferrell, 1995). In a hospital-based study, the risk for pressure ulcers increased with the client's age (Pernege, et al., 1998).

A serum albumin level of less than 3.5 grams per deciliter is used to justify a diagnosis of malnutrition for Medicare and Medicaid. It was also the most frequently found indicator for pressure ulcers in nursing home residents (Gilmore et al., 1995).

Protein intake has been the subject of many studies. One found that changes in the area of pressure ulcers correlated with dietary protein intake but not with serum albumin levels (Hill, Cooper, and Robson, 1994). Another reported that clients who consumed the most protein (24 percent of kilocalories) and kilocalories (30 to 40 per kilogram) showed the greatest healing of their ulcers. Particular amino acids were investigated in relation to nitrogen balance. During 6 days of bed rest, healthy subjects supplemented with branched chain amino acids lost less nitrogen in the urine than control subjects (Breslow, Hallfrisch, and Goldberg, 1991; Stein et al., 1999). This is of relevance because individuals who might have been out of bed before developing pressure ulcers are likely to be on bed rest after developing them, and the inactivity itself might impair optimal utilization of the protein consumed.

Another study showed a significant reduction in surface area of pressure ulcers with vitamin C supplementation without demonstration of a measurable vitamin C deficiency (Osterweil, Wendt, and Ferrell, 1995). Topical application of essential fatty acids to the skin for 21 days reduced the development of pressure ulcers: 5 percent of the experimental group compared to 27 percent of the control group. In addition, the ulcers of the control group were more extensive, and two clients developed more than one ulcer (Declair, 1997).

Although zinc functions in collagen synthesis that contributes to wound healing, zinc supplementation has been shown to be beneficial only in clients with clinical zinc deficiency. Diagnosing deficiency is particularly problematic since no consistent relationship between dietary zinc and plasma levels has been established. In addition, zinc supplementation has caused both stimulation and suppression of the immune system in elderly clients (Ausman and Russell, 1999).

Provision of a nutritionally complete diet provides the best condition for recovery and healing, whereas supplementing with specific nutrients to clients who are not clinically deficient has little effect on pressure ulcer healing (Thomas, 1997). Clients at risk of malnutrition are not identified and treated as often as one might suppose. Of 34 eating-dependent nursing home residents, 70 percent were underweight, 26 percent were hypoalbuminemic, 50 percent were anemic, and 38 percent had pressure ulcers. Despite those indications for nutritional intervention, only 35 percent received a multivitamin supplement and 3 percent a trace mineral supplement (Rudman et al., 1995). For clients at risk for or suffering from pressure ulcers, efforts to ensure adequate intake of all essential nutrients through meals, balanced meal-replacing supplements, and vitamin-mineral supplements should receive priority attention.

Nutritional support is only a part of the overall strategy to combat pressure ulcers. The other risk factors must be controlled and diligent nursing care provided to effectively prevent or treat this serious complication.

a liquid breakfast preparation. Protein–energy malnutrition was reversed in one study by serving as much of a favorite food, ice cream, as the client wanted (Winograd and Brown, 1990).

No scientific evidence has been offered to support the benefit of meal-replacement supplements as snacks for healthy older people (Morley, 1997), although the successful marketing of such products indicates that mature adults are open to changing their dietary habits. Women over age 50 who were aware of the link between calcium intake and bone disease consumed 76 milligrams more calcium per day than women who were unaware of the relationship. The mean intakes of 625 milligrams for the aware women and 510 milligrams for the unaware women were not even close to the 1998 RDA of 1200 milligrams (Tepper and Nayga, 1998), however. The need for education in this population is significant.

Increasing physical activity according to the client's ability offers benefits beyond weight control. Physical activity helps to prevent heart disease and hypertension, improves bone mineral density, enhances balance and strength for activities of daily living, and promotes restful sleep. Many individuals, however, report never having been advised to exercise by their health-care providers. An intervention to enable the client to see improvement (or the need for improvement) is the keeping of an activity log (Jones and Jones, 1997).

The nurse's role in nourishing the hospitalized older client undergoing diagnostic tests is discussed in Clinical Application 13–4. Obtaining adequate food for such a client may tax the nurse's ingenuity because of both timing issues and the need to entice a fatigued and perhaps fearful client to eat.

CLINICAL APPLICATION 13–3

Learning to Eat with Dentures

Persons need to learn to use dentures one step at a time. The steps are in exactly the same order as those used by infants learning to eat. The person should first practice swallowing liquids with the dentures in place. After this is mastered, soft foods can be chewed. Lastly, the person should learn to bite regular foods with the dentures. Splitting up the learning process into manageable units helps to make this process less frustrating for the new denture wearer.

Nutrition Education for Adults

Because none of the age groups of adults is remarkable for complying with recommended food intake guides, some general suggestions for improvement are pertinent for most adults. Current issues relate to excessive intakes of food energy (kilocalories), fat (total, saturated, and cholesterol), alcohol, and sodium. Only for calcium and iron is the concern a deficiency (Life Sciences, 1995).

Knowledge is related to behavior and behavior change. Elderly people were shown to be more likely to drink 1 percent or skim milk if they had increased nutrition knowledge or were trying to reduce cholesterol intake. Other significant variables were higher income and being female (Elbon, Johnson, and Fischer, 1998). Teaching clients about the benefits of lower-fat milks and about products to control lactose intolerance when appropriate could assist them to improve their health status with little effort by the health-care provider. Because the true prevalence of lactose intolerance in the elderly is unknown (Ausman and Russell, 1999), and because dairy products are nutrient-dense, working with elderly clients to improve their intake is a good use of the health-care provider's expertise.

Use of a modified Nutrition Screening Initiative checklist identified 68 to 89 percent of elderly people served by congregate or home-deliv-

TABLE 13–7 Topics to be Assessed in the Elderly*

Oral Cavity Function
- Difficulty tasting, changes in taste perception
- Bleeding gums, dry mouth
- Difficulty chewing, toothaches, poorly fitting dentures
- Foods client is unable to eat

Meal Management
- Who shops? Where? Ease of making food decisions?
- Transportation problems?
- Budgeting a concern? Knowledge to make informed choices?
- Who cooks? Knowledge and skill level?
- Refrigeration, storage, and cooking facilities?
- Ability to manage containers: jars, cans, bottles

Psychosocial Factors
- Where are most meals eaten?
- Mealtime companions
- Recent change in living conditions?
- Satisfaction with situations?

*In addition to the normal assessment, that is, appetite or weight changes, bowel habits.

Table 13–8 Increasing Food Intake in the Elderly

Get the Person Ready for Meals
- Provide oral hygiene before meals to freshen and moisten mouth.
- Suggest smokers refrain for 1 hour before a meal to increase appetite.
- Manage the environment by removing unsightly supplies or noxious waste.
- Allow 90 minutes to elapse after a significant amount of supplement before serving the next meal.

Promote Social Interaction
- Encourage potluck meals with friends for those who live alone.
- Combine meal at senior center with an activity of interest.
- Encourage alert nursing home residents to choose compatible mealtime companions.
- Control the noise in the dining room to avoid overstimulating those with hearing aids.

Serve Food Attractively
- Vary textures, colors, flavors.
- To increase vegetable intake, offer raw, crisp-cooked, or marinated vegetables as appetizers.
- Use "good" dishes and flatware, centerpieces, tablecloths, or place mats.
- Provide enough nonglaring light so food can be seen clearly.

Provide Nutrient-Dense Foods
- Add powdered milk or ice cream to appropriate beverages and foods.
- Increase the eggs, milk, or cheese in recipes.
- Help client to select satisfactory meal-replacer supplements whether commercial canned products or instant-breakfast powders. When appropriate, offer 1 ounce every hour and use as "chaser" when administering medications.
- If additional kilocalories are needed, choose whole milk for beverages and cooking instead of reduced fat varieties.
- If milk-based products are unpalatable for the client, explore the use of clear liquid supplements that offer complete nutrition. (See Chapter 15.)

Obtain Outside Help
- Home health aide to shop, do basic fix-ahead preparations.
- Meals-on-Wheels for homebound.
- Food stamps, surplus commodity programs for those eligible.
- Instructional materials on food purchasing, storage, cooking from county extension services.

ered meal programs to be at moderate or high risk of malnutrition. The most frequent needs were nutrition counseling, drug/nutrient counseling, and dentition-related problems (Weddle, Wellman, and Bates, 1997). The tools provided in Appendix C can be used to identify learning needs of individual clients as well as to research the status of groups of clients.

In view of the recent changes in RDAs, recommending supplements for certain groups of people and instruction in the judicious use of those products might help clients modify their major risk factors. Vitamins D and B$_{12}$ and calcium supplements are recommended in the Modified

Food Pyramid for 70+ Adults. A note that users of supplements are generally more likely to have healthier lifestyles than nonusers frequently accompanies interpretations of nutritional findings. Daily use of supplements was highest among women, whites, those 75 years or older, those at or above poverty level, those with more than 12 years of schooling, former smokers, and those consuming less than one alcoholic beverage per week. Men and women who used supplements consumed diets lower in fat and higher in fiber and vitamins A and C, and women users had diets higher in vitamin E and calcium than nonusers (Slesinski, Subar, and Kahle, 1996). Of adults over the age of 60, 65 percent of supplement users were of high or middle socioeconomic status, and 87 percent were white. Those who had lower fat intakes and consistent exercise habits were also more likely to take supplements (Freeman et al., 1998).

Most adults could benefit from instruction in the key concepts of nutrition: balance, variety, and moderation. The alert nurse has an important contribution to make in identifying knowledge deficits and impaired health practices related to nutrition. This responsibility applies to all clients receiving nursing care, not only those with obvious nutrition-related medical diagnoses.

CLINICAL APPLICATION 13–4

Hospitalization of the Elderly

Except for obstetrical and pediatric clients, elderly clients dominate as consumers of health care. Eighty percent of the elderly, compared to 40 percent of individuals under the age of 65 years, have one or more chronic diseases. Frequently elderly clients are admitted to the hospital undernourished, but their situation also worsens during hospitalization. Nutritional depletion between admission and discharge (diagnosed by a decrease of 3.6 percent in midarm circumference) occurred in 27 percent of geriatric and internal medicine patients (average age of 79 years) and was correlated with anorexia (Incalzi et al., 1996).

Serving no food to a client because of diagnostic tests is starvation. The conscientious nurse obtains meals or feedings for a client who was **nil per os**, or NPO (i.e., "nothing by mouth") for breakfast and lunch. There is nothing magical about the times of 8 AM–12 NOON–6 PM for meals. The committed nurse will arrange for adequate nourishment for clients, despite scheduling difficulties. Dietary staff have no idea when an individual client is finished with tests for the day until notified by the nurse.

Summary

As a group, adult men have better diets, although less than half of them consume the recommended number of servings of fruit and dairy products. Women's diets parallel men's except that fewer than 50 percent of women consume the recommended servings of any food group. The lowest intake is from the dairy group, a fact that has important ramifications for prevention of osteoporosis.

Aging affects almost all body systems, but significant individual differences occur. Older skin is less capable of vitamin D synthesis than that of younger people. The senses deteriorate, leading to difficulty obtaining information from the environment. Loss of teeth, arthritis of the jaw, and slowing of gastrointestinal function may decrease intake and digestion of food and absorption of nutrients. The liver and kidneys become less capable of detoxifying and excreting wastes. Muscular strength diminishes, and in a significant minority of people the bones become osteoporotic. The nervous and endocrine controls become less effective, increasing the older client's risk for dehydration and diabetes mellitus. The cardiovascular and immune systems also are less likely to rebound quickly after stress than in a younger person.

Physical changes are not the only factors to be assessed. Changing social, economic, and physical circumstances affect the nutritional status of the elderly client. When a spouse dies, grief, depression, and poor appetite or lack of culinary skill often affect the survivor. Learning to live on Social Security benefits, a pension, and savings may place a strain on some elderly people.

Some of these factors may be difficult to elicit from the client during the history-taking. The multiple physiologic changes in the elderly client along with the occurrence of chronic diseases in this age group necessitates special care in assessment. Interaction of these many factors could exacerbate a marginal or subclinical deficiency or overdose into a major problem. Any of the cultural traditions associated with food could be important for psychosocial development. Enjoyment of food in the company of others offers opportunities to share one's knowledge and skill and to validate one's own life experiences.

Improving food intake in adults requires them to choose to upgrade their diets. Increasing their awareness and knowledge is the first step. Assisting them to set one or two achievable goals and to select acceptable strategies is likely to be more successful than simply dictating a plan to them (Wellness Tips 13–1).

Wellness Tips 13–1

Dairy Products
- To increase intake of calcium and vitamin D, use milk or cheese in sauces, desserts, casseroles, and beverages.
- Experiment with drinking milk as part of a meal and with lactase products if intolerance is perceived.
- Select low-fat products if appropriate for weight control.
- If intake of calcium remains low, consult with health-care provider about supplementation.
- If client is housebound, and consuming few vitamin D-fortified foods, consult with health-care provider about supplementation.

Fruits and Vegetables
- Tally the day's intake: 2 servings of fruit and 3 servings of vegetables are the minimums.
- Once the minimums are achieved, increase the total number of servings to 9.
- Select fruit for dessert or between meal snacks.
- Carry vegetables with you to work: snack packs of carrots, broccoli, etc.
- Add beans to dishes, for example, add some canned kidney beans to a tossed salad.

Eating Whole Grain
- Eat whole grain cereals, breads, pastas, and baked products. Look for "whole grain" listed as the first ingredient on the package.
- If current intake is solely refined grains, begin by substituting one whole grain product.
- Experiment with various products to find ones you like.
- Sprinkle wheat germ on cereal, casseroles, salads, and desserts.
- Substitute wheat germ for some of the nuts in a recipe.

Case Study 13–1

Mr. E is a 70-year-old widower who relies on public transportation. His home is two blocks off the bus route and eight blocks from the nearest supermarket. Mr. E has moderately painful knees from arthritis. He has been taking the bus to the supermarket every other day so that he could manage one package on the way home. He has confided to the nurse in his docctor's office that he is ready to "just give up. It's too much trouble to eat anymore." Mr. E's weight today is 160 lb, 5 lb less than last month.

Nursing Care Plan

Subjective Data	Dependent on public transportation
	Painful knees
	Verbalized discouragement with procuring food
Objective Data	Weight loss of 5 lb in past month
Nursing Diagnosis	NANDA: Altered Health Maintenance (North American Nursing Diagnosis Association, 1999, with permission)
	Related to impaired mobility outside of home, as evidenced by verbalization to nurse and weight loss of 5 lb in past month.

Desired Outcomes Evaluation Criteria	Nursing Actions/ Interventions	Rationale
NOC: Health Beliefs: Perceived Resources (Johnson, Maas, and Moorhead, 2000, with permission.)	NIC: Health System Guidance (McCloskey and Bulechek, 2000, with permission)	
Mr. E. will acknowledge need for assistance with meals to stop losing weight by end of visit today.	Discuss Mr. E's weight change with him. Determine what kind of assistance he would accept.	Clients are likely to change behaviors only if the new behavior is acceptable to them.
Given several options of community support, Mr. E will select one and begin to implement the change within 3 days.	Describe Senior Citizen Nutrition Program, Meals on Wheels, home health aide shopping service, and door-to-door Care-a-Van service. Explore social support available from family and less restricted friends.	Clients may know about these programs but prefer to remain independent. Allowing the client some time to choose makes the choice more his own.
	Nurse to follow up with telephone call in 3 days.	Following up with a telephone call shows the nurse is committed to working through this problem with Mr. E.

Critical Thinking Question

1. What additional data could be sought in a more comprehensive assessment?
2. What other areas could be investigated to help balance to Mr. E's need for assistance with his desire for independence?
3. As you read this case, how would you define the underlying problem?

 Study Aids

Subjects ·Internet Sites	
National Policy and Resource Center on Nutrition and Aging · · · · · · .http://www.fiu.edu/~nutreldr	
International Food Information Council ·.http://ificinfo.health.org/index2-4.htm	
USDA Continuing Survey of Food Intakes by Individuals · · · · · · · · .http://www.barc.usda.gov/bhnrc/foodsurvey/home.htm	
Nutrition Monitoring ·.http://www.cdc.gov/nchs/data/tronm.pdf	
Office of Disease Prevention and Health Promotion · · · · · · · · · · · ·.http://odphp.osophs.dhhs.gov/	
Compilation of information on nutrition and health · · · · · · · · · · · ·.http://www.arborcom.com	
	http://www.healthfinder.gov
Client education ·.http://www.nutritionnewsfocuc.com/archive/al/NuFrEldrly.html
	http://oznet.ksu.edu/ext_F&N/Nutlink/pages/ELDER.HTM
	http://www.aafp.org/patientinfo
Osteoporosis ·.http://www.nof.org	
Dementia ·.http://health.net.nz/alzheimers/relatedDementias.asp	
	http://www.aafp.org/patientinfo/dementia.html

Chapter Review

1. Which of the following items are of concern in the diets of adults because adults ingest too much of them?
    a. Calcium and caffeine
    b. Kilocalories and fat
    c. Iron and zinc
    d. Incomplete protein
2. The decrease in gastric acid that accompanies aging causes concern for the absorption of which of the following nutrients?
    a. Carbohydrate and water
    b. Fat and cholesterol
    c. Vitamins A and E
    d. Vitamin B_{12} and iron
3. A nurse making a home visit routinely screens for dehydration in elderly clients. Which of the following would the nurse assess?
    a. Body temperature and urine specific gravity
    b. Tongue condition, pulse rate, and muscle strength
    c. Skin turgor and heart and lung sounds
    d. Client's intake and output records
4. Which of the following conditions is likely to contribute to vitamin D deficiency in older adults?
    a. Atrophied skin, dislike for milk, and indoor life
    b. Lack of exercise, failing hearing and vision
    c. Slowed peristalsis, diminished secretion of intrinsic factor
    d. Achlorhydria and inability to chew meats
5. Ms. P is a 58-year-old retired cook who tells the clinic nurse she regrets not having had children and grandchildren. Which of the following activities might assist Ms. P to attain generativity?
    a. Editing a cookbook for her church group.
    b. Taking a class in ethnic cooking in preparation for her next trip.
    c. Serving on the Meals-on-Wheels advisory board.
    d. Volunteering to teach a special recipe at a local school.

Clinical Analysis

Ms. O is a 66-year-old retired schoolteacher who suffered a stroke 8 months ago. For the past 7 months she has resided in a nursing home. Ms. O has residual weakness on the right side. She has not mastered the use of tableware with her left hand. Her nurse is concerned because Ms. O weighs 125 pounds; she had weighed 135 pounds upon admission to the nursing home. The nursing assistants report that Ms. O takes a little of most foods but refuses to eat more than half of any of the foods.

1. The nurse discovers that a contributing factor in Ms. O's refusal to eat is embarrassment over her inability to control her lips. Which of the following outcomes would be appropriate in this case?
    a. Client will gain 5 pounds in the next 2 weeks.
    b. Client will consume 3/4 of the food served within 1 week.
    c. Client will feed herself with her left hand within the next 3 weeks.
    d. Client will consent to tube feeding.
2. Which of the following nursing actions is appropriate initially to minimize Ms. O's embarrassment?
    a. Allowing her to eat her meals alone in her room
    b. Ordering finger foods that she can eat with her left hand
    c. Assigning her to a table with other stroke patients who feed themselves
    d. Instructing the nursing assistants to feed Ms. O privately
3. Which of the following activities could reasonably be expected to increase Ms. O's appetite?
    a. Participating in a craft session before lunch
    b. Taking a nap before dinner
    c. Walking before lunch or dinner
    d. Watching television with her roommate after breakfast

Bibliography

Adam, O: Review anti-inflammatory diet in rheumatic diseases. Eur J Clin Nutr 49:703, 1995.

Alaimo, K, et al,: Food insufficiency exists in the United States: Results from the third national health and nutrition examination survey (NHANES III). Am J Public Health 88:419, 1998.

Albertson, AM, Tobelmann, RC, and Marquart, L: Folate consumption and the role of ready-to-eat cereal for American women aged 15 to 50 years. Top Clin Nutr 12:58, 1997.

Alexander, JW: Immunonutrition: The role of omega-3 fatty acids. Nutrition 14:627, 1998.

Ausman, LM, and Russell, RM: Nutrition in the elderly. In Shils, ME, et al, (eds): Modern Nutrition in Health and Disease ed 9. Lippincott, Williams and Wilkins, Philadelphia, 1999.

Bonjour, J-P, Schurch, M-A, and Rizzoli, R: Nutritional aspects of hip fractures. Bone 18:139S, 1996.

Breslow, RA, Hallfrisch, J, and Goldberg, AP: Malnutrition in tubefed nursing home patients with pressure sores. J Parenter Enteral Nutr 15:663, 1991.

Bush, LA, et al,: D-E-N-T-A-L: A rapid self-administered screening instrument to promote referrals for further evaluation in older adults. J Am Geriatr Soc 44:979, 1996.

Centers for Disease Control: Prevalence of overweight among children, adolescents, and adults—United States, 1988–1994. MMWR 46:199, 1997. Accessed at http://www.cdc.gov/ejpo/mmwr/preview/mmwrhtml/00046647.htm

Centers for Disease Control: Osteoporosis among estrogen-deficient women—United States, 1988–1994. MMWR 47:969, 1998. Accessed 08/25/1999 at http://cdc.gov/epo/mmwr/preview/mmwrhtml/00055690.htm

Cooper, C: The crippling consequences of fractures and their impact on quality of life. Am J Med 103(2A):12S, 1997.

Corti, M-C, et al: Serum albumin level and physical disability as predictors of mortality in older persons. JAMA 272:1036, 1994.

Crespo, CJ, et al,: Leisure-time physical activity among US Adults. Arch Intern Med 156:93, 1996.

Declair, V: The usefulness of topical application of essential fatty acids (EFA) to prevent pressure ulcers. Ostomy Wound Manage 43:48, 1997.

de Deckere, EA: Health aspects of fish and n-3 polyunsaturated fatty acids from plant and marine origin. Eur J Clin Nutr 52:749,1998.

Denney, A: Quiet music: An intervention for mealtime agitation? J Gerontol Nurs 23:16, 1997.

Elbon, SM, Johnson, MA, and Fischer JG: Milk consumption in older Americans. Am J Public Heatlh 88:1221, 1998.

Elmstahl, S, et al,: Malnutrition in geriatric patients: A neglected problem? Journal of Advanced Nursing 26:851, 1997.

Feskanich, D, et al,: Vitamin K intake and hip fractures in women: a prospective study. Am J Clin Nutr 69:74, 1999.

Freedman, ML, and Ahronheim, JC: Nutritional needs of the elderly: Debate and recommendations. Geriatrics 40:45, 1986.

Freeman, MS, et al,: Cognitive, behavioral, and environmental correlates of nutrient supplement use among independently living older adults. Journal of Nutrition for the Elderly 17:19, 1998.

Gilmore, SA, et al,: Clinical indicators associated with unintentional weight loss and pressure ulcers in elderly residents of nursing facilities. J Am Diet Assoc 95:984, 1995.

Gold, PE: Role of glucose in regulating the brain and cognition. Am J Clin Nutr 61(4 suppl):987S, 1995.

Grisso, JA, et al,: Risk factors for hip fracture in black women. The Northeast Hip Fracture Study Group. N Engl J Med 330:1555, 1994.

Groff, JL, Gropper, SS, and Hunt, SM: Advanced Nutrition and Human Metabolism. West Publishing Company, Minneapolis/St. Paul, 1995.

Hill, DP, Cooper, DM, and Robson, MC: Serum albumin is a poor prognostic factor for pressure ulcer healing in controlled clinical trials. Wounds 6:174, 1994.

Incalzi, RA, et al,: Energy intake and in-hospital starvation. A clinically relevant relationship. Arch Intern Med 156:425, 1996.

Incalzi, RA, et al,: Inadequate caloric intake: a risk factor for mortality of geriatric patients in the acute-care hospital. Age and Ageing 27:303, 1998.

Johnell, O: The socioeconomic burden of fractures: Today and in the 21st century. Am J Med 103(2A):20S, 1997.

Johnson, M, Maas, M, and Moorhead, S: Nursing Outcomes Classification (NOC), ed 2. Mosby, Philadelphia, 2000.

Jones, JM, and Jones, KD: Promoting physical activity in the senior years. J Gerontol Nurs 23:40, 1997.

Kayser-Jones, J, and Schell, E: The mealtime experience of a cognitively impaired elder: ineffective and effective strategies. J Gerontol Nurs 23:33, 1997.

Krall, EA, and Dawson-Hughes, B: Osteoporosis. In Shils, ME, et al, (eds): Modern Nutrition in Health and Disease ed 9. Lippincott Williams and Wilkins, Philadelphia, 1999.

Kremer, JM: Effects of modulation of inflammatory and immune parameters in patients with rheumatic and inflammatory disease receiving dietary supplementation of n-3 and n-6 fatty acids. Lipids 31 (Suppl):S-243, 1996.

Kuczmarski, RJ, et al,: Increasing prevalence of overweight among U.S. adults. JAMA 272, 205, 1994.

Lawrence, RC, et al,: Estimates of the prevalence of arthritis and selected musculoskeletal disorders in the United States. Arthritis Rheum 41:778, 1998.

Life Sciences Research Office, Federation of American Societies for Experimental Biology: Third Report on Nutrition Monitoring in the United States: Executive Summary. Washington, DC, 1995. Accessed 11/13/99 at http://www.cdc.gov/nchs/data/tronm.pdf

Martin, RH: The role of nutrition and diet in rheumatoid arthritis. Proc Nutr Soc 57:231, 1998.

Martin, WE: The oral cavity and nutrition. In Geriatric Nutrition 2 ed. Raven Press, Philadelphia, 1995.

McCloskey, JC, and Bulechek, GM: Nursing Interventions Classification (NIC), 3 ed. Mosby, Philadelphia, 2000.

Melhus, H, et al,: Excessive dietary intake of vitamin A is associated with reduced bone mineral density and increased risk for hip fracture. Ann Intern Med 129:770, 1998.

Meydani, M, and Meisler, JG: A closer look at vitamin E. Postgrad Med 102:199, 1997.

Meydani, SN, et al,: Vitamin E supplementation and in vivo immune response in healthy elderly subjects. JAMA 277:1380, 1997.

Morley, JE: Anorexia of aging and protein–energy undernutrition. In Morley, JE, Glick, Z, and Rubenstein, LZ (eds): Geriatric Nutrition ed 2. Raven Press, Ltd, New York, 1995.

Morley, JE: Anorexia of aging: Physiologic and pathologic. Am J Clin Nutr 66:760, 1997.

Morrisson, SG: Feeding the elderly population. Nurs Clin North Am 32:791, 1997.

National Live Stock and Meat Board: Eating in America Today, ed 2. Chicago, 1995.

Nelson, ME, et al,: Effects of high-intensity strength training on multiple risk factors for osteoporotic fractures. JAMA 272:1909, 1994.

Nicklas, TA, et al,: Impact of breakfast consumption on nutritional adequacy of the diets of young adults in Bogalusa, Louisiana: ethnic and gender contrasts. J Am Diet Assoc 98:1432, 1998.

North American Nursing Diagnosis Association: Nursing Diagnoses: Definitions and Classification 1999–2000, North American Nursing Diagnosis Association, Philadelphia, 1999.

Osterweil, D, Wendt, PF, and Ferrell, BA: Pressure ulcers and nutrition. In Morley, JE, Glick, Z, and Rubenstein, LZ (eds): Geriatric Nutrition ed 2. Raven Press, Ltd, New York, 1995.

Paganini-Hill, A, et al,: Exercise and other factors in the prevention of hip fracture: The Leisure World study. Epidemiology 2:16, 1991.

Payette, H, et al,: Predictors of dietary intake in a functionally dependent elderly population in the community. Am J Public Health 85:677, 1995.

Perkins, AJ, et al,: Association of antioxidants with memory in a multiethnic elderly sample using the Third National Health and Nutrition Examination Survey. Am J Epidemiol 150:37, 1999.

Perneger, TV, et al,: Hospital-acquired pressure ulcers: Risk factors and use of preventive devices. Arch Intern Med 158:1940, 1998.

Perrig, WJ, Perrig, P, and Stahelin, HB: The relation between antioxidants and memory performance in the old and very old. J Am Geriatr Soc 45:718, 1997.

Pfefferbaum, A, et al,: In vivo brain concentrations of N-acetyl compounds, creatine, and choline in Alzheimer Disease. Arch Gen Psychiatry 56:185, 1999.

Popkin, BM, Siega-Riz, AM, and Haines, PS: A comparison of dietary trends among racial and socioeconomic groups in the United States. N Engl J Med 335:716, 1996.

Quinn, C: The Nutrition Screening Initiative: Meeting the nutritional needs of elders. Orthop Nurs 16:13, 1997.

Ranieri, P, et al,: Determinants of malnutrition in a geriatric ward: Role of comorbidity and functional status. Journal of Nutrition for the Elderly 16:11, 1996.

Rose, D, and Oliveira, V: Nutrient intakes of individuals from food-insufficient households in the United States. Am J Public Health 87:1956, 1997.

Rousseau, ME: Dietary prevention of osteoporosis. Lippincott's Primary Care Practice 1:307, 1997.

Rudman, D, et al,: Observations on the nutrient intakes of eating-dependent nursing home residents: Underutilization of micronutrient supplements. J Am Coll Nutr 14:604, 1995.

Russell, RM, Rasmussen, H, and Lichtenstein, AH: Modified food guide pyramid for people over 70 years of age. J Nutr 129:751, 1999.

Ryan, C, Eleazer, P, and Egbert, J: Vitamin D in the elderly. Nutr Today 30:228, 1995.

Sahyoun, NR, et al,: Body Mass Index, weight change, and incidence of self-reported physician-diagnosed arthritis among women. Am J Public Health 89: 391, 1999a.

Sahyoun, NR, et al,: Estrogen replacement therapy and incidence of self-reported physician-diagnosed arthritis. Prev Med 28:458, 1999b.

Schiffman, SS: Taste and smell losses in normal aging and disease. JAMA 278:1357, 1997.

Slemenda, C: Prevention of hip fractures: Risk factor modification. Am J Med 103(2A):65S, 1997.

Slesinski, MJ, Subar, AF, and Kahle, LL: Dietary intake of fat, fiber and other nutrients is related to the use of vitamin and mineral supplements in the United States: The 1992 National Health Interview Survey. J Nutr 126:3001, 1996.

Stein, TP, et al,: Attenuation of the protein wasting associated with bed rest by branched-chain amino acids. Nutrition 15:656, 1999.

Subar, AF, et al,: Dietary sources of nutrients among US adults, 1989 to 1991. J Am Diet Assoc 98:537, 1998.

Sullivan, DH, Sun, S, and Walls, RC: Protein-energy undernutrition among elderly hospitalized patients: A prospective study. JAMA 281:2013, 1999.

Tepper, BJ and Nayga, RM: Awareness of the link between bone disease and calcium intake is associated with higher dietary calcium intake in women aged 50 years and older: Results of the 1991 CSFII-DHKS. J Am Diet Assoc 98:196, 1998.

Thomas, DR: Specific nutritional factors in wound healing. Adv Wound Care 10:40, 1997.

Tully, MW, et al,: The Eating Behavior Scale: A simple method of assessing functional ability in patients with Alzheimer's Disease. J Gerontol Nurs 23:9, 1997.

U.S. Department of Agriculture. Pyramid Servings Data. 1994–96 Continuing Survey of Food Intakes by Individuals. February 1999. Accessed 10/05/1999 at http://www.barc.usda.gov

Vellas, BJ, et al,: The roles of nutrition and body composition in falls, gait, and balance disorders in the elderly. In Morley, JE, Glick, Z, and Rubenstein, LZ (eds): Geriatric Nutrition ed 2. Raven Press, Ltd, New York, 1995.

Watson, J, and Jaffee, MS: Nurse's Manual of Laboratory and Diagnostic Tests ed 2. FA Davis, Philadelphia, 1995.

Weddle, DO, Wellman, NS, and Bates, GM: Incorporating nutrition screening into three Older Americans Act elderly nutrition programs. Journal of Nutrition for the Elderly 17:19, 1997.

Weinberg, AD, Minaker, KL, and the Council on Scientific Affairs, American Medical Association. JAMA 274:1552, 1995.

Winograd, CH, and Brown, EM: Aggressive oral refeeding in hospitalized patients. Am J Clin Nutr 52:967, 1990.

Food Management

LEARNING OBJECTIVES

After completing this chapter, the student should be able to:

1. Describe the conditions under which microbiologic food illnesses can occur.
2. Discuss the information on food labels.
3. Identify foods that are likely to harbor disease-producing microbiologic organisms.
4. Describe one systematic approach to identify nutritional hazards in a person's diet.
5. Teach clients how to prevent food-borne illnesses.

Effective meal management requires knowledge about food safety, including microbiological hazards, environmental pollutants, natural food intoxicants, and nutritional hazards. How food is handled between the time it leaves the farm and the time it reaches the dinner table affects our health and well-being. As health care moves from institutions to home care, health-care workers need to understand the vital importance to human well-being of safe and nutritious food.

Each American eats more than 10,000 pounds of food each year. Considering the number of people involved in the growth, distribution, preparation, and service of food, our food safety record is excellent. The United States food supply is as safe, wholesome, and nutritious as any in the world.

Food safety is a concern not just here in the United States but also worldwide. Some food handling and consumption behaviors that were practiced ten years ago are not considered safe today. New strains of pathogens or disease-producing organisms are continually evolving; in some cases these organisms have proven resistant to antibiotics. The development of resistant food-borne pathogens has been attributed to increased use of antibiotics in hospitals, outpatient facilities, and veterinary applications (Wegener et al., 1999). See Box 14–1 for many foods involved in recent outbreaks of food-borne illness.

The Food and Drug Administration (FDA) has developed a list of food safety problems. Problems are ranked in descending order of impor-

tance, based on the number of people affected by the problem and its severity:

1. Microbiologic hazards
2. Nutritional hazards
3. Environmental pollutants
4. Natural food intoxicants
5. Food additives

The most common food-borne illnesses are caused when bacteria and other microbiological microorganisms that are naturally present in the environment contaminate food and are allowed to grow because of improper food handling (Clark, 1999). This chapter discusses each of the FDA's food safety concerns.

Microbiologic Hazards

Many organisms in our environment cause disease, including bacteria and parasites, viruses and fungi. These microorganisms may be carried from one host to another by animals, humans, inanimate objects including food, and environmental factors, such as air, water, and soil. Many microorganisms cause disease. Under certain conditions, food can become a vehicle for disease transmission.

Most food-borne diseases infect the tissues of the digestive tract and cause gastric distress; symptoms range from mild to severe. Mild symptoms include gastric and intestinal distress with abdominal pain, nausea, vomiting, diarrhea, and cramps. Severe symptoms include dehydration, bloody stools, and neurological disorders.

Prevalence and Costs

Approximately 9000 Americans die each year from food-borne disease, and an estimated 80 million become ill (Williams, 1999). Young, old, pregnant, and immunocompromised clients (YOPI)—25 percent of the U.S. population—are at the greatest risk. Clinical Application 14–1 discusses clients with suppressed immune systems.

Bacterial Food-Borne Disease

Bacteria are everywhere and account for 90 percent of all food-borne disease. Doorknobs, countertops, hands, eyelashes, mouths, some water

Box 14–1 Selected Examples of Foods Involved in Recent Outbreaks of Food-Borne Illness

Food source never identified	9578 people affected, many of them children; 11 deaths; 20 to 30 people critically ill in Japan (Morganthau, 1997)
Cantaloupe, 1991	400 people ill with *Salmonella* in 23 states (Morganthau, 1997)
Hamburger, 1993	Two deaths, 600 people ill from *E. coli* in two states (100 deaths and 20,000 cases in the United States each year) (CDC*, 1999)
Alfalfa sprouts, 1995	242 people ill from *Salmonella* in 17 states (Morganthau, 1997)
Raspberries, 1996	1000 people in 20 states ill from *Cyclospora* (a parasite) (CDC*, 1999)
Eggs, 1996 (See Clinical Application Box 14–2)	250 people ill from *Salmonella* in one state (CDC*, 1999)
Unpasteurized apple juice, 1996	70 people ill from *E. coli* in two states (Cody et al., 1999)
Oysters, 1997	400 people in five states ill from Norwalk virus (CDC, 1999)
Strawberries, 1997	230 people ill with hepatitis A in one state (CDC, 1999)
Deli meat, 1998	79 people ill and 12 deaths from listerosis in 16 states (CDC, 1999)
Parsley 1998	264 people in 36 states and Canada ill from *Shigella sonnei* (CDC, 1999)

*CDC = Centers for Disease Control

supplies, and food are a few of the many places where bacteria can be found.

On one square inch of our bodies live as many as 10,000 bacteria. While a large number of bacteria cause disease, most are harmless and many are helpful. Bacteria that cause disease are called pathogens, and bacteria that are not harmful are called normal flora. Normal flora help keep pathogenic bacteria from multiplying as rapidly as they might otherwise.

Bacteria are hearty, and scientists have found colonies thriving 1,600 feet below sea level with neither oxygen nor sunlight (www.pfizer.com, accessed 3-2000). Given sufficient time and the right conditions, most bacteria adapt to a new environment in 2 hours. For this reason, control of bacterial growth is vital.

Conditions for Growth

Bacterial growth refers to an increase in the number of organisms. Under ideal conditions, cell numbers can double every half hour: one cell becomes two, two become four, and four become eight (in an hour and a half). A single bacterium can multiply to 33 million after 12 hours. Bacteria cannot be eradicated from our environment. The growth of bacteria, however, can be controlled. For this reason, it is important to understand the conditions that are necessary for bacteria to grow. The following conditions are necessary for microbiological food illness to occur:

- Source of bacteria—The bacteria must come in contact with the food.
- Food—The food must permit the bacteria to grow and increase in number or produce a poisonous toxin.
- Temperature—The temperature must be favorable for the growth of bacteria. The temperature range in which most bacteria multiply rapidly is 40°F to 140°F, the range that includes room temperature and body temperature (Fig. 14–1).

- Time—Enough time must elapse for bacteria to grow, produce a toxin, or both.
- Moisture—Bacteria need water to dissolve and digest food. Foods that contain water support the growth of bacteria better than do dehydrated foods.
- Ingestion—An unsuspecting person must eat the food or drink the beverage that contains the toxin or bacteria.

Bacteria are frequently odorless, tasteless, and colorless. Without laboratory analysis there is no way to tell whether or not a food will cause

CLINICAL APPLICATION 14–1

Food Safety and Immunosuppressed Clients

All clients receiving immunosuppressive agents need counseling on food safety and sanitation. These clients have an inability to fight infections, so a relatively small number of bacteria could cause illness. Immunosuppressive agents are drugs that interfere with the body's ability to fight infections. These drugs are used in tissue and organ transplantation procedures, such as a kidney transplant. They are also used in controlling certain diseases.

AIDS (acquired immune deficiency syndrome) is caused by a virus. This virus permits infections, malignancies, and nervous system disorders to develop out of control. According to the FDA, AIDS clients are 300 times more likely than healthy persons to contract a Salmonella infection if the organism is present. Preventing food illness from occurring in the first place will save these patients much expense and suffering. All AIDS clients need instruction on the importance of good handwashing and personal hygiene. Proper instruction on food selection, storage, and preparation is also indicated.

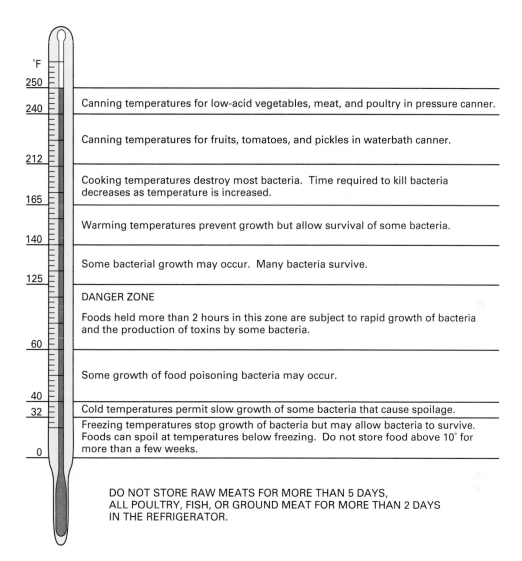

Figure 14–1:
A temperature guide to food safety (http://www.ars.usda/dgac)

illness. Bacterial food-borne diseases are traditionally subdivided into two groups, food infections and food intoxication. Table 14–1 lists pathogens of both groups, foods linked to these organisms, and manifestations.

Food Infections

A **food infection** is an illness caused by eating a food containing a large number of disease-producing bacteria. Symptoms of food infections usually start 12 to 36 hours after consumption of the offending food. Probably the best-known genus of bacteria causing food-borne illness is *Salmonella.* The infection, called **salmonellosis,** is transmitted by the consumption of contaminated foods or contact with an infected person. Some foods support the growth of *Salmonella* better than others. See Clinical Application 14–2 for guidelines on the safe handling of eggs, a common vehicle for salmonella transmission. Typhoid fever is caused by one type of *Salmonella* bacteria. This illness is spread by food and water

contaminated by feces and urine of clients and carriers. Figures 14–2 and 14–3 illustrate *Streptococci* and *Salmonella typhimurium.*

Other types of bacteria also cause food infections. *Campylobacter jejuni* is considered an emerging pathogen. This organism is carried in the intestinal tracts of cows, hogs, sheep, and poultry. Contaminated water or raw manure can spread the organism. For example, an animal can defecate on a vegetable garden and contaminate the produce. Foods found to be contaminated with *Campylobacter jejuni* include raw milk, fresh mushrooms, and raw hamburger. *Campylobacter* can be controlled by keeping food below 40°F or above 140°F and by maintaining good food-handling practices.

Another emerging pathogen is *Listeria.* This organism is problematic because the bacteria can grow slowly at refrigerator temperatures (32 to 34°F) and on moist surfaces. Cooking facilities must be kept clean and dry to prevent the growth of this organism. One household compound

Table 14–1 Pathogens, Common Food Vehicles and Symptoms

Pathogen	Common Food Vehicles	Symptoms
Salmonella/Food Infection	Raw eggs, raw milk, poultry, red meat, ground beef	Sudden onset of headache, abdominal pain, diarrhea, nausea and vomiting. Dehydration may be severe and fever is usually present. May develop into septicemia.
Listeria/Food Infection	Soft cheeses, deli meats, pâté, burritos, ice cream	Meningoencephalitis and or septicemia in newborns and adults and abortion in pregnant women.
Escherichia coli 0157:H7/Food Infection	Ground beef, other beef, raw milk, unpasteurized apple juice	May lead to acute hemorrhagic colitis (cramps, bloody diarrhea, nausea, vomiting, and fever). May result in hemolytic uremic failure or kidney failure
Campylobacter jejuni/Food Infection	Poultry, beef, raw eggs, water	An acute gastroenteritis of variable severity characterized by diarrhea, abdominal pain, malaise, fever, nausea, and vomiting. Guillain–Barre syndrome or meningitis has been seen in severe cases.
Norwalk Virus/ Food Infection	Raw shellfish and salad ingredients in the United States. Rehydrated cereals, grains, legumes, and nuts worldwide.	Usually a self-limited mild to moderate disease with nausea, vomiting, diarrhea, abdominal pain, headache, malaise, and low-grade fever.
Staphylococcus aureus/Food Intoxication	Poultry, processed meats, cheeses, ice cream, mixed dishes such as potato salad, and spaghetti	Wide variety of syndromes with manifestations such as skin lesions, lung or brain abscess, and endocarditis. May lead to Ritter Syndrome (an inflammatory skin disease seen in newborns, characterized by pustules that fill with a straw-colored fluid and become encrusted).
Clostridium botulinum/Food Intoxication	Improperly processed canned food Large masses of food with air-free center	Acute bilateral cranial nerve impairment and descending weakness or paralysis. Double vision, dysphasia, and dry mouth may be present. Vomiting, diarrhea, or constipation may be present initially.

effective in inhibiting or inactivating this organism is chlorine (bleach), one tablespoon per gallon of water.

Infection with *Clostridium perfringens* is characterized by intense abdominal cramps and diarrhea that usually begin 8 to 22 hours after consumption of the contaminated food or beverage. Careful control of a food's temperature and good personal hygiene help protect a person from infection.

Food Intoxication

Food intoxication is an illness caused by the consumption of a food in which bacteria have produced a poisonous toxin. One of the most common species of bacteria that produce a poisonous toxin is *Staphylococcus aureus*, often referred to simply as staph. Staph have been reported to be

in the nasal passages of 30 to 50 percent of healthy people and on the hands of 20 percent of all healthy people. Infected cuts, boils, and burns harbor this organism. Heat destroys the bacteria but not the toxins the bacteria already have produced. Because heat does not destroy the toxin, control of temperature alone will not provide protection. Prevention of staph poisoning must include good personal hygiene and keeping foods below 40°F or above 140°F.

Clostridium botulinum is another bacterium that produces a toxin. The resulting disease is **botulism**. The organism is found in soils throughout the world and can be found in the intestinal tracts of domestic animals. Vegetables grown in contaminated soil harbor this organism. Botulin, the toxin produced by *C. botulinum*, is so poisonous that a single ounce would be enough to kill the world's population. The spores of

CLINICAL APPLICATION 14–2

Guidelines for the Safe Handling of Eggs

- Prepare eggs individually. For example, individually prepared and immediately served poached, soft-cooked, and over-easy eggs with a partially set yolk are a low-risk way to eat eggs.

- Serve eggs soon after preparation. Do not hold longer than necessary. Do not cook, chill, hold, and reheat unless temperature is tightly maintained (below 50°F or greater than 140°F).

- Refrigerate eggs. Keep eggs at less than 45°F, both shell eggs and mixtures. Egg should not remain out of refrigeration for more than 1 hour.

- Do not use eggs with cracks or leaks. Inspect each egg individually.

- Use a pasteurized egg product if procedures require pooling or undercooked/raw eggs. Pasteurized is safer, but be aware that pasteurized eggs must also be handled with care. Time/temperature abuse is still a factor: They must be thawed under refrigeration or kept refrigerated—the egg is still a perfect medium for bacteria.

- Cook eggs adequately. Cooking for any amount of time reduces the number of bacteria present. In general, cook eggs until the white is set and the yolk begins to thicken. The white coagulates between 144°F and 149°F and the yolk between 149°F and 158°F. Eggs are pasteurized at 140°F for 3 1/2 minutes.

C. botulinum grow under anaerobic (without air) conditions. Canned foods are processed to be anaerobic; thus they provide an ideal medium for the growth of this bacterium. Home-canned, nonacid fruits and vegetables, faultily processed commercially canned tuna, and improperly packaged smoked fish all have transmitted botulism.

Botulism can be avoided by the proper processing and preparation of susceptible foods. Home canners should consult a reliable home-canning food guide regarding proper time, pressure, and temperature required to kill spores for each specific food. As an additional precaution, all home-canned foods should be boiled for at least 10 minutes prior to serving to destroy botulinal toxins (Box 14-2).

Norwalk virus is another emerging pathogen that can withstand freezing temperatures and also chlorine solutions. This organism is, however, susceptible to high temperatures (above 140°F). The best insurance against this pathogen is to eat foods hot. Other control measures include good personal hygiene and the purchase of food and water from reliable sources.

Bacterial Food-Borne Disease on the Rise

The risk of food-borne illness is increasing for several reasons including:

- The worldwide overuse of antibiotics. Antibiotics kill not only pathogens but also normal flora, which help keep the disease-producing organisms in balance. If an antibiotic is overused, it loses its effectiveness in killing disease-producing bacteria because in response to the antibiotic's "attack," some of the bacteria undergo genetic mutations that make them strong enough to fight off the action of the drug. Those stronger bacteria then flourish and become harder to kill than the bacteria that originally caused the problem (Gershoff, 1998).

  Some experts believe the overuse of antibacterial soap and sanitizing agents is leading to the development of bacteria that will be able to withstand the action of antibacterial agents. New strains of pathogens can evolve and become resistant to antibacterials in 90 days, yet it takes humans hundreds of thousands of years to build the immunity to fight them (Mishler, 1999). For this reason, some experts do not recommend the use of antibacterial soaps in low-risk situations, such as daily household use.

- In the United States, the average age of the population continues to increase as life expectancy increases. Older people are more susceptible to pathogenic bacteria than younger people; fewer organisms are needed to produce symptoms in older people.

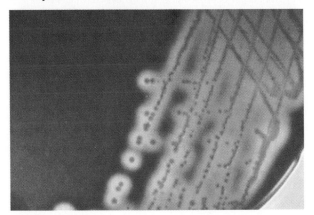

Figure 14–2:
Streptococci (from Thomas, CL (ed): Taber's Cyclopedic Medical Dictionary, FA Davis Publishing Co. p. 191, Philadelphia, 1997).

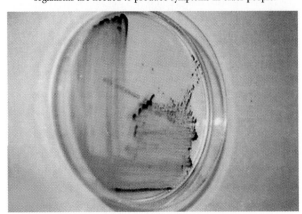

Figure 14–3:
Salmonella (from Thomas, CL (ed): Taber's Cyclopedic Medical Dictionary, FA Davis Publishing Co. p. 191, Philadelphia, 1997).

Box 14–2 Botulism and Mad Cow Disease

Outbreaks of serious disease have been linked to changes is food preparation and processing. In botulism, the anaerobic organism secretes a toxin in airtight food packages. The source has classically been considered to be home-canned, nonacid fruits and vegetables. But other sources have been found. Years ago in Alaska, botulism was traced to the substitution of plastic bags for clay pots in the preparation of a Native American dish. Similarly, smoked fish packaged in plastic bags rather than in waxed paper and wooden crates was identified as the source of the disease in Michigan. More recently, in 1994, the largest outbreak of botulism in the United States since 1978 was documented in El Paso, Texas. Thirty people who ate a potato-based dip in a Greek restaurant became ill, four of whom required mechanical ventilation. The source of the type A botulism toxin was found to be baked potatoes wrapped in aluminum foil and stored at room temperature for several days before they were incorporated into the dip.

Mad cow disease (bovine spongiform encephalopathy, BSE) in Britain has a similar history, but of disastrous dimension. BSE is one of several subacute degenerative diseases of the brain, invariably fatal, with very long incubation periods and no demonstrable inflammatory or immune response. A disease called scrapie is common in sheep, but a species barrier was thought to protect other animals and humans. In the 1970s the disease was spread to cattle through contaminated feed and supplements.

Infected brain, spinal cord tissue, or blood transmits the pathogen. A related affliction in humans, Creutzfeldt-Jakob disease (CJD), had been conveyed by contaminated neurosurgical instruments, dural grafts, corneal transplants, and pituitary hormones. Now a new variant of CJD (vCJD) has been identified and linked to ingestion of beef (Gale, 1998; Hillerton, 1998; Ironside, 1998; Will, 1998).

The causative agent is a prion, a proteinaceous infectious agent that is extremely difficult to destroy. It is resistant to heat, pressure cooking, ultraviolet light, irradiation, bleach, formaldehyde, and weak acids. Even autoclaving (a process that sterilizes by steam pressure) at 135°F for 18 minutes does not eliminate infectivity.

A change in the British processing of animal carcasses for animal feed in 1982 began the transmission of the infective agent to cattle. Deregulation of the industry allowed processing standards to fall. Four years later, the first case of BSE was confirmed in Britain. In 1988, the use of protein from ruminants was banned as a constituent of ruminant feed. Specific bovine organs were banned for use as food for humans in 1989 and as fertilizer in 1991. Various export bans were imposed from 1990 to 1994.

By March 1995, more than 146,000 confirmed cases of BSE were recorded in Britain. As a result, cohort animals have been slaughtered, more than 900,000 dairy bull calves have been culled from herds, and all cattle more than 30 months old have been removed from the human food chain. Since the incubation period is usually 3 to 6 years, and since British beef cattle are usually slaughtered at about 2 years of age, it was not certain that BSE is eradicated from the food chain. By 1998, eating meat from infected animals probably caused 24 human deaths from vCJD. Of these, 23 occurred in the United Kingdom and one in France (Fishbein, 1998).

The ultimate extent of the epidemic is unknown. Predictions cover a wide range: virtual extinction of BSE by the year 2000 (Hillerton, 1998) or 2001 (Bradley, 1998) to a high degree of uncertainty concerning the size of the vCJD epidemic through the years 2001 to 2003 (Ghani et al. 1998). The latter conclusion is based on a mathematical model showing that the minimum incubation period was about nine years and that at least 20 percent of the people with vCJD diagnosed through 1998 were exposed to the agent prior to 1986.

Progress has been made in protecting the food supply. Until now the presence of tissue from the central nervous system could not be detected in meat products. A new procedure to do so has been developed by Lucker et al. (1999).

What is clear from both the botulism and the spongiform encephalopathy outbreaks is that drastically altering proven food-processing procedures without verifying equivalent safety can be dangerous. In the cases of serious diseases, the hazard is substantial.

- Food production has become more centralized, an effect that has both good and bad ramifications. Food inspectors can more closely monitor the sanitation at food-processing plants, but a food-borne illness outbreak affects more people in wider geographical areas.

- Increased sensitivity of laboratory equipment has dramatically improved the ability to detect food-borne illness outbreaks and to trace the sources of these outbreaks.

- As the population becomes highly educated about food safety, illnesses that in the past might have been dismissed as "stomach flu" are increasingly being identified as food-borne illnesses.

- Many foods are imported from countries whose regulatory procedures are not as stringent as those in the United States.

- Consumers are eating more meals away from home and using more convenience foods. Both behaviors increase the number of individuals involved in food handling and the time food is held in the danger zones. For example, a frozen convenience food is held in the temperature danger zone (between 40 and 140°F) twice, once during assembly in the food-processing factory and a second time when the consumer is reheating it.

- Consumers are eating more raw food and more lightly grilled and sautéed foods, which are sometimes not cooked to proper temperatures.

Parasitic Infections

A **parasite** is an organism that lives within, upon, or at the expense of a living host without providing any benefit to the host. Several parasites can live in animals that human beings use for food. When a person eats an animal infected with a parasite, he or she also consumes the parasite and the result is illness. Two common parasites are *Trichinella spiralis* and tapeworms.

Trichinella Spiralis

Trichinella spiralis is a worm that becomes embedded in the muscle tissue of pigs. A pig may be fed meat from an animal that harbors the worm in its muscle. Some farmers still feed hogs table scraps that contain meat. The worm produces larvae that are protected from animal (including human) digestion. The larvae mature in the animal's stomach in 5 to 7 days. The adult worms then invade the lining of the small intestine, where they reproduce. The larvae enter the bloodstream of the animal and are carried to all parts of the body. They then penetrate the muscles, form cysts, and remain alive and infective for months. The cycle is completed when another animal eats the muscle containing the live *Trichinella spiralis* larvae.

When a human being eats the larvae, usually in undercooked pork, he or she develops **trichinosis**. The symptoms of trichinosis usually appear 9 days after the ingestion of the infected meat, but the time can vary from 2 to 28 days. This period of time is called the **incubation period**— the length of time it takes to show disease symptoms after exposure to the offending organism. The first symptoms, which mimic food poisoning, are nausea, vomiting, and diarrhea. When the larvae migrate into muscles, including the heart muscle, systemic symptoms develop that include fever, swelling of the eyelids, sweating, weakness, and muscular pain. Death due to heart failure may occur.

Tapeworms

Tapeworms are acquired by humans through the ingestion of raw seafood or undercooked beef and pork. Hogs and steers become intermediate hosts when they graze on sewage-polluted pastures. Tapeworm infestation can occur when human wastes contaminate freshwater streams and lakes, animal pastures, or feed. Symptoms of a tapeworm infection may be trivial or absent. In some people, the worms attach to the jejunum and hosts develop vitamin B_{12} deficiency, anemia, and massive infections with diarrhea. Obstruction of the bile duct or intestine can be another complication.

Viral Infections

A **virus** is a microscopic parasite that is entirely dependent on the nutrients inside host cells for its metabolic and reproductive needs. Viruses may invade the cells of people, animals, plants, and bacteria to survive and thereby cause disease. Food frequently serves as a vehicle for some viruses, including those that cause influenza and infectious hepatitis. Food can become contaminated in its growing environment or during processing, storage, distribution, or preparation.

Some viruses are found in the intestinal tract of infected humans. If an infected person neglects to wash his or her hands after defecation and then handles food, the virus can contaminate the food and be passed on to unsuspecting consumers. The disease varies from a mild illness lasting 1 to 2 weeks to a severely disabling disease lasting several months (Chin, 1999).

Hepatitis A Virus

The hepatitis A virus causes infectious hepatitis, a liver disease. This virus can be found in water that has been contaminated with raw sewage and in shellfish harvested from fecally contaminated water. During food processing, hepatitis A can be transmitted when polluted water is used or by fecal contamination from insects or rodents. Infected workers can transmit the virus through sandwiches, baked goods, or any other food that is handled. Thus there are three ways the virus can be spread: polluted water, insects and rodents, and infected food handlers. The onset of viral hepatitis A is abrupt with fever, malaise, anorexia, nausea, and abdominal discomfort. A few days later the client may develop jaundice

Substances Made Poisonous by Other Organisms

The consumption of toxic fish and plants can cause illness. Some molds can also produce disease (others are beneficial).

Toxic Seafood

The tissue of fish and shellfish can be naturally toxic to humans even when the fish is fresh. The fish may not show any outward signs of illness, and there is usually no way to tell whether the fish is toxic or not. Because most fish toxins are stable to heat, cooking does not destroy them. **Paralytic shellfish poisoning** outbreaks have been reported involving the consumption of poisonous clams, oysters, mussels, and scallops.

Ciguatera poisoning is a serious human intoxication caused by ingestion of any of over 400 species of marine fish (Shils, 1999). This intoxication results from eating certain fish that have consumed marine bacteria and algae associated with coastal reefs and nearby waterways. Fish eating the algae become toxic, and the effect is magnified through the food chain so that large predatory fish become the most toxic; this occurs worldwide in tropical areas (Chin, 1999). Coastal waters are routinely monitored for the presence of the organism that produces ciguatera. If excessive numbers of the organism are found, a "red tide" alert is made. The best prevention is to avoid eating fish caught during a red tide.

Scromboid fish poisoning is caused by the presence of undesirable bacteria. This poisoning occurs in fish such as tuna, mackerel, bonito, and skipjack. The bacteria produce a toxin on the flesh of fish after the fish have been caught. Scromboid fish poisoning can be prevented by the adequate refrigeration of freshly caught fish and the purchase of fish from reputable sources.

Molds

Molds are the most widely encountered microorganism. Molds are spread by air currents, insects, and rodents. Some molds are beneficial. For example, molds are used to manufacture several types of cheese and soy sauce. Like bacteria, molds are often involved in food spoilage and are a nuisance in the food industry. A number of molds grow well in cold storage but are easily destroyed by a mild heating process, at which temperatures of 140°F or higher are reached.

Molds grow on bread, cheese, fruits, vegetables, starchy foods, preserves, grains, and a wide variety of other products. *Aspergillus* molds produce a series of mycotoxins called aflatoxins that may be present in peanuts or peanut products, corn, and cottonseed meal (Shils, 1999). Many experts believe aflatoxins to be the most potent liver toxin and cancer-producing agent known.

Table 14–2 Food Handling Tips Related to Specific Agents and Susceptible Foods

Infective Agent and Susceptible Foods	Food Handling Tips
Salmonella species Meat, eggs, poultry, milk, and products made with these foods	Wash hands especially after defecation and after preparing uncooked meat, poultry, and eggs. Wash all surfaces and utensils that come in contact with meat, eggs, and poultry thoroughly Refrigerate prepared food in small containers. Thoroughly cook all foodstuffs from animal sources. Avoid recontamination within the kitchen after cooking. (For example, do not allow food that has been cooked to come into contact with utensils used in the preparation of raw meats.) Never serve raw eggs, fish, and undercooked meats (see Clinical Application 14–2). Do not allow infected people to handle food. Instruct children to wash their hands after handling pet turtles, ducklings, or chicks.
Typhoid fever Any food or water	Wash hands after urination and/or defecation. Avoid contaminated water and ice.
Staphylococcus aureus Bruised poultry, processed meats, cheeses, ice cream, mixed dishes such as potato salad and spaghetti	Personal hygiene: hand washing, avoid handling food when you have infected cuts, boils, and burns (see Figure 14–1). Temperature control: store food below 40°F or above 140°F (see Figure 14–2); do not eat food held at room temperature for longer than 4 hours.
Clostridium perfringens Meats, stews, gravies, large masses of food	Cool food rapidly in shallow containers that are no more than 4 in. deep. Heat all leftovers to at least 165°F. Hold all hot food above 140°F.
Clostridium botulinum Canned foods Large masses of food with an air-free center	Never taste food from a bulging container. Do not serve home-canned food to institutionalized clients. Follow manufacturer's directions when home canning and use only equipment that has been carefully cleaned. Avoid home-smoked fish. Do not store home-smoked fish in plastic bags.

The best advice is to discard moldy bread; even if no other mold is visible, mold may have penetrated the rest of the item. Mold on natural cheese can be safely removed and the remainder of the cheese eaten because the mold is not as likely to have penetrated the rest of the cheese. Food-handling tips related to microbiological hazards are summarized in Table 14–2.

Avoiding Nutrition Hazards

Nutrition hazards are the number-two safety risk according to the FDA. Although problems associated with an unbalanced diet occur frequently, clinical symptoms of illness are not as acute and severe as those arising from microbiologic hazards. Illness from food infection or food intoxication poses an immediate danger. The following sections cover food labeling laws and a method health-care workers can use to assist in the evaluation of a client's dietary status. Knowledge of these topics can help pre-

vent the nutritional hazards associated with consumption of an unbalanced diet.

The Food Label

Food labeling has been developed by the federal government to provide up-to-date, easier-to-use nutrition information (Figs. 14–4 and 14–5). The 1989 RDAs were still used by the food industry to calculate food labels as this text was prepared. Features of the food label include:

1. *Standardized Format:* Every label has the same layout and design; the nutrition information is entitled "Nutrition Facts." Some very small packages may use a simplified format.
2. *Serving Sizes:* All serving sizes listed on similar products are stated in consistently used household and metric measures to allow comparison shopping.
3. *Daily Values:* The bottom half of the "Nutrition Facts" panel shows either the minimum or maximum levels of nutrients people should

The Food Label at a Glance

Descriptors
The FDA has set specific definitions for:
- free
- light
- more
- good source
- high
- low
- reduced
- less

For fish, meat, and poultry:
- lean
- extra lean

Ingredients
are listed in descending order by weight, and the list is required on almost all foods, even standardized ones like mayonnaise and bread.

Health Claim
message referred to on the front panel is shown here.

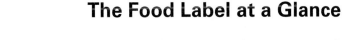

FROZEN MIXED VEGETABLES
IN SAUCE

- Low Fat
- Cholesterol Free
- Good Source of Fiber

See back panel for nutrition information

(See back panel for message on saturated fat and cholesterol and heart disease.)

NET WT. 8.9 oz. (252 g)

Ingredients: Broccoli, carrots, green beans, water chestnuts, soybean oil, milk solids, modified cornstarch, salt, spices.

"While many factors affect heart disease, diets low in saturated fat and cholesterol may reduce the risk of this disease."

Source: Food and Drug Administration 1993

Health Claims
can carry information about the link between certain nutrients and specific diseases. For such a "health claim" to be made on a package, FDA must first determine that the diet-disease link is supported by scientific evidence. At this time, FDA is allowing seven specific claims about the relationships between:

- fat and cancer risk
- saturated fat and cholesterol and heart disease risk
- calcium and osteoporosis risk
- sodium and hypertension risk
- fruits, vegetables, and grains that contain soluble fiber and heart disease risk
- fiber-containing grain products, fruits, and vegetables and cancer risk
- fruits and vegetables and cancer risk.

Figure 14–4:
The Food Label at a Glance. The food label must include descriptors, ingredients, and only certain allowed health claims in a standardized format. (From the Food and Drug Administration, 1993.)

consume each day for a healthful diet. For example, the value listed for carbohydrates refers to the minimum level, while the value for fat refers to the maximum level.

4. *Percent Daily Values:* The figures for percentage of daily values are based on a 2000-kilocalorie diet; this schema makes it easier for consumers to judge the nutritional quality of a food.

5. *Health Claims:* The Food and Drug Administration allows only seven specific claims about the relationships between:

- Fat and cancer risk
- Saturated fat and cholesterol and heart disease risk
- Calcium and osteoporosis risk
- Sodium and hypertension risk
- Fruits, vegetables, and grains that contain soluble fiber and heart disease risk
- Fruits and vegetables and cancer risk
- Soy protein included in a diet low in saturated fat and cholesterol and coronary heart disease

6. *Descriptors:* Terms like "low," "high," and "free" used on food labels must meet legal definitions. Free means less than 0.5 gram of fat per serving and tiny or insignificant amounts of cholesterol, sodium, and sugar. *Low* indicates 3 grams of fat (or less) per serving; also low in saturated fat, cholesterol, and/or kilocalories. *Lean* signifies less than 10 grams of fat, 4 grams of saturated fat, and 95 milligrams of cholesterol per serving. ("Lean" is higher in fat than

"Low.") *Extra Lean* means 5 grams of fat, 2 grams of saturated fat, and 95 milligrams of cholesterol per serving. ("Extra Lean" is lower in fat than "Lean" but not as low in fat as "Low.") *Light* (Lite) denotes 1/3 fewer kilocalories or 1/2 the fat of the original; no more than 1/2 the sodium of the higher-sodium version. *Cholesterol Free* means the item has less than 2 milligrams of cholesterol and 2 grams (or less) of saturated fat per serving. *High:* In order for a food to be listed as "High" in a particular nutrient, it must contain 20 percent or more of the Daily Value for that nutrient. *Good Source Of:* One serving of a food considered to be a good source of a vitamin, mineral, or fiber, contains 10 to 19 percent of the Daily Value for that particular vitamin, mineral, or fiber.

7. Ingredients are listed in descending order by weight. The ingredients list is required on almost all foods, even some standardized ones like ice cream, mayonnaise, and bread (see Figs. 14–4 and 14–5).

Evaluation of Dietary Status

Reviewing a client's reported intake or actual food consumption and comparing this amount to the Food Guide Pyramid can assist in the identification of some nutrients that may be lacking in a person's diet. Table 14–3 lists recommended number of servings needed each day according to sex, age, and physiological state (breast-feeding or pregnant). The following method of comparing a client's daily intake to the Food Guide Pyramid is suggested; answer these questions about the client.

The Food Label at a Glance

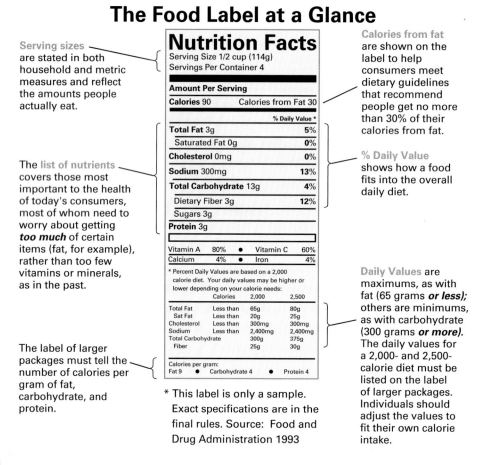

Serving sizes are stated in both household and metric measures and reflect the amounts people actually eat.

The list of nutrients covers those most important to the health of today's consumers, most of whom need to worry about getting *too much* of certain items (fat, for example), rather than too few vitamins or minerals, as in the past.

The label of larger packages must tell the number of calories per gram of fat, carbohydrate, and protein.

Nutrition Facts
Serving Size 1/2 cup (114g)
Servings Per Container 4

Amount Per Serving

Calories 90   Calories from Fat 30

% Daily Value *

Total Fat 3g — 5%
Saturated Fat 0g — 0%
Cholesterol 0mg — 0%
Sodium 300mg — 13%
Total Carbohydrate 13g — 4%
Dietary Fiber 3g — 12%
Sugars 3g
Protein 3g

Vitamin A 80% • Vitamin C 60%
Calcium 4% • Iron 4%

* Percent Daily Values are based on a 2,000 calorie diet. Your daily values may be higher or lower depending on your calorie needs:

		Calories 2,000	2,500
Total Fat	Less than	65g	80g
Sat Fat	Less than	20g	25g
Cholesterol	Less than	300mg	300mg
Sodium	Less than	2,400mg	2,400mg
Total Carbohydrate		300g	375g
Fiber		25g	30g

Calories per gram:
Fat 9 • Carbohydrate 4 • Protein 4

* This label is only a sample. Exact specifications are in the final rules. Source: Food and Drug Administration 1993

Calories from fat are shown on the label to help consumers meet dietary guidelines that recommend people get no more than 30% of their calories from fat.

% Daily Value shows how a food fits into the overall daily diet.

Daily Values are maximums, as with fat (65 grams *or less);* others are minimums, as with carbohydrate (300 grams *or more).* The daily values for a 2,000- and 2,500-calorie diet must be listed on the label of larger packages. Individuals should adjust the values to fit their own calorie intake.

Figure 14–5:
The Food Label at a Glance. The food label must include descriptors, ingredients, and only certain allowed health claims in a standardized format. (From the Food and Drug Administration, 1993.)

1. Did the client consume at least the recommended servings of grains for his or her sex, age, and physiological state? Nutrients supplied by this group include carbohydrate, folic acid, thiamin, iron, and niacin. A person who does not eat enough grains may be deficient in these nutrients. In addition, this nutrient group supplies fiber.

2. Did the client consume recommended servings of fruits? After counting the number of servings of fruits eaten, check for a reliable source of vitamin C (such as citrus, melons, and berries). It is difficult for a client to meet his or her vitamin C allowance without including fruits or some vegetables in the diet. Other nutrients in this group are fiber, iron, potassium, folic acid, carbohydrate, and other trace minerals. Remember that many fruits function as a "scrub brush" for the teeth and intestines.

   If an individual's diet is low in fruits, ask about his or her **dentition,** the status of a person's teeth. Inspect the client's mouth and observe how many teeth are missing. Does the client have oral pain when chewing? Is the client able to tolerate all food textures? The client may avoid eating a particular fruit (especially raw) because of chewing problems. The client may also have a problem with elimination.

3. Did the client consume the recommended number of servings of vegetables? After counting the servings of vegetables, check for a reliable source of vitamin A (such as broccoli, carrots, or other dark green or yellow vegetable). It is difficult for an individual to meet his or her vitamin A allowance without including some vegetables in the diet. Many of the comments listed under fruits also apply to the vegetable group. For example, elimination problems may be related to a poor dietary intake of fiber secondary to the exclusion of vegetables from the diet. A person may elect to omit raw vegetables from his or her diet because of poor dentition.

4. Did the client consume the appropriate amount of milk for his or her age, sex, and physiological state? If not, the diet may be lacking in calcium, vitamin D, and riboflavin. Double-check for other reliable sources of calcium such as cheese and foods made with milk.

5. Did the client consume the number of recommended servings from the meat group for his or her age and physiological state? If not, the diet may be lacking in protein, iron, and B-vitamins. Remember that the meat group also includes cheese, eggs, dried beans and legumes, and other protein-rich foods.

TABLE 14–3 How Many Servings Do You Need Each Day?

Calorie level*	about 1600	about 2200	about 2800
Bread group	6	9	11
Vegetable group	3	4	5
Fruit group	2	3	4
Milk group	2–3†	2–3†	2–3†
Meat group	2, for a total of 5 oz	2, fol- a total of 6 oz	3 for a total of 7 oz

*These are the calorie levels if your choose low-fat, lean foods from the five major food groups and use foods from the fats, oils, and sweets group sparingly.
†Women who are pregnant or breast-feeding, teenagers, and young adults to age 24 need three servings.
SOURCE: USDA: *Food Guide Pyyramid—A Guide to Good Eating.* Consumer Information Center, Pueblo, Colorado.

Environmental Pollutants

A great many people are concerned about environmental pollution. Although the problem is widespread, situations that pose a severe and immediate danger to health are uncommon. The U.S. Environmental Protection Agency (EPA) regulates the use of pesticides and sets tolerance levels to provide a high margin of safety in food. Issues in food preparation and processing are discussed in Box 14–2.

Chemical Poisoning

Chemical poisoning occurs when people eat toxic substances that may be intentionally or accidentally added to foods during growing, harvesting, processing, transporting, storing, or preparing foods. Two general types of chemical poisoning can occur. They are heavy-metal and chemical-product contamination pesticides.

Heavy Metals

Several metals can be toxic. Sources of metals in the soil include parts of rocks and minerals that have weathered to produce soil, water erosion of soil particles, metals as added ingredients or impurities in fertilizers, pesticides containing metals, metals in manure and sludge, and metals in airborne dust. The origin of airborne dust is industrial and mining waste, fossil fuel combustion products, radioactive fallout, pollen, sea spray, and meteoric and volcanic material. Airborne dust eventually settles to the ground and becomes part of the soil. Plants may grow normally but contain levels of selenium, cadmium, molybdenum, or lead that are toxic to humans.

The toxic action of metals is believed to be important in enzyme poisoning. For example, mercury, lead, copper, beryllium, cadmium, and silver have been found to inhibit the enzyme alkaline phosphatase. One function of alkaline phosphatase is in the mineralization process of bone. Some disease states associated with the consumption of toxic minerals include rickets and bone tumors. Lead ingestion with a subsequent elevation of blood lead levels has been linked to a variety of toxic effects including adverse neurologic, neurobehavioral, and developmental effects (Shils, 1999) (see Clinical Application 8–5 in Chapter 8).

Mercury is extremely toxic and is widely distributed over the surface of the earth. Episodes of serious poisoning include those in Minamata (1953 to 1960) and the Niigata area (1965) in Japan (Shils, 1999), in which large chemical plants poured industrial waste containing mercury into nearby bays. Area residents who ate fish from the bays complained of numbness of the extremities, slurred speech, unsteady gait, deafness, and visual disturbances. Mental confusion and muscular incoordination were apparent in all the clients.

Chemical Products

Chemical food-borne illness is also associated with chemical products such as detergents, sanitizers, pesticides, and other chemicals that may enter the food supply. After such toxins have been ingested, the symptoms of chemical poisoning appear in a few minutes to a few hours, but usually in less than 1 hour. Nausea, vomiting, abdominal pain, diarrhea, and a metallic taste are common complaints with chemical food-borne illnesses.

Consumers generally have many chemicals in their homes. When compounds such as detergents and cleaners are used for the wrong purpose or in excessive amounts, they can cause illness and death. Chemical poisoning can be prevented by:

1. Using each product for its intended use and in the amounts recommended
2. Reading the label before use
3. Keeping chemicals in their original containers
4. Never storing or transporting chemicals in containers used to store food. They may be mistaken for food or beverages (especially by children).

Pesticides are chemicals used to kill insects or rodents. Improperly used pesticides have caused poisonings when they were accidentally mixed with food. The use of pesticide-containing aerosols around foods and packaging materials and in food preparation areas can be dangerous.

Pesticide residues are of great concern to consumers. **Residues** are trace amounts of any substance remaining in a product at the time of sale. Three governmental agencies are involved in the regulation of products that enter the U.S. food supply:

- The Environmental Protection Agency (EPA)
- The Food and Drug Administration (FDA)
- The United States Department of Agriculture (USDA) Food Safety and Inspection Service (FSIS)

The EPA regulates the use of potentially harmful pesticides that are used in food production. Included among the duties of the EPA is the establishment of tolerance levels for pesticides.

The FDA, in addition to its other functions, regulates animal drugs, including food additives, herbicides, and environmental contaminants. The FSIS sets tolerance levels for these residues in edible foods. In setting a tolerance level, the FSIS determines the highest dose at which a residue causes no ill effects in laboratory animals, called the **tolerance level**. The tolerance level is then divided by a factor ranging from 100 to 1000 to account for possible differences between animals and humans.

The numbers used assume that humans are 10 times more sensitive than the most sensitive animal species tested. In addition, a further assumption is made that children and the elderly are 10 times as sensitive as others. This is the 100-fold safety factor (multiplying 10 times 10). A large margin of safety is built into residue limits established for compounds involved in the production of human food.

The Food Safety and Inspection Service (FSIS) enforces the residue limits in meat and poultry. The FDA is responsible for foods other than meat and poultry. When an illegal residue is found, the FDA can conduct an investigation and the FSIS can detain future shipments from the violating producer.

Natural Food Intoxicants

Many foods (unprocessed or uncooked) contain natural components that can harm health. All foods are made up of chemicals, some of which can alter the way the body uses nutrients. For example, phytates contained in grains decrease the bioavailability of zinc, calcium, iron, and manganese (Shils, 1999). Bioavailability is defined as the rate and extent to which an active drug or nutrient or metabolite enters the general circulation, permitting access to the site of action (Thomas, 1999).

Proteinase inhibitors found in many varieties of beans, peas, peanuts, and potatoes block the activity of enzymes such as trypsin and chymotrypsin (Shils, 1999). The literature on natural toxins in foods is extensive, and only a few examples can be discussed in this text.

Healthy people who eat well-balanced diets should not worry about natural food intoxicants. Illness from naturally occurring toxic compounds in foods is not common in this country. However, if an individual eats large amounts of a single food at one time, he or she may experience the effects of natural food intoxicants. The best protection against the effects of natural food intoxicants is to eat a wide variety of foods, thereby limiting exposure to any one toxic compound.

Food Additives

Additives may be introduced into food deliberately or accidentally. An **additive** is a substance added to food to increase its flavor, shelf life, characteristics such as texture, color, and aroma, and other qualities.

Intentional Use of Additives

Additives are intentionally added directly to food during processing for several reasons. For example, a preservative may be added to a bakery product to retard the growth of mold.

There are four reasons additives are intentionally used:

1. To maintain or enhance a food's nutritional value: frequently vitamins, minerals, and different forms of fiber are added to food.
2. To maintain a food's quality: many additives are used to prevent the growth of microorganisms and extend a product's shelf life. Some additives, called antioxidants, are used to prevent fats in food from deteriorating. Antioxidants are substances that prevent chemical breakdown by preventing or inhibiting the uptake of oxygen. Selected antioxidants may be effective in delaying some cancers' proliferation, mainly those related to fat metabolism, such as breast and prostate cancer.
3. To assist in processing, transporting, or holding a food: one additive that helps facilitate the processing of food is an **emulsifier**. An emulsifier helps to evenly distribute the molecules of two liquids that normally do not mix. Mayonnaise is an example of an emulsified product.

Table 14–4 Common Food Additives

Acidity control agents	Influence flavor, texture, and shelf life	Sodium bicarbonate Citric acid Hydrogen chloride Sodium hydroxide Acetic acid Phosphoric acid Calcium oxide
Antioxidants	Prevent discolorization Protect fats from rancidity	Vitamin C Vitamin E BHT and BHA
Flavors	Food enhancers	Hydrolyzed vegetable protein Black pepper Mustard Monosodium glutamate
Leavenening agents	To make dough rise	Sodium acid phosphate Sodium aluminum phosphate Monocalcium phosphate Yeast
Preservatives	To extend shelf life	Sulfur oxide Benzoic acid Propionic acid EDTA
Stabilizers and thickeners	To enhance texture	Sodium caseinate Gum arabic Modified starch Pectin

Baking soda and baking powder are other commonly used additives. These substances cause such products as cakes to rise and improve their texture and volume as well.

4. To improve the way a food tastes, looks, or smells: artificial colors, flavors, and sweeteners all fall into this category.

Types of common food additives are listed in Table 14–4.

Use of Steroids in Animal Production

The FDA has approved hormones or steroids for use in beef cattle and sheep. Currently, the only FDA-approved hormones for animal use are the anabolic (growth-promoting) steroid implants. Steroids are given to the animal in the form of implants, which are deposited underneath the skin on the backside of the animal's ear. Implants improve feed efficiency (the animal's ability to grow on a given amount of food), reduce the cost of meat production, and result in the production of carcasses with more lean meat and less fat. The implants are composed of natural or synthetic steroid sex hormones: estrogens, androgens, progestins, and combinations thereof (Ritchie, 1990).

Many consumers are concerned about the health hazards of eating beef and sheep with steroid residues. Hormone implantation results in some increase in the hormone content of beef tissue. Beef muscle from an implanted steer contains 0.022 nanograms per gram of steroids compared with 0.015 nanograms per gram in the muscle of nonimplanted steer (Ritchie, 1999). (A nanogram equals one billionth of a gram.) These numbers really do not mean much unless you compare them with the amount of the same steroid produced daily in the human body. Before puberty, a boy produces 41,000 nanograms of estrogen and progesterone daily. A pregnant woman produces 20 million nanograms.

These steroids are also naturally present in our food supply. A 3-ounce serving of potatoes contains 225 nanograms, and a 3-ounce serving of cabbage contains about 2000 nanograms of these steroids. The fact is that the hormone content of beef, whether from an implanted animal or not, contains very low levels of steroids, compared with levels naturally produced by the human body or naturally present in foods.

Accidental Use of Additives

Some additives enter the food supply accidentally. For example, chemicals may enter food through contact with surfaces that have been cleaned with chemical solutions.

Food-Handling Guidelines

Food-handling guidelines that can help decrease the risks of food-borne disease are presented in Box 14–3.

FOOD SELECTION The greater the variety of foods consumed, the less the likelihood of exposure to excessive amounts of contaminants from any single food item. Remember that contaminants of natural origin are present in foods.

FOOD STORAGE Proper storage of food helps ensure that there will be minimal contamination of the food from any source.

SANITATION AND PERSONAL HYGIENE The cleanliness of people involved in food handling and a clean working environment are essential to the prevention of food-borne disease. An unclean person cannot handle food in a sanitary fashion. Smoking and eating while preparing food may result in food contamination. Personal practices such as scratching the head, placing fingers in or about the mouth or nose, and sneezing may contaminate food. Frequent hand washing with soap is the best insurance against food contamination. In fact, the most common way sources of disease are transmitted from a food handler to food is by the hands. Needless to say, it is essential to always wash your hands after using the toilet (Fig. 14–6).

PREVENTING CROSS-CONTAMINATION Cross-contamination refers to the spreading of a disease-producing organism from one food to another. It can happen when a food preparer handles raw meat, eggs, or milk and then handles fruit, lettuce, or bread products that will be served uncooked. The cook transfers the offending substance or organism to the uncooked food item. Organisms can also be transferred to nonfood items such as a cooking utensil and then passed on to the food or a person.

SAFE FOOD PREPARATION Food is least protected during actual food preparation because of necessary handling, possible contamination from the environment, and the room's temperature. Food should always be pre-

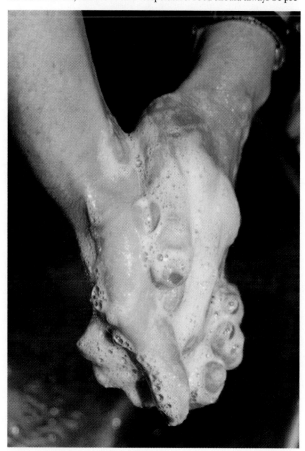

Figure 14–6:
This illustration demonstrates the amount of soap lather necessary to thoroughly cleanse the hands.

Box 14–3 Food Handling Guidelines

Shop Carefully

Make meat, fish, poultry, eggs, and refrigerated and frozen foods the last items you pick up in the grocery store. (These foods support the growth of bacteria better than other foods.)

Do not buy containers or packages that leak, dented cans, or expired foods.

Wrap hazardous items in plastic bags before placing them in the grocery cart.

Wrap produce in plastic baggies.

Buy frozen items that are rock solid (not partially thawed).

Use a cooler to transport hazardous items when the temperature is above 80°F.

Insist that items to be eaten raw (bread and produce) are not bagged with hazardous items.

Buy only the amount of deli meat that can be eaten in 1 to 2 days

If a prepared hot item is purchased, take it home and eat it or hold it above 140°F. Hold it for no longer than 2 hours.

Do not buy fish from unreliable sources.

Buy pasteurized fruit juices.

Storage

Keep the refrigerator, freezer, and storage cabinets clean.

Use pest control measures.

Store cleaning supplies away from food.

Do not store home-smoked fish in plastic airtight bags.

Use thermometers.

Store raw meats on the bottom shelf of the refrigerator.

Never store meats, fish, or poultry above fruits and vegetables.

Dispose of hazardous perishable items on a timely basis.

Cover and date food.

If the power goes out, keep the freezer closed except to add dry ice. Foods that contain ice crystals can be safely refrozen. When in doubt, throw it out!

Food Preparation

Avoid hand-to-food contact; use utensils.

Wash hands frequently.

Use a thermometer to check internal food temperatures:
- Meats and eggs 160°F.
- Leftovers and casseroles 165°F.
- Poultry 165°F.
- Ground meats 165°F (brown throughout).

Roast meats at oven temperatures of 300°F or above.

Cook with a constant heat source. Don't partially cook meat, fish, etc. at one time and then finish it later.

Clean work surfaces with soap and hot water before and after food preparation.

Carefully clean raw fruits and vegetables using warm water and a brush. Peel waxed fruit (wax makes it difficult to remove any residual pesticides).

Use roasting pans or covered containers to cook foods in the microwave to keep the steam in contact with the food. Rotate or stir food often; allow standing time and always use a thermometer when cooking foods in the microwave.

Cut mold from cheeses.

Food Display and Service

Serve food on clean platters.

Hold hot foods at 140°F or hotter if possible.

Hold cold foods at 40°F or colder.

If you cannot hold foods within these temperature ranges display and serve food for no longer than 2 hours and then discard leftovers.

Do not taste leftovers until after you reheat them to an internal temperature of 165°F.

Use a thermometer.

Never serve raw eggs, fish, or undercooked meats.

Preventing Cross Contamination

Keep work surfaces clean.

Think while cooking.

Never allow fresh bread, vegetables, and fruit to come in contact with hazardous items.

Clean chopping boards after the preparation of each menu item.

Use clean utensils to prepare each food item. Do not use the same utensil to both prepare and serve a hazardous food.

Always use a deep pan to store meats, fish, and poultry in the refrigerator to keep juices from dripping on other items.

Sanitation and Personal Hygiene

Do not smoke or eat while preparing food.

Frequently wash hands especially after defecation and after preparing hazardous foods.

Avoid touching body parts.

Wear clean clothes.

Avoid handling foods when ill with diarrhea, sore throat, cough, or when you have infected fingers, and other infectious signs.

Instruct children to wash their hands before touching food, especially after handling pet turtles, ducklings, or chickens.

Safe Cooling and Reheating

Thaw foods properly (in the refrigerator or under cold running water).

Use a microwave to thaw foods only as part of a continuous cooking process.

After thawing, cook food immediately.

Chill cooked foods rapidly in a shallow (2-inch deep container).

Do not let foods cool off at room temperature.

Pack lunches in insulated containers and freeze sandwiches.

Reheat leftovers to an internal temperature of 165°F.

pared with the least amount of hand contact. All work surfaces that come in contact with raw meats should be thoroughly cleaned using soap and hot water. Every attempt should be made to keep foods in the 40- to 140-degree temperature range for as short a time as possible.

SAFE COOLING AND REHEATING Food should be thawed properly; it can be done in refrigerated units at a temperature that should not exceed 40°F. It can also be accomplished under running water at a temperature of 70°F or below. Using the microwave oven to thaw food is a safe method as long as the thawing is part of a continuous cooking process. After thawing the food should be cooked immediately. All foods that have been cooked and then refrigerated should be reheated to a safe temperature of 165°F.

FOOD SERVICE AND DISPLAY Foods should be served, displayed, and held on clean plates at correct temperatures and should be discarded if held for longer than recommended. Proper cleanliness, an awareness of time, and temperature regulation are the most important ways the consumers can control the growth of bacteria. If the temperature is above 90°F foods should be held for no longer than one hour without refrigeration or heat. At cooler temperatures, hold the food for no longer than 2 hours. Hot foods should be held above 140°F and cold foods at 40°F or lower. Leftovers should be reheated to 165°F before they are tasted. Leftovers that are held outside these temperature ranges for longer than recommended times should be disdarded.

Summary

The United States food supply is as safe, wholesome, and nutritious as any in the world, but there are no guarantees that all food purchased and eaten in the country is safe. Thousands of substances besides nutrients are present in foods. Most of these substances are harmless in the amounts typically eaten if the food item is selected, stored, and prepared under recommended conditions. Many foods contain toxic substances naturally. Only in recent years have we been able to detect and measure these toxic substances. The human body appears able to safely handle small amounts of some toxic substances without injury.

The FDA ranks pathogenic (disease-causing) microorganisms as the most dangerous food-related public health threat. An individual is more likely to suffer from a food-borne illness due to microbiologic contamination than from any other source. Good food-handling methods can control most microbiologic hazards. Selecting a wide variety of foods, storing the foods appropriately, and preparing foods correctly all help prevent illness. Health-care workers should teach their clients about the use of food labels and the risks of microbiologic and residual chemical hazards of foods.

Nursing Care Plan

Subjective Data	Client stated she drinks an eggnog made with a raw egg each day.
	Client's daughter stated she makes her mother such a beverage.
Objective Data	Height: 5 ft, 0 in. Weight: adm 122 lb 100 percent RBW Age 95
Nursing Diagnosis	NANDA: Risk for Infection (North American Nursing Diagnosis Association, 1999, with permission.)
	Related to knowledge deficit as evidenced by client's statement, "I eat one raw egg each day," and the client's age.

Desired Outcomes Evaluation Criteria	Nursing Actions/ Interventions	Rationale
NOC: Risk Control (Johnson, Maas, and Moorhead, 2000, with permission.)	NIC: Nutrition Management (McCloskey and Bulechek, 2000, with permission.)	
The client will state that raw eggs can make one ill.	Provide verbal and written information to the client and the client's daughter on the relationship between food illness and *Salmonella* infections	Elderly clients are particularly at risk for salmonellosis.
	Have the client and the client's daughter state that raw eggs are hazardous.	Verbal recognition of a hazard is the first step in behavioral change.
The client will accept an eggnog made from pasteurized egg product.	Request the dietitian send an eggnog made with pasteurized egg product to client at bedtime each day.	The risk of salmonellosis from pasteurized eggs is lower than from raw eggs.
	Chart acceptance or rejection of the beverage.	Acceptance of the modified eggnog will increase long-term compliance.

Critical Thinking Question

1. What other areas of the home might you inspect to minimize the risk of a food-borne illness?

2. What clients need to take extra precautions to prevent a food-borne illness?

3. Do you think it is within the scope of practice for a nurse when making a home visit to discuss unsafe food practices?

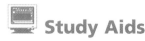

Study Aids

Subjects ....**Internet Sites**

General overview ....http://www.foodsafety.gov
accessed 4-2000

Food Guidelines ....http://www.ars.usda.gov/dgac
accessed 4-2000

Food-borne illness ....http://www.nalusda.gov/fnic/foodborne/foodborn.htm
accessed 4-2000

Food-borne incidence ....http://www.cdc.gov/od/oc/media
accessed 4-2000

BSE ....http://www.maff.gov.UK
accessed 4-2000

Chapter Review

1. Cold foods should be stored:
   a. at less than 50°F
   b. at less than 0°F
   c. at less than 40°F
   d. for no more than 6 hours outside the recommended temperature range.
2. The term "low" on a food label means the product contains:
   a. less than 3 grams of fat (or less) per serving; also low in saturated fat, cholesterol, or kilocalories
   b. ___ the fat of the original
   c. less than 10 grams of fat, 4 grams of saturated fat, and 95 milligrams ofcholesterol per serving
   d. more fat than a product labeled "Extra lean."
3. Foods commonly contaminated with Campylobacter are:
   a. Hard-cooked scrambled eggs
   b. Raw vegetables
   c. Canned foods
   d. Raw poultry
4. The best method to control the spread of food-borne illness is by:
   a. Wearing gloves when handling food
   b. Proper hand washing
   c. Taking food supplements
   d. Avoiding certain foods
5. A person who excludes all vegetables from the diet is likely to lack adequate:
   a. Vitamin A
   b. Fat
   c. Riboflavin
   d. Zinc

Clinical Analysis

1. Mr. P has brought his 35-year-old male companion who has a history of AIDS to the ambulatory care clinic for treatment for a sudden onset of headache, abdominal pain, diarrhea, nausea, and vomiting. The nurse should:
   a. Document all food consumed during the past seven days
   b. Inquire about food practices in the home
   c. Inspect Mr. P's passport for foreign travel in the past month
   d. Document the client's immunization status
2. A nurse is on the planning committee for the annual hospital picnic. One employee volunteers to make Texas-style chili at home and serve it at the picnic. The nurse has a responsibility to:
   a. Inquire how the chili will be made, transported, and held at recommended temperatures
   b. Taste the chili upon arrival at the picnic for safety
   c. Check the temperature of the chili upon arrival at the picnic
   d. Review the recipe for the potential use of unsafe ingredients
3. Mr. J is an 85-year-old man recently discharged from the hospital for a partial bowel obstruction that he had surgically repaired. His wife is getting ready to serve him eggnog made with raw eggs. The nurse should:
   a. Ignore the situation because that is not the purpose of the visit
   b. Inquire about any gastrointestinal pain Mr. J may have had
   c. Instruct the wife about the safe preparation of eggs
   d. Assess the amount of sugar used in the beverage

Bibliography

Almond, JW: Will bovine spongiform encephalopathy transmit to humans? Br Med J 311:1415, 1995.

Angulo, FJ, Getz, J, and Hendricks, KA: A large outbreak of botulism: The hazardous potato. J Infec Dis 178:172, 1998.

Bradley, R: An overview of the BSE epidemic in the UK. Dev Biol Stand 93:65, 1998.

Centers for Disease Control and Prevention: Outbreaks of *Shigella sonnei* Infection Associated with Eating Fresh Parsley–United States and Canada, July–August 1998. Morbidity and Morality Weekly Report. Printed and published by the Mass Med Soc 48:14; April 16, 1999.

Centers for Disease Control and Prevention: 1600 Clifton Road, MS D–25, Atlanta, GA, (accessed May 17, 1999) www.cdc.gov/od/oc/media/mmwrnews/n990312.htm.

Centers for Disease Control: Safer and Healthier Food. Morbidity and Morality Weekly Report. 48. 905–913. MMWR, 1999.

Chin, J (ed): American Public Health Department: Control of Communicable Disease Manual Ed 16. American Public Health Association, Washington, DC, 1999.

Clark, N (ed): What's your food safety I. Q.? Environmental Nutrition. New York, NY, 22:6. June 1999.

Cody, SA et al.: An outbreak of *Escherichia coli* 0157:h7 Infection from unpasteurized commercial apple juice. Ann Inter Med. 130:202, 1999.

Collee, JG: A dreadful challenge. Lancet 347:917, 1996.

Collinge, J, and Rossor, M: A new variant of prion disease. Lancet 347:916, 1996.

Fishbein L: Transmissible sponiform encephalopathies, hypotheses and food safety: An overview.. Sci Total Environ 217:71, 1998.

Food and Drug Administration: Focus on Food Labeling. Read the Label, Set a Healthy Table. FDA Consumer. DHHS Publication No. (FDA) 93–2262. Department of Health and Human Services, Public Health Services, Food and Drug Administration, 1993.

Food and Drug Administration: Federal Register, October 26, 1999. Vol. 64, no. 206, 57699–57733. Accessed 12/29/2000 at http://wm.cfsan.fda.gov.

Gale, P: Quantitative BSE risk assessment: Relating exposures to risk. Lett Appl Microbiol 27:239, 1998.

Gershoff, SN (eds): Antibacterial Overkill. Tufts University Health and Nutrition Newsletter. V. 16, No. 8, p. 1. Oct. 1998.

Ghani, AC et al.: Epidemiological determinants of the pattern and magnitude of the vCJD epidemic in Great Britain. Proc R Soc Lond B Biol Sci 265:2443, 1998.

Gore, SM: More than happenstance: Creutzfeldt–Jakob disease in farmers and young adults. Br Med J 311:1416, 1995.

Halpern, I, Neidle, D, and Ready, J: (accessed May 18, 1999), www.heathandsafety.org/food.html

Hillerton, JE: Bovine spongiform encephalopathy: Current status and possible impacts. J Dairy Sci 81:3042, 1998.

Institute of Food Science & Technology: (accessed May 18, 1999) www.easynet.co.uk/ifst/hottop1.htm.

Ironside, JW: Prion diseases in man. J Pathol 186:227, 1998.

Jackson Citizen Patriot: Investigators searching for source of contamination at meat plant. Jackson, MI p. A–7. Sunday, January 31, 1999

Johnson, M, Maas, M, and Moorhead, S: Nursing Outcomes Classification (NOC), ed 2. Mosby, Philadelphia. 2000.

Kimberlin, RH: Creutzfeldt–Jakob disease [Letter]. Lancet 347:65, 1996.

Lucker, E et al.: Development of an integrated procedure for the detection of central nervous tissue in meat products using cholesterol and neuron-specific enolase as markers. J Food Proc 62:268, 1999.

McCloskey, JC, and Bulechek, GM: Nursing Interventions Classification (NIC), 3 ed. Mosby, Philadelphia, 2000.

Mishler, T: What's the fuss about? Impact, Gordon Food Service. p. 21. May/June, 1999.

Mocsny, N: The spongiform encephalopathies: Prion diseases. J Neuroscience Nurs 30: 302, 1998.

Morganthau, T: E. Coli Alert. p. 30. Newsweek. Sept 1, 1997.

North American Nursing Diagnosis Association: Nursing Diagnoses: Definitions and Classification 1999–2000, North American Nursing Diagnosis Association, Philadelphia, 1999.

Ohio State University Extension Factsheet: (accessed May 18, 1999) http://www.ohioline.ag.ohio-state.edu/hyg-fact/5000/5569.html

Patterson, WJ, and Dealler, S: Bovine spongiform encephalopathy and the public health. J Pub Health Med 17:261, 1995.

Pfizer Inc: www.pfizer.com/rd/microbes/ecoli.html

Ridley, RM, and Baker, HF: The myth of maternal transmission of spongiform encephalopathy. Br Med J 311:1071, 1995.

Ritchie, HD: Agriculture on the stand: Are modern practices safe? Michigan State University, 1990 (unpublished paper).

Roberts, GW: Furrowed brow over mad cow. Br Med J 311:1419, 1995.

Schonberger, LB: New variant Creutzfeldt–Jacob disease and bovine sponiform encephalopathy. Infect Dis Clin North Am 12:111, 1998.

Shils, ME (ed): Modern Nutrition in Health and Disease, 9th edition. Williams and Wilkins, Baltimore, 1999.

Tabizi, SJ et al.: Creutzfeldt–Jakob disease in a young woman. Lancet 347:945, 1996.

Thomas, CL (ed): Tabers Cyclopedic Medical Dictionary, 18th edition. FA Davis, Philadelphia, 1997.

Tyler, KL: Risk of human exposure to bovine spongiform encephalopathy. Br Med J 311:1420, 1995.

United States Department of Agriculture: (accessed 4–2000), www.ars.usda.gov/dgac

Watson, L: Safety and Regulation of Plant Biotechnology. Plant Biotechnology, Monsanto St. Louis, Missouri, 1995.

Wegener, HC et al.: Use of antimicrobial growth promoters in farm animals and *Enterococcus faecium* resistance to therapeutic antimicrobial drugs in Europe. Emerg Infect Dis 5(3):329–35, May–June, 1999.

Will, RG et al.: A new variant of Creutzfeldt–Jakob disease in the UK. Lancet 347:921, 1996.

Will, RG: New variant Creutzfeldt–Jakob disease. Dev Biol Stand 93:79, 1998.

Williams, SR: Essentials of Nutrition and Diet Therapy. 7th edition. Mosby, St. Louis, 1999.

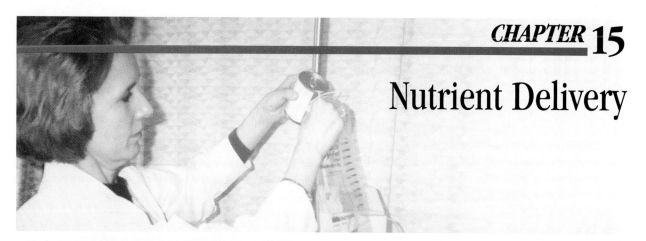

CHAPTER 15

Nutrient Delivery

Food services in health-care facilities have two major functions: the preparation and delivery of meals to clients and the nutritional care of clients. The nutritional care of clients includes three areas:

1. Assessing the client's need for nutrients
2. Monitoring the client's nutrient intake
3. Counseling the client about nutritional needs.

High-quality nutritional care saves the client and society health-care dollars and preventable hardship.

Food Service in Institutions

Nurses need to become familiar with some aspects of the food service in the organizations where they are employed. Specific duties of nurses are often related to meal service schedules.

Meal Service Patterns

Most institutions serve three meals to clients each day as well as several between-meal feedings. Feedings between meals are available for clients in need of extra nutrients, those who desire extra food, or those unable to consume sufficient kilocalories at the regular mealtimes.

It is important for nurses to know the times meals are served to clients. The dietary and nursing departments must coordinate their schedules so that clients receive their food while it is hot and attractive. The administration of medications sometimes must also be coordinated with meal-delivery schedules. Scheduling the client for diagnostic tests, blood work, and educational sessions should be coordinated with the meal service schedule.

Nutritional Care Services

Institutions vary in the types of nutritional services they offer clients. A large teaching hospital or medical center frequently has nutrition professionals on staff who specialize in the treatment of particular types of client. A critical care dietitian, for example, has special training to assess, plan, implement, and counsel clients in high-risk stages of trauma, disease, and conditions that affect nutritional support. In such settings, other health-care workers can rely on the critical care dietitian to provide technical support.

At the other end of the spectrum, in a small community hospital or a long-term care facility, a dietitian may be present only part time or as a consultant. In such circumstances, other health-care workers must plan to make the best use of the dietitian's services when he or she is available. In this situation the nursing staff assumes more responsibility for the nutritional care of clients.

Assessment, Monitoring, and Counseling

Nutritional care is a joint responsibility of the dietary and nursing departments. Assessing, monitoring, and counseling activities are usually done in collaboration.

Assessment

Some dietary departments screen clients for nutritional problems during admission. Clients found to be at a nutritional risk have a complete nutritional assessment, which usually includes the following:

1. Height, weight, and weight history
2. Laboratory test values

3. Food intake information
4. Potential food–drug interactions
5. Mastication and swallowing ability
6. Client's ability to feed himself or herself
7. Bowel and bladder function
8. Evaluation for the presence of pressure ulcers
9. Food allergies and intolerances
10. Any other factors affecting nutritional status, such as food preferences and cultural and religious beliefs about food
11. Determination of body composition
12. Presence of severe burns, trauma, infection, or other physiological stress that increases nutrient needs and is likely to prolong hospital stay.

In some health-care facilities, nurses are responsible for screening clients for nutritional problems. If the nurse finds a client at nutritional risk, she or he should make a referral to the dietitian.

Regulatory agencies of long-term care facilities require that clients have a nutritional assessment performed by a registered dietitian shortly after admission. The assessment identifies clients at nutritional risk. The care plan should reflect nutritional problems identified during the assessment.

Monitoring

All clients should be reassessed or monitored at appropriate intervals. Some clients in hospital intensive care units require continuous monitoring. Other clients require daily reassessment.

The client care conference is a productive means of monitoring clients. It is most effective if all health-care workers come prepared. Before the conference, information on the nutritional care of the client should be gathered including:

1. The client's initial nutritional assessment
2. The client's present body weight and weight history
3. A record of the client's recent food acceptances
4. Any changes in the client's medical condition
5. The client's diet order.

With this information in hand it is easy to determine most changes in the client's nutritional status. Weight loss is readily identified. A review of the client's food acceptance record, if available, can verify whether such a weight loss is likely a result of poor food intake.

Those clients whom health-care providers have determined to be at nutritional risk because of poor food intake should be treated; treatment may include a nutritional supplement, between-meal feedings, a the change in diet prescription, or a change in feeding status. If, for example, a client can no longer feed himself or herself, the client's feeding status would need to be changed from self-feed to assisted feeding. Monitoring the client's weight, laboratory values, and food intake is an important part of delivering high-quality nutritional care.

Counseling

All clients should be evaluated for nutritional counseling. The assumption that a client is not expected to be discharged and therefore is not entitled to education is unjustifiable. Educating the client about nutritional concerns helps the client assume responsibility for his or her own care, thus promoting self-esteem and a sense of worth.

Diet Manuals

Current accreditation standards (both long-term and acute care) require all institutions that provide health-care to have a diet manual available to all health-care workers. The diet manual defines and describes all diets used in the facility and includes information about the particular food service operation. What is included in a "soft diet" may vary slightly from one institution to another. For example, one soft diet may allow lettuce, whereas another does not. The diet manual is developed and approved jointly by all health-care professionals in a facility. Regional food preferences and the unique training of the facility's medical staff and other professionals influence the choice of food items allowed or avoided on special diets.

The administrative dietitian is usually responsible for initiating the selection of a diet manual or for writing the manual. Most aspects of the nutritional care given to clients are covered in such a manual, including nutritional supplements stocked by the pharmacy, purchasing, and dietary departments; dietary preparation for diagnostic procedures; kilocalorie count procedures; meal-service delivery schedules; client educational services; a listing of foods allowed, restricted, and avoided on the various diets; and nursing procedures to follow when transmitting a diet order.

When developing the manual, the dietitian usually consults with other department heads and members of the medical staff. After the manual is developed and written, it must be approved by the facility administrator and the medical staff. Physicians are usually requested to follow the manual when prescribing diets for clients. The medical staff, nursing department, and other professionals in the hospital can and do influence the nutritional care given to clients by participating in the diet manual approval process.

Diet Orders

The physician is responsible for prescribing a diet for the client. Just as you cannot administer a medication to a client without a medication order, you cannot serve a diet to a client without a written physician's diet order. One of the functions of the diet manual is to define a diet. The diet manual is the first place to look when clients request food items that are not being served to them. The diet manual may state, perhaps, that the food item is restricted or not allowed on the client's prescribed diet.

SPECIAL DIETS The purpose of a special or modified diet is to restore or maintain a client's nutritional status by manipulating one or more of the following aspects of the diet:

1. Nutrients such as protein, calcium, iron, sodium, potassium, and vitamin K may be increased, decreased, or eliminated.
2. Kilocalories may be either restricted or increased.
3. Texture or consistency of foods may be an issue. For example, only clear liquids may be served.
4. Use of seasonings such as pepper may be restricted or eliminated.

All modified diets are variations of the general diet; the client nonetheless needs all the essential nutrients. For this reason, each modified diet must be carefully planned to provide each of the essential nutrients or a documented reason for not providing one or more essential nutrients.

Table 15–1 Composition of Liquid Diets

Diet	Protein (g)	Fat (g)	Carbohydrate (g)	Sodium (mEq)	Potassium (mEq)	Kilocalories
Clear liquid	5	trace	70–95	65	20	375
Clear liquid with three 6-oz servings of Citrotein/Enlive	30	1	140–165	80	30	750
Full liquid	50	55	205	110	65	1500

SOURCE: Adapted from Pemberton, CM, et al.: Mayo Clinic Diet Manual: A Handbook of Dietary Practice, ed 6, BC Decker, Philadelphia, 1988, p 47.

Much confusion results when the terminology in the diet order is not the same as the terminology in the diet manual. For example, a low-salt diet may not be the same as a low-sodium diet as defined in the diet manual. Physicians may persist in ordering a low-salt or low-sodium diet, even though the diet manual requests that all sodium-restricted diets be ordered in units of sodium such as 2-gram sodium or 4-gram sodium.

Physicians may become confused because they have patients admitted at different facilities simultaneously. Many facilities have eliminated this confusion by defining a low-sodium and low-salt diet in the diet manual (the definitions for both low-salt and low-sodium diets differ markedly from one facility to another). Other vague diet orders are *salt-free, diabetic, regular diabetic, low-fat, fat-free,* and *as tolerated.* The nursing or dietetic staff should clarify all vague diet orders with the physician before the client is served. All health-care workers should become familiar with the terminology in the facility's diet manual.

Diet manuals are not usually designed to be used directly for client instruction. Much of the information in the diet manual is directed to physicians and other health-care workers to assist in the implementation of special diets. For example, many diet manuals describe indications and contraindications for use of a particular diet. An **indication** is the circumstance that indicates when the diet should be used. A **contraindica-**tion describes a circumstance when the diet should not be used. The diet manual also lists nutrients deficient in a particular diet. This type of information may alarm and confuse some clients.

COMMON DIET ORDERS Some common diet orders are for *clear liquid, full liquid, soft,* and *general* or *regular.* A clear liquid diet is any transparent liquid that can be poured at room temperature. Gelatin, some juices, broth, tea, and coffee are clear liquids. A clear liquid diet is nutritionally inadequate. Clear liquid complete nutritional supplements, however, are available. A full liquid diet is any liquid that can be poured at room temperature. Milk, custard, thinned hot cereals, all fruit juices, ice cream, and all items allowed on the clear liquid diet are allowed on most full liquid diets. The major difference between a clear liquid and a full liquid diet is that the latter contains milk and milk products (Table 15–1 and Boxes 15–1 and 15–2).

Soft diets vary greatly from one facility to another. For example, a mechanical soft diet is ordered when the client has only a few or no teeth (edentulous). A soft diet is ordered following surgery when easily digested foods are required. A facility that specializes in treating clients with eye, ear, nose, and throat disorders may have many types of soft diets. A pureed diet usually consists of foods that have been run through a blender or food

Box 15–1 Clear Liquid Diet

Description: The clear liquid diet provides energy and fluid in a form that requires minimal digestive action.

Indications: The clear liquid diet is prescribed when it is necessary to limit undigested food in the gastrointestinal tract, before bowel surgery, diagnostic imaging procedures, and colonoscopic examination. A clear liquid diet is also used during acute stages of illness to assist with fluid and electrolyte replacement and as a first step in oral alimentation following intravenous feeding, surgery, and gastrointestinal disturbances.

Adequacy: This diet is inadequate in all nutrients and should be used only in the short term.

Food Allowed

Coffee and tea
Carbonated beverages such as 7-Up and ginger ale
Fruit-flavored gelatin and popsicles
Apple, grape, or cranberry juice
Clear fat-free broth and bouillon
Sugar

Foods to Avoid

All other food and beverages

Recommended to Enhance Nutrition
Complete nutritional supplements such as Enlive (Ross) or Citrotein (Novartis)
High-protein broth and gelatin desserts are also available

Sample breakfast, lunch, and dinner menu
Clear apple, grape, or cranberry juice
Broth
Flavored gelatin
Coffee or tea
Sugar
Clear liquid complete nutritional supplement if client is on this diet for longer than two meals

---

Box 15–2 Full Liquid Diet

Description: The full liquid diet provides foods and beverages that are liquid or may become liquid at body temperature.

Indications: This diet is used as a progression between clear liquids and a soft diet and following oral surgery. Acutely ill clients with a chewing or swallowing dysfunction and clients with oral, esophageal, or stomach disorder who are unable to tolerate solid foods because of strictures or other anatomical disorders find this diet useful.

Adequacy: This diet can be adequate in all nutrients according to the 1989 Recommended Dietary Allowances. Special care needs to be taken to meet folacin, iron, thiamin, niacin, vitamin A, fiber, and kcalories allowances.

Foods Allowed	**Foods Not Allowed**
Beverages: Any beverage that pours at room temperature	All others
Breads, cereals, and grains: Cooked refined cereals (thinned or strained) such as cream of wheat	All others
Fruits: All fruit juices	All others
Vegetables: Any vegetable juice	All others
Meats: None	
Milk: Any	
Fats: Butter, margarine, cream, and oils	All others
Other: Custard, ice cream, flavored gelatin, sherbet, sugar, and Popsicles	All others and any made with coconut, nuts, or whole fruit

Special Notes:
The use of a complete nutritional liquid supplement is often necessary to meet nutrient allowances for clients who follow this diet for longer than 3 days. An oral supplement that contains fiber minimizes the potential for problems with constipation and abdominal cramping. However, liquid supplements with fiber are not indicated for all patients on full-liquid diets.

Sample Menu	*Lunch and Dinner:*
Breakfast: 1/2 cup fruit juice 1/2 cup cream of wheat 1 cup pasteurized eggnog Coffee, cream, and sugar	1/2 cup fruit juice 1/2 cup vegetable juice 1 cup strained cream soup 1/2 cup custard 8 oz. Ensure or Sustacal or similar product Coffee as desired

Snacks:
A complete nutritional supplement as needed to meet protein and kilocalorie allowances

---

processor to meet the consistency needs of the patient. Table 15–2 lists recommended foods on a pureed, mechanical soft, and soft diet.

A general or regular diet means that the client is on an unrestricted diet. Frequently, an "as tolerated" or "progressive" diet may be prescribed, which means that a clear liquid diet is to be served initially and the diet advanced (full liquid to soft to general) as the client is able to tolerate. The nurse is usually responsible for determining the client's tolerance for food just prior to tray delivery. This last-minute determination of

client tolerance is necessary for many clients because of fluctuating medical status.

Diets for Diagnostic Procedures
Many diagnostic procedures that require dietary preparation are performed in hospitals. It is important to follow the facility's diet manual when preparing a client for a diagnostic procedure.

POOR CLIENT PREPARATION Poor dietary preparation can force a client to have an expensive procedure repeated or postponed (Figure 15–1).

Table 15–2 Consistency Modifications—Recommended Foods

Food Group	Pureed Diet	Mechanical Soft Diet	Soft Diet
Soups	Broth, bouillon, strained or blenderized cream soup	Broth, bouillon, strained or blenderized cream soup	Broth, bouillon, cream soup
Beverages	All	All	All
Meat	Strained or pureed meat or poultry, cheese used in cooking	Ground, moist meats, or poultry, flaked fish, eggs, cottage cheese, cheese, creamy peanut butter, soft casseroles	Moist, tender meat, fish, or poultry, eggs, cottage cheese, mild flavored cheese, creamy peanut butter, soft casseroles
Fat	Butter, margarine, cream, oil, gravy	Butter, margarine, cream, oil, gravy, salad dressing	Butter, margarine, cream, oil, gravy, crisp bacon, avocado, salad dressing
Milk	Milk, milk beverages, yogurt without fruit, nuts, or seeds, cocoa	Milk, milk beverages, yogurt without seeds or nuts, cocoa	Milk, milk beverages, yogurt without seeds or nuts, cocoa
Starch	Cooked, refined cereal, mashed potatoes	Cooked or refined ready-to-eat cereal, potatoes, rice, pasta, white, refined wheat, light rye bread or rolls, graham crackers as tolerated	Cooked or ready-to-eat cereal, potatoes, rice, pasta, white, refined wheat, light rye or graham bread, rolls, or crackers
Vegetables	Strained or pureed, juice	Soft, cooked, without hulls or tough skin as in peas and corn, juice	Soft, cooked, vegetables, limit strongly flavored vegetables and whole-kernel corn, lettuce and tomatoes
Fruit	Strained or pureed, juice	Cooked or canned fruit without seeds or skins, banana, juice	Cooked or canned fruit, banana, citrus fruit without membrane, melon, juice
Desserts	Gelatin, sherbet, ice cream without nuts or fruit, custard, pudding, fruit ice, Popsicle	Gelatin, sherbet, ice cream without nuts or fruit, custard, pudding, fruit ice, Popsicle	Gelatin, sherbet, ice cream without nuts, custard, pudding, cake, cookies without nuts or coconut, fruit ice, Popsicle
Sweets	Sugar, honey, jelly, candy, flavorings	Sugar, honey, jelly, candy, flavorings	Sugar, honey, jelly, candy, flavorings
Miscellaneous	Seasonings, condiments	Seasonings, condiments	Seasonings, condiments

SOURCE: From Pemberton, CM, et al.: Mayo Clinic Diet Manual: A Handbook of Dietary Practice, ed 6, BC Decker, Philadelphia, 1988, p. 49, with permission.

Figure 15–1A is an x-ray from a poorly prepared client. Feces in the colon block the view of structures within the colon. Figure 15–1B shows the colon of a well-prepared client. In the absence of fecal material the entire length of the colon can be visualized.

Some x-ray procedures are not only expensive but also uncomfortable. The client must have the procedure repeated if necessary bodily structures cannot be visualized. Although the specific dietary preparation for x-ray studies of the colon may vary from one facility to another, dietary preparation usually is somewhat similar. The client should be instructed not to eat or drink anything after midnight on the day of the imaging study. In addition, the client may need to follow a clear liquid diet for 12 to 48 hours prior to the x-ray procedure.

Many clients undergo x-ray studies as outpatients. The nurse working in a physician's office is usually responsible for dietary instruction prior to these procedures. A reliable diet manual should be consulted before the scheduling of clients for such studies.

MISDIAGNOSIS: Poor dietary preparation can lead to a misdiagnosis. For example, a blood sample for a fasting blood glucose (FBS) test should be drawn on a **fasting** individual, that is, one who has not had any food (nor, sometimes, fluid) by mouth for at least 8 hours prior to the blood draw. If the client eats before the procedure, his or her blood glucose level may be elevated, and this elevation may cause a misdiagnosis of diabetes. A misdiagnosis may cause a client unnecessary anxiety and expense (Wellness Tip 15–1).

Importance of Nutritional Care

Malnutrition associated with acute and chronic disease is common in hospital settings. **Acute** means that the illness is characterized by a rapid onset, severe symptoms, and a short course. **Chronic** means that the illness has a long duration.

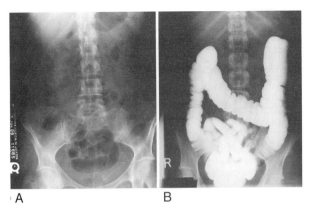

Figure 15–1:
(A) Image of a client who was poorly prepared for a barium enema. (B) Image of a client who was adequately prepared for a barium enema (courtesy of Dr. Russell Tobe)

The presence and importance of malnutrition has been increasingly recognized over the past 15 to 20 years. It is one of the most common conditions affecting the care of hospitalized clients. In one study, 200 of 500 clients were found to be malnourished on admission (McWhirtner, 1994). Many clients become increasingly more malnourished while in the hospital. Measurements of food intake in at-risk clients leave no doubt as to the main cause of hospital-induced malnutrition: many clients do not consume enough food (Dickerson, 1995).

Malnutrition is associated with a 25 percent morbidity and a 5 percent mortality. **Morbidity** is defined as the rate of being diseased. **Mortality** is defined as the death rate. A malnourished client is thus more likely to be sicker and run a higher risk of death than a well-nourished client with the same diagnosis. Because malnutrition affects morbidity and mortality, it is also associated with a prolonged hospital stay.

Iatrogenic Malnutrition

The term **iatrogenic malnutrition** was first used in 1974 (Butterworth and Blackburn, 1975). Iatrogenic malnutrition is a less offensive phrase than "induced malnutrition," that is, induced by a physician or an institution. Routine hospital practices such as extended periods of food or nutrient deprivation because of treatments, as well as diagnostic tests that interfere with the client's meal schedule or that cause a lack of appetite are related to the high prevalence of malnutrition. Drug therapy may also affect a client's appetite. Some drugs cause drowsiness, lethargy, nausea, and anorexia. Problems related directly to an illness, such as pain, unconsciousness, paralysis, vomiting, and diarrhea, can also interfere with eating.

Today many institutions have written policies and procedures for nurses and dietitians to follow to minimize the likelihood of iatrogenic

Wellness Tip 15–1

- When a physician prescribes a diagnostic procedure for any outpatient, ask about the need for special dietary preparation. This question may prevent a misdiagnosis or the need to have a costly procedure repeated.

CLINICAL APPLICATION 15–1

Methods for Nurses to Combat Iatrogenic Malnutrition

Nursing actions can affect the nutritional health of institutionalized clients. All of the following behaviors minimize the likelihood of malnutrition:

Recording height and weight

Regular communication among nurses, physicians, dietitians, and other health-care workers

Food tray viewing (monitoring) and documentation of client's food intake

Good food sanitation for oral and enteral feedings

Knowledge of the importance of good nutrition, nutritional supplements, and the composition of vitamin mixtures

Monitoring the length of time clients are NPO, on liquid diets, and on intravenous feedings of only glucose

Appreciation of the role of nutrition in the prevention and recovery from infection

Recognition of the increased nutritional needs due to injury or illness

Monitoring of stool frequency, urinary losses, losses by suction tubes, drainage, and so forth

Recording of weight at regular intervals

Monitoring of behavior patterns, vomiting, and any unusual comments clients make about food

Monitoring of client fluid intake and output.

---

malnutrition. The tasks nurses should perform to combat institutional malnutrition are discussed in Clinical Application 15–1.

Methods of Nutrient Delivery

Nutrients can be delivered to the client orally in foods or supplements, by tube feeding, or parenterally through veins. An **enteral tube feeding** means the feeding of an appropriate formula or liquid via a tube to a client's gastrointestinal tract. A **parenteral feeding** designates any intravenous route.

Oral Delivery

Most institutionalized clients are fed orally. All of the factors mentioned throughout this text influence whether or not the food items served are actually consumed by the client. Whenever possible, the client should be encouraged to eat foods, not only as an optimal way to obtain nutrients but also because it is beneficial for the client to continue to experience the normal psychologic and physical pleasure associated with eating.

The Menu

An institution's menu can be selective or nonselective. A selective menu is similar to a restaurant menu; clients can choose the specific menu items that appeal to them. Everyone has food likes and dislikes; what appeals to one client may not appeal to another. Clients eat best when they fill out their own menus, or a close significant other does so for them. Marking the menu is one way in which a client can participate daily in care planning.

Some institutions do not have a selective menu. Only one kind of meal is prepared and served to all clients. Food and labor required for institutions providing a selective menu is more expensive than for institutions providing a nonselective menu. However, many clients may fail to eat the food when the menu is nonselective.

Eating Environment

Health-care workers need to create as pleasant an environment as possible immediately before and during mealtime. The room should be checked for objectionable odors, sounds, and sights. Obviously, a full bedside commode or an emesis basin discourages eating. The client should be prepared to eat when the tray arrives. Cleaning the client's hands and face helps the client become more enthusiastic about eating. The client's bedside table should be cleared of all miscellaneous items so that the table can be used for the client's tray. Because all food loses and gains temperature quickly, unnecessary delays in serving the tray should be avoided. The client should be properly positioned to eat. This includes elevating the head of the bed (if condition permits) and positioning the bedside table to the correct height.

Some clients may find the odor of food offensive. For these clients it is best for the nurse not to uncover the food items directly in front of them, so as to minimize the risk of nausea.

Assisted Feeding versus Self-Feeding

Some clients must be fed. Food should be offered in bite-sized portions and in the order that the client prefers. Nurses should check the temperature of all hot liquids against the inside of their wrists before offering them to the client. Clients should not be rushed during feeding. Talking with the client while feeding makes mealtime more pleasant and signals to the client that he or she is not rushed. Sitting while feeding the client also indicates a willingness to spend time with the client and encourages relaxation.

Some nurses have found they can enhance a client's food intake by using the following technique:

- Sit behind the client.
- Place your right arm over the client's arm (if you and the client are right-handed).
- Place a fork or spoon with food in either the client's hand or your own hand (depending on the client's ability to do this maneuver).
- Guide the client's hand to his or her mouth.

This technique mimics normal eating behavior.

In a long-term care facility, it is important that a client's ability to feed himself or herself be reevaluated at regular intervals. Any client's condition can change, and health-care workers need to constantly be aware of any changes in the client's condition.

Assisting the Disabled Client

A client with a disability may require either total or partial assistance with eating. Partial assistance may include opening milk cartons and plastic bags containing condiments and eating utensils, buttering the bread, and cutting the meat. Visually impaired clients may be able to feed themselves once they are told where the food is placed on the plate. The usual technique is to describe food placement in terms of hours on a clockface.

Some clients can feed themselves but may be very slow, clumsy, and messy. A towel under the chin may assist in cleanup. Offering hot beverages in small amounts may minimize the likelihood of an accident.

Sometimes a particular quality of a food offered to clients may influence whether or not they can feed themselves; the consistency of food is one example. A thin liquid may cause some clients to choke. A thicker substance such as yogurt may be better tolerated. Some disabled people are able to manage finger foods such as French fries or hard-cooked eggs. It is best to learn the food tolerances and preferences of disabled clients by observation and simply by asking them what they can tolerate.

Health-care workers should encourage clients to remain as independent as possible in all the activities of daily living, including eating. If a client cannot feed himself or herself, an evaluation should be made. Some clients' inability to feed themselves may be related to neuromuscular disabilities. Many special eating devices have been developed to assist such clients. The occupational therapist has had special training in the selection and fitting of such eating devices.

Supplemental Feedings

Many clients are unable to consume sufficient kilocalories or nutrients because of anorexia or an increased need for nutrients. The first step with this type of client is to offer additional foods at or between meals. Any between-meal feedings must adhere to the client's diet order. A kilocalorie count should be started for poor eaters; kilocalorie counts are one method to monitor the effectiveness of nutritional care. If the client will not accept the supplemental feedings, another treatment approach may be needed.

Liquid supplementation is often useful; many clients accept liquids better than solids. Many debilitated clients seem to feel less full after drinking a beverage than after eating a comparable number of kilocalories and nutrients in foods. Liquid supplements can include milk, milk shakes, and instant breakfast drinks. Many different commercially prepared liquid formulas are available. Four different types of supplements are used as oral feedings: modular supplements, intact or "polymeric" formulas, elemental or "predigested" formulas, and disease-specific formulas.

MODULAR SUPPLEMENTS A **modular supplement** contains only one nutrient. Modular supplements are designed for clients who require the addition of only one nutrient. Moducal, Nutrisource CHO, Polycose, and Sumacal are supplements produced by different manufacturers that contain only carbohydrate. Medium-chain triglycerides supply only one form of lipid. Microlipid is another example of a of lipid supplement (see appendix). Modular supplements for protein include Pro Mod, Propac, Pro-Mix, and Casec. Modular supplements are available in a liquid or powder form and can be added to foods, other types of oral supplements, or tube feedings.

INTACT OR "POLYMERIC" FORMULAS An **intact** or **"polymeric" formula** is used when the gastrointestinal tract is functional and the client needs all of the essential nutrients in a specified volume. There are dozens of such products on the market. A complete supplement should always be used when the formula is the sole source of nutrition. Ensure, Sustacal,

---

Clinical Calculation 15–1 How Much Oral Supplement Is Indicated?

1. Place client on a kilocalorie count.
2. Calculate client's kilocalorie allowance.
3. Select an appropriate oral supplement for the client. Some hospitals allow clients to taste several supplements and choose the one most palatable to them.
4. Determine the difference between the client's recorded food intake and kilocalorie allowance.
5. Determine the kilocalorie concentration of the formula. This can be done by referring to either the appropriate table in the diet manual or the supplement's label. Usually formulas are between 1.0 to 2.0 kcal/mL.
6. Determine how many milliliters of formula are needed to meet the client's kilocalorie allowance.
7. Divide the total milliliters needed by the number of feedings to be offered.
8. Calculate the client's protein allowance (0.8 g/kg).
9. Check to make sure that the client's protein allowance will be met by the combination of recorded protein intake and volume to be provided in the supplement. Also check to make sure that the client will not be receiving more than twice the RDA for protein.

Example:

1. Assume that the client ate 550 kcal.

2. Assume that the client is a woman who weighs 60 kg, is 55 years of age, and is 5 ft 6 in. tall. (Review Chapter 6, "Energy Balance" if necessary to calculate kilocalorie allowance; the 30 kcal per kilograms was taken from the table in that chapter.)

Client needs approximately 30

kcal/kg = 30 kcal/kg x 60 kg

kcal allowance = 1800 kcal

3. Assume that the client has tasted several supplements and prefers Sustacal Liquid.
4. The client's kilocalorie allowance is 1800 kcal.

The client ate 550 kcal

The difference is 1250 kcal

5. Sustacal Liquid contains 1.0 kcal/mL (information obtained from the product's label).
6. The client needs 1250 mL of Sustacal Liquid.

$$\frac{1250 \text{ kcal}}{1 \text{ kcal/mL per milliliter}} = 1250 \text{ mL}$$

7. The client stated she would prefer to drink this feeding six times per day, some on each tray and at three between-meal feedings.

$$\frac{1250 \text{ mL}}{6 \text{ feedings}} = 210 \text{ mL per feeding*}$$

8. Assume from the client's recorded food intake that she is eating about 10 g of protein per day. A woman weighing 60 kg has a protein allowance of 0.8 g/kg.

60 kg x 0.8 g/kg = 48 g of protein

Subtract the 10 g eaten from trays –10

The supplement should provide at least 38 g of protein and no more than 86 g [(48 x 2)–10] of protein.[†]

9. Sustacal liquid contains 61 g of protein per 1000 mL or 0.061 g/mL.

1250 mL x 0.061 g/mL = 76.25 g of protein

The client's protein allowance will more than be met by 1250 mL of Sustacal Liquid and food, but will not exceed the 200% guideline.

*This product is available in both quarts and 240-mL units. Some institutions stock only 240-mL units and may prefer to dispense this feeding in 240-mL units. In this situation, divide 240 mL into 1250 mL. The client would need only 5.2 feedings per day. This would be offered to the client in four feedings of 240 mL for a total of 960 mL and one feeding of 290 mL to equal the 1250 mL.

[†]It is important that the feeding and food not provide more than twice the client's protein allowance. In this case, 48 x 2 = 96 g. As the client is eating about 10 g of protein per day and will consume about 76 g more in the supplement, her total protein intake would be approximately 86 g/day. This amount does not exceed twice her RDA for protein and is therefore acceptable.

Resource, and Meritene are examples of complete nutritional supplements. Some complete nutritional supplements are also designed for tube feedings; the consistency and flavor of a feeding designed to be tube-fed will probably not be acceptable to the client when fed orally.

Intact formulas differ from one another. Some contain lactose and some do not. Some provide fiber. The product may be a powder for reconstitution, a liquid, or a pudding. It may be flavored or unflavored. The percentages of kilocalories derived from carbohydrates, fats, and proteins may be different.

The carbohydrate, fat, and protein may be derived from various sources. For example, the protein source in Meritene is concentrated skim milk, while the protein source in Ensure is sodium and calcium caseinates and a soy-protein isolate. For many reasons the source of any of the three energy nutrients may be important. For example, Meritene,

Carnation Instant Breakfast, and Sustagen are not good supplements to use for a client with a lactose intolerance. Citrotein and Enlive are clear liquid polymeric formulas.

Commercial supplements should be used only after the client's requirements for nutrients have been assessed. Some health-care workers still think that if some is good, more is better and therefore encourage the client to consume greater amounts of oral supplement. Excess nutrients, however, are rarely beneficial. Not only do clients become frustrated because they cannot consume all of the supplement served to them, but to do so may be medically harmful. Many organs in the human body are in a stress situation in the poorly nourished client. Why subject the client's kidneys or liver to unnecessary work if the nutrients cannot be used efficiently? A suggested procedure to follow when determining the volume of an oral supplement to serve to a client is demonstrated in Clinical Calculation 15–1.

ELEMENTAL OR "PREDIGESTED" FORMULAS Another group of oral supplements includes **elemental or "predigested" formulas**. Examples of elemental or predigested formulas include Flexical, Vital, and Vivonex. The nutrients in these formulas are easier to digest or already partially digested. For example, maltrodextrins, corn syrup solids, oligosaccharides, and glucose polymers are rapidly hydrolyzed by maltase and oligosaccharidases, which are apt to be present in the small intestine in higher concentrations than lactase.

Protein is either partially or totally predigested. Partially predigested protein (small peptides) offer an advantage over totally predigested protein (single amino acids). Peptides and free amino acids do not inhibit each other's transport across the gastrointestinal tract, and absorption of nitrogen is actually improved by the inclusion of small peptides. Easier-to-digest fats include medium-chain triglycerides. Partially digested fats include monoglycerides and diglycerides.

Predigested formulas contain little lactose and residue and may be given orally or through a tube. These formulas are very expensive and are designed only for use with clients with limited gastrointestinal function or metabolic disorders. Because they are less palatable than intact feedings, client acceptance is sometimes a problem when they are administered orally.

DISEASE-SPECIFIC FORMULAS The last group of oral supplements includes those designed for clients with specific metabolic problems. For example, special formulas are available for clients with liver (Hepatic-Aid, Travasob Hepatic), pulmonary (Respalor, Pulmocare), and kidney disorders (Suplena, Amin-Aid, Travasob Renal). These special formulas are discussed in subsequent chapters.

Oral supplements are also used extensively to wean clients from both tube and parenteral feedings. Once a client ceases to consume foods orally, a transition period is always necessary to reacclimate the client back to oral feedings. This process can sometimes take a couple days to months. An enteral formula comparison chart can be found in the Appendix K.

Enteral Tube Feeding

Tube feedings are the second way nutrients can be delivered to clients. With some medical conditions oral feeding is impossible, insufficient, or impractical. Several common conditions in which a tube feeding is indicated are listed in Table 15–3.

Tube feedings, like oral supplements, can be made from table foods or purchased commercially prepared. If the client's finances are tight and the client has no impairment of digestion and absorption, he or she can be taught to prepare a tube feeding from table foods prior to discharge. Home-prepared tube feedings are less expensive than commercially prepared feedings, but more prone to contamination. Many of the commercial products described in the previous section can be used by tube-fed clients.

Gastrointestinal Function

The gastrointestinal tract should always be used to the extent possible. Oral supplements should be considered before tube feeding; tube feeding should

Table 15–3 Conditions Indicating a Tube Feeding*

Condition	Examples
Client has mechanical difficulties that make chewing and/or swallowing impossible or difficult	Obstruction of the esophagus, weakness or nausea, mouth sores, throat inflammation
Client has an intestinal disease and cannot digest or absorb food adequately	Malabsorption syndromes
Client refuses to eat or cannot eat	Anorexia nervosa, senile dementia
Client is unable to consume a sufficient amount of food because of clinical condition	Coma, serious infections, trauma victims, clients with large kilocalorie requirements

*Other conditions will be discussed in subsequent chapters.

always be considered before intravenous feeding. Tube feeding is safer, cheaper, and more physiological than intravenous feeding; in other words, it more nearly mimics normal feeding conditions. Nutrients should be supplied intact rather than predigested if the client has normal digestion. Intact nutrients are nutrients that are not predigested. With intact nutrients the body must keep producing all the secretions and enzymes necessary for digestion, thereby forcing the gastrointestinal tract to function.

Tube Placement

Feeding tubes can enter the body through the nose or through a surgically made opening. A **nasogastric (NG) tube** runs from the nose to the stomach. A **nasoduodenal (ND) tube** runs from the nose to the duodenum. A **nasojejunal (NJ) tube** runs from the nose to the jejunum. These types of tubes are designed for short-term use only because of client discomfort and tissue irritation.

When long-term tube feeding is needed or a tube cannot be inserted through the nose, an **ostomy,** or surgically created opening, is created. An **esophagostomy** is a surgical opening into the esophagus through which a feeding tube is passed. A **gastrostomy** is a surgical opening in the stomach through which a feeding tube is passed; this is the most common tube insertion method.

Percutaneous endoscopic gastrostomy or PEG tube placement is used for clients who require a feeding tube long term. A PEG tube can be placed percutaneously with the aid of an endoscope or surgically if the client is already undergoing abdominal surgery or has a condition that makes working with an endoscope difficult (Bliss and Lehmann, 1999). Percutaneous endoscopic jejunostomy (PEJ) tube placement is generally reserved for clients who are not candidates for a PEG. A client who has had a gastrectomy (stomach removal) procedure requires a PEJ tube placement.

A critical responsibility of nurses is assessment of feeding tube placement. The most reliable method of determining tube placement is radiography. Unfortunately, feeding tubes migrate (after x-ray) and may move out of the stomach or jejunum. Tube migration places the client at risk for aspiration because the tube may move into the trachea. The client is also at risk if he or she regurgitates the feeding. **Regurgitation** means to cause to flow backward. If the feeding backs up into the client's lungs, a lung infection can develop.

When a client has inhaled fluids regurgitated from the stomach, he or she may develop aspiration pneumonia. **Aspiration** is the state whereby a substance has been drawn up into the nose, throat, or lungs. One study showed a 28 percent occurrence of aspiration within a 30-day period after tube placement. Among clients most at risk of aspirating formula are the elderly and those who have an impaired lower esophageal sphincter, reflux disease, delayed gastric emptying, or a decreased cough or gag reflex (Bliss and Lehman, 1999). It is important to follow the procedure of the institution when inserting and measuring tube placement.

Many practitioners consider an analysis of the color and pH of fluid intentionally aspirated from a tube to be the second best method to assess tube placement. A pH-paper reading of between 0 and 4 indicates the tube is likely in the stomach and helps rule out inadvertent respiratory placement. Gastric fluid is most often grassy green, tan to off white, bloody, or brown (Metheny et al. 1998). Tracheobronchial fluid is usually off-white and heavily tinged with mucus. Although they are not infallible methods, pH and color analysis to assess tube placement but can offer valuable clues.

Contamination

Unfortunately, tube feedings provide an excellent environment for the growth of microorganisms. When a tube feeding becomes contaminated with bacteria, the client receiving the feeding may become ill and may suffer from gastrointestinal problems such as nausea, vomiting, or diarrhea. For this reason, many hospitals and nursing homes use only commercially prepared tube feedings (as opposed to those prepared in-house from table foods). Commercial feedings are packaged under sterile conditions. Most hospitals do not have a sterile area in their dietary departments. Even commercially prepared formulas can become contaminated if they are not handled safely after opening.

To prevent contamination, first check the can for the correct product, flavor, expiration date, and any signs of contamination such as swelling. If the can is swollen, notify your supervisor. Do not administer a feeding from a damaged can. Other cans in the same shipment should be checked for contamination.

Good personal hygiene is important. The following recommendations help reduce the possibility of contamination:

- Always wash your hands before opening the can.
- Wash the top of the can carefully before opening the can.
- Shake the can well before opening it.
- If a can opener is needed, be sure it is clean.
- Transfer the formula into a clean container.
- Use sterile, bottled, or boiled water to dilute the formula (if indicated).
- Label any remaining formula carefully with the client's name, room number, the date the formula was opened, the amount in the container, the name of the product, and other pertinent information. Other information may include whether the formula is diluted or contains medications, vitamins, or other additives.

- Store the formula in the refrigerator in a covered container. When a new supply of formula is received, place it in the rear of the storage area so that the older formula is used first.
- Once opened, most formulas should be discarded after 24 hours.

Administration

Tube feedings can be administered continuously, intermittently, or by bolus. Clogging of the tube occurs significantly more often with continuous rather than intermittent feedings (Galindo-Ciocon, 1993).

CONTINUOUS FEEDING Many professionals feel that **continuous feeding** is preferable to other methods. A continuous feeding is always recommended for formulas delivered directly into the small intestine. One recommended rate is 30 to 50 milliliters per hour, increasing daily by 25 milliliters per hour to the rate necessary to meet energy needs. This gradual increase in the formula's volume gives the client's gastrointestinal tract a chance to adjust to the formula and helps prevent many complications that occur in tube-fed clients. Safety precautions for continuous feedings include (1) flushing the tube with water every 4 to 6 hours and (2) allowing no more than a 4-hour hang time for each bag of formula unless the formula is packaged in a sterilized delivery system. These procedures help prevent contamination and bacterial growth. An infusion pump is necessary for precise control of a continuous feeding.

INTERMITTENT FEEDING An **intermittent feeding** means giving a 4- to 6-hour volume of feeding solution over 20 to 30 minutes. Clients tolerate intermittent feedings much better than bolus feedings because these feedings more closely approximate normal eating behavior. The tube needs to be flushed after each feeding to minimize bacterial growth and prevent contamination.

BOLUS FEEDING **Bolus feeding** means giving a 4- to 6-hour volume of feeding solution within a few minutes. A client is thus fed only four to six times per day. Feedings given by this method are frequently poorly tolerated, with clients complaining of abdominal discomfort, nausea, fullness, and cramping. Some clients, however, can tolerate bolus feedings after they have had a period of adjustment to the tube feeding. Bolus feedings are usually poorly tolerated for feedings that enter the intestines.

The adjustment period should follow the procedure described above, that is, the volume of feeding is slowly increased. Clients on bolus feedings should be instructed not to recline for at least 2 hours following the feeding. Tubes should be irrigated (flushed with water) after each bolus feeding to prevent contamination.

Potential Complications

Complications fall into three categories: mechanical, gastrointestinal, and metabolic. Table 15–4 reviews these complications of tube-fed clients and lists system-specific prevention strategies. Metabolic complications are discussed in later chapters.

Osmolality

The osmolality of a solution is based on the number of dissolved particles in the solution. The greater the number of particles, the higher the osmolality.

TABLE 15–4 Common Mechanical, Gastrointestinal, and Metabolic Complications of Tube-Fed Clients and Prevention Strategies

Complication	Prevention Strategy
Mechanical	
Tube irritation	Consider using a smaller or softer tube
	Lubricate the tube before insertion
Tube obstruction	Flush tube after use
	Do not mix medications with the formula
	Use liquid medications if available
	Crush other medications thoroughly
	Use an infusion pump to maintain a constant flow
	Feeding should not be started until tube placement is radiographically confirmed
Aspiration and regurgitation	Elevate head of client's bed greater than or equal to 30 degrees at all times
	Discontinue feedings at least 30 to 60 minutes before treatments where head must be lowered (e.g., chest percussion)
	If the client has an endotracheal tube in place, keep the cuff inflated during feedings
	Test pH of aspirate with pH paper or meter
	a. pH of tracheobronchial secretions is alkaline, >7.4
	b. pH of gastric secretions is acidic <5.0
	c. As the tube moves from the acid stomach to the alkaline duodenum, pH will change from acid to alkaline
	Place a black mark at the point where the tube, once properly placed, exits the nostril
Tube displacement	Replace tube and obtain physician's order to confirm with x-ray imaging
Gastrointestinal	
Cramping, distention, bloating, gas pains, nausea, vomiting, diarrhea*	Initiate and increase amount of formula gradually
	Bring formula to room temperature before feeding
	Change to a lactose-free formula
	Decrease fat context of formula
	Administer drug therapy as ordered, e.g., Lactinex, kaolin-pectin, Lomotil
	Change to formula with a lower osmolality
	Change to formula with a different fiber content
	Practice good personal hygiene when handling any feeding product
	Evaluate diarrhea-causing medications the client may be receiving (e.g., antibiotics, digitalis)
Metabolic	
Dehydration	Assess client's fluid requirements before treatment
	Monitor hydration status
Overhydration	Assess client's fluid requirements before treatment
	Monitor hydration status
Hyperglycemia	Initiate feedings at a low rate
	Monitor blood glucose
	Use hyperglycemic medication if necessary
	Select low-carbohydrate formula
Hypernatremia	Assess client's fluid and electrolyte status before treatment
	Provide adequate fluids
Hyponatremia	Assess client's fluid and electrolyte status before treatment
	Restrict fluids
	Supplement feeding with rehydration solution and saline
	Diuretic therapy may be beneficial
Hypophosphatemia	Monitor serum levels
	Replenish phosphorus levels before refeeding
Hypercapnia	Select low-carbohydrate high-fat formula
Hypokalemia	Monitor serum levels
	Supplement feeding with potassium if necessary
Hyperkalemia	Reduce potassium intake
	Monitor potassium levels

* The most commonly cited complication of tube feeding is diarrhea.

Table 15–5 Osmolality of Selected Formulas

Formula	Milliosmoles*/hg	Description
Stresstein	910	Elemental formula
Vivonex HN	810	Elemental formula
Ensure	450	Intact or polymeric
Isocal	300	Intact or polymeric

*Please note the wide range in osmolality of the various formulas.

At a given concentration, the smaller the particle size, the greater the number of particles present. Oral supplements and tube feedings with a high osmolality draw body fluid into the bowel, resulting in a fluid imbalance. The symptoms are diarrhea, nausea, and flushing. The osmolality of normal body fluids is approximately 300 milliosmoles per kilogram. Predigested nutrients have a higher osmolality than intact nutrients. An **isotonic** feeding has an osmolality of 300 milliosmoles, the same osmotic pressure as body fluids. Table 15–5 lists the osmolality of selected formulas.

Sensitivity to the osmolality of oral supplements and tube feedings varies greatly from one individual to another. A high-osmolality feeding can provide a more concentrated source of nutrients than a feeding of lower osmolality. All clients need a period of adjustment to a high-osmolality formula. The majority of clients are able to eventually develop a tolerance to a high-osmolality formula; some clients, however, are more likely to develop symptoms of an intolerance. These include debilitated clients, clients with gastrointestinal disorders, preoperative and postoperative clients, gastrostomy and jejunostomy clients, and clients whose gastrointestinal tract has not been challenged by food for a significant period of time.

Administration of Medications to a Tube-Fed Client

All health-care workers should be aware of potential drug–food interactions in order to minimize or prevent complications (see Chapter 17). Clinical Application 15–2 discusses suggested procedures for administering medications through feeding tubes. Medications can be physically incompatible with the tube feeding because of changes in the feeding's viscosity (thickness) or flow characteristics. Some medications may also cause the feeding to separate, granulate, or coagulate.

Monitoring the Tube-Fed Client

Nutritional status, fluid balance, and gastrointestinal tolerance all need to be monitored in tube-fed clients. Whether the client requires daily or weekly monitoring depends on client acuity, duration of feeding, and the practice in the individual facility.

Nutritional status monitoring begins with a comparison of the client's kilocalorie and protein allowances to the volume and composition of the nutritional product utilized. Initially the client's kilocalorie and protein allowances are not usually met because a tube feeding is usually started at a low volume to increase gastrointestinal tolerance. Changes in the client's medical status and treatment, physical activity, and tolerance to the tube feeding may continually alter the volume and kind of feeding the client requires. Thus, the kilocaloric and protein content of the tube feeding requires reassessment.

In stable clients, serum levels of sodium, blood urea nitrogen, hemoglobin, and albumin are indicators of fluid status (Skipper, 1998). Fluid intake and output need to be recorded daily. Fluid intake should be

---

CLINICAL APPLICATION 15–2

Procedures for Administering Medications through Feeding Tubes

Procedures for the administration of medications through feeding tubes may vary slightly from one institution or facility to another. The following suggested procedures, however, are common in most facilities:

1. If possible, administer drugs in liquid form.

2. If the drug is not available in liquid form, consult with the pharmacist; he or she may be able to procure a liquid form or similar drug provided by the American Society of Hospital Pharmacists in Pediatric Extemporaneous Formulation List of the manufacturer's suggestions.

3. Exercise caution when calculating equivalent liquid doses. Many liquid dosage forms are intended for pediatric use and the dose of the drug must be adjusted appropriately for adults.

4. Administer crushed tablets only when no other alternatives are available.

5. If crushed tablets are administered, crush the tablet to a fine powder and mix with water. Do not crush any tablet on the list of oral drugs that should not be crushed. Do not crush drugs with a sustained-release action or an enteric coating. If in doubt, consult with the pharmacist.

6. Administer each drug separately. Do not mix all the medications for one dosing time. Flush with at least 5 mL (1 tsp) of water between each medication.

7. Flush the tube with at least 30 mL of water before giving the medication and before restarting the tube feeding.

8. To avoid causing gastric irritation and diarrhea, drugs that are hypertonic or irritating to the cells that line the gastrointestinal tract, such as potassium chloride, should be diluted in at least 30 mL of water prior to administration.

9. If the medication is ordered to be added to the feeding, observe the feeding after the addition for any reaction or precipitation. Shake the solution thoroughly. Label the feedings with at least the name and amount of they drug added, the time, date, and your initials.

10. Drugs usually administered with meals to avoid gastric irritation, such as indomethacin, should also be diluted with water prior to administration .

11. Sustained- or slow-release formulations of drugs that are used for once-daily dosing may need to have divided dosing schedules when administered in liquid form.

Adapted from Wright, 1986, p. 33.

---

at least 500 cc greater than output in clients who are neither overhydrated nor underhydrated. This 500-cc surplus is needed to cover insensible losses in feces and from the skin and lungs. Clinical signs of hydration status include skin turgor, presence of axillary sweat, condition of the mucous membranes, and the presence or absence of edema. Constipation is

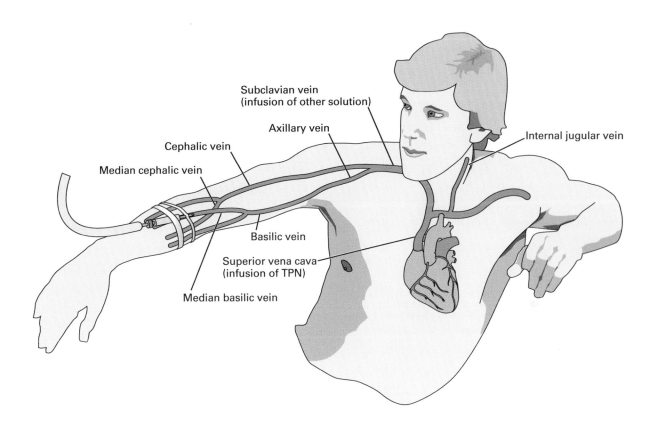

Subclavian vein
(infusion of other solution)

Axillary vein

Cephalic vein

Median cephalic vein

Internal jugular vein

Basilic vein

Superior vena cava
(infusion of TPN)

Median basilic vein

Figure 15–2:
Correct placement of a peripherally placed central catheter (PICC). (Courtesy of F.A. Davis, adapted from Phillips with permission.)

another possible sign of dehydration. Critically ill clients are usually over-hydrated, whereas stable clients are often dehydrated (Skipper, 1998).

Gastrointestinal tolerance can be assessed by the absence or presence of diarrhea, bowel sounds, nausea, distention, and vomiting. The type of feeding delivered, the volume given, or the delivery rate can cause diarrhea. Diarrhea is frequently caused by medications. Antibiotics, laxatives, H_2 receptor blockers, and antacids with magnesium can cause stools to become watery. Medications that contain sorbital can also have a laxative effect (Burnham, 2000).

Gastric residuals are usually measured several times daily. Because elevated residuals indicate delayed gastric emptying and a potentially increased risk for aspiration, feedings are advanced only when gastric residuals are within acceptable limits (150 to 200 ml) (Skippper, 1998). Measurement of gastric residuals in a stable alert client who has a well-established tolerance to the tube feeding is usually not necessary. Feedings continuously dripped into the intestines do not normally produce a gastric residue because there is no place for the fluid to collect.

Home Enteral Nutrition

Many clients on tube feedings are being discharged from hospitals and nursing homes. Most hospitals and nursing homes that discharge clients on home enteral nutrition (HEN) have a **nutrition support service.** The delivery of effective nutritional support requires a team effort. Team members usually include the physician, pharmacist, nurse clinician, dietitian, and social worker. Team functions vary from one facility to another. Members of nutrition support teams assess, monitor, and educate clients. Some nutrition support service team members also arrange for client follow-up in outpatient clinics or in the home.

Parenteral Nutrition

Parenteral nutrition in which nutrients are delivered to the client through the veins (intravenously) is the third means of feeding. **Peripheral parenteral nutrition** (PPN) means to feed the client via a vein away from the center of the body (Fig. 15–2). In **total parenteral nutrition** (TPN) the client is fed via a central vein. TPN and PPN can be used to provide partial or total daily nutritional requirements. Clients who cannot or should not be fed through the gastrointestinal tract are some of the candidates for TPN and PPN. See Box 15–3 for appropriate indications for the use of PPN and TPN.

Peripheral Parenteral Nutrition (PPN)

Intravenous (IV) feeding (peripheral parenteral nutrition, PPN) is routine in most healthcare institutions. IV solutions, usually containing water, dextrose, electrolytes, and occasionally other nutrients, are used to maintain fluid, electrolyte, and acid–base balance. Intravenous solutions do contain kilocalories. The calculation of the kilocalorie content of an intravenous solution is demonstrated in Clinical Calculation 15–2.

Box 15–3 Indications for Peripheral Parenteral Nutrition (PPN) and Total Parenteral Nutrition (TPN)

PPN

PPN is an effective method of nutritional support for clients with mild to moderate nutritional deficiencies who are unable to receive enteral nutrition or for whom the central venous route is inaccessible or undesirable. Specifically, PPN is indicated for clients:

- Who are expected to be NPO 5 days
- Who have inadequate GI function expected to last 5 to 7 days
- Who are making the transition to an oral diet or tube feeding
- In whom central venous access is contraindicated
- Who are malnourished and expected to be NPO for several days
- Who have energy and protein requirements that can be met with PPN (1800 kcalories per day or less)

TPN

Potential candidates for TPN include those clients who are anticipated to require nutritional support for longer than 10 days or who have an increased requirement for energy, such as clients:

- Who need preoperative preparation but are severely malnourished
- Who have postoperative surgical complications
- Who have inflammatory bowel disease
- Who have inadequate oral intake or malabsorption

Clinical Calculation 15–2 Calculation of Kilocalories in IV Solutions

D_5W means 5 percent dextrose in water. The subscript following the D tells you the percent of dextrose in the solution. Other common concentrations of sugar and water are $D_{10}W$ and $D_{50}W$.

A 5 percent concentration of dextrose means 100 mL of water contains 5 g of dextrose. A 10 percent concentration of dextrose means 100 mL of water contains 10 g of dextrose. A 50 percent concentration of dextrose means 100 mL of water contains 50 g of dextrose. A simple proportion should be used to calculate the number of kilocalories in any given volume of a solution.

The formula is:

$$\frac{\text{percent of concentration}}{100 \text{ mL}} = \frac{\times \text{ grams of dextrose}}{\substack{\text{volume of solution} \\ \text{client received}}}$$

For example, a client has received 1000 mL of D_5W:

$$\frac{5 \text{ gram of dextrose}}{100 \text{ mL}} = \frac{\times \text{ grams of dextrose}}{1000}$$

$$= 50 \text{ grams of dextrose}$$

Proportions are solved by cross-multiplication and division: (5 g × 1000 mL) divided by 100 mL = 50 g of dextrose. One gram of carbohydrate given intravenously provides a 3.4 kcal, thus 50 g × 3.4 kcal/g = 170 kcal.

Amino acids and fat can be supplied peripherally. To prevent ketosis, intravenous lipid emulsions should contribute no more than 60 percent of the total kilocalories provided. Dextrose concentrations are limited to approximately 10 percent, because peripheral veins cannot withstand concentrations greater than 900 milliosmoles per kilogram (Moore, 1993). Thus, PPN has often failed to provide adequate kilocalories and other nutrients for repair and replacement of losses. PPN has been used to supplement a partially successful enteral nutrition program.

A new system for PPN (called all-in-one or three-in-one) has been developed that allows a higher osmotic load (1200 to 1350 milliosmoles per liter) to be delivered peripherally. Lipids, amino acids, and dextrose are all incorporated in one container. Tolerance of this higher osmotic admixture in peripheral veins might be attributed to the buffering and dilution effects of intravenous fats in combination with the higher pH of the amino acid solutions and the addition of heparin to the admixture (Hoheim et al. 1990).

The ratio of nonprotein to protein kilocalories, important in peripheral feedings, is discussed in Chapter 24.

Total Parenteral Nutrition (TPN)

When nutrients are infused into a central vein, parenteral nutrition is often referred to as total parenteral nutrition (TPN) or **hyperalimentation.** Hyperalimentation is actually a misnomer because it implies that the solution exceeds nutritional requirements. The **superior vena cava,** one of the largest-diameter veins in the human body, is often used for TPN. Total parenteral nutrition can deliver greater nutrient loads, because the blood

flow in the superior vena cava rapidly dilutes these solutions 1000-fold. Concentrations for both dextrose and amino acids are determined by the client's needs. See Clinical Calculation 15–3 for an explanation and demonstration of the calculation of a sample TPN solution.

INSERTION AND CARE OF TPN LINE The physician inserts the TPN line usually through the subclavian vein and into the superior vena cava. It can be inserted at the client's bedside using strict aseptic technique. The TPN solution is a sterile mixture of dextrose, amino acids, lipid emulsion, electrolytes, vitamins, trace elements, and other additives. The pharmacist usually prepares the TPN solution. Careful attention is required to provide vitamins and minerals to clients maintained on TPN to prevent problems such as Wernicke–Korsakoff syndrome (Chapter 7).

Total parenteral nutrition has both advantages and disadvantages. Central TPN should not be carried out without experienced personnel and proper facilities. One disadvantage of TPN is that it takes a highly trained staff to provide safe administration and close monitoring, and the solution itself is costly. This makes the therapy very costly. The nurse is responsible for assessing, monitoring, and educating the client destined for home TPN. The clinical dietitian on the TPN team usually has an advanced degree and special training. The dietitian is responsible for constant nutrition assessment, monitoring, interpretation of data, and calculating formula needs with the physician.

MONITORING Careful administration of the TPN solution is important. Most reputable institutions have a strict protocol that must be followed by all health-care professionals. (A **protocol** is a description of steps to be followed when performing a procedure.) Protocols vary widely from one

---

Clinical Calculation 15–3 Calculation of a Sample TPN Solution/TPN Energy Nutrient Content

TPN solutions are usually packed in 500-cc bags. Pharmacists prefer to use dextrose and amino acids in 500-cc bags and vary the concentration of the nutrients to achieve the appropriate nutritional parameters. For example, a 500-cc bag of dextrose mixed with a 500 cc bag of amino acids equals 1000 cc. Lipids are usually provided as 250 cc of 20 percent lipid (1/2 bag) or 500 cc (one bag) of 10 percent lipid. The client's needs for kilocalories, protein, and fat can be accommodated by individualizing the concentration of each energy nutrient. For example, dextrose can be ordered from 5 to 70 percent, noted as "D_5, D_{40}, D_{50}," etc. Commonly used concentrations of amino acids are 5 percent, 8.5 percent, and 10 percent.

NUTRITIONAL VALUES USED IN COMPUTATIONS OF TPN SOLUTIONS

Dextrose	= 3.4 kcal/g
20 percent lipid	= 2.0 kcal/cc
10 percent lipid	= 1.1 kcal/cc
Protein	= 4.0 kcal/g
1 g of nitrogen	= 6.25 g protein

Calculate the total kilocalories, nonprotein kilocalories, grams of nitrogen, calorie/nitrogen ratio, and percent kilocalories from fat in 500 cc D_{50}, 500 cc 10 percent amino acids, and 250 cc 10 percent lipid.

Dextrose	Percent concentration $\times$ volume = grams of dextrose	$0.50 \times 500 = 250$ g dextrose
	Grams of dextrose $\times$ 3.4 kcal/g = kcal of solution	250 g dextrose $\times$ 3.4 kcal/g = 850 kcal
Amino acids	Percent concentration $\times$ volume = grams of protein	0.10×500 cc = 50 g protein
	Grams of protein $\times$ kcal/g = protein kcal	50 g protein $\times$ 4 kcal/g = 200 kcal
Lipids	Kcal/cc $\times$ volume in cc = fat kcal	1.1×250 cc = 275 kcal
Total kilocalories	Add kcal from dextrose, protein, and lipid	$850 + 200 + 275 = 1325$ kcal
Percent kilocalories from fat	Kcal from fat divided by total kcal = percent fat kcal	275 . 1325 = 21 percent fat

institution to another. Most TPN protocols include a slow start, a strict schedule, close monitoring, instructions for increasing the volume, maintenance of a constant rate, and instructions for a slow withdrawal. The solution may require adjustment, which can be made by increasing or decreasing any or all of the nutrients. Careful monitoring of the client's response to TPN and taking corrective measures when needed are essential for safe administration of these solutions.

Many metabolic complications are possible with TPN. Rapid shifts of potassium, phosphorus, and magnesium intracellularly result in a lowering of their concentrations in the serum. The TPN solution may need to be altered if there is a drop in the serum values of these electrolytes. Providing glucose in excess of kilocaloric needs can result in several problems, including carbon dioxide retention with respiratory difficulty. High glucose content of TPN solutions also leads to hyperglycemia. Therefore, glucose levels should be assessed regularly. Liver function test results will become abnormal after an excess glucose load. Excess glucose may lead to hyperlipidemia and fatty deposits in the liver.

The avoidance of metabolic complications directly related to a glucose overload is one reason TPN clients need to be monitored closely. These complications can be avoided by providing only an appropriate and not an excessive amount of kilocalories. In addition, an initial slow infusion at low concentrations prevents complications. Box 15–4 lists general recommendations for TPN monitoring.

TRANSITION AND COMBINATION FEEDINGS Clients need a transition period from TPN to oral feedings. Some physicians prefer to wean clients from TPN by using tube feeding. Other physicians prefer to avoid the tube and wean clients orally. In the latter case, as the client's oral intake

Box 15–4 Monitoring TPN

Initial Assessment
- Vital signs (respiration, pulse, temperature)
- Body weight and height
- Serum electrolytes, glucose, creatinine, blood urea nitrogen levels
- Serum magnesium, calcium, phosphorus levels
- Serum triglycerides and cholesterol levels
- Liver function tests
- Serum albumin and prealbumin
- Complete blood count
- Energy (estimated or measured), protein, fluid, and micronutrient needs

Routine every 4 to 8 hours
- Vital signs

Every 24 hours
- Weight
- Fluid intake and output
- Serum electrolytes, glucose, creatinine, blood urea nitrogen levels; daily for 5 days or until stable; then twice a week

Weekly
- Serum ammonia, SGOT, serum calcium, phosphorus, magnesium, total protein, and albumin
- Complete blood count
- Reassessment of actual oral, enteral, and TPN intake

Other monitors may be indicated depending on the client's clinical condition.

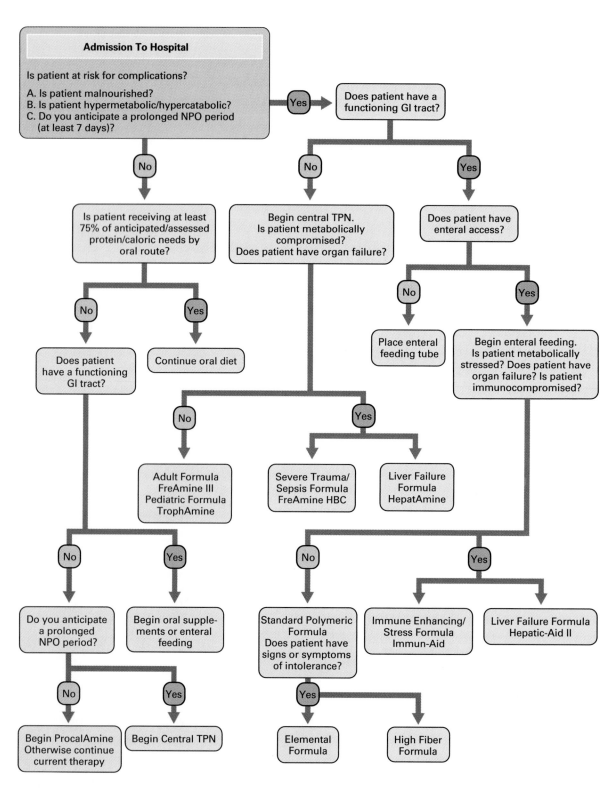

Figure 15–3:
Nutrition Support Decision Tree (Courtesy of B. Baun Medical Inc.)

increases, the TPN solution is gradually withdrawn. Expect clients who have been on TPN for a significant period of time to experience some difficulty with oral feedings. They may need much encouragement to eat.

One of the problems with TPN is that the gastrointestinal tract does not have to work during its administration. Consequently the gastrointestinal tract will have undergone some atrophy. Oral foods should be offered slowly during the weaning process. Some physicians avoid this problem by allowing some clients to consume a clear liquid or light diet while on TPN, if their condition permits.

HOME PARENTERAL NUTRITION Increasingly, clients are being discharged on TPN. These clients need adequate follow-up by either the hospital or a community home health agency.

Summary

The nutritional care of clients is a joint responsibility of the dietary and nursing departments. All nurses who work in institutions need to know not only how meals are distributed to clients but also current meal-service schedules, which affect the administration of medications and the scheduling of clients for procedures. Nutritional care includes three areas: assessing the client's need for nutrients, monitoring nutrient intake, and counseling clients about nutritional needs.

Nutrients can be delivered to clients orally, via tube feeding, or parenterally. See Figure 15–3 for a nutritional support decision tree. One principle is followed when selecting a feeding route: if the gastrointestinal tract works, use it to maximum capability. Every means should be attempted to assist clients to eat orally and independently. Oral feedings should be considered before tube feeding. Tube feeding should be considered before intravenous feeding. Intravenous feeding can be delivered peripherally or centrally. Clients on either tube feedings or intravenous feedings need to be closely monitored.

Case Study 15–1

P was brought in to the emergency room by ambulance with his mother. The mother stated her son was hit by a car while riding his bike. P is 11 years old, 4 ft 11 in. tall, and weighs 89 lb. The client's mother stated her son was well prior to the accident. In the emergency room it was observed that both his eyes were surrounded by contusions, his throat and the left side of his face were swollen. Communication with the client was at first minimal because it was painful for him to speak. An intravenous solution of D_5W was started in the emergency room. He was also shown to have a fractured femur. Surgery was required to reset the bone. The physician determined that traction would be necessary. P was expected to require traction, and thus hospitalization, for 3 to 5 weeks.

Five days later, P is still having problems swallowing. He has not progressed beyond sips of clear liquids. The kilocalorie count shows an average daily intake of 395 kcal, with only 8 g of protein for the past 3 days. P appears to be in pain when he swallows and has choked twice on larger sips of the clear liquids. The client speaks only in single words or short sentences. It is still painful for him to talk. The swelling in his esophagus has decreased enough to allow the insertion of a small silicone feeding tube. The physician has ordered a nasogastric feeding tube with Enrich. The order reads:

Day 1 Continuous drip 50 mL/h 1/2 strength
Day 2 Continuous drip 50 mL/h 3/4 strength
Day 3 Continuous drip 50 mL/h full strength
Day 4 Continuous drip 84 mL/h full strength

Enrich contains 1.1 kcal/mL and 39.7 g of protein per 1000 mL. P may have ice chips and small amounts of clear liquids in addition to the tube feeding as desired. The physician states, "The client will remain on a tube feeding until he can consume his kilocalorie requirement orally. This client requires adequate nutrition to enable the femur to heal properly." P is not expected to be discharged on a home enteral tube feeding. His prognosis is good and he is expected to make a full recovery.

The physician inserts the nasogastric tube because of the swelling in the esophagus and the danger of a perforation. The nurse assists at the client's bedside. The client holds the nurse's hand tightly as the tube is inserted. He has a worried look on his face, increased facial perspiration, and increased pulse/respirations during the procedure.

Nursing Care Plan

Subjective Data	Client held hand tightly during nasogastric tube insertion and appeared worried, apprehensive, and jittery.
Objective Data	Client is a trauma victim who showed increased perspiration and increased pulse/respirations during the tube insertion procedure.
Nursing Diagnosis	NANDA: Fear (North American Nursing Diagnosis Association, 1999)
	Related to enteral nutrition therapy and situational crisis as evidenced by tension during tube insertion and increased pulse/respirations and perspiration.

Desired Outcomes Evaluation Criteria	Nursing Actions/ Interventions	Rationale
(NOC) (Johnson, Maas, and Moorhead, 2000)	Diarrhea Management (NIC) (McCloskey and Bulechek, 2000)	
The client will state he needs the food in the tube feeding to heal his leg until he is eating better.	Explain enteral nutrition therapy procedures as performed.	A tube feeding is unfamiliar to most clients. Knowledge about the procedure may relax the client.
	As the client's condition permits, be available for listening and talking. Encourage the client to acknowledge and express feelings.	The client needs to vent his feelings about both the tube feeding and the situational crisis (the accident).

Critical Thinking Question

1. What would you do if the client pulled out the tube after insertion?
2. How would you re-assess the client's continued need for a tube feeding?
3. How should this client be monitored while on the tube feeding?

Study Aids

Subjects	Internet Sites
Tube feedings	http://www.medscape.com
	http://www.med.upenn.edu/criss/perm/helptube.html
	http://www.nyer.com/protocol.htm
Ethical considerations Position paper, American Dietetic Association	http://www.eatright.org/alegal.html
American Society of Enteral and Parenteral Nutrition	http://www.clinnutr.org/homepage
Continuing education course for nurses on enteral tube feedings	http://medcominc.com/CE_Feeding_Tubes.htm
Abstracts from the *American Journal of Clinical Nutrition*	http://www.ajcn.org

Chapter Review

1. Modular formula feedings:
   a. Always have a low osmolality
   b. Are designed for clients with malabsorption
   c. Contain a limited number of nutrients
   d. Are always predigested
2. A(n) ___ provides all of the essential nutrients in a specified volume.
   a. Intact or polymeric formula
   b. Modular feeding
   c. Intravenous feeding
   d. Elemental or predigested formula
3. Careful administration of total parenteral nutrition includes all the following except:
   a. A slow start
   b. Close monitoring
   c. Abrupt withdrawal
   d. A strict schedule
4. Diarrhea in a tube-fed client is most likely to be caused by the following:
   a. A continuous infusion feeding
   b. A bolus feeding
   c. A fluid deficit
   d. Insufficient kilocalories
5. Which of the following is *not* a recommended procedure for administering medications through a tube feeding?
   a. Mix all the medications together, crush thoroughly, mix with water, and add to the formula.
   b. If at all possible, use medications in the liquid form.
   c. Flush the tube with at least 30 milliliters of water prior to giving the medication and before resuming the tube-feeding formula.
   d. If a medication is ordered to be added to the formula, observe the feeding after the addition for any reaction or precipitation.

Clinical Analysis

1. Mr. J, 58 years old, visits his physician with a complaint of abdominal pain. He is scheduled for a diagnostic work-up, which will include a **barium enema** (x-ray study of his colon). Prior to this procedure, the nurse should instruct the client to:
   a. Eat a large breakfast on the day of the examination, such as orange juice, cereal, toast, scrambled eggs, and milk.
   b. Drink ample fluids on the morning of the examination, including at least 12 ounces of juice, 1 cup of gelatin, and broth.
   c. Take nothing orally after midnight on the day of the examination and consume only gelatin, clear broth, tea, coffee, and grape, apple, or cranberry juice on the day before the examination.
   d. Drink milk, juices, and coffee and eat only strained cream soups, ice cream, and gelatin on the day before the examination and take nothing orally after midnight.
2. Ms. L has a jejunostomy. She was discharged from the hospital last week after receiving instructions on home care from the nutrition support service. The local pharmacy is out of the Vivonex formula she has been instructed to use. As the nurse, you recommend that:
   a. She substitute Ensure
   b. She substitute Polycose
   c. She contact the Nutrition Support Service for instructions
   d. She substitute an intact or polymeric formula
3. Mr. W has been receiving a tube feeding of Ensure via nasogastric tube for 3 weeks via a bolus infusion. He has just started to have loose stools (300 milliliters each × 6 today). You should first suspect the following to be responsible for the diarrhea:
   a. A new medication added to his treatment plan
   b. Bacterial contamination
   c. Intolerance to the bolus delivery method
   d. Lactose intolerance

Bibliography

Bliss, DZ, and Lehmann, S: Tube feeding: Administration tips. RN. Vol 62, No. 8, 29, August, 1999.

Burnham, TH (ed): Drug Facts and Comparisons. Wolters Kluwer Co. St. Louis, Feb., 2000.

Butterworth, CE: The skeleton in the hospital closet. Nutrition Today 9:8, 1975.

Butterworth, CE, and Blackburn, GL: Hospital malnutrition and how to assess the nutritional status of a patient. Nutrition Today 10:8, 1975.

Davis, AE, et al.: Preventing feeding-associated aspiration. MEDSURG Nurs. 4:111, 1995.

Dickerson, J: The problem of hospital-induced malnutrition. Nurs Times 91:44, 1995.

Fater, KH: Determining nasogastric feeding tube placement. MEDSURG Nurs 4:27, 57, 1995.

Galindo-Ciocon, DJ: Tube feeding: Complications among the elderly. J Gerontol Nurs 19:17, 1993.

Hoheim, TA, et al.: Clinical experience with three-in-one admixtures administered peripherally. Nutr Clin Prac 5:118, 1990.

Johnson, M, Maas, M, and Moorhead, S: Nursing Outcomes Classification (NOC), ed. 2, Mosby, Philadelphia, 2000.

McCloskey, JC, and Bulechek, GM: Nursing Interventions Classification (NIC), ed. 3, Mosby, Philadelphia, 2000.

McWhirtner, JP: Incidence and recognition of malnutrition in hospital. Br Med J 308:946, 1994.

Methany, N, et al.: Testing feeding tube placement: Ausculation vs. pH method. AJN 98:5, 37 to 42, 1998.

Moore, MC: Pocket Guide to Nutrition and Diet Therapy. CV Mosby, St Louis, 1993.

North American Nursing Diagnosis Association: Nursing Diagnoses: Definitions and Classification 1999–2000, North American Nursing Diagnosis Association, Philadelphia, 1999.

Pagana, KD, and Pagana, TJ: Diagnostic Testing and Nursing Implications. CV Mosby, St Louis, 1992.

Pemberton, CM, et al.: Mayo Clinic Diet Manual: A Handbook of Dietary Practice, ed. 6. BC Decker, Philadelphia, 1988.

Phillips, LD: Manual of Intravenous Therapy. Philadelphia. F.A. Davis, 1994.

Skipper, A: Dietitian's Handbook of Enteral and Parenteral Nutrition. Aspen Publications, Gaithersburg, Maryland, 1998.

The Quality Assurance Committee of the American Dietetic Association: Suggested Guidelines for Nutrition Management of the Critically Ill Patient. American Dietetic Association, Chicago, 1984.

Wolfsen, HC, et al.: Tube dysfunction following percutaneous gastrostomy and jejunostomy. Gastrointest Endosc 36:3, 261–262, 1990.

Wright, B: Enteral feeding tubes as drug delivery systems. Nutr Supp Serv 6:33, 1986.

CHAPTER 16

Complementary Medicine: Botanical Remedies and Ergogenic Aids

LEARNING OBJECTIVES

After completing this chapter, the student should be able to:

1. Compare and contrast the regulatory processes for products sold in the United States as dietary supplements with those for products marketed as drugs.
2. List examples of adverse effects from five commonly used complementary medicines.
3. Identify interactions that can occur between botanical remedies and prescription and over-the-counter medications.
4. Use neutral questions when assessing a client's intake of supplements.
5. Discuss the use of special dietary supplements by athletes.

This chapter discusses two categories of complementary medicine, botanical remedies and ergogenic aids (substances that supposedly enhance athletic performance). Both are sold in the United States as dietary supplements for reasons described in this chapter. Examples of the wide range of products being sold are discussed here, but they do not constitute a comprehensive review of the market. The fact that a particular item is discussed does not imply endorsement. With these products, more than with over-the-counter or prescription medications, the watchword is "let the buyer beware," as the cases described amply demonstrate.

Botanical Remedies

Although the term "herbal medicine" is commonly used to describe the use of plant products sold as dietary supplements, some experts have objected to this phrase. Strictly speaking, an herb is a flowering plant whose stems above the ground are not woody (Stashower and Torres, 1995), and a shrub is a woody plant smaller than a tree, usually with permanent stems branching from or near the ground. Both herbs and shrubs are used as medicinal sources, including mainstream medicines. Here the term "botanical medicine" is used to mean the use of plant products that are not regulated as drugs in the United States but are sold as nutritional supplements.

Botanical products have been used to treat illnesses for centuries. Some of these products have been refined and synthesized to become drugs marketed by pharmaceutical companies. Digitalis originally was derived from purple foxglove. Morphine came from the opium poppy, quinine from cinchona bark, and aspirin from willow bark. Reserpine from snakeroot, a centuries-old Hindu remedy for snake bite, mental illness, and anxiety, was not accepted into Western medicine until the 1940s when it came to be used as a tranquilizer and an antihypertensive drug. Plants directly provide about 25 percent of currently used drugs; another 25 percent are chemically altered natural products (Sheehan, 1998).

All of these drugs can be used to treat illness, but they can also produce illness if misused or unwisely used. As discussed in Chapters 7 and 8, excessive ingestion of vitamins and minerals can produce disease just as insufficient amounts can. A basic premise of toxicology is that no chemical substance is absolutely safe; therefore, no chemical substance should be considered entirely harmless (Omaye, 1998). It follows then, that believing any substance to be safe simply because it is "natural" is a major error of logic.

In the relatively recent past, ingredients of medicines were kept secret, the same medicine was sold to treat or cure multiple unrelated illnesses, and certain medicines were distributed by unlicensed peddlers. Even among medical practitioners, revealing the contents of the prescription and giving client educational information are relatively new developments. Thirty or forty years ago, nurses were expected not to reveal to a client the name of the medicine he or she was receiving.

With botanical products, nature keeps some of the ingredients secret. Not all the constituents of these products have been identified. Therefore, when ingesting one of them, a person takes not only the active ingredient that is purported to have a medicinal effect but also other substances in the plant tissue as well. Among these other substances may be defensive chemicals the plant has evolved to protect itself from predators (Sheehan, 1998).

Regulation of Pharmaceuticals and Dietary Supplements

Laws of various countries treat drugs and dietary supplements differently. Even within the United States, some states regulate certain substances more stringently than do others. To the extent permitted by law, the Food and Drug Administration (FDA) is responsible for regulating pharmaceuticals and dietary supplements. In Germany, a similar agency, Commission E, has that responsibility.

Food and Drug Administration

Although the FDA oversees the safety of botanical products sold as dietary supplements, the rules governing their testing, processing, and labeling are vastly different from the rules governing prescription and over-the-counter drugs. Before receiving permission to market a new drug, the pharmaceutical company must conduct rigorous tests on animals and on people in randomized, double-blind clinical trials. Randomization requires that participants be assigned by coin toss or equivalent unbiased method to receive the investigative drug or not. **Double-blind** trials are experiments in which neither the subject nor the investigator knows whether a subject is receiving the treatment or a placebo.

Even after approval by the FDA, each company is granted the exclusive right or patent to manufacture the drug for a limited time only, after which other drug companies may copy, manufacture, and sell it. The patent application process is very long and expensive and is one reason sellers of botanical products give for not applying for a patent. Naturally occurring substances and laws of nature may not be patented. The process by which such a substance is purified or manufactured may be the subject of a process patent claim if it is new and non-obvious.

In 1994, Congress removed dietary supplements from the labeling provisions of the Nutrition Labeling and Education Act of 1990. Under the provisions of the Dietary Supplement Health Education Act of 1994, referred to by the acronym DSHEA, dietary supplements can be sold unless shown by the FDA to be unsafe, adulterated, or labeled in a misleading manner. The burden of proof in this case rests with the FDA, not with the manufacturer, and no prior notice from the manufacturer of intent to sell is required. The manufacturer must merely notify the FDA within 30 days after putting the product on the market.

Despite a long history of use, little is known about toxicity of botanical medicines. Most such knowledge is acquired from acute cases of toxicity sporadically reported.

Under DSHEA, a dietary supplement is defined as any product taken by mouth that contains a "so-called 'dietary ingredient' " (Center for Food Safety, 1999) and

1. Contains one or more nutrients, herbs, botanicals, or a concentrate, metabolite, or constituent extract from the ingredients previously mentioned
2. Is in the form of a supplement (meaning pill, tablet, capsule, liquid, or powder)
3. Is not represented as a food or sole item of a meal or the human diet
4. Includes a similar new drug or biologic approved under previous legislation and not currently being investigated (Food Institute, undated).

DSHEA does not limit the serving size or the amount of nutrients in any form of dietary supplement, but its regulations spell out the nature of the claims made for a product on the label and its format.

The following types of statements are allowed:

1. Benefits related to classic nutrient deficiency disease and disclosure of the prevalence of the disease
2. Description of the nutrient or dietary ingredient intended to affect the structure or function of the body
3. Characterization of the mechanism of action
4. Description of general well-being from consumption of the nutrient or dietary ingredient (Food Institute, undated).

In addition, the following information must be prominently displayed on the label: "This statement has not been evaluated by the Food and Drug Administration. This product is not intended to diagnose, treat, cure or prevent any disease."

By contrast, the rules for labeling the nutrient content of foods in the United States are much more stringent than those applied to dietary supplements. Substantiation through research or scientific agreement is needed for information to be permitted on a food label. The standard for the structure or function claim is that it be truthful and not misleading.

German Commission E

Filling a role in Europe similar to that of the FDA in this country, German Commission E is a governmental regulatory agency that has evaluated the safety and **efficacy** of botanicals based on clinical trials, cases, and scientific literature. Although admitting that herbal remedies in Germany must meet purity standards not presently in force in the United States, critics of the German system point to a double standard regarding proof of efficacy or effectiveness.

The standard of proof accepted by German Commission E for herbal remedies is set lower than for conventional drugs (Angell and Kassirer, 1999). Hundreds of preparations have been licensed in Germany by Commission E and are regulated as over-the-counter or prescription medications (Barrett, Kiefer, and Rabago, 1999). Since 1978, German Commission E has published more than 320 monographs on botanical products. This information has been translated into English by the American Botanical Council (whose website called HerbalGram is listed at the end of this chapter). Someone considering the use of botanical preparations should review the evidence presented by German Commission E and the American Botanical Council before deciding. Other suggestions for clients regarding the use of dietary supplements are given in the appendix.

Botanicals Are Big Business

In 1997, people in the United States spent $3.24 billion for botanical therapy (Klepser and Klepser, 1999). A telephone survey revealed that 12.1 percent of the respondents in 1997 had used herbal medicine in the previous 12 months, compared with 2.5 percent in 1990. That increase in usage is much greater than that in vitamin megadosing, which went from 2.4 percent of respondents in 1990 to 5.5 percent in 1997. Of the 44 percent of adults who said they regularly take prescription medicines, 18.4 percent reported the concurrent use of at least one botanical product, a high-dose vitamin, or both (Eisenberg et al., 1998).

The most popular botanical product in the United States is echinacea, with $300 million in annual sales. In 1997, U. S. sales of *Ginkgo biloba* totaled $240 million and of St. John's wort $200 million (O'Hara et al., 1998).

A survey of 136 patrons of two health-food stores revealed that they took a total of 805 supplements; 84.3 percent took supplements to prevent a health problem. Most of the customers were white (94.1 percent), female (75.7 percent), had at least one year of college education (70.6 percent), had health insurance (95.6 percent), and had a regular physician (85.3 percent) who typically was not consulted about dietary supplements (Eliason et al., 1997).

Areas of Concern with Botanicals

Because the FDA's responsibility begins only after the products have been packaged and marketed, the maintenance of quality is the responsibility of the manufacturer. Two major areas of concern with botanicals involve the lack of standardization of the products and the potential for contamination with dangerous substances.

Lack of Standardization

The potency of botanical products can vary with the climate and soil conditions and with the life cycle of the plants from which they come. Great differences in the quantities of active ingredients have been found, depending on the source, the species and part of the plant used, storage conditions (Borins, 1998), inclusion of look-alike plants, time of harvest, method of processing, and country of origin. Furthermore, it is not safe to assume that naturally occurring plant constituents are maintained at equivalent levels of biological activity when extracted, dried, and compacted into pills (American Dietetic Association, 1999).

Even worse, botanical products can come to market not containing the ingredients on the label. For example, researchers examined 50 commercial ginseng products sold in pharmacies or reputable stores for natural remedies in 11 countries and found that 6 of them did not contain any specific ginsenosides (Cui et al., 1994). Brand-name products with ingredients within 20 percent of the labeled amount are reported by brand name on a web page, Consumerlab (listed at the end of the chapter).

A traditional Chinese botanical product, jin bu huan (JBH; *Lycopodium serratum*), is used as a sedative and analgesic. Three unrelated children in Colorado, 13 months to 30 months of age, accidentally ingested 7 to 60 tablets of this remedy. All of the children experienced central nervous system depression and recovered after treatment in emergency rooms. Analysis of the tablets in all three cases revealed substances from the plant genus *Stephania* but none from *Polygala* as the label indicated. In this case, because the package insert also stated various medical indications for the product, it fell under the drug regulating authority of the FDA. (Centers for Disease Control, 1993b).

The same situation, tablets containing components of the genera *Stephania* and *Corydalis* but not *Polygala,* led to acute hepatitis in two women, ages 24 and 66 years, who ingested 4 to 16 tablets per week for 2 to 3 months. A third woman was treated for acute hepatitis, having purchased jin bu huan from the same store as the other two women had used, but the contents of the third woman's tablets were not reported (Centers for Disease Control, 1993a).

Potential for Contamination with Dangerous Substances

The desired botanical product may be contaminated with toxic substances. For example, within four days in March of 1994, the New York City Department of Health investigated 7 cases of **anticholinergic** poisoning in members of 3 different families. (Anticholinergic drugs inhibit the transmission of parasympathetic nerve impulses, making them useful drugs to reduce smooth-muscle spasms, dilate the pupil of the eye, and decrease gastrointestinal and bronchial secretions.)

In New York City, symptoms of toxicity appeared in these 10- to 40-year old clients within 2 hours of drinking tea made from leaves labeled "Paraguay tea" purchased commercially. Laboratory tests confirmed the presence of the anticholinergic drugs atropine, scopolamine, and hyoscyamine in these particular leaves, which are not present in the holly tree supposedly used for Paraguay tea. The investigation pinpointed the one grocery store handling the tea from a distributor who purchased the leaves from a farmer, had it shipped in bulk to New York, and packaged it for sale (Centers for Disease Control, 1995).

In another case, mixtures of herbs for "internal cleansing" led to digitalis poisoning in two women. Each sought medical treatment for nausea, vomiting, and palpitations. The first patient experienced nausea and severe vomiting within 24 hours of beginning the cleansing program but continued the regimen for 2 additional days. She discontinued the program but then restarted it at reduced dosage 2 days before seeking treatment in the emergency room for nausea, irregular heartbeat, and hot flashes. The second patient began the cleansing program 5 days before admission, discontinued it after 3 days, and sought medical care for visual disturbances, shortness of breath, and chest pressure in addition to nausea, vomiting, and palpitations.

An investigation by the FDA revealed the ingredient labeled plantain contained cardiac glycosides. The two women had consumed the same brand-name product with the same lot number. The raw material was traced to the supplier. Approximately 2700 kilograms (3 tons) of the plantain had been imported from Germany over a 2-year period. More that 150 manufacturers, distributors, and retailers received potentially contaminated plantain. Thirteen voluntary recalls were initiated by manufacturers and distributors. Eight firms received warning letters from the FDA, which issued 2 press releases and posted warnings for consumers on the FDA web site (Slifman et al., 1998).

A 43-year-old man sought treatment for abdominal pain. He received an extensive medical work-up including multiple blood tests, urine tests, abdominal and chest radiographs, abdominal ultrasounds, an upper gastrointestinal series with barium, gastroscopy, and colonoscopy. Finally the cause of his problem was determined to be lead poisoning. The source of the lead was tablets of "Indian plants," dispensed in an unlabeled plastic container by a person he consulted for his diabetes. Beginning with two tablets per day, the man had increased his intake to 8 tablets per day. Each tablet was found to contain 10 milligrams of lead (Beigel, Ostfeld, and Schoenfeld, 1998).

An asymptomatic case of lead poisoning was discovered in a 33-year-old Cambodian woman, but not her husband or their two children, when they attended a lead-screening clinic sponsored by a nursing school. The investigators concluded that the source of the lead was the red dye in "Koo So Pills" or "Koo Sar Pills" (the label and the package insert did not agree) she had taken at the rate of 6 per day for 7 days per month for 3 to 4 years for menstrual cramps (Centers for Disease Control, 1999).

Another incidental finding occurred when Chinese herbal balls were confiscated by the U.S. Fish and Wildlife Service in a case of alleged endangered-species violations. The herbal balls were subsequently tested for contaminants. These were factory-produced products manufactured in China that were supposed to contain herbs and honey to be consumed as a tea. Of the nine herbal balls tested, eight contained arsenic and mercury and one contained just arsenic (Espinoza, Mann, and Bleasdell, 1995).

The California Department of Health Services screened Asian patent medicines collected from retail herbal stores for undeclared pharmaceuticals and heavy metal contaminants. Of 243 samples tested for pharmaceuticals, 7 percent contained undeclared pharmaceuticals, the most common being ephedrine, chlorpheniramine, methyltestosterone, and phenacetin. Of the 251 samples tested for heavy metals, 10 percent contained lead, 14 percent contained arsenic, and 14 percent contained mercury. These contaminants were not found in trace amounts. The United States Pharmacopoeia limits the presence of heavy metals in most oral pharmaceuticals to 30 parts per million (ppm) with lower limits for lead, arsenic, and mercury (Box 16–1). These contaminated samples had means of 54.9 ppm of lead, 14,553 ppm of arsenic, and 1046 ppm of mercury (Ko, 1998).

Potentially Safe Botanical Products

Nine botanical products that have been judged to be relatively safe are reviewed next. Professors of pharmacy categorized seven herbal remedies as potentially safe: Asian ginseng, feverfew, garlic, ginkgo, saw palmetto, St. John's wort, and valerian (Klepser and Klepser, 1999). Echinacea and ginger are also discussed because of their popularity in the United States and appearances in medical literature. Four of these products, garlic, ginger, ginseng, and valerian, are on the FDA Generally Recognized As Safe list (the GRAS list) (O'Hara et al., 1998).

Any substance, even pure water, can be unsafe in excessive amounts or for particular people in certain situations. Clinical judgment is necessary for the practitioner seeking to help the client. Knowledge and caution are necessary for the client to weigh the risks and benefits of botanical therapy (Fig. 16–1).

Box 16–1 Standards for Drugs

The United States Pharmacopeia (USP), legally recognized since 1906, is a compendium of standards for drugs issued and revised periodically by a national committee of pharmacists, pharmacologists, physicians, chemists, biologists, and other allied personnel. Official drugs listed therein must meet standards of purity and strength as determined by chemical analysis or animal responses to specified doses.

The National Formulary (NF) is a list of drugs of established usefulness that are not listed in the U.S. Pharmacopeia. The NF was originally issued by the American Pharmaceutical Association but since 1980 has been published by the U.S. Pharmacopeial Convention.

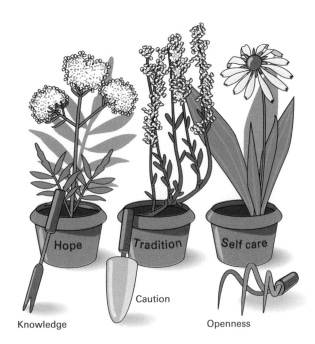

Figure 16–1:
Many people use botanical products because of their cultural traditions seeking a measure of self-care and hope. Those who use botanical products, however, need to cultivate knowledge and caution in their choices. They also should practice openness with their healthcare provider.

Asian Ginseng (Panax ginseng)

Asian ginseng is used in Germany as a tonic to combat lassitude, debility, and lack of energy and concentration (Klepser and Klepser, 1999). The active ingredients, known as ginsenosides, are present in varying quantities in different parts of the plant, with highest concentration believed to be in the root. At least 28 ginsenosides have been isolated, each of which produces unique effects on the central nervous system, the cardiovascular system, and other body systems. Some ginsenosides' effects are direct opposites of other ginsenosides' effects (Klepser and Klepser, 1999). Although other preparations of ginseng are not even classified in the genus *Panax*, much of the literature discusses ginseng as a homogeneous generic product. About 5 to 6 million people in the United States use products labeled "ginseng" (Sheehan, 1998).

Cautions: It is recommended that ginseng not be used by children, pregnant women, and persons with hypertension, psychological imbalances, headaches, heart palpitations, insomnia, asthma, inflammation, or infections with high fever. Severe hypotension upon withdrawal of the herb has been reported (Sheehan, 1998). *Adverse effects* include hypertension, euphoria, restlessness, nervousness, insomnia, skin eruptions, edema, and diarrhea. Ginseng may exert an estrogen-like effect in postmenopausal women, resulting in diffuse breast nodularity and vaginal bleeding. Vaginal bleeding was reported following the use of ginseng face cream for one month (Miller, 1998). *Drug Interactions:* Concomitant use with anticoagulants and nonsteroidal anti-inflammatory drugs (NSAIDs) should be avoided (Miller, 1998).

Echinacea (Echinacea purpurea, Echinacea pallida)

Parts of *Echinacea purpurea, Echinacea pallida* have been approved by German Commission E for limited uses (Echinacea, 1999). Between 1919 and 1950 echinacea was listed in the National Formulary (Box 16–1). In Germany, echinacea is dispensed through 2 million physicians' prescriptions per year (Barrett, Kiefer, and Rabago, 1999).

Echinacea is considered helpful for bolstering the immune system, especially for colds, flu, and chronic upper respiratory or urinary tract infections, but the opposite effect, immunosuppression, has been reported with long-term use (Capriotti, 1999). Echinacea was judged to be effective in reducing symptoms of the common cold in a sample of 246 individuals (Brinkeborn, Shah, and Degenring, 1999), but not effective in preventing colds or decreasing their duration in 108 individuals (Grimm and Muller, 1999).

Cautions: A person with allergies, especially to members of the composite family (aster, chrysanthemum, daisy, dandelion, goldenrod, marigold, ragweed, St. John's Wort, sunflower, thistle, and zinnia), should consult his or her healthcare provider before taking this herb. Echinacea is not recommended for longer than 8 weeks of use orally or 3 weeks parenterally. The healthcare provider should be consulted before taking echinacea if the client is a child or a woman who is pregnant, planning to become pregnant, or lactating (Echinacea, 1999). *Adverse Effects:* May cause liver toxicity, especially when used with other hepatotoxic drugs. May decrease the effectiveness of corticosteroids (American Society of Anesthesiologists, 1999). The most common complaint is of an unpleasant taste.

Feverfew (Tanacetum parthenium)

Encapsulated leaves of feverfew have been approved by the Canadian Health Protection Branch to prevent migraine headaches. Its mechanism of action is unknown. Some randomized, double-blind, placebo-controlled trials have shown feverfew to be effective in preventing migraines, but Vogler, Pittler, and Ernst (1998) conclude that clinical effectiveness of feverfew in the prevention of migraine has not been established beyond reasonable doubt. Variations in preparations used in trials make comparisons difficult (O'Hara et al., 1998).

Cautions: Feverfew should be avoided in pregnancy, lactation, for children under 2 years of age, and persons allergic to plants in the daisy family (Asteraceae). *Adverse Effects:* Gastrointestinal ulcers or canker sore occur in 5 to 15 percent of users, and abrupt cessation may cause rebound headache (American Society of Anesthesiologists, 1999). *Drug Interactions:* Feverfew may interact with anticoagulants and potentiate the antiplatelet effect of aspirin (Klepser and Klepser, 1999).

Garlic (Allium sativum)

German Commission E indicates garlic for the support of dietary measures for treating hyperlipoproteinemia and to prevent arteriosclerosis. Over a 4-year period, high-dose garlic powder reduced the increase in arteriosclerotic plaque volume by 5 to 18 percent (Koscielny et al., 1999), whereas a 12-week study of 25 patients showed no effect of garlic oil on cholesterol or serum lipoproteins (Berthold, Sudhop, and von Bergmann, 1998). Optimal effects are achieved by consuming raw cloves or enteric-coated tablets because the purported active ingredient is degraded by crushing, heat, and acid (O'Hara et al., 1998).

Garlic is known to inhibit platelet function and to increase levels of two antioxidant enzymes. A case of spontaneous spinal epidural hematoma was attributed to the 87-year-old man's consumption of 4 cloves of garlic daily for an unreported length of time to prevent heart disease (Rose et al., 1990). Although randomized trials have been reported, researchers admit the characteristic odor of garlic is difficult to hide for the purposes of double-blind studies.

Cautions: Allergies have been reported (Perez-Pimiento et al., 1999). *Adverse effects:* Garlic has been reported to cause heartburn, flatulence, sweating, lightheadedness, and excessive menstrual flow (Klepser and Klepser, 1999). The side effects of malodorous breath and skin can be moderated by consuming the garlic with protein or by taking **enteric-coated** tablets that dissolve in the intestine rather than the stomach (O'Hara et al., 1998). *Drug Interactions:* Garlic may potentiate anticoagulants' effects (Glisson, Crawford, and Street, 1999).

Ginger (Zingiber officinale)

The ancient Greeks and Romans used ginger as a digestive aid, as did people in East Indian and Chinese cultures. Sailors have used ginger for motion sickness. Western versions of the medicinal herb include ginger ale, ginger beer, and ginger tea. The root of this plant has been shown to reduce nausea and vertigo better than placebo. Its mechanism of action affects the stomach, rather than the central nervous system (Miller, 1998) where it improves gastroduodenal motility (Micklefield et al., 1999).

One study of 120 gynecologic laparoscopy clients, however, discerned no significant differences in postoperative nausea and vomiting for placebo, ginger, droperidol, or ginger plus droperidol (Visalyaputra et al., 1998). Ginger is also being investigated as a cancer preventive agent (Vimala, Norhanom, and Yadav, 1999). *Adverse Effects:* Ginger prolongs bleeding times. Other side effects are heartburn and diarrhea. *Drug Interactions:* Avoid using ginger with anticoagulant drugs (Miller, 1998).

Ginkgo (Ginkgo biloba)

In Germany, ginkgo is prescribed for treatment of cerebral circulatory disturbances and dementia and for peripheral arterial insufficiency. Its extract dilates arteries, inhibits arterial spasms, and decreases blood viscosity. In 7 of 8 clinical studies, statistically and clinically significant effects of ginkgo on cerebral insufficiency were shown as compared with placebo. An application to the treatment of dementia has been proposed (Le Bars et al., 1997). Ginkgo also significantly increased the blood flow velocity to the eye, suggesting a possible use in clients with glaucoma (Chung et al., 1999).

Adverse Effects: Four individuals have had spontaneous bleeding while taking gingko. A 70-year-old man bled into the anterior chamber of the eye 1 week after adding ginkgo to his aspirin regimen following coronary artery bypass surgery. A 78-year-old woman, stabilized on warfarin for 5 years after coronary bypass surgery, sustained a left **parietal** hemorrhage after using ginkgo for 2 months. A 72-year-old woman developed a **subdural hematoma** after taking ginkgo for 6 to 7 months. A 33-year-old woman suffered bilateral subdural hematomas after taking it for 2 years (Cupp, 1999). *Drug Interactions:* Taking gingko with aspirin or any nonsteroidal anti-inflammatory drug (NSAID) or anticoagulants is ill-advised. Ginkgo may also diminish the effectiveness of anticonvulsant drugs and potentiate the risk of seizures with medications known to decrease the seizure threshold, such as tricyclic antidepressants (Miller, 1998). The most commonly reported adverse effects of ginkgo are gastric disturbances, headache, dizziness, and vertigo. One case is reported of seizures and loss of consciousness after ingestion of 50 gingko seeds (Klepser and Klepser, 1999).

Saw Palmetto (Serenoa repens)

The German Commission E has indicated saw palmetto to decrease difficulties with urination associated with benign prostatic hypertrophy. Its mechanism of action is unknown, but it may inhibit the binding of dihydrotestosterone to androgen receptors in prostate cells or inhibit the enzyme responsible for converting testosterone to dihydrotestosterone. Compared with finasteride, saw palmetto produces similar improvement in urinary tract symptoms and urinary flow but with fewer adverse effects (Wilt et al., 1998). Teas made with saw palmetto are probably ineffective, because the active components are insoluble in water (Klepser and Klepser, 1999).

Cautions: Pregnant women and children should not take saw palmetto. *Adverse effects:* headache, nausea, and upset stomach. *Drug Interactions:* None have been reported, but the prudent person would avoid concurrent use of other hormonal therapies (Miller, 1998).

St. John's Wort (Hypericum perforatum)

In use as a treatment for psychiatric disorders since the 15th century, St. John's wort is indicated by German Commission E as supportive treatment for anxiety and depression. Its mechanism of action is unknown, but at least 13 active ingredients have been isolated (Klepser and Klepser, 1999). Theories have been suggested that St. John's wort may act as a monoamine oxidase inhibitor (MAOI) or a selective serotonin reuptake inhibitor. The dietary implications of MAOIs are discussed in the next chapter, but evidence thus far indicates food restriction is not necessary for clients taking St. John's wort (Miller, 1998).

In a 6-week trial, an extract of St. John's wort was judged to be equivalent to 20 milligrams of fluoxetine per day in relieving mild to moderate depression in elderly clients (Harrer et al., 1999). Similarly, in an 8-week trial, an extract of St. John's wort was judged to be more effective than imipramine and more effective than placebo (Philipp, Kohnen, and Hiller, 1999). After evaluating 4 clinical trials, Josey and Tackett (1999) concluded that St. John's wort was as effective as antidepressant medications and more effective than placebo.

Cautions: St. John's wort should be avoided in pregnancy because of its **abortifacient** action. It also may cause allergy. See the discussion of echinacea for possible sources of cross-reactivity. Because photosensitivity is common with the use of this botanical preparation, people taking it may need to protect themselves from exposure to the sun. A case report of subacute toxic neuropathy was attributed to demyelination of cutaneous axons due to singlet oxygen and free radicals produced from hypericins' exposure to light of (Bove, 1998). *Adverse reactions:* St. John's wort is reported to cause gastrointestinal irritation, tiredness, and restlessness. *Drug Interactions:* Interference with the action of warfarin (Yue, Bergquist, and Gerten, 2000) and indinavir, a protease inhibitor used to treat HIV infection (Lumpkin and Alpert, 2000) have been reported. Two cases of rejection of transplanted hearts (11 and 20 months after surgery) due to interference with the metabolism of cyclosporin were attributed to

beginning the use of St. John's wort, self-prescribed and prescribed by a psychiatrist, three weeks before symptoms appeared (Ruschitzka et al., 2000). The cases involving indinavir and cyclosporin were possibly due to induction of the cytochrome P450 metabolic pathway, (see Chapter 17). There is also a possibility of interactions with serotonin-reuptake inhibitors. St. John's wort may prolong the effects of anesthesia (American Society of Anesthesiologists, 2000). Use with other drugs causing photosensitivity should be avoided (Miller, 1998).

Valerian (Valeriana officinalis)

With a history dating to ancient Greece and Rome (Yager, Siegfreid, and DiMatteo, 1999), valerian has official pharmacopoeial status in Europe, where it is most commonly used as an ingredient in botanical medicines. Valerian exemplifies the dilemma of dealing with botanical products. Valerian's variety of components may correct numerous causes of insomnia, but that very variety and the instability of constituents creates problems with standardization (Houghton, 1999). Valerian is recommended by German Commission E to manage restlessness and nervous disorders of sleep. Its mode of action affecting the central nervous system is incompletely understood.

Some 44 constituents of valerian have been isolated. Compared with placebo, valerian significantly improved sleep quality in habitually poor or irregular sleepers. It has not been observed to change sleep stages (Miller, 1998).

Adverse Effects: headaches, hangover, excitability, insomnia, uneasiness, cardiac disturbances, ataxia, decreased sensibility, hypothermia, hallucinations, and increased muscle relaxation (Klepser and Klepser, 1999). Cardiac complications and delirium have been associated with withdrawal (Garges, Varia, and Doraiswamy, 1998). *Drug Interactions:* Since valerian prolongs thiopental- and pentobarbital-induced sleep, it should not be used with barbiturates (Miller, 1998).

A summary of the main uses of the nine botanical products mentioned above and situations in which they should be avoided appear in Table 16–1. Use with anticoagulants and during pregnancy are the most frequent contraindications cited. The absence of such a warning should not be construed as evidence of safety, however. Sufficient data as yet may not have been gathered.

When Things Go Wrong

Sometimes the use of home remedies goes terribly wrong, often because of human error, as in the following cases.

Choosing Toxic Plants

Chaparral (*Larrea tridentata*) is an evergreen desert shrub found in the southwestern United States and Mexico that has been used to treat a number of diseases and to prevent conception (Sheehan, 1998). Federal investigation of 18 reported cases of liver toxicity confirmed that chaparral ingestion caused 13 of them. Twelve of the 13 clients had ingested tablets or capsules from various manufacturers; the other person consumed chaparral as a tea. Cessation of ingestion of chaparral resulted in resolution in 11 clients. The remaining 2 underwent liver transplantation. The pathophysiology of chaparral-associated liver toxicity is unclear, but the 2 clients requiring liver transplantation took chaparral capsules for longer

Table 16–1 Commonly Used Botanicals' Main Uses and Avoidance Situations

PRODUCT	MAIN USE*	AVOID WITH
Asian ginseng (*Panax ginseng*)	To combat lack of energy	Anticoagulants NSAIDs Pregnancy
Echinacea (*E. purpurea, E. pallida*)	To bolster the immune system	Allergies to the daisy family Pregnancy Lactation
Feverfew (*Tanacetum parthenium*)	To prevent migraine headaches	Allergies to the daisy family Anticoagulants Aspirin Pregnancy
Garlic (*Allium sativum*)	To treat hyperlipoproteinemia	Anticoagulants Allergies
Ginger (*Zingiber officinale*)	To aid digestion and treat motion sickness	Anticoagulants
Ginkgo (*Ginkgo biloba*)	To improve cerebral circulation	Anticoagulants Aspirin NSAIDs
Saw palmetto (*Serenoa repens*)	To decrease urination difficulty	Other hormonal therapies Pregnancy
St. John's wort (*Hypericum perforatum*)	To support treatment for anxiety and depression	Allergies to the daisy family: anticoagulants, cyclosporin, indinavir Pregnancy (**abortifacient**) Serotonin-reuptake inhibitors Drugs causing photosensitivity
Valerian (*Valeriana officinalis*)	To manage restlessness and disorders of sleep	Barbiturates

*As listed in Canada or Germany. U.S. labeling may be re-worded.

than a year, compared with the other clients, who reported having ingested it for 2.8 to 24 weeks (Sheikh, Philen, and Love, 1997).

One of the individuals who received a liver transplant after being poisoned with chaparral went through extensive blood tests, an abdominal ultrasound, and CT scan. The latter reveal gallbladder pathology. An exploratory laparotomy was performed. Severe acute hepatitis was diagnosed by liver biopsy. At that point, the client's husband revealed that she had ingested 2 capsules of chaparral daily for 10 months, along with a pinch of garlic powder and a tea made from nettle and chickweed. Three weeks before admission, the client had developed symptoms of flu and *increased* her dose of chaparral to 6 capsules per day (Gordon et al., 1995). Two Canadian patients also developed acute hepatitis after ingesting chaparral leaf, one for 2 months and one for 3 months, but recovered after discontinuing use of the botanical product (Batchelor, Heathcote, and Wanless, 1995).

Misidentifying Plants

A 72-year-old woman became ill after drinking a tea she thought to be made of borage leaves. She developed nausea, vomiting, diarrhea, flickering in her eyes, and palpitations. Her electrocardiogram showed intermittent atrioventricular blockage. Her blood levels of digitoxin and digoxin were 133.5 ng/mL and 3.93 ng/mL (toxic >25 ng/mL and >2.4 ng/Ml), respectively. Symptomatic treatment was all that was necessary. The cause

was attributed to her gathering foxglove leaves, mistaking them for borage (Brustbauer and Wenisch, 1997).

In a similar case, an 18-month-old boy developed liver disease after consuming a tea supposedly made with peppermint and coltsfoot (*Tussilago farfara*) since 3 months of age. Conservative treatment led to a complete recovery within two months. Analysis of the leaves indicated that the parents had gathered alpendost (*Adenostyles alliariae*), mistaking it for coltsfoot (Sperl et al., 1995).

Tragedy resulted from giving Hispanic infants tea from homegrown "mint" plants The first infant's mother did not reveal the use of "mint" tea until the 2nd hospital day. After the 8-week-old infant died, autopsy revealed liver necrosis, hemorrhagic kidneys, left adrenal hemorrhage, bilateral lung consolidation, and diffuse cerebral edema with ischemic necrosis. The second infant, 6 months old, had been given the tea 3 times a week since he was 3 months old. Laboratory testing of the leaves from the involved plants and the infants' sera confirmed the source of the poison to be pennyroyal oil, a highly toxic agent used by herbalists to induce menstruation or abortion.

The second infant received some "mint" tea the evening before admission when he had vomited and had a fever. Although the second infant lived, he was left with liver and brain dysfunction. Medical opinion was that he tolerated the pennyroyal oil until he seemed to develop a viral infection, which precipitated the acute illness (Bakerink et al., 1996).

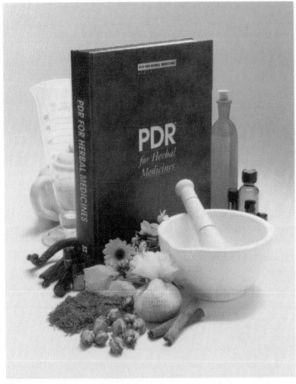

Bringing Science to Herbal Medicine

Physician's Desk Reference®
Introduces

PDR® for Herbal Medicines

The First Authoritative Herbal Guide
for Healthcare Professionals

Figure 16–2:
The 1st edition of the Physicians' Desk Reference for Herbal Medicines was published in 1998. (Courtesy of Medical Economics Company.)

Increasing the Dose

A uterine stimulant, blue cohosh (*Caulophyllum thalictroides*), was prescribed by a midwife as follows. Beginning 1 month before her due date, the pregnant woman was to take one tablet daily to induce uterine contractions. The woman took 3 tablets per day for 3 weeks. Spontaneous onset of labor resulted in precipitous delivery one hour later. The amniotic fluid was slightly stained with meconium. Within 20 minutes of birth, the infant became cyanotic and required mechanical ventilation. An electrocardiogram revealed an acute myocardial infarction.

He was extubated at 21 days of age and discharged from the hospital at 31 days of age. At 2 years of age, he displayed normal growth and development despite cardiomegaly and mildly reduced left ventricular function for which he received digoxin. The long-term prognosis was guarded. Congenital anomalies were ruled out and the cause for this newborn's heart attack was attributed to the blue cohosh that contains an alkaloid known to produce toxic effects on the myocardium of laboratory animals (Jones and Lawson, 1998).

A Prudent Course

Several issues arise when health-care providers assist clients who are attempting to maximize their health. The fact that many botanical products have been used for centuries does not negate the dangers cited in this chapter. Clearly in this market, "let the buyer beware" holds true. Aside from changing the law, what can be done to protect clients?

Thorough assessment is vital. In several of the worst cases cited, the fact that herbal remedies were used did not come to light until late in the treatment cycle. Did health-care providers ask the clients about use of botanical products? If so, was it done in a manner that permitted them to reveal their practices without being ridiculed or condemned?

Education is essential. Without disparaging a client's background, the health-care provider must counter the ill-advised attitude that "Everything natural is safe." Substances strong enough to produce the effects attributed to botanical preparations are medicines, no matter what the law currently allows for distribution. Such substances should be treated with respect. Use of childproof containers should be encouraged.

Health-care providers also must educate themselves about botanical products. The *Physicians' Desk Reference for Herbal Medicines,* shown in Figure 16–2, contains 1244 pages with prescribing information for over 600 herbs (Gruenwald, 1998). Keeping abreast of medical literature is as important in this field as in any other. Staying alert to press releases and general news items about botanical medicine helps health-care providers keep up to date.

Awareness of the dangers is essential. More than one source has recommended that the following botanicals be avoided: borage, chaparral, comfrey, ephedra, germander, kombucha, lobelia, pennyroyal, sassafras, and wormwood (Baker, 1999; Brody, 1999; Klepser and Klepser, 1999; and Sheehan, 1998).

So many people are taking botanical products that the American Society of Anesthesiologists (1999) issued a warning to consumers of herbal medicine to stop taking the products 2 to 3 weeks before scheduled surgery. Possible interactions cited were an unintended deepening of anesthesia and problems with bleeding and blood pressure.

A general nursing process approach to botanical use is given in Clinical Application 16–1.

Ergogenic Aids

Athletes in training, attempting to build a competitive edge, often alter their dietary intake and consume various supplements. This section summarizes some of these actions and cites scientific opinion as to the safety and effectiveness of the practices. Before using any of these supplements, the athlete, with the advice of the health-care provider, parents, and coach, should evaluate the supplement:

1. Is the link between the purported aid and known physiology and biochemistry logical?
2. Has the use been critiqued in peer-reviewed journals?

The Nursing Process and Botanical Remedies

Ask clients these questions about botanical use

Assessment: What kinds of herbal products, dietary supplements, or other natural remedies do you take?

Do you find the recommended dose satisfactory?
Are you taking any prescription or over-the-counter medications for the same purpose?
Have you used this product before? For how long?
Where do you obtain these products?
Is anyone else in your household taking botanical products?
Are you allergic to any plant products?
Are you pregnant, planning to become pregnant, or breast-feeding?

Analysis: Look up botanical remedies in the PDR for Herbal Medicines or on the Internet at http://www.rxlist.com if necessary.

Identify problem areas.

Planning: Prioritize problems to be addressed as to seriousness.

Products with known toxic effects.
Products given to children.
Home-grown plant materials.
Products with interactions to drugs the client is receiving

Implementation: Document findings in the record.

Offer educational advice to the client and document it.
If long-term studies establishing the safety of a product are lacking, encourage client to limit use to several weeks.
Multiple products for the same effect can lead to trouble.
Discourage use of botanical products for infants, children, pregnant women, and elderly without professional medical advice.
If the client wishes to use these products, reinforce the need to abide by recommended doses and to consistently use the same reputable supplier.
Encourage client to monitor for side effects and report them to health-care provider or the FDA's MEDWATCH at 1-800-FDA-1088 or on the Internet at http://www.fda.gov/medwatch/report/consumer/consumer.htm

Evaluation: Follow up the actions of the client at each visit.

Are there new symptoms?
Have the products, brands, doses been changed?
Have any products been stopped or new ones added?
Does the client think the products are effective?
Why or why not?

Adapted from Cirigliano and Sun, 1998; Cupp, 1999; Glisson, Crawford, and Street, 1999; and Yager, Siegfried, and DiMatteo, 1999.

3. What are the safety, ethical, and legal consequences of using the aid? (Butterfield, 1996).

The last item includes the rules of athletic conferences and the International Olympic Committee.

The use of ergogenic aids for improved physical prowess has roots in ancient history. Athletes and soldiers in the past consumed selected animal parts to acquire some of the animal's strength, speed, or agility. Ergogenic aids are intended to increase the potential for work output. Most ergogenic aids can be categorized as energy sources, cellular components, recovery aids, or anabolic enhancers (Applegate, 1999). Some clearly fall into the classes of nutrients discussed in Unit 1 of this text, whereas others do not, although they may be substances with physiological functions. For the sake of uniformity, the ergogenic aids included here will be categorized either as nutrients corresponding to those discussed in Unit 1 or as nonnutrients.

Nutrients

Various investigators have tested the effects on physical performance of altering ingestion of carbohydrate, protein, or antioxidant vitamins. Additionally, procedures to maximize water retention have been researched. Unfortunately, it is often impossible to obtain the amounts of nutrients recommended as ergogenic aids through food (Applegate, 1999).

Carbohydrates

Consuming carbohydrates immediately before or after exercise augments performance by increasing muscle glycogen stores, delaying fatigue, and enhancing recovery. An endurance athlete's carbohydrate consumption should be at least 60 percent of kilocaloric intake normally and 70 percent of energy intake for several days prior to competition. Ingesting carbohydrate 3 to 6 hours before exercise enhances performance (Applegate, 1999).

A short-term study has shown that ingesting carbohydrate following resistance training can decrease muscle protein degradation and urea nitrogen excretion, thereby promoting a more positive nitrogen balance (Kreider, 1999). Similar studies using carbohydrate and protein supplements produced a modest but significant increase in growth hormone levels and suggested the combination of nutrients might hasten the rate of muscle recovery during intense training (Kreider, 1999).

High-kilocalorie snacks to promote weight gain and muscle growth are effective for the former but not so desirable for the latter. Typically only 30 to 40 percent of the weight gained is fat-free mass, and thus the use of such snacks is not a strategy recommended for the average athlete (Kreider, 1999).

Protein and Amino Acids

Protein and amino acid supplementation may aid anabolism and increase strength (Applegate, 1999). Athletes involved in intense training may have greater protein needs than sedentary individuals (1.3 to 2 grams per kg per day, compared with 0.8 gram for sedentary people) but increasing protein intake beyond that level does not increase muscle growth (Kreider, 1999). The recommendation for athletes is to consume 12 to 15 percent of kilocaloric intake as protein, an intake that is possible through a normal diet that maintains energy balance.

GLUTAMINE Glutamine is an important fuel for some cells of the immune system and may have specific immunostimulatory effects. Oral glutamine, compared with placebo, appeared to have a beneficial effect on the incidence of infections reported by runners after a marathon (Castell and Newsholme, 1998). There is some evidence that this amino acid supplement promotes muscle growth and decreases exercise-induced immunosuppression, thus decreasing incidence of upper respiratory infections, but long-term studies have not been conducted. (Kreider, 1999).

Levels of plasma amino acids, mainly glutamine, were decreased in Olympic athletes suffering from chronic fatigue and infection. Inadequate protein intake appeared to be a factor, because 7 of the 12 athletes in the chronic fatigue group had restricted dietary intake of dairy products and animal protein (Kingsbury, Kay, and Hjelm, 1998).

BRANCHED-CHAIN AMINO ACIDS (BCAA) Leucine, isoleucine, and valine are branched-chain amino acids that make up about one third of muscle protein (Mero, 1999). Significant decreases in levels of plasma leucine follow exercise sessions. Theoretically, supplementation with branched-chain amino acids (BCAA) during intense training could reduce exercise-induced muscle damage and consequently lead to greater gains in fat-free mass (Kreider, 1999). Leucine or its metabolite, beta-hydroxy beta-methylbutyrate (beta-HMB), has been reported to increase fat-free mass in college football players and in elderly men and women; no significant difference was found between it and placebo in two other studies (Kreider, 1999). The effectiveness of individual amino acids as ergogenic aids requires further research with well-controlled studies (Applegate, 1999).

Dietary Antioxidants

The potential for antioxidants to enhance recovery from exercise is related to their ability to detoxify free radicals, which are produced during strenuous exercise. Evidence thus far supports the concept that supplemental dietary antioxidant intake protects against oxidative stress due to exercise and perhaps also enhances recovery and minimizes muscle soreness (Applegate, 1999).

Nonnutrients

Among the ergogenic aids promoted for athletes are several substances that occur in the human body as a result of metabolism, one commonly ingested foreign substance, caffeine, and the drug ephedrine. The United States Olympic Committee (USOC) has banned many drugs including over-the-counter cold medications that contain stimulants. The lists are accessible at its website (listed at the end of this chapter).

Bicarbonate

Muscular activity generates lactic acid as a waste product with consequent lowering of blood pH. The drop in pH is thought to inhibit the resynthesis of ATP and to inhibit muscle contraction. One physiological buffer is bicarbonate. Sodium bicarbonate (baking soda) has been shown to be an effective ergogenic aid during exercise lasting approximately 1 to 7 minutes (Applegate, 1999). McNaughton, Dalton, and Palmer (1999) showed sodium bicarbonate to be significantly more effective than placebo or no intervention in decreasing fatigue during 60-minute cycling sessions.

Even this common household item, baking soda, can be dangerous, producing alkalosis when overused. While not currently banned by the

International Olympic Committee, its use may eventually be judged a violation of the doping rule (Applegate, 1999).

Creatine

Creatine is a nonprotein substance synthesized in the body from the amino acids arginine, glycine, and methionine. When combined with phosphate, the resulting compound, phosphocreatine, serves as a storage form of energy that is released with anaerobic muscle contraction. Increasing the supply of creatine supposedly would increase muscle creatine and phosphocreatine concentration, leading to a higher rate of ATP resynthesis (Mujika and Padilla, 1997). Endogenous synthesis produces 1 to 2 grams of creatine per day, while dietary fish and meat provide another 1 to 2 grams. Creatine is eliminated by its irreversible conversion to creatinine at a rate of approximately 1 to 2 grams per day (Juhn and Tarnopolsky, 1998a).

Supplementation with oral creatine has shown inconsistent effects on athletic performance. One suggested reason for the divergence is that the initial levels of muscle creatine concentrations vary from individual to individual. For this reason, individuals with lower initial muscle creatine levels showed the best response (Juhn and Tarnopolsky, 1998a). Evidence in support of that theory came from a study of untrained subjects performing repeated exercises in the laboratory. They received ergogenic effects from creatine supplementation, whereas highly trained athletes performing single competition-like tasks did not (Mujika and Padilla, 1997). Performances that were enhanced by creatine supplementation were those involving high-intensity tasks lasting less than 30 seconds (Williams and Branch, 1998).

Creatine supplementation does result in weight gain that initially is the result of water retention. An increase in muscle mass is postulated with longer use. The weight gain is a mixed blessing, however. In running and swimming events, creatine supplementation was not ergogenic, causing increased elapsed time in a 6-kilometer run, a side effect probably related to the weight gain. For researchers, the weight gain complicates the task of designing double-blind, placebo-controlled studies (Juhn and Tarnopolsky, 1998a).

Although short-term use of creatine (less than 28 days' time) at recommended doses has not been shown to cause significant adverse effects, the involved studies were small and incomplete as to calculation of sample size required to obtain significance. Additionally, despite its presence in the heart, brain, and testes, creatine's effects on those organs and on the kidney and liver have not been investigated (Juhn and Tarnopolsky, 1998b). Creatine supplementation is legal and not construed as doping (Williams and Branch, 1998).

Steroids

Nonprescription steroids to enhance body-building are sold as dietary supplements. The use of the supplements is forbidden by the International Olympic Committee, the National Collegiate Athletic Association, and the National Football League, but not by the National Basketball Association, the National Hockey League, or major league baseball.

In the body, these products are converted to testosterone, the male sex hormone. The recommended dose of one of these products, androstenedione, is considered weak, but many athletes do not confine themselves to the recommended doses (Schnirring, 1998).

Table 16–2 Side Effects of Testosterone and Associated Drugs

MALE	ADOLESCENT	FEMALE
Acne	Severe facial and body acne	Acne
Enlarged breasts*	Premature closure of growth centers of long bones which may result in stunted growth*	Clitoral hypertrophy*
Premature balding		Decreased breast tissue
Blood clotting disorders		Deepened voice*
Testicular atrophy		Menstrual irregularities
Decreased sperm counts		Hirsutism (Excessive hair growth on face and body)*
Prostatic hypertrophy		
Kidney and liver dysfunction		Kidney and liver dysfunction*
Liver tumors		Flushing
Undesirable changes in lipoprotein and cholesterol levels		Diaphoresis (sweating)
		Vaginitis
Increased aggression and sexual appetite		
Depression and paranoia		

*May be permanent

(Adapted from Blue and Lombardo, 1999; Nursing 2000; Schnirring, 1998; U.S. Olympic Committee, 1997).

The lists of side effects of androgenic anabolic steroids, whether prescription or over-the-counter, is long and should give the prospective user pause (Table 16–2). Wives and girlfriends of users of androgenic anabolic steroids may be at risk for severe injury because of the user's increased aggression (Blue and Lombardo, 1999).

Glycerol

Glycerol is an alcohol that is a component of fats. The pharmaceutical grade of glycerol is called glycerin(e). It is used to moisten chapped skin, as an ingredient in suppositories for constipation, and as a sweetening agent in medications. Taken orally, it acts as an osmotic diuretic to reduce intracranial pressure and intraocular pressure.

As an ergogenic aid, glycerol has been tested as a means of hyperhydration to prevent dehydration. Although oral glycerin does enhance fluid retention, its effectiveness in improving athletic performance is controversial and largely unsubstantiated (Wagner, 1999). Appropriate hydration without glycerol is recommended, however. Dehydration is implicated in the occurrence of muscle cramps (Levin, 1993; Stamford, 1993).

Caffeine

Caffeine dosing before exercise delays the onset of fatigue and may enhance performance of high-intensity exercise. Proposed mechanisms for improving work output include caffeine's function as a central nervous system stimulant and through an alteration in fuel utilization. Caffeine is thought to increase fat oxidation and reduce carbohydrate use, thus sparing glycogen and delaying fatigue. Despite its ready availability, caffeine has side effects and causes some drug interactions.

Although the International Olympic Committee limits the amount of allowable caffeine in the urine to 12 micrograms per milliliter, individuals ingesting amounts of 3 to 9 milligrams per kilogram of body weight have not exceeded the limit (Applegate, 1999). Gauging the effects is problematic, however, because the onset and duration of the drug's effects are unknown (Nursing 2000). For a 154-lb (70 kg) athlete, 3 to 9 milligrams per kilogram of body weight would amount to 210 to 630 milligrams of caffeine, the amount in 12 to 37 ounces of brewed regular coffee.

Ephedrine

Another central nervous system stimulant, ephedrine, is available over-the-counter in nutritional supplements for body-builders and other athletes. Eating disorders and disorders of body image were especially prevalent among ephedrine users. In addition, of 36 female weightlifters, 7 (19 percent) displayed frank ephedrine dependency (Gruber and Pope, 1998). About 500 reports of adverse effects from ephedrine-containing dietary supplements, including 8 deaths, were received in less than 2 years in the state of Texas. One of the fatal coronary occlusions occurred in a 44-year-old man, an active swimmer and tennis player, who received the dietary supplement from his physician as a substitute for coffee and cocoa. The client discontinued those beverages, consumed the dietary supplement at recommended dosages, and died 3 weeks later (Centers for Disease Control, 1996).

Adverse reactions to ephedrine include the symptoms of headache, dizziness, insomnia, and nausea as well as the signs of tremor, fainting, vomiting, hypertension, heart palpitations, and convulsions. Medical diagnoses resulting from ephedrine-containing dietary supplements include myocardial infarction and stroke, which were the causes of death in 7 of the 8 cases reported. Adverse reactions vary and are not always proportional to the dose consumed. Approximately 21 states have passed regulations that are stricter than those of the federal government (Centers for Disease Control, 1996), and the United States Olympic Committee has banned ephedrine use by its athletes (November 1999).

Making Wise Decisions

Athletes often make tremendous sacrifices in the pursuit of excellence. Their drive and dedication is admirable, but rash judgments about the substances they take into their bodies is not. Clients need guidance in gathering and evaluating evidence about the safety and efficacy of nutritional supplements marketed for athletes. If an athlete chooses to take a nutritional supplement, the recommended dose should be used. More is not better. Physicians and dietitians specialize in sports medicine to help the athlete's decision making. One such physician cautions that nutritional supplements have not been tested in or approved for use by children or adolescents and that their use in this population should be approached with trepidation (Metzl, 1999).

Basic nutrition principles hold true for athletes as well as less active people. Increased kilocalories because of the activity, consuming proportionate protein, and drinking adequate water are appropriate approaches to athletic training. Extra snacks of sports drinks, fruit juices, low-fat milk, yogurt, whole-grain cereal, fruit, and pretzels are good choices to increase kilocaloric intake in a healthful manner.

A particular problem occurs in sports for which body size or weight is crucial. The deaths of collegiate wrestlers trying to "cut weight" were discussed in Chapter 9. Other activities with weight consideration that might lead to unwise dieting are gymnastics, cross country track, crew (rowing), and dance.

Summary

Botanical remedies are plant products sold as dietary supplements. Under United States law as of this writing, they are exempt from many of the regulations governing prescription and over-the-counter medications. Although the FDA oversees the safety of botanicals, the responsibility for proving a product is *unsafe* is the *government's*. With prescription and nonprescription drugs, in contrast, the *manufacturer* must demonstrate the medicine is *safe*.

Botanical products are commonly used in Germany, based on evaluation by German Commission E. Those evaluations have been published and often are consulted in the search for reliable information.

Often adults taking prescription medicines also use botanical products or high-dose vitamins, or both, frequently without the knowledge of their health-care provider. Areas of concern with botanical products are the lack of standardization and quality control and the contamination of the products with dangerous substances. Even botanicals that are considered reasonably safe should sometimes be avoided. The drug interaction most often cited for the botanicals discussed in the chapter was with anticoagulants.

Wellness Tips 16–1

- If a person is interested in botanical or ergogenic products, several steps are necessary to minimize risks:
  1. Accumulate as much information as possible. Investigate the credibility of the source of the information.
  2. Be careful. Proceed slowly. Use single-ingredient supplements in preference to mixtures. Use for a short time only.
  3. Discuss the program with the primary care provider.
  4. Do not use in infants, children, pregnant women, or the elderly.
  5. Be a minimalist. These substances are taken with the expectation of medicinal results. They are not harmless because they are "natural."

Although not as systematically monitored as prescription and over-the-counter drugs, adverse effects from botanical products are investigated, usually when the client becomes acutely ill after consuming a product. If a person wishes to use botanical products, he or she should avoid products with known toxic effects, investigate suppliers' reputations, take only the recommended dose and only for several weeks, and be as alert for side effects as one would be with prescription or over-the-counter medications. The health-care provider should be consulted *before* infants, children, pregnant women, and the elderly are given botanical products (Wellness Tips 16–1).

Ergogenic aids are supplements intended to improve athletic performance. As with botanical products, the data supporting the use of many of the aids are sparse, and long-term studies have yet to be performed. The results of many laboratory studies have not been confirmed by athletes in competition. Just because an item is available over the counter does not mean it is safe. Although there is agreement that athletes require additional protein, it can be obtained through a balanced diet that includes sufficient energy for their needs.

The greatest danger is the taking of androgenic anabolic steroids because of their severe and permanent side effects, especially in children and adolescents. Health-care providers should educate themselves about botanical products and ergogenic aids, query clients about their use of these supplements, and assist clients in making wise decisions by discussing their risks and benefits.

Case Study 16–1

Ms. P is a 25-year-old Caucasian woman who is attending a well-baby clinic. Her infant is 2 months old, in good health, and achieving satisfactory weight gain on breast milk. Ms. P, her husband, and two other children recently moved to this area, and her previous health-care providers are unavailable to her.

During her intake interview she relates that, aside from relations with her mother-in-law who now resides within a few miles of Mr. and Ms. P, the family is adjusting well. Ms. P becomes teary-eyed when describing the situation. The mother-in-law offers multiple suggestions that Ms. P is uncomfortable about implementing, but she is beginning to run out of excuses. Of greatest concern is the mother-in-law's insistence that the baby be given "mint tea" to settle its stomach when it regurgitates. Thus far, Ms. P has resisted the suggestion, but Mr. P is losing patience with her "stubbornness" since his mother successfully raised 11 children, and "what's a little tea going to hurt?"

Nursing Care Plan

Subjective Data	Verbalized uncertainty about choices
	Verbalized feelings of distress about situation
	Delayed decision making and implementation
Objective Data	Visibly upset and teary-eyed discussing her plight
Nursing Diagnosis	NANDA: Decisional Conflict (North American Nursing Diagnosis Association, 1999, with permission.) concerning infant care practices
	Related to conflicting advice from tradition-based mother-in-law and health-care providers

Nursing Care Plan *(Continued)*

Desired Outcomes Evaluation Criteria	Nursing Actions/ Interventions	Rationale
NOC: Decision Making (Johnson, Maas, and Moorhead, 2000, with permission.)	NIC: Decision Making Support (McCloskey and Bulechek, 2000, with permission.)	
Identifies relevant information	Provide or reinforce information about infant feeding.	American Academy of Pediatrics recommends breast-feeding without supplements of any kind. Regurgitation is very common until 6 months of age and does not indicate pathology that needs treatment.
Recognizes contradiction with others' desires	Help client formulate her reasons to explain to husband and mother-in-law.	Regular tea decreases iron absorption. "Mint" tea, especially from homegrown leaves, has been toxic to infants.
	Role-play the encounter if the client wishes.	Practice stating one's position and counterarguments can help a person maintain focus and composure in the actual situation.
Acknowledges social context of the situation	Assist client to identify persons whose opinions the mother-in-law would respect to encourage collaborative efforts to benefit the child.	Expanding the context to acknowledge all the adults involved are attempting to provide the best care they can for the infant may transform the situation beyond a battle of wills.
	Support client as she tries to maintain her role as primary caregiver of the infant.	Reinforce the fact that she has made good decisions regarding her older children.

Critical Thinking Questions

1. Identify potential compromises that might be made in this situation.
2. How do you visualize the mother-in-law? Does that image affect how you would approach this situation?
3. Devise a Plan B for the possibility that the sample Nursing Care Plan is not successful.

 # Study Aids

Subjects	Internet Sites
Botanical Remedies	http://www.herbalgram.org
	http://www.herbal-ahp.org
	http://www.libraries.uc.edu/lloyd
	http://www.herbs.org
	http://www.cpmcnet.columbia.edu/dept/rosenthal
	http://www.healthy.net/herbalists
	http://www.nnlm.nlm.nih.gov/pnr/uwmhg
	http://www.ars-grin.gov/duke
	http://www.wam.umd.edu/~mct/Plants/herbalism.html
	http://www.usda.gov/fnic/IBIDS
	http://www.rxnews.com
	http://www.asahq.org/PublicEducation/herbal.html
	http://www.ard-grin.gov/nfrisb
Sports Medicine	http://www.sportsci.org
	http://www.usoc.org/inside/in_1_3_7_3.html
	http://www.physsportsmed.com
	http://www.gssiweb.com

Continued on next page

Study Aids (continued)

Subjects	Internet Sites
Dietary Supplements	http://odp.od.nih.gov/ods/
	http://vm/cfsan.fda.gov/~dms/
	http://www.fda.gov/bbs/topics/FACTSHEETS/fs_diet1.html
	http://foodnet.fic.ca/industry/appii.html
	http://vm.cfsan.fda.gov/~dms/ds-oview.html
Quality Assurance	http://www.consumerlab.com
	http://www.rnlist.com
	http://usp.org
	http://www.quackwatch.com
	http://www.ftc.gov/opa/1999/9906/opcureall.htm
Food and Drug Administration	http://www.fda.gov/medwatch/report/hcp.htm
(for health-care providers and consumers to report adverse effects to drugs, medical devices, medical foods, and dietary supplements)	http://www.fda.gov/medwatch/report/consumer/consumer.htm

Chapter Review

1. Which of the following statements is true of botanical medicines?
   a. One brand is as good as another, since manufacturing is regulated by the government.
   b. These naturally occurring substances are inherently safer than prescription medicines.
   c. Many people are willing to try them to improve their health status.
   d. The rules governing their production and marketing are the same as for over-the-counter medications.

2. For which of the following clients would the nurse follow up immediately if the child's mother relates that she gives the child herbal tea?
   a. A 2-month-old
   b. An 18-month-old
   c. A 3-year-old
   d. A 4-year-old

3. If a person wishes to drink herbal tea, which of the following products would be the safest to consume?
   a. Tea from plants grown at home
   b. Tea sold in a grocery store with a food nutrition label
   c. Tea purchased in bulk from a health food store
   d. Tea ordered over the Internet

4. Which class of medications is likely to interact with the most botanicals discussed in the chapter?
   a. Barbiturates
   b. Anticoagulants
   c. Hormones
   d. Vitamins

5. For which of the following items is there most agreement that athletes require increased amounts compared with more sedentary individuals?
   a. Protein
   b. Creatine
   c. Glycerol
   d. Anabolic steroids

Clinical Analysis

1. Maria G. is pregnant with her third child. She tells the clinic nurse that she takes some herbal products "to keep my strength up and get me through the day." Which of the following products would raise the greatest concern for the nurse?
   a. Natural vitamin C
   b. Ginger
   c. St. John's wort
   d. Valerian

2. Which of the following responses by the nurse would be most helpful to maintaining a positive relationship with Maria?
   a. "Who told you to take herbal medicines?"
   b. "Let me write those herbs down on your chart. How do you spell them?"
   c. "Does your doctor know you are taking these herbs?"
   d. "It's not just herbs. Most medicines should be avoided in pregnancy to be on the safe side."

3. Theresa is a freshman member of a college golf team. After fainting on the 16th hole, she was taken to the health clinic for treatment. The admission assessment by the nurse should include height, weight, blood pressure, and
   a. Food preferences
   b. Theresa's knowledge of the Food Guide Pyramid
   c. History of recent travel
   d. Use of botanical products and supplements

Bibliography

American Dietetic Association: Position on functional foods. J Am Diet Assoc 99:1278, 1999.

American Society of Anesthesiologists. Anesthesiologists warn: If you're taking herbal products, tell your doctor before surgery. Press release 5/26/99. Accessed 5/16/2000 at http://www.asahq.org/PublicEducation/herbal.html

American Society of Anesthesiologists: What you should know about your patients' use of herbal medicines. Professional Information dated 3/21/2000. Accessed 5/16/2000 at http://www.asahq.org/ProfInfo/herb/herbbro.html

Angell, M, and Kassirer, JP: Drs. Angell and Kassirer reply [letter]. N Engl J Med 340:566, 1999.

Applegate, E: Effective nutritional ergogenic aids. Int J Sport Nutr 9:229, 1999.

Baker, J: Be smart, beware. AARP Bulletin, May 1999, 14.

Bakerink, JA, et al.: Multiple organ failure after ingestion of pennyroyal oil from herbal tea in two infants. Pediatrics 98:944, 1996.

Barrett, B, Kiefer, D, and Rabago, D: Assessing the risks and benefits of herbal medicine: An overview of scientific evidence. Altern Ther Health Med 5:40, 1999.

Batchelor, WB, Heathcote, J, and Wanless, IR: Chaparral-induced hepatic injury. Am J Gastroenterol 90:831, 1995.

Beigel, Y, Ostfeld, I, and Schoenfeld, N: A leading question. N Engl J Med 339:827, 1998.

Berthold, HK, Sudhop, T, and von Bergmann, K: Effect of a garlic oil preparation on serum lipoproteins and cholesterol metabolism: A randomized controlled trial. JAMA 279:1900, 1998.

Blue, JG, and Lombardo, JA: Steroids and steroid-like compounds. Clinics in Sports Medicine 18:667, 1999.

Borins, M: The dangers of using herbs. Postgraduate Medicine 104:91, 1998.

Bove, GM: Acute neuropathy after exposure to sun in a patient treated with St. John's wort. Lancet 352:1121, 1998.

Brinkeborn, RM, Shah, DV, and Degenring, FH: Echinaforce and other Echinacea fresh plant preparations in the treatment of the common cold. A randomized, placebo controlled, double-blind clinical trial. Phytomedicine 6:1, 1999.

Brody, JE: Americans gamble on herbs as medicine. NY Times, February 9, 1999.

Brustbauer, R, and Wenisch, C: [Bradycardiac atrial fibrillation after consuming herbal tea] Eng abst. Dtsch Med Wochenschr 122:930, 1997.

Butterfield, G: Ergogenic aids: Evaluating sport nutrition products. Int J Sport Nutr 6:191, 1996.

Capriotti, T: Exploring the "herbal jungle." MedSurg Nursing 8:53, 1999.

Castell, LM, and Newsholme, EA: Glutamine and the effects of exhaustive exercise on the immune response. Can J Physiol Pharmacol 76:524, 1998.

Center for Food Safety and Applied Nutrition. Overview of Dietary Supplements. U.S. Food and Drug Administration, May 1997, Updated April 1999. Accessed 8/2/1999 at http://vm.cfsan.fda.gov/~dms/ds-oview.html

Centers for Disease Control: Adult lead poisoning from an Asian remedy for menstrual cramps—Connecticut, 1997. MMWR 48:27, 1999. Accessed 8/11/1999 at http://www.cdc.gov/epo/mmwr/preview/mmwrhtml/00056277.htm

Centers for Disease Control: Adverse events associated with ephedrine-containing products—Texas, December 1993–September 1995. MMWR 45:689, 1996. Accessed 5/15/2000 at http://www.cdc.gov/epo/mmwr/preview/mmwrhtml.00043335.htm

Centers for Disease Control: Anticholinergic poisoning associated with an herbal tea—New York City, 1994. MMWR 44:193, 1995. Accessed 9/28/1999 at http://www.cdc.gov/epo/mmwr/preview/mmwrhtml/00022295.htm

Centers for Disease Control: Jin Bu Huan toxicity in adults—Los Angeles, 1993. MMWR 42:920, 1993a. Accessed at http://www.cdc.gov/epo/mmwr/preview/mmwrhtml/00022295.htm

Centers for Disease Control: Jin Bu Huan toxicity in children—Colorado, 1993. MMWR 42:633, 1993b. Accessed 10/21/1999 at http://www.cdc.gov/epo/mmwr/preview/mmwrhtml/00021421.htm

Chung, HS, et al.: Ginkgo biloba extract increases ocular blood flow velocity. J Ocul Pharmacol Ther 15:233, 1999.

Cirigliano, M, and Sun, A: Advising patients about herbal therapies [letter]. JAMA 280, 1565, 1998.

Cui, J, et al.: What do commercial ginseng preparations contain? [letter]. Lancet 344:134, 1994.

Cupp, MJ: Herbal remedies: adverse effects and drug interactions. Am Fam Physician 59:1239, 1999.

Echinacea. Rxlist, 1999. Accessed 10/22/99 at http:///www.rxlist.com/cgi/alt/echinacea

Eisenberg, DM, et al.: Trends in alternative medicine use in the United States, 1990–1997. JAMA 280:1569, 1998.

Eliason, BC, et al.: Dietary supplement users: Demographics, product use, and medical system interaction. J Am Board Fam Pract 10:265, 1997.

Espinoza, EO, Mann, M-J, and Bleasdell, B: Arsenic and mercury in traditional Chinese herbal balls [letter]. N Engl J Med 333:803, 1995.

Food Institute of Canada. Appendix II: Dietary Supplement and Health Education Act of 1994, undated. Accessed 10/10/1999 at http://foodnet.fic.ca/industry/appii.html

Garges, HP, Varia, I, and Doraiswamy, PM: Cardiac complications and delirium associated with valerian root withdrawal [letter]. JAMA 280:1566, 1998.

Glisson, J, Crawford, R, and Street, S: Review, critique, and guidelines for the use of herbs and homeopathy. Nurs Pract 23:44, 1999.

Gordon, DW, et al.: Chaparral ingestion. JAMA 273:489, 1995.

Grimm, W, and Muller, HH: A randomized controlled trial of the effect of fluid extract of Echinacea purpurea on the incidence and severity of colds and respiratory infections. Am J Med 106:138, 999.

Gruber, AJ, and Pope, HG: Ephedrine abuse among 36 female weightlifters. Am J Addict 7:256, 1998.

Gruenwald, J (ed): Physicians Desk Reference for Herbal Medicines. Medical Economics, Oradell, NJ, 1998.

Harrer, G, et al.: Comparison of equivalence between St. John's wort extract LoHyp-57 and fluoxetine. Arzneimittelforschung 49:289, 1999.

Houghton, PJ: The scientific basis for the reputed activity of valerian. J Pharm Pharmacol 51:505, 1999.

Johnson, M, Maas, M, and Moorhead, S: Nursing Outcomes Classification (NOC), ed 2. Mosby, Philadelphia, 2000.

Jones, TK, and Lawson, BM: Profound neonatal congestive heart failure caused by maternal consumption of blue cohosh herbal medication. J Pediatr 132:550, 1998.

Josey, ES, and Tackett, RL: St. John's wort: A new alternative for depression? Int J Clin Pharmacol Ther 37:111, 1999.

Juhn, MS, and Tarnopolsky, M: Oral creatine supplementation and athletic performance: A critical review. Clin J Sport Med 8:286, 1998a.

Juhn, MS, and Tarnopolsky, M: Potential side effects of oral creatine supplementation: A critical review. Clin J Sport Med 8:298, 1998b.

Kingsbury, KJ, Kay, L, and Hjelm, M: Contrasting plasma free amino acid patterns in elite athletes: Association with fatigue and infection. Br J Sports Med 32:25, 1998.

Klepser, TB, and Klepser, ME: Unsafe and potentially safe herbal therapies. Am J Health-Syst Pharm 56:125, 1999.

Ko, RJ: Adulterants in Asian patent medicines. N Engl J Med 339:847, 1998.

Koscielny, J, et al.: The antiatherosclerotic effect of Allium sativum. Atherosclerosis 144:237, 1999.

Kreider, RB: Dietary supplements and the promotion of muscle growth with resistance exercise. Sports Med 27:97, 1999.

Le Bars, PL, et al.: A placebo-controlled, double-blind, randomized trial of an extract of Ginkgo biloba for dementia. JAMA 278:1327, 1997.

Levin, S: Investigating the cause of muscle cramps. The Physician and Sportsmedicine 21:111, 1993.

Lumpkin, MM, and Alpert, S: FDA Public Health Advisory Feb. 10, 2000. Accessed 1/5/2001 at http://www.fda.gov/cder/drug/advisory /stjwort.htm

McCloskey, JC, and Bulechek, GM: Nursing Interventions Classification (NIC), 3 ed. Mosby, Philadelphia, 2000.

McNaughton, L, Dalton, B, and Palmer, G: Sodium bicarbonate can be used as an ergogenic aid in high intensity, competitive cycle ergometry of 1 h duration. Eur J Appl Physiol 80:64, 1999.

Mero, A: Leucine supplementation and intensive training. Sports Med 27:347, 1999.

Metzl, JD: Strength training and nutritional supplement use in adolescents. Curr Opin Pediatr 11:292, 1999.

Micklefield, GH, et al.: Effects of ginger on gastroduodenal motility. Int J Clin Pharmacol Ther 37:341, 1999.

Miller, LG: Herbal medicinals. Arch Intern Med 158:2200, 1998.

Mujika, I, and Padilla, S: Creatine supplementation as an ergogenic aid for sports performance in highly trained athletes: A critical review. Int J Sports Med 18:491, 1997.

North American Nursing Diagnosis Association: Nursing Diagnoses: Definitions and Classification 1999–2000, North American Nursing Diagnosis Association, Philadelphia, 1999.

Nursing 2000 Drug Handbook. Springhouse Corporation, Springhouse, PA, 2000.

O'Hara, MA, et al.: A review of 12 commonly used medicinal herbs. Arch Fam Med 7:523, 1998.

Omaye, ST: Safety facets of antioxidant supplements. Top Clin Nutr 14:26, 1998.

Perez-Pimiento, AJ, et al.: Anaphylactic reaction to young garlic. Allergy 54:626, 1999.

Philipp, M, Kohnen, R, and Hiller, K: Hypericum extract versus imipramine of placebo in patients with moderate depression: Randomised multicentre study of treatment for eight weeks. Brit J Med 319:1534, 1999. Accessed 5/16/2000 at http://www.bmj.com/cgi/reprint /319/7224/1534.pdf

Rose, KD, et al.: Spontaneous spinal epidural hematoma with associated platelet dysfunction from excessive garlic ingestion: A case report. Neurosurgery 26:280, 1990.

Ruschitzka, F, et al: Acute heart transplant rejection due to Saint John's wort. Lancet 355:548, 2000.

Schnirring, L: Androstenedione et al.: Nonprescription steroids. The Physician and Sportsmedicine 26:15, 1998.

Sheehan, DM: Herbal medicines, phytoestrogens and toxicity: Risk:benefit considerations. Proc Soc Exp Biol Med 217:379, 1998.

Sheikh, NM, Philen, RM, and Love, L: Chaparral-associated hepatotoxicity. Arch Intern Med 157:913, 1997.

Slifman, NR, et al.: Contamination of botanical dietary supplements by Digitalis lanata. N Engl J Med 339:806, 1998.

Sperl, W, et al.: Reversible hepatic veno-occlusive disease in an infant after consumption of pyrrolizidine-containing herbal tea. Eur J Pediatr 154:112, 1995.

Stamford, B: Muscle cramps. The Physician and Sportsmedicine 21:115, 1993.

Stashower, ME, and Torres, RZ: Chaparral and liver toxicity [letter]. JAMA 274:871, 1995.

United States Olympic Committee: Drug Control Education. Inside the USOC, updated May 1997. Accessed 10/19/1999 at http://www.usoc.org/inside/in_1_3_7_3.html

United States Olympic Committee Drug Control Administration: USOC Guide to Prohibited Substances and Methods. November 17, 1999. Accessed 5/15/2000 at http://www.usoc.org/inside/drugadmin.html

Vimala, S, Norhanom, AW, Yadav, M: Anti-tumour promoter activity in Malaysian ginger rhizobia used in traditional medicine. Br J Cancer 80:110, 1999.

Visalyaputra, S, et al.: The efficacy of ginger root in the prevention of postoperative nausea and vomiting after outpatient gynecological laparoscopy. Anesthesia 53:506, 1998.

Vogler, BK, Pittler, MH, and Ernst, E: Feverfew as preventive treatment for migraine: A systematic review. Cephalalgia 18:704, 1998.

Wagner, DR: Hyperhydrating with glycerol: Implications for athletic performance. J Am Diet Assoc 99:207, 1999.

Williams, NH, and Branch, JD: Creatine supplementation and exercise performance: An update. J Am Coll Nutr 17:216, 1998.

Wilt, TJ, et al.: Saw palmetto extracts for treatment of benign prostatic hyperplasia: A systematic review. JAMA 280:1604, 1998.

Yager, J, Siegfreid, SL, and DiMatteo, TL: Use of alternative remedies by psychiatric patients: Illustrative vignettes and a discussion of the issues. Am J Psychiatry 156:1432, 1999.

Yue, Q-Y, Bergquist, C, and Gerden, B: Safety of St John's wort [letter]. Lancet 355:575, 2000.

Unit **III**
Clinical Nutrition

CHAPTER 17

Food, Nutrient, and Drug Interactions

LEARNING OBJECTIVES
After completing this chapter, the student should be able to:

1. Explain the importance of proper scheduling of medications in relation to food intake.
2. Identify two groups of clients likely to experience food–drug interactions.
3. Recognize certain food and drug interactions discussed in the text.
4. Describe four ways in which nutrients and drugs can interact and give an example of each.
5. Discuss one potentially life-threatening food–drug interaction and design nursing interventions to avoid this possibility.
6. Name several drug–nutrient interactions that affect water balance in the body.

This chapter explains and gives examples of the different ways in which drugs interact with foods (including beverages), nutrients (including nutrient formulas and supplements), and the non-nutrient components of foods. An interaction is the process of one substance affecting another. The food or nutrient can enhance the action of a drug or inhibit it. Similarly, a drug can facilitate the body's use of nutrients or impede it. In no sense is the discussion exhaustive. The drugs discussed here illustrate the broad range of interactions and do not necessarily reflect the preferred treatment for the conditions mentioned. In all cases, pharmaceutical references should be consulted when administering medications.

A drug is a substance, other than a food, that is intended to affect a structure or function of the body. As used in this text, the term drug includes alcohol and both prescription and over-the-counter drugs. As is the usual practice in medical literature, the **generic names** of drugs are used here.

The Effects of Drugs on Nutritional Status

Any person who takes a drug risks potentially harmful effects from food and drug interactions. Nutritional status can be affected because these interactions might alter (1) food intake, (2) the absorption of nutrients or drugs, (3) the metabolism of nutrients or drugs, or (4) the excretion of nutrients or drugs. Some known interactions are considered clinically desirable because they help control a disease process. For example, by restricting a client's dietary vitamin K, the effect of warfarin, an anticoagulant, is prolonged. Many effects that result from food and drug interactions are undesirable. These include nutritional deficiencies, growth retardation in children, loss of disease control, and acute toxic reactions. Some individuals, especially the elderly, are at higher risk than others for suffering unwanted effects.

Identifying Clients at High Risk

Persons at highest risk for food and drug interactions are those who (1) take many drugs, including alcohol; (2) require long-term drug therapy; or (3) have poor or marginal nutrition. These and other risk-increasing factors are listed in Clinical Application 17–1. The elderly are particularly vulnerable because they are more likely to have several of the risk factors mentioned. Persons 65 years of age and older make up about 12 percent of the population but take approximately 30 percent of all prescribed and over-the-counter (OTC) medications (Smith, 1995).

Over one-third of 311 retirement community residents reported using alcohol with a high-risk medication. Half the residents who reported some alcohol intake also took antihypertensive drugs, perhaps without knowing that alcohol alone exacerbates hypertension. Over one-quarter of these residents used aspirin, and one-fifth took other nonsteroidal anti-inflammatory drugs (NSAIDs) that, taken with alcohol, can cause increased bleeding time and gastric inflammation and bleeding (Adams, 1995). Individuals receiving these medications are likely to be on long-term regimens, further increasing the risk of adverse effects (Fig. 17–1). The elderly are also more prone to food–drug interactions as a result of self-medication, noncompliance with prescribed regimens, and changes in their needs associated with aging. Clinical Application 17–2 lists factors that should trigger investigation of the client's risk of drug-nutrient interactions.

Minimizing Food and Drug Interactions

Known adverse outcomes of food and drug interactions can be offset by changes in drug dosage, diet, or both. Because drugs often increase or

Factors Increasing the Risk of Drug–Nutrient Interactions

The risk of a drug-nutrient interaction is increased if a client:

- *Is malnourished*
- *Consumes alcohol*
- *Takes a high-potency vitamin or mineral supplement*
- *Is receiving many drugs*

or if the client's drugs:

- *Are given with meals*
- *Are instilled into a feeding tube*
- *Are prescribed long-term to control chronic disease*
- *Are known to cause malabsorption or have antinutrient effects*

In any of the above situations,

- *a careful search of pharmacology literature,*
- *a thorough assessment, and*
- *an ongoing effort to monitor the client's status are appropriate.*

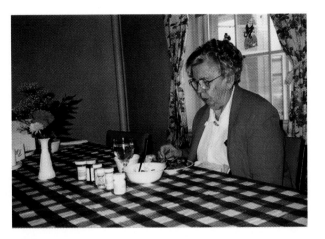

Figure 17–1:
This woman has several risk factors for drug–nutrient interactions. She is elderly, is on a multiple drug regimen, and takes some of her medications with a meal.

decrease the absorption of nutrients, it may be necessary to change (1) the route of administration, (2) the dose of a drug, (3) the time interval between doses, and/or (4) whether or not the drug is administered with food. For example, therapeutic drug levels may not be achieved or may take longer to build up in the body if less of the drug is absorbed because of an interaction with food. This could prolong a disease or prevent its cure. Dosage adjustments often minimize such effects.

Certain foods or nutrients (including supplements) may be (1) added to the diet, (2) deleted from the diet, or (3) required in increased or reduced amounts to counterbalance adverse nutrient-drug interactions. For example, protein inhibits the absorption of phenytoin, an anticonvulsant drug, whereas carbohydrate increases its absorption. Depending on the desired therapeutic effect, dietary intake of protein and/or carbohydrate may be modified. Food and drug interactions can be complex, especially if the client is on a multiple-drug regimen or is at high risk for other reasons. Health care professionals need a sound knowledge of potential food and drug interactions and the ability to apply their knowledge in practice. Physicians, dietitians, pharmacists, and nurses share responsibility for being aware of and for preventing or controlling such interactions

Screening Clients at Risk of Drug–Nutrient Interactions

Further nutritional assessment may be in order if the client:

1. Reports a recent weight change
2. Abuses alcohol
3. Consumes a modified diet including one characterized by significant changes in protein content
4. Takes medication with meals
5. Has a worsening of signs and symptoms of the disease
6. Displays laboratory values indicating nutrient depletion
7. Receives medications known to interfere with nutrition

(Lasswell, et al., 1995). The clinical pharmacist can be a valuable ally of the nurse when scheduling medications for optimal effect. Likewise, nurses may ask a clinical dietitian to assess a client's risk for food–drug interactions. Because of the multitude of medications available and the complexity of potential interactions, most health care organizations use computer-generated client profiles that include all the medications the client is to receive and thereby can identify interactions. A good reference library on the clinical unit also helps provide information.

The Effects of Drugs on Foods and Nutrients

Drugs can (1) affect food intake, (2) alter the absorption of nutrients through both luminal and mucosal effects, (3) modify the metabolism of nutrients, and (4) increase or decrease the excretion of certain nutrients.

The Effects of Drugs on Food Intake

Even before food is ingested, drugs can affect food intake. Several drugs increase or decrease appetite, interfere with the senses of taste and smell, or cause gastric irritation. Food is sometimes used to temper these and other side effects of drugs.

Decreased Appetite

Central nervous system stimulants, including dextroamphetamine and methylphenidate, both used in the treatment of narcolepsy or the management of attention deficit disorder (ADD), have the effect of depressing the desire for food. One of the side effects of these stimulants in children is slowed growth. Dextroamphetamine is more likely to interfere with growth than is methylphenidate. Antineoplastic drugs (agents that prevent the development, growth, or proliferation of malignant cells) are well known for causing a loss of appetite (**anorexia**). Other side effects, including severe nausea, vomiting, and **stomatitis**, exacerbate anorexia. Examples of such antineoplastic drugs are bleomycin, plicamycin, and vincristine. Poor appetite can also result from drugs that cause a dry mouth. Many antihistamines, including brompheniramine and diphenhydramine, decrease saliva output, thereby causing decreased appetite. Bulk-forming laxatives containing psyllium may reduce appetite because of a feeling of abdominal fullness.

When assessing a client with a weight-loss history or one taking drugs known to cause food and drug interactions, nurses should review the client's drug regimen. Both physician-prescribed and self-prescribed drugs and nutritional supplements are pertinent to include in a nutritional assessment.

Increased Appetite

Some antidepressants, such as doxepin, may promote appetite and lead to marked weight gain. Another such drug, bupropion, can either increase or decrease appetite. Medroxyprogesterone, a female hormone used as an oral contraceptive and in cyclic hormone therapy after menopause, also increases appetite. This hormone occurs naturally in the second half of the menstrual cycle and in pregnancy (to support the growth requirements of the mother and fetus). To minimize the effect of increased appetite, if weight gain is not desired, several nursing interventions might be appropriate. Instructing the client to increase the fiber content of the diet, especially with fruits and vegetables, and encouraging the client to drink 6 to 8 glasses of water daily, to eat slowly, and to chew food thoroughly are strategies that may prove helpful.

Changes in Taste or Smell

The senses of taste and smell influence how one responds to foods. Some drugs alter the perception of these senses, making foods and beverages taste bitter, metallic, or unpleasant. Although this usually leads to a decreased appetite, some individuals try to rid themselves of the sensation by eating constantly. Acetylsalicylic acid (ASA), more commonly known as aspirin, is a drug used to control pain or to reduce fever. It also is taken in small daily doses to decrease the risk of heart attacks. One gram of aspirin, about three adult-dose tablets, increases the taste perception of bitterness. An anti-infective reserved for tuberculosis and other serious infections, streptomycin, is excreted in the saliva. One result is a metallic or bitter taste, even when the drug is administered by intramuscular injection.

Lithium carbonate, an antimanic drug, causes a metallic taste sensation. Other common side effects of this drug related to nutritional intake are dry mouth, anorexia, nausea, vomiting, and diarrhea. Lithium carbonate also has serious interactions with a person's fluid and electrolyte balance (discussed later).

Penicillamine, a drug given for rheumatoid arthritis and for **Wilson's disease**, in which a genetic defect prevents excretion of copper, causes a loss of taste and smell. The drug binds with copper so that it can be excreted by the kidney. The loss of taste and smell is caused by zinc deficiency because penicillamine also binds with zinc, causing its excretion. The angiotensin-converting enzyme (ACE) inhibitors, such as captopril, used to treat hypertension cause a loss of taste perception. A postulated mechanism of action is decreased salivary magnesium concentration (Utermohlen, 1999). Nursing interventions that may help a client with taste changes include providing good oral hygiene before meals and avoiding bitter foods in favor of the other taste sensations—sweet, sour, or salty.

Gastric Irritation

Drugs that cause gastric irritation are often taken with food to reduce this side effect. Aspirin can cause gastric bleeding and over time can lead to

anemia. Taking aspirin with food, milk, crackers, or a full glass of water reduces the likelihood of stomach irritation. Other NSAIDs and potassium chloride are also associated with gastric irritation.

The Effects of Drugs on Nutrient Absorption

Drugs can affect the absorption of nutrients in several ways. Drug-induced alterations in absorption are categorized according to two general mechanisms of action: luminal effects or mucosal effects.

Luminal Effects

Drug-induced changes within the intestine that affect the absorption of nutrients or drugs without altering the intestine itself are called **luminal effects**. These drug-induced changes may affect peristalsis, pH, or the formation of complexes.

PERISTALSIS Laxatives may interfere with the absorption of nutrients and other drugs because they stimulate peristalsis and thus cause a rapid transit time of intestinal contents. Long-term use may result in physical dependence and electrolyte imbalances. Two laxatives, bisacodyl and phenolphthalein (common ingredients in over-the-counter preparations), interfere with the uptake of glucose, water, calcium, sodium, and potassium by the cells.

A relatively short period of malabsorption with diarrhea may interfere with the absorption of vitamin K. This interference in turn enhances the activity of warfarin, especially if the person's intake of green vegetables has been sparse. Clients taking warfarin who experience diarrhea or decreased food intake should have their prothrombin times or INRs (International Normalized Ratios) monitored more frequently than usual and warfarin dosages adjusted accordingly (Smith, Aljazairi, and Fuller, 1999).

Other drugs may slow peristalsis and thus cause a slow transit time. The long-term use of either docusate sodium, a stool softener, or chlorpromazine, an antipsychotic drug, results in the increased absorption of cholesterol, an undesirable side effect in most clients.

CHANGES IN pH The absorption of weakly acidic drugs takes place in the stomach, whereas the absorption of neutral and alkaline drugs takes place in the small intestine. Drug-induced changes in the pH of these sites influence the absorption of both nutrients and drugs. For example, an acid pH is necessary for folic acid absorption. It is also required for intrinsic factor to combine with vitamin B_{12} (extrinsic factor) for the absorption of vitamin B_{12}. Because long-term antacid or potassium chloride therapy neutralizes gastric acidity, the result is a decrease in the absorption of thiamin, folic acid, and vitamin B_{12}. The histamine H_2 receptor antagonists, such as cimetidine, and the gastric acid-pump inhibitor omeprazole also decrease vitamin B_{12} absorption because of altered gastric pH (Utermohlen, 1999). Antacids and potassium also decrease the absorption of iron because an acid medium is necessary to convert ferric iron (Fe^{3+}) to ferrous iron ($2+$), the more absorbable form.

FORMATION OF COMPLEXES Sometimes, foods or nutrients bind with or form complexes with drugs. This combining can increase, decrease, or prevent the absorption of one or the other.

Cholestyramine, a lipid-lowering agent, binds with bile salts, which increases the excretion of cholesterol. Unfortunately, it may also bind with the fat-soluble vitamins A, D, E, and K. These vitamins are then excreted along with the cholesterol. Because vitamin K is not stored in the body in significant amounts, cholestyramine therapy can lead to a deficiency of prothrombin and result in hemorrhage. However, water-soluble forms of these vitamins are available for patients who need them. Cholestyramine also interferes with the absorption of folic acid, vitamin B_{12}, calcium, and iron, necessitating vigilant monitoring of the client's nutritional status. Mineral oil, a lubricant, is sometimes used as a laxative. The fat-soluble vitamins dissolve in the indigestible oil and are excreted as are calcium and phosphorus. Therefore, taking mineral oil on a long-term, daily basis is undesirable. In addition, children and elderly adults with relaxed cardiac sphincters are at risk for aspiration pneumonia if they regurgitate the mineral oil. These untoward side effects as well as recommended dietary interventions (see Chapter 22) should be taught to clients seeking advice regarding treatment of constipation.

Mucosal Effects

The luminal effects do not affect the tissues or organs. In contrast, **mucosal effects** are drug-induced changes that affect the absorption of nutrients or drugs by damaging or altering tissue structures. Mucosal effects include decreased digestive enzymes, damaged intestinal mucosa, and inhibited transport mechanisms.

DECREASED DIGESTIVE ENZYMES Hundreds of enzymes are involved in digestion. Many drugs, including alcohol, can destroy the structural integrity of digestive organs by damaging tissues. This usually causes decreased enzyme production, resulting in poor nutrient absorption. Long-term alcohol consumption damages the pancreas, decreasing enzyme production. Thus the breakdown of amino acids and fats, chiefly governed by the action of pancreatic enzymes, is slowed or insufficiently completed. The result is reduced or poor absorption of amino acids and fats.

DAMAGED INTESTINAL MUCOSA A number of drugs contribute to the malabsorption of other drugs by their damaging effect on the intestinal mucosa. Some drugs produce general malabsorption, and other drugs are more specific and decrease the absorption of only certain nutrients. Alcohol abuse causes several changes in the intestinal mucosa that lead to the malabsorption of many nutrients. Most commonly affected are thiamin and magnesium, but folic acid, niacin, and pyridoxine also may be malabsorbed.

Because neomycin, an anti-infective agent, inhibits protein synthesis in bacteria, it is sometimes used to reduce the bacterial count in the bowel before intestinal surgery. Changes produced in the intestinal mucosa by neomycin lead to the decreased absorption of fat; vitamins A, D, and K; folic acid; and vitamin B_{12}. This malabsorption is not likely to cause problems when the drug is used short-term.

Gastrointestinal tract cells, because of their short life and rapid turnover, are killed by many antineoplastic drugs, such as methotrexate. Methotrexate administration therefore results in the malabsorption of vitamin B_{12}, folic acid, and calcium.

Colchicine, an antigout drug, may cause generalized malabsorption because it damages the intestinal mucosa. The consequences are inhibited absorption of vitamin B_{12}, folic acid, and calcium. In addition, colchicine reduces the absorption of fat, lactose, and carotene.

INHIBITED TRANSPORT MECHANISMS Several nutrients have to be helped across the intestinal membrane to the bloodstream. A number of drugs impair the absorption of nutrients through their effects on the transport mechanism. For example, the sedative/hypnotic drug glutethimide impairs the transport of calcium.

Phenytoin, a drug used to control epileptic seizures or heart rhythm irregularities, is structurally similar to folic acid. They compete for the same receptors in the small bowel (Berg, et al, 1995). Other antiepileptic drugs have the same potential, and major fetal malformations have been documented in 4 to 8 percent of epileptic mothers compared with 2 to 4 percent of mothers without epilepsy. Whether women taking antiepileptic drugs require a larger supplement of folic acid than other women is unknown, but spacing of doses of the antiepileptic drug throughout the day is recommended to control blood levels (Morrell, 1998). Reduced folic acid absorption also occurs with sulfasalazine, an anti-inflammatory agent used to treat ulcerative colitis. The decrease in absorption is caused by the inhibited transport of folic acid.

The Effects of Drugs on Nutrient Metabolism

Many drugs alter the metabolism of nutrients. Two commonly prescribed classes of drugs, corticosteroids and beta-adrenergic blocking agents, change the way the body uses energy nutrients. Drugs also disrupt vitamin metabolism through a variety of mechanisms.

Alteration of Energy Nutrient Metabolism

Beta-adrenergic blocking agents, such as atenolol and metoprolol, are given for hypertension and **angina pectoris**. These drugs decrease **lipolysis** and muscle **glycogenolysis**, thus decreasing the amount of fat and glucose available for energy. The mechanism by which protein is altered is unclear, but the end result of long-term treatment with beta-blockers may be increased body fat, decreased fat-free mass, and a resting energy expenditure reduction of 8 to 17 percent (Lamont, 1995).

Corticosteroids are hormones that are produced by the adrenal gland. Pharmaceutical doses of these drugs are given for their anti-inflammatory effects. The side effects of the drug are signs and symptoms like those of Cushing's syndrome, a disease that results from oversecretion of corticosteroids. The metabolism of all the energy nutrients is affected. Corticosteroids stimulate the conversion of fat and protein to glucose. Hyperglycemia results, or preexisting diabetes is worsened. Corticosteroids increase the catabolism of the matrix of the bone, inhibit the osteoblasts from building new bone, and prevent the liver from processing vitamin D. When this lack of vitamin D results in insufficient calcium absorption by the intestine, parathyroid hormone causes withdrawal of calcium from the bones and osteoporosis results. Similar protein wasting affects the skin and skeletal muscle, producing easy bruising and weakness. Corticosteroids also cause a redistribution of fat deposits to the trunk, the back of the neck, and the face so that the person eventually develops a "moon face" and/or a "buffalo hump."

Interference with Vitamin Metabolism

Although vitamins have specific and singular functions in the body, several mechanisms can interfere with their proper metabolism. The same vitamin may be affected by different drugs at various phases of its metabolism.

Anti-infective drugs destroy intestinal bacteria, which synthesize vitamin K (Conly and Stein, 1994). Sometimes buttermilk or yogurt with active bacterial cultures is effective in replacing the intestinal bacteria.

Table 17–1 Dietary Restrictions for Oral Anticoagulant Therapy

Avoid	One Serving Per Day, 1 Cup Raw or 1/2 Cup Cooked	Check with Prescriber If Large Increases or Decreases
Kale (except garnish)	Broccoli	Green vegetables
Parsley (except garnish)	Brussels sprouts	Garbanzo beans
Natto (Japanese)	Spinach	Lentils
	Turnip or other greens	Soybeans or soybean oil
		Liver
		Green tea

A group of enzymes called cytochrome P450 (CYP450), found in all body cells except red blood cells and skeletal muscle cells, helps metabolize fat-soluble vitamins, steroids, fatty acids, and other substances and helps detoxify drugs and environmental pollutants. Twelve genetically determined families of **cytochrome P450 enzymes** have been identified in humans. Three of these families are involved with most of the drug transformations carried out in the liver. Some antiepileptic drugs stimulate these enzymes and appear to be associated with vitamin K deficiency, which can lead to hemorrhagic diseases in the newborn. One recommendation is to provide a pregnant woman receiving antiepileptic drugs with a vitamin K supplement during the last month of pregnancy (Morrell, 1998).

The molecular structure of warfarin, an anticoagulant drug, resembles that of vitamin K. Warfarin achieves its therapeutic effect by "fooling" the liver into using it in place of vitamin K to manufacture prothrombin. Warfarin also interferes with the synthesis of clotting factors VII, IX, and X. Eating large amounts of foods high in vitamin K during anticoagulant therapy with warfarin decreases or may even negate the desired effect of the drug. Clients should not stop eating foods containing vitamin K, but they should avoid large variations in the amounts eaten. A problem might arise if they eat a lot of green leafy vegetables one day and then none for the following several days. Dry green tea leaves have as much vitamin K per gram as broccoli, cabbage, spinach, lettuce, Brussels sprouts, and turnip greens (Groff, Gropper, and Hunt, 1995). A case of interaction with warfarin was reported in a 44-year-old client who had been stabilized on the drug but who later drank one-half to one gallon of green tea per day (Taylor and Wilt, 1999). An additional side effect of warfarin therapy involves the function of vitamin K in bone metabolism. Clients receiving long-term warfarin therapy have been shown to have decreased bone mineral density (Sato et al., 1997). Table 17–1 summarizes instructions for clients taking warfarin products.

Methotrexate, an antineoplastic agent, is an antagonist of folic acid. It successfully destroys cancer cells because they too require folic acid for DNA replication. In the process, the efforts of normal body cells to divide are also impaired.

Both the antituberculosis drug isoniazid and the antiparkinson agent levodopa form a complex with vitamin B_6. The kidney then excretes this complex in the urine, rather than returning it to the bloodstream. Individuals most at risk for peripheral neuritis from vitamin B_6 deficiency are clients who are pregnant or elderly or who have diabetes, alcoholism, or uremia (Utermohlen, 1999). An additional consequence of vitamin B_6 deficiency is an inability to convert tryptophan to nicotinic acid, resulting in a niacin deficiency (Kelly et al., 1998). Supplemental pyridoxine may be added to a levodopa regimen to correct a vitamin B_6 deficiency, but this will decrease the effectiveness of levodopa.

Phenytoin, an anticonvulsant, interferes with the liver's processing of vitamin D. Clients receiving long-term therapy need an estimated 15 to 25 micrograms of vitamin D daily to prevent rickets or osteomalacia.

Effects of Drugs on Nutrient Excretion

Drugs usually cause excessive excretion, rather than retention, of nutrients. Drugs can act on the excretion of nutrients in four ways: they can (1) compete with nutrients for binding sites, (2) form chemical bonds with the nutrient, (3) deplete the nutrient supply in the body's tissues, and (4) interfere with the kidneys' reabsorption of the nutrient into the bloodstream.

Competition for Binding Sites

Many drugs circulate in the bloodstream attached to plasma proteins. These plasma proteins serve a similar function in relation to some nutrients. The plasma protein and its hitchhiker drug or nutrient form a large particle. Sometimes there are too few binding sites on the plasma proteins for all of the drug or nutrient. When that happens, excess drug or nutrient accumulates as free, small particles in the bloodstream. The kidney is likely to excrete these small particles rather than to restore them to the bloodstream. One common drug that interferes in this manner with a nutrient is acetylsalicylic acid, or aspirin. It displaces folic acid from its plasma protein. The kidney then excretes the folic acid in the urine.

A client with low levels of serum albumin as a result of malnutrition is at risk for drug toxicity with drugs that are usually highly bound to albumin. The drug that is bound to protein is inactive, whereas the unbound drug circulating in the blood is active and able to exert its intended therapeutic effect. Examples of drugs with an affinity to bind to protein are salicylates, warfarin, and thiopental (Yaffe and Sonawane, 1997). Figure 17–2 illustrates two results of the competition between drugs and foods or nutrients for protein binding sites.

Formation of Chemical Bonds

To combat heavy-metal poisoning, an antidote drug is administered that combines chemically with the metal. The drug plus the metal then is excreted harmlessly. As with many treatments, the drug is not specific and will combine with nutrients as well as the noxious heavy metal, such as lead or mercury. An example of this type of interaction involves penicillamine. It forms a stable bond with zinc, copper, iron, and other metals, causing excessive excretion and thus possibly leading to deficiencies.

Depletion of Nutrients in Tissues

As part of its overall catabolic effect, the anti-inflammatory glucocorticoid prednisone depletes tissues of ascorbic acid. The ascorbic acid accumu-

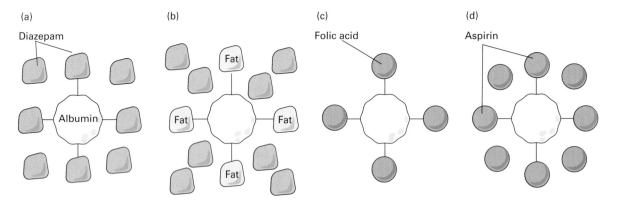

Figure 17–2:
In sketch (a), 4 molecules of diazepam are bound to the albumin molecule leaving the other 4 molecules of diazepam free to leave the bloodstream for the central nervous system. In sketch (b), fat displaces the diazepam from the albumin molecule so that all 8 molecules of diazepam are immediately free to exert sedative effects on the central nervous system. In sketch (c), 4 molecules of folic acid are attached to the albumin molecule able to circulate through the kidney intact. In sketch (d), aspirin displaces the folic acid from the albumin molecule and the separate molecules of folic acid are likely to be excreted in the urine.

lates in the blood and is excreted. Because ascorbic acid is necessary for the healing of wounds, one side effect of prednisone and other corticosteroids is poor wound healing.

When alcohol is present, folic acid "leaks" from the liver into the bloodstream, allowing for excessive excretion in the urine. This interaction can lead to folic acid deficiency.

Interference with Reabsorption by the Kidney

Many diuretic agents prevent normal reabsorption of sodium into the bloodstream within the kidney. This increases the amount of sodium excreted by the kidney into the urine. Along with the sodium, water is excreted. Often the drug's action is not specific enough to dispose of sodium alone. Many diuretics also cause loss of potassium. Sometimes the client must take pharmacologic doses of potassium chloride to prevent hypokalemia. One diuretic, furosemide, produces calcium loss in addition to potassium loss by the same mechanism. In contrast, other diuretics for example, amiloride, spironolactone, and triamterene, are potassium sparing, eliminating the need for supplementation. In a study of drug-nutrient interactions, between 11 and 36 percent of long-term care facility clients were shown to be at risk for hyperkalemia or hypokalemia, states in which the serum potassium is outside the normal range (Lewis, Frongillo, and Roe, 1995). Table 17–2 summarizes the effects of drugs on foods and nutrients. Figure 17–3 shows some of the nutritional effects related to changes in the gastrointestinal tract caused by medications.

The Effects of Foods and Nutrients on Drugs

Foods and nutrients can decrease, delay, or increase the absorption of drugs. They can also cause alterations in drug metabolism.

The Effects of Foods on Drug Absorption

The interaction of food with a drug can be used to therapeutic advantage in some cases. In other situations, knowledge of interactions helps the healthcare team schedule meals and medication doses to the best advantage of the client.

Decreased or Delayed Absorption

Food, non-nutrient components of foods, or nutrients in food may decrease or delay the absorption of drugs. Drug bioavailability may vary as much as 50 percent, depending on the drug–meal relationship (Lewis, Frongillo, and Roe, 1995). Food delays the absorption of cortisone, a glucocorticoid used as an anti-inflammatory drug. Taking cortisone with food produces a more consistent blood level of the drug than taking it without food. Other factors, such as a drug's susceptibility to acid degradation or its ability to form insoluble complexes, also influence whether a drug is administered with food or between meals.

Food in the stomach, acidic fruit or vegetable juices, and carbonated beverages increase gastric acidity. Anti-infective drugs particularly susceptible to acid degradation are penicillin G, cloxacillin, and ampicillin. An acid medium breaks down these drugs, resulting in a less effective blood level. To diminish such acid degradation, these anti-infective drugs are best administered between meals. Conversely, individuals with less gastric acid, for example, young infants and the elderly, may achieve higher blood levels of these drugs than intended.

Drugs formulated to dissolve in the intestine rather than in the stomach are **enteric-coated**; an acid-resistant shell covers the active ingredient (Fig. 17–4). The stomach environment normally is acid and the duodenum's is alkaline. Milk raises the pH of the stomach, making it more alkaline. Taking enteric-coated drugs with milk allows the coating to dissolve early and thereby decreases the action of the drug. Some formulations of erythromycin, an anti-infective drug, are enteric-coated and should not be taken with milk. Alcohol and hot beverages can also cause premature erosion of the enteric-coating on drugs.

Table 17–2 The Effects of Drugs on Nutrients

Drug Group	Drug	Effects/Action on Nutrient	Mechanism of Action
		ALTERATION IN FOOD INTAKE	
Analgesic	Acetylsalicylic acid	Decreases appetite	Altered taste; gastric irritation
Antineoplastic	Bleomycin, plicamycin, vincristine	Decreases appetite	Side effects: anorexia, nausea, vomiting, stomatitis
Antihistamine	Brompheneramine, diphenhydramine	Decreases appetite	Side effect: dry mouth
Laxative	Psyllium	Decreases appetite	Gives feeling of fullness
Antidepressant	Bupropion	Increases/decreases appetite	Side effects
CNS stimulant	Dextroamphetamine, methylphenidate	Decreases appetite	Depressed desire for food
Antidepressant	Doxepin	Increases appetite	Side effect
Antimanic	Lithium carbonate	Decreases appetite	Altered taste; Side effects: dry mouth, anorexia, nausea, vomiting
Hormone	Medroxyprogesterone	Increases appetite	Natural effect of hormone
Chelating agent	Penicillamine	Decreases appetite/overeating	Altered taste and smell
Anti-infective	Streptomycin	Decreases appetite/overeating	Altered taste
Antihypertensive	Captopril	Decreases appetite	Loss of taste sensation
		ALTERATION IN NUTRIENT ABSORPTION	
Alcohol	Ethanol	Decreases absorption of amino acids, fat, thiamin, folic acid, niacin, pyridoxine, and magnesium	Decreased enzyme production, damaged intestinal mucosa
Histamine H_2 receptor antagonist	Cimetidine	Decreases vitamin B_{12} absorption	Reduced gastric acidity
Gastric acid-pump inhibitor	Omeprazole	Decreases vitamin B_{12} absorption	Reduced gastric acidity
Antacid	Aluminum hydroxide, calcium carbonate magnesium hydroxide	Decreases absorption of folic acid, vitamin B_{12} and iron	Reduced gastric acidity
Electrolyte therapy	Potassium	Decreases absorption of folic acid, vitamin B_{12}, and iron	Reduced gastric acidity
Laxative	Biscodyl, phenolphthalein	Interferes with uptake of glucose, potassium, calcium, sodium, and water	Increased peristalsis
Lipid-lowering agent	Cholestyramine	Interferes with absorption of vitamins A, D, K, B_{12}, folic acid, and the mineral calcium	Formation of complexes
Antigout agent	Colchicine	Malabsorption of vitamin B_{12}, folic acid, calcium; reduces absorption of fat, lactose, and carotene	Damaged intestinal mucosa
Stool softener	Docusate sodium	Increases absorption of cholesterol	Altered peristalsis
Sedative/hypnotic	Glutethamide	Leads to calcium deficiency	Impaired transport mechanism
Antineoplastic,	Methotrexate	Decreases absorption of vitamin B_{12}, folic acid, and calcium	Damaged intestinal mucosa
Laxative	Mineral oil	Decreases absorption of vitamins A, D, E, and K, calcium, and phosphorus	Formation of complexes
Anti-infective	Neomycin	Decreases absorption of fat, fat-soluble vitamins, vitamin B_{12}, lactose, iron, sucrose, sodium, potassium, and calcium	Damaged intestinal mucosa

(continued on next page)

Table 17–2 The Effects of Drugs on Nutrients (continued)

Drug Group	Drug	Effects/Action on Nutrient	Mechanism of Action
Anticonvulsant	Phenytoin	Reduces absorption of folic acid	Inhibited intestinal enzymes
Anti-inflammatory agent	Sulfasalazine	Reduces absorption of folic acid, iron	Inhibited transport mechanism
ALTERATION IN NUTRIENT METABOLISM			
Alcohol	Ethanol	Amino acids poorly utilized	Damaged intestinal mucosa
Anticonvulsant	Phenytoin	Folic acid and vitamin D deficiency	Impeded conversion of vitamin D to intermediate form
Anti-infective	Broad spectrum antibiotics	Decreases vitamin K synthesis	Destruction of intestinal bacteria
Beta-adrenergic blockers	Atenolol, metoprolol	Increases body fat; decreases fat-free mass and REE	Decreased lipolysis and muscle glycogenolysis
Glucocorticoids	Cortisone, hydrocortisone, methylprednisolone, prednisone	Decreases glucose tolerance; produces tissue wasting, osteoporosis, "moon face," and/or "buffalo hump"	Protein catabolism; mobilization of fats; conversion of fat and protein to glucose
Hormone	Estrogen/progesterone	Folic acid, vitamin B_6 and vitamin B_{12} deficiencies; altered serum lipid and triglyceride levels	Multiple mechanisms
Antiepileptic	Phenytoin	Hemorrhagic disease in newborn	Interference with vitamin K metabolism through stimulation of cytochrome P450 enzymes
Antitubercular	Isoniazid	Vitamin B_6 deficiency leading to niacin deficiency	Increased urinary excretion
Antiparkinson agent	Levodopa	Vitamin B_6 deficiency leading to niacin deficiency	Increased urinary excretion
Antineoplastic	Methotrexate	Folic acid deficiency	Folic acid antagonist
Anticoagulant	Warfarin	Depletes vitamin K	Interference with synthesis of clotting factors
ALTERATION IN NUTRIENT EXCRETION			
Analgesic	Acetylsalicylic acid	Increases excretion of folic acid	Competition for binding sites
Alcohol	Ethanol	Increases excretion of folic acid	Nutrient not retained in liver
Diuretic	Furosemide	Increases excretion of sodium, potassium, and calcium	Interference with reabsorption by kidneys
Chelating agent	Penicillamine	Increases excretion of metals: zinc, copper, and iron	Formation of chemical bonds
Glucocorticoid	Prednisone	Increases excretion of vitamin C	Catabolism of tissues

Tetracycline, an anti-infective agent, combines with the salts of iron, magnesium, aluminum, and calcium to form insoluble compounds. The drug and the nutrient thus bound are both unavailable for absorption. For this reason, tetracycline should not be administered within 1 to 3 hours of taking iron supplements or eating iron-containing foods (red meat, egg yolks), milk or other dairy products, or antacids containing magnesium, aluminum, and/or calcium. Another class of anti-infective drugs, the fluoroquinolones, including ciprofloxacin, combine with calcium, iron, and zinc, resulting in decreased absorption of the anti-infective drugs to such an extent as to produce treatment failures (Gregg, 1999).

Amino acids compete for intestinal absorption with levodopa, a drug used in the management of Parkinson's disease. A separation of 3 hours between administration of levodopa and ingestion of high-protein food improves absorption. A high-protein meal also inhibits the transfer of levodopa across the blood–brain barrier. Clients with Parkinson's disease may find that daytime restriction of protein intake gives them a higher level of functioning. Consuming their required protein at bedtime is a compensatory strategy (Utermohlen, 1999). Protein also competes for absorption with methyldopa (an antihypertensive), delays the action of phenytoin (an anticonvulsant), and inhibits the absorption of theo-

phylline, a bronchodilator used to treat asthma and chronic obstructive pulmonary disease.

A high-fiber meal decreases the absorption of digoxin, a drug used to treat congestive heart failure and certain cardiac arrhythmias by slowing and strengthening cardiac contractions. The pectin in apples and jelly reduces the absorption of acetaminophen, an analgesic.

Fatty meals inhibit the absorption of zidovudine, an antiretroviral drug used in the management of human immunodeficiency virus (HIV) infections (Gregg, 1999).

Increased Absorption

Foods and nutrients may also increase or facilitate the absorption of drugs. Some drugs are affected in one or more ways by one or more nutrients. Levodopa, discussed earlier, has a second interaction with food. Although protein delays the absorption of levodopa, carbohydrate facilitates it. Giving levodopa with carbohydrate-rich snacks improves the absorption of the drug. Similarly, protein delays the anticonvulsant action of phenytoin, but the presence of carbohydrate increases the absorption.

In general, protein inhibits the absorption of theophylline, a bronchodilator given for asthma or chronic obstructive pulmonary disease, but

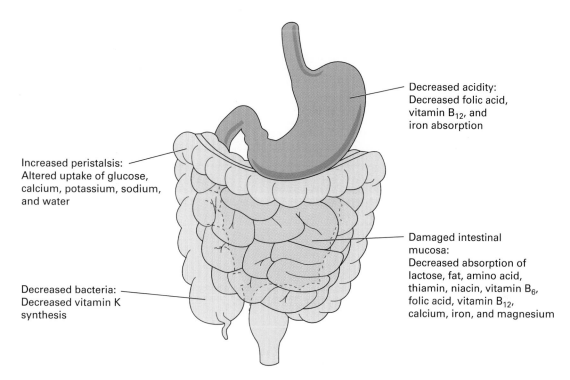

Decreased acidity:
Decreased folic acid,
vitamin B$_{12}$, and
iron absorption

Increased peristalsis:
Altered uptake of glucose,
calcium, potassium, sodium,
and water

Damaged intestinal
mucosa:
Decreased absorption of
lactose, fat, amino acid,
thiamin, niacin, vitamin B$_6$,
folic acid, vitamin B$_{12}$,
calcium, iron, and magnesium

Decreased bacteria:
Decreased vitamin K
synthesis

Figure 17–3:
Both therapeutic effects (decreased gastric acidity and increased peristalsis) and side effects (damaged intestinal mucosa and decreased colon bacteria) can adversely affect nutrient utilization.

fat or carbohydrate accelerates its absorption. Various preparations of controlled-release theophylline, however, responded differently in relation to food intake (Utermohlen, 1999), so administration information for the specific product should be sought.

Fatty foods enhance the absorption of griseofulvin, an antifungal drug. For a person on a low-fat diet, the drug can be administered either in a **micronized** form or in a low-fat suspension. The pharmacist can suspend the drug in a small amount of corn oil.

The Effects of Foods on Drug Metabolism

Foods can alter the metabolism of drugs. One metabolic food–drug interaction, described in the following section, can be life-threatening.

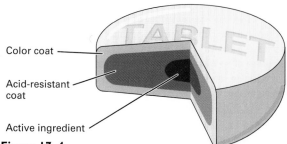

Color coat

Acid-resistant
coat

Active ingredient

Figure 17–4:
Enteric-coated tablet. Substances that penetrate the acid-resistant coating defeat the purpose of this type of tablet. (From Clayton, BD, and Stock, YN, 1989, p. 56, with permission.)

Monoamine Oxidase Inhibitors

The usual abbreviation for this group of drugs is **MAOI (monoamine oxidase inhibitor)**. Several antidepressants are MAO inhibitors, and some other drugs produce similar reactions (see the drugs listed in Table 17–3).

MECHANISM OF DRUG ACTION These drugs prevent the breakdown of tyramine and dopamine, chemicals necessary for proper functioning of the nervous system. The drugs' therapeutic effect is to increase the concentration of epinephrine, norepinephrine, serotonin, and dopamine in the central nervous system, thus counteracting depression.

In the peripheral nervous system, MAO inhibitors also prevent the release of the norepinephrine that builds up in the nerves. The stores of norepinephrine become especially high in the nerves that regulate the size of blood vessels. The result is a decreased ability to constrict peripheral blood vessels. The vasodilation thus produced leads to hypotension. To compound the situation, the drugs also inhibit the body's normal response to a low blood pressure, an increased heart rate. Thus the individual displays the unusual combination of hypotension and bradycardia.

EFFECT OF FOODS ON MAO INHIBITORS Some foods contain **tyramine**, a metabolic intermediate product in the conversion of the amino acid tyrosine to epinephrine. Foods that contain degraded protein, such as aged cheese, are high in tyramine. When a client on MAO inhibitors consumes foods or beverages high in tyramine, the drugs prevent the normal breakdown of tyramine. As a consequence, the tyramine oversupply leads to excessive epinephrine, producing hypertension. Sometimes the blood pressure is severely elevated, which can cause intracranial hemorrhage.

Table 17–3 Tyramine-Restricted Diet

Description	Indication	Adequacy
Restricts food with naturally high levels of tyramine.	Used when clients receive drugs classified as monoamine oxidase inhibitors (MAOs) and those with MAO activity. *Antidepressants*: Phenelzine; Tranylcypromine *Anti-infectives*: Furazolidone; Isoniazid *Antineoplastics*: Procarbazine *Antiparkinson*: Selegiline	Adequate in all nutrients according to the current Recommended Dietary Allowance if the individual makes appropriate food choices.

Description	To Avoid	To Use Moderately
Breads and cereals	None	None
Fruit and vegetables	Avocados Bananas Figs Broad (fava) beans Chinese pea pods Eggplant Italian flat beans Mixed Chinese vegetables	None
Dairy	Aged cheese (brick, blue, brie, cheddar, Camembert, Swiss, Romano, Roquefort, mozzarella, Parmesan, provolone) Yogurt	Gouda cheese Processed American cheese
Meat and fish	Any canned meat Beef or chicken liver Sausage (bologna, salami, pepperoni, summer) Fish (caviar, dried fish, salt herring)	
Beverages	Ale, beer, sherry, red and white wines	Coffee, colas, hot chocolate (1–3 cups per day)
Other	Chocolate, bouillon and other protein extracts, meat tenderizer, soy sauce, yeast concentrates	

As with many substances, individuals responses to tyramine vary. Several factors interact to determine the severity of reaction: (1) the amount of tyramine ingested, (2) the dose of the MAO inhibitor, (3) client susceptibility, and (4) the time between the drug dose and a tyramine-containing meal.

TYRAMINE-RICH FOODS Many foods contain enough tyramine to create problems for clients receiving MAO inhibitors. These include foods and beverages such as cheese, beer, and Chianti wine, in which aging is used to enhance flavor. The amount of tyramine varies even in different samples of a particular food. Table 17–3 describes the tyramine-restricted diet. Because this interaction can be life-threatening, the best advice to give a client is to avoid all foods capable of causing problems, even though a small amount of the food, or a given batch of a product, might be safe. New formulations of antidepressant MAO inhibitors, such as moclobemide, are more selective in targeting the central nervous system and do not require severe dietary restrictions (Utermohlen, 1999).

Effects of Other Nutrients

Certain nutrients increase the amount of a drug in the bloodstream, thus increasing or decreasing the risk of toxicity. For example, fat displaces the antianxiety drug diazepam from **protein binding sites**, thus increasing the amount of unbound drug circulating in the bloodstream. This increased serum concentration leads to increased activity of the drug.

Normal potassium and calcium levels are necessary for adequate muscle function, including that of the heart. Hypokalemia or hypercal-cemia increases the risk of toxicity from digitalis. Clients receiving digitalis and loop diuretics, a common combination, require careful monitoring.

A flavonoid compound in grapefruit juice, tentatively identified as naringin, may inhibit the metabolism of calcium channel blockers used to combat hypertension. Consequently, the drug's action is extended. Grapefruit juice increases bioavailability of felodipine, nifedipine, nitrendipine, and nisoldipine. Normally, the liver extensively metabolizes these drugs immediately after absorption into the portal circulation from the intestinal tract, leaving only a portion of the original dose available in the systemic circulation (Schultz, n.d.). This process is called the **first-pass effect**. A similar effect of increased bioavailability is seen when grapefruit juice is administered with cyclosporin, an immunosuppressive drug given to prevent rejection of transplanted organs as well as in severe rheumatoid arthritis (Ioannides-Demos et al., 1997). Eliminating grapefruit juice can thwart the interaction, or it may be used to enhance blood levels of a particular drug by administering it with grapefruit juice. Anticipation of the effects and consistency in administration are the keys to successful treatment. Table 17–4 summarizes the effects of foods and nutrients on drugs.

Occasionally, a food or beverage contains a drug that produces untoward effects. For example, a woman was seen in a dermatology clinic for a persistent rash, worsened by sunlight. She habitually drank 500 milliliters of tonic water daily. Tonic water is a carbonated mixer that contains lemon, lime, sweeteners, and quinine, a drug used to treat malaria and nocturnal leg cramps. The amount of quinine in the water, 40 milligrams

Table 17–4 The Effects of Foods and Nutrients on Drugs

Effect	Type of Food/Nutrient	Action on Drug
Decrease in absorption	Amino acids in proteins	Inhibit absorption of levodopa, methyldopa, and theophylline; delay action of phenytoin
	Acidic juices, carbonated beverages	Degrade penicillin G, cloxacillin, and amphicillin
	Milk	Increases pH of stomach, causing premature erosion of enteric coatings
	Calcium in dairy products	Combines with tetracycline to impair absorption
	Foods high in calcium, iron, or zinc (dairy products, red meat)	Combine with fluoroquinolones such as ciprofloxacin to decrease absorption
	High-fiber meal	Decreases absorption of digoxin
	Alcohol, hot beverages	Cause premature erosion of enteric coatings
	Pectin in jelly, apples	Reduces absorption of acetaminophen
	Carbohydrate	Decreases absorption of isoniazid
	Fatty foods	Inhibit absorption of zidovudine
Increase in absorption	Carbohydrate	Enhances absorption of levodopa, phenytoin, and theophylline
	Fatty foods	Enhance absorption of griseofulvin
Altered metabolism	Caffeine	Enhances effect of theophylline
	Fat	Enhances activity of diazepam
	Tyramine-containing foods	May cause hypertensive crisis when combined with MAO inhibitors
	Grapefruit juice	Increases bioavailability of calcium channel blockers and cyclosporin

in 500 milliliters, was much less than that given pharmacologically to adults. Among quinine's side effects, however, is a skin rash. Once the woman stopped drinking tonic water, her skin problem was cured (Wagner, Diffey, and Ive, 1994).

Effects of Non-nutrient Intakes

Although it is not a nutrient, caffeine should be included in a dietary assessment. Caffeine increases the effect of theophylline and stimulants. In some users, caffeine produces effects similar to those of other psychoactive substances characterized by dependence: tolerance, withdrawal symptoms, persistent desire for the substance or unsuccessful efforts to control its use, and continued use despite knowledge of persistent physical or psychological problems related to its use (Strain et al., 1994).

Another non-nutrient marketed as a food supplement is Ma-huang. This is the main plant source of ephedrine, a drug with central nervous system stimulating effects, which is used in many over-the-counter deconges-

tants and diet aids. In one case, a man took increasing amounts of an herbal diet supplement containing Ma-huang over a 2-month period for weight control. He became uncharacteristically restless, sleepless, argumentative, and aggressive and was so disorganized at work that he was given a leave of absence. Discontinuation of the herbal supplement and a prescribed sedative returned him to normal in 3 days (Capwell, 1995). The amount of Ma-huang in the supplement was never ascertained. As discussed in Chapter 16, manufacturers of food supplements are not bound by the same regulations as manufacturers of prescription and over-the-counter drugs.

The Body's Homeostatic Mechanisms Affect Drug Levels

In addition to nutritional status, the status of the person's acid–base balance and fluid and electrolyte balance affects the excretion of drugs. To consider either acid–base balance or fluid and electrolyte balance in isolation risks oversimplifying the body's functions. The functions of these two regulatory systems are interwoven.

Acid–Base Balance

The kidneys play a major role in maintaining the normal composition of the blood and tissue fluid. The contents of urine, therefore, reflect the metabolic state of the body. The end products of the foods that are consumed and the drugs that are taken make the urine either more acid or more alkaline. Freshly voided urine usually has an acid pH, averaging about 6.0.

Alkaline Urine

Large amounts of citrus juices, greater than 1 liter per day (Smith, 1995), or a vegetarian diet causes the urine to become alkaline. When the body is producing alkaline urine, the kidneys take longer to excrete alkaline drugs. Higher levels of the drugs remain in the bloodstream for a longer period. Examples of alkaline drugs are the cardiac antidysrhythmic quinidine, the tricyclic antidepressant imipramine, and amphetamine stimulants. If the client's metabolism causes an alkaline urine, these drugs have more pronounced and prolonged effects. Clients treated with these drugs should neither change the amounts of citrus juice they consume nor become vegetarians without consulting the physician.

The opposite effect occurs when a person's metabolism produces alkaline urine and the drugs are acidic. The kidney excretes acidic drugs faster than usual if the urine is alkaline. One acidic drug that should spring to mind immediately is acetylsalicylic acid, or aspirin. Another acidic drug is the barbiturate phenobarbital, commonly used as an anticonvulsant. The kidney excretes both of these drugs faster than normal if the patient is producing an alkaline urine.

Acid Urine

Large doses of ascorbic acid (vitamin C) make the urine more acidic. Vitamin C is sometimes given specifically for the purpose of acidifying the urine. For example, a urinary pH of 5.5 or less is necessary for the urinary anti-infective drug methenamine to be effective. In an acid urine, the drug becomes ammonia and formaldehyde, both bactericidal chemicals.

Sulfonamides are antimicrobial drugs that are often given for urinary tract infections. One of the possible side effects of sulfonamides is **crystalluria**, crystallization of the drug in the urinary tract. Although some drugs crystallize more readily than others, these drugs are more likely to crystallize in concentrated or acid urine. For this reason, clients should be instructed to drink ample fluid. It may also be necessary to deliberately alkalinize the urine with another drug or diet modification to prevent crystallization. Table 17–5 summarizes the effects of urinary pH on the excretion of drugs.

Table 17–5 Effects of Urinary pH on Drugs

	Alkaline Urine	Acid Urine
Increased excretion	Acetylsalicylic acid Phenobarbital	Amphetamines Imipramine Quinidine
Decreased excretion	Amphetamines Imipramine Quinidine	Acetylsalicylic acid
Necessary for adequate effect	Sulfonamides	Phenobarbital Methenamine

Fluid and Electrolyte Balance

A person's fluid and electrolyte status also interacts with drugs. Potassium intake, sodium and water intake, and licorice can cause serious imbalances in fluid and electrolyte status in certain situations.

Salt Substitutes and ACE Inhibitors

The angiotensin converting enzyme (ACE) inhibitors lower blood pressure by preventing conversion of angiotensin I to angiotensin II, thereby decreasing aldosterone secretion and increasing excretion of sodium and water. (See Fig. 9-5.) Clients receiving ACE inhibitors such as captopril, enalapril, and lisinopril should be monitored for hyperkalemia. The excessive serum potassium may be related to potassium sparing diuretics or salt substitutes. One client had to be resuscitated following cardiac arrest before the contribution of a salt substitute to his hyperkalemia became apparent (Ray, Dorman, and Watson, 1999).

Sodium, Fluids, and Lithium Carbonate

Both sodium intake and increased fluid intake affect the antimanic drug lithium carbonate. This drug is absorbed, distributed, and excreted with sodium. Therefore, decreased sodium intake with decreased fluid intake may lead to lithium retention. Conversely, increased sodium intake and increased fluid intake increase the excretion of lithium and decrease its antimanic effect, thus worsening signs and symptoms of mania. Because of this important interaction, clients who take lithium are taught to monitor the concentration or **specific gravity** of their urine.

Licorice

Licorice, a flavoring agent, contains glycyrrhizic acid, which, when metabolized, inhibits an enzyme that controls the conversion of cortisol to cortisone in the kidney. As little as "a couple of twists" per day can counteract the effects of diuretics and increase the mineralocorticoid effects of corticosteroids (Utermohlen, 1999). When eaten in excess, licorice can cause sodium and water retention, hypertension, hypokalemia, and alkalosis. Control of hypertension took 8 months for a 49-year-old woman who, unbeknownst to her physician, consumed large quantities of a licorice-flavored sweet. Licorice is used to flavor many foods, some chewing tobacco, chewing gum, alcoholic beverages, and some laxatives, and therefore a person may be unaware of ingesting it (Dellow, Unwin, and Honour, 1999).

Responsibilities of Healthcare Professionals

The Joint Commission on the Accreditation of Healthcare Organizations mandates that clients be given information on the medications they receive, including potential dietary interactions. Although the dietitian is charged with this responsibility, the successful completion of the task requires cooperation from the healthcare team. Charting Tips 17–1 lists the principles for charting client teaching.

Institutionalized clients do not necessarily receive maximum therapeutic effects from their medications. Researchers found that only 50 percent of 424 doses of three cardiac medications (hydralazine, phenytoin, and propranolol) were administered correctly on a full stomach, and only 53 percent of 101 doses of captopril were correctly given on an empty stomach. In the 24 hours studied, only 15 percent of 153 clients received all their medication doses correctly timed with meals. This last group included the only client whose physician's order specified taking the drug before meals (Strong et al., 1991). Managing a medication regimen is a challenging but worthwhile effort. The consequences of improper scheduling can be treatment failure, toxicity, and/or increased expense.

Charting Tips 17–1

- Record the client's knowledge at the start of your teaching
- Identify information discussed.
- Indicate evidence, such as verbalization or recitation, that indicates client understood your teaching.
- Whenever possible, give the client a choice. If the client makes a choice, chart the decision as the client's.
- Document educational materials given to the client.

Summary

This chapter has only touched the surface of the subject of food and drug interactions. For every drug included in the discussion here, many others had to be omitted. Commonly prescribed drugs and those that have significant interactions with foods are included, as are various modes of food and drug interactions.

Persons at highest risk for food–drug interactions are those who (1) take many drugs, including alcohol; (2) require long-term drug therapy; or (3) have poor or marginal nutrition. All clients should be instructed about how to prevent or manage possible interactions (Wellness Tips 17–1). Food–drug interactions can affect (1) food intake, (2) absorption of nutrients or drugs, (3) metabolism of nutrients or drugs, and (4) excretion of nutrients or drugs.

Medications influence food intake by decreasing or increasing appetite, causing taste changes, or provoking gastric irritation. Drugs affect nutrient absorption through luminal or mucosal effects and impact nutrient metabolism through many mechanisms. Medications affect the excretion of nutrients by competing for binding sites, forming chemical bonds, depleting nutrients in tissues, and interfering with kidney reabsorption. In addition, foods and nutrients can affect drug levels and actions by increasing or decreasing absorption and altering the medica-

Wellness Tips 17–1

- Learn as much as possible about proper administration of medications in relation to food intake.
- Be especially cautious about combining medications with alcohol intake.
- If a medication with known nutrient interactions is necessary long-term, discuss appropriate proactive nutritional interventions with the healthcare provider.
- Follow the package directions regarding the maximum use of over-the-counter medications.
- If several healthcare providers are prescribing medications, be sure each knows the entire regimen being followed, including dietary intake.
- Maintain a balanced, varied, and moderate diet.

tion's metabolism. Three particularly important nutrient–drug interactions are those of tyramine-containing foods with MAO inhibitors, of sodium and water with lithium carbonate, and of vitamin K with warfarin. Also at risk are clients in unstable acid–base or fluid and electrolyte balance and those with alterations in serum proteins.

Case Study 17–1

Mrs. S. a 72-year-old client, is being seen by the home health nurse to reaffirm her suitability for independent living. She has a history of congestive heart failure for which she has been successfully treated with digoxin 0.125 mg daily for the past 6 months. Mrs. S takes the tablet with her usual breakfast of orange juice and tea.

Recently she has had difficulty with constipation. Obtaining information on bowel hygiene on her own, she decided to improve her nutritional intake by adding a high-fiber cereal to her breakfast.

After 1 week, her constipation has been relieved, but she now is becoming fatigued easily. When climbing a flight of stairs she finds it necessary to rest twice en route. The nurse asked Mrs. S to weigh herself. Mrs. S reported she had gained 5 lb in 2 weeks. Based on the above data and her observations, the home health nurse prepared a nursing care plan. The portion of it pertinent to food and drug interactions appears below.

Nursing Care Plan

Subjective Data	Easily fatigued
	Short of breath < 1 flight of stairs
	History of constipation, relieved by addition of high-fiber cereal to diet
	Medications—digoxin, 0.125 mg daily in morning with breakfast.
Objective Data	Alert, oriented, cooperative. Vital signs normal except pulse 90 beats per minute. Weight gain—5 lb over 2 weeks.
Nursing Diagnosis	NANDA: Knowledge deficit (North American Nursing Diagnosis Association, 1999, with permission.)
	Related to food-drug interaction as evidenced by beginning signs of heart failure

Desired Outcomes Evaluation Criteria	Nursing Actions/ Interventions	Rational
NOC: Knowledge: Diet (Johnson, Maas, and Moorhead, 2000, with permission.)	NIC: Teaching: Prescribed Diet (McCloskey and Bulechek, 2000, with permission.)	
Client will revise medication or meal schedule immediately to maximize effectiveness of digoxin.	Teach client to separate digoxin from high-fiber foods.	High-fiber foods decrease the absorption of digitalix preparations.

Critical Thinking Questions

1. What additional assessment data could impact the resolution of this situation?
2. In what way might this scenario develop such that the nurse should contact the client's physician during the home visit?
3. How would you approach the follow-up care of this client?

Study Aids

Subjects	Internet Sites
Food, Nutrient, and Drug Interactions	http://www.nclnet.org/fooddruord.html
	http://www.pharmacy.ab.umd.edu/~umdi/grape.htm
General Drug Information	http://www.usp.org
	http://www.pharminfo.com
	http://www.rxlist.com
	http://www.medscape.com/druginfo
	http://www.fda.gov
	http://www.wvjolt.wvu.edu/v2i1/simmons.htm
	http://www.intmed.mcw.edu/drug.html
Epilepsy	http://www.efa.org
	http://www.aesnet.org
	http://neuro-www.ngh.harvard.edu/forum
Vitamin K in Foods	http://www.nal.usda.gov/fnic/foodcomp/Data/Other/pt104.pdf

Chapter Review

1. Which of the following clients is at greatest risk for food–drug interaction?
   a. A 50-year-old man with no current disease who takes one baby aspirin daily to prevent heart disease
   b. A 75-year-old woman taking medication for several chronic diseases
   c. A 39-year-old man who usually consumes two cocktails before dinner
   d. A 25-year-old pregnant woman who is taking a prenatal vitamin supplement and calcium tablets

2. How do food and drugs interact?
   a. Drugs may affect food intake.
   b. Either may affect the absorption of the other.
   c. Certain foods and drugs specifically interfere with the metabolism of the other.
   d. Nutrients and drugs can increase or decrease the rate of excretion of one another.
   e. All of the above are true.

3. It is recommended that levodopa be taken with carbohydrate-rich snacks but separated from any high-protein meal by 3 hours because:
   a. Glucose from the carbohydrate aids in the distribution of the drug.
   b. Carbohydrate causes the release of insulin, which is necessary for the absorption of levodopa.
   c. Amino acids compete with levodopa for absorption.
   d. Levodopa is likely to sensitize the person to various proteins.

4. A client taking lithium is most likely to experience increased mania with:
   a. Decreased fluid intake and decreased sodium intake.
   b. Decreased fluid intake and increased potassium intake.
   c. Increased sodium intake and decreased potassium intake.
   d. Increased sodium intake and increased fluid intake.

5. Individuals taking the anticoagulant warfarin must be counseled to consume no more than one serving per day of:
   a. Broccoli or spinach
   b. Vegetable oils
   c. Kale and parsley
   d. Dried apricots and dates

Clinical Analysis

Mr. AS is being admitted to a long-term care facility. He is a 45-year-old post-trauma client. The motor vehicle accident in which he became paralyzed below the waist also killed his wife and daughter. The accident occurred 6 months ago. In the meantime, he has been treated at a rehabilitation center. He is depressed and freely sharing his feelings of guilt and loss. The depression has interfered with his progress toward rehabilitation. After many trials of various antidepressants, he is now receiving phenelzine. The following questions relate to his care.

1. To ensure that everyone caring for Mr. AS is alerted to potential complications related to his drug therapy, the nurse begins a nursing care plan. The nursing diagnosis that best states this problem as described by the data is:
   a. Coping, ineffective individual: related to deaths of family members as evidenced by expressions of grief and guilt.
   b. Risk for altered tissue perfusion, cerebral, related to inappropriate diet combined with phenelzine therapy
   c. Knowledge deficit related to potential food–drug interaction between tyramine-containing foods and monoamine oxidase inhibitor
   d. Bowel elimination, altered: related to paraplegia as evidenced by involuntary passage of stool.

2. Close attention to Mr. AS's diet is essential. Which of the following foods will he have to avoid completely?
   a. Baked beans, dates, and roast beef
   b. Sugar, molasses, and maple syrup
   c. Bologna, cheddar cheese, and wine
   d. Green beans, whole-wheat bread, and oranges

3. When teaching nursing assistants about the dietary restrictions needed by Mr. AS, the nurse should be sure the nursing assistants understand that:
   a. The potential complication can be life-threatening.
   b. Mr. AS is to be kept unaware of the seriousness of his condition.
   c. As time goes on, the forbidden foods can be added to the diet slowly, one at a time.
   d. If Mr. AS does not cooperate in his dietary care, his paralysis is likely to worsen.

Bibliography

Adams, WL: Potential for adverse drug-alcohol interactions among retirement community residents. J Am Geriatr Soc 43:1021, 1995.

Berg, MJ, et al.: Folic acid improves phenytoin pharmacokinetics. J Am Diet Assoc 95:352, 1995.

Capwell, RR: Ephedrine-induced mania from an herbal diet supplement [Letter]. Am J Psychiatry 152:647, 1995.

Clayton, BD, and Stock, YN: Basic Pharmacology for Nurses, ed 9. CV Mosby, St. Louis, 1989.

Conly, J, and Stein, K: Reduction of vitamin K_2 concentrations in human liver associated with the use of broad spectrum antimicrobials. Clin Invest Med 17:531, 1994.

Dellow, EL, Unwin, RH, and Honour, JW: Pontefract cakes can be bad for you: Refractory hypertension and liquorice excess. Nephrol Dial Transplant 14:218, 1999.

Gregg, CR: Drug interactions and anti-infective therapies. Am J Med 106:227, 1999.

Groff, JL, Gropper, SS, and Hunt, SM: Advanced Nutrition and Human Metabolism, ed 2. West Publishing Company, Minneapolis/St. Paul, 1995.

Ioannides-Demos, LL, et al.: Dosing implications of a clinical interaction between grapefruit juice and cyclosporine and metabolite concentrations in patients with autoimmune diseases. J Rheumatol 24:49, 1997.

Johnson, M, Maas, M, and Moorhead, S: Nursing Outcomes Classification (NOC), ed 2. Mosby, Philadelphia, 2000.

Kelly, MP, et al.: A diagnostically reasoned case study with particular emphasis on B_6 and zinc imbalance directed by clinical history and nutrition physical examination findings. Nutrition in Clinical Practice 13:32, 1998.

Lamont, LS: Beta-blockers and their effects on protein metabolism and resting energy expenditure. J Cardiopulm Rehabil 15:183, 1995.

Lasswell, AB, et al.: Family medicine residents' knowledge and attitudes about drug–nutrient interactions. J Am Coll Nutr 14:137, 1995.

Lewis, CW, Frongillo, EA, and Roe, DA: Drug-nutrient interactions in three long-term care facilities. J Am Diet Assoc 95:309, 1995.

Morrell, MJ: Guidelines for the care of women with epilepsy. Neurology 51(Supp l4):S21, 1998.

McCloskey, JC, and Bulechek, GM: Nursing Interventions Classification (NIC), ed 3. Mosby, Philadelphia, 2000.

North American Nursing Diagnosis Association: Nursing Diagnoses: Definitions and Classification 1999–2000, North American Nursing Diagnosis Association, Philadelphia, 1999.

Ray, KK, Dorman, S, and Watson, RDS: Severe hyperkalaemia due to the concomitant use of salt substitutes and ACE inhibitors in hypertension: A potentially life threatening interaction. J Hum Hypertens 13:717, 1999.

Sato, Y, et al.: Long-term oral anticoagulation reduces bone mass in patients with previous hemispheric infarction and nonrheumatic atrial fibrillation. Stroke 28:2390, 1997.

Schultz, N, with Mays, DA (eds): Did you drink your grapefruit juice this morning? Accessed 11/21/1999 at http://www.pharmacy.ab.umd.edu/~umdi/grape.htm

Smith, CH: Drug–food/food–drug interactions. In Morley, JE, Glick, Z, and Rubenstein, LZ (eds): Geriatric Nutrition, ed 2. Raven Press, New York, 1995.

Smith, JK, Aljazairi, A, and Fuller, SH: INR elevation associated with diarrhea in a patient receiving warfarin. Ann Pharmacother 33:301, 1999.

Strain, EC, et al.: Caffeine dependence syndrome. JAMA 272:1043, 1994.

Strong, A, et al.: Drug administration in relation to meals in the institutional setting. Heart Lung 20:39, 1991.

Taylor, JR, and Wilt, VM: Probable antagonism of warfarin by green tea. Ann Pharmacother 33:426, 1999.

Utermohlen, V: Diet, nutrition, and drug interactions. In Shils, ME, et al. (eds): Modern Nutrition in Health and Disease, ed 9. Lippincott Williams and Wilkins, Philadelphia, 1999.

Wagner, GH, Diffey, BL, and Ive, FA: "I'll have mine with a twist of lemon" Quinine photosensitivity from excessive intake of tonic water [Letter]. Br J Dermatol 131:734, 1994.

Yaffe, SJ, and Sonawane, BR: Drug therapy and the role of nutrition. In Walker, WA, and Watkins, JB: Nutrition in Pediatrics, ed 2. BC Decker, Hamilton, Ontario, 1997.

CHAPTER 18

Weight Control

LEARNING OBJECTIVES

After completing this chapter, the student should be able to:

1. List basic principles of energy imbalance.
2. Discuss the effects of weight loss on the body.
3. Identify the medical, psychological, and social problems associated with too much and too little body fat.
4. Discuss the federal guidelines for the identification, evaluation, and treatment of overweight and obesity in adults.
5. Describe the symptoms commonly exhibited by a client with anorexia nervosa and/or bulimia.
6. Evaluate at least three fad diets used for weight reduction

Weight management and control are issues for many people. Obesity accounts for more than $68 billion in direct health care expenses each year, consuming more than 6 percent of the total U.S. healthcare expenditures (Wolf, 1998). Obesity is now considered epidemic not only in the United States but also worldwide (Popkin and Doak, 1998). Alarm about the increased prevalence of overweight and obesity in the United States prompted the federal government to publish the first guidelines on the identification, evaluation, and treatment of overweight and obesity in the United States (National Institutes of Health, 1998).

This chapter discusses: (1) terminology and classification, (2) the prevalence of energy imbalance, (3) basic scientific principles of energy metabolism and body composition, (4) consequences of obesity, (5) theories about obesity, (6) federal Guidelines on the Identification, Evaluation, and Treatment of Overweight and Obesity, and (7) reduced body mass. The goal of this chapter is to provide a foundation to enable the evaluation of further research and treatment options.

Terminology and Classification

The classification of an individual as underweight, normal weight, overweight, mildly obese, moderately obese, or severely or extremely obese historically has been difficult for the scientific community. How a person is classified often determines whether treatment is indicated and the kind of treatment that is appropriate. Obesity and, to a lesser extent, overweight are characterized by an excess accumulation of body fat. Height-weight tables, for lack of a better method, have been widely used historically to assist the health care community in the classification of overly fat clients. Athletes and athletic clubs frequently use percent body fat for individual evaluation. The National Institutes of Health recommends the use of body mass index (BMI) by health care professionals. Height-weight tables, percent body fat, and body mass index are discussed separately in the following sections, along with the merits and limitations of each method.

Height and Weight

Percent body weight is computed from height-weight tables. The Metropolitan Life Insurance Company produced the first height-weight table in 1942. The original purpose of this table was to determine life insurance rates based on life expectancy studies. People who weighed more than the amounts recommended on the tables either paid higher premiums or were rejected when they applied for life insurance. The medical community adopted these tables for health purposes.

The term *ideal body weight* means a person's weight as compared to the weight in the Ideal Height Weight Table. The Metropolitan Life Insurance Company released the Ideal Height Weight Table in 1943. The term *desirable body weight* means a person's weight as compared to the weight shown on the Desirable Height-Weight Table, which the Metropolitan Life Insurance Company released in 1959. The data used to compile these tables were based on extensive mortality studies of insured lives conducted by the Association of Life Insurance Medical Directors of America and Society of Actuaries.

In 1983, the Metropolitan Life Insurance Company issued a new table. This table is based on mortality data collected from the 1979 Build Study. Data collected showed that a modest increase in weight (2–13 pounds) did not result in a decreased life expectancy. Thus, the weights in the 1983 table are about 2–13 pounds heavier than those in the 1959 table in each sex, frame size, and height category. The weights on this table are not necessarily based on a healthy body weight but on death rates. In this text, the 1983 Height-Weight Table is used.

Much controversy exists concerning which height-weight table best meets the health needs of the population. In fact, many other organizations and researchers have developed their own height-weight tables because of a dissatisfaction with the Metropolitan Life Insurance Company's tables. It is important to realize that height-weight tables of the Metropolitan Life Insurance Company are based on mortality (death rates), which are not necessarily the weights at which people are healthy, perform their jobs optimally, or even look their best. Height-weight tables cannot replace a thorough body audit, an accurate diet history, information about exercise patterns, or measurement of a client's body fat content.

Percent Reasonable Body Weight

Mild, moderate, and severe obesity are often expressed in terms of percent reasonable body weight (RBW). *Overweight* is often used to mean 10–20 percent above RBW. *Obese* is often used to mean more than 20 percent above reasonable body weight. The obese client may be classified further as:

- mildly obese: 20–40 percent overweight, or 120–140 percent reasonable body weight (RBW)
- moderately obese: 41–100 percent overweight, or 141–200 percent RBW
- severely obese: greater than 100 percent overweight, or 200 percent RBW

All researchers and the medical community do not universally accept the classification of the degree of obesity by this method. However, some members of the medical community use this method in medical record documentation.

Percent Body Fat

The terms *overweight* and *obesity* are used to describe excessive accumulations of body fat that are detrimental to health and well-being. Although an RBW expressed as a percent over 120 percent or a body mass index in excess of 30 kg/m^2 may alert the healthcare worker that the client may be overly fat, this is not always foolproof. Two examples are discussed next to illustrate this concept.

First, consider a 5-foot 4-inch female (without shoes) with a medium frame weighed with indoor clothing. According to the 1983 Metropolitan Height and Weight Table for Adults, she should weigh 127–141 pounds. Let's review the calculation of RBW. Subtract 127 pounds from 141 pounds for a difference of 14 pounds. Divide 14 pounds by 2 for an answer of 7 pounds. Add 7 pounds to 127 pounds for a sum of 134 pounds. A weight of 134 pounds is this client's RBW. Let's say this client weighs 134 pounds. Her RBW would be 100 percent. Can we automatically conclude that this client is not obese? The answer is no. The optimal fat content for females is 18–22 percent. A more accurate definition of *obesity for females* is a fat content greater than 33 percent. A person at her reasonable body weight is metabolically obese if her body fat content exceeds 33 percent. The female in this example may have all the health risks of obesity even at 100 percent RBW if her body fat content exceeds 33 percent. Some researchers believe that a percent body fat of 30 classifies a person as obese. The medical and scientific communities do not universally accept the definitions of obesity.

Second, consider a 5-foot 9-inch male (without shoes) with a medium frame size weighed with indoor clothing. According to the Metropolitan Height and Weight Table for Adults, this individual should weigh 158–180 pounds. The same process can be used to derive his reasonable body weight. First, subtract 158 pounds from 180 pounds for an answer of 22 pounds. Next divide 22 pounds. by 2 for an answer of 11 pounds. Add 11 pounds to 158 pounds to calculate his RBW, which is 169 pounds. Let's say this client weights 225 pounds. That weight, 225 pounds, divided by 169 pounds equals 133 percent. Can we automatically classify this client as moderately obese? The answer is again no. This client may have a body fat content of only 15 percent. Remember, the optimal fat content for males is 15–19 percent. This individual may be a trained athlete and the excess weight the result of increased muscle mass. A fat content in excess of 25 perdent is considered *obese for males*. Some researchers dispute this numerical value and believe it should be lower.

At least half of body fat is located subcutaneously (just beneath the skin). Therefore, the measurement of skinfold thickness is commonly used to estimate a person's body fat content. In this chapter, the four-site

---

Clinical Calculation 18–1 Calculating Body Fat Content Using the Four-Site Technique

Worksheet for Calculating Percent Body Fat Using Skin Calipers

Skinfold Measurements	1	2	3	=	Total ÷ 3 = Average
Biceps	___ +	___ +	___	= ___	___
Triceps	___ +	___ +	___	= ___	___
Subscapular	___ +	___ +	___	= ___	___
Suprailiac	___ +	___ +	___	= ___	___
Total value of the average of four sites:					___

Procedure to Calculate Percent Body Fat Using Skin Calipers in Adults

1. Take skinfold measurements directly on the skin, not through clothing.
2. Pick up and hold the skinfold with one hand while measuring it with calipers held by the other hand.
3. Take three measurements at each of the four sites. Then average the three measurements of each skinfold to arrive at a final figure.

- Biceps measure the muscle belly of the biceps. This will generally be a point on the straightened arm just opposite the nipple.
- Triceps
- Subscapular measure on the back just under the shoulder blade.
- Suprailiac measure approximately 1 in above the hip bone.

4. Add the averages of all skinfold sites to arrive at a total skinfold measurement.
5. To determe the percent body fat, compare the total measurement with the values in the appropriate Body Fat and Skinfolds table located in Appendix E.

(Adapted, courtesy of Jan Wohgulmuth, PT, Director of Physical Therapy at Doctor's Hospital of Jackson, Michigan)

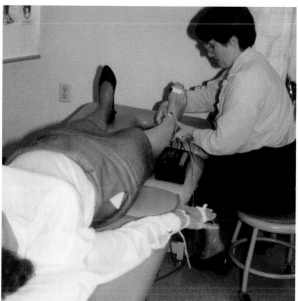

Figure 18–1:
The measurement of a client's percent body fat using bio-electrical impedance. This method is widely used by athletes to measure changes in body composition as a result of training. For example, a decrease in percent body fat and a stable body weight indicate an increase in muscle mass.

measurement technique to determine percent body fat is discussed. This technique requires minimal calculations.

The work sheet in Clinical Calculation 18–1 can be used to calculate a client's percent body fat using skin calipers. A total of twelve measurements should be taken at four different sites. The three numbers obtained at each site are added together and averaged to give a value of one number per site. All these numbers are added together and compared to the number on a standard table to determine the client's percent body fat. A standard table is provided in appendix E. This procedure takes time and requires accurate measurements.

Other techniques to estimate body fat involve underwater weighing, tissue x-rays, ultrasound, electrical conductivity, electrical impedance, computed tomographic scans, and magnetic resonance imaging scans. Electrical impedance is widely used in athletic clubs and gyms (Fig. 18–1). The other procedures are expensive and not available in clinical settings. Limitations include less accuracy in extremely obese persons, states of overhydration and underhydration, hormone abnormalities, and the need for a qualified technician; these are of limited usefulness for persons trying to lose weight.

Body Mass Index

A client's **body mass index (BMI)** is his or her body weight in kilograms divided by height in meters squared. BMI can be determined without doing any calculations by using a body mass index chart (Table 18–1). The BMI is an indicator of optimal weight for health and is different from lean body mass or percent body fat calculations because it considers only height and weight. A BMI of 20–25 kilograms per meter squared is normal. Overweight clients have a BMI of 25–30. Obese clients have a BMI above 30 (National Institutes of Health, 1998). Severe or extreme obesity is characterized by a BMI above 40. The BMI can also be used to estimate relative risk for disease compared to people of normal weight. Table 18–2 classifies overweight and obesity by BMI. The National Institutes of Health (NIH) recommends and encourages all health care professionals to use BMI to classify clients as underweight, normal weight, overweight, and so on in clinical settings.

Table 18–1 Body Mass Index Chart

Height (inches)	19	20	21	22	23	24	25	26	27	28	29	30	31	32	33	34	35
							Body Weight (pounds)										
58	91	96	100	105	110	115	119	124	129	134	138	143	148	153	158	162	167
59	94	99	104	109	114	119	124	128	133	138	143	148	153	158	163	168	173
60	97	102	107	119	118	123	128	133	138	143	148	153	158	163	168	174	179
61	100	106	111	116	122	127	132	137	143	148	153	158	164	169	174	180	185
62	104	109	115	120	126	131	136	142	147	153	158	164	169	175	180	186	191
63	107	113	118	124	130	135	141	146	152	158	163	169	175	180	186	191	197
64	110	116	122	128	134	140	145	151	157	163	169	174	180	186	192	197	204
65	114	120	126	132	138	144	150	156	162	168	174	180	186	199	198	204	210
66	118	124	130	136	142	148	155	161	167	173	179	186	192	198	204	210	216
67	121	127	154	140	146	153	159	166	172	178	185	191	198	204	211	217	223
68	125	131	138	144	151	158	164	171	177	184	190	197	203	210	216	223	230
69	128	135	142	149	155	162	169	176	182	189	196	203	209	216	223	230	236
70	132	]39	146	153	160	167	174	181	188	195	202	209	216	222	229	236	243
71	136	143	150	157	165	172	179	186	193	200	208	215	222	229	236	243	250
72	140	147	154	162	169	177	184	191	199	206	213	221	228	235	242	250	258
73	144	151	159	166	174	182	189	197	204	212	219	227	235	242	250	257	265
74	148	155	163	171	179	186	194	202	210	218	225	233	241	249	256	264	272
75	152	160	168	176	184	192	200	208	216	224	232	240	248	256	264	272	279
76	156	164	172	180	189	197	205	213	221	230	238	246	254	263	271	279	287

(continued on next page)

Table 18–1 Body Mass Index Chart (continued)

Height (inches)	36	37	38	39	40	41	42	43	44	45	46	47	48	49	50	51	52	53	54
								Body Weight (pounds)											
58	179	177	181	186	191	196	201	205	210	215	220	224	229	234	239	244	248	353	258
59	178	183	188	193	198	203	208	212	217	222	227	232	237	242	247	252	257	262	267
60	184	189	194	199	204	209	215	220	225	230	235	240	245	250	255	261	266	271	276
61	190	195	201	206	211	217	222	227	232	238	243	248	254	259	264	269	275	280	285
62	196	202	207	213	218	224	229	235	240	246	251	256	262	267	273	778	284	289	295
63	203	208	214	220	225	231	237	242	248	254	259	265	270	278	282	287	293	299	304
64	209	215	221	227	239	238	244	250	256	262	267	273	279	285	291	296	302	308	314
65	216	292	228	234	240	246	252	258	264	270	276	282	288	294	300	306	312	318	324
66	223	229	235	241	247	253	260	266	272	278	284	291	297	303	309	315	322	398	334
67	230	336	242	249	255	261	268	274	280	287	293	299	306	312	319	399	331	338	344
68	236	243	249	256	262	269	276	282	289	295	302	308	315	329	328	335	341	348	354
69	243	250	257	263	270	277	284	291	297	304	311	318	324	331	338	349	351	358	365
70	250	257	264	271	278	285	292	299	306	313	320	327	334	341	348	355	362	369	376
71	257	265	272	279	286	293	301	308	315	322	329	338	343	351	358	365	379	379	386
72	265	272	279	287	294	302	309	316	324	331	338	346	353	361	368	375	383	390	397
73	272	280	288	295	302	310	318	325	333	340	348	355	363	371	378	386	393	401	408
74	280	287	295	303	311	319	326	334	342	350	358	365	373	381	389	396	404	419	420
75	287	295	303	311	319	397	335	343	351	359	367	375	383	391	399	407	415	423	431
76	295	304	312	320	328	336	344	353	361	369	377	385	394	402	410	418	496	435	443

To use the table, find the appropriate height in the left-hand column. Move across to a given weight. The number at the top of the column is the BMI at that height and weight. Pounds have been rounded off.

Waist Circumference

Although BMI and waist circumference are frequently correlated, this is not always the case. For example, a person with thin arms and legs may have a low BMI and a high waist circumference. Because an individual with abdominal obesity is at a greater health risk than an individual with gluteal-femoral obesity, the panel recommends that the waist circumference be used to assess abdominal fat content. Men with a waist circumference greater than 40 inches, or 102 cm, and women with a waist circumference greater than 35 inches, or 88 cm, are at a high risk. A high waist circumference with a high BMI increases disease risk. In some populations, waist circumference is a better indicator of relative disease risk than is BMI; examples include Asian-Americans and persons of Asian descent living elsewhere. Waist circumference also assumes greater value at older ages. Individuals with a BMI greater than 35 kg /m² do not usually need to have their waist circumference measured because it usually is greater than the 40 and 35 inches.

Table 18–2 Classification of Overweight and Obesity by Body Mass Index (BMI)

	Obesity Class	BMI (kg/m²)
Underweight		<18.5
Normal		18.5 to 24.9
Overweight		25.0 to 29.9
Obesity	I	30.0 to 34.9
	II	35.0 to 39.9
Extreme Obesity	III	≥40

Source: National Institutes of Health: Clinical Guidelines on the Identification, Evaluation, and Treatment of Overweight and Obesity, 1998.

Prevalence of Overweight and Obesity

Prevalence means the total number of cases of a specific disease in an existing population at a certain time. The most recent NHANES III surveys, conducted from 1988 to 1994, reported that approximately 59 percent of men and 50 percent of women in the United States are either overweight or obese. Using the BMI definition for obesity, 20 percent of men and 25 percent of women are obese (National Institutes of Health, 1998), and an additional 39 percent of men and 25 percent of women are overweight (Fig. 18–2). The development of excess body weight is strongly influenced by age, sex, and economic, racial, and ethnic factors. For example, minority females are the most likely to be obese, with a 37 percent prevalence in non-Hispanic black female populations and a 33 percent prevalence in Mexican-American women.

Many experts are concerned about the incidence and prevalence of obesity in the nation's children. **Incidence** is defined as the frequency of occurrence of any event or condition over time and in relation to the population in which it occurs. Asian children have the lowest incidence of obesity. Native Americans have the highest incidence of obesity. Several studies suggest that one-third or more infants in the Western industrialized world are too heavy. Estimates for schoolchildren vary between 6 and 15 percent. Adolescent rates have been calculated at 20 to 30 percent (Pi-Sunyer, 1999). Clinical Application 18–1 discusses tips for weight control in young children.

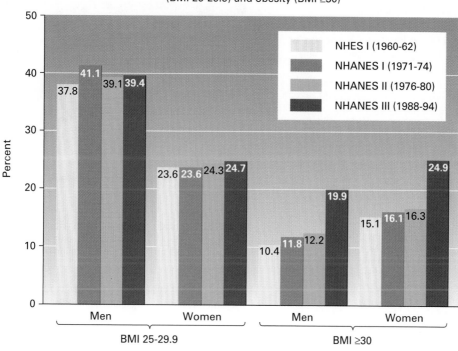

Figure 18–2:
Age-Adjusted Prevalence of Overweight (BMI 25 to 29.9) and Obesity (BMI ≥30)

Basic Science of Energy Imbalance

Nutrition is a science supported by a research base. The scientific method to understanding anything involves recognizing a problem, formulating a hypothesis (or question), accumulating data that answer the question, and analyzing the findings, as distinguished from an intuitive approach. As healthcare providers, we have a responsibility to understand the basic science behind the information we disseminate. The federal government's guidelines are based on science. The recommendations are based on evidence that has been replicated or a joint consensus of expert judgement (National Institutes of Health, 1998). Nursing students are encouraged to take a course in scientific methodology to learn how to evaluate scientific research. The science of nutrition is based on peer-reviewed research that can be replicated. Yet, all scientific information should be critically read and evaluated.

Energy Imbalance

Energy imbalance results when the number of kilocalories eaten does not equal the number used for energy. An individual can determine whether food intake is meeting energy needs by monitoring his or her weight. If more kilocalories are eaten than are used by the body, weight gain will occur. If fewer kilocalories are eaten than are used by the body (and protein intake is adequate), weight loss will occur. (A low protein intake over an extended period will eventually lead to fluid retention and a subsequent weight gain from the fluid retained. In this situation, energy imbalance is difficult to ascertain by body weight alone.) In cases in which a single healthcare provider or a group with access to the medical record follows the progress of a client for an extended time, energy balance can be assessed by monitoring the normally hydrated client's weight history.

There are two basic principles of energy imbalance. First, it takes a specific number of kilocalories to gain or lose a pound of body fat. Second, the body stores energy and uses stored energy in a highly specific manner.

The Five-Hundred Rule

To lose 1 pound of body fat per week, an individual must eat 500 kilocalories fewer per day than his or her body *expends* for 7 days. To gain 1 pound of body fat per week, the individual must eat 500 kilocalories more per day for 7 days than his or her body expends. The gain or loss of body fat need not occur during the course of a week; the kilocalorie surplus or deficit may occur over a month or year. The principle is the same. The total number of kilocalories required to gain or lose a pound of body fat is 3500. Wellness Tip 18–1 discusses one implication of the five-hundred rule.

Body Fat Stores

Excess kilocalories from any source (fat, carbohydrate, or protein) are stored as body fat in adipose tissue. The human body is able to store adi-

CLINICAL APPLICATION 18–1

Tips for Weight Control in Young Children

Obesity in young children is frequently genetic but it can be minimized by sound health habits. Following is a list of health habits that should be encouraged in young overweight children:

1. The more hours spent watching television, the heavier the child. For this reason, viewing time should be restricted to no more than 2 hours per day.
2. The more physical activity, the leaner the child. Thus the child should be encouraged to engage in all forms of physical activity. Examples of appropriate activity for very young children include ballet lessons, tricycle or bicycle riding, walking daily with another family member, swimming lessons, and sledding. Try to cultivate the enjoyment of year-round athletic activities in the child. See Figure 18–3.
3. The length of time the child spends chewing food may decrease the number of kilocalories the child spontaneously eats. Always serve fresh fruits and vegetables with every meal, including breakfast. Examples of low-kilocalorie snacks that require chewing include cut-up apples, peaches, pears, carrots, cucumbers, and green peppers.
4. Fat is the most concentrated source of calories. Try to limit the child's fat intake. Foods that contain fat include all meat, fish, and poultry. It is best to restrict the amount and the kind of meat, fish, and poultry eaten by the overweight child. The amount of meat a child should eat is frequently calculated by the dietitian. Some dairy products also are high in fat. The child should be encouraged to consume nonfat dairy products such as skim milk, partly skimmed cheeses, diet cheeses, and nonfat yogurt. Other sources of fat include salad dressings, margarine, nuts, seeds, oil, bacon, avocado, cream cheese, and sour cream.
5. Teach the child to be aware of what he or she eats.
6. Encourage the child to eat slowly. For example, serve a hot soup at the beginning of a meal. The child will have to wait for the soup to cool before it can be consumed.
7. Try not to make the child feel guilty about his or her weight problem. Again, recent research has shown that massive obesity in children is partly genetic. The child is not totally responsible for his or her present body weight. Try to be kind, patient, and considerate but firm.
8. Small daily decreases in energy expenditure may be significant over the course of a year. Lifestyle behaviors such as the use of television remote controls, telephone extensions, and garage door openers all decrease energy expenditure.
9. Fast food meals are positively associated with energy intake (Jeffrey, 1988).

Wellness Tip 18–1

- Too many kilocalories from any source of carbohydrates, fat, and/or protein promote weight gain.

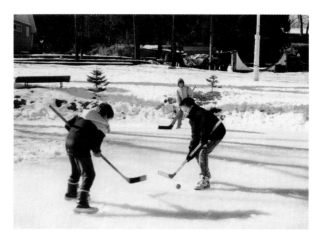

Figure 18–3:
Tips for Weight Control in Children (cited in Clinical Application 18–1.) Youngsters who engage in year-round sports activities are better able to maintain their weight than others.

pose fat tissue in unlimited amounts. This can lead to overweight and, eventually, **obesity**. During a kilocalorie deficit, the body first seeks the energy necessary to sustain body functions in glycogen stores, which are limited. When a kilocalorie deficit occurs for longer than about 1 day, the body seeks the energy necessary to sustain its functions in both body fat stores (adipose tissue) and body protein stores (organ and muscle mass).

Energy Imbalance and Body Composition

Weight loss affects body composition, and body composition affects health. The human body's two largest components are fat and lean body mass that includes protein. Protein is stored primarily in muscle tissue, organs, and certain body chemicals. Preservation of lean body mass and optimal health goes hand in hand. A loss of structural body content (e.g., heart and respiratory muscles, kidney, liver, body chemicals) is undesirable. Exercise can preserve and somewhat increase lean body mass. Weight gain increases body fat content. Weight loss decreases both body fat and lean body mass. An understanding of the difference between body fat content and lean body mass content is crucial to understanding the science of energy imbalance. The health benefits of weight loss are all related to a loss of body fat, and not a loss of lean body mass.

Loss of Fat Versus Loss of Water and Protein

Most people, especially the overweight, can lose only about 2 pounds of body fat a week by eating less. Any weight loss beyond that is probably due to loss of water and/or lean muscle tissue. There is always some loss of body protein along with body fat during weight loss. This is because lean body mass is more metabolically active and therefore burns more kilocalories than fat tissue. The loss of body protein from reduced food intake alone is greater than the loss of body protein from a combination of reduced food intake and regular exercise. Also, the greater the rate of weight loss, the more organ and muscle mass is lost. For example, Table

Table 18–3 Example of the Yo-Yo Effect—Weight Loss and Regain

Patient Information	Weight		
	Before Dieting	After Dieting for 2 Weeks	After Regain
Body weight (pounds)	217	204	217
Body fat (pounds)	70	66	79
Percent body fat	32.2 percent	32.2 percent	36 percent
Lean body mass lost		2.5 lb muscle and organ mass	
		6.5 lb water	
		4 lb fat	
		13 total lb*	

*Does not take into account that most people regain more weight than they originally lost.
Fat and lean body mass are inversely proportional. As one goes up, the other goes down. Water composition is directly proportional to lean body mass. About 72–73 per cent of lean body mass is water. Over a 12-week period on the diet, about 15 lb of muscle and organ mass (not including water) may be lost.

18–3 considers the client who loses 13 pounds of body weight over a 2-week period by diet alone.

Variation with the Severity of Obesity

Weight loss affects body composition of lean and obese people differently. The amount of lean body mass an individual loses during weight reduction depends on the degree of severity of his or her obesity. Obese animals tolerate starvation better than thin ones, and the same is true of humans (Forbes, 1999). "Tolerate" means that they conserve body protein during weight loss. This means overweight and mildly obese individuals are at a higher risk of becoming protein-depleted during rapid weight loss. Rapid weight loss (0.5–1.0 pounds per day), if sustained for many weeks, is associated with an excessive loss of lean body mass and protein depletion of the heart (Van Itallie, 1988). Malnutrition of the heart muscle can lead to sudden death. As individuals lose more and more fat during rapid weight loss, their ability to conserve lean body mass decreases. Thus, the length of time an individual diets as well as his or her beginning total body fat content has an impact on the amount of lean body mass lost.

Success Rates for Weight Loss

Weight cycling and type of diet can influence the weight loss success rate. Studies suggest that starvation and self-imposed dieting result in binge eating once food becomes available. Also, psychological manifestations, such as preoccupation with food and eating, increased emotional responsiveness and dysphoria (excessive anguish and depression) as well as distractibility (Polivy, 1996).

Weight Cycling

An individual who loses weight rapidly has difficulty maintaining weight loss. This is partly due to the loss of lean body mass (LBM). Because it takes fewer kilocalories to support fat than protein tissue, weight regain occurs. Most weight regained is in the form of body fat. Any weight regained is usually all body fat. When a client gains and loses weight repeatedly, it is called **yo-yo dieting** or **weight cycling**.

Consequences of Obesity

The problems of obesity can lead to many adverse consequences. The distribution of body fat affects a person's susceptibility to medical problems, and the psychological ramifications of obesity are significant. Clients are often enmeshed in a tangle of cultural, religious, emotional, societal, and perceptual issues. Many clients find great difficulty in breaking the cycle of behaviors that contribute to obesity. A greater understanding of each issue equips the healthcare provider with the tools necessary to educate and encourage overweight and obese clients.

Social

The social consequences of obesity are connected to cultural expectations and the documented prejudice many obese people experience.

Cultural Expectations

"Culture," in this context, refers to the convictions of a given people during a given period. Currently, many Americans are preoccupied with leanness. Leanness is perceived as being attractive and desirable. Fatness is perceived as being unattractive and undesirable. Yet what is and has been considered attractive has changed over time. Leanness has not always been the preferred body build. For example, during the 1800s, the overly fat body was considered the most attractive. Carrying excess weight meant that the person was well-to-do, that he or she could afford to overeat. Many experts think that our society is slowly changing perceptions of what is attractive. For example, women with well-developed muscles are perceived as being more attractive to many than her lean, not-so-muscular counterpart. The increased numbers of female bodybuilders demonstrate this attitudinal change.

In the United States, obese people have been under intense pressure to lose weight. This is evidenced by the $30 billion being spent on weight-reduction programs and special foods each year (Rosenbaum, 1999). In an effort to be more attractive, many obese clients try to lose weight. Over time, however, most people regain the weight they have lost and often regain an additional few pounds over and above their original weight. Thus, a self-defeating cycle begins.

Prejudice Documented

Several classic studies show that obese persons are the objects of prejudice and unfair discrimination. In a 7-year follow-up study of women 16–24 years old, obese women were less likely to have been married and had less schooling, lower incomes, and higher rates of household poverty than those with other chronic medical conditions (Gortmaker et al., 1993;

Box 18–1 Psychological Consequences of Food Restriction

Food restriction either voluntary or involuntary has consequences. Xenophon in ancient Greece described a "ravenous hunger" in soldiers who had been deprived of food during a military campaign (Stunkard, 1993). During World War II Keyes, et al. studied the effects of semistarvation on subjects (Keyes, et al. 1950). Cocina and Dixon studied the effects of food deprivation on rats (Cocina and Dixon, 1983). In all of these studies, the subjects responded to food deprivation with extraordinarily similar behaviors. First, restrained eaters did not necessarily have much, if any, long-term weight loss. Second, restraining one's eating makes one highly susceptible to bouts of excessive eating even after restrictions are lifted. Third, study subjects exhibited cognitive and emotional changes when food was restricted including: heightened emotional responsiveness; cognitive disruptions, including distractibility; and a focus on food and eating (Polivy, 1996).

Healthcare providers need to caution clients about the consequences of restrained eating. Overweight clients need to be helped to give up their weight reduction diets and to be advised to eat balanced healthful diets. Obese clients need to be taught to incorporate their favorite foods into more moderate levels of intake and to increase their physical activity. A reduction in counterproductive "restraint" seems likely to produce both physical and psychological well-being (Polivy, 1996).

Canning and Mayer, 1966). Healthcare workers should try to understand their own feelings about fatness, obesity, and obese persons. All too often, healthcare workers insult obese clients without being aware of it. For example, comments made in front of clients, such as "It will take three of us to move this client," are hurtful. Clients benefit when healthcare workers are sensitive to their psychological needs. Above all else, nurses should treat obese clients with respect, kindness, and patience.

Psychological

Obesity can be associated with a range of psychological problems, which may also result from food restriction (Box 18–1). On important psychological consequence of obesity is body image disturbances.

Body Image Disturbances

Body image is the mental picture a person has of himself or herself. A disturbed body image can manifest itself in two ways. First, people with distorted body images are usually dissatisfied with their bodies. Chronic complaints, demands for extra attention, and frequent negative statements made by clients about the way they look may be signs of an underlying body image disturbance. Second, persons with distorted body images frequently do not view their bodies realistically. For example, people may view themselves as having certain body parts larger than they actually are. A later section in this chapter discusses clients with anorexia nervosa, a mental health disorder, who frequently have body image disturbances. Very thin clients who have this condition frequently view themselves as overweight despite valid evidence to the contrary.

A classic study showed that body image disturbances are not found in emotionally healthy obese individuals (Stunkard and Mendelson, 1961). Body image disturbances are most common in young women of the middle and upper-middle classes who have been obese since childhood. Many of them have a generalized neurotic disturbance and their parents and peers have criticized them for their obesity (Stunkard and Burt, 1967; Stunkard and Mendelson, 1961).

Medical

Obesity is considered a major health problem in the United States and is also considered a chronic medical condition. Excessive body weight has been associated with nonfatal disease risks and chronic disease.

Life Expectancy

The relationship between life expectancy and severe obesity is clear: a severely obese client has a shorter life expectancy than his or her lean counterpart. Less clear is the relationship of overweight and less severe obesity to life expectancy. Some researchers are questioning whether obese clients do have a shorter life expectancy.

Recently a prospective study of more than one million adults in the United States was published (Calle et al., 1999). This study found a high body mass index was associated with an increased risk of death from all causes at all ages among men and women who had never smoked and had no history of disease. The lowest death rates were found at body masses between 23.5 and 24.9 in men and 22.0 and 23.4 in women. Death rates increased throughout the range of moderate and severe overweight for both men and women but less so for blacks, particularly black women. The risk of death increased with an increasing body mass index in all age groups and for all categories of the causes of death.

The risk of death is directly related to body mass index (BMI). Men and women with a BMI of about 30 or more had roughly 50 to 100 percent higher mortality than those with a body mass index below about 25. People with body mass values between 25 and 30 had an increased mortality rate of about 10 to 25 percent (Williamson, 1999). About 20 percent of the U.S. adult population has a body mass index of 30 or more (Flegal et al., 1998). Mortality rate is also elevated in persons with a low BMI (usually below 20) as well as in persons with a high BMI (World Health Organization, 1995).

Disease Risk

Obesity is associated with many chronic diseases. Obesity is strongly linked to heart disease as well as high blood pressure, high cholesterol levels, and noninsulin-dependent diabetes mellitus. Obesity is also associated with sleep apnea, gallbladder disease, fatty liver, lung function impairment, endocrine abnormalities, childbearing and childbirth complications, trauma to the weight-bearing joints, excessive protein in the urine, **dysphoria**, and increased hemoglobin concentration. Overweight men have higher rates for colorectal and prostate cancer, and overweight women have higher rates for cancer of the ovary and of the breast.

Many nonfatal risks are also associated with obesity. A nonfatal risk is a hazard that does not decrease life expectancy but does decrease the quality of life for an individual. Back and joint pain is one example of a nonfatal health risk. Much research is under way to determine whether weight loss can prevent chronic diseases; however, once **co-morbidity** factors are present, lifestyle strategies should be directed toward the improvement of metabolic parameters associated with the co-morbidity (Franz, 1998). Poor blood glucose levels were more closely associated with heart disease among clients with diabetes than was body weight. Therefore, healthcare providers may need to carefully consider whom they treat for obesity and why. Most experts recommend weight reduction counseling for the prevention of weight gain. On the other hand, treatment efforts for obese clients with a co-morbidity such as diabetes should be directed at normalization of blood glucose and lipid levels first and weight reduction second.

The distribution of body fat affects risks. Abdominal obesity is more dangerous than gluteal-femoral obesity (Bjorntorp, 1986). In **abdominal obesity** the excess weight is between the client's chest and pelvis. Clients with abdominal obesity are said to be shaped like an apple. Clients with abdominal obesity are especially vulnerable to chronic disease risks associated with excessive body weight. In **gluteal-femoral obesity** the excess weight is around the client's buttocks, hips, and thighs. Clients with gluteal-femoral obesity are said to be pear-shaped. Clients with

gluteal-femoral obesity are not as susceptible to chronic disease risks associated with excessive body fat.

The treatment of obesity is an important means of controlling some major chronic and degenerative diseases. For example, blood pressure levels can be reduced by a diet high in fruits and vegetables and low in fat (Franz, 1998). Up to four servings of fruits and five servings of vegetables are recommended.

Factors that Influence Food Intake

Food choices and exercise patterns have a major influence on food intake. However, in recent years, numerous hormones and neuropeptides that stimulate or inhibit food intake through central or peripheral mechanisms have been identified and investigated in experimental models, as have molecules that affect metabolic rates and energy expenditure (Lowell and Spiegelman, 2000). Figure 18–4 illustrates multiple molecules and pathways involved in internal food intake regulation. In general, there is

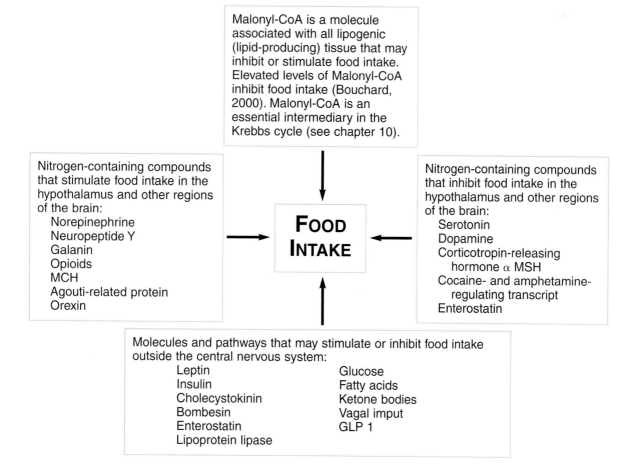

Figure 18–4:
The hormones, molecules, and pathways that influence food intake through central or peripheral mechanisms. Source: Adapted from Bouchard, C: Inhibition of food intake by inhibitors of fatty acid synthase. N Eng J Med. 343:25,. p.1889 December, 21, 2000.

Box 18–2 Frequently Asked Questions About Theories of Obesity

CAN A MALFUNCTIONING HYPOTHALAMUS CAUSE WEIGHT GAIN?

The brain partially controls hunger and satiety. The hypothalamus in the brain appears to be the center for weight control. Satiety is the feeling of satisfaction after eating. Appetite refers to the pleasant sensation based on previous experience that causes a person to seek food to eat. Hunger is the physical sensation caused by a lack of food, characterized by a dull or acute pain at or around the lower portion of the chest. A malfunctioning hypothalamus could cause an individual to receive incorrect hunger signals, thus stimulating continued eating and signaling weight gain. Appetite, satiety, and hunger may be incorrectly processed by a malfunctioning hypothalamus.

Various areas of the hypothalamus are sensitive to at least 13 neurochemicals, and these areas are involved in the regulation of hunger, eating, and satiety (Wooley and Hunt, 1998). The ventromedial nucleus and the lateral lobe in the hypothalamus are the two most significant areas. The ventromedial nucleus, which is activated by serotonin and antagonized by norepinephrine, mediates satiety. The lateral lobe, which is activated by norepinephrine and or dopamine and antagonized by serotonin, mediates hunger and thirst (Wooley and Hunt, 1998). Selective hypothalamic neurotransmitters are now being considered as medications to alter the brain sensation of hunger, appetite, and satiety. However, more research is necessary to better understand long-term and short-term effects of these medications.

IS OBESITY THE RESULT OF POOR METABOLISM?

Some obese individuals actually require fewer kilocalories for normal body functions than do lean individuals. Some obese individuals use kilocalories very efficiently and may have poor metabolism.

WHAT IS THE FUNCTION OF BROWN FAT, AND HOW DOES IT AFFECT OBESITY?

Brown fat, a special type of fat cell, accounts for less than 1 percent of total body weight. The function of brown fat is to burn kilocalories and release the energy as heat. Energy released as heat is not stored as body fat. Some obese people may have defective brown fat or less brown fat than lean people.

WHAT IS THE SET POINT THEORY?

The set point theory argues that each individual has a unique, relatively stable, adult body weight that is the result of several biologic factors. The obese person may have a higher set point than his or her lean counterpart.

WHY SHOULD THE NUMBER OF FAT CELLS IN THE BODY INFLUENCE WEIGHT?

Obese individuals have many more fat cells than do their lean counterparts. A kilocalorie deficit can reduce the fat in each cell but cannot break down the entire cell. Once manufactured, a fat cell exists until death. Empty fat cells pressure the reduced obese person to fill the depleted cells. The reduced obese person must learn to constantly ignore internal hunger signals. Although obese individuals are able to do this for a short period, long-term adaptation to hunger pains is difficult.

ARE THERE ANY ENZYMES IN THE METABOLIC CHAIN THAT CONTRIBUTE TOWARD OBESITY?

Lipoprotein lipase is an enzyme that is involved in the uptake of fatty acids for the manufacture of fat in individual fat cells. Research has shown that the activity of this enzyme increases during weight reduction. This action makes the fat cell even more efficient in synthesizing fats.

REFERENCES

Lindpaintner, K: Finding an obesity gene—A rate of mice and men. N Engl J Med 332:679, 1995.
Rohner-Jeanrenaud, F,. and Jeanrenaud, B: Obesity, leptin, and the brain. N Engl J Med 334:324, 1996.

---

redundancy and counterbalance among these pathways so that, for instance, the inhibitory effect of one molecule is dampened by another. This complex redundancy and counterbalance makes the effective treatment of obesity complex. Perhaps in the future, as researchers learn more about the human energy balance system, more effective and safe treatments for energy imbalances may be available.

Theories about Obesity

Theories about obesity are plentiful (Box 18–2). The truth may be that any one of these theories is accurate for a specific client but that none is true for everyone. For example, research has shown that obese mice have a deficiency of the hormone leptin. Some researchers have referred to an obesity gene called ob gene. The ob gene produces leptin, a hormone that, if all is working correctly, helps to prevent obesity. Leptin is produced by the adipocytes and travels through the blood presumably to the hypothalamus. Leptin appears to act as an adipostat by signaling the brain regarding adipose tissue stores. Administration of exogenous leptin to deficient rodents leads to decreased food intake, increased metabolic activity, and weight loss (Shils, 1999). Many experts think leptin acts as an afferent satiety signal. There is a strong correlation among serum leptin concentrations, percentage body fat, and the body mass index. However, some obese mice have elevated levels of leptin in their serum. For this group of mice, the pathology is not a deficiency of leptin but perhaps a receptor or a postreceptor defect in the hypothalamus. Leptin studies have been done mostly in mice, not humans, and further research is necessary to provide a better understanding of the metabolic implications of the plasma leptin concentrations in humans.

Identical twins raised in different environments (adopted and non-adopted) have been studied extensively. From these studies, many experts believe obesity is about 33 percent genetic and 66 percent environmental (food and exercise behaviors) (Romsos, 1996). Keep the theories in Box 18–2 in mind when counseling a client who is overweight, obese, or underweight. There is more than one cause for the development and maintenance of obesity. However, body weight can be decreased by a modification of food and exercise behaviors. Health care professionals should not give up treating these clients. Overweight and obese clients in well-designed programs can achieve a weight loss of as much as 10 percent of baseline weight, a weight loss than can be maintained for a sustained period of time (1 year or longer) (National Institutes of Health, 1998).

Fad Diets

Many kinds of fad diets have come and gone. Typically, such diets limit the person to a few specific foods or food combinations. For example, one common fad diet recommends the consumption of a high fat content, and carbohydrates are restricted. This diet does not meet the recommendations of the American Heart Association, the American Cancer Society, and the American Dietetic Association and may be harmful. High fat intake has been associated with many chronic and degenerative diseases. Another example of a fad diet is the grapefruit diet. On this diet, the individual is allowed only grapefruit. Such a diet cannot possibly lead to a lifelong change in eating behaviors and is not nutritionally balanced.

A high-protein, low-carbohydrate diet for weight reduction is currently very popular. One version recommends a 40–45 percent protein, a 30–35 percent fat, and a 20–25 percent carbohydrate kilocaloric distribution. These diets tend to be high in saturated fat and cholesterol and low in vitamins A and C and thiamin and iron (Pi-Sunyer, 1999). Risk of heart disease increases because serum LDL cholesterol increases along with homocysteine (see Chapter 20). The National Cancer Institute believes the elimination of fruits, vegetables, whole grains, and beans may increase the risk of cancer. Athletic performance is reduced on a low-carbohydrate diet (www.foodandhealth.com) because a high-carbohydrate diet can enhance performance during strenuous athletic events. Rising blood pressure and elevated uric acid levels from too much protein may cause gout. Uric acid and calcium oxalate stones are more likely to form on a high-protein diet. Over time, excess protein intake, especially from animal sources, increases the loss of calcium in the urine, which may contribute to osteoporosis (www.foodandhealth.com).

Screening

How do health professionals decide whom to treat or not treat? Not all clients should be encouraged to lose weight. Repeating gaining and losing weight is harmful. Inappropriate weight loss methods, including repeated crash diets, can have damaging effects on physical health and psychological well-being.

Responsible weight loss programs screen clients for the following.

1. Is weight loss indicated for this client? Is the client internally motivated to lose weight? The basic motivation to undergo treatment must originate from the client.

2. What level of health supervision is necessary? Are clients screened for psychosocial conditions that would make weight loss inappropriate? Are clients at medical risk, requiring a physician's care?

3. What factors in the client's history and lifestyle are relevant to the weight loss program? For example, a weight loss program that costs a significant amount of money may not be affordable for low-income clients.

4. Does the diet attempt to adapt weight-reduction approaches to the needs of diverse client groups?

The best candidates for weight reduction are those who express the desire to change their total lifestyle. The client must be motivated enough to agree to participate in routine exercise program, follow a low-kilocalorie diet, and change lifelong food behaviors. A significant time investment on the client's part is necessary. Capacity to succeed is best demonstrated by deeds rather than words. For example, will the client attend all program sessions and self-monitor his or her food intake?

In addition, the best candidates for weight reduction are not under stress currently. Stressful life events such as a recent divorce, death of a significant other, or change in living situation or job status decrease the chances of success.

Most individuals associate weight loss with being more attractive. The association between weight loss and wellness is a secondary consideration. The health benefits of weight loss are related to a loss of body fat, not a loss of lean body mass. The individual who loses a high amount of lean body mass rather than fat derives minimal health benefits from weight loss.

Setting Realistic Goals

Nurses can assist clients in setting realistic goals for weight reduction. Often clients have an unrealistic weight loss goal. For example, the weight reduction diet may be planned to allow for a one pound per week weight loss. The client may expect to lose five pounds per week. A female client may expect to be able eventually to wear a size 5 dress as a result of dieting. This is not a realistic expectation for some clients with large bones.

All overweight clients should be educated to stop gaining weight. Healthcare workers provide a valuable service when they teach clients how to prevent weight gain.

Federal Guidelines on the Identification of Overweight and Obesity in Adults

There are clearly advantages to weight loss by overweight and obese clients. Chief among the reasons to avoid weight gain is to decrease the risk of disease and treat some persons who already have an obesity-related disorder. The treatment of energy imbalances depends on an understanding of the degree of overweight and obesity.

Advantages of Weight Loss

The panel that developed the federal clinical guidelines for the identification of overweight and obesity in adults focused on the medical benefits to be derived from weight loss. This panel recommended:

- Weight loss to lower blood pressure in overweight and obese persons with high blood pressure.
- Weight loss to lower elevated levels of cholesterol, low-density lipoprotein cholesterol, and triglycerides and to raise low levels of high-density lipoprotein cholesterol in overweight and obese persons with dyslipidemia (see Chapter 20).
- Some weight loss to lower elevated blood glucose levels in overweight and obese persons with type 2 diabetes.

Measurement of Degree of Overweight and Obesity

According to the federal guidelines, practitioners should use the body mass index and waist circumference to classify the degree of energy imbalance in clients. Body weight alone can be used to follow weight loss and to determine efficacy of treatment (National Institutes of Health, 1998). The reason the use of BMI is advocated in clinical practice is ease of measurement and cost.

Other Risk Factors

Persons with cardiovascular disease or diabetes mellitus with evident obesity should be evaluated for weight loss. The panel recognized that the decision to quit smoking should be given priority over weight loss.

Federal Guidelines on the Evaluation and Treatment of Overweight and Obesity

The federal guidelines address goals for weight loss, how to achieve weight loss, goals for weight maintenance, how to maintain weight loss, and special treatment groups.

Goals for Weight Loss

The initial goal of weight loss should be to reduce body weight by 10 percent from the baseline. With success, further weight loss can be attempted, if indicated. Safe weight loss occurs at about 1–2 pounds per week for a period of 6 months, with the subsequent strategy based on the amount of weight lost (National Institutes of Health, 1998).

How to Achieve Weight Loss

The panel explores a variety of weight loss options to achieve weight loss, including dietary therapy, physical activity, behavior therapy, combined therapy, pharmacotherapy, and weight loss surgery. The approach taken should depend on professional evaluation and the client's BMI, waist circumference, and other risk factors (National Institutes of Health, 1998).

Diet Therapy

A diet for weight loss would be reduced in total kilocalories but adequate in all nutrients. The diet should contain adequate protein, all essential vita-

mins and minerals, a small amount of fat, dietary fiber, and enough carbohydrate to prevent ketosis (Nonas, 1998). More specifically, the diet should provide at least 100 grams of carbohydrate, 25–35 grams of fiber, no more than 30 percent fat and 10 percent saturated fat, and the recommended daily allowance (RDA) for the essential nutrients. The meal plan should be one the client can and will follow. When clients are given a standardized meal plan on paper, weight loss is not usually successful. However, when behavior modification, nutritional counseling, and exercise recommendations support the meal plan, weight loss can be more successful.

Different clients need different types of meal plans or dietary directions. A few clients just want to be told what to eat and will follow through with appropriate behaviors. Some clients want and require simplified instructions. They do not want to invest the time in learning a complicated diet. A Food Pyramid Guide dietary plan may work well for this type of client (provided behavior modifications and the need for exercise are also discussed). Portion control needs to be emphasized with this approach. Reasonable portion sizes are indicated on most versions of Food Pyramid Guides.

A common tool used for teaching clients how to eat to lose weight is the American Diabetic and Dietetic Association's Exchange Lists. This approach has been successful for clients who want detailed information and are willing to invest the time required to learn food exchanges. This approach clearly spells out portion sizes. The ADA Exchange Lists are located in Appendix A. Sometimes clients are unable to change their food intake so drastically. In this situation, nutritional counselors should encourage clients to make major behavioral changes in their eating habits slowly. The goal in weight-reduction counseling is to help the client make permanent lifestyle changes. The current recommendation is that clients should be encouraged to change only one or two negative food behaviors at a time. For example, if the nutrition counselor recommends that the client substitute skim milk for whole milk, it is not wise to simultaneously discourage the use of sweets. The goal is to encourage permanent changes in eating behavior, so the client needs time to make the necessary adjustments. With this in mind, perhaps it is best to review one exchange list at a time with some clients. After the client has changed negative behaviors associated with one exchange list, recommendations can be suggested to change negative behaviors associated with another exchange list. Changing a negative behavior usually take several weeks. Priority should be given to eliminating foods in the fat, milk, and meat lists that are high in fat and in which the client overindulges. An average woman will lose weight on a 1200-kilocalorie diet. Larger women and most men will lose weight on a 1500-kilocalorie diet.

Physical Activity

Population studies conducted in the United States, Great Britain, and France have suggested that the rapidly increasing prevalence of obesity in recent decades may be largely due to increasing sedentary behaviors, perhaps to a greater extent than dietary excesses (Weinser et al., 1998). The propensity to be physically inactive seems to be at least partly determined by genetics. Individuals with certain body builds may be genetically predisposed to engage in less spontaneous physical activity and to have relatively low energy requirements. However, physical activity behaviors also influence whether we stay lean or become obese. One study showed that within twin pairs, the twin who reported being more physically active was generally less obese than the more sedentary sibling (Samaras et al., 1999).

The panel recommends that physical activity is part of a comprehensive weight loss therapy and weight maintenance program because it: (1) modestly contributes to weight loss in overweight and obese adults, (2) may decrease abdominal fat, (3) increases cardiopulmonary fitness, and (4) may help with weight loss. The combination of a reduced-kilocalorie diet and increased physical activity is recommended because it produces weight loss, decreases abdominal fat, and increases cardiopulmonary fitness. Initially, moderate levels of exercise for 30–45 minutes 3–5 days per week should be encouraged. All adults should set a long-term goal to accumulate at least 30 minutes or more of moderate-intensity physical activity on most, and preferably all, days of the week. (National Institutes of Health, 1998). Wellness Tip 18–2 encourages exercise.

To identify those individuals at a major heart disease risk, a physician should screen all clients before exercise recommendations are made. Clients with known heart, lung, or metabolic disease should have a physician-supervised stress test before beginning an exercise program.

When following an exercise program, fluid intake should be adequate. Individuals should drink water before, during, and after exercise. Close attention should be paid to thirst to prevent dehydration. Four ounces of water every 15 minutes is usually sufficient, but at very high temperatures this may not be adequate. The thirst mechanism may not be adequate to prevent dehydration in many elderly persons and in individuals involved in heavy exercise during hot weather. Such persons need to be taught to drink water even if they are not thirsty.

Behavior Modification

Behavior modification is a useful adjunct when incorporated into treatment for weight loss and weight maintenance. A client's motivation to enter weight-loss therapy and his or her readiness to implement the weight-control plan require evaluation. Permanent weight loss can result only from a permanent change in eating and exercise behaviors. The behavioral strategies most commonly applied in weight-reduction programs include self-monitoring, stimulus control, slowed-down eating, a reward system, and cognitive behavior modification. Table 18–4 lists specific techniques used to help clients modify their behaviors. See Wellness Tip 18–3.

SELF-MONITORING Clients keep their own food records, track their body weights, and record exercise completed during self-monitoring. Many clients come to regard self-monitoring of their food intake as the single most helpful strategy in a weight-reduction program. Recording of food intake seems to work best when clients know they must turn in the records to their nutritional counselor.

Requiring clients to monitor their weight once a week is also a helpful behavioral strategy. When clients are gaining weight, they tend to avoid scales and mirrors (Foreyt, 1996). Requiring clients to weigh themselves

Table 18–4 Weight Control: Behavior Modification Techniques

Self-Monitoring
- Keep a food diary and record all food intake.
- Keep a weekly graph of weight change.
- Keep an exercise diary.

Stimulus Control
- At home, limit all food intake to one specific place.
- Plan food intake for each day.
- Rearrange your schedule to avoid inappropriate eating.
- Sit down at a table while eating.
- At a party, sit a distance from snack foods, eat before you go, and substitute lower kilocalorie drinks for alcohol.
- Decide beforehand what you will order at a restaurant.
- Save or reschedule everyday activities for times when you are hungry.
- Avoid boredom; keep a list of activities on the refrigerator.

Slowed-Down Eating
- Drink a glass of water before each meal. Drink sips of water between bites of food.
- Swallow food before putting more food on the utensil.
- Try to be the last one to finish eating.
- Pause for a minute during your meal and attempt to increase the number of pauses.

Reward Yourself
- Chart your progress.
- Make an agreement with yourself or a significant other for a meaningful reward.
- Do not reward yourself with food.

Cognitive Strategies
- View exercise as a means of controlling hunger.
- Practice relaxation techniques.
- Imagine yourself ordering a side salad, diet dressing, low-fat milk, and a small hamburger at a fast-food restaurant.
- Visualize yourself enjoying a fresh apple in preference to apple pie.

helps to keep them on their eating plan. Clients should also be asked to record their exercise in a notebook. Again, the notebook should be reviewed regularly in the training program.

STIMULUS CONTROL **Stimulus-control** strategies are designed to help clients rearrange their lifestyle to reduce the chances of inappropriate eating habits. Clients are taught to examine their behaviors to determine which ones may trigger them to eat inappropriately. For example, a truck driver may eat two doughnuts every morning for breakfast because he or she drives past the bakery on the way to work. The nutritional counselor may recommend that this client take a different route to work to reduce the probability of his or her buying doughnuts.

Wellness Tip 18–2

- Everyone should set a long-term goal to accumulate 30 minutes or more of moderate-intensity physical activity on most days of the week.

Wellness Tip 18–3

- To lose weight, keep a food diary. Behavior modification in combination with exercise helps prevent weight gain and promote weight loss.

SLOWED-DOWN EATING Some overweight and obese people eat very rapidly. It takes approximately 20 minutes from the time food has been eaten for the brain to receive the message that food has been consumed. An individual can consume many extra kilocalories in 20 minutes. These clients are frequently taught a number of behavioral techniques to slow down their eating.

REWARD SYSTEM Many clients respond better to any type of suggested behavioral change when they are working for specific rewards. In one program, for example, a client earns tokens whenever he or she performs a desirable behavior. The tokens are redeemable at the hospital's gift shop for merchandise.

COGNITIVE STRATEGIES Many weight-reduction programs include cognitive strategies. The goal of cognitive strategies is to increase the client's knowledge of his or her eating behaviors so that he or she can develop skills to cope with inappropriate behaviors. Teaching the client to relax is one type of cognitive strategy. The use of imagery is another, for example, asking clients to imagine themselves coping successfully with anxiety-arousing events.

Pharmacotherapy

Weight-loss drugs approved by the FDA may be used as part of a comprehensive weight-loss program including diet and physical activity for clients with a BMI greater than or equal to 30 with no concomitant obesity-related risk factors or diseases according to the new federal guidelines. For clients with a BMI greater than or equal to 27 with concomitant obesity-related risk factors or diseases, medications may also be indicated. Drugs should never be used without lifestyle modification (National Institutes of Health, 1998). Drug therapy for obesity should be continually monitored for efficacy and safety and discontinued if the client does not lose weight. Table 18–5 lists weight-loss medications, actions, and adverse effects. Many researchers have come to the conclusion that long-term treatment, including pharmacotherapy, may be necessary for many obese clients (Poston, 1998). However, few medications approved by the FDA are available for long-term treatment of obesity, they do not work for all individuals, and on average they induce only modest weight loss (Yanorski and Yanorski, 1999).

Weight Loss Surgery

Weight loss surgery is an option in carefully selected clients with clinically severe obesity (BMI ≥40, or ≥35 with co-morbid conditions) when less invasive methods of weight loss have failed and the client is at high risk for obesity-associated morbidity or mortality (National Institutes of Health, 1998).

Many different surgical procedures have been and are being used to treat obesity. The removal of fat tissue through a vacuum hose is called **liposuction**. **Lipectomy** is surgical removal of adipose tissue. Both of these procedures are done more for cosmetic reasons than for weight control. A **jejunoileal bypass** involves the removal of a part of the small intestine. Clients lose weight after this procedure because they cannot absorb all the food they eat, although this places these clients at a nutritional risk. All gastric (stomach) procedures either route food around (bypass) or through only part of the stomach (reduction). Diagrams of **gastric stapling** and **gastric bypass (roux-en-Y)**, two common procedures, are shown in Fig. 18–5. When the stomach is smaller or reduced, only a limited amount of food can be consumed at one feeding. This induces weight loss from reduced kilocalorie intake. Clinical Application 18–2 discusses problems that clients often encounter after gastric surgery for weight reduction and suggests general guidelines for these clients to follow. Clients should be followed carefully postoperatively due to risks for deficiencies such as iron, folacin, and vitamin B_{12}. Clients are also at risk for maladaptive eating behavior (Fahey and Miller, 1997).

The results that can be expected from gastric surgery procedures should always be spelled out to clients. No permanent effects can be promised, and having the surgery does not mean that afterward the client can overeat indefinitely without weight gain. Ninety percent of weight loss occurs in the first year, and clients often begin to gain again in the second and third years. Only a minority achieve a weight as low as 125 percent of HBW. The procedure should be viewed as a tool to be used in conjunction with behavioral training—the small pouch helps clients learn to reduce the amount of food consumed and slows down their intake. After the first year, due to stretching of the pouch or intestinal adaptation, much of the effect of the surgery can be negated and the lost weight ay be regained.

Goals for Weight Loss Maintenance

Weight regain often occurs after weight loss. A program of dietary therapy, physical activity, and behavior therapy enhances the likelihood of weight loss maintenance. Drug therapy can also be used according to the guidelines published by the National Institutes of Health; however, drug safety and efficacy beyond 1 year of total treatment have not been established.

Table 18–5 Weight Loss Drugs+

Drug	Action	Adverse Effects
Dexfenfluramine*	Serotonin reuptake inhibitor	Valvular heart disease
Fenfluramine*	Serotonin releaser	Primary pulmonary hypertension
		Neurotoxicity
Sibutramine	Norepinephrine, dopamine and serotinin reuptake inhibitor	Increase in heart rate and blood pressure
Orlistat±	Inhibits pancreatic lipase, decreases fat absorption	Decrease in absorption of fat-soluble vitamins
		Soft stools and anal leakage
		Possible link to breast cancer

+Ephedrine, caffeine, and fluoxetine have also been tested for weight loss, but are not approved for use in the treatment of obesity.
 Mazindol, phentermine, benzphetamine, and phendimetrazine are approved for only short-term use for the treatment of obesity.
*FDA approval withdrawn
±FDA approval pending

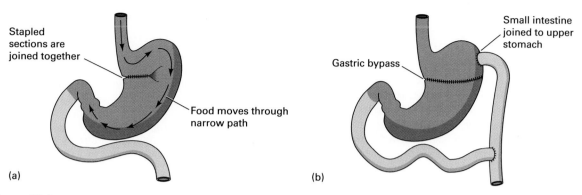

Figure 18–5:
Illustrations of two common surgical procedures used to treat obesity: (A) gastric stapling and (B) gastric bypass

CLINICAL APPLICATION 18–2

Complications of Gastroplasty and Gastric Bypass

There are many potential acute complications of gastric surgery for weight reduction. These include:

1. Nausea, vomiting, bloating, and/or heartburn: These signs and symptoms can be caused by overeating, not chewing food well, eating too quickly, drinking cold or carbonated beverages, using drinking straws, or eating gassy foods.
2. Staple disruption (for gastric stapling procedures): The result of loosened staples is that a larger intake of food is necessary before satiety can be achieved. Excessive food intake or vomiting can cause the staples to become disrupted.
3. Obstruction: An obstruction is the blockage of a structure. In this case, a blockage can occur close to the area stapled. A frequent cause of obstruction is poorly chewed food. The result is stomach pain, nausea, and vomiting.
4. Dumping syndrome: Intake of concentrated sweets and large quantities of fluids cause quick dumping of food into the small intestine. Abdominal fullness, nausea, diarrhea 15 minutes after eating, warmth, weakness, fainting, racing pulse, and cold sweats are symptoms of this syndrome.
5. Among the long-term risks is osteoporosis, due to decreased calcium absorption

Guidelines for the Client Following Gastric Surgery for Weight Reduction

The client who has had gastric surgery for weight reduction may find the following general guidelines helpful:

1. Eat three to six small meals per day.
2. Eat slowly.
3. Chew food thoroughly.
4. Eat very small quantities.
5. Stop eating when full.
6. Drink most fluids between meals.
7. Select a balanced diet.
8. Take a multivitamin-multimineral supplement.
9. Exercise regularly.

How Weight Loss Is Maintained

The literature suggests using weight loss and weight maintenance therapies that provide a greater frequency of contacts between clients and practitioners over the long term. This can lead to more successful weight loss and weight maintenance (National Institutes of Health, 1998).

Obese clients who successfully lost weight and kept the lost weight off report the following (Foreyt, 1993):

- Clients who have kept off excess body weight report they have at least 30 minutes of moderate exercise each day, have a strong social support network, lost the weight gradually over a 6-month period, changed their attitudes toward their body weight, and made realistic lifestyle changes.
- They eat smaller portion sizes.
- They avoid food high in fat.
- Seventy-seven percent of clients who kept food records kept off previously lost weight versus 29 percent who did not keep food records.
- They eat a minimum of 35 servings of fruits and vegetables per week.
- They undereat two days per week.
- Nutritional portioned foods (Weight Watchers or Healthy Choice TV dinners and diet beverages) as meal replacements were widely used by successful dieters.
- The most frequently reported exercise was walking.
- The more structured the weight loss program was, the more successful the participants were.

The Role of Nutrition Educators

All healthcare workers become confused about their role as nutrition educators. Appropriate roles for nutrition educators include:

- Provide accurate information.
- Warn against dangerous practices such as self-imposed starvation diets that eliminate one or more of the major food groups and encourage the intake of only one food group.
- Guide clients to understand the risks and benefits of weight loss and weight-loss programs, products, medicines, procedures.
- Teach clients to evaluate the risks and benefits for themselves.
- When appropriate, refer clients to healthcare professionals, including physicians and dietitians.

• In states where there are regulations, assist in efforts to enforce these standards for safe weight loss.

Special Treatment Groups

The federal panel discussed three groups of people that merit special consideration: smokers, older adults, and culturally diverse groups. All smokers, regardless of their weight status, should first quit smoking. Prevention of further weight gain should be encouraged. If weight gain occurs, it should be treated through diet, physical activity, and behavior therapy, maintaining the primary emphasis on abstinence from smoking (National Institutes of Health, 1998). Weight reduction in older adults should be guided by an evaluation of the potential benefits of weight loss for day-to-day functioning and reduction of the risk of future cardiovascular events, as well as the client's motivation to lose weight. Care should be taken in this group to ensure that any weight loss program minimizes the likelihood of adverse effects on bone health or other aspects of nutritional status. A standard approach to weight loss may work differently in different cultural groups, a factor that must be considered when setting expectations about treatment outcomes. For example, female subjects who participated in one study indicated that weight control methods and socioenvironmental context in which they conduct their lives merits attention (Tyler, Allan, and Alcozer, 1997).

Prevention of Overweight and Obesity

The current epidemic of obesity is partially caused by an environment that promotes excessive food intake and discourages physical activity (Hill and Peters, 1998). Prevention of excess body fat is the key to a healthy body weight. Clinical Application 18–3 offers some ways to prevent and control excess body fat. Figure 18–6 illustrates the crucial need to provide opportunities for children to engage in enjoyable physical activity.

The Client with Reduced Body Mass

Clients with a reduced body mass are as difficult, if not more difficult, to treat as overly fat clients. Body fat has important roles in insulation and protection of body organs. A client with a low body fat content usually has a loss of lean body mass as well, and loss of this functioning tissue concerns clinicians. Women cease to ovulate and menstruate when the percent of body fat falls below a certain level. The client may experience cardiac abnormalities and become more prone to infections. These clients are at risk for osteoporosis in the long term.

Classification

Methods similar to those used to diagnose overly fat clients can be used to diagnose clients with reduced body mass. A person whose weight is more than 15 percent below a reasonable body weight (RBW) may be classified as underweight. A man with a body fat content less than 15 percent and a woman with a body fat content less than 18 percent may be classified as having a reduced body mass. A BMI less than 20 percent may indicate that the client has a reduced body mass.

CLINICAL APPLICATION 18–3

Prevention and Control of Excess Body Fat

Weight maintenance is the key to weight control. How can we as healthcare workers help out clients to achieve and maintain a healthy body weight?

We know it takes more kilocalories to support body protein content than body fat content. Healthcare workers should first encourage patients to exercise more to increase their body protein content. Many experts believe that our society's increasingly sedentary lifestyle may be responsible for the increasing prevalence of obesity.

Second, eating fat is fattening. Here are some reasons to avoid dietary fat:

1. Teaspoon for teaspoon, fat contains more kilocalories than either carbohydrate or protein.

2. There is very little energy cost to convert fat in food to body fat. Carbohydrates in food must be converted to fat before carbohydrate can be stored in fat cells. This conversion requires an expenditure of kilocalories. Kilocalories used to convert carbohydrate in food to body fat are not stored as body fat.

3. Once a fat cell has been manufactured, there is no evidence that it can ever be broken down; it exists until death. When dieting, a person can reduce the amount of fat in each fat cell but not break down the cell completely. Some researchers believe that an empty fat cell sends a message to the reduced-obese person's brain to eat. The reduced-obese/overweight person must learn to cope with a message constantly coming from the brain to eat. This is another reason why it is very difficult for a client to keep weight off permanently. Prevention of weight gain is the easiest way to maintain a reasonable body weight.

Third, a low-fiber intake may predispose a client to obesity. Fiber has a high satiety value. Obesity is uncommon among the populations of countries where a high proportion of dietary kilocalories is consumed as starchy vegetables. Educating clients to eat the recommended six servings of starch and five to nine servings of fruits and vegetables may help clients achieve satiety. Many starches, fruits, and vegetables contain appreciable amounts of fiber. There is some evidence that fiber consumption may predict weight gain more strongly than total or saturated fat consumption (Ludwig et al., 1999).

Adherence to a low-fat and low-fiber diet will not always result in a permanent weight loss. An individual can still gain weight on a low-fat diet if he or she overeats foods high in carbohydrates. Portion control is important. For some people, the most valuable information on the food label is the serving size.

To summarize, the healthcare worker can educate clients to (1) exercise more, (2) eat less fat, (3) eat more fiber, and (4) use portion control.

One method to determine whether a client is eating enough food is to monitor his or her food intake. Kilocalorie intake is monitored by recording actual food consumption and calculating the kilocalories eaten.

Eating Disorders

Eating disorders may be caused by psychological factors and may result in nutritional problems. Many experts are concerned about the prevalence of anorexia nervosa and bulimia.

Anorexia Nervosa

Anorexia nervosa is a medical condition that results from self-imposed starvation. Symptoms include:

1. Loss of 20–40 percent of usual body weight (UBW); refer to Clinical Calculation 18–2 to calculate UBW
2. Decreased resting energy expenditure (REE)
3. **Amenorrhea** (cessation of menstruation)
4. Constipation
5. Excessive hair loss
6. Abnormal sleeping patterns
7. Preoccupation with food
8. Body image disturbance
9. Misconception about physical status
10. Intake of only 500–800 kilocalories per day
11. Slow eating
12. Increased physical activity
13. Social isolation
14. Intense fear of becoming obese
15. Poor muscle tone

This disorder may be life threatening. Among females, the disorder begins before age 20 in one-half and three-fourths before age 21. This disorder occurs 8–12 times more frequently in females than males (Huse and Lucas, 1999). The client may resort to a variety of devices to lose weight, including starvation, vomiting, and laxative use.

Bulimia

Bulimia is much more common than anorexia nervosa, especially during adolescence and young adulthood. The mean age for females at diagnosis was 23 years. The prevalence rates have been as high as 9 percent (Huse and Lucas, 1999). The condition is rare in males. Bulimics binge and purge.

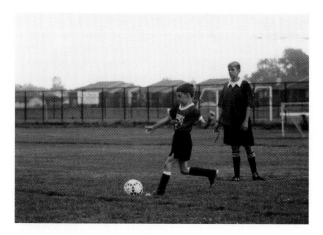

Figure 18–6:
The parents who provide their child with the opportunity to engage in physical activity have given that child a special gift with life-long benefits.

Consequences

Long-term follow-up of studies indicates that excessive leanness is associated with increased mortality and decreased life expectancy. However, the causes of mortality are different from those associated with excess weight. An excessively lean person is almost twice as likely to succumb to respiratory diseases such as tuberculosis. In addition, these clients have greater difficulty maintaining body temperature during cold weather. Infections and disturbances of the gastrointestinal tract are more likely in an underweight person, as is fragile bone structure and osteoporotic changes.

Causes

A person may be underweight because of genetic factors or because of a long-term or recent weight loss. As part of the nutrition screening process, the healthcare worker should ask the client about any change in body weight. A good question is, "Have you experienced any undesired weight loss?" If the client responds yes, it is important to determine the time frame of the weight loss. However, a response such as "I have always been lean" indicates a lifetime pattern and may reveal that the client's leanness is genetic. A response of, "No, I intentionally lost weight" may reveal an anorexic client.

Rapid Loss Increases Risk

The greater the rate of weight loss, the more the client is at a nutritional risk. **Rate** means loss per unit of time. For example, a 20-pound weight loss in 2 weeks is an excessive weight loss. Such a client has lost a large amount of lean body mass. However, a 20-pound weight loss during a 20-week period could be attributed mostly to a loss of body fat with a minimal loss of lean body mass. If the client began with surplus body fat stores, a loss of 20 pounds may not place this client at a high nutritional risk. If the client had a reduced body mass, even a slow weight loss may place him or her at a nutritional risk.

Not all changes in body weight are caused by insufficient kilocalorie intake. For example, a client may lose several pounds of body weight over the course of a single day as a result of diuretic therapy. The weight loss in this instance would be due to water loss, and not to body fat or protein loss.

Clinical Calculation 18–2 Percent Usual Body Weight

The healthcare worker can calculate the client's percent usual body weight (UBW). The formula is:

$$\frac{\text{Present weight}}{\text{Usual weight}} \times 100$$

A 5 percent weight loss in 1 month may not be significant. However, a 5 percent weight loss over a week may be significant. The kcal deficit may be related to a recent change in medication, an underlying but as yet undiagnosed condition, a recent change in living situation, or not taking the time to eat.

Binging involves the consumption of as much as 5000 to 20,000 kilocalories per day. **Purging** is the intentional clearing of food out of the system by vomiting and/or using enemas, laxatives, and diuretics. Athletes such as ballerinas and gymnasts sometimes are bulimic. The female triad is a serious syndrome comprising three interrelated components: (1) disordered eating, (2) amenorrhoea, and (3) osteoporosis (Wast, 1998).

Treatment of Eating Disorders

There are many approaches to treatment of eating disorders, including nutritional counseling, behavioral therapy, family therapy, and group ther-apy. It is important to help the client discover the reason he or she chooses to eat, not eat, binge, or purge. Some of these clients have symptoms including a fixation on food, weight, physique, or exercise (Zerbe, 1999). Some clients are admitted to the hospital for treatment. Careful recording of kilocalories consumed is indicated. Sometimes nurses are asked to sit with these clients and watch them eat. These clients may attempt to hide food in their clothes, mouth, bedding, or anywhere else. It is sometimes necessary for the nurse to accompany these clients to the bathroom. Clients with eating disorders have been known to flush their food down the toilet. For these reasons, the physicians of such clients often order daily weighing.

Summary

Energy imbalance results from an inequality of energy intake and expenditure. The reason an individual eats more or fewer kilocalories than needed to maintain a stable body weight is now only partially understood. Weight loss decreases *both* body fat and lean body mass. Care needs to be taken to minimize the loss of lean body mass during weight reduction. Exercise should be encouraged because it helps minimize the loss of lean body mass. In June 1998, the first federal guidelines on the identification, evaluation, and treatment of overweight and obesity in adults were published. Exercise, a well-balanced diet, and behavior modification are all essential components of a sound weight-reduction program. Medications and surgical interventions may be indicated for individuals who meet the criteria set by the guidelines. Treating the client who has a reduced body mass is a concern for healthcare workers.

Case Study 18–1

The client arrives at the physician's office for a routine blood pressure check. Her blood pressure is 150/95. Her medications are 100 mg Lopressor bid and 10 mg atace qd. The client works nights as a cashier at a service station and days at a dry cleaner. Her BMI is 28. She recently had a stress test that was considered normal. The doctor would like the client to lose weight to help lower her blood pressure.

Nursing Care Plan

Subjective Data	Client stated, "I can barely afford my blood pressure medication and the doctor has encouraged me to lose about 14 pounds. I know I need to eat less and exercise more. I need to spend less money on medications. I completed the sixth grade in school." A food frequency record showed that Mrs. R usually eats four times each day. Her usual pattern includes 3 cups of low fat milk, 8 starches (mostly refined), 1 serving of vegetables, 1 fruit, 6 to 8 ounces of meat, 5 fats, 1 dessert, and an occasional beer. She eats fast food two nights each week and has pizza weekly for lunch.
Objective Data	Blood pressure 150/95; Height 5 ft 6 in. BMI 28; waist circumference 36; stress test was normal
Nursing Diagnosis	Altered nutrition: more than body requirements (NANDA) as evidenced by client's statements and a BMI of 28 and a waist circumference of 36

Desired Outcomes Evaluation Criteria	Nursing Actions/ Interventions	Rational
NOC: Knowledge: Diet (Johnson, Maas, and Moorhead, 2000, with permission.)	NIC: Teaching: Prescribed Diet (McCloskey and Bulechek, 2000, with permission.)	
Increase physical activity	Recommend Mrs. R monitor her exercise behaviors and try to walk at least 20 minutes three times per week and increase to seven days per week as able.	Self-monitoring of lifestyle behaviors promotes behavioral change. The most sedentary individuals receive the most health benefit from even small amounts of exercise.
Consume foods in appropriate portions following the Food Pyramid Guide.	Review food pyramid model with Mrs. R with emphasis on whole grains and fruits and vegetables and the avoidance of fats. Review portion sizes indicated on this teaching tool.	The Food Pyramid Guide is a good tool to use for clients with a lower reading level and promotes a high-fiber, low-fat diet.
Will enlist a supportive person to walk with her or talk to when tempted to eat.	Assist client to identify such a person among her relatives and friends.	A strong social support system fosters success.
Client will state why a weight loss of 1 to 2 pounds a week may reduce her blood pressure.	Explain to client that the rate of weight loss is important and why.	A 1- to 2-pound per week weight loss will minimize the loss of lean body mass. Self-starvation rarely results in long-term weight loss for overweight clients.

Critical Thinking Question

1. What foods does this client need to eat less and what foods does she need to eat more?
2. What would you tell the client if after one week she gained a pound even though she had given up her daily dessert and had increased her vegetable intake to 5 servings each day?
3. What other dietary modifications would you recommend?

Study Aids

Subjects	Internet Sites
Obesity: State of-the-Art Update	http://www.cyberounds.com/conferences/nutrition/conferences/0498/conference.html, accessed April 1999
Clinical Guidelines on the Identification, Evaluation, and Treatment of Overweight and Obesity in Adults	http://www.nhlbi.nih.gov/nhlbi/cardio/obes/prof/guidelns/ob, accessed May 2000
North American Association for the Study of Obesity	http://naaso.org, accessed May 2000
Weight reduction program with emphasis on physical activity	http://www.shapeup.org, accessed May 2000
Food and Communications	http://www.foodandhealth.com, accessed May 1999
American Dietetic Association	http://eatright.org, accessed, May 2000

Chapter Review

1. To lose 2 pounds of body fat per week, an individual must eat _____ fewer kilocalories each day for 7 days without a change in energy expenditure.
   a. 1000
   b. 1500
   c. 2000
   d. 2500
2. A very rapid rate of weight loss (1 pound per day) in an adult who is slightly overweight:
   a. Usually encourages permanent changes in behavior
   b. May lead to sudden death in some clients
   c. Will preserve lean body mass
   d. Fosters long-term weight maintenance
3. An obese client should be enrolled in a weight management program and meet the following criteria before medications are tried:
   a. BMI of 20 and a waist circumference of 30 inches
   b. Waist circumference in a male of at least 35 inches and a BMI of 27
   c. A BMI of 27 and no concomitant obesity-related risk factors
   d. BMI of 30 or greater and a waist circumference of at least 35 inches in a female
4. A client with anorexia nervosa.
   a. has an increased resting energy expenditure
   b. frequently complains of constipation
   c. is not likely to have a body image disturbance
   d. typically seeks the company of others
5. An elderly overweight smoker should first be encouraged to:
   a. Lose weight
   b. Quit smoking
   c. Lose weight and quit smoking using any means possible
   d. Evaluated to determine if weight loss is indicated and bone health is adequate

Clinical Analysis

1. Mrs. R is a 40-year-old mother of three. She has arthritis in both knees. She weighs 180 pounds, has a medium frame, and is 5 feet, 3 inches tall. Her BMI is 32. Her physician has told her to lose weight to help reduce her knee pain. According to Mrs. R she never thought she was overweight until she was 24 years old. At this time, her weight started increasing. When she weighed 140 pounds, she started to diet. One time she lost a total of 25 pounds, which she promptly regained plus an additional 5 pounds. The client described four additional weight cycles. Mrs. R claims she cannot exercise because "it is too painful on my knees." She has tried every conceivable type of diet, including a comprehensive medically supervised weight-control program. Mrs. R states that for the past year, no matter how little she eats, she cannot lose weight even on a 1200-kilocalorie diet. Mrs. R:
   a. Apparently knows a great deal about low-kilocalorie foods, because she has successfully lost weight before
   b. Knows very little about foods, because she always regained the weight she lost
   c. Lacks motivation, because she has an inability to follow through with the appropriate behavior
   d. Should be discouraged from further attempts to control her weight
2. Mrs. M had a slow weight gain for about 10 years. She asks for advice concerning how to best manage her weight. Mrs. M lives a sedentary lifestyle, eats three well-balanced meals each day, and enjoys going out to dinner with her husband one night each week. Her BMI is 27. Mrs. M would most likely benefit from:
   a. Decreasing her meal frequency
   b. Increasing her physical activity
   c. Taking a medication to lose weight
   d. Not going out to dinner with her husband each week
3. Mr. P wants to lose weight and has a BMI of 30 and a waist circumference of 41. Initially, the nurse should advise Mr. P to:
   a. Follow a 1200-calorie diet
   b. Ask his doctor for a medication to assist in weight reduction
   c. Self-monitor and write down his food intake and physical activity
   d. Refer client to a surgeon for an evaluation

Bibliography

Bjorntorp, P: Fat cells and obesity. In Brownell, KD, and Foreyt, JP (eds): Handbook of Eating Disorders: Physiology, Psychology, and Treatment of Obesity, Anorexia, and Bulimia. Basic Books, New York, 1986.

Bouchard C: Inhibition of Food Intake by Inhibitors of Fatty Acid Synthase. N Eng J Med 343–25, December 2000.

Calle, EE, et al.: Body-Mass Index and Mortality in a Prospective Cohort of US Adults. N. Engl J Med. 341(15):1097, 1999.

Canning, H, and Mayer, J: Obesity: Its possible effect on college acceptance. N Engl J Med. 275:1172, 1966.

Coscina, DV, and Dixon, LM: Body weight regulation in anorexia nervosa: Insights from an animal model. In Darby, PL, Garfield, PE, Garner, DM, et al. (eds): Anorexia Nervosa: Recent Developments. Allan R. Liss, New York, 1983.

Donnelly, JE, et al.: Preventing childhood obesity. Food and Nutrition News. National Live Stock and Meat Board. 67:1, 1995.

Faherty, JP, and Miller, E: Management of the overweight patient. Family Practice Recertification. 19(8):45, August 1997.

Flegal, KM, et al.: Overweight and obesity in the United States: Prevalence and trends.1960–1994. Int J Obesity 341:427, 1998.

Forbes, GB: Body Composition. In Shils, ME, Olson, JA, Shike, M, Ross, AC (eds): Body Composition. Modern Nutrition in Health and Disease, ed. 9. Williams and Wilkins, Baltimore, 1999.

Forety, JP, and Goodrick, G: Evidence of success for behavior modification in weight loss and control. Ann Intern Med 119:698, 1993.

Frantz, MJ: Managing obesity in patients with comorbidities. The Obesity Epidemic. J Am Diete Assoc 98(10, suppl 2):s39, October 1998.

Ginsburg-Feller, F: Growth of adipose tissue in infants, children, and adolescents: Variations in growth disorders. Int J Obes 5, 1981.

Gortmaker, SL, et al.: Social and economic consequences of overweight in adolescence and young adulthood. N Engl J Med 329:1008, 1993.

Hill, JO, and Peters, JC: Environmental contributions to the obesity epidemic. Science. 280 (5368):1371, May 1998.

Huse, P, and Lucas, AR: Behavioral Diorders Affecting Food Intake: Anorexia Nervosa, Bulimia Nervosa, and other Psychiatric Conditions. In Shils, ME, Olson, JA, Shike, M, and Ross, AC (eds): Modern Nutrition in Health and Disease. Williams and Wilkins, Baltimore, 1999.

Jefferey, RW: Epidemic obesity in the United States: Are fast food and television viewing contributing? Am J Public Health. 2:27., February 1988.

Johnson, M, Maas, M, and Moorhead, S: Nursing outcomes Classification (NOC), ed 2. Mosby, Philadelphia, 2000.

Keyes, A, Brozek, J, Mickelson, O, et al.: The Biology of Human Starvation. 2 vols. University of Minnesota Press, Minneapolis, 1950.

Klesges, RC, Shelton, ML, and Klesges, LM: Effects of television on metabolic rate: Potential implications for childhood obesity. Pediatrics 91:281, 1993.

Kuczmarski, RJ, Carrol, MD, Flegal, KM, and Troiano, RP: Varying body mass index cutoff points to describe overweight prevalence among AUS Adults: NHANES III (1988 to 1994) Obes Res 5:542, 1997.

Lindpaintner, K: Finding an obesity gene—a tale of mice and men. N Engl J Med 332:679, 1995.

Lowell, BB, and Spiegelman, BM: Toward a molecular understanding of adaptive thermogenesis. Nature 404:652–60, 2000.

Ludwig, DS, et al.: Dietary fiber, weight gain, and cardiovascular disease risk factors in young adults. JAMA 282(16):1539-46, October 1999.

McCloskey, JC, and Bulechek, GM: Nursing Interventions Classification (NIC), ed 3. Mosby, Philadelphia, 2000.

National Dairy Council: Weight Management: A Summary of Current Theory and Practice. National Dairy Council, Rosemont, IL, 1985.

National Institutes of Health and National Heart, Lung, and Blood Institute: Clinical Guidelines on the Identification, Evaluation, and Treatment of Overweight and Obesity in Adults. Bethesda, MD, June 1998.

National Institute of Health Consensus Development Panel: Health Implications of Obesity. Ann Intern Med 103:1073, 1985.

National Research Council: Diet and Health Implications for Reducing Chronic Disease Risk. Report of the Committee and Diet and Health, Food and Nutrition Board, Commission on Life Sciences. National Academy Press, Washington DC, 1989.

Nonas, CA: A model for chronic care of obesity through dietary treatment. The Obesity Epidemic. J. Am Diete Assoc 98(suppl 2):10, October 1998.

North American Nursing Diagnosis Association: Definitions and Classification 1999–2000, North American Nursing Association, Philadelphia, 1999.

Pate, RR: Physical activity and public health: A recommendation from the Centers of Disease Control and Prevention and the American College of Sports Medicine. JAMA 273:402, 1995.

Pi-Sunyer, FX: In Shils, ME, Olson, JA, Shike, M, and Ross, AC (eds): Obesity. Modern Nutrition in Health and Disease. Baltimore, Williams and Wilkins, 1999.

Popkin, BM, and Doak, CM: The obesity epidemic is a worldwide phenomenon. Nutr Rev 56(4 pt 1):106, April 1998.

Poston, WS II, et al.: Challenges in obesity management. South Med J. 8:710-20, Aug 1998.

Polivy, J: Psychological consequences of food restriction. J Am Diete Assoc 96:589, 1996.

Pyle, RL, Mitchell, JE, and Eckert, ED: Bulimia: A report of 34 cases. J Clin Psychiatry 42:60, 1981.

Rippe, JM: The obesity epidemic: Challenges and opportunities. J Am Diete Assoc 98(10, suppl 2):5, October 1998.

Rohner-Jeanrenaud, F, and Jeanrenaud, B: Obesity, leptin, and the brain. N Engl J Med 334:324, 1996.

Romsos, DR: Efficiency of energy retention in genetically obese animals and in dietary-induced thermogenesis. Fed Proc 40:2524, 1981.

Romsos, D: "Gene-Whiz" The Obesity/Gene Connection. (Unpublished lecture) 23rd Annual Nutrition Conference. Michigan State University, East Lansing, MI, March 6, 1996.

Rosenbaum, M, et al.: Obesity. N Engl J Med. 337:336, 1997.

Russell, RM: Nutrition. JAMA 273:1699, 1995.

Samaras, K, et al.: Genetic and environmental influences on total-body and central abdominal fat: the effect of physical activity in twin females. Ann Intern Med 130:873, 1999.

Stunkard, AJ, and Burt, V: Obesity and body image II: Age of onset of disturbances in the body image. Am J Psych 123:1443, 1967.

Stunkard, AJ, and Mendelson, M: Disturbances in body image of some obese persons. J Am Diet Assoc 38:328, 1961.

Thomas, CL: Tabers Cyclopedic Medical Dictionary, ed 18. FA Davis, Philadelphia, PA, 1993.

Turner, RC, et al.: RR for the United Kingdom Prospective Diabetes Study Group. Risk factors for coronary artery disease in non-insulin dependent diabetes mellitus: United Kingdom prospective diabetes study (UKPDS: 23) MJ 316:823-28, 1998.

Tyler, DO, Allan, JD, and Alcozer, FR: Weight loss methods used by African American and Euro-American women. Research in Nursing and Health. 20(5):413, 1997.

US Department of Health and Human Services: PHS, NHANES III. Antropometric Procedures Video. US Government Printing Office Stock Number 017-022-01335-5. US GPO, Public Health Service, Washington DC, 1996.

Van Itallie, TB: Obesity. In Jeejeebhoy, KN (ed): Current Therapy in Nutrition. BC Decker, Toronto, Canada, 1988.

Wadden, T, and Stunkard, A: Social and psychological consequences of obesity. Ann Int Med 103:1062, 1985.

Walker, BR, Ballard, IM, and Gold, JA: A muticenter study comparing marindol and placebo in obese patients. J Int Med Res 5:85, 1977.

Wast, RV: The female athlete. The triad of disordered eating, amenorrhea, and osteoporosis. Sports Med 2: 63, August 1998.

Weinsier, RL, et al.: The etiology of obesity: Relative contribution of metabolic factors, diet, and physical activity. Am J Med. 105:145, 1998.

Williamson, DF: The prevention of obesity. N Engl J Med. 341:1140, 1999.

Wooley, BH, and Hunt, JK: Managing obesity: A comprehensive approach. US Pharmacist. Reprint. North Mount Olive, New Jersey, September 1998.

World Health Organization. Physical Status: The use and interpretation of anthropometry. Report of WHO Expert Committee. World Health Organ Tech Rep Ser 854:1-452, 1995.

www.foodandhealth.com, accessed May 2000.

Yanovski, JA, and Yanovski, SZ: Recent advances in basic obesity research. JAMA 282(16):1504, October 1999.

Zerbe, KJ: Anorexia nervosa. When the pursuit of bodily perfection becomes a killer. Postgrad Med 1:161, January 1999.

CHAPTER 19

Diet in Diabetes Mellitus and Hypoglycemia

LEARNING OBJECTIVES

After completing this chapter, the student should be able to:

1. Define and classify diabetes mellitus and describe the treatment for each type.
2. Discuss the goals of nutritional care for persons with diabetes mellitus.
3. List nutritional guidelines for illness, exercise, delayed meals, alcohol, hypoglycemic episodes, vitamin/mineral supplementation, and eating out for people with diabetes.
4. Describe dietary treatment for reactive hypoglycemia as compared to diabetes mellitus.

This chapter introduces the importance of nutrition in diabetes and hypoglycemia. These two diseases are associated with insulin secretion and/or resistance to insulin accompanied by characteristic long-term complications. Diabetes mellitus is caused by the low secretion and/or utilization of insulin. Hypoglycemia is caused by excessive secretion of insulin. Diabetes mellitus has been diagnosed in approximately 16 million people, or 5.9 percent, of the population in the United States. An additional 4–5 million individuals are believed to have undiagnosed diabetes. Each year about 800,000 new cases are diagnosed. This equals more than 2000 people per day or 90 people per hour (Peterson and Vinicor, 1998). Wellness Tip 19–1 discusses the importance of early diagnosis of diabetes. Nationally, diabetes is the seventh leading cause of death. Hypoglycemia is much rarer than diabetes mellitus. Nutrition is integral to the management of diabetes.

Wellness Tip 19–1

- Approximately half of all individuals with diabetes are undiagnosed. Do you or any of your family members have any of the signs or symptoms of this disease? Early detection and treatment of diabetes reduces morbidity and mortality.

Definition and Classification

Diabetes mellitus is characterized by the passage of sweet urine, excessive urine production, thirst, excessive hunger, and, in some cases, weight loss. Records from the ancient Greeks described this condition as early as the first century A.D. Diabetes mellitus can be defined as a group of disorders with measurable persistent hyperglycemia. **Hyperglycemia** means an elevated level of glucose in the blood. Definitions and classifications for the various subclasses of diabetes mellitus have been standardized. The following sections define and classify the major types of diabetes.

Definition

Diabetes is diagnosed and defined by laboratory analysis. Fasting glucose levels of at least 126 milligrams per deciliter (mg/dL) on two occasions are required for a diagnosis of diabetes in nonpregnant adults. Random blood glucose (RBG) greater than 200 mg/dLplus classic symptoms (increased urination, increased thirst, weight loss) is also an established method to diagnose diabetes in adults and children. Random means the blood sample is tested without regard to time of day, prior diet, and physical activity. Refer to Clinical Application 19–1 for an explanation of other tests used for diabetes.

Classification

There are two major forms of diabetes: **type 1 and type 2** (note the use of Arabic numerals). The American Diabetes Association recommends the use of three additional categories to classify diabetes: secondary diabetes, impaired glucose tolerance (IGT), and gestational diabetes.

Type 1

Type 1 diabetes has also been called insulin-dependent diabetes mellitus (IDDM), juvenile onset diabetes, and Type I diabetes. All of these terms are still used in medical records. Patients with this disorder cannot survive without daily doses of insulin because the pancreas does not produce sufficient insulin for glucose uptake. This results in elevation of blood glucose. These variations in blood glucose levels make these patients prone to two conditions. The first condition is **ketoacidosis**. The signs of ketoacidosis are hyperglycemia and excessive ketones. Ketoacidosis is discussed further later in this chapter. The second condition is **hypoglycemia**, or a low blood glucose level. Type 1 diabetes can occur at any

CLINICAL APPLICATION 19–1

Laboratory Tests for Diabetes

Several types of biochemical tests are discussed below: fasting blood sugar, glucose tolerance test, urine tests, and glycolated hemoglobin.

Fasting Blood Sugar

A measurement of a fasting blood sugar (FBS) is performed routinely on most diabetic clients. In preparation, the client should be instructed not to eat or drink for 8 to 12 hours before the test. Water is the exception, as it will not interfere with test results. The test ideally should be done after at least 3 days of unrestricted diet (≥150 gms carbohydrate per day) and unlimited physical activity. The individual should remain seated and not smoke throughout the test. If the client usually takes insulin or a hypoglycemic agent, the medication should not be taken or given until the blood test is done. Normal FBS should be 70 to 110 mg/dL. A finding of 140 mg/dL on two occasions is diagnostic of diabetes mellitus.

Glucose Tolerance Test

In the glucose tolerance test, a measured amount of glucose is given orally or intravenously after a fasting blood sugar sample has been drawn. Blood samples are then drawn at specified intervals. The client's ability to process glucose can be evaluated by this means. A blood glucose value above or equal to 200 mg/dL at 2 hours and at least one other sample at less than 2 hours are required for the diagnosis in nonpregnant adults. A normal 2-hour blood sample would have an upper level of 140 mg/dL. Values between 140 and 200 mg/dL are indicative of impaired glucose tolerance.

Clients may need to discontinue certain drugs for 3 days prior to the test. Also, a high-carbohydrate diet of 300 g of carbohydrate per day should be followed for the same period. The client should be given written instructions explaining the pretest dietary requirements. An inadequate diet prior to the glucose tolerance test may diminish carbohydrate tolerance and cause high glucose levels, creating a false-positive result. During the test, the client should not be permitted to have anything by mouth except water. Tobacco, coffee, and tea can alter the test results.

Urine Tests

For most people, when blood glucose reaches 180 to 200 mg/100 mL, the kidneys begin to spill glucose into the urine. This point of spillage is called the **renal threshold**.

At one time, this test was assumed to reflect the glucose content of the blood, but the renal threshold varies from individual to individual. The renal threshold may also change in a given individual with decreasing kidney function. Although urine tests are used as screening tests, they are less reliable than the blood glucose tests available for home use.

Urine Acetone

As a consequence of the body's inability to metabolize glucose, fat is partially broken down for energy. The intermediate products of fat breakdown are ketone bodies. These ketone bodies build up in the blood because the quantity of fat being catabolized exceeds the body's capacity to process these intermediate products effectively. As this occurs, ketone bodies begin to spill into the urine. One of the ketone bodies is acetone, which can be measured in the urine. The presence of acetone in the urine is called **ketonuria**. Ketonuria is a sign that the diabetes is out of control. Clients are often taught to test for urinary ketones if their blood glucose level exceeds 240 mg/dL. When a client exhibits ketonuria, the physician should be consulted for changes in the diet prescription or insulin dosage.

Glycosylated Hemoglobin (HbAic)

Glucose attaches to the hemoglobin molecule in a one-way reaction throughout the 120-day life of the red blood cell. In a high-glucose environment, a greater percentage of the hemoglobin is glycosylated. This blood test is performed on a random blood sample; the client does not have to fast. The result is not influenced by exercise or diabetic drugs.

Because the **glycosylated hemoglobin** value reflects the average blood glucose level for the preceding 2 to 3 months, it is a good test of the effectiveness of long-term therapy. A client cannot follow the prescribed regimen for just a few days prior to a doctor's visit and claim otherwise. Glycosylated hemoglobin will be 4 to 8 percent of the total hemoglobin in adults without diabetes. In clients with diabetes, a value of 7 percent indicates good control of the disease, and greater than 8 percent is considered high.

A HbAic is recommended at least two times a year for those in good control and more often if the HbAic is greater than 8 percent or when there is a change in the treatment plan.

age, although its usual onset is during childhood. Five to ten percent of people with diabetes have type 1. The onset of this disorder is usually abrupt, and the condition is difficult to control.

Type 2

Type 2 diabetes has also been called noninsulin-dependent diabetes mellitus (NIDDM), adult onset diabetes, and type II diabetes. Persons with type 2 are not insulin dependent or prone to ketoacidosis. However, some of them do use insulin because of persistent hyper-

glycemia. Clients with this condition can manufacture some insulin but do not make a sufficient amount or cannot use insulin efficiently. Typically, the noninsulin-dependent diabetic client develops his or her condition after age 45 (www.diabetes-midon.org, accessed May 2000). Most of these clients are obese, and weight reduction usually improves their ability to process glucose. Excess body fat seems to be related to a decrease in the number of cell receptor sites. About 90–95 percent of all people with diabetes in the United States have type 2. The prevalence of type 2 diabetes is markedly increased among Native Americans,

Table 19–1 Insulin-Dependent and Noninsulin-Dependent Diabetes Mellitus

	Type 1	Type 2
Cause	Beta cells damaged	Tissues resist insulin
Most common age at onset	Under 20 years	Over 45 years
Medication	1. Insulin injections OR	1. None OR
	2. Insulin injections and oral agents	2. Oral agents OR
		3. Some individuals may require insulin injections to attain optimal blood glucose levels.
Usual body build	Thin, underweight	Obese
Nutrition therapy	Integration of insulin therapy, activity, and food intake	Achievement of near normal glucose, lipid, and blood pressure goals.
	Consistent timing of food intake	Weight loss is desirable and possible with some clients.

African Americans, Hispanic Americans, and Pacific Islanders. The cultural implications of these statistics were discussed in the Chapter 2. The onset of this disorder is gradual. The condition is usually easier to control than type 1. Table 19–1 summarizes the differences between types 1 and 2.

Other Specific Types

Most diabetes results from a primary failure of insulin production and/or use, but diabetes can occur as a result of a variety of disorders, including pancreatitis, cystic fibrosis, surgical removal of the pancreas, Cushing's disease, or pharmacological doses of glucocorticoids (e.g., prednisone) or other hormones or drugs. The term **secondary diabetes** is sometimes used when one of these disorders is responsible for the hyperglycemia. The diabetes may be resolved if the cause is alleviated. If the cause is not correctable, secondary diabetes is treated similarly to other forms of diabetes.

IMPAIRED GLUCOSE TOLERANCE(IGT) IMPAIRED FASTING GLUCOSE (IFG) Impaired glucose tolerance (IGT) and impaired fasting glucose (IFG) are terms that refer to a metabolic state intermediate between normal and glucose homeostasis and diabetes. Individuals who have a fasting glucose level of greater than 110 mg/dL but less than 126 mg/dL on more than two occasions meet the criteria for IGT or IFG. IGT may represent a step in the development of types 1 and 2 diabetes. In fact, 25 percent of clients with IGT later develop diabetes mellitus.

GESTATIONAL DIABETES Gestational diabetes (GDM) is the term for glucose intolerance in pregnancy. Women who are diagnosed as diabetic before pregnancy are not classified as having gestational diabetes. Clinical Application 19–2 discusses diabetes mellitus in pregnancy. Gestational diabetes is diagnosed slightly differently from other forms of diabetes. After an oral glucose load, diagnosis of gestational diabetes is made if two plasma values equal or exceed the following (www.diabetes-midon.org, accessed, May 2000):

Fasting:	105 mg/dL
1 hour:	190 mg/dL
2 hours:	165 mg/dL
3 hours:	145 mg/dL

The condition usually disappears after childbirth. However, women who have had gestational diabetes are at an increased risk for developing type 2 diabetes as they age.

Normal Nutrient Metabolism

An understanding of diabetes mellitus is based on knowledge of the pancreas, the organ that produces insulin. It is also important to understand the cellular sources of glucose, the normal blood glucose curve, and the functions of insulin and other hormones. All of these are discussed in the following sections of this chapter.

Anatomy of the Pancreas

The pancreas is a gland that lies behind the stomach. It has both exocrine and endocrine secretions. The exocrine functions of the pancreas include the flow of enzymes into the intestine through ducts. Endocrine secretions (hormones) flow directly into the bloodstream.

Clusters of cells in the pancreas called the **islets of Langerhans** produce three hormones. These islets contain three types of cells: alpha, beta, and delta. The alpha cells produce **glucagon**, the beta cells produce insulin, and the delta cells produce **somatostatin** (Fig. 19–1). Special sensors at junctions of the three types of cells monitor levels of blood glucose and stimulate the release of the appropriate hormone.

Functions of Insulin

Insulin is the only hormone that lowers blood glucose. A person normally secretes insulin in response to an elevated blood glucose level. Insulin decreases blood glucose by accelerating its movement from the blood into the cells. As glucose enters the cells, it may be metabolized to yield energy, may be stored as glycogen, or may be converted to fat (Table 19–2). The ultimate fate of glucose once it is inside the cell depends on body need and the amount of glucose that enters the cell. The cells' energy needs will be met first. If cells have available glucose over and above immediate energy needs, the excess glucose is stored as glycogen. Insulin stimulates the storage of glucose as glycogen. Once the glycogen stores are filled to capacity, any remaining glucose is converted to fat. The body can store about 0.4 pound of glycogen, which is equal to 800 kilocalories (Matthews, 1999).

CLINICAL APPLICATION 19–2

Diabetes in Pregnancy

Pregnancy raises blood insulin levels in all women. It is an adaptive mechanism. Early in pregnancy, the woman's body cells store energy. Later, the woman's tissues become insulin resistant so that the fetus can draw on energy stores when the woman is fasting.

When the pregnant woman has or develops hyperglycemia, the mother's blood glucose crosses the placenta but her insulin does not. Then the fetus produces more insulin, which increases his/her fat deposition. Women with diabetes have large babies for this reason.

Perinatal mortality of infants born to women with diabetes is higher than that of infants of women who do not have diabetes. Ketosis in early pregnancy can produce congenital malformations, central nervous system disorders, and low intelligence. With strict control of the diabetes, however, 97 percent of the fetuses survive, compared with 98 to 99 percent born to women without diabetes.

Insulin resistance is greater in the morning in pregnant women. For this reason, usually only 39 grams of CHO are planned into the breakfast meal plan. There is a heightened tendency for maternal ketosis during fasting, and the possible adverse effects of ketones on the fetus suggest that periods of fasting during pregnancy should be avoided. Small, frequent feedings throughout the day are recommended. A bedtime snack that contains between 15 and 45 grams of CHO is recommended to minimize an accelerated production of ketones, which has been known to occur during sleeping. Clients should be reminded not to skip meals. Following is a summary of these recommendations:

- Breakfast: 30 grams of CHO
- Lunch and dinner: 60 grams of CHO
- Snacks: between 15 and 45 grams of CHO (dependent on the client's energy allowance based on individual assessment)
- Recommend bedtime snack for all clients
- Include protein and fat at each meal (amount dependent on client's energy allowance based on individual assessment)

Nutritional regulation is central to management of diabetes in pregnant women. During pregnancy the most commonly recommended kilocalorie distribution is: 40 to 45 percent carbohydrate, 20 to 25 percent protein, and 30 to 40 percent fat. This is not the same kilocalorie distribution commonly used in nonpregnant diabetic individuals.

The treatment goal is to prevent hypoglycemia, defined as fasting plasma concentrations of 70 to 90 mg/dL and 2-hour postprandial plasma glucose levels of less than 140 mg/dL. Some medical experts believe that this goal is too rigid because hypoglycemia during early pregnancy may be teratogenic. Hypoglycemic agents have been shown to cause significant risk to the fetus. In most instances, women are advised to discontinue use of hypoglycemic agents before conception. If medication is necessary to control hyperglycemia, insulin is safer for the fetus.

Early pregnancy loss and congenital malformations can be minimized by optimal medical care and client education before conception in women with diabetes. Contraception, timing of conception, control of metabolic state, self-management techniques, assessment of diabetic complications, and other medical complications should be discussed with the female client of child-bearing age. The desired outcome of glycemia control in the preconception phase of care is to lower glycohemoglobin so as to achieve maximum fertility and optimal embryo and fetal development (American Diabetes Association, 1996a). Preconception counseling is best accomplished by a multidisciplinary team approach including a diabetologist; internist or family practice physician; obstetrician; and diabetes educators, including nurses, registered dietitians, social workers, and other specialists as necessary. Self-management skills essential for control during pregnancy include (Position Paper of the American Dietetic Association, 1996a):

- Using an appropriate meal plan
- Timing of meals and snacks
- Planning physical activity
- Choosing time and site of insulin injections
- Using carbohydrate and glucagon for hypoglycemia
- Reducing stress, coping with denial
- Testing capillary blood glucose
- Self-adjusting insulin doses

Insulin influences the metabolism of protein and fat. Insulin stimulates entry of amino acids into cells and enhances protein formation. It also enhances fat storage in adipose tissue and indirectly inhibits the breakdown of fat for energy. If the body has ample glucose available for energy, protein and fat need not be broken down to meet energy needs. If the body does not have glucose available for energy, it will use dietary protein or break down internal body protein stores to meet its immediate need for energy.

Insulin levels fluctuate in the blood. Normally, blood insulin levels increase as the blood glucose level increases. A high level of insulin in the blood signals the cells not to break down stores for energy (Table 19–3). An anabolic, or building, state exists when metabolism is normal and glucose and insulin levels are high. Normally insulin levels decrease

as the blood sugar level decreases. A low level of insulin in the blood indirectly signals the body to begin to break down body stores for glucose. A catabolic, or breaking-down, state exists when metabolism is normal and glucose and insulin levels are low. Figure 19–2 illustrates glucose use by the cells.

Other Hormones

Glucagon and somatostatin assist in coordinating the storage and mobilization of the energy nutrients (carbohydrate, fat, and protein). Glucagon increases blood glucose levels and stimulates the breakdown of body protein and fat stores. Somatostatin acts locally within the islets of Langerhans to depress the secretion of both insulin and glucagon. Evidence has shown that these hormones may not be at optimal levels in some clients with diabetes.

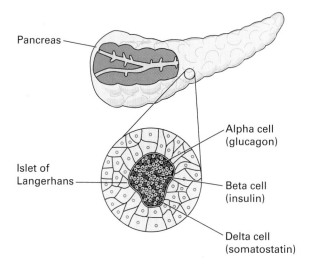

Figure 19–1:
View of the pancreas and an enlarged islet of Langerhans. Alpha cells secrete glucagon, beta cells secrete insulin, and delta cells secrete somatostatin.

Cellular Sources of Glucose

The cells obtain glucose from both the food that is eaten and internal glucose stores. Almost all of the carbohydrate eaten (except fiber), about 50 percent of the protein eaten, and about 10 percent of the fat eaten will enter the blood as glucose. The internal body stores that can be converted to glucose are glycogen, some protein, and the glycerol portion of triglycerides. Body fat is stored as triglycerides in adipose tissue. To understand diabetes, it is necessary to know how the body coordinates all internal and external sources of glucose to maintain a normal blood glucose range.

Blood Glucose Curve

Given the vital need for every cell to have an uninterrupted supply of energy, the human body has evolved to allow an uninterrupted energy supply to reach cells without continuous eating. A normal blood glucose range is usually about 70–110 mg/dL. (Some laboratories assign a normal blood glucose range of 80–120 mg/dL.) The difference is the result of the type of equipment the laboratory uses, and not the glucose content of the blood.) The blood glucose level increases after eating and decreases in the fasting state. Figure 19–3 illustrates the normal blood glucose curve.

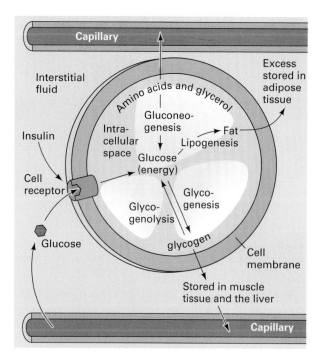

Figure 19–2:
Insulin is necessary for glucose to gain entry into a cell. Once inside the cell, glucose can meet several fates: glucose can be burned as energy or stored as glycogen or the glycerol portion of a fat molecule or some amino acids can be broken down into glucose. Some amino acids will be converted to glucose if the cell requires glucose.

Causes of Diabetes

The causes of diabetes include genetic factors, lifestyle, and viral infections. Although these causes are explained separately for the sake of clarity, in reality they are often interconnected.

Genetic Factors

Some of the susceptibility to diabetes is genetic. Researchers have discovered that people with type 1 diabetes have certain genes associated with

Table 19–2 Metabolic Activities Promoted by Insulin

Activity	Name of Metabolic Pathway
Movement of glucose into cells	None
Energy production from glucose	Glycolysis
Manufactuure of glycogen	Glycogenesis
Fat formation from carbohydrate and protein	Lipogenesis

Note: "Genesis" means building up.

Table 19–3 Metabolic Activities Inhibited by a High Level of Insulin

Activity	Name of Metabolic Pathway
Movement of glucose from noncarbohydrate sources, e.g., glycerol and amino acids	Gluconeogenesis
Release of glucose from glycogen	Glycogenolysis
Breakdown of fat from adipose tissue	Lipolysis

Note: "Genesis" means building up.

Normal blood glucose levels

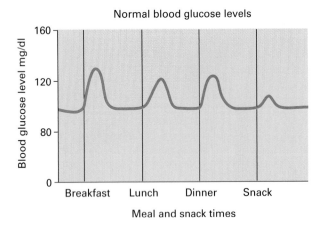

Figure 19–3:
A person's blood glucose level normally goes up after food consumption and then down between feedings.

their immune response. These particular genes are often found in children with type 1 diabetes. However, not everyone with these genes develops clinical diabetes. Before diabetes becomes apparent, this genetic susceptibility is often triggered by the individual's lifestyle or other environmental factors. These factors cause a series of events that results in damage to or destruction of the pancreatic beta cells. Inheritance is even more prominent in the development of type 2 than in type 1 diabetes, as the next section describes.

Insulin Resistance

A person may be genetically susceptible to **insulin resistance**. Insulin resistance occurs when both an individual's glucose and blood insulin levels are elevated. Insulin may not be released at the right times and/or be unable to assist the movement of glucose into the cells because of a lack of receptor sites. Before glucose can enter the cells, the insulin must first attach itself to specific receptor sites on the cells' outer surfaces. Persons with type 2 diabetes may lack enough receptor sites, have faulty receptor sites, or have postreceptor defects. Excess body fat seems to be related to a decrease in the number of receptor sites. Type 2 diabetes is often associated with insulin resistance.

Lifestyle

A healthy lifestyle is particularly important for the *prevention* of diabetes in genetically susceptible clients. Excessive body fat, inactivity, and stress are risk factors for diabetes as highlighted in Wellness Tip 19–2. Up to 90 percent of clients with type 2 diabetes have a higher than recommended percent of body fat. A loss of body fat alone is sometimes sufficient to balance the insulin produced with a modified food intake. At least a dozen studies have demonstrated that weight loss reduces insulin resistance and increases peripheral glucose uptake (Maggio and Pi-

Wellness Tip 19–2

- Excess body fat, inactivity, and stress are lifestyle choices that can increase the risk of diabetes. Type 2 diabetes can sometimes be prevented with good lifestyle choices.

Sunyer, 1997). Inactivity is a lifestyle risk factor that predisposes one to diabetes. Sometimes emotional or physical stress is the stimulus that causes hyperglycemia. The body's stress response involves the release of epinephrine from the adrenal glands. One action of epinephrine is to raise the blood sugar level so the person has energy for the "fight or flight" response.

Viral Infections

Links have been noted between viral epidemics and the onset of diabetes. During the late fall and winter months, a disproportionate number of cases of type 1 diabetes are diagnosed. Because these seasons are also associated with peak occurrence of childhood viral diseases, it is possible that a causal connection exists between viral epidemics and the onset of type 1 diabetes.

Antibodies to pancreatic islet cells have been found in some people with diabetes. Type 1 diabetes is usually an autoimmune disease that is characterized by the presence of a variety of autoantibodies on the surface of or within the beta cells of the pancreas. Individuals with more than one autoantibody (i.e., ICA, IAA, GAD, IA-2) are at a high risk for type 1 diabetes (www.medscape.com/, accessed May 2000). In **autoimmune diseases**, the body cannot recognize its own cells but rather treats them as foreign invaders. The event that provokes this process usually is a viral infection. These elevated antibodies may be detected in about 90 percent of clients prior to the diagnosis of diabetes. Physicians order laboratory tests to check the levels of these antibodies in clients' blood. If the levels are elevated, the physician can inform the client of his or her situation. It is inappropriate to inform a client of a highly probable prognosis unless treatment options are presented at the same time. However, after speaking to a client, physicians frequently will request other health care professionals to explain in detail to the client the treatment options.

Signs and Symptoms of Diabetes

The classic triad of signs and symptoms includes **polyuria**, increased urination; **polydipsia**, increased thirst; and **polyphagia**, increased appetite and weight loss. The triad is most commonly seen in type 1 diabetes. The following section describes these and other signs and symptoms commonly seen in persons with diabetes.

Classic Triad

In diabetes, glucose cannot optimally move from the intravascular space across a cell membrane into the intracellular space. This is why the diabetic person's blood glucose level remains elevated after eating. Under normal circumstances, the blood glucose level does not increase excessively because excess glucose undergoes glycolysis and is readily converted to adipose tissue or stored as glycogen inside the cell. As the glucose-rich blood circulates through the kidneys, these organs reabsorb all the glucose of which they are capable. After this point is reached, glucose enters the urine. **Glycosuria** means an abnormally high amount of glucose in the urine. As the glucose exits the body in the urine, water is pulled out also as a result of the osmotic effect of glucose. This results in

Wellness Tip 19–3

- Keep your eyes working by keeping your blood pressure and blood glucose under control. Diabetes is the leading cause of adult blindness in the United States. Often no symptoms appear before damage occurs.

polyuria, or a large urine output. The large loss of water causes excessive thirst and polydipsia and prompts the person to drink fluids.

When glucose is not available for energy inside the cells, the body begins to break down protein and fat for energy. In untreated type 1 diabetes, the body's cells are starving. These starving cells send a message to the brain to turn on the person's appetite. The person responds by eating to satisfy the craving for food. The third symptom or sign of diabetes is polyphagia, an abnormal increase in appetite. Polyphagia, polyuria, and polydipsia are the three classic signs or symptoms reported or seen in clients with diabetes.

Other Signs and Symptoms

The abnormal carbohydrate metabolism of diabetes and its effects on the body's tissues cause other problems. Weight loss is more commonly seen in clients with type 1 diabetes than in clients with type 2. Blurred vision is common in both types. The need for good eye care is discussed in Wellness Tip 19–3. Fatigue is frequently seen in these clients. High glucose levels impair white blood cell functioning, thus increasing the client's susceptibility to infection. Commonly involved agents are *Staphylococcus aureus* and *Candida albicans* involving the skin and mucous membranes. Recurrent furuncle (boil, caused by localized infection), **vaginitis** (inflammation of the vagina), or bladder infections in a client may stimulate testing for diabetes. Poor wound healing is related to decreased circulation. Circulatory problems in men may manifest as impotence.

Complications

Both acute and chronic complications occur with diabetes mellitus. Acute complications require immediate care. Chronic complications include diseases of the eye, kidneys, heart, and nervous system. Chronic complications are responsible for the increased death rate among individuals with diabetes and the diminished quality of life that many of these clients experience.

Acute Clinical Situations

Three acute complications are seen in clients with diabetes: **diabetic ketoacidosis (DKA)**, hyperglycemic hyperosmolar nonketotic syndrome, and **hypoglycemia**.

Ketoacidosis

Individuals with type 1 diabetes who experience a profound insulin deficiency may progress to the condition of ketoacidosis. The three main precipitating factors in ketoacidosis are a decreased or missed dose of insulin, an illness or infection, or uncontrolled disease in a previously undiagnosed person. Ketoacidosis is a complex, life-threatening condition that demands emergency treatment. The predominant clinical manifestations of dehydration, acidosis, and electrolyte imbalances and general principles of treatment are discussed next.

DEHYDRATION Without insulin, glucose cannot be transferred across the cell membranes into the cells. A greatly increased number of glucose molecules (300–800 mg/dL) in the blood exert an osmotic effect, causing water to move from within the cells to the intravascular space and producing cellular dehydration. The body excretes the excess water, glucose, and electrolytes in the urine.

ACIDOSIS Unaware that the problem is not lack of glucose, but lack of insulin, the body proceeds to increase blood glucose by mobilizing protein and fat from the tissues to be converted to glucose by the liver. Because the human body can use only the glycerol portion of the triglyceride molecule for glucose, the fatty acid portion is processed into ketones. Normally the ketones are metabolized and excreted as carbon dioxide and water. Under conditions of ketoacidosis, however, the body cannot metabolize this overload of ketones rapidly enough to maintain homeostasis, and thus the client has excessive ketones in the blood (ketonemia) and spills ketones in the urine (ketonuria). Acetone is one of the ketone bodies for which urine is tested. The ketone bodies are acid, and thus the term ketoacidosis.

The body can initiate several homeostatic mechanisms as it attempts to correct the acidosis. It decreases the level of carbonic acid in the blood by increasing the excretion of carbon dioxide through involuntary deep, gasping rapid breaths called **Kussmaul respirations**. The client's breath has a fruity odor from the ketonemia. The kidney increases the hydrogen ion content or acidity of the urine it excretes. Buffering of hydrogen can occur in the cells also, where it displaces potassium to the extracellular fluid.

ELECTROLYTE IMBALANCES Clients with severe ketoacidosis may excrete 6.5 liters of fluid and 400–500 milliequivalents of sodium, potassium, and chloride in 24 hours. A fluid loss of 15 percent of body weight is not unusual. Most critical in the treatment of electrolyte imbalances in diabetic ketoacidosis is the body's level of potassium. As the cells are being catabolized for fuel, the intracellular potassium is transferred to the intravascular space. Serum potassium levels can be low, normal, or elevated in the person with ketoacidosis, depending on the body's current coping mechanism. Regardless of the serum concentrations of potassium and sodium, the pathological process of diabetic ketoacidosis depletes these electrolytes. Either hypokalemia or hyperkalemia can lead to cardiac arrhythmias and must be carefully managed in clients with ketoacidosis.

TREATMENT Clients with severe diabetic ketoacidosis are critically ill. Treatment includes supplemental insulin, fluid and electrolyte replacement, and medical monitoring. Serum electrolyte levels change dramatically once treatment commences. Intensive care is necessary to provide the careful monitoring and frequent adjustments in therapy required as the fluids and electrolytes are being replaced. Intravenous regular insulin will permit the use of carbohydrate for energy and will halt the body's excessive use of fat, which has produced the ketone bodies. Insulin drives glucose back into the cells. Potassium, too, moves from the intravascular space to the intracellular space, necessitating frequent measurement of the serum levels of both glucose and potassium. When the client recovers, identification of the precipitating factor for the ketoacidosis and education focused on preventing additional occurrences are essential.

Hyperglycemic Hyperosmolar Nonketotic Syndrome

The four signs of **hyperglycemic hyperosmolar nonketotic syndrome** (HHNS) are blood glucose level greater than 600 mg/dL, absence of or slight ketosis, plasma hyperosmolality, and profound dehydration. This life-threatening emergency is usually seen in the elderly or people with undiagnosed type 2 diabetes. HHNS is like DKA except that the insulin deficiency is not as severe, so increased **lipolysis** (the breakdown of body lipid stores) does not occur. Because these clients do not have symptoms of vomiting, nausea, and acidosis brought on by severe ketosis, as do clients with type 1 diabetes, they often do not seek prompt medical help. Their blood sugar levels are higher and their dehydration more severe than is seen in ketoacidosis.

In these clients, prolonged osmotic diuresis and dehydration secondary to hyperglycemia lead to decreased renal blood flow and allow the blood glucose to reach very high levels. Medications that cause an increase in blood glucose levels, chronic disease, and infection may contribute to this condition. Examples of medications that cause hyperglycemia with diabetes include corticosteroids, such as hydrocortisone and prednisone; thiazide diuretics, such as lasix, hydrodiuril, and naturetin; dilantin; and estrogens. Treatment includes correction of the electrolyte imbalance, hyperglycemia, and dehydration.

Hypoglycemia

In both type 1 and type 2 diabetes (treated with medications), an individual can develop hypoglycemia. Hypoglycemia may be caused by too much insulin (accidental or deliberate); too little food intake; a delayed meal; excessive exercise; alcohol (especially in the fasting state); and/or medications such as oral hypoglycemic agents. Symptoms may include confusion, headache, double vision, rapid heartbeat, sweating, hunger, seizure, and coma. The treatment of hypoglycemia is discussed later in this chapter.

Chronic Complications

Clients with both type 1 and type 2 diabetes of sufficient duration are vulnerable to serious complications involving the eyes, kidneys, and nervous system. Diabetic **retinopathy** is a disorder that involves the retina. Diabetes is a leading cause of blindness and of visual loss in the adult U.S. population. The blurred vision reported by these clients is related to retinopathy. These clients are also at a higher risk for cataracts.

Diabetic neuropathy is a chronic complication of diabetes mellitus. Clients may complain of a lack of sensation in their extremities. They may puncture, cut, or burn their feet and not feel any pain. A wound may become infected and heal poorly. Gangrene, or tissue death, may follow. The treatment for gangrene is amputation. Neuropathy can affect gastric or intestinal motility, erectile function, bladder function, cardiac function, and vascular tone (Nathan, 1993). **Gastroparesis** (paralysis of the stomach) may occur and alter the absorption of meals, which makes glycemic control problematic. Cardiovascular disease is more common in these clients. There is increasing epidemiological evidence that hyperglycemia is not only associated with but also predicts coronary heart disease events, strokes, and mortality from heart disease (Kuusisto et al., 1994).

Diabetic **nephropathy**, or kidney disease, is another common complication in diabetic clients. Tragically, some clients with diabetes do not take the threat of chronic complications seriously until much damage has occurred.

Treatment

The current medical goal is to *normalize* the blood glucose throughout the day, which goes far beyond what has been clinical practice in the past. A normal blood glucose level is less than or equal to 109 mg/dL before a meal and less than 140 mg/dL 2 hours after a meal. Realistic target levels for individuals with diabetes treated intensively are 70–140 mg/dL before meals, less than 180 mg/dL 2 hours after meals, and glycosylated hemoglobin within 1 percent of normal. A landmark study known as the Diabetes Control and Complications Trial (DCCT) in individuals with IDDM demonstrated that intensive control of blood glucose levels delays the onset and slows the progression of diabetic retinopathy, nephropathy, and neuropathy (Diabetic Control and Complications Trial Research Group, 1993).According to this study's results, people with type I diabetes who followed a tightly controlled regimen, compared with those who followed a standard regimen, showed reductions of approximately:

- 76 percent in progression of diabetic retinopathy
- 54 percent in albuminuria (albumin in the urine, which may be a sign of renal impairment)
- 36 percent in microalbuminuria (a more sensitive indicator of protein in the urine, which may be an early warning of renal impairment)
- 60 percent in rates of neuropathy

A tightly controlled regimen is not without problems, however. Among these is an increased incidence of insulin-induced hypoglycemic episodes. A more recent study showed that clients undergoing intensive diabetes treatment do not face deterioration in the quality of their lives, even while the rigor of their diabetes care is increased (The Diabetes Control and Complication Trial Research Group, 1996). This evidence has been further strengthened by a recent report from the United Kingdom Prospective Diabetes Study (UKPDS), which demonstrated that intensive therapy for type 2 diabetes significantly lowered the rate of diabetes-related events (UK Diabetes Prospective Diabetes Study Group, 1998).

All healthcare workers should assist the general population in the early detection of diabetes and prevention of complications. As Figure 19–4 emphasizes, the three cornerstones of the management of diabetes after diagnosis are physical activity, medication, and nutritional management. Self-monitoring of blood glucose levels enables the client to assess how each of these factors interacts. Blood glucose monitoring, physical activity, medication, and diet are discussed next.

Self-Monitoring of Blood Glucose

Many individuals monitor their own blood glucose levels with a device called a blood glucose meter. This procedure is called **self-monitoring of blood glucose** (SMBG). Individual response to medication, diet, and exercise can be determined with this advanced technology. SMBG can be performed using a single drop of blood. The client obtains the drop of blood from a finger with either a lancet or a spring-loaded device. The blood sample is placed in the meter, and the test results are available in less than 1 minute. The client can then adjust insulin dose and food and exercise behaviors accordingly. Many experts consider SMBG to be the most important development in diabetes management since the discovery of insulin.

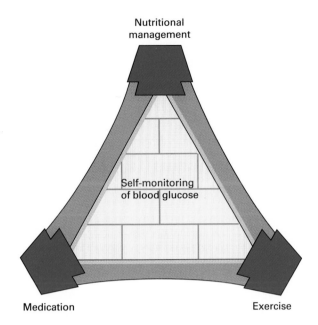

Figure 19–4:
Nutritional management, medication, and exercise are the three components of treatment for diabetes. Each of these cornerstones has an influence on blood glucose levels. An individual can identify how each of these cornerstones impacts his or her blood glucose level by self-monitoring blood glucose.

SMBG has allowed clients to try to normalize their blood glucose levels throughout the day. Healthcare workers need to carefully teach clients how to interpret the results of SMBG (Fig. 19–5). Continual reassessment of the client's technique and blood glucose records is necessary to guide treatment decisions. To evaluate the need for changes in diet or medications, monitoring should be done at least twice a day; four times a day for 3 days each week is preferable for clients who are stable. If near-normalization of blood glucose is the treatment goal, SMBG must be done four to eight times daily (before and 2 hours after each meal and/or snack). During acute illness, more frequent self-monitoring is indicated.

Physical Activity

Exercise plays a key role in the management of diabetes. All individuals with diabetes who exercise should be encouraged to follow these guidelines:

1. Wear proper footwear, and use other protective equipment if necessary.
2. Avoid exercise in extremely hot and cold environments.
3. Inspect feet daily and after exercise for open areas, blisters, punctures, swelling, and redness; report any of these signs to the physician immediately.
4. Avoid exercise during periods of poor metabolic control (blood glucose levels that are <60 or >240 mg/dL levels).
5. Wear a diabetes ID badge or bracelet.

6. Carry a source of glucose in case of a decrease in blood glucose, as exercise decreases blood glucose levels.

Exercise and Type 2 Diabetes

Physical activity is widely endorsed for persons with type 2 diabetes. Physical activity increases the number and binding capacity of insulin receptors, assists in lowering blood glucose levels, and reduces insulin requirements in persons who use insulin. Improved blood lipid levels occur in some clients who engage in regular exercise. This helps delay or prevent the cardiovascular disease complications often seen in these clients. Exercise also assists in weight control and improves muscle strength and flexibility.

Aerobic exercise should be encouraged at 50–70 percent maximum heart rate and of at least 40 minutes duration to promote breakdown of body fat. Daily exercise is recommended, but three times a week is considered the minimum required to aid blood glucose management. Current research suggests that three 10-minute exercise sessions provide a substantial health benefit especially for the sedentary individual. The strategy to break down activity sessions into shorter, more frequent increments may be helpful to clients who have difficulty being physically active.

Exercise and Type 1 Diabetes

The American Diabetes Association strongly endorses an exercise program for people with type 1 diabetes because of the potential to improve cardiovascular fitness and psychological well-being. Exercise involves some risk for individuals with type 1 diabetes because it changes insulin requirements in sometimes unpredictable ways more than 24 hours after the exercise. Retinopathy, neuropathy, and renal disease may worsen in some clients with type 1 diabetes who exercise. Blood pressure may also become elevated. For this type of client, self-monitoring of blood glucose should be incorporated into a modified exercise program tailored to individual client needs and limitations. The client should demonstrate the ability to self-treat a hypoglycemic episode.

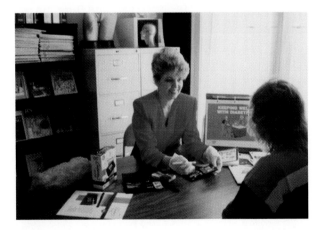

Figure 19–5:
Client learning how to self-monitor her blood glucose levels. Note that the nurse is wearing personal protective equipment: gloves.

Exercise, SMBG, and Food Intake

Type 1 clients with diabetes who do exercise and all type 2 clients who engage in nonroutine exercise should monitor their blood glucose levels before, during, and after exercise. If the blood glucose level is greater than 100 mg/dL before exercise, there is usually no need for additional food if the planned exercise is of short duration and low intensity. Exercise of long duration and high intensity generally requires more kilocalories. Snacks that contain an additional 15–30 grams of carbohydrate-containing food should be ingested for every 30–60 minutes of exercise (Franz, 1987). Good choices for snack foods include fruit, starch, and milk exchanges. To prevent wide swings in blood glucose levels, care should be taken not to overeat. Too much food will cause the blood glucose level to go up too high and subsequently to drop too low. Exercise is best done 60–90 minutes after meals when the blood glucose level is highest.

Medications

Two types of medications are used with diabetic clients: insulin and oral hypoglycemic agents. Clients with type 1 diabetes require insulin. Clients with type 2 diabetes may not require any medication or may need to have an oral hypoglycemic agent or insulin prescribed. Frequently, clients with type 2 diabetes are able to discontinue the medication after a loss of body fat.

Insulin

Almost all the insulin used in the United States is human. Human insulin is manufactured by recombinant-DNA technology (biosynthetic). Human insulin (Humulin) produces few allergic reactions. Insulin cannot be taken orally because the gastrointestinal tract enzymes would digest it before absorption. Insulin must be administered by needle either **subcutaneously** (beneath the skin) or intravenously (IV). Only regular insulin is given IV. The substances used to delay absorption of intermediate- and long-acting insulins are not designed for IV administration. Regular insulin is usually administered IV only for the severely hyperglycemic or hospitalized client.

Insulin can also be administered with an insulin pump. These pumps are designed to provide a small inflow of insulin continuously and large inflows before eating, thus mimicking normal insulin secretion. Continuous subcutaneous insulin infusion (CSII) or insulin pumps have been available for nearly 20 years, but only recently have they been widely used.

Medications are described according to the onset, peak, and duration of action. Insulin is categorized as rapid-acting, intermediate-acting, or long-acting. Table 19–4 lists the times of onset, peak, and duration of insulin. Variation in duration makes it possible to inject insulin in a pattern that is as close as possible to normal insulin activity. Ideally, the medication is planned around the diet, not vice versa. Most experts know that it is far easier to change a medication than a food behavior.

A new insulin approved by the FDA in early 2000, Lantus, has no pronounced peaks and remains at a relatively constant level over 24 hours. This medication has the potential to greatly facilitate the treatment of diabetes.

Oral Hypoglycemic Agents

Oral hypoglycemic agents lower blood glucose levels in type 2 diabetes. These drugs stimulate insulin release from the pancreatic beta cells, reduce glucose output from the liver, and increase the uptake of glucose in tissues. Many new oral agents are being prescribed in the United States, and many more are in development (Table 19–5). Recently, oral agents and insulin administered simultaneously have been used successfully to treat type 1 diabetes. Commonly prescribed oral hypoglycemic agents include glipizide, glyburide, glimiperide, metformin, acarbose, and tolazamide. Oral agents are increasingly being used in combinations. Many of the new oral agents work on different cell receptor sites. For example, metformin and acarbose can be added to sulfonylurea (e.g., glimiperide, glyburide) with an additional 0.5–2 percent reduction in HbAic level (Zimmerman and Hagan, 1998).

Table 19–4 Times of Onset, Peak, and Duration of Action for Rapid-Acting, Intermediate-Acting, and Long-Acting Insulin

Insulin	Times in Hours		
	Onset	Peak	Duration
Rapid-acting*			
Regular intravenously			
Regular subcutaneously	0.17 to 0.5	1.25 to 0.5	0.5 to 1
	0.5 to 1	2 to 4	8 to 12
Intermediate-acting			
Lente subcutaneously	1 to 2.5	7 to 15	24
NPH subcutaneously	1 to 1.5	4 to 12	24
Long-acting			
Ultralente Subcutaneously	4 to 8	10 to 30	>36
Lantus**			

*Humulin R, Iletin R, Novolin R, and Velosulin R are all names of rapid-acting insulins. Semilente is also classified as a rapid-acting insulin, although its onset is 1.0–1.5 hours. The peak is 5–10 hours and the duration is 12–16 hours. Thus, semilente is slower to act, peaks more slowly, and has a longer duration than other rapid-acting insulins

**Lantus is a long-acting insulin that is designed to be given at HS. Lantus has no pronounced peaks with a relatively constant level over 24 hours. The FDA approved Lantus in early 2000.

Table 19–5 Diabetes Oral Medications and Major Actions

Classification	Major Actions	Generic Name (Trade name)	Comments
Sulfonylureas	Stimulate insulin release by the pancreas and may help decrease liver glucose production	Glipizides (Glucotrol) Glyburide (Glynase, Micronase, and Diabeta)	Glipizide must be taken on an empty stomach Glyburide can be taken with food or on an empty stomach. Low toxicity. Use caution with elderly.
Biguanides	Decrease liver production of glucose. Increase glucose uptake into tissues.	Metformin (Glucophage)	Given in 2–3 doses per day with meals. Not metabolized. Often used in combination with sulfonylureas
Meglitinide	Stimulates immediate insulin release from pancreas as needed for meals.	Repaglinide (Pradin)	Given in 2–4 doses per day 15–30 minutes before meals
Alpha-Glucosidase Inhibitors	Slow the rate of digestion of starches and complex sugars.	Acarbose (Precose) Miglitol	Given in 3 doses per day with meals. 98% not absorbed. Rest excreted by kidneys.

Source: Adapted from *Quick Reference Guide to Diabetes for Health Care Prodividors* by Michigan Diabetes Outreach Network. www.Diabetes-midon.org and *Sodon Sentinal*, Vol. 4, Issue 4 by Michigan Diabetes Outreach Network.

Medical Nutritional Management

Diabetes is directly related to how the body uses food. Nutrition is thus an essential component of management for all persons with diabetes. Studies have shown that clients report improved health, better control of body weight, improved control of blood glucose and lipid levels, and improved use of insulin when they adhere to dietary recommendations. The goals of nutritional care for persons with diabetes are the control and prevention of complications. This involves the promotion of normal nutrition and dietary modification to control blood glucose and lipid levels. Clients' nutritional goals need to be determined individually. There is **no** "diabetic diet" or "ADA diet," but several meal-planning approaches are widely endorsed by the American Diabetes and the American Dietetic associations.

The next sections describe the overall goals of nutritional care, the need to individualize nutritional care to meet each client's goals, assessment of client readiness to change negative eating behaviors, survival skills needed by all clients with diabetes, and various meal-planning approaches that are widely used for these clients.

Nutritional Goals

The goal of medical nutritional therapy is to educate the person with diabetes to make changes in food and exercise habits that lead to improved metabolic control. Specifically, the client needs assistance with:

1. The attainment and maintenance of near-normal blood glucose levels as feasible by the coordination of food intake, endogenous and exogenous insulin and/or hypoglycemic agents, and with physical activity. This is a challenge in some clients who have fluctuating endogenous insulin production.
2. The attainment and maintenance of optimal serum lipid levels

3. Provision of adequate kilocalories to

   - attain and maintain a healthy body weight for adults and normal growth and development for children
   - recovery from illnesses
   - to meet the metabolic needs of pregnancy and lactation

4. The prevention and treatment of the acute and chronic complications of diabetes, such as renal disease, autonomic neuropathy, hypertension, and cardiovascular disease
5. Improvement of overall health through good nutrition. *The Food Guide Pyramid and Dietary Guidelines for Americans* illustrate and summarize nutritional guidelines for all Americans, including people with diabetes.

Goal Priority

The medications prescribed, the type of diabetes the individual has, and the client's desire to change behavior determine goal priority. A high priority for the person taking insulin is to facilitate consistency in the timing of meals and snacks to prevent wide swings in blood glucose. This requires coordination among exercise, insulin, and food intake. A high priority for the individual with type 2 diabetes is achieving glucose, blood pressure, and lipid goals. To achieve these goals, diet is a cornerstone of treatment. Although weight reduction for these clients usually improves short-term glycemic levels and long-term metabolic control, traditional weight loss strategies have not been effective in achieving long-term weight loss. The client's motivation to lose weight needs to be carefully assessed by the health care educator.

Meal Frequency

Meal spacing is more crucial in type 1 than in type 2 diabetes. Consistent timing and meal size assist in stabilization of blood glucose levels in type

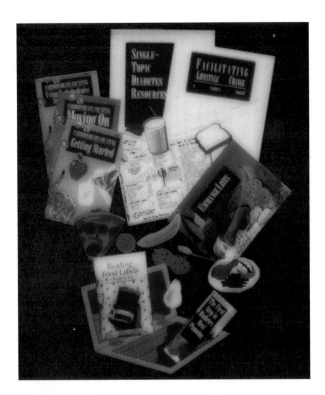

Figure 19–6:
Teaching materials available from the American Diabetes and American Dietetic Associations. (1996, The American Dietetic Association, New Meal Planning Approaches. Used with permission.)

1 diabetes. In general, people with diabetes benefit from eating on a regular basis (every 4–5 hours) while awake.

Client Readiness to Change Behavior

Food behaviors are difficult to change. Although some clients with diabetes do successfully change or alter food behaviors to enhance their outcomes, many clients do not, will not, or cannot change harmful food behaviors. Modification of harmful behaviors involves progression through five stages: precontemplation, contemplation, preparation, action, and maintenance. Individuals typically recycle through these stages several times before terminating negative behaviors. Following is a brief description of each of these stages:

1. *Precontemplation:* individuals exhibit no intention to change behavior in the foreseeable future.
2. *Contemplation:* individuals know they have a problem and they are seriously thinking about overcoming the harmful behavior but are not ready to take action.
3. *Preparation:* individuals plan to take action in the near future, may have taken action unsuccessfully in the past, and may report small behavioral changes.
4. *Action:* individuals modify their behavior, experiences, and/or environment to overcome the harmful behavior. This stage requires considerable commitment of time and energy.

5. *Maintenance:* individuals continue to work to prevent relapse and to consolidate gains.

Healthcare workers can assist clients in the precontemplation and contemplation stages by attempting to raise patients' consciousness about the benefits of behavioral change. Stimulus control and reinforcement also help patients become more aware of the need to alter behaviors (see Chapter 18, Weight Control). The most difficult problems posed by clients for the health educator are at the precontemplation phase (Jacobson, 1993).

The healthcare educator needs to carefully consider how much information the client desires and how ready he or she is to change food behaviors. An educational tool that takes 3–4 hours to review with a client is inappropriate for someone who is willing to devote just a few minutes to learning about his or her diet. In contrast, the client who wants to learn everything he or she can about self-care will not be satisfied with an elementary meal plan. See Figure 19–6 for an illustration of the wide variety of meal-planning resources available for use by these clients.

Survival Skills

The American Diabetes and Dietetic associations recommend that the newly diagnosed client initially learn basic "survival skills." See Box 19–1 for information the client needs to know immediately. Appendix L has handouts on survival skills for clients on medication and treated by diet alone. Once the client has demonstrated an understanding of this basic knowledge, a firm foundation has been set for the acquisition of additional, more individualized information.

Meal-Planning Approaches

There are about a dozen appropriate meal-planning approaches. The most elementary approaches include *The Food Guide Pyramid, Dietary Guidelines for Americans*, and *The First Step in Diabetes Meal Planning*. Any one of these meal-planning approaches is considered survival-skill level information. After the client has demonstrated an understanding of the meal-planning approach initially used by the health educator, the use of a more advanced approach should be considered. The client will achieve optimal blood glucose and lipid control with a more sophisticated meal-planning approach. Two of the more widely used, more advanced meal-planning systems are discussed next. Various meal-planning approaches are discussed in Box 19–2.

THE EXCHANGE LISTS OF THE AMERICAN DIETETIC AND THE AMERICAN DIABETES ASSOCIATIONS This approach to meal planning, introduced in Chapter 2, Individualized Nutritional Care, teaches the learner about food composition. Usually the registered dietitian reviews this approach with the client and then the nurse reinforces the dietitian's teaching. The educator needs to anticipate spending a total of 1–2 hours to thoroughly explain this approach to a client (Fig. 19–7). This can best be accomplished in two or more sessions. *The Exchange Lists of the American Dietetic and American Diabetes Associations* is used to calculate energy nutrient distribution.

ENERGY NUTRIENT DISTRIBUTION Total energy requirements for the individual with diabetes do not differ from those for individuals without diabetes. Therefore, please refer to Chapter 6, Energy Balance, to determine the total kilocalorie requirement for a person. The distribution of

Box 19-1 Survival Information for the Client With Diabetes

Initial education for the client with diabetes should include basic knowledge that will facilitate the maintenance of acceptable (safe) blood glucose levels. Individuals with diabetes must come to accept responsibility for self-management and the need for ongoing education. Survival skills are typically reviewed with these clients during the first educational session.

1. Diabetes is caused by a lack of insulin and/or an inability to use the insulin the body produces. There is no cure for diabetes, but it can be controlled through diet, exercise, and medications.
2. An acceptable blood glucose is 70 to 110 mg/dL before meals and less than 200 mg/dL two hours after meals. The client is said to be adequately controlled if the blood glucose level is between these numbers relative to the time meals are eaten. Better control can be possible with more finely controlled blood glucose levels.
3. Monitoring and recording blood glucose levels can be done with a blood glucose monitor. All individuals with diabetes are encouraged to monitor their blood glucose levels. Hospital nurses and dietitians, home healthcare agencies, and healthcare workers in physicians' offices can teach the client how to monitor blood glucose levels.
4. Nutrition is an important part of blood glucose control. The Food Pyramid provides an initial acceptable dietary guide of what foods should be eaten. Foods chosen from the Food Pyramid guide should be divided into three or more equal feedings. Carbohydrate-containing foods are especially important to distribute evenly throughout the day. It is important to eat at regular times each day, to avoid skipping meals, and to eat about the same amount each day. Try to limit fat, salt, sugar, and alcohol intake. Portion control is important. Alcohol consumption on an empty stomach may cause a low blood glucose reaction. Try to increase intake of fruits, vegetables, and whole grains.
5. Exercise is beneficial for most people with diabetes, however, before beginning any exercise program, consult the doctor. Exercise is the most beneficial when the blood glucose is below 200 mg/dL. Regular exercise is more beneficial than sporadic exercise and best done 60 to 90 minutes after eating.
6. An understanding of the peak, onset, and duration of any medication used to treat a high blood glucose is important. Good insulin injection technique (if applicable) is essential.
7. A high blood glucose (greater than 240 mg/dL) is potentially dangerous, especially if untreated. Always check the urine for ketones if the blood glucose is more than 240 mg/dL. Contact the physician if the blood glucose is greater than 240 mg/dL and the urine is positive for ketones.
8. A blood glucose of less than 60 mg/dL is dangerous and may lead to confusion, disorientation, and coma. Signs of a low blood glucose include: sweating, slurred speech, headache, weakness, tremors, hunger, nervousness, tingling of the lips, and rapid heart beat. In the event these signs are noted, immediately:
   1. Check the blood glucose, if low proceed to step 2
   2. Take 1/2 cup of fruit juice OR 1/2 cup of milk OR 6 hard candies
   3. Wait 15 minutes and then recheck the blood glucose
   Repeat the process if the blood glucose is less than 100 mg/dL.
9. Over the long term, diabetes can lead to foot problems, including infection and amputation. Check the feet (and legs) daily. Look for sores, redness, infection, drainage, swelling, or bruises. Report problems to the doctor early. Keep the feet clean and dry. Never go barefoot. Protect any area where sensation is lost.
10. Have an annual examination with a board certified ophthalmologist (a doctor specializing in eye care). Diabetes is the leading cause of adult blindness in the United States. Often there are no symptoms before damage occurs.
11. The person with diabetes should wear a personal identification bracelet or necklace.

energy nutrients refers to the percentage of total kilocalories that should be derived from carbohydrate, fat, and protein. Distribution also refers to the division of carbohydrate, fat, and protein among the day's meals/feedings. Clinical Calculation 19–1 shows how the percentage of energy nutrients is converted to grams of carbohydrate, fat, and protein and distributed throughout the day's meals/feedings. The next three sections elaborate on energy nutrient distribution.

CARBOHYDRATE Complex carbohydrate should ideally provide the majority of kilocalories in the diet, or about 55–60 percent of the total kilocalories. Many complex carbohydrates are also excellent sources of dietary fiber. Water-soluble fibers found in fruits, oats, barley, and legumes can influence glucose and insulin levels by smoothing out the postprandial (after eating) glucose curve, thereby helping to lower plasma lipid levels. The American Diabetes Association recommends a fiber intake of between 20 and 35 grams per day for clients with diabetes (Anderson, 1999). Complex carbohydrates also provide many needed vitamins. A limited amount of carbohydrate, or about 5 percent of the total carbohydrate, may be derived from simple carbohydrates (single or double sugars found in simple sugars, fruits, some starches, and milk). In general, people with diabetes need to eat consistent amounts of carbohydrates (from milk, meat, bread/starches) at meals, especially if using insulin.

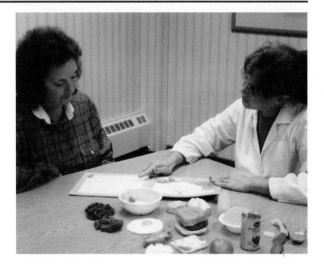

Figure 19–7:
A diabetes educator providing nutritional counseling. The use of food models facilitates the learning process and teaches portion control.

Box 19–2 Meal-Plannning Approaches

Approach	Comments	Availability
Food Pyramid	Initial phase of teaching Provides a basic foundation in normal nutrition. Does not emphasize meal consistency.	A colorful version is available from the National Dairy Council, 10255 West Higgins Road, Suite 900, Rosemont, IL 60018-4233 1-708-803-2000
Dietary Guidelines	Initial phase of teaching Provides a basic foundation in normal nutrition, 40 pages in length. Does not emphasize meal consistency.	United States Department of Agriculture Home & Garden Bulletin #232, Local Cooperative Extension Office
The First Step in Diabetes Meal Planning	Initial phase in teaching Combines Food Pyramid and Dietary Guidelines, and provides information on meal consistency in a simplified format.	The American Dietetic Association, 216 West Jackson Boulevard, Suite 800, Chicago, IL 60606-6995 1-800-366-1655
CHO Counting Level I Level II Level III	Progressive teaching tool that leads to maximum control of blood glucose and lipid levels. Decreased emphasis on balance and variety.	The American Dietetic Association, 216 West Jackson Boulevard, Suite 800, Chicago, IL 60606-6995 1-800-366-1655
Month-O-Meals	Each book contains 28 complete and interchangeable menus for breakfast, lunch, dinner, and snacks. Excellent approach for the client who "just wants to be told what and when to eat."	The American Dietetic Association, 216 West Jackson Boulevard, Suite 800, Chicago, IL 60606-6995 1-800-366-1655
Exchange Lists of the American Dietetic and the American Diabetes Associations	Allows the health-care educator to distribute all of the energy nutrients. More emphasis on the importance of eating a balanced diet than the CHO counting approach. Time consuming to learn and teach	The American Dietetic Association, 216 West Jackson Boulevard, Suite 800, Chicago, IL 60606-6995 1-800-366-1655

Clinical Application 19–3 discusses the glycemic index of foods. Note that glucose has a high glycemic index, honey has a low glycemic index, and sucrose falls somewhere between them. White bread, potatoes, and cornflakes all have a higher glycemic index than sucrose. Thus, it is incorrect to tell a client that sucrose and honey cause the blood glucose level to increase faster or higher than an equal amount of carbohydrate from some complex carbohydrates. A client may ask why a particular food that contains starch causes the blood glucose level to increase rapidly, and knowledge of the glycemic index of that particular food may help answer the client's question. Clients who monitor their blood glucose levels have many such questions and look to all healthcare professionals for information.

The Food Guide Pyramid and Dietary Guidelines for Americans also recommend that the bulk of kilocalories be derived from complex carbohydrate and that only minimal amounts of simple sugars be consumed. Simple sugars are empty kilocalories that contain almost no vitamins, minerals, and fiber.

Clinical Calculation 19–1 How to Distribute the Energy Nutrients and Calculate a Diet Using the Exchange System

In the following example, an 1800-kcal diet is being converted to 55 percent carbohydrate, 20 percent protein, and 25 percent fat.

$$1800 \text{ kcal} \times 0.55 = 990 \text{ kcal} \div 4 \text{ kcal/g} = 248 \text{ g carbohydrate}$$
$$1800 \text{ kcal} \times 0.20 = 360 \text{ kcal} \div 4 \text{ kcal/g} = 90 \text{ g protein}$$
$$1800 \text{ kcal} \times 0.25 = 450 \text{ kcal} \div 9 \text{ kcal/g} = 50 \text{ g fat}$$

In the following example, 248 g of carbohydrate, 90 g of protein, and 50 g of fat are converted to a 1/5, 2/5, 1/5, and 1/5 distribution. Each fraction represents one meal: thus 1/5 of the energy nutrients are to be provided each at breakfast, supper, and the evening snack; 2/5 of the energy nutrients are to be provided at the noon meal. Please note: 1/5 equals 20 percent and 2/5 represents 40 percent.

$$248 \text{ g of carbohydrate} \times 0.20 = 50 \text{ g} \times 3 \text{ meals } 150$$
$$248 \text{ g of carbohydrate} \times 0.20 = 99 \text{ g} \times 1 \text{ meals} = \frac{99}{249}$$
$$90 \text{ g of protein} \times 0.20 = 18 \text{ g} \times 3 \text{ meals } 54$$
$$90 \text{ g of carbohydrate} \times 0.40 = 36 \text{ g} \times 1 \text{ meal} = \frac{36}{90}$$

Because only a small percentage of dietary fat enters the bloodstream as glucose, normally fat is not calculated into the distribution. Lunch (2/5 distribution) would contain about 99 g of carbohydrate and 36 g of protein. Each of the other meals (1/5 distribution) would contain about 50 g of carbohydrate and 18 g of protein.

The next step is to determine the number of exchanges to be provided from each of the six exchange groups. There is no exact method used to determine this step. Usually the client is consulted to determine the amount of nonfat milk, fruits, vegetables, and so forth that he or she would be willing to consume. An effort should be made to calculate the diet with at least the recommended servings given in the Food Pyramid guide. Many healthcare workers determine the amount of nonfat milk, fruits, and vegetables to be provided first. This is followed by the grams of carbohydrate to be contributed by these groups. The remaining carbohydrate is then allocated to the starch group.

The protein is determined by first calculating the amount previously provided by nonfat milk, vegetables, and starches; the remaining protein is then allocated to meat exchanges. The fat is determined by first calculating the amount previously provided by the meat exchanges; the remaining fat is then allocated to fat exchanges. The calculations and meal plan for our sample 1800 kcal with 55 percent carbohydrate, 20 percent protein, and 25 percent fat with a 1/5, 2/5, 1/5, and 1/5 distribution appear in Table 19–6.

PROTEIN. The need for protein in the diabetic population is the same as for the general population. For example, the adult RDA of 0.8 gram per kilogram of protein, or approximately 12–20 percent of total kilocalories, is indicated. Excessive amounts of dietary protein should be avoided in people with diabetes, just as members of the general population should avoid it. The concept that excessive dietary protein may have a health risk is discussed in the Chapter 5 on protein.

FAT. The American Diabetes Association recommends that total fat be less than 30 percent of total kilocalories. Note again, this is similar to the Dietary Guidelines for Americans. Ten percent of fat should come from polyunsaturated fat, 10 percent from saturated fat, and 10 percent from monounsaturated fat. In addition, cholesterol should ideally be kept below 300 mg per day.

Some people with diabetes have better glucose control on high monounsaturated fat diets (40–45 percent of the kcalories). If a diet is 40–45 percent fat, the carbohydrate content of the diet drops to 35–45 percent. This contradicts the general guideline given earlier in the chapter that the ideal complex carbohydrate level for the person with diabetes should be about 55–60 percent of total kilocalories. Diabetes is a complicated disease, and some patients with diabetes benefit from a highly individualized approach to diet manipulation. Some patients with hypertriglyceridemia and elevated LDL cholesterol levels respond better to a 40–45 percent high monounsaturated fat diet (Nuttall and and Chasuk, 1998). This is why the percent of kilocalories from fat and the kind of fat consumed by persons with diabetes merit consideration. This concept requires rigid compliance. Individual evaluation by a registered dietitian is necessary to assess feasibility.

Not all clients with diabetes have these lipid abnormalities. In epidemiological studies, an increased plasma triglyceride and low HDL cholesterol have been associated with an increased risk for clinically apparent

Table 19–6 Sample 1800-Kilocalorie Diabetic Diet*

DIVISION OF ENERGY NUTRIENTS AND EXCHANGES

Exchange List	Number of Daily Exchanges	Protein (90 g)	Fat (50 g)	Carbohydrate (218 g)	Breakfast	Lunch	Dinner	HS
Skim milk	2	16	0	24	1/2	1		1/2
Starch	11	33	0	165	2	4	3	2
Fruit	3	0	0	45	1	1	0	1
Vegetable	3	6	0	15	0	2	1	0
Meat	5	35	25	0	1	2	1	1
Fat	5	0	25	0	1	1	2	1

MEAL PLAN AND SAMPLE MENUS

Meal Pan	Sample Menu 1	Sample Menu 2
Breakfast		
1/2 skim milk	1/2 cup skim milk	1/2 cup skim milk
2 starch	2 slices of toast	1 cup of oatmeal
1 fruit	1/2 cup orange juice	1/2 banana
1 meat	1/4 cup low-cholesterol egg substitute	1 low-fat sausage link
1 fat	1 tsp margarine	2 pecans
Lunch		
1 skim milk	1 cup skim milk	1 cup skim milk
4 starch	1 1/3 cup brown rice	2 slices of bread†
		1 cup broth-type vegetable soup and 3 ginger snaps
1 fruit	1 apple	1/2 cup pineapple juice
2 vegetables	1 cup green beans	1/2 cup asparagus and 1 cup raw carrots
2 meat	2 oz stir-fried chicken	2 slices low-fat cheese†
1 fat	1 tsp oil	1 tsp margarine†
Dinner		
3 starch	1 lg baked potato	1/4 10-in pizza, thin crust and 2 bread sticks (4 x 1/2 in)
1 vegetable	1/2 cup broccoli‡	Sliced tomato
Free vegetable	Lettuce salad	Lettuce salad
1 meat	1 oz ground beef	(on pizza)
2 fat	2 tbsp sour cream‡	(on pizza)
	1 tbsp French dressing	1 tbsp Italian dressing
Free	Coffee	Diet soft drink
HS		
1/2 skim milk	1/2 cup skim milk	1/2 cup skim milk
2 starch	1 1/2 oz pretzels	6 cups hot-air popped popcorn
1 fruit	15 grapes	1 peach
1 meat	1 oz low-fat cheese stick	1 tbsp Parmesan cheese
1 fat	2 walnuts	1 tbsp diet margarine

*The calculations and meal plan based on 55 percent carbohydrate, 20 percent protein, and 25 percent fat with a 1/5, 215, 1/5, and 1/5 distribution.
†Cheese sandwich.
‡Potato toppings.

cardiovascular disease in people with diabetes. Overall, cardiovascular disease is at least two to three times more common in patients with type 2 diabetes (Nuttall and Chasuk, 1998).

CARBOHYDRATE COUNTING In 1995, the American Diabetes and Dietetic associations introduced carbohydrate counting, a new menu-planning concept. Carbohydrate counting refers to a teaching tool that includes three progressive levels of difficulty, achievement, and self-care to be mastered by the client. These three progressive levels are designated Level I, Level II, and Level III. They are summarized in Box 19–3. Because carbohydrate is assumed to be the main factor affecting postprandial blood glucose elevation, priority is given to counting the total amount of carbohydrate consumed at one meal and/or snack as opposed to the

CLINICAL APPLICATION 19-3

Glycemic Index

Different food sources that contain equal amounts of carbohydrate have been found not to have an equal impact on blood glucose levels. The **glycemia index** of food attempts to classify foods according to their impact on blood glucose. The higher the glycemic index value, the higher the blood glucose would be expected to rise after ingestion of the food.

Foods high in water-soluble fiber, in the raw state, high in binders, and eaten as part of a mixed meal reduce the glycemia response. Dairy products, pasta, dried peas, and legumes are examples of foods with a low glycemic index. Potatoes, some cereals, and bread are examples of foods with a high glycemic index.

Food is usually eaten as mixed nutrient sources. For example, spaghetti is usually eaten with tomato sauce or as part of a meal. Because a mixed meal tends to dilute the glycemia index of any one of the meal's constituents, the glycemia index is rarely taught in clinical practice. However, some highly motivated and well-educated people with diabetes are beginning to use information about the glycemic index of foods to assist in meal planning. Thus it is important to understand this concept. The following table compares effects of foods based on equal amounts of carbohydrate, not serving sizes or energy content. By convention, white bread is assigned a value of 100.

Food	Glycemic index
Glucose	138
Potato, russet, baked	135
Cornflakes	119
White bread	100
White table sugar (sucrose)	86
Rice	83
Banana	79
All-bran cereal	73
Spaghetti	66
Dried peas	56
Apple	53
Ice cream	52
Milk	49
Honey (fructose)	30

source of the carbohydrate. Diabetes educators use Level I, then Level II, and possibly Level III as a client masters the previously taught level. The advantages of the carbohydrate-counting meal plan concept include single-nutrient focused, more precise matching of food and insulin, flexible food choices, a potential for improved blood glucose, and client-controlled treatment. Challenges for the client who uses this system may include the need to weigh and measure food, maintenance of extensive food records, monitoring of the blood glucose before and after eating, the need to calculate grams of carbohydrate consumed, the need to maintain healthful eating, and weight management.

Knowledge of carbohydrate counting is often a prerequisite before consideration for insulin pump therapy. It is also a prerequisite for clients who want to learn how to calculate insulin:carbohydrate ratios. This type of teaching is usually done by a certified diabetes educator (CDE) and is considered Level III teaching.

The rationale for carbohydrate counting is a carbohydrate = a carbohydrate = a carbohydrate or one starch exchange = one fruit exchange = one milk exchange. One carbohydrate unit (or exchange) is about 15 grams of carbohydrate with an acceptable range of 8–22 grams per carbohydrate choice. Food labels, tables of food composition, and *Exchange Lists for Meal Planning* are some of the tools clients can use to determine the carbohydrate content of a particular food. Following is a typical meal plan for a client who has been taught to count carbohydrates:

Breakfast: 3 carbohydrates (range 38 to 52 grams)
  Example: 1 whole bagel and 8 ounces (oz) skim milk
Lunch: 3 carbohydrates (range 38 to 52 grams)
  Example: 8 oz. regular cola and 1 fresh orange and 1 slice whole wheat bread
Dinner: 3 carbohydrates (range 38 to 52 grams)
  Example: 1 1/2 cups pasta
Snack: 1 carbohydrate (8 to 22 grams)
  Example: 8 ounces skim milk

Most healthcare workers (including students) underestimate the amount of time a client must be willing to spend to learn the carbohydrate counting. The American Diabetes and the American Dietetic associations estimate that clients need between 90 and 180 minutes to master one level of this menu-planning system (The American Diabetes and the American Dietetic Associations, 1995). Client visits (usually three) should be spread over several months. One study documented that patients who received three sessions with a registered dietitian experienced significant improvements in glucose control (FBG and HbA1c), serum cholesterol, and weight (Franz, et al, 1995). However, clients learn new information and change eating behaviors at different rates. Each client benefits from an individualized teaching plan. The need for lifelong learning should be emphasized.

Protein and fat intake are not counted with this meal planning system but should be given some consideration. Clients are usually counseled to eat about the same amount of protein each day and choose foods that are low in fat. For example, based on an individualized assessment, a client may be counseled to choose a food that provides approximately 3 grams of fat or less for each carbohydrate (15 grams). Thus, if a client is considering a canned entrée containing 30 grams of carbohydrate, he or she knows the food is not a good choice if it contains more than 6 grams of fat (Zeman and Ney, 1996).

Special Considerations

Persons with diabetes frequently ask questions about nutritional problems related to vitamin and mineral supplementation, alcohol, acute illness, eating out, and delayed meals. The following sections discuss these nutrition-related problems.

Vitamin and Mineral Supplementation

There is no evidence that people with diabetes benefit from vitamin or mineral supplementation solely because they have diabetes. Two minerals commonly mentioned in relation to diabetes are chromium and magnesium. Chromium deficiency has been related, hypothetically, to develop-

Box 19–3 Carbohydrate Counting			
Title	Level I	Level II	Level III
Food Pyramid	Getting Started	Moving On	Intensive Diabetes Management Using Carbohydrate/ Insulin Ratios
Educational concepts	Foods that should be eaten Importance of eating on time Use of foods to counteract hypo-glycemia	Rationale for meal plan Expands on the selection of healthy foods Provides additional tips for meal planning	Sets the stage for self-management skills that provide flexibility and best control of diabetes The nutrient con-tent of food Interpretation of food labels Use of dietetic foods and sweeteners Advice for dealing with fast food, eating out, and parties
Client goals	Carbohydrate die-tary consistency Flexible food choices	Adjust food, medi-cation, and activ-ities based on patterns from client daily records.	Adjust insulin dose using ratio of carbohydrate/ insulin dosage
Intended audiences	Type 1 Type 2 GDM	Person on diet only, oral agents, or insulin who has mastered basics of carbohydrate counting	People on intensive therapy People who have mastered insulin adjustment and supplementation
Primary distribu-tion channels	Physician's offices Hospitals HMOs Clinics with regis-tered dietitians on staff	Settings with a reg-istered dietitian or certified diabetes educator who has diabetes training and experience	Settings with health-care team trained in intensive insulin therapy

ment of diabetes in humans for years, but persuasive studies in Western people are not available that recommend chromium supplementation for diabetic individuals. Most people with diabetes are not chromium defi-cient, and thus chromium supplementation cannot be routinely recom-mended (Anderson, 1999). Similarly, magnesium should be used as a dietary supplement only if hypomagnesemia (low levels of magnesium in the blood) is demonstrated (Anderson, 1999).

Individuals on very-low-calorie diets (less than 800 kilocalories) or pregnant women may need a vitamin and mineral supplement. Any disease condition that normally affects the ingestion, digestion, absorption, metab-olism, and excretion of nutrients may require a supplement as it would for the person without diabetes.

Alcohol

The moderate use of alcohol does not adversely affect diabetes in the well-controlled client. Recommendations follow (American Diabetes Association, 1994):

For insulin users:

- Limit to two drinks per day.
- Drink only with food.
- Do not cut back on food.
- If history of alcohol abuse, abstain.
- Abstain during pregnancy.

For noninsulin users:

- Substitute for fat kilocalories.
- Limit to promote weight loss or maintenance.
- Limit with elevated triglycerides.
- If there is a history of alcohol abuse, abstain.
- Abstain during pregnancy.

Nutrition During Acute Illness Episodes

Acute illness affects everyone, including the person with diabetes. Colds and flu-like symptoms can be fatal for some people with dia-

Table 19–7 Easily Consumed Carbohydrate Containing Foods for "Sick Days"

Food	Amount	Grams of Carbohydrate
Regular cola	1/2 cup	13
Ginger ale	3/4 cup	16
Milk	1 cup	12
Apple juice	1/2 cup	15
Grape juice	1/3 cup	15
Orange juice	1/2 cup	15
Pineapple juice	1/2 cup	15
Prune juice	1/3 cup	15
Regular gelatin	1/2 cup	20
Sherbet	1/2 cup	30
Tomato juice*	1/2 cup	5

*High in sodium.

betes unless precautions are taken. Secretion of both glucagon and epinephrine increases during illness and contributes to an increase in blood glucose levels. This may lead to a loss of glucose, fluid, and electrolytes. Dehydration, electrolyte depletion, and a loss of nutrients may follow. Acute illnesses can lead to DKA in IDDM and to HHNS in NIDDM.

Dehydration is more rapid when electrolytes and fluids are not replaced. Vomiting, diarrhea, and fever all result in fluid loss. During acute illness, the individual should be instructed to monitor his or her blood glucose level every 2–4 hours until the symptoms subside. Urine ketone levels should be checked. The following guidelines are recommended (www.diabetes-midon.org, accessed May 2000):

- If the blood glucose is over 250 mg/dL: drink kilocalorie-free, caffeine-free liquids in place of a meal. Also, consume additional liquids from kilocalorie- and caffeine-free sources.
- If the blood glucose is between 180 and 250 mg/dL: drink or eat 15 grams of CHO in place of a meal (one carbohydrate). Also, consume additional liquid from kilocalorie- and caffeine-free sources.
- If the blood glucose is under 180 mg/dL: drink or eat usual mealtime CHO amount. Also, consume additional liquid from kilocalorie- and caffeine-free sources.
- When the glucose drops to less than 100 mg/dL and vomiting persists, immediate attention is required. Hospitalization may be necessary.

Increased fluids reduce the risk of dehydration. Clients who are vomiting or nauseated and are unable to tolerate regular food drink liquids that contain carbohydrate and/or electrolytes (Table 19–7). A general guideline is that approximately 15 grams of carbohydrate should be consumed every 1–2 hours. Some clients have an individually calculated sick-day menu based on the carbohydrate content of their regular diet.

Other meal-planning tips that may prove helpful during periods of acute illness include (1) increasing water intake, even for clients who can eat regular food; (2) eating smaller, more frequent feedings; and (3) eating soft, easily digested foods.

Eating Out and Fast Foods

The best advice for persons with diabetes who enjoy eating out is that they know their meal-planning system and order small. For example, an individual counting carbohydrates and eating a small hamburger at McDonald's with a side salad, diet dressing, and a glass of skim milk would count:

3 carbohydrates	Grams of CHO
2 starches (hamburger bun)	30
1 milk	12
Total	42

The individual can always mix 4 ounces of orange juice with diet soft drinks for a fruit punch beverage if he or she needs an additional 15 grams of carbohydrate.

Hypoglycemia in Diabetes Mellitus (The 15-15 Rule)

The immediate treatment goal for a glucose level of less than 60 mg/dL is to increase blood glucose to within a normal level as rapidly as possible. Take care not to overtreat hypoglycemia. If the client is monitoring his or her blood glucose level, at the first sign or symptom of hypoglycemia he or she should measure the blood glucose level. If the blood glucose level is less than 60 mg/dL, 15 grams of carbohydrate should be consumed. Fifteen grams of carbohydrate are equal to 2–3 glucose tablets, 6–10 Lifesavers candy, or 4–6 ounces of juice. Fifteen minutes later, he or she should measure the blood glucose a second time. This is called the 15-15 rule. The process may need to be repeated a second time to achieve a blood glucose level between 70 and 110 mg/dL; check laboratory's normal range. Treat with 15 grams of carbohydrate, wait 15 minutes, and retest. If the reaction is not resolved, treat again. Overtreatment can be avoided by adherence to the 15-15 rule. Clients who do not test their blood glucose levels should be taught to do so.

Clients should be advised to carry a source of carbohydrate with them at all times. A snack should be consumed if a meal or snack is delayed (preplanned or not preplanned) by a half hour or more. At least one significant other should be instructed about hypoglycemia and the 15-15 rule.

Teaching Self-Care

Persons with diabetes ultimately treat themselves. The better educated the individual is about diabetes, the greater the likelihood of his or her avoiding the acute and chronic complications of this disease. Many public health departments, hospitals, and clinics hold classes for clients with diabetes. Newly diagnosed clients with diabetes need to learn survival skills. Healthcare workers often have to repeat instructions several times before the client understands the survival skills being taught. Because of the genetic predisposition toward diabetes, many newly diagnosed clients have relatives who have suffered from the acute and chronic complications of diabetes. Hearing about such complications firsthand often creates fear in newly diagnosed clients. They need time to accept their condition. Occasionally, it may take as long as a full year before clients can grasp the principles of self-care. This is especially difficult for children (see Clinical Application 19–4). During hospitalization, it is extremely difficult to effectively educate clients. Follow-up with a certified diabetes educator (CDE) and a registered dietitian (RD) is crucial.

CLINICAL APPLICATION 19–4

Children with Diabetes

Kilocalorie allowances are based on a person's weight. As a rough estimate, a 1-year-old child needs 1000 kcal per day. For older children, 100 kcal per year of age are added to the daily intake. For a 9-year-old child, this would equal 1900 kcal. Typically, 55 percent of the total kilocalories should be consumed as carbohydrate. 1900 kcal multiplied by 55 percent equals 1045 kcal. To convert kilocalories from carbohydrate to grams of carbohydrate divide by 4. 1045 kcal divided by 4 kcal/g equals 260 g of carbohydrate.

How these grams of carbohydrate are divided among the day depends on the child's prescribed medications and lifestyle. Let's assume the child eats three meals and two snacks (at mid-afternoon and bedtime) and takes one dose of basal insulin in the morning and three doses of regular insulin, one before each meal.

The diet could be planned to provide 20 percent of the carbohydrate at each feeding. Twenty percent of 260 g of carbohydrate equals 52 g or 3 1/2 carbohydrate choices. The child and the child's parents would be instructed to provide about 52 g of carbohydrate at each feeding.

As long as the child eats balanced meals that provide all the essential nutrients, the source of the carbohydrate is not important. Scientific evidence has shown that the use of sucrose as part of the meal plan does not impair blood glucose control in individuals with type I and type II diabetes (American Dietetic Association, 1994). A typical menu for the child follows:

Grams of Carbohydrate Breakfast	Acceptable range 46 to 60
1/2 cup of Honey Nut Cheerios	12 (package label)
3/4 cup skim milk	9 (exchange value)
1/2 cup orange juice	15 (exchange value)
1 slice toast	15 (exchange value)
1 tsp peanut butter	0
Total carbohydrates	51
Lunch	
Ham and cheese sandwich with 2 slices of bread	30 (exchange value)
1 apple	15 (exchange value)
3/4 cup skim milk	9 (exchange value)
Carrot sticks	0 (free with this system)
Total carbohydrates	54
Mid-Afternoon Snack	
3/4 cup apple juice	23 (exchange value)
13 animal crackers	25 (exchange value)
Total carbohydrates	48
Dinner	
1/8 15-in cheese pizza	39 (table of food composition)
6 oz regular cola	20 (table of food composition)
Total	59
Bedtime Snack	
1/2 cup skim milk	6 (exchange value)
Raw broccoli with dip	0 (free with this system)
10 (1 1/2 oz) whole-wheat crackers (no added fat)	30 (exchange value)
1/2 oz jelly beans	14 (table of food composition)
Total carbohydrates	50
Total carbohydrates for the day	262

Hypoglycemia

Hypoglycemia, caused by increased endogenous insulin production (hyperinsulinism), is rarer than diabetes mellitus. Hyperinsulinism is most likely caused by islet cell tumors or, less often, by reactive hypoglycemia. Hypoglycemia that occurs 1–3 hours after a meal and resolves spontaneously with the ingestion of carbohydrate is often termed reactive hypoglycemia.

The dietary management of reactive hypoglycemia consists of avoiding simple carbohydrates and sometimes taking small, frequent feedings. The meal plans for diabetes offer a reasonable guide to meal planning. Table 19–8 is a 1-day meal plan for this type of diet.

Summary

Diabetes mellitus is caused by an undersecretion or underutilization of insulin and/or receptor or postreceptor defects. Diabetes is actually a group of disorders with a common sign of hyperglycemia. The two major types of diabetes are type 1 and type 2. Impaired glucose tolerance or impaired fasting glucose, secondary diabetes, and gestational diabetes are other categories of this disease. Persons with diabetes suffer from acute and chronic complications. Treatment involves medication, nutrition management, and exercise. Nutrition is a fundamental part of treatment. Hypoglycemia, a rarer condition than diabetes, is caused by oversecretion of insulin and is also treated with dietary manipulation.

Table 19–8 Sample Meal Plan for Hypoglycemic Diet

Exchange Group	Sample Menu	Exchange Group	Sample Menu
Morning		*Mid-afternoon*	
1 fruit	1/2 cup unsweetened orange juice	1 meat	1 oz low-fat cheese
1 starch	3/4 cup whole-grain cereal	1 starch	4 whole-grain crackers
1 meat	1 low-fat cheese or	*Evening*	
1/2 skim milk	1/2 cup skim milk	2-4 meat	2-4 oz lean meat
Free	Decaffeinated coffee	1 starch	1/2 cup potato or pasta
Mid-morning		1 vegetable	1/2 cup vegetable
1 meat	1 tbsp peanut butter	1 fat	Lettuce salad with dressing
1 starch	4 whole-grain crackers	1 fruit	1 piece fresh fruit
Noon		Free	Decaffeinated coffee or tea
Chefs salad		*Bedtime*	
2–4 meat	2–4 oz lean meat	1 starch and	1/2 sandwich (1 slice whole-grain
1 vegetable	Lettuce, tomatoes, and	1 meat	bread and 1 oz lean meat)
1 fat	Dressing	1 vegetable	Fresh vegetables
1 fruit	1 small piece fresh fruit	Free	Decaffeinated beverage
1 skim milk	1 cup skim milk		
1 starch	2 breadsticks (4 × 1/2 in		

Case Study 19–1

Mrs. S, a 45-year-old black woman, was admitted to the hospital with medical diagnoses of type 2 diabetes and cellulitis of the left leg. Her admitting height was 5 ft. 5 in. and weight 200 lb (BMI = 33.5). Wrist measurement shows Mrs. S has a large frame. Vital signs were temperature 98.6°F, pulse 70 beats per minute, respirations 16 per minute, and blood pressure 160/95.

Mrs. S reported a gradual increase in her weight since her third child was born 20 years ago. That baby weighed 12 lb. Two previous pregnancies produced infants weighing 10 and 11 lb. She has no known allergies.

None of the children live at home. Mrs. S lives with her husband, who works as a construction laborer. She has been seasonally employed as a hotel maid at a nearby resort. Health insurance coverage is sporadic. They have a new insurance policy now.

Mrs. S is the oldest of six children. Her father died of a heart attack at age 60. Her mother died of a stroke at age 62 following 15 years of treatment for diabetes mellitus. The sister who is closest to Mrs. S in age developed diabetes mellitus 3 years ago and is being treated with oral medication. Their youngest sister was diagnosed as an insulin-dependent diabetic at age 18 following an episode of mumps.

Mrs. S reports a good appetite and a fluid intake of about 3 quarts per day. Her favorite beverage is iced tea with sugar and lemon. She does most of the grocery shopping and cooking.

Mrs. S hit her left ankle with the screen door about 2 months ago. The resulting sore has not healed but has gotten worse. Mrs. S knows that a sore that does not heal is a sign of cancer, which is why she sought medical attention. The ankle now has an open lesion 5 cm in diameter over the lateral ankle bone. The entire foot is swollen to twice the size of the right foot. The bandage over the sore had greenish-yellow drainage on lt.

A random blood glucose test in the doctor's office 3 hours after her last meal was 400 mg/dL. Her urine glucose was negative for ketones. Before she left the office, the physician told Mrs. S she has type 2 diabetes mellitus.

The physician prescribed the following care for Mrs. S:
- Bed rest with left leg elevated
- Bedside commode
- Diet assessment and teaching
- Multivitamin, 1 capsule, daily
- Culture and sensitivity of drainage from left leg
- Cefuroxime, 250 mg, orally every 12 h
- Warm, moist dressing to left leg ulcer four times per day
- Fasting blood sugar (FBS), electrolytes in AM

The admitting nurse constructed the following Nursing Care Plan for Mrs. S.

Nursing Care Plan

Subjective Data	Family history of diabetes mellitus
	Large appetite
	Large fluid intake
	Delay in seeking medical attention
Objective Data	Obesity (BMI = 33.5))
	Newly diagnosed type 2 diabetes
	Possible hypertension (only one reading given)
	Open lesion 5 cm diameter over left lateral ankle; purulent discharge
Nursing Diagnosis	Health Maintenance, altered related to inappropriate self-care (North American Nursing Diagnosis Association, 1999) as evidenced by delay in seeking medical attention

Desired Outcomes Evaluation Criteria	Nursing Actions/ Interventions	Rationale
Knowledge: Treatment Regimen (NOC) (Johnson, Maas, and Moorhead, 2000)	Teaching: Disease Process (NIC) (McCloskey and Bulechek, 2000)	
Client will verbalize self-care measures related to type 2 by hospital discharge.	Refer to dietitian for nutritional assessment and education.	The cornerstone of treatment of type 2 is weight loss. Although any weight loss will help, to reach a healthy weight, Mrs. S needs to lose 51 lb. A dietitian's expertise is needed.
	Review survival skills with client (see Appendix for client teaching tool).	The American Diabetes Association recommends all patients with diabetes learn survival skills if they do not know this core information.
Client will verbalize willingness to continue nursing/medical regimen after discharge.	Refer to social worker for sources of medical attention when uninsured.	Social workers are most familiar with community resources.
	Teach principles of wound care, including effect of high blood sugar on infection.	If Mrs. S understands that high blood sugar feeds the bacteria causing the infection, she may be more willing to work hard to control the diabetes.
	Reinforce dietitian's instruction. Have Mrs. S state the Dietary Guidelines and the reason why they are important.	Knowledge usually precedes behavior change.
	Have Mrs. S describe the meal plan she follows.	Short periods of instruction are most effective; frequent review of the material will help the client master it.
	Ask physician to discuss exercise regimen when the blood sugar is under control.	Mrs. S needs a prescribed exercise program suited to her level of conditioning.

Critical Thinking Questions

1. The client would like to learn how to monitor her own blood glucose levels (as the nurses do) before discharge. How would the nurse, in the role of client advocate, arrange for this to be done? Why is a physician's written order important?

2. The client's fasting blood glucose level has decreased steadily during her 3-day hospitalization. On the morning of discharge, the FBS was 150 mg/dL. The client stated, "It has come down enough. Now, I don't need to worry about the diabetes any longer." How would you respond?

3. Why is a referral to a certified diabetes educator crucial for this client?

Study Aids

Subjects . . . .**Internet Sites**

American Diabetes Association . . . . .http://www.diabetes.org, accessed May 2000

American Association of Diabetes Educators . . . . .http://www.aadenet.org, accessed May 2000
An association dedicated to the needs of diabetes educators

American Dietetic Association . . . . .http://www.eatright.org, accessed May 2000
Offers links to other sites

Center for Chronic Disease Control's Diabetes and . . . . .http://www.cdc.gov/nccdphp/ddt/ddthome.htm accessed May 2000
Public Health Resource

Setting insulin doses . . . . .http://www.diabetesnet.com/math/1500.html, accessed May 2000

Report on the Expert Committee on the Diagnosis and   http://www.medscape.com/ADA/DC/2000/v23.n01s/
Classification of Diabetes Mellitus   pnt-dc23s10.01html, accessed May 2000

Custom Cuisine: mail order meals for clients with diabetes . . . . . . .http://www.c-cuisine.com, accessed May 2000

Diabetes and Medicare benefits . . . . .http://www.medicare.gov, accessed May 2000

Information on managing diabetes . . . . .http://www.lilly.com/diabetes/, accessed May 2000

Michigan Diabetes Outreach Network . . . . .http://www.diabetes-midon.org, accessed May 2000

Chapter Review

1. If a client has a history of ketoacidosis, he or she most likely has diabetes.
   a. Type 1
   b. Type 2
   c. Pituitary
   d. Gestational

2. The following statement is true:
   a. Acute illness lowers blood glucose levels.
   b. Fluid and electrolyte replacement is essential during episodes of acute illness in all persons with diabetes.
   c. Persons with diabetes who have an acute illness require a vitamin and mineral supplement.
   d. Persons with diabetes should never eat forms of simple sugar.

3. Dietary guidelines for people with diabetes include:
   a. One serving of alcohol daily
   b. Consume no more than 2000 milligrams of sodium each day.
   c. Restrict fat intake to less than 10 percent of total kilocalories.
   d. Consume at least 20 to 35 grams of fiber each day.

4. For most clients, the cornerstone of treatment of type 2 diabetes is:
   a. Stress management
   b. Meal planning
   c. Strict adherence to five planned meals per day
   d. Hypoglycemic drugs

5. The diet for reactive hypoglycemia includes the following features:
   a. Small, frequent meals with restricted simple sugars
   b. Three meals with ample simple sugars and high in complex carbohydrate
   c. Four to six small meals that are high in fat
   d. Three high-carbohydrate meals that are moderate in fat

Clinical Analysis

Ms. N, a 14-year-old, was diagnosed one year ago with type 1 diabetes mellitus. Her blood sugar levels have been stable on an intermediate-acting insulin and a 370-gram CHO diet. The teenager is now being seen in the doctor's office for routine follow-up. The nurse is reviewing Ms. N's knowledge of self-care.

1. To assess knowledge, the nurse asks how the client would handle a day when the client could not eat solid foods. Which of the following answers would show understanding of the usual procedure?
   a. Skip insulin that day.
   b. Call the doctor after missing one meal.
   c. Replace the carbohydrates in the meal plan with liquids containing equal amounts of carbohydrate.
   d. Take half her usual insulin dose and double the usual fluid intake.

2. The client plays volleyball for the high-school team and is moderately active during practices and games. SMBG records indicate a daily glucose level of between 120 and 140 mg/dL prior to the time she usually plays volleyball. Which of the following behaviors are appropriate for her before playing?
   a. No additional food is indicated.
   b. Increase intake by 15 grams of carbohydrate.
   c. Decrease intake by 15 grams of carbohydrate.
   d. Increase intake by one vegetable exchange and one fat exchange.

3. The client states, "I am getting tired of pricking my finger several times a day. Why can't I manage my diabetes with urine testing like my grandmother?" Which of the following responses by the nurse would be most appropriate?
   a. "The urine test is more accurate in older people."
   b. "The point at which sugar is spilled in the urine varies even for one individual. Therefore, the blood test is more accurate."
   c. "Urine tests are more costly."
   d. "The blood test is the newest thing. Your grandmother's doctor must be old-fashioned."

Bibliography

Anderson, JW: Nutritional Management of Diabetes Mellitus. In Shils, ME, Olson, JA, Shike, M, Ross, CA (eds): Modern Nutrition in Health and Disease, ed 9. Baltimore, Williams and Wilkins, 1999.

American Diabetes Association: Maximizing the Role of Nutrition in Diabetes Management. American Diabetes Association, Alexandria, VA, 1994.

American Diabetes Association: Position statement American Diabetes Association: Diabetes mellitus and exercise. Diabetes Spectrum 19:530, 1996a.

American Diabetes Association: Position statement American Diabetes Association: Nutrition recommendation and principles for people with diabetes mellitus. Diabetes Care 19(suppl 1):516, 1996b.

American Dietetic Association: Manual of Clinical Dietetics, ed 4. American Dietetic Association, Chicago, 1992.

Black, JM, and Matassarin-Jacobs, E.: Luckmann and Sorenson's Medical-Surgical Nursing, ed 4. WB Saunders, Philadelphia, 1993.

Boyko, EJ, Lipsky, BA: Infection and diabetes. In Harris, MI, Cowie, CC, Stern, MP, Boyce, EJ, Reiber,GE, and Bennett, PH (eds): Diabetes in America, ed 2. U,S, Govt. Printing Office, (NIH pub). No 095-1468) pp 485–499, Washington DC, 1995.

Committee on Diet and Health Food and Nutrition Board Commission on Life Sciences National Research Council: Diet and Health. National Academy Press, Washington DC, 1989.

Deglin, JH, and Vallerand, AH: Davis's Drug Guide for Nurses, ed 4. FA Davis, Philadelphia, 1995.

Diabetes Control and Complication Trial Group: Influence of intensive treatment on quality-of-life outcomes in the diabetes control and complications trial. Diabetes Care 19:195, 1996.

Diabetes Control and Complication Trial Group: The effect of intensive treatment of diabetes on the development and progression of long-term complications in insulin-dependent diabetes mellitus. New Engl J Med 329:977, 1993.

Franz, MJ: Exercise and the management of diabetes mellitus. J Am Diet Assoc 87:872, 1987.

Franz, MJ, et al.: Nutrition principles for the management of diabetes and related complications. Diabetes Care 17:490, 1994.

Franz, MJ, et al.: Effectiveness of medical nutrition therapy provided by dietitians in the management of noninsulin-dependent diabetes: A randomized, controlled clinical trail. J Am Diete Assoc. 95:1009, 1995.

Golden, SH, et al.: Perioperative glycemic control and risk of infectious complications in a cohort of adults with diabetes. Diabetes Care 22:1408, 1999.

Guyton, AC: Textbook of Medical Physiology, ed 7. WB Saunders, Philadelphia, 1986, p. 932.

Kuusisto, J, et al.: NIDDM and its metabolic control predict coronary heart disease in elderly subjects. Diabetes 43:960, 1994.

Jacobson, AM: Commentary. Diabetes Spectrum 6:36, 1993.

Johnson, M, Maas, M, and Moorhead, S: Nursing Outcomes Classification (NOC), ed 2. Mosby, Philadelphia, 2000.

Maggio, C and Pi-Sunyer, X: The prevention and treatment of obesity: Application to type-2 diabetes. Diabetes Care. 20:1744, 1997.

Matthews, DE: Protein and Amino Acids. In Shils, ME, Olson, JA, Shike, M, and Ross, CA (eds): Modern Nutrition in Health and Disease, ed 9, Baltimore, Williams and Wilkins, 1999.

McCloskey, JC, and Bulechek, GM: Nursing Interventions Classification (NIC), ed 3. Mosby, Philadelphia, 2000.

Michigan Diabetes Outreach Network: Quick Reference Guide to Diabetes for Health Care Providers. SODON (Southern Michigan Outreach Diabetes Network): Southern Michigan Diabetes Outreach Network Newsletter Vol. 4, Issue 4. Coldwater, MI, November 1999.

Nathan, DM: Long-term complications of diabetes mellitus: New Engl J Med 328:1676, 1993.

North American Nursing Diagnosis Association: Nursing Diagnoses: Definitions and Classification 1999–2000, North American Nursing Diagnosis Association, Philadelphia, 1999.

Nuttall, FQ, and Chasuk, RM: Nutrition and the management of type 2 diabetes. J Family Practice. 47(5 suppl), 1998.

Pagana, KD, and Pagana, TJ: Mosby's Diagnostic and Laboratory Test Reference, ed 2. Mosby, St. Louis, 1995.

Pastors, JG: Nutritional Care of Diabetes. Nutrition Dimension Inc., San Marcos, FL, 1992.

Pemberton, CM, et al.: Mayo Clinic Diet Manual, ed 6. BC Decker, Philadelphia, 1988.

Peterson, KA, and Vinicor, F: Strategies to improve diabetes care delivery. J Family Practice 47(5 suppl), 1998.

Position paper of the American Dietetic Association. Nutrition recommendations and principles for people with diabetes mellitus. J Am Diet Assoc 94:504, 1994.

Position paper of the American Diabetes Association: Preconception care of women with diabetes. Diabetes Care 19(suppl):525, 1996a.

Prochaska, JO, DiClemente, Norcross: In search of how people change: Application to addictive behavior. Diabetes Spectrum 6:25, 1993.

UK Prospective Diabetes Study Group: Intensive blood-glucose control with sulphonylurea or insulin compared with conventional treatment and the risk of complications in patients with type 2 diabetes. (UKPDS 33). Lancet 352:837, 1998.

www.diabetes-midon.org accessed 11-16-99.

www.medscape.com/ADA/DC/2000.v23no01s.01/pnt-dc23s01.01.html

www.lilly.com/diabetes/

Zeman, FJ, and Ney, DM: Applications in Medical Nutritiona Therapy. Merril, Columbus, 1996.

Zimmerman, BR, and Hagen, MD: An evaluation of new agents in the treatment of type 2 diabetes. Am J Family Practice 47(5), November 1998.

CHAPTER 20

Diet in Cardiovascular Disease

LEARNING OBJECTIVES

After completing this chapter, the student should be able to:

1. Discuss the relationship of diet to the development of cardiovascular disease.
2. Distinguish between type II and type IV hyperlipoproteinemias as to aggravating factors and dietary modifications.
3. Identify strategies that are likely to reduce the risk of cardiovascular disease.
4. Describe the 2-gram sodium diet.
5. List several flavorings and seasonings that can be substituted for salt on a sodium-restricted diet.

The cardiovascular system includes not only the heart and blood vessels but the blood-forming organs as well. This chapter discusses common diseases of the heart and blood vessels that can be influenced by diet modification. Conditions resulting from faulty blood forming are included in other chapters. Iron-deficiency anemia is discussed in Chapter 8 on minerals and pernicious anemia in Chapter 7 on vitamins and Chapter 11 on pregnancy. Nutritional care of leukemia clients is included in Chapter 23, Diet in Cancer.

Occurrence of Cardiovascular Disease

Diseases of the cardiovascular system include 3 of the 15 most common causes of death in the United States. Diseases of the heart (coronary, hypertensive, and rheumatic) occupy first place with an age-adjusted death rate in 1997 of 130.5 per 100,000 population, accounting for 726,974 deaths. Cerebrovascular disease is third with a death rate of 25.9, accounting for 159,791 deaths, and atherosclerosis is fifteenth with a rate of 2.1 per 100,000 population. Each of these death rates has declined between 1979 and 1999, heart disease by 34.6 percent, cerebrovascular disease by 37.7 percent, and atherosclerosis by 63.2 percent (Centers for Disease Control, 1999b).

Heart disease has been the leading cause of death in the United States since 1921. As is apparent from Figure 20–1, the death rate from heart disease peaked in 1950 at 307.4 per 100,000. The death rate began declining even before the advances in coronary care and current medications were available. However, the decreases in death rates for heart disease are not evenly distributed throughout the population. For example, during 1985–1996, the death rate for white men declined 29 percent but for American Indian/Alaskan Native women only 10 percent (Centers for Disease Control, 1999a). An analysis of countries with declining death rates attributed two-thirds of the decline to coronary-event rates and one-third to changes in case fatalities (Kuulasmaa et al., 2000).

Stroke has been the third leading cause of death since 1938. The southeastern United States is known as the "Stroke Belt." Age-adjusted death rates for cerebrovascular diseases for South Carolina, Arkansas, Mississippi, Georgia, Tennessee, North Carolina, the District of Columbia, and Louisiana are the highest reported except for American Samoa, Guam, and the Virgin Islands (Centers for Disease Control, 1999c). The only risk factor for stroke predominant in the Southeastern states is physical inactivity, but insufficient data from several states limits what conclusions can be drawn (Hahn, Heath, and Chang, 1998). Throughout the United States, non-Hispanic blacks had approximately four times the risk of stroke mortality as non-Hispanic whites at ages 35–54 and three times the risk at ages 55–64. Suggested reasons for the ethnic differences include greater prevalence of risk factors for stroke, such as obesity, uncontrolled hypertension, physical inactivity, poor nutrition, diabetes, and smoking, as well as barriers to health care, such as lack of health insurance, inadequate transportation, and unfamiliarity with early warning signs of stroke (Centers for Disease Control, 2000).

Underlying Pathology

Two major pathological conditions contribute to cardiovascular disease. One is atherosclerosis, the most common form of **arteriosclerosis**. The second is hypertension, which is discussed here as contributing to pathology and later in the chapter as a risk factor for cardiovascular disease.

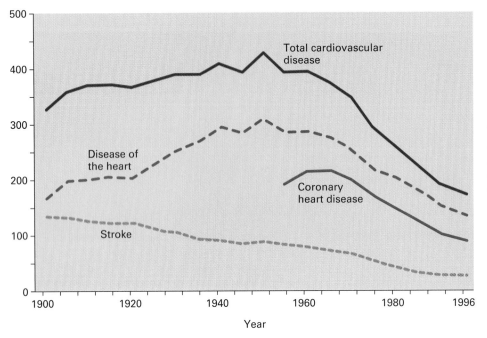

Figure 20–1:
Age-adjusted death rates per 100,000 population for total cardiovascular disease, diseases of the heart, coronary heart disease, and stroke, by year—United States, 1900–1996. (Centers for Disease Control, 1999a)

Atherosclerosis

In **atherosclerosis** fatty deposits of cholesterol, fat, or other substances accumulate inside the artery. Initially, the deposited material, or plaque, is soft, but later it becomes fibrosed or hard. This disease process interferes with the pumping of blood through the artery in two ways: (1) the deposits gradually make the lumen smaller and smaller and (2) the fibrosis makes it progressively harder for the artery to constrict or dilate in response to the tissues' needs for oxygenated blood (Fig. 20–2). When the lumen, or opening through the artery, is 70 percent blocked by atherosclerotic plaque, the person is likely to show symptoms of impaired circulation distal to the obstruction. The atherosclerotic process begins early in life. People 15–34 years old, autopsied after trauma or accidents, were found to have increased fatty and fibrous arterial lesions, which were more extensive in the older victims. More extensive lesions were also associated with higher serum LDL cholesterol levels (Fisher, Van Horn, and McGill, 1997).

Because half of myocardial infarction clients do not have abnormal blood lipids (both discussed below), other factors that might affect a person's risk profile are being explored. One of these is serum homocysteine because homocysteinemia has been reported to be an independent risk factor for atherosclerosis. Homocysteine is discussed in Clinical Application 20–1. Another factor that has recently been associated with atherosclerosis is inflammation. One marker of inflammation, plasma C-reactive protein, an abnormal protein produced by the liver in response to acute inflammation, has been extensively investigated in relation to atherosclerosis. This test distinguished women at high risk of cardiovascular disease even when their lipid profiles were in the normal range (Ridker et al., 2000) and reaffirmed early findings on men (Koenig et al., 1999; Ridker et al., 1997). This confirmation of an inflammatory process in atherosclerosis expands the rationale for the use of aspirin to prevent cardiovascular disease. In addition to its anticoagulant properties, it is an anti-inflammatory agent. Various infective agents are also under investigation as contributing to inflammation in cardiovascular disease (Mattila et al., 1998; Roivainen et al., 2000).

Hypertension

Blood pressure is the force exerted against the walls of the arteries by the pumping action of the heart. It is recorded in two numbers, such as 120/80. The top number, **systolic pressure**, is the pressure when the heart beats. The bottom number, **diastolic pressure**, is the pressure between beats. Both pressures are reported in millimeters of mercury (mm Hg).

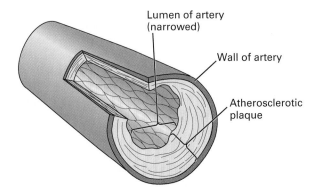

Figure 20–2:
Buildup of atherosclerotic plaque within an artery. Note both the narrowed diameter and the roughness within the lumen. (From Scanlon and Sanders, p. 284, with permission.)

CLINICAL APPLICATION 20–1

Homocysteine and Atherosclerosis

History

Thirty years ago, extensive atherosclerosis was found on autopsy of individuals with elevated plasma homocysteine levels due to errors of metabolism. This autosomal recessive genetic disease, homocystinuria, occurs in about 1 of 200,000 live births. When untreated, homocystinuria results in thromboembolic events in 50 percent of the patients and a mortality rate before the age of 30 of 20 percent (Nygard et al., 1997).

Correlational Studies

Even among individuals without homocysteinuria, a link has been found between plasma homocysteine levels and atherosclerosis. More than 75 clinical and epidemiologic studies have shown a relation between total homocysteine levels and coronary artery disease, peripheral artery disease, stroke, or venous thrombosis (Nygard et al., 1997). Even mild hyperhomocysteinemia is associated with increased risk of arteriosclerotic disease and stroke (Selhub and D'Angelo, 1997). In the Physician's Health Study, men whose homocysteine levels were only 12 percent above the upper limit of normal had three times the risk of myocardial infarction (Stampfer et al., 1992). A prospective study of patients with angiographically confirmed coronary artery disease found a strong, graded relation between plasma homocysteine levels and overall mortality (Nygard et al., 1997). Homocysteine levels were found to be positively correlated with severe coronary atherosclerosis, with no clear cutoff point below which there was no increased risk (Verhoef et al., 1997).

Pathology

Homocysteine is an amino acid produced as the essential amino acid methionine is catabolized. Homocysteine is not ingested and normally not detectable in the plasma or urine because it is processed intracellularly (Klor et al., 1997). Hyperhomocysteinemia, in the absence of kidney disease, indicates faulty metabolism due to vitamin deficiency (folate, B_{12}, B_6) or a genetic defect (Selhub and D'Angelo, 1997). There is no conclusive evidence that increasing methionine or animal protein intake results in chronically higher concentrations of homocysteine in the blood of individuals with adequate intakes of vitamins B_6, B_{12}, and folic acid (Evans et al., 1997). Vitamin deficiencies, on the other hand, are exacerbated by a diet high in animal protein, a rich source of methionine (Welch, Upchurch, and Loscalzo, 1997).

No unifying hypothesis explains the atherogenic and thrombogenic effects of plasma homocysteine (Refsum et al., 1998). The exact mechanism of homocysteine's pathology is unknown, but vascular damage seems to be key (Klor et al., 1997). Human and animal studies have demonstrated that homocysteine damages endothelial cells and predisposes the person to platelet adhesion, activation, and subsequent thrombus formation (Welch, Upchurch, and Lascalzo, 1997). Homocysteine facilitates the generation of hydrogen peroxide, which is toxic to the vascular endothelium, producing oxidative damage to LDL cholesterol and endothelial cell membranes (Miller, 1996), but this toxic effect occurs only in the presence of copper (Klor et al., 1997).

Multiple causes are suggested for mild hyperhomocysteinemia. Enzyme deficiencies involving the metabolism of vitamins B_6, B_{12}, and folic acid have been researched. Other possible etiologic factors include age, gender, renal disease, some drugs and vitamin intake (Shimakawa et al., 1997). Plasma concentrations of folate and the coenzyme form of vitamin B_6 and the level of folate intake were inversely associated with carotid artery stenosis after adjustment for age, sex, and other risk factors (Selhub et al., 1995).

Severe, genetic hyperhomocysteinemia, regardless of the causative enzyme defect, is almost always associated with premature and aggressive vascular disease (Graham et al., 1997). Approximately half the individuals who are homozygotes for cystathionine beta-synthase deficiency suffer a thromboembolic event by age 29 (Shimakawa et al., 1997).

Dietary/Supplementary Associations

Higher intakes of folic acid and vitamins B_{12} and B_6 have been linked to lower risk of vascular disease. Individuals who took supplements containing folic acid, cobalamin, or pyridoxine had 0.38 relative risk of atherosclerotic vascular disease (cardiac, cerebral, or peripheral) compared with nonusers of vitamin supplements. Note was made, however, that the subjects who took vitamins may also have been more conscientious about their health habits in other ways (Graham et al., 1997). Women who reported taking at least four multiple vitamin capsules a week for 5 or more years had the lowest risk of coronary heart disease in the Nurses' Health Study (Rimm et al., 1998).

Over an 8-week period, supplementation with vitamins B_6 and B_{12} and folic acid decreased homocysteine levels 27.9 percent in men with mild homocysteinemia. The effect was most noticeable in those whose folate concentrations at baseline were lowest (Woodside et al., 1998).

Recommendations

Careful laboratory procedures are essential if plasma homocysteine is to be used to assess cardiovascular risk. Fasting blood samples are recommended because a protein-rich meal may cause an increase of 15–20 percent in homocysteine levels. Additionally, the posture of the subject during the blood draw should be standardized because it affects albumin concentration, which in turn determines protein-bound homocysteine (Refsum et al., 1998).

One group of researchers recommended that estimation of total plasma homocysteine levels be part of a vascular disease risk assessment (Graham et al., 1997). Other researchers avoid blanket recommendations because not all patients with heart disease, but only about 20–30

Continued on next page

CLINICAL APPLICATION 20–1 (cont.)

percent of them (Miller, 1996), have elevated homocysteine levels. Furthermore, although six prospective studies showed an association between homocysteine and cardiovascular disease risk, another five studies did not, leading to the conclusion that until clinical trials are conducted, homocysteine levels cannot be considered predictive of cardiovascular disease (Malinow, Bostom, and Krauss, 1999). Almost two-thirds of the cases of high serum homocysteine concentrations in the United States are associated with low concentrations of folate, vitamin B_{12}, or both (Selhub et al., 1999). The present state of knowledge allows the possibility that homocysteine may be only a marker of atherosclerosis (Christen et al., 2000) or of folate status, and other unknown mechanisms may explain the lower rates of coronary heart disease associated with higher intakes of folate and vitamin B_6 (Rimm et al., 1998).

Randomized clinical trials are needed to determine whether lowering homocysteine levels through supplementation with folic acid and vitamins B_6 and B_{12} reduces the occurrence of atherothrombotic vascular disease. Recent fortification of grain with folic acid, although initiated to prevent neural tube defects during pregnancy, may coincidentally reduce hyperhomocysteinemia. A comparison of blood samples from groups of middle-aged and older adults showed that those tested after fortification was implemented had plasma folate levels that were 117 percent higher than people whose blood was drawn before fortification. The prevalence of high homocysteine concentrations was 48 percent less in the after-fortification group also (Jacques et al., 1999).

The dearth of definitive answers to the significance of homocysteine levels in the blood illustrates the difficulty of researching biological events in a changing environment. For individuals who elect to monitor their homocysteine levels, clear and cautious interpretation by the health care provider is essential. Meanwhile, avoiding smoking, maintaining desirable cholesterol levels, and controlling weight and blood pressure are recommended to reduce the risks of cardiovascular disease.

Diagnosis of Hypertension

Hypertension, which affects about 50 million people in the United States, is defined as blood pressure of 140/90 or higher on at least three occasions on different dates. The category also includes persons taking antihypertensive medication. Several readings are taken on different days to eliminate the possibility of excitement or nervousness causing a transient hypertension. Hypertension is classified as Stages 1, 2, or 3 (Table 20–1). A person with hypertension may not feel sick, so blood pressure screening is often offered as a community service (Fig. 20–3). Along with temperature, pulse, and respirations, blood pressure is a vital sign. The National Stroke Association recommends blood pressure checks for all clients at every physician visit (Gorelick et al., 1999).

Types of Hypertension

Depending on the cause of the hypertension, it is labeled primary or secondary. About 90 percent of hypertensive clients have primary or **essen-**

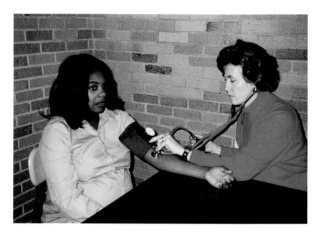

Figure 20–3:
Hypertension is a silent killer. Blood pressure monitoring is a part of most health system visits. Even children are occasionally hypertensive.

tial hypertension. There is no single, clear-cut cause for this high blood pressure.

Secondary hypertension occurs in response to another event or disease process in the body. One such event is pregnancy, during which pregnancy-induced hypertension may occur. Medications also can cause secondary hypertension. Birth control pills that contain progesterone stimulate the production of renin, which may result in an elevation in blood pressure. As detailed in Chapter 17, the combined intake of **monoamine oxidase (MAO) inhibitors** and tyramine-rich foods or beverages can cause hypertension. Secondary hypertension also can result from diseases of the kidney, adrenal glands, or nervous system.

Positive Feedback Cycle

Many cardiovascular conditions have interlocking causative factors. The interaction between atherosclerosis and hypertension is referred to as a **positive feedback cycle**. In this situation, the presence of the second condition worsens the first. Atherosclerosis narrows the lumen of the arteries, and the smaller opening increases the blood pressure. Then the higher blood pressure forces more lipids into the arterial wall, worsening the atherosclerosis, and the cycle is repeated.

End Result of Pathology

Most people do not have either atherosclerosis or hypertension. More commonly, they have both conditions. Although many organs are likely to

Table 20–1 Classification of Blood Pressure for Adults Age 18 and Over

Category	mmHg Systolic		mmHg Diastolic
Optimal	<120	and	<80
Normal	<130	and	<85
High-normal	130–139	or	85–89
Hypertension			
Stage 1	140–159	or	90–99
Stage 2	160–179	or	100–109
Stage 3	> or = 180		> or = 110

be damaged by atherosclerosis and hypertension, the major concern is the effect on the heart and brain, as described in the next sections on coronary heart disease and cerebrovascular disease.

Coronary Heart Disease

When the coronary arteries that supply the heart muscle with blood become blocked, the result is coronary heart disease (CHD) or coronary artery disease (CAD), which affects 12.2 million people in the United States. If the blockage is temporary, due to increased activity and the body's increased demand for oxygen, the person may experience **angina pectoris**, or severe pain and a sense of constriction about the heart. Rest and the administration of vasodilating medications commonly produce relief, but changes in diet and lifestyle are necessary to stave off heart damage. However, if the vessel is blocked by atherosclerotic plaque; by a **thrombus**, a blood clot that develops in one of the coronary arteries; or by an **embolus**, a circulating mass of undissolved matter, the heart tissues beyond the point of obstruction receive no oxygen or nutrients. When this happens, the person exhibits signs and symptoms of a **coronary occlusion**, or a heart attack. When the blood supply cannot be restored quickly, myocardial cells in the affected area die. The medical diagnosis then becomes **myocardial infarction** (MI). Acute myocardial infarction occurs in 1.5 million people in the United States annually, causing death in one-third of cases (Spencer, Carson, and Crouch, 1999).

Congestive Heart Failure

Congestive heart failure (CHF) affects an estimated 4 million Americans. Each year 200,000 people die of CHF (Brady, Rock, and Horneffer, 1995), but the mortality rate has been declining since 1971. The prevalence of heart failure increases steadily with increasing age, from less than 1 percent in 35-year-olds to over 8 percent in 75-year-olds (National Institutes of Health, 1997).

Congestive heart failure occurs when the heart is unable to maintain adequate circulation of the blood. CHF results from an injury or a reduction in function of the heart muscle. Causes may be atherosclerosis, hypertension, myocardial infarction, rheumatic fever, or a birth defect. When the heart cannot keep up with the demands on it, a sequence of events sets up another positive feedback cycle.

The right side of the heart collects the blood returning from the body and pumps it to the lungs to excrete carbon dioxide and absorb oxygen. If the right ventricle is failing, usually due to lung disease, the blood backs up into the veins that empty into the right atrium, and the client has the signs of peripheral edema. As a result of fluid volume excess and edema of the small bowel, the client suffers from anorexia and nausea.

The left side of the heart receives the oxygenated blood from the lungs and pumps it out to the body. If the left ventricle is failing, usually following a myocardial infarction, the blood that cannot be pumped effectively to the body backs up in the blood vessels of the lungs. Next the fluid from the blood is forced into the lung tissue. The client will display shortness of breath and moist lung sounds and will expectorate frothy pink sputum.

In addition, if the heart cannot pump enough to maintain blood pressure, the body implements the reninresponse. Angiotensin II constricts the blood vessels, raising blood pressure. Aldosterone causes the kidney to conserve sodium, and with it, water. More fluid fills the blood

vessels. The higher blood pressure pushes this fluid out into the interstitial spaces, causing edema.

Obviously, one side of the heart cannot function for long if the other side is failing. Nevertheless, the health-care worker learns to look for signs of heart failure in the extremities in right-sided failure or in the lungs in left-sided failure.

Cerebrovascular Accident

When a blood vessel in the brain becomes blocked by atherosclerosis, the tissue supplied by that artery dies. This is the most common cause of cerebrovascular accidents, or strokes, in the United States. Strokes also can be caused by an embolus or a ruptured blood vessel. Cerebrovascular accidents, affecting 4.4 million people in the United States, are usually secondary to atherosclerosis, hypertension, or a combination of both. Strokes are also related to coronary heart disease. The risk of ischemic stroke is 31 percent in the first month following a myocardial infarction (Gorelick et al, 1999).

Peripheral Vascular Disease (PVD)

This is a broad classification of diseases affecting arteries and veins distal to the heart. Atherosclerosis is a major causative factor of peripheral vascular disease (PVD), affecting an estimated 2.4 million Americans (Grace, Crosby, and Ventura, 1995). Signs and symptoms vary depending on the vessels affected, the extent of the damage, and the duration of the problem. The effects of peripheral vascular disease range from limitation of activities to amputation of digits or extremities due to gangrene.

Risk Factors in Cardiovascular Disease

The occurrence of cardiovascular disease in a person cannot be predicted with certainty. Many attributes and behaviors interact to produce the illness.

Unchangeable Risk Factors

Age, sex, race, family history, and personal medical history can be predictive of atherosclerosis and hypertension in some people. None of these risk factors can be modified to prevent disease.

Age, Sex, and Race

Age-related changes account for many cardiovascular events. For example, hypertension usually develops at about age 50 to 60 and coronary atherosclerosis occurs more frequently in individuals over the age of 40. Sex-related occurrence of coronary heart disease is readily apparent as risk increases in males after age 45 and females after age 55. Until menopause, women have less atherosclerosis and coronary heart disease than men. Estrogen affects lipid metabolism, as will be discussed later. Women past menopause and younger diabetic women are stricken with coronary heart disease just as often as men are.

Hypertension is twice as common in blacks as in whites. Also, blood pressure shows steeper increases with advancing age in blacks than in whites (Melby, Toohey, and Cebrick, 1994).

Table 20–2 Inherited Hyperlipoproteinemias

| | | | | Increased Plasma Values | | | | |
| | | | | Lipoprotein | | | Lipid | |
Type	Frequency	Inheritance Pattern	Aggravated by	Chylomicrons	VLDL	LDL	Cholesterol	Triglycerides
I	Very rare	Autosomal recessive	Fat	X				X
IIA	Common	Autosomal dominant	Fat		X		X	
IIB	Common	Autosomal dominant	Fat		X	X	X	X
III	Uncommon	Multifactorial	CHO	Remnants			X	X
IV	Very common	Autosomal dominant	CHO		X			X
V	Rare	Autosomal recessive	Fat and CHO	X	X		X	X

Adapted from Dietary Management, 1980, and Fauci et al., 1998.

Family and Prior Medical Histories

A family history of premature coronary heart disease in a parent or sibling increases a person's risk of the disease. Premature coronary heart disease has been defined as occurring in a male under the age of 50 or a female under age 60 (Williams and Bollella, 1995).

Of special concern are the inherited **hyperlipoproteinemias**, or increased lipoproteins and lipids in the bloodstream (Table 20–2). One of these hyperlipoproteinemias, type IV, is very common and is often associated with **noninsulin-dependent diabetes mellitus** (NIDDM). Some of the other types are seen less often. All six types have a connection to food intake of fats, carbohydrates, or both. Blood plasma values vary in each condition. For example, type I hyperlipoproteinemia is aggravated by fat, and the chylomicrons are elevated because they carry exogenous triglycerides that cannot be broken down. Thus, plasma triglyceride levels are elevated as well.

Type II hyperlipoproteinemia results from a single gene defect in the cell receptor that binds circulating low-density lipoproteins. It is an autosomal dominant characteristic. Individuals with this defect have a rate of coronary heart disease 25 times that of the normal population. In addition, clients with type IIA hyperlipoproteinemia generally develop heart disease 15 years earlier than the rest of the population. Some even suffer heart attacks in infancy and childhood.

In addition to the inherited disorders of lipid metabolism, hyperlipoproteinemia can develop secondary to other conditions and environmental factors such as diet. Diabetes mellitus, alcohol consumption, oral contraceptives, kidney disease, liver disease, and hypothyroidism can either cause or aggravate existing lipid disorders.

A person's medical history is pertinent when evaluating risks of cardiovascular disease. The risk of heart attack rises more sharply after surgical menopause (removal of the ovaries) than after natural menopause. A person who has already suffered a stroke has an increased risk of a subsequent stroke.

Changeable Risk Factors

Unlike age, sex, race, and family or personal history, some risk factors for cardiovascular disease can be modified. The major changeable risk factors are hypertension, serum cholesterol, obesity, diabetes mellitus, physical inactivity, cigarette smoking, and alcohol intake. These are discussed in the following sections.

Hypertension

Approximately 30 to 40 million adults in the United States have high blood pressure, and 2 million new cases are diagnosed annually. The prevalence steadily increases with age, as the blood vessels become less resilient due to atherosclerosis, and 4 percent of 18- to 29-year-old persons have hypertension compared to 65 percent of individuals 80 years and older (National High Blood Pressure Education Program, 1993). Very old persons may account for many of the cases because estimates of hypertension in younger adults are decreasing. In 1960–1962, 37 percent of people 20 to 74 years old in the United States were estimated to have hypertension compared to 23 percent in 1988–1994 (Centers for Disease Control, 1999a).

Unfortunately, only about 70 percent of people with pressures greater than 140/90 are aware of it, and about 50 percent of them are being treated, with about 25 percent adequately controlled. A decrease of just 2 mm Hg in systolic pressure is estimated to have the potential to reduce annual mortality from stroke by 6 percent and from coronary heart disease by 4 percent.

Two dietary influences have been related to hypertension: high salt intake and low intakes of potassium, calcium, and magnesium.

HIGH SALT INTAKE Age-related increases in blood pressure are related to salt intake. Blood pressure values increase with age everywhere but in extremely remote areas of the world and are significantly related to sodium intake. Decreasing sodium intake by 2300 milligrams will decrease systolic blood pressure by 3 to 6 mm Hg (Elliott et al., 1996). Although sodium has been identified as the major influence on blood pressure, it does not increase blood pressure when administered with anions other than chloride (Kotchen and Kotchen, 1999). Moreover, not everyone is equally responsive to salt intake. Clinical trials showed greater effectiveness of sodium restriction in hypertensive subjects than in normotensive subjects. Decreases in systolic and diastolic pressures averaged 5 and 3 millimeters of mercury in the former but only 2 and 1 millimeters of mercury in the latter (National High Blood Pressure Education Program, 1993). Individuals most likely to benefit from salt restriction include African-Americans, older people, and clients with hypertension or diabetes. African-Americans excrete sodium less efficiently than Caucasians (Kotchen and Kotchen, 1999). An intake goal of 6 grams of sodium chloride (containing about 2.4 grams of sodium) is considered reasonable by the National Institutes of Health (1997).

LOW POTASSIUM, CALCIUM, AND MAGNESIUM INTAKES Low intakes of these three minerals have been associated with hypertension, the major modifiable risk factor for stroke. Diets containing less than 600 milligrams of calcium daily are most clearly associated with hypertension, and dietary

Table 20–3 Desirable Serum Cholesterol Levels (mg/dL) in Children and Adults

	Ages 2 to 19 years*	Ages >20 years
Total cholesterol	<170	<200
Low-density lipoprotein	<110	<130
High-density lipoprotein	>45	>35

*Recommended by Williams and Bollella, 1995.

calcium is also inversely related to systolic blood pressure in young children (Kotchen and Kotchen, 1999). Griffith and colleagues (1999) analyzed 42 clinical trials and reported that calcium supplementation resulted in very small reductions in systolic (1.44 mm Hg) and diastolic (0.84 mm Hg) blood pressure. Similarly, Whelton and He (1999) analyzed 33 clinical trials and reported that potassium supplementation reduced mean blood pressure, 4.4 mm Hg systolic and 2.45 mm Hg diastolic. High potassium intake produces a greater reduction in blood pressure in African-Americans than in Caucasians and in individuals with a high salt intake (Kotchen and Kotchen, 1999). Increased risk of stroke was associated with lower potassium, magnesium, and cereal fiber intakes (Ascherio et al., 1998).

As is commonly is seen in nutrition studies, an intake of certain foods can be correlated with an increase or reduction of disease, but individual nutrients when tested are not. It may be the individual nutrient selected to be tested has a small effect alone but works in conjunction with other nutrients or that the substance in the food causing the effect has not been identified. Obtaining adequate dietary intake from food, not supplements, is recommended (National Institutes of Health, 1997).

Elevated Blood Cholesterol

Despite its categorization as a risk factor for cardiovascular disease, cholesterol serves vital functions in the body. It is a component of the nerve tissue of the brain and spinal cord, of the tissues of the liver, the adrenal glands, and the kidneys, and of bile. Cholesterol is a precursor of adrenal hormones and the sex hormones. Blood cholesterol levels, however, are frequently measured to promote health and prevent disease. The recommended frequency is every five years in healthy people.

Among 2- to 11-year-old children, 25 percent are reported to have borderline high cholesterol. Table 20–3 lists compares desirable serum cholesterol levels in children and adults. It is recommended that a child's risk of CHD be evaluated by family history between the ages of 2 and 6 and updated regularly (Williams and Bollella, 1995). Certain groups of children with elevated blood cholesterol would be missed in the process: urban African-American adolescents (Rifai et al., 1998), children with incomplete family health histories, children in single-parent families, and children whose parents have not had their cholesterol checked (Dennison, Jenkins, and Pearson, 1994). Children who have elevated serum cholesterol levels have to be managed carefully so that sufficient food is provided to support growth. Universal screening of children for hypercholesterolemia is not recommended (Committee on Nutrition, 1992).

RELATIONSHIP TO PATHOLOGICAL CHANGES Serum cholesterol levels are directly associated with CHD mortality in the United States and Northern Europe (Verschuren et al., 1995) and with atherosclerosis and CHD risk. Cholesterol-lowering clinical trials using **angiograms** show improved coronary perfusion. For every 1 percent reduction in serum cholesterol, a person decreases his risk of CHD by 2 percent. Even so, cholesterol-lowering alone is unlikely to reduce CHD mortality in the United States and Northern Europe to the level of Mediterranean and Japanese people (Verschuren et al., 1995).

RELATIONSHIP TO DIET The liver manufactures about 1000 milligrams of cholesterol daily. Only foods of animal origin contain cholesterol, but the body's ability to process cholesterol impacts serum lipid levels. An estimated two-thirds of the population is able to compensate for increased dietary cholesterol by manufacturing less of it. This ability to compensate, or its lack, is thought to be genetically determined (Howell, 1997).

Consumption of substances other than dietary cholesterol can also influence serum cholesterol levels. Trans unsaturated fatty acids in vegetable oil products have been identified as more potent risk factors for cardiovascular disease than saturated fat. About 63 to 75 percent of the intake of trans fatty acids is derived from baked goods, fried fast foods, and other prepared foods, rather than from margarines (Ascherio, Katan, and Stampfer, 1999). Trans fats have been shown to raise LDL levels and lower

Table 20–4 Functions and Significance of Various Lipoproteins

Lipoprotein	Normal Value in 12- to 14-Hour Fasting Specimen	Function	Clinical Significance
Chylomicrons	0	Transport exogenous triglycerides from intestines to blood stream	Present in blood only after a meal
VLDL	13–32 mg/dL	Main transporter of endogenous triglyceride	Synthesized by liver and small intestine from free fatty acids, glycerol, and carbohydrate
LDL	38–40 mg/dL	Transports cholesterol to body cells	Major form of lipoprotein in atherosclerotic lesions. The higher the LDL level, the greater the risk of CHD
HDL	20–48 mg/dL	Transports cholesterol from body cells to liver to be excreted	Synthesized by liver and intestines. The higher the HDL level, the lower the risk of CHD; aerobic exercise increases HDL level in men but only slightly in women

---

Box 20–1 Research on Antioxidants in Cardiovascular Disease

Attempts to understand the effects of antioxidants on cardiovascular disease have involved vitamins and flavonoids. Often several studies are necessary to clarify the process of disease prevention or progression. Sometimes the research produced results contrary to those expected.

Animal subjects fed antioxidants showed regression in their atherosclerotic lesions (Fuller and Jialal, 1994). In laboratory experiments, the antioxidant vitamins are expended in a particular order: C, E, and beta-carotene (Frei, 1994). High dietary intake of these vitamins was inversely correlated with coronary heart disease in 5133 Finnish men and women (Abbey, Noakes, and Nestel, 1995). Higher vitamin E intake was associated with a lower incidence of CHD (Rimm et al., 1993; Stampfer et al., 1993), with reduced risk of heart attacks in persons with heart disease (Stephens et al., 1996) and with lower coronary mortality (Knekt et al., 1994; Kushi et al., 1996). The vitamin E reciprocally sparing mineral selenium was lower in the blood of acute myocardial infarction clients than in healthy controls.

Beta-carotene intake through vegetables and fruit was inversely related to cardiovascular mortality and to incidence of myocardial infarction. Men in the placebo group of a hyperlipidemia study with the highest total serum carotenoid levels (of which beta-carotene is only 25 percent) had a relative risk of CHD events of 0.64 compared to men with the lowest serum carotenoid levels (Morris, Kritchevsky, and Davis, 1994). Supplements of beta-carotene alone were not effective in reducing cardiovascular disease (Hennekens et al., 1996).

Antioxidant flavonoids, found in vegetables, fruits, tea, and wine inhibit oxidation of LDL and reduce thrombotic tendency in laboratory experiments. A high flavonoid intake in elderly men, mainly from tea, onions, and apples, was associated with lower mortality from CHD (Hertog et al., 1993). A similar association was found for women, but not men, in Finland (Knekt et al., 1996), and an association between more tea drinking and less aortic atherosclerosis was documented in the Netherlands (Geleijnse et al., 1999). After 25 years of follow-up in a cross-cultural study, intake of flavonoids was inversely associated with CHD mortality and explained about 25 percent of the variance in CHD rates in seven countries (Hertoeg et al., 1995).

Giving supplemental vitamin E and/or beta-carotene to smokers, however, produced unexpected increases in mortality: from hemorrhagic stroke in those receiving vitamin E and from lung cancer and ischemic heart disease in those receiving beta-carotene (Alpha-Tocopherol, 1994). Similarly, supplementing smokers or asbestos workers with beta-carotene and retinyl palmitate was followed by increased risk of death from lung cancer and cardiovascular disease (Omenn et al., 1996). No known physiologic mechanism can explain these findings (Olson, 1999).

Rather than expecting a single nutrient to alter the occurrence of disease, it is now thought that antioxidants work together to produce the effects related to food consumption. Supplementation with tocopherol reduced in vitro oxidation by 50 percent and vitamin C by 15 percent, but together the reduction was 78 percent (Niki et al., 1995). Moreover, oxidation is a physiological process. For instance, some oxidation products act against invading bacteria so that providing large doses of antioxidants could upset the body's defenses.

The declining heart disease rate has been correlated with increased fruit and vegetable consumption in the United States, a safe means of achieving optimal blood concentrations of antioxidants. The American Heart Association advises that the most prudent and scientifically supportable recommendation for the general population is to consume a balanced diet with emphasis on antioxidant-rich fruits and vegetables and whole grains (Tribble, 1999).

HDL levels. Trans fatty acids are not specified on food labels, but a proposal by the FDA would include trans fatty acids on labels by the year 2002.

Coffee intake has shown mixed effects on cholesterol, perhaps varying because of the brewing techniques. Unfiltered coffee (common in Scandinavia and Turkey) contains cafestol that potently raises serum VLDL and LDL levels by an unknown mechanism (van Tol et al., 1997). Instant coffee has been filtered in the manufacturing process, and many coffeemakers require filters.

LIPOPROTEINS AS RISK FACTORS Fats cannot dissolve in water but are bound to proteins for transportation in the bloodstream. These fat-carrying complexes are called lipoproteins. There are four main classes of lipoproteins: **chylomicrons, very low-density lipoproteins** (VLDL), **low-density lipoproteins** (LDL), and **high-density lipoproteins** (HDL). Table 20–4 summarizes the functions, significance, and normal laboratory values of these four classes of lipoproteins. Further research is revealing lipid subfractions including Lp(a) and small, dense LDL to be significant risk factors for cardiovascular disease (Gotto, 1998).

The higher the LDL, the greater is the risk of CHD. Therefore, the primary target of cholesterol-lowering regimens is the LDL cholesterol. The goals of therapy are to lower the LDL value to (1) below 160 milligrams per deciliter if fewer than two other risk factors for cardiovascular disease are present or (2) below 130 milligrams per deciliter if two or more other risk factors are present (Expert Panel, 1993). LDL cholesterol is deposited into macrophages in the endothelial wall on its way to becoming part of atherosclerotic plaque. Two types of LDL receptors have been identified in the macrophages. One type recognizes unoxidized LDL and limits the amount taken into the cell. The other type recognizes oxidized LDL but does not stop its entry into the cell (Spencer, Carson, and Crouch, 1999). Because it is thought that oxidized LDL is more atherogenic than unoxidized LDL, much current research involves antioxidants. Box 20–1 summarizes some of these conflicting findings.

Conversely, the higher a person's HDL level, the lower is the risk of coronary heart disease. A high HDL level (60 mg/dL or more) negates one other risk factor in tallying a person's risk. A low HDL value of less than 35 mg/dL is added as a risk factor. Increased HDL levels related to exercise have been clearly demonstrated in men, but the findings are less clear in premenopausal women because levels of HDL vary with the phases of the menstrual cycle (Hartung, 1995). Genetic factors account for about half the variation in the serum HDL cholesterol levels in the population (Grundy, 1999).

Obesity

People who are overweight have two to six times the risk of developing hypertension as people with a healthy body weight. An estimated 50 percent of hypertension could be prevented by weight control. The location of the body fat is significant: abdominal fatness is related to cardiovascular disease and diabetes mellitus more than is gluteal-femoral fatness. Even a 20-pound weight loss is estimated to lower systolic blood pressure by 6.3 mm Hg and diastolic by 3.1 mm Hg (Kotchen and Kotchen, 1999).

Excess body fat is a cause of hypertension and coronary heart disease. The Nurses Health Study showed that the risk of coronary heart disease in middle age increased by 2.6 to 3.6 percent in these women for every kilogram of weight gain after age 18. Using the BMI as the criterion, the risk of coronary heart disease was 20–77 percent greater for women with a BMI between 23 and 24.9 compared to women with a BMI less than 21. For women with a BMI of 29 or more, the risk was 3.5 times that of the women with a BMI of 21 (Willett et al., 1995).

For stroke also, the Nurses Health Study showed steadily increasing risk with a greater BMI. Compared to women with a BMI less than 21, those with a BMI of 27 had a relative risk of ischemic stroke of 1.75, up to a relative risk of 2.37 for a BMI of 32 or higher (Rexrode et al., 1997).

Diabetes Mellitus

At any given cholesterol level, diabetic persons have a two to three times higher risk of atherosclerosis than other people. Diabetic women lose the preventive advantages usually associated with premenopausal women regarding cardiovascular risk.

Insulin is required to maintain adequate levels of **lipoprotein lipase**, an enzyme that breaks down chylomicrons. When lipoprotein lipase is inadequate, chylomicrons and VLDL particles accumulate in the blood. After the diabetes is controlled, serum lipid levels decrease. Lipoprotein lipase is more active in physically active subjects and increases with exercise. This factor is very important in the management of Type II (NIDDM) diabetes. Another example of altered physiology is described in Box 20–2, relating undernutrition in utero to increased risk for diabetes mellitus and cardiovascular disease in adulthood.

Physical Inactivity

Activity is inversely related to blood pressure independent of being overweight in both sexes and across all ages. Hypertension is less prevalent in active adults than in age-matched subjects for whites and blacks, for both sexes, and for younger and older persons. Increasing physical activity has been shown to decrease both systolic and diastolic pressures by 6 to 7 mm Hg (National High Blood Pressure Education Program, 1993). Thus, moderately intense physical activity, such as brisk walking for 30–45 minutes on most days of the week, is recommended. Sporadic bouts of intense exercise in mostly sedentary individuals are not advised because of the stress it would place on the body.

Cigarette Smoking

Smoking may cause an increase in blood pressure at the time, possibly due to a release of vasoactive substances, but whether long-term smoking causes chronic hypertension is less clear (Parmley, 1997). Smokers have lower levels of HDL even when weight is held constant. An estimated

430,000 deaths are caused annually by tobacco use, including 174,000 from heart disease (Parmley, 1997). Within a year of smoking cessation, the cardiovascular benefits are apparent (National Institutes of Health, 1997), and within 2 years, the risk of myocardial infarction approaches that of a nonsmoker (Parmley, 1997).

Alcohol Consumption

In small amounts, alcohol seems to cause vasodilation, whereas at high doses it acts as a vasoconstrictor. The mechanism by which alcohol affects blood pressure has not been established (Kotchen and Kotchen, 1999). Individuals consuming 1 to 2 drinks per day have lower blood pressure than nondrinkers, but blood pressure is positively correlated with an alcohol intake of three or more drinks per day, independent of age, BMI, and cigarette smoking. In an estimated 5–7 percent of cases, hypertension is attributed to an alcohol intake of three or more drinks per day (National High Blood Pressure Education Program, 1993).

The association between alcohol and hypertension is not universal, but an estimated 30–60 percent of alcoholics have hypertension. When hospitalized for detoxification, the average alcoholic's systolic blood pressure decreases by 20 mm Hg. Alcohol has been found to induce strokes, even in normotensive clients. A high intake of alcohol also increases serum triglyceride levels.

Persons who consume one or two alcoholic drinks per day have about a 30–50 percent reduced risk of coronary heart disease compared to individuals who abstain from alcohol. Approximately one-half of this effect is attributed to increased HDL levels (Pearson, 1996).

Box 20–2 Fetal Nutrition and Cardiovascular Disease in Adulthood

Studies have connected low birth weight, thinness, and short body length at birth with high death rates from cardiovascular disease and high prevalence of Type II (NIDDM) diabetes mellitus (Barker, 1999). The associations are seen in small for gestational age (SGA) babies, rather than premature infants, and are independent of social class or lifestyle. Babies who are thin at birth tend to be insulin resistant as adults and have a high prevalence of diabetes mellitus, hypertension, and hyperlipidemia as adults. Studies with laboratory animals have confirmed these relationships. A few studies show relationships in humans as well. For example, in a study of men and women through age 71, at all ages beyond infancy people with lower birth weights had higher blood pressure (Law et al., 1993). In another study, Jamaican children's systolic blood pressure was demonstrated to be inversely related to their birth weight (Forrester et al., 1996).

It is suggested that undernutrition during gestation alters the relationships between glucose and insulin and between growth hormone and insulin-like growth factors. In this way, the fetus adapts to its environment to permit survival, but its changed physiology makes it susceptible to cardiovascular disease in later life (Barker et al., 1993).

Table 20–5 Major Risk Factors for Cardiovascular Disease

RISK FACTOR	CORONARY HEART DISEASE	CEREBROVASCULAR DISEASE
Unchangeable		
Age	80 percent of deaths due to CHD occur in persons 65 years of age or older. Men's heart attacks occur at a younger age than women's do.	Risk doubles each decade after age 55
Gender	Men have greater risk of CHD than women. Even after menopause, when women's risk of CHD increases, their death rate is still lower than men's.	Incidence and prevalence about equal; more than 50 percent of deaths occur in women
Race		African-Americans, Hispanics, and Asian-Pacific Islanders have greater risk than Caucasians
Heredity	Parental history increases risk. Primary hyperlipoproteinemia genetically derived.	Increases risk
Prior Medical History	Risk of heart attack rises more sharply after surgical menopause (oophorectomy) than after natural menopause.	Previous stroke increases risk
Changeable		
Hypertension	Increases workload of heart. Hypertension is more severe in African-Americans and thus increases risk.	Major modifiable risk factor. Reducing diastolic pressure 5–6 mm Hg reduces stroke risk by 42 percent.
High Blood Cholesterol	Risk increases as serum levels rise. Reducing cholesterol levels by 20 percent has produced a 33 percent reduction in coronary mortality.	
Obesity	Truncal obesity increases risk even without additional risk factors. Excess weight increases workload of heart, raises LDL cholesterol and triglyceride levels, and lowers HDL cholesterol level. Middle-aged women with BMIs between 23 and 25 had a 50 percent increase in risk of coronary heart disease. Men aged 40–65 years old with BMIs between 25 and 29 had a 72 percent increased risk.	Truncal obesity increases risk even without additional risk factors.
Diabetes Mellitus	Greatly increases risk, even when glucose levels under good control. About two-thirds of people with diabetes die of heart or blood vessel disease.	Greatly increases risk, even when glucose levels are under good control.
Physical Inactivity	Moderate-intensity activity beneficial; more vigorous activity increases benefit. Exercise can help control cholesterol, diabetes, and obesity. In some persons, exercise moderates hypertension.	
Cigarette Smoking	Doubles the risk. Biggest risk factor for sudden cardiac death (within an hour of heart attack). Smoking cancels the premenopausal advantage women have over men in the risk of heart disease. Secondhand smoke increases risk for nonsmokers.	Nicotine and carbon monoxide damage the cardiovascular system. Smoking plus using birth control pills greatly increases risk.
Alcohol Intake	Persons who consume alcohol moderately (less than 1 drink/day for women or 2 drinks/day for men) have lower risk of heart disease than nondrinkers. Heavy consumption causes hypertension.	More than 1 drink/day for women or 2 drinks/day for men and binge drinking can lead to stroke. Alcohol probably increases risk of hemmorhagic stroke but decreases risk of ischemic stroke.

Compiled from American Heart Association, 2000b and 2000d; Eckel, 1997; Gorelick et al., 1999; Klatsky, 1998; Pearson, 1996; Shepard et al., 1995.

Several of the major risk factors for cardiovascular disease not only exert individual effects but also contribute to a cascade effect. For instance, race and physical inactivity affect obesity, and all three factors impact blood pressure. Major risk factors for coronary heart disease and cerebrovascular disease appear in Table 20–5.

Prevention of Cardiovascular Disease

Prevention of cardiovascular disease depends on minimizing a person's changeable risk factors. Because of the cascade effect, a single change may affect several risk factors. Dietary modifications to prevent cardiovascular disease include careful selection of fat-containing foods, possible inclusion of soybean products, a hypertension-focused intervention called the DASH diet, control of alcohol intake, and use of specialty foods.

Dietary Fat

People in the United States have changed their sources of animal protein between 1977 and 1987. Red meat consumption decreased from 91 to 73 pounds per person per year. Chicken consumption increased from 30 to 43 pounds and seafood from 13 to 15 pounds in the same period (Denke, 1994). To implement the Food Pyramid guide recommendations, meats, fish, and poultry should be baked, broiled, or grilled, not fried. Legumes are an excellent meat substitute and contribute soluble fiber.

Not all animal fat is equally threatening to one's heart and blood vessels. Eskimos following their traditional diet eat a lot of animal fat; they also have a low rate of CHD. Many researchers attribute this to the high omega-3 fatty acid content of the fish Eskimos eat. Omega-3 fatty acids have been shown to reduce serum triglyceride levels, but the recommended source is fish, not fish oil supplements (Ahmed, Clasen, and Donnelly, 1998). Cold water ocean fish, some cold water inland fish, and some other foods contain omega-3 fatty acids in varying amounts. These fatty acids help decrease serum triglycerides, while lowering total cholesterol and blood pressure. Fish that contain omega-3 fatty acids include herring, mackerel, rainbow trout, salmon, sardines, swordfish, and tuna. Risk of death from CHD was shown to be 25 percent less in health professionals eating some fish versus those eating none at all. One or two servings a week seems to achieve maximum results (Katan, 1995). In a 30-year study, fish intake of 1.25 ounces per day reduced risk of death from coronary heart disease by 38 percent (Daviglus et al., 1997). Not all research is easily interpreted. Clinical Application 20–2 describes apparent paradoxes in diet and diseases in different countries. Other food sources of omega-3 fatty acids are butternuts, soybeans, flaxseed, and walnuts.

Fruits and Vegetables

Consumption of greater amounts of fruits and vegetables was shown to be associated with lower risk of ischemic stroke. Average servings of 5.1 among the men in this study and 5.8 among the women reduced the risk of stroke 31 percent compared to individuals who consumed the least number of servings. Up to a maximum of six, each additional serving of fruit or vegetable, excluding potatoes and legumes, reduced the risk of

ischemic stroke 4 percent among the men and 6 percent among the women (Joshipura et al., 1999).

Soybeans

The cholesterol-lowering benefits derived from soy products are being researched. A meta-analysis of 38 controlled clinical trials in which intake of soy protein averaged 47 grams per day showed decreases in total cholesterol of 9.3 percent, in LDL cholesterol of 12.9 percent, and in triglycerides of 10.5 percent (Anderson, Johnstone, and Cook-Newell, 1995). Consumption of a Step I Diet with soy protein compared to animal protein decreased LDL cholesterol significantly (Wong et al., 1998) and soy supplements significantly decreased total cholesterol by 6 percent and LDL cholesterol by 7 percent in perimenopausal women (Washburn et al., 1999). Other studies have reported disadvantages. Compared to casein, soy protein temporarily raised **lipoprotein (a)**, a genetic variant of LDL that is an independent risk factor for coronary artery disease (Nilausen and Meinertz, 1999). An untoward effect of texturized vegetable protein in a metabolic ward study was a highly significant reduction in HDL cholesterol and a significant increase in serum triglyceride while achieving only a borderline significant reduction in LDL cholesterol (Duane, 1999).

Comparing coronary heart disease rates in Japan with those of Western countries stimulated some of the interest in soy as a healthful component of the diet. Even cursory examination of the typical diets, however, shows divergent practices in addition to the consumption of soy. For instance, the Japanese may substitute soy for foods high in saturated fat. The Japanese diet is higher in complex carbohydrates than Western diets. The evidence suggests that soy may be a useful complement to the traditional dietary means of lowering serum cholesterol levels. The FDA has approved a health claim stating that eating 25 grams of soy protein daily as part of a low-fat, low-cholesterol diet may reduce the risk of cardiovascular disease. Because soy has led to increased tumor activity in animals with estrogen-dependent tumors, however, individuals at high risk for such tumors should discuss their plans with their primary healthcare provider before adding large amounts of soy to their diet (Birt, 2000). Figure 20–4 shows a Soy Food Guide Pyramid featuring some soy products.

The DASH Diet

An 11-week clinical feeding trial of individuals with systolic blood pressure of less than 160 mm Hg and diastolic pressures from 80 to 95 mm Hg showed that dietary modification is effective in reducing blood pressure. The trial was named *Dietary Approaches to Stop Hypertension*, thus called the "DASH Diet." After 3 weeks on a *Control Diet*, low in fruits, vegetables, and dairy products with fat content typical of the United States, the participants were randomly assigned to continue on the *Control Diet* or to receive a *Fruits and Vegetables Diet* or a *Combination Diet* for 8 weeks. The *Fruits and Vegetables Diet* was similar to the *Control Diet* except that it provided more fruits and vegetables and fewer snacks and sweets. The *Combination Diet* was rich in fruits, vegetables, and low-fat dairy foods and had reduced amounts of total fat, saturated fat, and cholesterol than either of the other two diets. The potassium, magnesium, and calcium levels of the *Control Diet* were at about the 25th percentile of U.S. consumption, whereas those minerals in the *Fruits and Vegetables Diet* and the *Combination Diet* were close to the 75th percentile.

CLINICAL APPLICATION 20–2

The Limits of Population Studies

In the 1960s, the lowest rates of heart disease reported among seven countries were in Japan and Greece. People in those two countries were poles apart in fat consumption: 10 percent of kilocalories in Japan and 40 percent on the island of Crete. But the Greeks derived less than 10 percent of kilocalories from animal protein and 33 percent of their kilocalories from olive oil, which is 82 percent monounsaturated. Diets high in monounsaturates enhance the resistance of LDL cholesterol to oxidation, whereas polyunsaturates are more susceptible to oxidation (Hiser, 1995).

Since 1976, a decrease in cardiovascular mortality in men and women was experienced in Spain, despite increased intakes of dairy products and meat, particularly pork and poultry. If attention focused only on those foods, the rationale for the decreased mortality would be missed. Most of the decrease in cardiovascular mortality was due to a decline in stroke mortality. Improved hypertension control, including decreased intake of salt and salt-cured foods, is thought to have influenced this trend. Other contributing factors were increased consumption of fruit and fish, reduction in cigarette smoking, and expanded access to clinical care, including a major increase in the use of aspirin as a platelet inhibitor (Serra-Majem et al., 1995).

Consumption of red wine is credited with conferring some protection against coronary heart disease. The "French Paradox" refers to that country's second lowest coronary heart disease mortality rate among 21 countries, in the face of its rank as having the highest alcohol intake and the highest wine intake. Other studies have shown a maximum protective effect of alcohol against CHD at one to two drinks per day. Higher alcohol intake is progressively associated with higher risks of cardiovascular disease and other causes of mortality. A 12-year study of French men indeed found a decrease in cardiovascular mortality of 30 percent associated with a daily intake of 48 grams of alcohol, mostly wine. In contrast, mortality by cancer and violent death was increased compared with that of abstainers (Renaud and Gueguen, 1998).

It is suggested that antioxidant flavonoids in red wine, not the alcohol, contribute to wine's protective effect against heart disease (Hertog et al., 1993; van Poppel et al., 1994) by inhibiting the copper-catalyzed oxidation of LDL (Frankel et al., 1993). Purple grape juice reduced LDL susceptibility to oxidation in clients with coronary artery disease (Stein et al., 1999) and reduced platelet aggregation in healthy people (Keevil et al., 2000). Given the potential for abuse, proposing alcohol as a preventive measure against heart disease is perilous, but purple grape juice would be acceptable to many people for whom alcohol intake poses significant risks.

Men in eastern Finland have one of the highest recorded incidences of mortality from CHD. An association was reported between high levels of stored iron (as assessed by serum ferritin levels or ratio of serum tranferrin receptor to serum ferritin) and increased risk for acute myocardial infarction (Salonen et al., 1992; Tuomainen et al., 1998). Iron overload thus was hypothesized to cause the higher occurrence of CHD in men compared to women. A study in Greece also correlated high dietary iron intake with increased risk of coronary artery disease in men and women 60 years of age or older (Tzonou et al., 1998). A more detailed study found no association between total iron intake and risk of myocardial infarction after adjustment for age and sex but did find high dietary intake of heme iron associated with occurrence of and mortality from myocardial infarction (Klipstein-Grosbusch, 1999), and a reanalysis of Salonen's data associated increased iron intake with increased consumption of red meat (American Heart Association, 2000a).

Yet another interpretation of the north-south differential in mortality rates from cardiovascular disease involves the effect of sunlight on the skin. Cholesterol levels rise in populations with increasing distance from the equator. Even within Scotland and Northern Ireland, CHD mortality rates are generally higher in the north than in the south. This theory states that as people are exposed to less sunlight, less vitamin D is synthesized, allowing more of the substrate to be manufactured into cholesterol. Vitamin D is thereby regarded as an inhibiting factor of coronary heart disease along with antioxidants (Grimes, Hindle, and Dyer, 1996).

Thus evidence accumulates slowly and must be interpreted cautiously. The many correlations found in large studies do not prove causation and may not be clinically useful. Frequently, watchful waiting is the better strategy than lurching from one test to another or one intervention to another before confirmatory research is reported. In human beings, multiple factors are likely interacting to produce the result observed. Investigations into genetics and bacterial infections and their relationships to cardiovascular disease are ongoing

---

Weight reduction did not confound the results because kilocalories were adjusted to maintain weight. Likewise the three types of diets each contained about 3 grams of sodium, and individuals were permitted no more than three caffeinated beverages and no more than 2 standard alcoholic beverages (see below) per day. Reported intakes of alcohol were similar across all the diets.

After 8 weeks, compared to those consuming the *Control Diet*, persons on the *Fruits and Vegetables Diet* showed reductions in systolic blood pressure of 2.8 mm Hg if normotensive and 7.2 mm Hg if hyper-

tensive. The corresponding reductions in diastolic pressures were 1.1 mmHg and 2.8 mm Hg. After 8 weeks, compared to those consuming the *Control Diet*, persons on the *Combination Diet* showed reductions in systolic blood pressure of 5.5 mm Hg if normotensive and 11.4 mm Hg if hypertensive. The corresponding reductions in diastolic pressure were 3.0 mm Hg and 5.5 mm Hg (Appel et al., 1997). The *Combination Diet* was subsequently named the DASH Diet.

An outstanding feature of this trial was its emphasis, not on limiting or restricting foods, but on increasing intake of certain foods. Commonly

Daily Soyfood Guide Pyramid

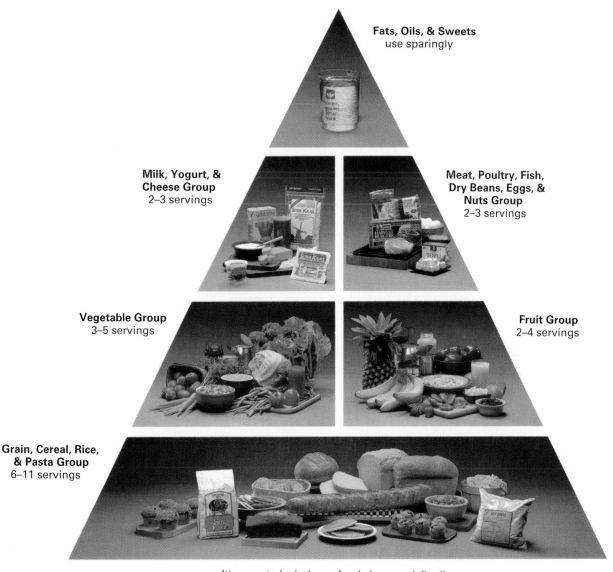

It's easy to include soyfoods in your daily diet.

Figure 20–4:
Daily Soyfood Guide Pyramid. Soy products include oil, milk, cheese, yogurt, beans, burgers, tofu, grits, and flour. (Indiana Soybean Development Council, with permission.)

Table 20–6 The DASH Diet

Food Group	Daily Servings	Serving Sizes	Examples and Notes	Significance of Food Group to DASH Diet
Grains and Grain Products	7–8	1 slice bread 1/2 cup dry cereal 1/2 cup cooked cereal, rice, or pasta	Whole wheat bread, English muffin, pita bread, bagel, cereals, grits, oatmeal	Major sources of energy and fiber
Vegetables	4–5	1 cup raw leafy 1/2 cup cooked 6 oz. Juice	Tomatoes, potatoes, carrots, peas, squash, broccoli, turnip greens, collards, kale, spinach, artichokes, sweet potatoes, beans	Rich sources of potassium, magnesium, and fiber
Fruits	4–5	6 oz. juice 1 medium fruit 1/4 cup dried fruit 1/2 cup fresh, frozen, or canned fruit	Apricots, bananas, dates, oranges, grapefruit, mangoes, melons, peaches, pineapples, prunes, raisins, strawberries, tangerines	Important sources of potassium, magnesium, and fiber
Low Fat or Nonfat Dairy Foods	2–3	8 oz. milk 1 cup yogurt 1.5 oz. cheese	Skim or 1 percent milk, skim or low fat buttermilk, nonfat or low-fat yogurt, part skim mozzarella cheese, nonfat cheese	Major sources of calcium and protein
Meats, Poultry, and Fish	2 or fewer	3 oz. cooked meat, poultry, or fish	Select only lean; trim away visible fat, broil, roast, or boil instead of frying; remove skin from poultry	Rich sources of protein and magnesium
Nuts, Seeds, and Legumes	4–5 per week	1.5 oz. or 1/3 cup nuts 1/2 oz. or 2 tbsp seeds 1/2 cup cooked legumes	Almonds, filberts, mixed nuts, peanuts, walnuts, sunflower seeds, kidney beans, lentils	Rich sources of energy, magnesium, potassium, protein, and fiber
Fats and oils	2.5	1 tsp.	Canola, olive, peanut oils	Contain mainly monounsaturated fatty acids

Adapted from National Institutes of Health, 1997, and the ADA Exchange Lists, Appendix A.

available foods, not specialty foods containing fat substitutes, were used throughout the trial. As is shown in Table 20–6 and Figure 20–5, the major differences between the basic Food Guide Pyramid and the DASH Diet are:

- an increase of 1 daily serving of vegetables,
- an increase of 1–2 daily servings of fruits, and
- inclusion of 4–5 servings *per week* of nuts, seeds, and beans.

The example is based on a 2000-kilocalorie diet. Individuals requiring more or less energy intake would need to make proportionate adjustments.

Alcohol

National U.S. guidelines for hypertension prevention and management are more specific regarding alcohol intake than was the DASH trial. Clients should limit alcohol to no more than 1 ounce of ethanol (24 ounces of beer or 10 ounces of wine or 2 ounces of 100-proof whiskey) per day. Women and lighter-weight men, however, should limit intake to half this amount (National Institutes of Health, 1997). Canadian guidelines are the same for men but somewhat more liberal for women, specifying two standard drinks per day or 14 per week for men and 9 per week for women (Campbell et al., 1999).

Specialty Foods

More and more foods are packaged bearing health claims. Whole-grain foods high in soluble fiber may claim to reduce the risk of heart disease *in a low-fat diet*. Many popular foods are marketed in light or fat-free versions. Other products contain new ingredients to produce a health benefit. One example is the formulation of table spreads and salad dressings with plant sterols. These compounds in plants, which structurally resemble cholesterol but are not absorbed in the human body to any extent, actually inhibit the absorption of cholesterol. Food products containing plant

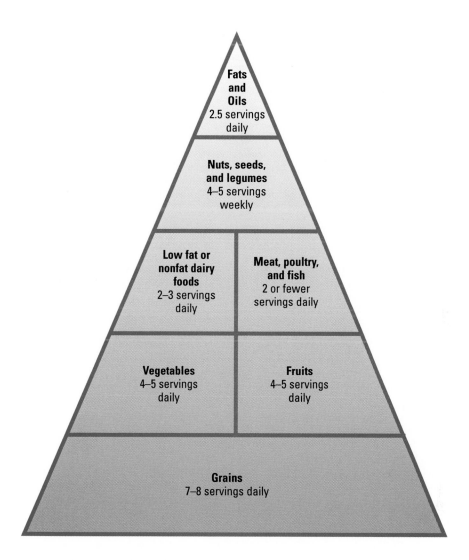

Figure 20–5:
The Dash Diet, featuring increased amounts of fruits and vegetables compared to the Basic Food Guide Pyramid and specifying servings of nuts, seeds, and beans, has been shown to reduce hypertension. The numbers of servings are based on a 2000-kilocalorie diet. (Adapted from National Institutes of Health, 1997.)

sterols have been useful, either alone (Miettinen et al., 1995) or along with low-fat diets (Hallikainen and Uusitupa, 1999), in reducing LDL cholesterol. Monitoring for side effects of plant sterols is recommended. Decreases in alpha- and beta-carotene levels have been reported. There is one contraindication to the use of plant sterols. In a rare inherited metabolic disease (40 reported cases) called sitorsterolemia, plant sterols are absorbed at a high rate and are not removed effectively by the liver, resulting in premature atherosclerosis (Plat and Mensink, 1998).

Dietary Modifications in Cardiovascular Disease

The major dietary modifications for clients with cardiovascular disease involve reductions in cholesterol and sodium. In addition to weight con-

trol, sodium restriction may be effective for some clients with hypertension. Dietary intervention is recommended for 6 weeks in cases of mild hypertension before other treatments are instituted. Although clinical trials often isolate specific nutrients or foods to test, a diet prescription most likely will use a multipronged approach.

Cholesterol-lowering Diets

Dietary modification to lower blood lipid levels produces the greatest reduction in persons with higher initial values for total cholesterol, LDL cholesterol, and triglycerides (Ahmed, Clasen, and Donnelley, 1998).

The Step I and Step II Diets

Dietary modification for hyperlipoproteinemia is well structured. The Step I diet is a strict interpretation of the recommended dietary intake for

Table 20–7 Description of the Step I and Step II Diets

Nutrient*	Recommended Intake as a Percent of Total Kilocalories	
	Step I Diet	Step II Diet
Total fat	30% or less	30% or less
Saturated	7 to 10%	Less than 7%
Polyunsaturated	Up to 10%	Up to 10%
Monounsaturated	Up to 15%	Up to 15%
Carbohydrate	55% or more	55% or more
Protein	Approximately 15%	Approximately 15%
Cholesterol	Less than 300 mg per day	Less than 200 mg per day
Total kilocalories	To achieve and maintain desired weight	To achieve and maintain desired weight

*Excluding kilocalories from alcohol

Kilocalories/Day	Recommended Grams of Fat Based on Total Kilocalories		
	Total Grams of Fat	Step I Diet Grams of Saturated Fat	Step If Diet Grams of Saturated Fat
1200	40 or less	9–13	Less than 9
1500	50 or less	12–17	Less than 12
1800	60 or less	14–20	Less than 14
2000	67 or less	16–22	Less than l6
2200	73 or less	17–24	Less than 17
2500	83 or less	19–28	Less than 19
3000	100 or less	23–33	Less than 23

Reproduced with permission
American Heart Association World Wide Web Site
www.americanheart.org/Heart_and_Stroke_A_Z_Guide/stepl.html, 2000
Copyright American Heart Association

Americans, whereas the Step II diet reduces saturated fat to 7 percent of kilocalories and limits cholesterol to less than 200 milligrams per day. The nurse usually reviews the Step I diet with the client in the physician's or clinic office. If, after 3 months, no significant change is seen in serum cholesterol levels, the client should be referred to a registered dietitian for instruction in the Step II diet. Ongoing instruction and follow-up have produced the best results.

One analysis of instruction in the Step I diet by registered dietitians achieved a 13 percent reduction in total cholesterol and 15 percent in LDL cholesterol in 8 weeks (Sikand, Kashyap, and Yang, 1998). Not all efforts are that successful. A meta-analysis of community-based studies showed a 3 percent reduction for the Step I Diet and 6 percent for Step II (Tang et al., 1998).

Only after 6 months of intensive dietary therapy and counseling should drug therapy be considered for clients without evidence of coronary heart disease (Ahmed, Clasen, and Donnelly, 1998). If used, drug therapy is added to dietary therapy, not substituted for it. Clients with established CHD or atherosclerotic disease should begin immediately on the Step II diet (Expert Panel, 1993).

The Step I and Step II diets are profiled in Table 20–7, and detailed instructions on cholesterol-lowering diets are listed in Table 20–8. More stringent restriction of energy to 25–22 percent of kilocalories from fat in a yearlong study did not produce appreciably better LDL cholesterol levels than diets containing 26–27 percent of energy from fat and had the disadvantage of raising triglyceride levels significantly (Knopp et al., 1997). The American Heart Association's Nutrition Committee recommends that

adults consume no less than 15 percent of kilocalories as fat to decrease risk of deficiencies of fatty acids, vitamins, and other nutrients. Similarly, the American Academy of Pediatrics recommends a fat intake of no less than 20 percent of kilocalories for children older than 2 years (Fisher, Van Horn, and McGill, 1997).

Rationale for Selection of Foods
Clients should be taught healthy choices and portion control, not that any foods are good or bad. Some of the reasons certain foods should be limited are given below.

FAT Monounsaturated fats may significantly lower LDL and cholesterol as well as protect against blood clots. Any oil contributes substantial kilocalories. See Figure 20–6 for information on a new source of monounsaturated fatty acids.

Reducing saturated fat intake decreases serum cholesterol more than reducing dietary cholesterol. Using nonfat or low-fat dairy products rather than higher fat ones can reduce fat intake by as much as 90 percent. This is an especially important strategy because milk fat contains more cholesterol-raising fatty acids than meat fat does (Grundy, 1999). Cooking methods affect the fat in meat. For instance, warm water rinsing of cooked, crumbled ground beef containing 30 percent fat reduced its fat content by 33–52 percent (Love and Prusa, 1992). Other techniques to reduce fat in meat are shown in Figure 20–7.

A dietary trial of survivors of myocardial infarction was stopped after an average of 27 months because the experimental group had a 73 per-

Table 20–8 Cholesterol-Lowering Diets

Description	Indication	Adequacy
These diets limit lipids. The Step 1 diet is strict interpretation of the Food Pyramid. The Step 2 diet is more restrictive.	These diets are prescribed when clients have elevated serum cholesterol.	The diets are adequate in all nutrients with the possible exception of iron because of the restriction on red meat. If the client is also on a sodium restricted diet, imitation cheese, bacon, and eggs may exceed the prescription. Clients must be encouraged to consume enough energy to maintain a healthy body weight.

Food Group	Recommended	Use Sparingly

Milk
Step 1:
  3 servings/day
Step 2:
  2 servings/day
	Skim milk, 1 percent milk, cultured buttermilk, evaporated skim or nonfat milk
	Nonfat or low-fat yogurt and frozen yogurt
	Low-fat soft cheese
	  Farmer and pot labeled no more than 2 to 6 g of fat/oz
	1 percent or 2 percent fat cottage cheese
		Whole milk, regular, evaporated, condensed
		Cream: half-and-half, most nondairy creamers
		Real or nondairy whipped cream
		High-fat cheeses: Neufchatel, Brie, American, feta, mozzarella, cheddar, muenster
		Cream cheese
		Ice cream
		Sour cream
		Custard-style yogurt
		Whole-milk ricotta

Breads and Cereals
Step 1:
  4-7 servings/day
Step 2:
  5-8 servings/day
	Breads: whole wheat, rye, pumpernickel, pita, white, bagels, English muffins, sandwich buns, dinner rolls, rice cakes made without whole milk, eggs, or butter
	Low-fat crackers: sticks, rye crisp, saltines, zwieback
	Hot cereals, most dry cold cereals
	Pasta: noodles, macaroni, spaghetti
	Rice
	Dried peas and beans, split peas, black-eyed peas, chick peas, kidney beans, navy beans, lentils, soybeans, low-fat tofu
		Croissants, butter rolls, sweet rolls, Danish pastry, doughnuts
		Most snack crackers: cheese crackers, butter crackers, crackers containing saturated fat
		Granola-type cereal containing saturated fat
		Egg noodles
		Pasta and rice made with cream, butter, or cheese sauce

Fruits & Vegetables
Steps I and 2:
  3 fruit servings/day
  4 vegetable servings/day
	Fresh, frozen, canned, or dried	Those prepared with butter, cream, or cheese sauce

Meat, Poultry, Fish, Shellfish *Steps I and 2:* 6 oz/day	Lean meat with fat trimmed: Beef—round, sirloin, chuck, loin Lamb—leg, arm, loin, rib Pork—tenderloin, leg, shoulder Veal—all except ground Poultry without skin Fish, shellfish Refer to very lean meat and substitutes list	Prime grade Fatty meat: Beef—corned, brisket, short ribs, regular ground Pork—spare ribs Goose, domestic duck Organ meats: liver, sweetbread brain, kidney Sausage, bacon Regular luncheon meats Frankfurters Caviar, roe

Continued on next page

Table 20–8 Cholesterol-Lowering Diets (Continued)

Food Group	Recommended	Use Sparingly

Eggs
Step 1:
   3 yolks/week
Step 2:
   2 yolks/week
	Eggwhites
	Cholesterol-free egg substitutes
		Egg yolks except as specified

Fats and Oils
Step 1:
   4-6 servings/day
Step 2:
   5-7 servings/day
	Monounsaturated (preferred): Peanut, olive, canola (rapeseed)
	Polyunsaturated: Corn, safflower, sunflower, sesame, soybean
	Margarine or shortening high in unsaturated fatty acids: tub, diet, liquid, stick with <2 g of saturated fat/tbsp
	Mayo, salad dressing high in unsaturated fats
	Low-fat dressings
		Saturated oils and fat: butter, lard, bacon fat, coconut, palm, and palm kernel oils
		Margarine or shortening high in saturated fatty acid
		Dressings made with egg yolk

Desserts and Miscellaneous *Step 1 and 2:* 2 servings/day	Low-fat frozen desserts: sorbet, sherbet, Italian ice, frozen yogurt, popsicles Angel food cake Low-fat cookies: fig bars, gingersnaps Low-fat candy: hard candy, jelly beans Low-fat snacks: pretzels, plain popcorn Nonfat beverages: carbonated drinks, juices, tea, coffee	High-fat frozen desserts: ice cream, frozen tofu High-fat cakes: most store-bought, pound, frosted cakes Store-bought pie Most store-bought cookies Most candy Chips made with saturated fat Buttered popcorn High-fat beverages: frappes, milkshakes, floats, eggnogs

Sample Menus, Step 1	
Breakfast	**Lunch and Dinner**
1/2 grapefruit 1/2 cup oatmeal 1 bagel 2 tsp. reduced fat margarine 1/2 cup skim milk Coffee	3 oz chicken or fish, baked without skin Wild rice Three bean salad with olive oil and vinegar Dinner roll with honey 1/2 cup steamed asparagus Angel food cake with strawberries 1 cup skim milk Herb tea

cent reduction in risk of re-infarction or death compared to the control group (de Lorgeril et al., 1994). The experimental group's diet contained more bread, more vegetables, more fish, less red meat (replaced by poultry), and fruit every day. Olive or canola oils and canola margarine were the only fats used for salad and food preparation. Despite the significant differences in outcomes, no difference between groups was shown in serum cholesterol, triglycerides, or HDLs. The protective effect was attributed to alpha-linolenic acid, a precursor of n-3 long-chain fatty acids that has been inversely associated with risk of fatal coronary heart disease (Zambon et al., 2000). The canola oil margarine given to the experimental group during the study contained 8 times the alpha-linolenic acid found in olive oil. Likewise, substituting walnuts for 35 percent of the energy obtained from monounsaturated fat in a low-fat diet produced greater reductions in total cholesterol, LDL cholesterol, and lipoprotein(a) levels with the walnut diet than with the basic low-fat diet (Zambon

et al., 2000). The low-fat diet emphasized grains, vegetables, fish, and olive oil, and limited red meat and eggs. Here, too the effect was attributed to alpha-linolenic acid in the 8–11 walnuts consumed each day. Substitution is the key factor. While on the walnut-augmented diet, these hypercholesterolemic men and women consumed less olive oil than when they were on the low-fat diet.

Sometimes a dietary change to improve health has unexpected consequences, as happened when hydrogenated vegetable oils were substituted for saturated fats. Hydrogenation increases the amount of trans fatty acids in the product (see illustration of trans fatty acid in Chapter 4, Fats). Intake of trans fatty acids was directly related to the risk of CHD in women (Willett et al., 1993) and to risk of myocardial infarction in both men and women (Ascherio et al., 1994). The latter increased risk was significant only for clients consuming more than 2 1/2 pats of margarine per day compared to those consuming less than 1 pat per day. Liquid or soft (tub) margarines generally have lower trans

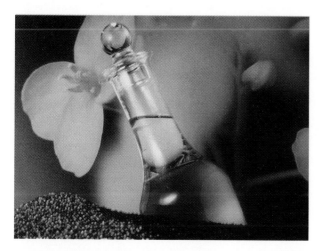

Figure 20–6:
CA-NO-LA (Canadian Oil) is derived from a variation of rapeseed developed by traditional plant breeding. It is high in monounsaturated fatty acids. (Photograph compliments of Canada's Canola Industry, used with permission.)

fatty acid content than hard (stick) margarines, but even hard margarines have less cholesterol-raising potential than butter (Expert Panel, 1994).

FIBER Soluble fiber lowers serum cholesterol by binding with it, promoting fecal elimination. Examples of foods high in soluble fiber are legumes, oats, barley, broccoli, apples, and citrus fruits. A diet supplemented with oat bran reduced the LDL levels by an additional 6 percent in children with hypercholesterolemia (Williams, 1995). After adjusting for other risk factors, a 10-gram increase in dietary fiber was associated with a 44 percent decrease in MI. Further analysis indicated cereal fiber, rather than vegetable or fruit fiber, was the main reason for the reduction (Rimm et al., 1996). Adding 3 grams per day of soluble fiber from oat bran can reduce total cholesterol by 5–6 milligrams per dL (Ahmed, Clasen, and Donnelly, 1998).

Many investigators have reported the effects of a soybean diet on blood lipids. Under the strict control of a metabolic ward as well as under outpatient conditions, a 22–25 percent reduction in LDL levels was achieved in hypercholesterolemic clients. The diet is not effective for normocholesterolemic individuals and is not markedly effective for hypercholesterolemic clients whose cholesterol levels have already been reduced by standard diets. The mechanism suggested to explain the effect of soy is that soy protein stimulates LDL receptors that are chronically depressed in persons with hypercholesterolemia (Sirtori et al., 1995). To expand the use of the soybean diet, the search for more palatable soy products is ongoing (Klein, Perry, and Adair, 1995).

SUGAR In persons with elevated serum triglycerides, a high-sucrose intake further increases triglyceride levels. Almost any recipe can be satisfactorily made with two-thirds to three-fourths the usual sugar. Increasing the amounts of vanilla extract and cinnamon will give the impression of sweetness.

Diet Tailored to Types of Hyperlipoproteinemia

Because of altered physiology, clients with the different types of hyperlipoproteinemia may need modified cholesterol-lowering diets. The dietitian

works with clients to maximize compliance. Although some of the clients may need cholesterol-lowering drug therapy, adjunct dietary therapy is likely to reduce the amount of medication required. Cholesterol-lowering drugs are recommended in addition to, not instead of, dietary modification.

Beyond the general recommendations to lower saturated fat consumption, clients with hyperlipoproteinemia need more stringent diets. All of these clients who are overweight are urged to lose the excess weight. Alcohol raises triglyceride and HDL levels but has minimal effect on LDL cholesterol (Ahmed, Clasen, and Donnelly, 1998) and therefore is restricted in certain types of hyperlipoproteinemia. Refer again to Table 20–2 in relation to the following diet modifications for the different types of hyperlipoproteinemias.

TYPE I This person is deficient in the enzyme triglyceride lipase. The serum chylomicrons are elevated because they carry the exogenous triglyceride in the bloodstream after meals. To treat this condition, food sources of triglyceride are restricted. Usually a 20- to 30-gram fat diet is prescribed, which generally limits the person to 3–4 ounces of lean meat per day and results in a diet deriving less than 10 percent of energy from fat (Grundy, 1999).

TYPE IIA This diet contains less than 200 milligrams of cholesterol per day. LDL and cholesterol elevations characterize Type IIA hyperlipoproteinemia. Polyunsaturated and monounsaturated fats should outnumber saturated fats by a factor of 1.5 or 2 to 1.

TYPE IIB This diet is the same as for Type IIA, plus limitation in alcohol and high-carbohydrate foods, especially simple sugars. In Type IIB hyperlipoproteinemia, triglyceride levels are elevated, whereas in Type IIA they are not. Alcohol and carbohydrate stimulate triglyceride production and therefore are to be restricted. Usually the diet is calculated to provide only 40 percent of the kilocalories from carbohydrate.

TYPE III Carbohydrate aggravates Type III hyperlipoproteinemia. Here dietary carbohydrate is limited to 35–40 percent of kilocalories. Because

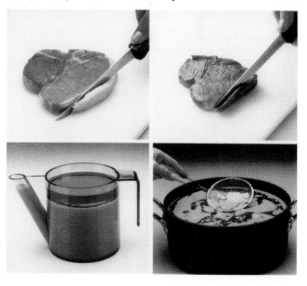

Figure 20–7:
Selecting lean meat, trimming off visible fat, and skimming fat from meat juices reduce the amount of fat consumed. (From the National Live Stock and Meat Board, 444 North Michigan Avenue, Chicago, IL 60611, with permission.)

triglycerides are elevated, alcohol and sugar should be restricted. If cholesterol levels continue to be high after weight loss, dietary cholesterol should be moderately reduced.

TYPE IV This very common hyperlipoproteinemia also is aggravated by carbohydrate. Therefore only 35–40 percent of kilocalories should come from carbohydrate. Triglycerides are elevated, so sugar intake should be limited. Alcohol should be consumed at a rate of not more than 1–2 ounces per week, if at all.

TYPE V This hyperlipoproteinemia is characterized by high serum levels of both chylomicrons and VLDL. Most clients with Type V hyperlipoproteinemia display insulin resistance in the liver that apparently contributes to the production of VLDL. To control the chylomicronemia, a very-low-fat diet is prescribed. Obese clients are urged to lose weight and increase activity to decrease production of VLDL by the liver. Despite compliance with the dietary restrictions, some clients require triglyceride-lowering medications (Grundy, 1999).

Because all hyperlipoproteinemias are not the same, neither are the dietary treatments. Nurses should be informed about the differences and not assume that all clients with hyperlipoproteinemia receive the same diet prescription. For best results, the clinical dietitian should individualize the diet with the client.

Sodium-Controlled Diets

As many as one-third of mild hypertensive cases can be controlled with sodium restriction, usually a 2-gram sodium diet. Results may not be apparent for up to 8 weeks. The preference for salty foods is learned and culturally transmitted, even when heavy salting is no longer necessary for preservation of food. After 3 months on a sodium-restricted diet, most individuals lose their appetite for salt. Box 20–3 lists the legal definitions for sodium and salt descriptions on labels.

Unseen contributions to sodium intake may come from other beverages, over-the-counter medications, and drinking water. Table 20–9 lists sodium content of beverages. Many toothpastes and mouthwashes contain significant

amounts of sodium and should not be swallowed. Over-the-counter medications that may contain significant amounts of sodium include analgesics, antacids, antibiotics, antitussives, laxatives, and sedatives.

The American Heart Association recommends a limit of 20 milligrams of sodium per liter of water as a standard for persons who require a restricted sodium diet. As much as 42 percent of the nation's water supply exceeds this amount (Korch, 1986). Many municipal water supplies are softened, which can increase the water's sodium content excessively. Sodium in city water supplies has varied from 1.2 milligrams per liter in Seattle to 100 milligrams per liter in Phoenix. Many households have water softeners in their homes that increase the water's sodium content. Consideration should also be given to the sodium content of specialty bottled waters. "Mineral waters" contain from 8 to 172 milligrams of sodium per liter. "Read the label" is appropriate advice here. Clients who require a diet containing less than 2 grams of sodium may elect to use bottled, distilled, deionized, or demineralized water for drinking and cooking in order to consume preferred sodium-containing foods. Many dietitians work with clients to develop individualized diet plans. Some clients prefer a daily allotment of salt in a shaker to be used as desired. If this strategy is adopted, the foods high in sodium must be limited to a greater extent than for a standardized sodium-controlled diet.

A number of salt substitutes are available. Many of them use potassium instead of sodium. These may be unsuitable for clients with kidney disease or those taking potassium-sparing diuretics or ACE inhibitors. Clients should consult their health care providers about employing salt substitutes. These products are for table use only. Salt substitutes are not appropriate for cooking because they turn bitter.

In clinical practice, diet orders such as "no-added-salt diet" or "low-sodium diet" require clarification. Usually, a facility's diet manual defines the terms. A "no-added-salt diet" may be calculated as 4 grams of sodium and a "low-sodium diet" as 2 grams in one facility but at different levels in another. Diet prescriptions should be written in milligrams of sodium to achieve the desired result. Table 20–10 describes diets with various levels of sodium control. Figure 20–8 shows some of the seasonings permitted on a sodium-controlled diet.

Table 20–9 Sodium Content of Beverages*

	Regular		Diet	
Beverage†	Sodium (mg)	Kilocalories	Sodium (mg)	Kilocalories
Club soda			75	0
Coffee	4	0		
Cola	15	151		
With aspartame			21	2
With saccharin			75	2
Gatorade	39	123		
Ginger ale	25	125	130	4
Kool-Aid	0	150		
With aspartame			0	6
Lemonade	12	150		
Lemon-lime soda	41	149	70	4
Pepper-type	38	151	70	0
Root beer	49	152	170	4
Tea	2	0		

*Serving size is 12 fluid ounces
†Sodium content may vary. depending on the source of water.

Box 20–3 Labeling Regulations for Sodium Content Descriptions

Term	Legal Definition
Free	Less than 5 mg of sodium per serving.
Salt Free	Must meet the criteria for free.
Very Low* Sodium	Less than 35 mg of sodium per serving. For meals and main dishes: 35 mg or less per 100 g.
Low* Sodium	Less than 140 mg of sodium per serving. Meals and main dishes: 140 mg or less per 100 g.
Reduced or Less	This term means that a nutritionally altered product contains 25 percent less sodium than the regular, or reference, product. However, a reduced claim can't be made on a product if its reference food already meets the requirement for a "low" claim.
Light in sodium or Lightly salted	May be used on food in which the sodium content has been reduced by at least 50 percent compared to an appropriate reference food.
Unsalted or No Added Salt	Must declare "This is not a sodium free food" on information panel if the food is not sodium free.

*Synonyms for low include "little," "few," and "low source oil "

Other Modifications

Clients taking potassium-wasting diuretics may require dietary or supplemental potassium. The choices become more complex when the client is also on a sodium-controlled diet. In general, fruits are high in potassium and low in sodium. Another adjunct source of supplemental potassium is a salt substitute.

After a heart attack, the client may be in shock. One adaptive response of the body is to slow gastrointestinal function. Thus the client should receive nothing by mouth while shock persists. Fluid is given intravenously to maintain fluid balance and to keep an access site open for intravenous medications. As the client recovers, the diet usually progresses from a 1000- to 1200-kilocalorie liquid diet to a soft diet of small, frequent meals. Large meals can increase the workload of the heart. Food is served at a moderate temperature. Very hot or very cold foods are thought to produce irregular heart rhythms.

Clients should avoid caffeine after heart attacks. Normal people have been observed to have serious **arrhythmias** after 9 or more cups of coffee or tea, whereas persons with histories of abnormal rhythms showed the same effects after 2 cups. Drinking more than 10 cups of caffeinated coffee per day was found to be a risk factor for sudden cardiac arrest in persons with coronary artery disease (de Vreede-Swagemakers et al., 1999). Women who drank more than 5 cups of any type of coffee per day had an increased risk of myocardial infarction whether they smoked or not (Palmer et al., 1995). Hypertensive clients should use caffeine in moderation because it increases blood pressure.

For clients in congestive heart failure, the diet order may read "as tolerated." Successfully nourishing them presents a challenge. Based on body weight, anthropometic measures, and plasma protein status, 50–68 percent of clients with congestive heart failure are malnourished. These clients frequently are anorectic due to unwelcome dietary changes, visceral congestion, and depression, but the loss of lean body mass exceeds that expected from anorexia alone (Hughes and Kostka, 1999). Food for the client with congestive heart failure should be nutrient-dense, easily eaten, and easily digested. An hour's rest before meals conserves energy.

Large meals, which would exert upward pressure on the chest, are undesirable. Liquid formulas can be used to provide nutrients while moderating the feeling of fullness. It may be necessary to supplement with water-soluble vitamins and minerals that are likely to be lost with the excretion of excess fluid.

Clients who have had a stroke may have chewing or swallowing problems. Often, thicker rather than thinner liquids are easier for a person with swallowing difficulty to manage. Nurses feeding clients with hemiplegia should place the food on the unaffected side of the tongue. Turning the client's head toward the weak side while sitting upright may help with swallowing. In addition, stroke clients may be aphasic and unable to communicate their needs or desires. A speech therapist is skilled in adaptive devices and restorative therapy for clients with dysphagia and aphasia.

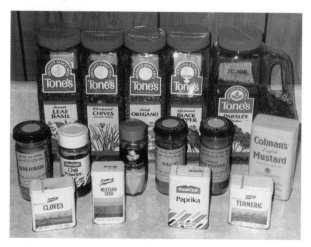

Figure 20–8:
These are just a few of the many condiments and seasonings that are available to the client who needs to restrict sodium intake.

Table 20–10 Sodium-Controlled Diets

Description	Indication	Adequacy	
These diets control sodium intake to prescribed levels.	Clients with hypertension, congestive heart failure, fluid-retaining kidney or endocrine disease, or other edematous conditions.	The 500 mg and 250 mg diets may be deficient in some nutrients.	
Soups	LS*	LS	LS	LS
Milk	2 cups	2 cups	1 cup	LS
Bread	3 slices	3 slices	LS	LS
Cereal	1 serving	LS	LS	LS
Fruits	Free	Free	Free	Free
Egg	1	1	1	1
Meat/substitutes	6 oz	5 oz	4 oz	4 oz
Vegetables	LS	LS	LS	LS
Desserts	1 serving	LS	LS	LS
Margarine	5 tsp	3 tsp	3 tsp	LS
Condiments	LS	LS	LS	LS

*Any food in the following LS list.

Food Group	Lower in Sodium (LS)	Higher in Sodium
Milk	Commercially made low-sodium milk Low-sodium cheese	All milk from animals Yogurt Regular cheese Commercial milk products
Breads and cereals	Bread and crackers prepared without salt Rice, barley, and pasta without added salt Baked goods made without salt, baking soda, or baking powder Unsalted cooked cereal Puffed rice, puffed wheat, shredded wheat Cornmeal, cornstarch	Commercial mixes Frozen bread dough Regular crackers Instant rice and pasta mixes Instant and quick cooking cereals Commercial stuffing and casserole mixes Self-rising flour and cornmeal Baked goods and quick breads made with salt, baking soda, baking powder, or egg white
Fruits	Fresh, frozen, dried, or canned fruit without added sodium All fruit juices	Crystallized or glazed fruit Maraschino cherries Dried fruit with sodium preservatives
Vegetables	Fresh, frozen without salt, low-sodium canned vegetables except those listed at right	Canned and frozen vegetables and juices Sauerkraut
Meat, poultry, fish, shellfish	Fresh, frozen, or canned low-sodium meat and poultry Low-sodium luncheon meats Eggs Low-sodium peanut butter Fresh fish Canned low-sodium tuna and salmon	Real and imitation bacon Luncheon meat Chipped or corned beef Smoked or salted meat or fish Kosher meat Frozen and powdered egg substitutes Regular peanut butter Brains kidney, clams, lobster, crab, oysters, scallops, shrimp, and other shellfish
Fats and oils	Cooking oil Unsalted butter, margarine, salad dressings, and shortening	Salted butter and margarine Commercial salad dressings

(Table continued on following page)

Table 20–10 Sodium-Controlled Diets (Continued)

Food Group	Lower in Sodium (LS)	Higher in Sodium
Desserts and miscellaneous	Alcohol Coffee, coffee substitutes Lemonade Tea Low-sodium candy Unflavored gelatin Jam, jelly, maple syrup, honey Unsalted nuts and popcorn	Regular canned or frozen soups Soup mixes Salted popcorn, nuts, potato chips, snacks Instant cocoa or powdered drink mixes Canned fruit drinks Commercial pastry, candy, cakes, cookies, gelatin desserts
Condiments and seasonings	Sweet: Allspice, Almond extract, Anise seed, Apricot nectar, Baking chocolate, Cardamon, Cinnamon, Coriander, Ginger, Lemon extract, Lemon juice, Mace, Maple extract, Mint, Nutmeg, Orange extract, Orange juice, Peppermint extract, Pineapple, Pineapple juice, Unsalted pecans, Vanilla extract, Unsalted walnuts, Walnut extract Tangy: Basil, Bay leaves, Caraway seeds, Cayenne pepper, Chili powder, Chives, Cloves, Curry powder, Dill weed, Garlic, Garlic powder (not salt), Green pepper, Horseradish without salt, Marjoram, Mustard powder (not prepared), Mustard seed, Onion powder (not salt) Onions, Oregano, Paprika, Parsley, Pepper, Poppy seed, Rosemary, Sage, Savory, Sesame seeds, Tarragon, Thyme, Turmeric	Any salt Barbecue sauce Bouillon cubes or granules Catsup Chili sauce Tartar sauce Horseradish sauce Meat extracts, sauces, and tenderizers Kitchen Bouquet Gravy and sauce mixes Monosodium glutamate Prepared mustard Olives Pickles Saccharin, other sugar substitutes containing sodium Soy sauce Teriyaki sauce Worcestershire sauce

Sample Menus for 2 g Sodium Diet

Breakfast	Lunch and Dinner
1/2 cup orange juice 1/2 cup shredded wheat 2 slices toast 2 tsp margarine 1 tbsp strawberry jam 1 cup 1 percent milk Sugar Coffee	3 oz chicken breast, turkey, or fish baked in lemon Juice Baked potato 2 tsp margarine 1/2 cup broccoli Tossed salad with homemade oil and vinegar dressing 1 dinner roll 1/2 cup sherbet 1 cup 1 percent milk (day's total = 2 cups) Tea

Summary

Cardiovascular diseases are responsible for more deaths in the United States than are diseases of any other body system. Some of the causative factors, such as age, gender, race, and family and medical history, are beyond a person's control. Other risk factors can be modified.

Underlying pathology in cardiovascular diseases involves both atherosclerosis and hypertension. Each reinforces the other in a vicious circle, often leading to coronary heart disease, congestive heart failure, or stroke.

The major changeable factors for cardiovascular disease are hypertension, cholesterolemia, obesity, diabetes mellitus, physical inactivity, cigarette smoking, and excessive alcohol intake (Wellness Tips 20–1).

Additional risk factors that affect hypertension are excessive salt intake and low intakes of potassium, calcium, and magnesium. Closely linked to cardiovascular diseases are specific elevations of blood lipids and lipoproteins. The most common hyperlipoproteinemia is type IV. It is aggravated by carbohydrate intake, which must be limited as part of the treatment.

Dietary modifications in cardiovascular disease most often involve cholesterol-lowering or sodium-controlling measures. Other qualities of the diet may require adjustment, such as potassium intake and the amount, timing, and texture of meals.

Wellness Tips 3–2

- Know your risk for cardiovascular disease. Not knowing is scored against you in the American Heart Association quiz.
- To begin, select one risk factor to change that has the potential to significantly influence your risk profile.
- Make a commitment to modifying that risk factor. Solicit assistance from family and friends.
- Implement one strategy at a time.
- Stay alert to reports of effective strategies. Wise and satisfying selections are facilitated when so many products are available.
- Lengthen your time frame to encompass the rest of your (healthy) life.

Case Study 20–1

Mr. Z is a 59-year-old white man who was admitted to the acute care hospital with a diagnosis of possible myocardial infarction. Subsequent testing proved Mr. Z did not have an infarction. His medical diagnoses are myocardial ischemia and type IV hyperlipoproteinemia. He is being readied for discharge to home.

Mr. Z is vice president for sales of a large manufacturing company. His business activities involve luncheon and dinner meetings at which alcohol consumption is common. He stated he has "at least one cocktail, usually two" with lunch and with dinner.

The clinical dietitian visited Mr. Z to instruct him on the diet prescribed by the physician. After the dietitian left, Mr. Z said to the nurse, "That diet is impossible for my situation. She just doesn't understand the business world. I don't believe there's anything wrong with my heart, anyway. It was just indigestion."

Providing client care is a dynamic process. Based on the above information, the nurse added the following modifications to Mr. Z's nursing care plan.

Nursing Care Plan

Subjective Data	Reported alcohol intake of 2 to 4 oz per day
	Perceived incompatibility of prescribed diet with lifestyle
	Stated disbelief in medical diagnosis
Objective Data	Elevated blood VLDL and triglyceride
Nursing Diagnosis	NANDA: Noncompliance (North American Nursing Diagnosis Association, 1999)
	Related to denial of illness and negative perception of treatment regimen as evidenced by statements to nurse.

Desired Outcomes Evaluation Criteria	Nursing Actions/ Interventions	Rationale
NOC: Health beliefs (Johnson, Maas, and Moorhead, 2000, with permission.)	NIC: Decision Making Support (McCloskey and Bulechek, 2000, with permission.)	
Client will acknowledge consequences of noncompliant behavior by time of hospital discharge.	Review pathophysiology of hyperlioproteinemia and atherosclerosis with client.	Mr. Z is a competent adult. He is able to make his own choices. Repeating the information on atherosclerosis is an attempt to be sure his choice to reject the treatment regimen is informed.
	Analyze with the client the possibility of partial compliance.	Perhaps the many changes required are overwhelming Mr. Z. One or two alterations might be acceptable as a starting point.
	Obtain client's permission to discuss discharge instructions with significant other.	Enlisting a support person might, over time, give Mr. Z reason to reconsider his decision.
	Inform physician of extent of intended noncompliance.	This is a change in the client's mental condition. It is appropriate to notify the physician and record it on the client's medical record.

Critical Thinking Questions

1. How could additional assessment data regarding family history be helpful in interpreting this client's reaction? Would you expect his reaction to be different if the diagnosis of myocardial infarction had been confirmed?
2. What additional interventions have the potential to achieve the stated outcome before hospital discharge?
3. How would you plan for the follow-up care for this client?

Study Aids

Subjects	Internet Sites
Hypertension	.http://www.nhlbi.nih.gov/guidelines/hypertension/jnc6card.htm
	http://www.nhlbi.nih.gov/guidelines/hypertension/jncintro.htm
Coronary Heart Disease	.http://www.americanheart.org/ Heart_and_Stroke_A_Z_Guide/riskfact.html
	http://www.doh.gov.uk/nsf/coronary.htm
	http://www.mayohealth.org/mayo/pted/htm/coronary.htm
	http://www.cdc.gov/nccdphp/cvd/womensatlas
Stroke	.http://stroke-site.org
	http://www.strokeassociation.org
	http://www.stroke.org
	http://www.americanheart.org/ Heart_and_Stroke_A_Z_Guide/riskfact.html
DASH Diet	.http://dash.bwh.harvard.edu
	http://www.nih.gov/news/pr/apr97/Dash.htm
Cholesterol	.http://rover.nhlbi.nih.gov/chd/
	http://www.nhlbi.nih.gov/health/prof/heart/index.htm#chol
	http://www.nhlbi.nih.gov/about/ncep/ncep_pd.htm
	http://www.hmscweb.com/NCEPguidelines.htm
	http://solar.rtd.uk.edu/~esmith/cholest.html
	http://www.aafp.org/afp/980501ap/ahmed.html
Soy	.http://www.talksoy.com
	http://soyfood.com
Plant stanol esters	.http://www.benecolphysician.com
	http://www.benecol.com
General client information	.http://www.aafp.org/healthinfo
	http://healthanswers.com
Health Resources for Latinos, blacks, American Indians & . . . . Alaska natives, Children, Religions, and the Stroke Belt	.http://www.nhlbi.nih.gov/health/prof/heart/latino/latin_pg.htm
	http://www.nhlbi.nih.gov/health/prof/heart/other/r_chdbk.htm
	http://www.nhlbi.nih.gov/health/prof/heart/other/na_bkgrd.htm
	http://www.nhlbi.nih.gov/health/prof/heart/other/jumpstrt.htm
	http://www.nhlbi.nih.gov/health/prof/heart/other/church.htm
	http://www.nhlbi.nih.gov/health/prof/heart/other/sb_spec.htm
Interactive sites: Quizzes, Risk Assessment	.http://www.americanheart.org/risk/quiz.html
	http://nhlbi.nih.gov/health/public/heart/other/hh_iq_ab.htm
	http://www.nhlbi.nih.gov/heart/obesity/pa_1q-ab.htm
	http://www.chd-taskforce.com
Web sites with search capability	.http://www.nal.usda.gov/fnic/etext/fnic.html
	http://www.healthfinder.gov
	http://www.nhlbi.nih.gov/about/nhaap
	http://www.americanheart.org

Chapter Review

1. The underlying pathological processes in cardiovascular disease are:
    a. Atherosclerosis and hypertension
    b. Coronary occlusion and obesity
    c. Diabetes mellitus and cerebrovascular accidents
    d. Kidney failure and congestive heart failure
2. The first action a hypertensive client should take to lower blood pressure is to:
    a. Restrict fluid to 1500 milliliters per day
    b. Eliminate saturated fat from the diet
    c. Lose weight if necessary
    d. Limit sodium intake to 1 gram per day
3. Soluble fiber also helps to lower blood cholesterol levels. Which of the following are good sources of soluble fiber?
    a. Broccoli and prunes
    b. Whole-wheat bread and grapes
    c. Green beans and raspberries
    d. Oats and legumes
4. Which of the following seasonings are permitted on a sodium-controlled diet?
    a. Catsup, horseradish mustard, and tartar sauce
    b. Chili powder, green pepper, and caraway seeds
    c. Celery seeds, seasoned meat tenderizer, and teriyaki sauce
    d. Dry mustard, garlic, and Worcestershire sauce
5. A high sucrose intake is related to cardiovascular disease because:
    a. Many cardiac clients have a genetic deficiency of sucrase.
    b. A high-sugar diet causes hyperactivity and hypertension.
    c. Excess sugar has to be excreted, causing premature aging of the kidney.
    d. Sucrose is positively related to triglyceride levels in the body.

Clinical Analysis

Mr. T is a 55-year-old black man being seen in a health clinic for hypertension. His blood pressure was 150/102 three months ago when he was first diagnosed. It has remained below that level but has not returned to normal. Today his blood pressure is 146/100.

Mr. T is 5 feet 9 inches tall and weighs 173 pounds. He has a medium frame. When first diagnosed, he weighed 178 pounds. A weight-loss diet with no added salt was prescribed, but progress has been slow.

Now the physician is prescribing a 2-gram sodium diet and starting Mr. T on a mild potassium-wasting diuretic. The clinic nurse is responsible for instructing the client.

1. Before he or she instructs Mr. T, which of the following actions by the nurse would best ensure his compliance with the diet?
    a. Doing a financial analysis to see if Mr. T can afford the special foods on his new diet
    b. Finding out which favorite foods Mr. T would have most difficulty giving up
    c. Listing the possible consequences of hypertension if it is not controlled
    d. Asking to see Mrs. T to instruct her on the preparation of foods for the new diet
2. Which of the following breakfasts would be best for Mr. T?
    a. Applesauce, raisin bran, 1 percent milk, and a bagel with cream cheese
    b. Canned pears, cornflakes, whole milk, and a cholesterol-free plain doughnut
    c. Cooked prunes, instant oatmeal, 2 percent milk, and raisin toast with margarine
    d. Orange juice, shredded wheat, skim milk, and whole-wheat toast with jelly
3. Mr. T has agreed to limit his alcohol intake to two drinks per week. He asks the nurse to recommend beverages compatible with his diet. Which of the following is the best choice?
    a. Tomato juice and bouillon
    b. Buttermilk and club soda
    c. Plain tea and fruit juice
    d. Gatorade and lemonade

Bibliography

Abbey, M, Noakes, M, and Nestel, PJ: Dietary supplementation with orange and carrot juice in cigarette smokers lowers oxidation products in copper-oxidized low-density lipoproteins. J Am Diet Assoc 95:671, 1995.

Ahmed, SM, Clasen, ME, and Donnelly, JE: Management of dyslipidemia in adults. Am Fam Physician 57:2192, 1998.

Alpha-Tocopherol, Beta-Carotene Cancer Prevention Study Group. The effect of vitamin E and beta-carotene on the incidence of lung cancer and other cancers in male smokers. N Engl J Med 330:1029, 1994.

American Heart Association: Iron and heart disease. 2000a. Accessed 6/5/2000 at http://www.americanheart.org/Heart_and_Stroke_A_Z_Guide/iron.html

American Heart Association: Risk factors and coronary heart disease. 2000b. Accessed 6/6/2000 at http://www.americanheart.org/Heart_and_Stroke_A_Z_Guide/riskfact.html

American Heart Association, Step I and Step II Diets. 2000c. Accessed 6/5/2000 at http://www.americanheart.org/Heart_and_Stroke_A_Z_Guide/step1.html

American Heart Association: Stroke risk factors. 2000d. Accessed 6/6/2000 at http://www.americanheart.org/Heart_and_Stroke_A_Z_Guide/Strokeri.html

Anderson, JW, Johnstone, BM, and Cook-Newell, ME: Meta-analysis of the effects of soy protein intake on serum lipids. N Engl J Med 333:276, 1995.

Appel, LJ, et al.<AU3>: A clinical trial of the effects of dietary patterns on blood pressure. N Engl J Med 336:1117, 1997.

Ascherio, A, et al., 1998: Intake of potassium, magnesium, calcium, and fiber and risk of stroke among US men. Circulation 98:1198, 1998.

Ascherio, A, et al.: Trans-fatty acids intake and risk of myocardial infarction. Circulation 89:94, 1994.

Ascherio, A, Katan, MB, and Stampfer, MJ: Trans fatty acids and coronary heart disease. N Engl J Med 340:1994, 1999.

Barker, DJ, et al.: Fetal nutrition and cardiovascular disease in adult life. Lancet 341:938, 1993.

Barker, DJP: Fetal origins of cardiovascular disease. Ann Med 31 (Suppl 1):3, 1999.

Birt, DF: The straight story on soy. American Institute for Cancer Research Newsletter, issue 67, page 5, Spring, 2000.

Brady, JA, Rock, CL, and Horneffer, MR: Thiamin status, diuretic medications, and the management of congestive heart failure. J Am Diet Assoc 95:541, 1995.

Campbell, NR, et al.: Lifestyle modifications to prevent and control hypertension. CMAJ 160 (9 Suppl):S1-6, 1999.

Centers for Disease Control: Age-specific excess deaths associated with stroke among racial/ethnic minority populations—United States, 1997. MMWR 49:94, 2000. Accessed 3/1/2000 at http://www.cdc.gov/epo/mmwr/preview/mmwrhtml/mm4905a2.htm

Centers for Disease Control: Decline in deaths from heart disease and stroke—United States, 1900–1999. MMWR 48:649, 1999a. Accessed 11/6/1999 at ftp://ftp.cdc.gov/pub/Publications/mmwr/wk/mm4830.pdf

Centers for Disease Control: Mortality patterns—United States, 1997. MMWR 48:664, 1999b. Accessed 11/6/1999 at ftp://ftp.cdc.gov/pub/Publications/mmwr/wk/mm4830.pdf

Centers for Disease Control: Number of deaths, death rates, and age-adjusted death rates for major causes of death for the United States, each division, each state, Puerto Rico, Virgin Islands, Guam, and American Samoa, 1997. National Vital Statistics Reports 47:82, 1999c. Accessed 12/9/1999 at http://www.cdc.gov/nchs/fastats/pdf/47_19t24.pdf

Christen, WG, et al.: Blood levels of homocysteine and increased risks of cardiovascular disease. Arch Intern Med 160:422, 2000.

Committee on Nutrition, American Academy of Pediatrics: Statement on Cholesterol. Pediatrics 90:469, 1992.

Daviglus, ML, et al.: Fish consumption and the 30-year risk of fatal myocardial infarction. N Engl J Med 336:1046, 1997.

de Lorgeril, M, et al.: Mediterranean alpha-linolenic acid-rich diet in secondary prevention of coronary heart disease. Lancet 343:1454, 1994.

Denke, MA: Role of beef and beef tallow, an enriched source of stearic acid, in a cholesterol-lowering diet. Am J Clin Nutr 60(suppl):1044S, 1994.

Dennison, BA, Jenkins, PL, and Pearson, TA: Challenges to implementing the current pediatric cholesterol screening guidelines into practice. Pediatrics 94:296, 1994.

de Vreede-Swagemakers, JJ, et al.: Risk indicators for out-of-hospital cardiac arrest in patients with coronary artery disease. J Clin Epidemiol 52:601, 1999.

Dietary Management of Hyperlipoproteinemias. A Handbook for Physicians and Dietitians. U.S. Department of H.E.W., Bethesda, MD, 1980.

Duane, WC: Effects of soybean protein and very low dietary cholesterol on serum lipids, biliary lipids, and fecal sterols in humans. Metabolism 48:489, 1999.

Eckel, RH: Obesity in heart disease. Circulation 96:3248, 1997. Accessed 6/5/2000 at http://www.americanheart.org/Scientific/statements/1997/119701.html

Elliott, P, et al.: Intersalt revisited: Further analyses of 24-hour sodium excretion and blood pressure within and across populations. Br Med J 312:1249, 1996.

Evans, RW, et al.: Homocyst(e)ine and risk of cardiovascular disease in the multiple risk factor intervention trial. Arterioscler Thromb Vasc Biol 17:1947, 1997.

Expert Panel on Detection, Evaluation and Treatment of High Blood Cholesterol in Adults (Adult Treatment Panel II): Second report of the Expert Panel on Detection, Evaluation and Treatment of High Blood Cholesterol in Adults (Adult Treatment Panel II). Circulation 89:1329, 1994.

Expert Panel on Detection, Evaluation and Treatment of High Blood Cholesterol in Adults: Summary of the second report of the National Cholesterol Education Program (NCEP) Expert Panel on Detection, Evaluation and Treatment of High Blood Cholesterol in Adults (Adult Treatment Panel II). JAMA 269:3015, 1993.

Fauci, AS, et al.: Harrison's Principles of Internal Medicine Companion Handbook. McGraw-Hill, New York, 1998.

Fisher, EA, Van Horn, L, and McGill, HC: Nutrition and children. Circulation. 95:2332, 1997. Accessed 6/5/2000 at http://www.americanheart.org/Scientific/statements/1997.059702.html

Forrester, TE, et al.: Fetal growth and cardiovascular risk factors in Jamaican schoolchildren. BMJ 312:156, 1996. Accessed 12/13/1999 at http://www.bmj.com/cgi/content/full/312/7024/156

Frankel, EN, et al.: Inhibition of oxidation of human low-density lipoprotein by phenolic substances in red wine. Lancet 341:454, 1993.

Frei, B: Reactive oxygen species and antioxidant vitamins: Mechanisms of action. Am J Med (suppl 3A)97:3A–5S, 1994.

Fuller, CJ, and Jialal, I: Effects of antioxidants and fatty acids on low-density-lipoprotein oxidation. Am J Clin Nutr 60(suppl):1010S–3S, 1994.

Geleijnse, JM, et al.: Tea flavonoids may protect against atherosclerosis. Arch Intern Med 159:2170, 1999.

Gorelick, PB, et al.: Prevention of a first stroke: A review of guidelines and a multidisciplinary consensus statement from the National Stroke Association. JAMA 281:1112, 1999.

Gotto, AM Jr: The new cholesterol education imperative and some comments on niacin. Am J Cardiol 81:492, 1998.

Grace, ML, Crosby, FE, and Ventura, MR: Nutritional education for patients with peripheral vascular disease. J Health Educ 25:142, 1995.

Graham, IM, et al.: Plasma homocysteine as a risk factor for vascular disease. JAMA 277:1175, 1997.

Griffith, LE, et al.: The influence of dietary and nondietary calcium supplementation on blood pressure: An updated metanalysis of randomized controlled trials. Am J Hypertens 12(1 Pt 1):84, 1999.

Grimes, DS, Hindle, E, and Dyer, T: Sunlight, cholesterol and coronary heart disease. QJM 89:579, 1996.

Grundy, SM: Nutrition and diet in the management of hyperlipidemia and atherosclerosis. In Shils, ME, et al. (eds): Modern Nutrition in Health and Disease, ed 9. Lippincott Williams and Wilkins, Philadelphia, 1999.

Hahn, RA, Heath, GW, and Chang, M-H: Cardiovascular disease risk factors and preventive practices among adults—United States, 1994: A behavioral risk factor atlas. MMWR 47:35, 1998. Accessed 5/30/2000 at http://www.cdc.gov/epo/mmwr/preview/mmwrhtml/00055888.htm

Hallikainen, MA, and Uusitupa, MIJ: Effects of 2 low-fat stanol ester-containing margarines on serum cholesterol concentrations as part of a low-fat diet in hypercholesterolemic subjects. Am J Clin Nutr 69:403, 1999.

Hartung, GH: Physical activity and high density lipoprotein cholesterol. J Sports Med Phys Fitness 35:1, 1995.

Hennekens, CH, et al.: Lack of effect of long-term supplementation with beta carotene on the incidence of malignant neoplasms and cardiovascular disease. N Engl J Med 334:1145, 1996.

Hertog, MGL, et al.: Dietary antioxidant flavonoids and risk of coronary heart disease: The Zutphen Elderly Study. Lancet 342:1007, 1993.

Hertog, MGL, et al.: Flavonoid intake and long-term risk of coronary heart disease and cancer in the Seven Countries Study. Arch Intern Med 155:381, 1995.

Hiser, E: The Mediterranean diet and cardiovascular disease. J Cardiopulm Rehabil 15:179, 1995.

Howell, WH: Diet and blood lipids. Nutr Today 32:110, 1997.

Hughes, C, and Kostka, P: Chronic congestive heart failure. In Shils, ME, et al. (eds): Modern Nutrition in Health and Disease, ed 9. Lippincott Williams and Wilkins, Philadelphia, 1999.

Jacques, PF, et al.: The effect of folic acid fortification on plasma folate and total homocysteine concentrations. N Engl J Med 340:1449, 1999.

Johnson, M, Maas, M, and Moorhead, S: Nursing Outcomes Classification (NOC), ed 2. Mosby, Philadelphia, 2000.

Joshipura, KJ: Fruit and vegetable intake in relation to risk of ischemic stroke. JAMA 282:1233, 1999.

Katan, MB: Fish and heart disease: What is the real story? Nutrition Reviews 53:228, 1995.

Keevil, JG, et al.: Grape juice, but not orange juice or grapefruit juice, inhibits human platelet aggregation. J Nutr 130:53, 2000.

Klatsky, A: Alcohol and cardiovascular diseases: A historical overview. Novartis Foundation Symposium 216:2, 1998.

Klein, BP, Perry, AK, and Adair, N: Incorporating soy protein into baked products for use in clinical studies. J Nutr 125:666S–74S, 1995.

Klipstein-Grosbusch, et al.: Dietary iron and risk of myocardial infarction in the Rotterdam Study. Am J Epidemiol 149:421, 1999.

Klor, HU, et al.: Nutrition and cardiovascular disease. Eur J Med Res 2:243, 1997.

Knekt, P, et al.: Antioxidant vitamin intake and coronary mortality in a longitudinal population study. Am J Epidemiol 139:1180, 1994.

Knekt, P, et al.: Flavonoid intake and coronary mortality in Finland: A cohort study. Br Med J 312:478, 1996.

Knopp, RH, et al.: Long-term blood cholesterol-lowering effects of a dietary fiber supplement. Am J Prev Med 17:18, 1999.

Knopp, RH, et al.: Long-term cholesterol-lowering effects of 4 fat-restricted diets in hypercholesterolemic and combined hyperlipidemic men. JAMA 278:1509, 1997.

Koenig, W, et al.: C-reactive protein, a sensitive marker of inflammation, predicts future risk of coronary heart disease in initially healthy middle-aged men: results from the MONICA (Monitoring Trends and Determinants in Cardiovascular Disease) Augsberg Cohort Study, 1984 to 1992. Circulation 99:237, 1999.

Korch, GC: Sodium content of potable water: Dietary significance. J Am Diet Assoc 86:80, 1986.

Kotchen, TA, and Kotchen, JM: Nutrition, diet, and hypertension. In Shils, ME, et al. (eds): Modern Nutrition in Health and Disease, ed 9. Lippincott Williams and Wilkins, Philadelphia, 1999.

Kushi, LH, et al.: Dietary antioxidant vitamins and death from coronary heart disease in postmenopausal women. N Engl J Med 334:1156, 1996.

Kuulasmaa, K, et al.: Estimation of contribution of changes in classic risk factors to trends in coronary-event rates across the WHO MONICA Project populations. Lancet 355:675, 2000.

Law, CM, et al.: Initiation of hypertension in utero and its amplification throughout life. BMJ 306:24, 1993.

Love, JA, and Prusa, KJ: Nutrient composition and sensory attributes of cooked ground beef: Effects of fat content, cooking method, and water rinsing. J Am Diet Assoc 92:1367, 1992.

Malinow, MR, Bostom, AG, and Krauss, RM: Homocyst(e)ine, diet, and cardiovascular diseases. Circulation 99:178, 1999. Accessed 6/5/2000 at http://www.americanheart.org/Scientific/statements/1999/019901.html

Mattila, KJ, et al.: Role of infection as a risk factor for atherosclerosis, myocardial infarction, and stroke. Clin Infec Dis 26:719, 1998.

McCloskey, JC, and Bulechek, GM: Nursing Interventions Classification (NIC), 3 ed. Mosby, Philadelphia, 2000.

Melby, CL, Toohey, ML, and Cebrick, J: Blood pressure and blood lipids among vegetarian, semivegetarian, and nonvegetarian African Americans. Am J Clin Nutr 59:103, 1994.

Miller, AL: Cardiovascular disease: Toward a unified approach. Alternative Medicine Review 1:132, 1996.

Miettinen, TA, et al.: Reduction of serum cholesterol with sitostanol-ester margarine in a mildly hypercholesterolemic population. N Engl J Med 333:1308, 1995.

Morris, DL, Kritchevsky, SB, and Davis, CE: Serum carotenoids and coronary heart disease. JAMA 272:1439, 1994.

National Institutes of Health. The DASH diet. Press Release 4/3/97. Accessed 5/30/2000 at http://www.nih.gov/news/pr/apr97/Dash.htm

North American Nursing Diagnosis Association: Nursing Diagnoses: Definitions and Classification 1999–2000, North American Nursing Diagnosis Association, Philadelphia, 1999.

National High Blood Pressure Education Program: Working Group Report on Primary Prevention of Hypertension. National Institutes of Health (No. 93-2669), Bethesda, MD, 1993.

National Institutes of Health: The sixth report of the Joint National Committee on Prevention, Detection, Evaluation, and Treatment of High Blood Pressure. NIH Publication 98-4080, Bethesda, MD, 1997. Accessed 12/9/1999 at http://www.nhlbi.nih.gov/guidelines/hypertension/jncintro.htm

Niki, E, et al.: Interaction among vitamin C, vitamin E and beta-carotene. Am J Clin Nutr 62:1322S, 1995.

Nilausen, K, and Meinertz, H: Lipoprotein (a) and dietary proteins: Casein lowers lipoprotein (a) concentrations as compared with soy protein. Am J Clin Nutr 69:419, 1999.

Nygard, O, et al.: Plasma homocysteine levels and mortality in patients with coronary artery disease. N Engl J Med 337:230, 1997.

Olson, JA: Carotenoids. In Shils, ME, et al. (eds): Modern Nutrition in Health and Disease, ed 9. Lippincott Williams and Wilkins, Philadelphia, 1999.

Omenn, GS, et al.: Effects of a combination of beta-carotene and vitamin A on lung cancer and cardiovascular disease. N Engl J Med 334:1150, 1996.

Palmer, JR, et al.: Coffee consumption and myocardial infarction in women. Am J Epidemiol 141:724, 1995.

Parmley, WW: Nonlipoprotein risk factors for coronary heart disease: Evaluation and management. Am J Med 102(2A):7, 1997.

Pearson, TA: Alcohol and heart disease. Circulation 94:3023, 1996. Accessed 6/6/2000 at http://www.americanheart.org/Scientific/statements/1996/1116.html

Plat, J, and Mensink, RP: Safety aspects of dietary plant sterols and stanols. Postgraduate Medicine A Special Report November:32, 1998.

Refsum, H, et al.: Homocysteine and cardiovascular disease. Annu Rev Med 49:31, 1998.

Renaud, S, and Gueguen, R: The French paradox and wine drinking. Novartis Found Symp 216:208, 1998.

Rexrode, KM, et al.: A prospective study of body mass index, weight change, and risk of stroke in women. JAMA 277:1539, 1997.

Ridker, PM, et al.: C-reactive protein and other markers of inflammation in the prediction of cardiovascular disease in women. N Engl J Med 342:836, 2000.

Ridker, PM, et al.: Inflammation, aspirin, and the risk of cardiovascular disease in apparently healthy men. N Engl J Med 336:973, 1997.

Rifai, N, et al.: Failure of current guidelines for cholesterol screening in urban African-American adolescents. Pediatrics 98:383, 1998.

Rimm, EB, et al.: Dietary iron intake and risk of coronary disease among men (abstract). Circulation 87:692, 1993.

Rimm, EB, et al.: Folate and vitamin B$_6$ from diet and supplements in relation to risk of coronary heart disease among women. JAMA 279:359, 1998.

Rimm, EB, et al.: Vegetable, fruit, and cereal fiber intake and risk of coronary heart disease among men. JAMA 275:447, 1996.

Roivainen, M, et al.: Infections, inflammation, and the risk of coronary heart disease. Circulation 101:252, 2000.

Salonen, JT, et al.: High stored iron levels are associated with excess risk of myocardial infarction in Eastern Finnish men. Circulation 86:803, 1992.

Scanlon, VC, and Sanders T: Essentials of Anatomy and Physiology, ed 2. FA Davis, Philadelphia, 1995.

Selhub, J, and D'Angelo, A: Hyperhomocysteinemia and thrombosis: Acquired conditions. Thromb-Haemost 78:527, 1997.

Selhub, J, et al.: Association between plasma homocysteine concentrations and extracranial carotid-artery stenosis. N Engl J Med 332:286, 1995.

Selhub, J, et al.: Serum total homocysteine concentrations in the Third National Health and Nutrition Examination Survey (1991–1994): Population reference ranges and contribution of vitamin status to high serum concentrations. Ann Intern Med 131:331, 1999.

Serra-Majem, L, et al.: How could changes in diet explain changes in coronary heart disease mortality in Spain? The Spanish paradox. Am J Clin Nutr 61(suppl):1351S–9S, 1995.

Shepherd, J, et al.: Prevention of coronary heart disease with pravastatin in men with hypercholesterolemia. N Engl J Med 333:1301, 1995.

Shimakawa, T, et al.: Vitamin intake: A possible determinant of plasma homocysteine among middle-aged adults. Ann Epidemiol 7:285, 1997.

Sikand, G, Kashyap, ML, and Yang, I: Medical nutrition therapy lowers serum cholesterol and saves medication costs in men with hypercholesterolemia. J Am Diet Assoc 98:889, 1998.

Sirtori, CR, et al.: Soy and cholesterol reduction: Clinical experience. J Nutr 125:598S, 1995.

Spencer, AP, Carson, DS, and Crouch, MA: Vitamin E and coronary artery disease. Arch Intern Med 159:1313, 1999.

Stampfer, MJ, et al.: A prospective study of plasma homocyst(e)ine and risk of myocardial infarction in US physicians. JAMA 268:877, 1992.

Stampfer, MJ, et al.: Vitamin E consumption and the risk of coronary disease in women. N Engl J Med 328:1444, 1993.

Stein, JH, et al.: Purple grape juice improves endothelial function and reduces the susceptibility of LDL cholesterol to oxidation in patients with coronary artery disease. Circulation 100:1050, 1999.

Stephens, NG, et al.: Randomized controlled trial of vitamin E in patients with coronary disease: Cambridge Heart Antioxidant Study (CHAOS). Lancet 347:781, 1996.

Tang, JL, et al.: Systematic review of dietary intervention trials to lower blood total cholesterol in free-living subjects. BMJ 316:1213, 1998. Accessed 12/12/1999 at http://www.bmj.com/cgi/content/full/316/7139/1213.

Tribble, DL: Antioxidant consumption and risk of coronary heart disease: Emphasis on vitamin C, vitamin E, and beta-carotene. Circulation 99:591, 1999.

Tuomainen, TP, et al.: Association between body iron stores and the risk of acute myocardial infarction in men. Circulation 97:1461, 1998.

Tzonou, A, et al.: Dietary iron and coronary heart disease risk: A study from Greece. Am J Epidemiol 147:161, 1998.

van Poppel, G, et al.: Antioxidants and coronary heart disease. Ann Med 26:429, 1994.

van Tol, A, et al.: The cholesterol-raising diterpenes from coffee beans increase serum lipid transfer protein activity levels in humans. Atherosclerosis 132:251, 1997.

Verhoef, P, et al.: Plasma total homocysteine, B vitamins, and risk of coronary atherosclerosis. Arterioscler Thromb Vasc Biol 17:989, 1997.

Verschuren, WMM, et al.: Serum total cholesterol and long-term coronary heart disease mortality in different cultures. JAMA 274:131, 1995.

Washburn, S, et al.: Effect of soy protein supplementation on serum lipoproteins, blood pressure, and menopausal symptoms in peri-menopausal women. Menopause 6:7, 1999.

Welch, GN, Upchurch, GR, and Loscalzo, J: Homocysteine, oxidative stress, and vascular disease. Hospital Practice 15:81, June 1997.

Whelton, PK, and He, J: Potassium in preventing and treating high blood pressure. Semin Nephrol 19:494, 1999.

Willett, WC, et al.: Intake of trans fatty acids and risk of coronary heart disease among women. Lancet 341:581, 1993.

Willett, WC, et al.: Weight, weight change, and coronary heart disease in women. JAMA 273:461, 1995.

Williams, CL: Importance of dietary fiber in childhood. J Am Diet Assoc 95:1140, 1995.

Williams, CL, and Bollella, M: Guidelines for screening, evaluating, and treating children with hypercholesterolemia. J Pediatr Health Care 9:153, 1995.

Wong, WW, et al.: Cholesterol-lowering effect of soy protein in normocholesterolemic and hypercholesterolemic men. Am J Clin Nutr 68(6 Suppl):1385S, 1998.

Woodside, JV, et al.: Effect of B-group vitamins and antioxidant vitamins on hyperhomocysteinemia: A double-blind, randomized, factorial-design, controlled trial. Am J Clin Nutr 67:858, 1998.

Zambon, D, et al.: Substituting walnuts for monounsaturated fat improves the serum lipid profile of hypercholesterolemic men and women. Ann Intern Med 132:538, 2000.

CHAPTER 21

Diet in Renal Disease

LEARNING OBJECTIVES

After completing this chapter, the student should be able to:

1. Identify the major causes of acute and chronic kidney failure.
2. List the goals of nutritional care for a client with kidney disease.
3. List the nutrients commonly modified in the dietary treatment of kidney disease.
4. Discuss the relationship among kilocaloric intake, dietary protein utilization, and uremia.
5. Discuss the nutritional care of clients with kidney disease in relation to their medical treatment.

Diet therapy for clients with kidney disease depends on an understanding of the normal function of the kidneys and basic concepts of pathophysiology of renal diseases. (**Renal** means pertaining to the kidneys.) The nutritional care of clients with renal disease is complex. These clients frequently must learn not just one diet in which one to seven nutrients are controlled but several different diets as their medical condition and the treatment approach change. The failure to adhere to necessary diet changes can result in death. One aspect of working with clients with renal disease is that inattentiveness to dietary restrictions can be objectively measured in weight changes or changes in blood chemistry.

This first part of this chapter discusses the internal structure and functions of the kidneys. Common kidney diseases, major forms of treatment available for clients, and the dietary treatment for renal disease are then presented. A brief discussion of urinary calculi and urinary tract infections concludes the chapter.

Anatomy and Physiology of the Kidneys

Internal Structure

The functioning unit of the kidney is the **nephron**. Each kidney contains about a million nephrons. Figure 21–1 shows an individual nephron. Each nephron has two main parts. The first part, **Bowman's capsule**, is the cup-shaped top of the nephron. Inside Bowman's capsule is a network of blood capillaries called the **glomerulus** (plural, *glomeruli*). The second part of the nephron is the **renal tubule**. (A **tubule** is a small tube or canal.) The renal tubule is the rope-like portion of the nephron. This rope-like structure ends at the collecting tubule. Several nephrons usually share a single **collecting tubule**.

Functions

The kidneys assist in the internal regulation of the body by performing the following functions:

1. *Filtration:* The kidneys remove the end products of metabolism and substances that have accumulated in the blood in undesirable amounts during the filtration process. Substances removed from the blood include urea, creatinine, uric acid, and urates. Undesirable amounts of chloride, potassium, sodium, and hydrogen ions are also filtered from the blood. The **glomerular filtration rate** (GFR) is the amount of fluid filtered each minute by all the glomeruli of both kidneys and is one index of kidney function. This is normally about 125 milliliters per minute (Fig. 21–2).

2. *Reabsorption:* Previously filtered substances (e.g., water and sodium) needed by the body are reabsorbed into the blood in the tubules.

3. *Secretion of Ions to Maintain Acid–Base Balance:* Secretion is the process of moving ions from the blood into the urine. Secretion allows for the amount of a particular substance to be excreted in the urine in concentrations greater than the concentration filtered from the plasma in the glomeruli. The kidneys regulate the balance between bicarbonate and carbonic acid by the secretion and exchange of hydrogen ions for sodium ions, which are used to form base.

4. *Excretion:* The kidneys eliminate unwanted substances from the body as urine.

5. *Renal Control of Cardiac Output and Systemic Blood Pressure:* The kidneys adapt to changing cardiac output by altering resistance to blood flow both at the beginning of the glomerulus and at the end.

6. *Calcium, Phosphorus, and Vitamin D:* The kidneys produce the active form of vitamin D, **calcitriol**. Activated vitamin D regulates

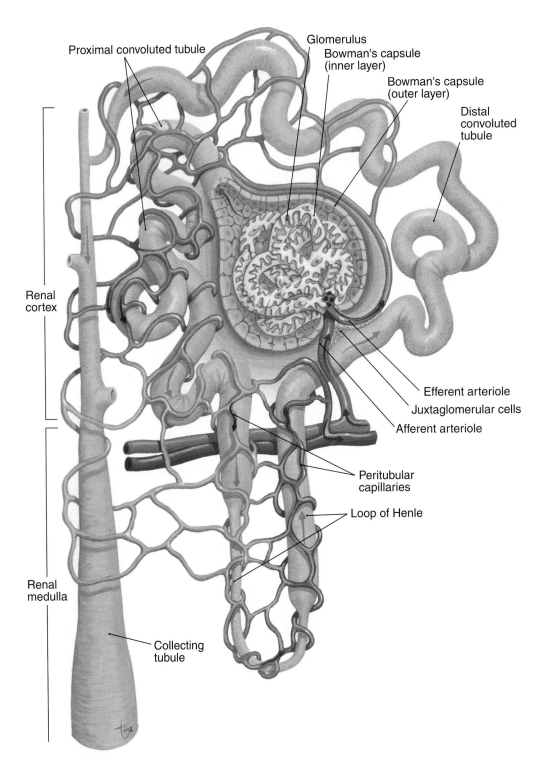

Figure 21–1:
A nephron with its associated blood vessels. The arrows indicate the direction of blood flow. (Courtesy of FA Davis from: Scalon, VC, and Saunders, T: Essentials of Anatomy and Physiology, ed. 3. FA Davis Publishing Co., Philadelphia, 1998.)

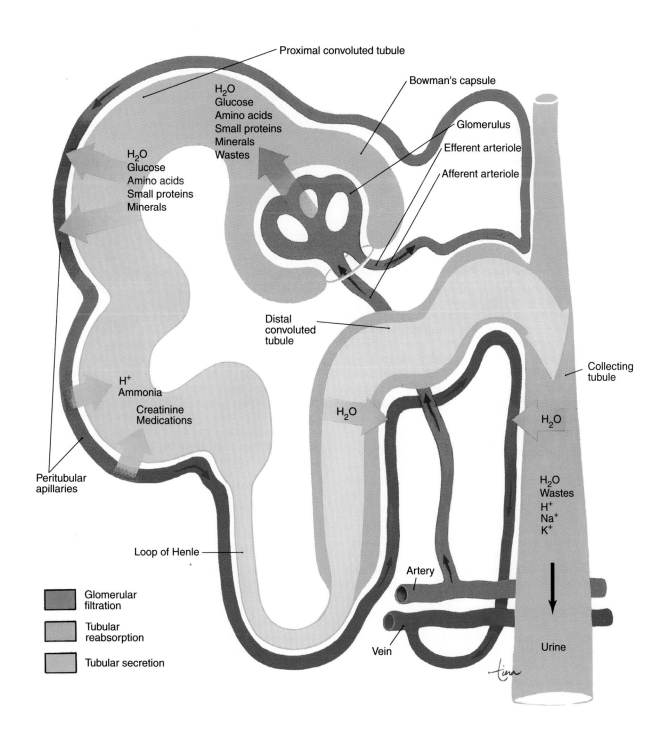

Figure 21–2:
Schematic representation of glomerular filtration, tubular reabsorption, and tubular secretion. The renal tubule has been uncoiled, and the peritubular capillaries are shown adjacent to the tubule. (Courtesy of FA Davis from: Scalon, VC, and Saunders, T: *Essentials of Anatomy and Physiology,* ed. 3. FA Davis Publishing Co., Philadelphia, 1998.)

the absorption of calcium and phosphorus from the intestinal tract and assists in the regulation of calcium and phosphorus levels in the blood.

7. *Erythropoietin:* The kidneys produce a hormone called **erythropoietin**, which stimulates maturation of red blood cells in bone marrow.

Kidney Disease

Because the kidneys perform so many different metabolic functions, kidney disease has serious consequences. This section of the text discusses the causes of kidney disease and describes several common kidney disorders.

Causes

Renal disease can be caused by many factors, including trauma, infections, birth defects, medications, chronic disease (e.g., atherosclerosis, diabetes, hypertension), and toxic metal consumption. Diabetic nephropathy is the most common cause of renal failure. A physiological stress such as a myocardial infarction or an extensive burn can precipitate renal disease by decreasing the perfusion of the kidney or markedly increasing catabolism. Clinical Application 21–1, which describes the renal response after myocardial infarction, describes the effect of reduced renal blood flow. Catabolism causes an increase in nitrogenous products and potassium; these must be excreted, thus overworking the kidneys. Renal disease is a feared complication of many pathologies and treatments including radiocontrast materials used in diagnostic procedures, some antibiotics, and some pain medications.

Obesity increases the risk of renal disease. Losing weight reduces the severity of diabetes and hypertension, the two leading causes of kidney failure, and helps prevent those conditions in people who haven't developed them (Blumberg, 1999). Normalization of blood glucose and lipid levels along with blood pressure control also decrease the risk of renal disease. There is some evidence that a habitually high intake of dietary protein (greater than 1.6 grams/kg body weight) can cause kidney damage. These are among the reasons that all clients should be encouraged to follow the diets prescribed for them and faithfully take prescribed medications.

Glomerulonephritis

A general term for an inflammation of the kidneys is **nephritis.** This is the most common type of kidney disease. Inflammation of the glomeruli is called **glomerulonephritis**, which can be either acute or chronic. This condition often follows scarlet fever or a streptococcal infection of the respiratory tract. Young children and young adults are often victims. Symptoms include nausea, vomiting, fever, hypertension, blood in the urine **(hematuria)**, a decreased output of urine **(oliguria)**, protein in the urine **(proteinuria)**, and edema. Recovery is usually complete. However, in some clients the disease progresses and becomes chronic. This leads to a progressive loss of kidney function. Some clients develop **anuria**, which is a total lack of urine output. Without treatment, this condition is fatal.

CLINICAL APPLICATION 21–1

Renal Response after a Myocardial Infarction

Immediately after a heart attack or MI, blood flow through the systemic circulation is diminished. Systemic circulation refers to the blood flow from the left part of the heart through the aorta and all branches (arteries) to the capillaries of the tissues. Systemic circulation also includes the blood's return to the heart through the veins. Following a heart attack, blood flow to the myocardium, or heart muscle, is decreased, and myocardial function is impaired. Less blood is thus delivered to the tissues. The kidneys sense the decreased cardiac output and try to compensate by reabsorption of additional water. This may lead to a fluid overload and edema. Most clients after a MI are on fluid restriction for this reason.

Specific Tubular Abnormalities

A structural problem in the renal tubules may result in abnormal reabsorption or lack of reabsorption of certain substances by the tubules. The effect of a tubular abnormality is that the blood is not effectively cleansed.

Nephrotic Syndrome

The result of a variety of diseases that damage the glomeruli capillary walls is called **nephrotic syndrome**. Signs of nephrotic syndrome include proteinuria, severe edema, low serum protein levels, anemia, and hyperlipoproteinemia. Usually the higher the hyperlipoproteinemia, the greater is the proteinuria. The disease is caused by the degenerative changes in the kidneys' capillary walls, which consequently permit the passage of albumin into the **glomerular filtrate**. Water and sodium are retained. Edema is sometimes so severe that it masks tissue wasting due to the breakdown of tissue protein stores. The degree of malnutrition is hidden until the excess fluid is removed.

Nephrosclerosis

A hardening of the renal arteries is known as **nephrosclerosis**. This condition is caused by arteriosclerosis and results in a decreased blood supply to the kidneys. This leads to hypertensive kidney disease and can eventually destroy the kidney.

Progressive Nature of Kidney Failure

Kidney disease can be acute or chronic. In **acute renal failure**, the kidneys stop working entirely or almost entirely. Acute renal failure occurs suddenly and is usually temporary. It can last for a few days or weeks.

Chronic renal failure occurs when progressively more nephrons are destroyed until the kidneys simply cannot perform vital functions. Chronic renal failure occurs over time and is usually irreversible.

As individual nephrons are damaged, the remaining nephrons work harder to maintain metabolic homeostasis. As each functional nephron's workload is increased, the nephron becomes more susceptible to work overload and damage. The normal composition of the blood is altered when the remaining functional nephrons cannot assume any additional workload. Serum levels of **blood urea nitrogen** (BUN), creatinine, and uric acid become elevated. In some clients, even though the underlying condition (e.g., diabetes mellitus, hypertension) is treated, chronic renal disease may lead to **end-stage renal failure**. During end-stage renal failure, most or all of the kidneys' ability to produce urine and regulate blood chemistries is severely compromised.

Often, the first sign of chronic renal failure is sodium depletion. This occurs when the kidneys lose their ability to reabsorb sodium in the tubule. Symptoms associated with sodium depletion include a reduction of renal blood flow, dehydration, lethargy, decreased glomerular filtration rate (GFR), uremia (see next section), and client deterioration. The client's blood pressure and body weight drop. Urine volume may be increased initially in chronic renal failure. A loss of body fat and protein content is responsible for the weight loss. The client's serum albumin level may fall as protein is lost in the urine.

As kidney function further deteriorates, some of these symptoms reverse. The kidneys lose the ability to excrete sodium. When this occurs, symptoms include sodium retention, overhydration, edema, hypertension, and CHF. The body can excrete little or no urine.

The GFR gradually declines in chronic renal failure. Most clients with a GFR below 25 milliliters per minute will eventually require either dialysis or transplantation, regardless of the original cause of failure.

If these measures were not implemented, **uremia** would develop. Uremia is the name given to the toxic condition associated with renal insufficiency. Uremia is produced by the retention in the blood of nitrogenous substances normally excreted by the kidneys. The uremic client manifests many symptoms in virtually every body system as toxic waste products build up in the blood. The client may complain of fatigue, weakness, and decreased mental ability. The client's muscles may twitch and cramp. Anorexia, nausea, vomiting, and **stomatitis**, an inflammation of the mouth, may be present. Sometimes clients complain of an unpleasant taste in the mouth. To further complicate matters, gastrointestinal ulcers and bleeding are common. All of these symptoms have a direct effect on the client's willingness to eat.

Healthcare professionals have known for many decades that clients with chronic renal disease who have sustained a loss of GFR often continue to lose renal function until they develop terminal renal failure. Much research is ongoing to find a way to halt the progression of chronic renal failure. A high-protein diet, a high-phosphorus diet, a high-fat or -cholesterol diet, a high vitamin C intake, and a vitamin D overdose are among the nutrition related causes of progressive renal failure (Kopple, 1999). For this reason, dietary intervention is now instituted simultaneously with the initial diagnosis.

Treatment for Renal Disease

Renal functions cannot be assumed by another organ. There is no cure for chronic renal failure. However, many clients can be treated with dialysis (an artificial kidney) and/or a kidney transplant. Artificial kidneys have been used for about 45 years to treat clients with severe kidney failure.

Dialysis

Dialysis means the passage of solutes through a membrane. Two functions of the kidneys are (1) the removal of waste products and (2) the regulation of fluid and electrolyte balance. By removing waste products from the blood and assisting in the maintenance of fluid balance, dialysis reduces the symptoms of uremia, hypertension, edema, and the risk of CHF.

Dialysis is usually started when the client develops symptoms of severe fluid overload, high potassium levels, acidosis, or symptoms of uremia. Dialysis cannot restore the lost hormonal functions of the kidney. In addition, dialysis cannot correct the anemia that occurs because of a lack of erythropoietin. Some dialysis clients still need treatment for hypertension.

Hemodialysis

During **hemodialysis**, blood is removed from the client's artery through a tube, is forced to flow over a semipermeable membrane where waste is removed, and then is rerouted back into the client's body through a vein. Before dialysis can be initiated, an access site that allows blood to be removed from the body and replaced back into the body at the time of dialysis must be surgically created. Figure 21–3 illustrates a client undergoing a hemodialysis treatment. A solution called the **dialysate** is placed on one side of the semipermeable membrane, and the client's blood flows on the other side. The dialysate is similar in composition to normal blood plasma. The client's blood has a higher concentration of urea and electrolytes than the dialysate has, so these substances diffuse from the blood into the dialysate. The dialysate also contains glucose, and the more glucose the dialysate contains, the more fluid will move from the blood into the dialysate by osmosis. This process pulls extra fluid from the blood. The composition of the dialysate varies according to the requirements of each client.

Hemodialysis treatments usually last 3–5 hours and are administered three times per week. Some clients are taught to perform their own dialysis treatments at home. Dialysis is not as effective as normal kidney function because blood cleansing occurs only when clients are attached to artificial kidneys. Normal kidneys clear the blood 24 hours a day 7 days a week.

Peritoneal Dialysis

The **peritoneum** is the lining of the abdominal cavity. During **peritoneal dialysis**, the dialysate is placed directly into the client's abdomen. The

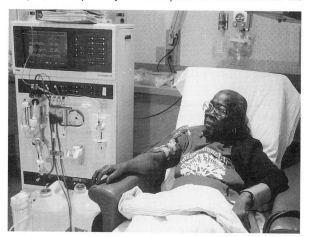

Figure 21–3:
Client undergoing hemodialysis at dialysis center. (Courtesy of FA Davis, from Williams, LS, and Hopper, PD: Understanding Medical and Surgical Nursing, FA Davis, Philadelphia, 1999.)

dialysate enters the body through a permanent catheter placed in the abdominal cavity. The peritoneum thus functions as the semipermeable membrane.

INTERMITTENT PERITONEAL DIALYSIS Between 1 and 2 liters of fluid are introduced into the abdominal cavity during intermittent peritoneal dialysis. The fluid is allowed to remain in the abdomen for about 30 minutes and then is drained from the body by gravity. One complete exchange takes about an hour. This process is repeated until the blood urea nitrogen level drops.

CONTINUOUS AMBULATORY PERITONEAL DIALYSIS **Continuous ambulatory peritoneal dialysis** (CAPD) is the dialysis method chosen by many clients. This is a form of self-dialysis. About 1 liter of dialysate is introduced into the abdominal cavity. The fluid remains in the cavity for 4–6 hours while the waste products diffuse into the dialysate. The dialysate is then replaced with a new solution. Clients can move about and pursue their activities of daily living during CAPD. The term continuous means that the client is dialyzing constantly. The advantage of CAPD is that the client's blood levels of sodium, potassium, creatinine, and nitrogen are kept within a much more stable range. Large shifts in fluid balance are also avoided. The decision about which treatment approach is best for an individual is based on medical condition, lifestyle behaviors, and personal preference. For example, a client with poor personal hygiene would not be a good candidate for CAPD because of a high risk for infection with this approach.

Kidney Transplant

A kidney transplant can restore full renal function. Immunosuppressants to prevent rejection of the transplanted kidney are necessary. Some commonly used immunosuppressants are azathioprine, corticosteroids, and/or cyclosporine. These medications have many side effects, including diarrhea, nausea, and vomiting, which influence nutrient intake and absorption.

Nutritional Care of the Renal Client

The nutritional needs of clients with renal diseases are changing constantly. The reason for the change is that the disease state and treatment approach are not static. Clients with kidney disease require constant assessment, monitoring, and counseling. In addition, it is an ongoing challenge to provide quality nutritional care to these clients, who frequently must be coaxed to eat. Anorexia, nausea, and vomiting are frequent complaints. It is common for the dietitian to see these clients more than once each day for nutritional problems during hospitalization.

Malnutrition

Malnutrition in hemodialysis clients is associated with increased morality and morbidity. One study cited moderate to severe malnutrition in 34 percent of study participants (Kuhlmann et al.,1997). Among the reasons for the malnutrition are increased catabolism, metabolic derangement, decreased food intake, and low-economic status. Oral supplements, tube feedings, intravenous feedings, and intradiaylytic parenteral nutrition have all been used to treat the protein-energy malnutrition seen in these clients.

Intradiayltic parenteral nutrition involves the administration of lipids, glucose, and amino acids into the peritoneal cavity.

Goals of Nutrition Therapy

Well-planned nutritional management is a fundamental part of any treatment plan for renal disease. Every client with renal disease requires an individualized diet based on the following goals:

1. Attain and maintain optimal nutritional status
2. Prevent net protein catabolism
3. Minimize uremic toxicity
4. Maintain adequate hydration status
5. Maintain normal serum potassium levels
6. Control the progression of renal osteodystrophy (discussed later)
7. Modify diet to meet other nutrition-related concern, such as diabetes, heart disease, gastrointestinal tract ulcers, and constipation
8. Retard the progression of renal failure and postpone the initiation of dialysis

No single diet is appropriate for all renal clients. Every client requires an individual assessment.

Dietary Components

Several basic components need to be monitored and, if possible, controlled in renal diets. These components are:

- Kilocalories
- Protein
- Sodium
- Potassium
- Phosphorus and calcium
- Fluid
- Saturated fat and cholesterol
- Iron, vitamins, and minerals

The need to restrict or encourage the consumption of any of these nutrients changes according to the client's medical status and treatment approach. For example, it may not be necessary for a client to control his or her phosphorus intake at one time but vital at another time.

Kilocalories

The intake of kilocalories is often increased for clients with renal disease. Clients on high-kilocalorie diets are usually given all the simple carbohydrates and monounsaturated and polyunsaturated fats they will eat. The end products of fat and carbohydrate catabolism are carbon dioxide and water. Neither of these dietary constituents imposes a burden on the client's compromised excretory ability. Inadequate nonprotein kilocalories will, however, encourage tissue breakdown and aggravate the uremia. Clients with renal insufficiency need 35–40 kcal/kg per day. The use of a specialized oral supplement such as *ReNeph LP/HC* (LP = low protein; HC = high kilocalorie) by Ross Laboratories is one example of an appropriate oral supplement for clients who are unwilling to eat enough food. An adequate intake of kilocalories is crucial to the success of the dietary treatment.

Some individuals with diabetes mellitus and renal diseases still need to have their blood sugar levels controlled. For these clients, it may or may not be advisable to increase simple carbohydrates. The need to control their blood sugar is sometimes a secondary concern. In some cases, the primary nutritional goal is to decrease the uremia. Uremic diabetic clients may have relatively high amounts of sugar planned in their diets.

Some renal clients require an alternate feeding route to attain and maintain optimal nutritional status. Accordingly, some physicians order a peripheral intravenous infusion of lipids to supplement oral feedings. Total parenteral nutrition solutions for renal clients are commercially available.

Protein

A primary goal of nutritional therapy in renal clients is control of nitrogen intake. Control may mean an increase or decrease of dietary protein as the client's medical condition and treatment approach change. In addition, the kind of protein fed to the client may be important. Some physicians prescribe a diet of high-biological-value protein when the client has an extremely high BUN level. Eggs, meat, and dairy products are examples of foods that contain protein of high biologic value.

Recently, the benefits of a vegetarian diet for patients with renal failure have proven useful. Studies using human and animal models suggest that some plant proteins may increase survival rates and decrease proteinuria, glomerular filtration rate, renal blood flow, and histologic renal damage compared to nonvegetarian diets (American Dietetic Association, 1997). Vegetarian diets by nature are higher in potassium and phosphorus because of all the vegetables, whole grains, and fruits they contain. The goal is to eat the right combination of plant proteins while keeping potassium and phosphorus under control. A referral to a renal dietitian is indicated for these patients. Protein restrictions are effective only if the client also consumes adequate kilocalories. Beginning renal insufficiency is usually referred to as a predialysis situation and requires a restriction or modification of protein intake.

The treatment approach selected by the client and the physician influences protein requirements. Hemodialysis clients sometimes need increased protein because hemodialysis results in a loss of 1–2 grams of amino acids per hour of dialysis. A client on CAPD has an even higher protein need because he or she dialyzes continuously. During dialysis, protein passes out of the blood with the waste products and into the dialysate fluid. When the dialysate fluid is discarded, a significant amount of protein is lost from the body. A high-protein diet is necessary to replenish these losses.

Sodium

The desirable sodium intake for renal clients depends on individual circumstances and is usually determined by repeated measurements of sodium in the serum and in the urine (if any). The sodium intake of many clients with renal failure must be restricted to prevent sodium retention in the body with consequent generalized edema.

The disease that precipitated the renal failure plays a role in determining the need for a sodium restriction. Because glomerulonephritis, for example, is more likely to produce hypertension and fluid retention, sodium restriction is often necessary. Low levels of sodium, absence of edema, and normal or low blood pressure often characterize other renal diseases, such as pyelonephritis. **Pyelonephritis** is an inflammation of the central portion of the kidney. In this situation, sodium intake can be higher than in the other groups of diseases but is individualized to the client's needs.

Potassium

Dietary potassium, like sodium, needs to be evaluated on an individual basis. **Hypokalemia** (low blood potassium level) needs to be avoided because it introduces the danger of cardiac arrhythmias and eventually cardiac arrest. Tables 21–1 and 21–2, respectively, list foods that are high and low in potassium. Salt substitutes are very high in potassium and should be avoided by most renal clients. It is important to recognize that a water softener may be a source of dietary potassium (Graves, 1998). The need to restrict potassium generally increases in clients with decreased urinary output.

The potassium content of fruits and vegetables varies according to the form in which they are eaten and the method of food preparation. For example, 1/2 cup of canned pears in heavy syrup has a potassium content of about 80 milligrams, and one fresh pear has a potassium content of about 210 milligrams. Potassium is water soluble. For this reason, some renal clients on very low potassium diets are taught to use large amounts of water when preparing vegetables and to discard the water after cooking. This decreases the potassium content of the vegetables. Unfortunately, it also decreases the water-soluble vitamins in the food. This is one reason that most renal clients need vitamin supplements. Clients should be taught to eat the fruits or vegetables in the form given on the list.

Phosphorus, Vitamin D, and Calcium

Phosphorus, vitamin D, and calcium are all normally balanced in the body. In clients with kidney disease, vitamin D cannot be activated. This leads to a low serum calcium level. At the same time, the kidneys cannot excrete phosphorus. This leads to an elevated serum phosphorus level. When the serum calcium level drops, calcium is released from the bones because of the increased secretion of **parathyroid hormone** (PTH). PTH is

Table 21–1 High-Potassium Foods to Avoid	
Dairy products	(In excess of 2 cups per day)
Meats	(In excess of 6 oz per day)
Starches	Bran cereals and bran products
Fruits	Avocado
	Bananas
	Orange, fresh
	Mango, fresh
	Nectarines
	Papayas
	Dried prunes
	(All others if eaten in excess of allowance)
Vegetables	Bamboo shoots
	Beet greens
	Baked potato, with skin
	Sweet potato fresh
	Spinach, cooked
	(All others if eaten in excess of allowance)
Others	Chocolate, cocoa
	Molasses
	Salt substitute
	Low-sodium broth
	Low-sodium baking powder
	Low-sodium baking soda
	Nuts

Table 21–2 Low-Potassium Foods and Beverages*

Gum drops
Hard, clear candy
Nondairy topping
Honey
Jams and jellies
Jelly beans
Lollipops
Marshmallows
Suckers
Sugar
Lifesavers
Chewing gum
"Poly-Rich" (nondairy creamer)
Cornstarch

Low-Potassium Beverages
Carbonated beverages
Lemonade
Limeade
Cranberry juice
Popsicles (1 stick—60 mL of fluid)
Hawaiian punch
Kool-Aid

Low-Potassium Unsweetened Beverages
Diet carbonated beverages
Diet lemonade
Diet Kool-Aid

*Note: Foods with sugar should not be eaten freely by diabetics.

secreted in an effort to correct the calcium imbalance. This chain of events may lead to renal osteodystrophy, which is a complication of chronic renal disease. **Renal osteodystrophy** leads to faulty bone formation.

Control of the blood levels of calcium and phosphorus involve three treatment approaches. First, clients with hypocalcemia and hyperphosphatemia are currently given calcitriol, the activated form of vitamin D. The second treatment approach is a dietary phosphorus restriction. Third, calcium supplements, a high-calcium diet, or both are frequently prescribed if the serum phosphorus is under control.

Phosphorus is found mainly in:

- Dairy products
- Dried beans and peas, such as kidney beans, split peas, and lentils
- Nuts and peanut butter
- Beverages such as cocoa, beer, and cola soft drinks

Clients on protein-restricted diets generally do not eat enough phosphorus to cause hyperphosphatemia. Clients on chronic renal dialysis with a more liberal protein intake may need to limit the intake of foods high in phosphorus.

Fluid

Predialysis (renal-insufficiency) and dialysis clients generally must restrict fluid intake because their kidneys can no longer excrete excess fluid. Fluids need to be allocated between meals and medications. Table 21–3 lists guidelines to follow for distributing fluids between meals and medications. Clients on hemodialysis are restricted to 500–1000 milliliters plus 24-hour urinary output. This allows for some fluid gain between dialysis treatments. For predialysis clients, fluids are usually restricted to 500 milliliters plus output. For clients on CAPD, fluid restriction is "as tolerated" according to their daily weight fluctuations and blood pressure.

Saturated Fat and Cholesterol

Clients with renal disease frequently have hyperlipoproteinemia. High serum lipid levels increase the progression of renal disease, which contributes to an increased risk of cardiovascular disease. Total cholesterol levels may be increased up to tenfold (American Dietetic Association, 1992). This is believed to be especially a problem in clients with nephrotic syndrome, diabetes, and/or an **LCAT deficiency**. LCAT is an enzyme that transports cholesterol from tissues to the liver for removal from the body. Most clients with an LCAT deficiency develop progressive glomerular injury.

Table 21–3 Guidelines for Fluid-Restricted Clients

If the Fluid Restriction Is:	Use This Amount of Fluids with Meals:	Use This Amount of Fluids with Medications:
1000 mL (4 cups)*	600 mL (2 1/2 cups)	400 mL (1 1/2 Cups)
1200 mL (5 cups)	700 mL (3 cups)	500 mL (2 cups)
1500 mL (6 cups)	1000 mL (4 cups)	500 mL (2 cups)
2000 mL (8 cups)	1000 mL (4 cups)	1000 mL (4 cups)

All foods contain some fluids, but it is especially important to count the following as part of the fluid allowance:

Milliliters of fluid per 1/2 Cup

Water	120	All juices	120	Watermelon	100
Coffee	120	Soda-pop	120	Sherbet	65
Tea	120	Ice	60	Ice cream	40
Sanka	120	Gelatin	100	Ice milk	40
Milk	120	Soup	120	Popsicle	80

*Approximate

Box 21–1 General Dietary Recommendations for Renal Patients

Dietary Component	Renal Insufficiency	Hemodialysis	Perztoneal Dialysis
Protein (g/kg HBW)*	0.6–0.8†	1.1–1.4	1.2–1.5
Energy (kcaSkg HBW)	35–40	30–35	25–35
Phosphorus (mg/kg HBW)	8–12‡	≤17§	≤17
Sodium (mg/day)	1000–3000	2000–3000	2000–4000
Potassium (mg/kg HBW)	Typically not restricted	40	Typically not restricted
Fluid (midday)	Typically not restricted	500–750 plus daily urine output or 1000 if anuric	≥2000
Calcium (mg/day)	1200-1600	Depends on serum level	Depends on serum level

*HBW = healthy body weight.
†The upper end of this range is preferred for patients with diabetes or malnutrition. Suggested protein intake for persons with nephron syndrome is 0.8 to 1.0 g/kg HBW.
‡Intake of 5 to 10 mg phosphorus per kilogram HBW is frequently quoted in the scientific literature, but 5 mg/kg HBW is practical only when used in conjunction with a very low-protein diet supplemented with specially formulated commercial feedings.
§It may not be possible to meet the optimum phosphorus prescription on a higher protein diet.

Source: Monsen, ER: Meeting the challenge of the renal diet. Copyright The American Dietetic Association. Reprinted by permission from Journal of the American Dietetic Association 93:638, 1993.

Significant hypertriglyceridemia is often present in clients with a history of renal disease. The nutritional care of clients with elevated triglycerides (type 4 hyperlipoproteinemia) includes a modified fat diet and a modification of carbohydrate intake. Clients are usually counseled to avoid saturated fat and to increase their intake of polyunsaturated and monounsaturated fat. Thirty to 35 percent of the total kilocalories are provided as fat because excessive carbohydrate could worsen the hypertriglyceridemia (Moore, 1993). Simple sugars and alcohol are usually limited for the same reason.

Iron

The anemias seen in clients with renal disease may be due to a lack of erythropoietin; a decreased oral iron intake, which often occurs as a result of dietary restriction; or blood loss. *Epoetin alfa*, a pharmaceutical form of erythropoietin, may be used to increase red blood cell production and thereby correct the anemia. The treatment for iron-deficiency anemia is oral or parenteral iron products and an increase in dietary sources of iron. A diagnosis of iron-deficiency anemia can be made by a laboratory measure of ferritin. **Ferritin** is the storage form of iron found primarily in the liver. A small amount of ferritin circulates in the blood and reflects the amount of iron in body stores. A laboratory value of less than 12 micrograms per liter suggests iron deficiency.

Nutritional therapy with iron supplements consists of 210 milligrams of ferrous iron salts per day divided among three to four doses. Absorption is enhanced when iron supplements are taken on an empty stomach or with vitamin C.

Vitamin and Mineral Supplementation

Chronically uremic patients are prone to deficiencies of water-soluble vitamins unless supplements are given (Kopple, 1999). Losses are most notable with pyridoxine, ascorbic acid, and folic acid (Wolfson, 1988). Supplementation of these nutrients is recommended for

clients on dialysis. Fat-soluble vitamins are not lost in the dialysate, and supplementation is not indicated except with vitamin D for another reason (see previous discussion). Because the body's ability to excrete excess fat-soluble vitamins is compromised, toxicity is a potential problem.

National Renal Diet

The American Dietetic Association and the National Kidney Foundation introduced the National Renal Diet in the fall of 1993. Because the dietary management of renal disease is tailored to the stage of disease and treatment approach, six meal-planning systems were developed. They are renal insufficiency without diabetes, renal insufficiency with diabetes, hemodialysis without diabetes, hemodialysis with diabetes, peritoneal dialysis without diabetes, and peritoneal dialysis with diabetes. These national meal-planning systems offer standardized guidelines for nutrition intervention and client education.

Each system provides food lists and calculation figures (derived from the average nutrient content of foods included in each list). Although the food lists developed for the client booklets were patterned after the *ADA Exchange Lists*, the varied nutritional requirements of clients with renal disease at different stages of treatment necessitated creation of specific food lists for each treatment modality. Box 21–1 shows the General Dietary Recommendations for Renal Patients by treatment approach. In addition, separate calculation figures and food lists were devised for clients with diabetes receiving each treatment modality, because foods high in sugars were excluded from the food lists for clients with diabetes.

Box 21–2 is an example of the calculation of a diet for a client receiving hemodialysis without diabetes (one of the six meal-planning systems). A case study and sample meal plan are shown. Box 21–3 is a condensed food list for the client with chronic renal failure who is receiving hemodialysis treatments. A sample menu derived from the

Box 21–2 Calculating the Renal Diet: Hemodialysis Case Study

AVERAGE CALCULATION FIGURES FOR RENAL DIETS (NO DIABETES)*

Food Choices	Energy kcal	PRO g	CHO g	Fat g	Na mg	K mg	P mg
Milk	120	4	8	5	80	185	110
Nondairy milk substitute	140	0.5	12	10	40	80	30
Meat	65	7	...	4	25	100	65
Starch	90	2	18	1	80	35	35
Vegetable							
Low potassium	25	1	5	tr	15	70	20
Medium potassium	25	1	5	tr	15	150	20
High potassium	25	1	5	tr	15	270	20
Fruit							
Low potassium	70	0.5	17	...	tr	70	15
Medium potassium	70	0.5	17	...	tr	150	15
High potassium	70	0.5	17	...	tr	270	15
Fat	45	...	...	5	55	10	5
High-calorie	100	tr	25	...	15	20	5
Salt	...	...	...		250	...	...

CASE EXAMPLE:

The client is a 55-year-old man who works full-time and has a sedentary lifestyle. He is 5 ft. 10 in. tall, has a medium frame, and weighs 68 kg. His ideal and usual weight is 76 kg. During the past 6–9 months, he has been anorectic and has had intermittent nausea and episodes of vomiting. He receives 4 hours of hemodialysis 3 times per week. His predialysis blood chemistry values were blood urea nitrogen, 22.50 mmol/L (63 mg/dL); sodium, 135 mmol/L (135 mEq/L); potassium, 4.0 mmol/L (4.0 mEq/L); phosphorus, 2.0 mmol/L (6.2 mg/dL); calcium, 2.25 mmoVL (9.0 mg/dL); and albumin, 33 g/L (3.3 g/dL). His urine output ranges between 800 and 1000 mL per day.

DAILY RENAL DIET PLAN GOALS

Nutrient	Level	Rationale
Energy (kcal)	3000	40 kcal/kg HBW
Protein (g)	91	1.2 g/kg HBW
Sodium (mg)	2000	Control fluid weight gain
Potassium (mg)	3000 (75 mEq)	≤40 mg/kg HBW
Phosphorus (mg)	300	≤17 mglkg HBW
Fluid (mL)	1500–1750	750mL plus urine output

SAMPLE CALCULATION OF RENAL DIET PLAN FOR HEMODIALYSIS

Food Choices	Choices no.	Energy kcal	PRO g	Na mg	K mg	P mg
Milk	1	120	4	80	185	110
Nondairy milk substitute	1	140	0.5	40	80	30
Meat	9	585	63	225	900	585
Starch	10	900	20	800	350	350
Vegetable	2	50	2	30	...	40
Low potassium		...	...	...	...	...
Medium potassium	(1)	...	...	...	150	...
High potassium	(1)	...	...	...	270	...
Fruit	3	210	1.5	...	...	45
Low potassium		...	...	...	...	...
Medium potassium	(1)	...	...	...	150	...
High potassium	(2)	...	...	...	540	...
Fat	10	450	...	550	100	50
High-calorie	5	500	...	75	100	25
Salt	1	...	...	250	...	...
Totals		2955	91	2050	2825	1235

*Because control of fat and carbohydrate intake is not a priority for all patients, practitioners may include their calculation in the meal plan on a case-by-case basis. Table abbreviations: PRO = protein, CHO = carbohydrate, Na = sodium, K = potassium, P = phosphorus, tr = trace, HBW = healthy body weight.

Source: Monsen, ER: Meeting the challenge of the renal diet. Copyright The Arnerican Dietetic Association. Reprinted by permission from Journal ofthe American Dietetic Association 93:638, 1993.

Box 21–3 Condensed Renal Food Lists for Chronic Renal Failure, Hemodialysis

MILK LIST

Approximate Nutrient Content: 4 g protein, 120 kcal, 80 mg sodium (Na), 185 mg potassium (K), 110 mg phosphorus (P)

Item	Amount
Milk	1/2 cup
Alterna (low-sodium milk substitute)	1 cup
Cream cheese	3 tbsp

NONDAIRY MILK SUBSTITUTES

Approximate Nutrient Content: 0.5 g protein, 140 kcal, 40 mg Na, 80 mg K, 30 mg P

Liquid nondairy creamer, polyunsaturated	1/2 cup
Dessert topping, nondairy, frozen	1/2 cup

MEAT LIST

Approximate Nutrient Content: 7 g protein, 65 kcal, 25 mg Na, 100 mg K, 65 mg P

Low-cholesterol egg substitute	1/4 cup
Lean beef, pork, poultry	1 oz
Unsalted canned tuna	1/4 cup

STARCH LIST

Approximate Nutrient Content: 2 g protein, 90 kcal, 80 mg Na, 35 mg K, 35 mg P

Bread (white, light rye, sourdough)	1 slice
Saltines, unsalted	4
Puffed wheat	1 cup
Rice, cooked	1/2 cup
Angel Food Cake	1 oz

VEGETABLE LIST

Approximate Nutrient Content: 1 g protein, 25 kcal, 15 mg Na, 20 mg P; serving size is 1 1/2 cup unless otherwise noted; prepared or canned without salt

Low Potassium (0–100 mg K)	
Lettuce, all varieties	1 cup
Cucumber, peeled	
Medium Potassium (101 to 200 mg K)	
Carrots	1 small, raw
Corn	1/2 ear
Broccoli	1/2 cup
High Potassium (201–350 mg K)	
Tomato	1 medium
Potato, baked	1/2 medium
Spinach, ckd.	

(Continued on next page)

---

condensed renal food list and the sample daily meal plan are shown in Table 21–4.

Nutrient Guidelines for Adults with Renal Disease

As you can see, the nutritional care of renal clients is complex. Table 21–5 summarizes clinical situations, dietary interventions, and the rationale for nutrient control.

Renal Disease in Children

Growth failure is commonly seen in children with chronic renal failure treated with dialysis, but it is not an inevitable complication. Inadequate kilocaloric consumption and/or metabolic acidosis are reasons for the poor growth. These children often need to have their sodium, potassium, and protein intake rigidly controlled, and this may contribute to poor food

intake. Anorexia and emotional disturbances are also contributing factors. Suggestions for improving children's intake include involving the children in selecting and preparing foods (insofar as possible); serving meals in an appealing, attractive manner (e.g., serving contrasting colors and textures of foods, using decorative tableware and dishes); serving small, frequent meals; ensuring that the child has someone with him or her at mealtime; and planning special mealtime events such as picnics (even if they have to be held in the hospital playroom).

Kidney Stones

Kidney stones may be found in the bladder, kidney, ureter, or urethra. During urine formation, the urine moves from the collecting tubules into the renal pelvis. From the **renal pelvis**, the urine moves down the **ureter**

Box 21–3 Condensed Renal Food Lists for Chronic Renal Failure, Hemodialysis (Continued)

FRUIT LIST

Approximate Nutrient Content: 0.5 g protein, 70 kcal, 15 mg P; serving size is 1/2 cup, unless otherwise noted

Low Potassium (0–100 mg K)
   Applesauce
   Pears, canned
Medium Potassium (101–200 mg K)
   Apple, fresh   1 small
   Watermelon   1 cup
High Potassium (201–350 mg K)
   Orange juice
   Pear, fresh   1 medium

FAT LIST

Approximate Nutrient Content: trace protein, 45 kcal, 55 mg Na, 10 mg K, 5 mg P

Unsaturated Fats
   Margarine   1 tsp
   Mayo   1 tsp
Saturated Fats
   Coconut   2 tbsp
   Powdered coffee whitener   1 tbsp

HIGH-KILOCALORIE CHOICES

Approximate Nutrient Content: 100 kcal, 15 mg Na, 20 mg K, 5 mg P

Carbonated beverages, fruit flavors, root beer   1 cup
Kool-Aid   1 cup
Lemonade   1 cup
Tang   1 cup
Gum drops   15

---

and into the urinary bladder. Finally, urine passes from the bladder down the urethra and exits the body. A stone, also called a **urinary calculus**, is a deposit of mineral salts held together by a thick, syrupy substance. A urinary calculus can block the movement of urine out of the body. Symptoms of a blockage include sudden severe pain with chills, fever, **hematuria** (blood in the urine), and an increased desire to urinate. A kidney stone can also pass out of the body with the urine.

Causes

The cause of most kidney stones is unknown. Some possible causes include an abnormal function of the parathyroid gland, disordered uric acid metabolism (as in gout), an excessive intake of animal protein, and immobility. At higher risk for kidney stones are men, people with a sedentary lifestyle, and Asians and Caucasians. Typically, kidney stones occur in clients who are between ages 30 and 50. A determination of the stone's composition may lead to a restriction of dietary substrates (the substance acted on). Frequent dietary substrates of kidney stones are oxalic acid and purines.

Treatment

All clients with kidney stones should be advised to drink sufficient water to keep the urine volume above 2 liters per day. About 3000 milliliters or 13 cups of water per day are necessary to produce this amount of urine. The primary reason for increasing fluid intake is to prevent formation of concentrated urine, in which crystals are more likely to combine and precipitate.

Oxalates

A diet that excludes foods high in oxalates (see Clinical Application 21–2) is frequently prescribed for clients with kidney stones if laboratory analysis shows a surgically removed or passed stone to be high in oxalates.

Calcium

Historically, if laboratory analysis of a surgically removed or passed stone was found to be high in calcium, a low-calcium diet was prescribed (600 milligrams per day). Today it is known that kidney stones are not usually caused by dietary calcium. In most individuals, kidney stones are usually less of a problem with an increased calcium intake than with a decreased calcium intake. A high-calcium diet binds the oxalate of dietary origin in the gastrointestinal tract and prevents its absorption, thereby reducing urinary oxalate formation (Weaver and Heanly, 1999).

Uric Acid Stones

Stones composed of uric acid are sometimes a complication of gout. **Gout** is a hereditary metabolic disease that is a form of arthritis. One symptom of gout is inflammation of the joints. The metabolism of uric acid is related to dietary purines. **Purines** are an end product of protein digestion. Thus, a purine-restricted diet is often prescribed for gout. Table 21–6 shows foods that are high, moderate, and low in purines. Many physicians do not prescribe a low-purine diet for the treatment of gout because the condition can be more effectively controlled by medications.

Table 21–4 Chronic Renal Failure, Hemodialysis Meal Plan and Sample Menu

Meal Plan	Sample Menu	Meal Plan	Sample Menu
Breakfast		*Afternoon Snack*	
1 nondairy milk substitute	1/2 cup liquid nondairy creamer, polyunsaturated	1 high-kilocalorie	1 cup Kool-Aid
		Supper	
1 high-potassium fruit	1/2 cup orange juice	1 high-potassium vegetable	1/2 cup ckd. drained spinach
2 starches	1 cup puffed wheat and 1 slice light rye toast	1 high-potassium fruit	1 fresh pear
1 meat	1/4 cup low-cholesterol egg substitute	2 starches	1/2 cup rice and 1 oz angel food cake
2 fats	2 tsp margarine	4 meat	4 oz broiled chicken breast
Morning Snack		2 fats	2 tsp margarine (used on chicken)
1 high-kilocalorie	1 cup Tang	1 high-kilocalorie	1 cup root beer
Lunch		*Bedtime Snack*	
1 medium-potassium vegetable	1 small raw carrot	1 milk	1/2 cup low-fat milk
1 medium-potassium fruit	1 small apple	2 starches	8 unsalted saltine crackers
2 starches	2 slices of sourdough white bread	1 meat	1/4 cup unsalted canned tuna
4 meats	4 oz unsalted lean beef	2 fats	2 tsp mayo (for tuna salad)
2 fats	2 tsp mayo	1 high-kilocalorie	1 cup limeade
1 high-kilocalorie	1 cup lemonade		

Table 21–5 Clinical Situation, Dietary Intervention, and Rationale for Nutrient Control

Clinical Situation	Rationale	Intervention
Proteinuria	Protein lost in urine	Increase dietary protein
CAPD	Protein lost in dialysate	Increase dietary protein
Elevated BUN and creatinine (Uremia)	Body unable to excrete waste generated from protein metabolism in the amounts eaten and/or catabolized	Decrease dietary protein Increase nonprotein kilocalories Emphasis on proteins with high biologic value
Edema (Anuria)	Body unable to reabsorb and excrete sodium and fluid in the amounts consumed	Fluid restrictions Sodium restriction
Hyperkalemia	Body unable to excrete potassium	Potassium restriction
Hyperphosphatemia	May be related to an inability to activate vitamin D Body unable to excrete the amounts of phosphorus consumed and absorbed	Phosphorus restriction Phosphate binders
Low ferritin levels	Iron deficiency; may be caused by blood loss and/or poor food intake	Increase kilocalories Increase nutrient density Iron supplements Vitamin C enhances iron absorption and should be consumed with meals
Poor growth, especially in children	Insufficient energy	Increase kilocalories to spare protein
Low number of red blood cells with normal ferritin level	Inability to manufacture erythropoietin	Epoetin alfa supplement
Elevated triglyceride levels	Common in renal patients	Type 4 hyperlipoproteinemia diet with modifications in fat and carbohydrate intake

CLINICAL APPLICATION 21–2

Foods High in Oxalic Acid

Beverages	mg/100 g
coffee, instant dry	143.0
tea, brewed	12.5
Fruits	
blackberries, raw	12.4
gooseberries, raw	19.3
plums, raw	11.9
Grains	
bread, whole-wheat	20.9
Vegetables	
beets, raw	72.2
beets, boiled	109.0
carrots, boiled	1 4.5
green beans, raw	43.7
green beans, boiled	29.7
rhubarb, raw	537.0
rhubarb, stewed	447.0
spinach, boiled	571.0
Miscellaneous	
cocoa, dry	623.0
Ovaltine, powder	45.9

Values taken from Pennington, JAT, and Church, HN: Food Values of Portions Commonly Used, 14th ed. Harper & Row Publishers, NY.

Table 21–6 Purines in Food

GROUP A: HIGH CONCENTRATION (150–1000 mg/100 g)	
Liver	Sardines (in oil)
Kidney	Meat extracts
Sweetbreads	Consomme
Brain	Gravies
Heart	Fish roes
Anchovies	Herring

GROUP B: MODERATE AMOUNTS (50–150 mg/100 g)	
Meat, game and fish other than those mentioned in Group A	
Fowl	Asparagus
Lentils	Cauliflower
Whole-grain cereals	Mushrooms
Beans	Spinach
Peas	

GROUP C: VERY SMALL AMOUNTS NEED NOT BE RESTRICTED IN DIET OF PERSONS WITH GOUT	
Vegetables other than those mentioned above	
Fruits of all kinds	Coffee
Milk	Tea
Cheese	Chocolate
Eggs	Carbonated beverages
Refined cereals, spaghetti, macaroni	Tapioca
Butter, fats, nuts, peanut butter*	Yeast
Sugars and sweets	
Vegetable soups	

*Fats interfere with the urinary excretion of urates and thus should be limited when attempting to promote excretion of urlc acid.

Source: From Thomas, CL (ed): Taber's Cyclopedic Medical Dictionary, ed 17. FA Davis, Philadelphia 1993, p 1643, with permission.

Surgery

Surgery is sometimes necessary to remove large kidney stones. Surgical removal of the stones prevents infection, reduces pain, and prevents a loss of kidney function.

Urinary Tract Infections

One form of **urinary tract infection** (UTI) is **cystitis**, an inflammation of the bladder. This condition is prevalent in young women. Recurrent UTI means that the individual has three or more bouts of infection per year. A general nutrition measure includes acidifying the urine by taking large doses of vitamin C. One study found the regular intake of a cranberry juice beverage reduced the frequency of bacteriuria with pyuria in older women (Avorn et al., 1994), and another small study confirmed this (Haverkorn, and Mandigers, 1994). Cranberry juice contains a substance with biologic activity that inhibits the growth of E. coli in the urinary tract (Fig. 21–4). Clients with UTIs should be encouraged to drink ample fluids.

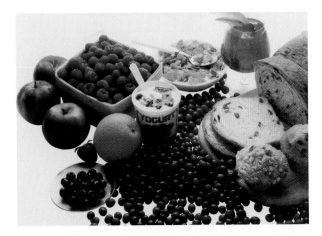

Figure 21–4:
Cranberry juice can be effective in decreasing the severity of urinary tract infections in the elderly. Cranberries contain a chemical compounds called proanthocyanides that seem to stunt the growth of E. coli, preventing it from adhering to the walls of the bladder and kidney. (Courtesy of Ocean Spray Cranberries.)

Summary

The basic functional unit of the kidney is the nephron. Millions of nephrons work together to form urine and remove unnecessary substances from the blood. Glomerular filtration rate (GFR) is a measure of kidney function. The kidneys also are the site where vitamin D_3 (calcitriol) and erythropoietin are activated. Kidney failure can be acute or chronic. Chronic renal disease is progressive. Much research is aimed at finding a way to stop the downward spiral of GFR in clients who are diagnosed with chronic renal failure. Current research is focused on the role of dietary protein and phosphorus in the progression of kidney failure. Treatment for kidney failure is dialysis or a kidney transplant.

Nutritional management of clients with renal disease is a fundamental part of treatment. Clients with kidney disease require constant assessment, monitoring, and counseling. The dietary components that may need modification are kilocalories, protein, sodium, potassium, phosphorus, fluid, cholesterol, and saturated fat. Vitamin and mineral supplements are often prescribed. Frequently, the diet these clients follow must be further modified as their medical condition and treatment approach changes. A National Renal Diet has been developed for these clients.

Some nutritional intervention is necessary for clients with kidney stones and UTIs. The fluid intake of these clients should be high. Usually, clients with kidney stones need to avoid foods that contain substances likely to form stones.

Case Study 21–1

Mr. U a 95-year-old man, was admitted to the hospital from his doctor's office for a shunt implantation with subsequent hemodialysis planned. A college graduate, he is employed as an engineer. His medical record indicates that he had an episode of acute glomerulonephritis about 10 years ago. He contracted the disease after a streptococcal throat infection. At that time his symptoms were hematuria, oligaluria, proteinuria, hypertension, and edema. He was discharged on a 4-g sodium diet.

Mr. U now complains of swollen ankles, headaches, and fatigue. He reports to have had a 10-lb weight gain over the past 6 weeks. His usual body weight is 170 lb; he is 5 ft. 10 in. tall and has a large frame. He now weighs 181 lb. His blood pressure is 155/99. Laboratory test results follow:

Test	Results	Normal Range
BUN	75 mg/dL	9–25 mg/dL
Creatinine	2 mg/dL	0.6–1.5 mg/dL
Serum phosphorus	4.4 mg/dL	3.0–4.5 mg/dL
Serum calcium	3.5 mgldL	3.5–5.0 mg/dL
Hemoglobin	6 mg/dL	14–18 g/dL
Hematocrit	19 percent	42–52 percent
Potassium	4.0 mEq/L	3.5–5.0 mEq/L
Albumin	3.5 g/dL	3.5–5.5 g/dL
Urine volume	900 mL/day	1000–1500 mL
Proteinuria	1 +	None
GFR	10 mL/min	125 mL/min
Cholesterol	280 mg/dL	<200 mg/dL
Triglycerides	140 mg/dL	40–150 mg/dL

The doctor has prescribed a 60-g protein, 2000-kcal, 2-g sodium, low-saturated fat, low-cholesterol diet and a fluid restriction of output plus 500 mL. Hemodialysis is ordered for three times a week. His medications include docusate sodium, furosemide, a multivitamin, vitamin B_6, and folic acid. Mr U stated that the protein, fluid, saturated fat, and cholesterol restrictions are new to him.

Nursing Care Plan

Subjective Data	Client complains of headaches, swollen ankles, and fatigue.
Objective Data	Client has an elevated BUN, phosphorus, blood pressure, and creatine. The client also has edema; a decreased GFR, hemoglobin, and hematocrit; and a decreased urinary output.
Nursing Diagnosis	Fluid Volume Excess (NANDA) related to renal insufficiency as evidenced by client complaints of headaches, swollen ankles, fatigue, and decreased urinary output, edema formation, and hypertension. (North American Nursing Diagnosis Association, 1999)

Desired Outcomes Evaluation Criteria	*Nursing Actions/ Interventions*	*Rationale*
(NOC) Fluid Balance (Johnson, M, and Maas, M, 2000)	(NIC) Fluid Management (McCloskey, J, and Bulechek, GM, 2000)	
The client will demonstrate a stabilized fluid balance with a calculated fluid intake and a measured fluid output. Vital signs will progress toward the normal range.	Measure urinary output q shift (q = every) and fluid intake	Client's urinary output may vary, and fluid intake must be adjusted accordingly.

Continued on next page

Nursing Care Plan (Continued)

Desired Outcomes / Evaluation Criteria	Nursing Actions/ Interventions	Rationale
	Plan fluid intake with client; monitor fluid intake and body weight.	Fluid intake must be controlled to prevent excessive edema and control blood pressure. Daily weight is the best measure of fluid balance.
	Monitor BUN/creatinine results, as needed.	The client is currently unable to excrete waste generated from protein metabolism in amounts eaten and/or catabolized. As the client begins dialysis treatments, the BUN/creatinine levels should decrease, and the protein content of the diet will need to be adjusted accordingly.
	Monitor blood pressure, pulses, and lung sounds q 4 hours.	The client's fluid volume excess and decreased GFR may increase secretion of renin and raise blood pressure.
	Encourage adequate kilocalorie intake.	The diet will not be effective in controlling BUN/creatinine levels unless adequate kilocalories are consumed.
The client wIl verbalize knowledge of condition and therapy regimen.	Discuss necessary changes in lifestyle and assist client to incorporate disease management into activities of daily living.	Because the client has a chronic disease, long-term compliance with the treatment approach will be necessary.
	Teach client to measure urinary output.	The client will need to learn to measure his own urinary output.
	Teach client to measure fluid intake daily; fluid intake should be 500 mL plus urinary output in milliliters.	The client will need to learn how to calculate his daily fluid intake based on his urinary output and insensible losses of fluid.
	Discuss with client the relationships of his symptoms (headaches, swollen ankles, fatigue) and signs (edema; decreased GFR, hemoglobin, hematocrit, urinary output; and elevated BUN/creatinine) to treatment approaches (hemodialysis and dietary restrictions).	Relating signs and symptoms to the client's treatment approach will assist him in understanding his treatment regimen.
	Refer to the dietitian for dietary teaching.	The client's needs will best be met if referral to the dietitian is made as soon as possible. A diet as complicated as this client's will require several hours of instruction. Information is usually better retained if small amounts of information are given at frequent intervals.
	Discuss with the client the importance of regular hemodialysis treatments.	Failure to receive regular hemodialysis treatments will result in an excessive fluid gain and abnormal laboratory values between treatments. Subsequent efforts to remove this excess fluid may result in a dangerous drop in blood pressure during the dialysis treatment.
The client will demonstrate behaviors consistent with dietary program.	Monitor client's food intake.	The best method to evaluate whether the client has learned his dietary restrictions is to monitor food intake.

Critical Thinking Question

1. Explain the relationship of each dietary modification to the signs and symptoms Mr. U is experiencing.
2. Mr. U eats only about half his needed kilocalories. What should you do?
3. Mr. U develops a stomach ulcer. What should you recommend?
4. Mr. U decides he would like to try CAPD. How would his diet probably change?

Study Aids

Subjects . . . . .Internet Sites

USDA Food Composition . . . . .http://www.nal.usda.gov/fnic/foodcomp, accessed May, 2000

The Nephron Information Center . . . . .http://www.nephron.com, accessed May, 2000

National Kidney Foundation . . . . .http://www.kidney.org, accessed May, 2000

Treatment Choices . . . . .http://www.lifeoptions.org/nlnh/9-10.html, accessed May, 2000

Renal Diets . . . . .http://www.andrew.cmu.edu/user/sorensen, accessed May, 2000
Computer program

American Dietetic Association . . . . .http://www.eatright.org, accessed May, 2000

Renal Diets . . . . .http://www.azstarnet.com/~bsmith/tools/getting_started.htm, accessed May, 2000

Chapter Review

1. Which of the following is not always a nutritional goal for a child with renal disease?
   a. Promote normal growth and development
   b. Maintain current hydration status
   c. Minimize uremic toxicity
   d. Stimulate client well-being
2. Kidney disease cannot be caused by:
   a. Consumption of toxic metals
   b. Habitual consumption of water
   c. Consumption of a diet habitually high in protein
   d. Trauma
3. Kilocalories usually need to be increased in protein-restricted diets because an adequate kilocalorie intake:
   a. Assists in the control of serum potassium
   b. Is necessary to prevent renal anemia
   c. Controls and prevents osteodystrophy
   d. Spares protein
4. The _____ intake from food is not monitored in renal clients.
   a. Vitamin D
   b. Fluid
   c. Protein
   d. Sodium
5. The most important nutritional consideration in treating clients with kidney stones is to:
   a. Limit calcium intake.
   b. Restrict all end products of protein metabolism.
   c. Restrict all food sources of calcium, oxalic acid, and purines.
   d. Increase fluid intake.

Clinical Analysis

1. Bill, age 10, has acute glomerulonephritis. His mother explains that Bill had a streptococcal infection 1 week prior to the illness. When planning Bill's care, the nurse recognizes that he needs help in understanding his diet. Bill's restrictions will include:
   a. A low-fat diet
   b. A calcium restriction
   c. Measuring urine output (if any) daily and planning his fluid intake
   d. A high-protein diet
2. Mr. Jones, a 49-year-old mechanic, has been admitted to the hospital with diagnosis of renal failure. Mr. Jones has been following a 40-gram protein, 2-gram sodium, 2-gram potassium, 1000-milliliter fluid restriction for the past 5 years. Mr. Jones is scheduled for surgery tomorrow to have a permanent fistula implanted for hemodialysis. Mr. Jones's nutritional needs will most likely change after he is maintained on hemodialysis to include:
   a. More oranges, bananas, and baked potatoes.
   b. More lean meat, eggs, low-fat milk, low-fat cheeses, soymilk, tofu, and peanut butter
   c. Less starches, breads, and cereals.
   d. Less margarine, oil, and salad dressings.
3. Mr. Jones is found to have an elevated serum phosphorus level after 6 months on hemodialysis. He should:
   a. Restrict his intake of dairy products.
   b. Restrict his intake of red meats.
   c. Increase his intake of sugar, honey, jam, jelly, and other simple sugars.
   d. Discontinue his phosphate binders.

Bibliography

American Dietetic Association: Manual of Clinical Dietetics, ed 5. American Dietetic Association, Chicago, 1996.

American Dietetic Association: Position of the American Dietetic Association: Vegetarian Diets. J Am Diet Assoc 97:1317, 1997.

Avorn, J, et al.: In reply [letter]. JAMA 272:589, 1994.

Avorn, J, et al.: Reduction of bacteriuria and pyuria after ingestion of cranberry juice. JAMA 271:751, 1994.

Blumberg, JB: More than one in four adults at risk for kidney failure. Tufts University Health and Nutrition Newsletter. 17:4. Pf.8, June 1999.

Fougue, D: Causes and interventions for malnutrition in patients undergoing maintenance dialysis. Blood Purif 15:112, 1997.

Graves, JW: Hyperkalemia due to a potassium-based water softener. NEJM. 1790, December 1998.

Guyton, AC, and Hall, JE: Textbook of Medical Physiology, ed. 9. WB Saunders, Philadelphia, 1995.

Gylys, BA, and Wedding, ME: Medical Terminology: A Systems Approach, ed. 4. FA Davis, Philadelphia, 1999.

Haverkorn, MJ, and Mandigers, J: Reduction of bacteriuria and pyuria using cranberry juice [letter]. JAMA 272:590, 1994.

Johnson, M, Maas, M, and Moorhead, S: Nursing Outcomes Classification (NOC), ed. 2. Mosby, Philadelphia, 2000.

Klahr, S, et al.: The effects of dietary protein restriction and blood-pressure control on the progression of chronic renal disease. N Engl J Med 330:877, 1994.

Kopple, JD: Renal Disorders and Nutrition. In Shils, ME, Olson, JA, Shike, M, and Ross, CA (eds): Modern Nutrition in Health and Disease, ed. 9. Williams and Wilkins, Baltimore, 1999.

Kopple, JD: McCollum award lecture, 1996: Protein-energy malnutrition in maintenance dialysis patients. Am J Clin Nutr 65:1544, 1997.

Kuhlmann, MK, et al.: Malnutrition in hemodialysis patients. Self-assessment, medical evaluations and "verifiable" parameters. Med Klin 1:13, Jan 15, 1997.

McCloskey, JC, and Bulechek, GM: Nursing Interventions Classification (NIC), 3 ed. Mosby, Philadelphia, 2000.

Monsen, ER: Meeting the challenge of the renal diet. J Am Diet Assoc 93:6, 1993.

Moore, MC: Pocket Guide to Nutrition and Diet Therapy, ed 2. Mosby Year Book, St Louis, 1993.

National Kidney Foundation: Nutrition and Changing Kidney Function. Publication no. 04-01CM. National Kidney Foundation, Inc., New York, 1999.

North American Nursing Diagnosis Association: Nursing Diagnosis: Definitions and Classifications 1999–2000, North American Nursing Diagnosis Association, Philadelphia, 1999.

Pennington, JAT, Bowes, AD, and Church, HN: Bowers and Churches Food Values of Portions Commonly Used, ed. 17. Lippincott and Wilkins Publishers. Baltimore, 1997.

Scalon, VD: Essentials of Anatomy and Physiology, ed. 3. FA Davis, Philadelphia, 1998.

Weaver, CM, and Heaney, RP: Calcium. In Shils, ME, Olson, JA, Shike, M, and Ross, CA (eds): Modern Nutrition in Health and Disease. ed 9. Williams and Wilkins, Baltimore, 1999.

Williams, LS, and Hopper, PD: Understanding Medical and Surgical Nursing. FA Davis, Philadelphia, 1999.

Wolfson, M: Use of water-soluble vitamins in patients with chronic renal failure. Semin Dialysis 1:28, 1988.

Zeller, K, et al.: Effect of restricting dietary protein on the progression of renal failure in patients with insulin-dependent diabetes mellitus. N Engl J Med 324:78, 1991.

CHAPTER 22

Diet in Gastrointestinal Disease

LEARNING OBJECTIVES

After completing this chapter, the student should be able to:

1. Distinguish the dietary preparation for gastrointestinal surgery from dietary preparation for surgery on other body systems.
2. Identify nutritional deficiencies that may accompany diseases or treatment of the gastrointestinal tract.
3. Describe nutritional deficiencies associated with steatorrhea.
4. List several nutritional consequences of cirrhosis of the liver.
5. Discuss dietary modifications for common gastrointestinal diseases treated medically and surgically.

Many disorders that affect the gastrointestinal tract and its accessory organs (liver, gallbladder, and pancreas) influence the nutritional status of clients. Most surgical procedures impact gastrointestinal tract function and require special dietary measures, both preoperatively and postoperatively. This chapter discusses diet modifications for surgical clients and for clients with common gastrointestinal diseases.

Dietary Considerations with Surgical Clients

Postoperatively, the healing process requires increased amounts of protein, vitamins C and K, and zinc, along with adequate amounts of other nutrients. Vitamin C is necessary for collagen formation; vitamin K for blood clotting; and zinc for tissue growth, bone formation, skin integrity, cell-mediated immunity, and generalized host defense.

Protein depletion causes increased risk of infection and shock. Protein is essential for the manufacture of antibodies and white blood cells, which help the body to fight infection. Hypoalbuminemia (low serum albumin) prevents the return of interstitial fluid to the venous system, decreasing intravascular fluid. This results in an increased risk of shock because of low intravascular volume. Local edema, which accompanies any trauma, including surgery, hampers circulation and healing. A low serum albumin level increases the time needed to reduce edema. The serum albumin level, then, becomes a useful and readily available measure of protein status. Clinical Application 22–1 elaborates the possible consequences of malnutrition in surgical clients.

Preoperative protein energy malnutrition was identified in 38 percent of clients undergoing abdominal surgery for benign conditions. Of these clients, 75 percent developed postoperative complications, compared with 22 percent of well-nourished clients (Dannhauser, Van Zyl, and Nel, 1995). Mild to severe malnutrition affected 39 percent of patients undergoing gastrointestinal or orthopedic surgical procedures, about two-thirds of whom received nutritional support (Bruun et al., 1999).

Persons with gastrointestinal disease are at special risk when facing surgery because such diseases interfere with nutrition. In cases involving gastrointestinal surgery, the gastrointestinal tract is incised and sutured, so postoperative feeding is postponed to allow healing. Clients with postoperative complications following gastrointestinal surgery were shown to be four times more likely to have been severely malnourished preoperatively as those without complications. Signs of severe malnutrition in this study were subcutaneous tissue loss and muscle wasting, often with edema, and ongoing weight loss of 10 percent or more of body weight (Detsky, Smalley, and Chang, 1994). A more complicated prognostic nutritional index (PNI) uses serum albumin, serum transferrin, triceps skinfold, and cutaneous delayed hypersensitivity in a formula to predict the risk of operative complications. In clients identified as high risk, 7 days of preoperative TPN was shown to produce a sixfold reduction in major sepsis (Mullen, 1981). In contrast to this multifaceted assessment tool, analysis of hospital records revealed that just 59 percent of gastrointestinal and orthopedic surgical charts even contained an entry on the client's body weight (Bruun et al., 1999).

Special notice should be given to surgical clients with liver disease. The liver has many functions, some of which are reviewed in Table 22–1. Because of the liver's role in metabolizing and detoxifying drugs, clients with liver disease must be carefully managed when surgery is necessary.

CLINICAL APPLICATION 22–1

Surgical Clients with Rampant Dental Caries

Within a period of weeks, three clients on a gynecological surgical unit suffered postoperative wound disruptions. Each disruption was a dehiscence, a separation of the wound edges. Dehiscence occurs most frequently between the fifth and twelfth postoperative days. Risk factors for dehiscence include obesity, malnutrition, dehydration, abdominal distention, increased abdominal pressure from improper deep breathing and coughing, and infection.

All three clients had at least one of the risk factors. One client ran a postoperative fever, which could have been caused by infection or dehydration. The other two clients had such severely carious teeth it would have been difficult for them to chew in the months before surgery. They probably were malnourished.

It is suggested that nurses refer preoperative clients with marked dental caries to the dietitian for nutritional assessment. Carious teeth can cause and be caused by poor eating habits.

Drugs may accumulate in the bloodstream because the liver cannot metabolize them. Moreover, some anesthetics, analgesics, and anti-infectives are toxic to the liver.

Preoperative Nutrition

Before elective surgery is undertaken, nutritional deficiencies should be identified and corrected. Many obese clients are instructed to lose weight to reduce the risks of surgery. If the client is anemic, an iron preparation can be prescribed. Other nutrients can be provided as needed. At least 2–3 weeks are required for objective evidence of the effectiveness of nutritional therapy. All surgical clients should receive instruction in the weeks before surgery.

If general anesthesia is to be employed, the stomach should be empty to prevent aspiration of gastric contents into the lungs. The usual procedure is to have the client take nothing by mouth (NPO) during the 8 hours before surgery even though clear fluids generally leave the stomach after 2 hours. A project to increase awareness of anesthesia practitioners to excessive fasting by preoperative clients reduced the mean fasting time for orthopedic clients from 11.9 to 6.5 hours. It is recommended that the anesthesia department prescribe the latest time a client may consume food

Table 22–1 Liver Functions

Related to	Produces/Processes	Stores	Breaks down
Carbohydrate	Glucose from galactose and fructose Glucose from glycogen Glucose from glycerol and protein	Glycogen	
Fat	Fat from glucose Cholesterol Fatty acids and glycerol from cholesterol, phospholipids, and lipoproteins Lipoproteins Water-soluble bilirubin (from fat-soluble) Bile	Fat	
Protein	Albumin Some globulins Prothrombin Fibrinogen Transferrin Enzymes to convert ammonia to urea		
Vitamins	Retinol-binding protein Other transport proteins Activates thiamine Activates pyridoxine Processes vitamin D	A, D, E, K Thiamin Riboflavin Pyridoxine Folic acid B_{12} Biotin	
Minerals		Iron	
Other			Worn-out red blood cells Acetaminophen Alcohol Aldosterone Bacteria Barbiturates Estrogen Glucocorticoids Morphine Progesterone Some anesthetics

and fluids preoperatively, rather than limiting everyone's intake beginning at midnight (Jester and Williams, 1999).

Surgery of the gastrointestinal tract demands additional bowel preparation. Anti-infectives such as neomycin sulfate, which remain predominantly in the bowel, may be given to kill intestinal bacteria. A low-residue diet for 2–3 days will minimize the feces left in the bowel. A low-residue diet reduces the fecal bulk by reducing food residue. Residue is the total solid material in the large intestine after digestion. A low-residue diet usually consists of foods that are easily digested and absorbed. Table 22–2 details a low-residue diet.

Postoperative Nutrition

Intravenous fluids are continued after surgery. The usual minimum replacement is 2 liters of 5 percent glucose in water in 24 hours. This amount contains 100 grams of glucose and delivers 340 kilocalories. Although this will not meet a person's resting energy expenditure, it will prevent ketosis. Previously well-nourished adults generally have nutrient reserves for 3–4 days of semistarvation. To prevent excessive muscle protein from being used for energy, adequate nourishment should be delivered to the client within 3 days.

To avoid abdominal distention, oral feedings ordinarily are delayed until peristalsis returns and is detected with a stethoscope. Another sign of peristalsis is the passage via the rectum of **flatus** (gas). Ambulation as

Table 22–2 Low-Residue Diet

Description	Indications	Adequacy
The low-residue diet limits milk and milk products and excludes any food made with seeds, nuts, and raw or dried fruits and vegetables. The purpose of the diet is to decrease colonic contents.	The diet can be used for severe diarrhea, partial bowel obstruction, and acute phases of inflammatory bowel diseases. Preoperatively the diet is used to minimize fecal volume and residue. Postoperatively the diet is used in the progression to a general diet. Long-term use of the diet is not recommended since it may aggravate symptoms during nonacute phases of disease.	Strict reduction in milk and milk products, vegetables, and fruits may necessitate supplementation of calcium, vitamin C, folate, and other nutrients.

Food Group	Choose	Decrease
Milk	2 cups/day Mild cheese	Strong cheese
Breads and cereals	White bread Refined cereals: cream of wheat, cream of rice, puffed rice, Rice Krispies, corn flakes Crackers without whole grains or seeds Rice, noodles, macaroni, spaghetti	Whole-grain breads Bread made with seeds, nuts, or bran Cracked wheat bread Whole-grain rice or pasta
Fruits	Juice without pulp Ripe banana Cooked or canned apples, apricots, Royal Anne cherries, peaches, pears Strained fruit	Prunes and prune juice Fruits not on "allowed" list Dried fruit
Vegetables	Juice without pulp Lettuce Cooked or canned asparagus, green and wax beans, beets, carrots, eggplant, pumpkin, spinach, acorn squash, seedless tomatoes, tomato sauce or puree, white or sweet potatoes without skin Strained vegetables	Vegetables not on "allowed" list Dried peas and beans Potato skins or chips Fried potatoes
Meat, poultry, fish, shellfish, eggs	Lean tender meat without grease: ground or well-cooked (roasted, baked, or broiled) beef, lamb, ham, veal, pork, poultry, organ meats, fish Eggs except fried	Tough, fried, or spiced meats Fried eggs

(Continued on next page)

Table 22–2 Low-Residue Diet (Continued)

Food Group	Choose	Decrease
Fats and oils	Smooth peanut butter Butter, oils Cream (deduct from milk allowance) Margarine	All other nuts Coconut Olives

Desserts and miscellaneous	Plain dessert made with allowed
	    foods: fruit, ices, sherbet, ice
	    cream, gelatin
	Candy: gum drops, hard candy, jelly
	    beans, plain chocolate,
	    marshmallows, butterscotch
	Honey, sugar, molasses
	Salt, pepper, ground seasonings
	Plain gravy
	Milk sauces (deduct milk allowance)
	Mayonnaise
	Coffee, decaffeinated coffee
	Jelly
	Tea
	Soda
		Popcorn
		Seeds of any kind
		Whole spices
		Chili sauce
		Rich gravy
		Vinegar
		Alcohol
		Jam, marmalade

Sample Menu

Breakfast	*Lunch/Dinner*
Strained grapefruit juice	Baked halibut with clear lemon juice
Cream of wheat	Twice baked potato (no onions)
Poached egg	Candied sweet potato (no nuts or whole spices)
White bagel with butter and honey	Canned pear and banana on lettuce
1/2 cup milk	French bread and margarine
Coffee	Rice pudding (no raisins; deduct milk from allowance)

permitted helps clients pass the flatus and avoid uncomfortable distention. **Paralytic ileus** is a complication of abdominal surgery and other traumatic events or diseases. Peristalsis ceases, and secretions and gas accumulate in the bowel, leading to distention and vomiting. Removal of secretions by suction is the usual treatment. In some situations, even clients with paralytic ileus after gastrointestinal surgery have been successfully fed with an isotonic polymeric formula via a tube in the proximal small intestine (Edington, Kon, and Martyn, 1997).

Clients are usually progressed from clear liquids to full liquids, a soft diet, and then a regular diet as soon as possible. The progression time varies with the client and surgical procedure. It may be hours or days. If "diet as tolerated" is ordered, the client should be asked what foods sound appealing. Sometimes, a full dinner tray when the client does not feel well "turns off" the small appetite he or she has. After gastrointestinal surgery, oral food and fluids are deferred longer than with other surgeries to allow healing. Giving the exact amount of food or fluid prescribed is important. More is not better if the client's stomach or intestine has been sutured. It is not advisable to give red liquids, such as gelatin or cranberry juice, after surgery on the mouth and throat to so that vomitus is not mistaken for blood or vice versa.

Surgical removal of a part of the gastrointestinal tract, such as the stomach, duodenum, jejunum, or ileum, may result in malabsorption of specific nutrients, as illustrated in Figure 22–1. For example, intrinsic factor, which is secreted by the stomach, carries vitamin B_{12} to the ileum for absorption. Iron absorbed from the duodenum and the jejunum is necessary for hemoglobin synthesis. Glucose, amino acids, fat- and water-solu-

ble vitamins, calcium, and magnesium, all absorbed in the jejunum, are necessary for metabolism. Bile salts are absorbed in the ileum. Although the loss of bile salts in the feces may seem harmless, the body ordinarily recycles these salts over and over in the management of fats. Prolonged impaired absorption of bile salts can result in failure to absorb fat and fat-soluble vitamins.

Disorders of the Mouth and Throat

Varied conditions such as dental caries, oral surgery, surgery of the head and neck, fractured jaw, or cancer chemotherapy or radiation therapy can cause difficulty with chewing and swallowing. Often the client requires a feeding tube as discussed in Chapter 15, Nutrient Delivery. Suggestions to manage dysphagia are described in Chapter 10, Digestion, Absorption, Metabolism, and Excretion.

Disorders of the Esophagus

The sole purpose of the esophagus is to conduct food to the stomach, but it sometimes malfunctions. Achalasia, gastroesophageal reflux, and hiatal hernia are types of esophageal disorders.

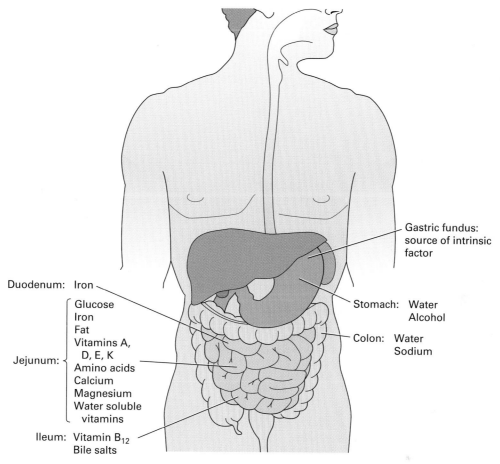

Figure 22–1:
The chief sites of absorption for various nutrients. Disease or resection of an area will increase the risk of deficiency of specific nutrients. (Adapted from Scanlon, VC, and Sanders, T: Student Workbook for Essentials of Anatomy and Physiology, ed 2. FA Davis, Philadelphia, 1995, p 252, with permission.)

Achalasia

Failure of the gastrointestinal muscle fibers to relax where one part joins another is called **achalasia**. Often this term is applied to the **cardiac sphincter**, which separates the stomach from the esophagus. Sometimes the condition is termed *cardiospasm*. The cause of achalasia is unknown. Very hot or cold foods may trigger esophageal spasm, and anxiety seems to aggravate the condition. Symptoms are described as "something sticking in my throat" and a feeling of fullness behind the breastbone (sternum). Vomiting may occur with achalasia, and aspiration of vomitus can cause pneumonia.

In mild cases, avoiding spicy foods and minimizing dietary bulk may be effective. Diets for these clients require much individual attention. Rarely does one achalasia client have intolerances for the same foods as another client. Plenty of liquids with small, frequent meals may help. Treatment of more severe cases involves stretching the cardiac sphincter or surgically incising it to enlarge the passage.

Gastroesophageal Reflux Disease (GERD)

Some regurgitation of stomach contents into the esophagus occurs in normal individuals. Usually the presence of stomach contents in the esophagus stimulates esophageal contractions that return the refluxed material to the stomach. If excessive reflux occurs, either in frequency or volume, or if the esophagus fails to contract in response to stomach contents, the individual has **gastroesophageal reflux disease** (also called *acid-reflux disorder*). Gastroesophageal reflux can usually be managed without surgery. This regurgitation is common in infancy and disappears with age, often to reappear in old age due to poor muscle tone of the cardiac sphincter. In infants, usually no treatment is undertaken unless there is evidence of aspiration of food into the respiratory tract or of failure to thrive. In adults, the most common underlying cause of gastroesophageal reflux is hiatal hernia, which is discussed in the next section. Other conditions associated with GERD due to increased abdominal pressure are obesity and pregnancy. Some experts believe that gastroesophageal reflux may be caused by failure of the car-

Table 22–3 Diet for Gastroesophageal Reflux and Hiatal Hernia

Description	Indications	Adequacy
The diet is designed to minimize reflux through timing of intake, texture control, limiting fat, and exclusion of sphincter relaxants and gas-forming foods. Adjunctive treatment involves positioning	Esophageal reflux, hiatal hernia, esophageal ulcers, esophagitis, esophageal strictures, heartburn.	The diet may not meet the RDAs for vitamin C and iron in the premenopausal woman.

Food Group	Choose	Decrease

Meal pattern	6 small meals
	1/2 cup liquid with meals
	Other liquids
	   >1 1/2 hours after meals
	   > 1/2 hour before meals
		Eating within 3 hours of bedtime

Adjunction therapy	Elevate head of bed 6 in. Relax at mealtime Consider weight loss if needed	Lying down in the hour after eating
Food Group		
Milk	Skim milk, buttermilk, evaporated skim milk Skim milk cheese Cottage cheese Low-fat yogurt	Other milk Hot chocolate
Breads and cereals	White and whole-grain breads Plain rolls, biscuits, and muffins Plain crackers Any cereals except those on "Decrease" list Rice Pasta	Pancakes, waffles, French toast Doughnuts, sweet rolls, nut breads Granola-type cereals with nuts and/or coconut
Fruits	Mild juices Any fruits except those on "Decrease" list	Avocado Raw apples and melons Orange, grapefruit, and tomato juices
Vegetables	Any vegetables except those on "Decrease" list	Creamed or fried vegetables Hashed brown potatoes Broccoli, brussels sprouts, cabbage, cauliflower, cucumber, dried peas or beans, onions, green pepper, rutabagas, sauerkraut, turnips
Meat, poultry, fish, shellfish eggs	6 oz/day lean beef, pork, ham, lamb, liver, veal, fish, skinless poultry/day Eggs	Sausage, bacon, frankfurters, luncheon meats, canned meats and fish, duck, goose
Fats and oils	3 tsp/day: oil, butter, margarine, mild salad dressing 2 tbsp of the following may substitute for 1 tsp of fat: light cream, sour cream, nondairy cream Vegetable pan sprays as desired Low-fat salad dressings	Fried foods Gravies and sauces Cream Salad dressing Shortening, lard, or oils in excess of allowance Nuts, peanut butter

(Continued on next page)

Table 22–3 Diet for Gastroesophageal Reflux and Hiatal Hernia (Continued)

Food Group	Choose	Decrease
Desserts and miscellaneous	Plain cakes and cookies Gelatin, popsicles Sherbet and pudding made with skim milk Caffeine-free carbonated beverages Decaffeinated tea Fat-free broth, boullion, consomme Soup made from allowed foods Cream soup made with skim milk Sugar, honey, syrup, molasses Jam, jelly, preserves Plain candy Salt Condiments and spices in small amounts Vanilla Vinegar	Ice cream, ice milk Pie, pastry Butter cake and icings Chocolate, coconut, cream, cream cheese, whipped cream, nuts, peppermint, spearmint Caffeinated beverages Decaffeinated coffee Tea Alcohol Potato chips Candy containing chocolate, nuts, coconut, or peppermint Popcorn Snack chips Pickles, relish Catsup, chili sauce Mustard Steak sauce

Sample Menu

35 Minutes Before Breakfast
2 glasses of water

Breakfast
1/2 banana
1/2 cup oatmeal
1/2 cup skim milk
1 slice toast with Jam

Midmorning Snack
1/2 cup pineapple Juice
3 graham crackers

35 Minutes Before Meal
2 glasses of water

Lunch/Dinner
3 oz skinless chicken breast baked in lemon juice
1/2 baked potato with 1 tbsp sour cream
1/2 cup whole kernel corn
3 small celery sticks
Hard roll with 1 tsp margarine
1/2 cup decaffeinated tea

35 Minutes Before Snack
2 glasses of water

Midafternoon/Evening snack
1 cup low-fat yogurt

diac sphincter to operate properly. The stomach is normally protected from hydrochloric acid by a thick layer of mucus. Because the esophagus is not so protected, repeated bouts of gastroesophageal reflux can lead to esophagitis and ulcer formation that, when healed, may cause a stricture at the site of the scar tissue. The prominent symptom of gastroesophageal reflux is heartburn with pain occurring behind the sternum, or breastbone. Sometimes the pain radiates to the neck and the back of the throat. Lying down or bending over may increase reflux and aggravate the pain. If the passage becomes narrowed, dysphagia may become bothersome.

Treatment involves a number of conservative measures. Small, frequent meals often help. Protein is associated with tightening of the cardiac sphincter and is used in normal amounts in the diet. Foods often avoided because they relax the sphincter are fat, alcohol, caffeine, peppermint, spearmint, and chocolate. Smoking also relaxes the sphincter. Decaffeinated coffee and pepper are frequently avoided because they stimulate gastric secretion. Acidic juices, such as citrus juices and tomato juice, may be irritating.

A change in eating behaviors and lifestyle may assist in the control of gastroesophageal reflux. Chewing food thoroughly, not eating within 3 hours of bedtime, and sitting upright for 2 hours after meals may increase food tolerance. Liquids may accompany meals unless the client with GERD reports early satiety or distention. Raising the head of the bed 6–8 inches enables gravity to help keep stomach contents contained. Symptoms of overweight clients have decreased with weight loss (Fraser-Moodie et al., 1999). Table 22–3 details a diet for gastroesophageal reflux.

Hiatal Hernia

The *esophageal hiatus* is the opening in the diaphragm through which the esophagus is attached to the stomach. A **hiatal hernia** is a protrusion of the stomach through the esophageal hiatus into the chest cavity (Fig. 22–2). The symptoms of hiatal hernia are similar to those of gastroesophageal reflux, and its medical treatment is the same. Persistent symptoms despite conservative treatment might lead the client to elect surgical repair of the hernia.

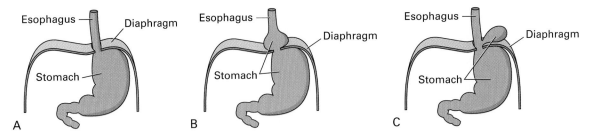

Figure 22–2:
In hiatal hernia, the upper part of the stomach squeezes into the chest cavity through the esophageal opening in the diaphragm. (A) Normal anatomy, (B) sliding hiatal hernia, (C) paraesophageal or rolling hiatal hernia. (From Williams and Hopper, p 579, with permission.)

Disorders of the Stomach

Disorders of the stomach often require diet modification and in some cases, surgery. The following sections discuss two common disorders, gastritis and peptic ulcers, and one disorder mainly associated with diabetes mellitus, gastroparesis.

Gastritis

Inflammation of the stomach is **gastritis**. Common causes of gastritis are the chronic use of aspirin and alcohol abuse. Other conditions that result in gastritis are food allergies, food poisoning, infections, radiation exposure, and stress. Symptoms of gastritis are anorexia, nausea, a feeling of fullness, and epigastric pain. Figure 22–3 illustrates the abdominal quadrants and regions used to record signs and symptoms revealed during the assessment process. Signs of gastritis are vomiting and eructating (belching).

The dietary treatment plan for gastritis includes having the client:

1. Eat at regular intervals.
2. Chew food, especially fibrous food, slowly and thoroughly.
3. Avoid foods that cause pain.
4. Avoid foods that cause gas, especially vegetables in the cabbage family, including broccoli, cauliflower, and Brussels sprouts.
5. Avoid the following:
   - gastric irritants such as caffeine and alcohol
   - nonsteroidal anti-inflammatory drugs (NSAIDs) such as aspirin
   - strong spices, including nutmeg, pepper, garlic, and chili powder
6. Eat in a relaxed manner.

More often than not, discovering which foods are responsible for the pain and discomfort of gastritis is a trial-and-error process. Tolerances vary from person to person. Prolonged or recurrent gastritis deserves medical attention.

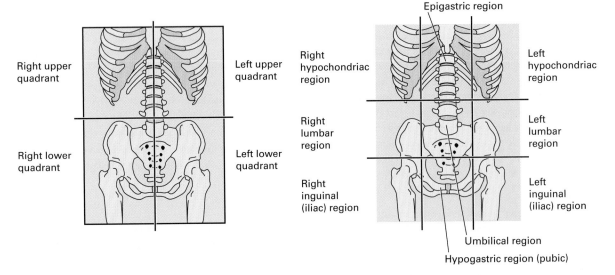

Figure 22–3:
Abdominal quadrants and regions of the abdomen are used to describe locations of signs and symptoms. (From Thomas, CL [ed]: Taber's Cyclopedic Medical Dictionary, ed 18. FA Davis, Philadelphia, 1997, pp 3, 4 by Beth Anne Willert, MS, Dictionary Illustrator, with permission.)

Delayed Gastric Emptying

This condition can be associated with certain prescription drugs as well as use of alcohol, tobacco, and marijuana. It can occur in anorexia nervosa and in malnutrition. Most frequently, however, delayed gastric emptying is seen in clients with diabetes mellitus associated with neuropathy, now thought to be chiefly mediated through the autonomic nervous system, and particularly the vagus nerve. The term used to denote this delayed gastric emptying is *diabetic gastroparesis*. One-fourth of clients requiring insulin for 10 years show evidence of delayed gastric emptying (Stenson, 1999). Treatment focuses on the cause of the disorder: removing offending drugs, intervening appropriately in malnutrition, and controlling hyperglycemia in clients with diabetes. Dietary interventions include increasing the liquids consumed (which leave the stomach sooner than solids) and reducing the fat ingested (which remains in the stomach longer than carbohydrate or protein).

Peptic Ulcers

Both gastric (stomach) and duodenal ulcers are called *peptic ulcers*. Peptic ulcers affect 10 percent of the world's population and men and women equally. Peptic ulcer disease is the primary cause of death of about 6500 persons annually in the United States and affects an estimated 25 million individuals in the United States during their lifetimes (Centers for Disease Control, 1997a). Duodenal ulcer incidence peaks in clients in their fifties and sixties and gastric ulcers in those between ages 60 and 80.

Pathophysiology

An ulcer client's mucosa is not sufficiently resistant to the acids secreted by the stomach. If just the superficial cells are involved, the lesion is called an **erosion**. If the muscular layer of the stomach or duodenum is involved, the person has an **ulcer**.

Gastric ulcers are more common on the lesser curvature or right side of the stomach than on the greater curvature. Duodenal ulcers account for 60 percent of all ulcers and are associated with increased acidity of the stomach. The majority of gastric and duodenal ulcers are related to infection with *Helicobacter pylori* (Soll, 1996). The organism occurs worldwide and is found in about 20–50 percent of adults in developed countries; however, only a small fraction of these people develop peptic ulcers.

The second most common form of peptic ulcer is related to the use of NSAIDs (Soll, 1996), and one-fourth of the cases of perforated peptic ulcer (see later) are attributed to the use of these drugs (Svanes, 2000). Long-term use of other medications such as potassium chloride and corticosteroids is also associated with ulcer formation. Smoking predisposes a person to ulcer formation and complicates treatment. Alcohol, coffee, and stress are suggested but unproven risk factors (Fauci et al., 1998). Nevertheless, in anticipation of the stress of critical illness, ICU clients are often treated prophylactically.

Signs and Symptoms

A gnawing, burning epigastric pain when the stomach is empty characterizes duodenal ulcer. This occurs 1–3 hours after eating or at night. With gastric ulcer, the pain is made worse by ingesting food or is unrelated to food intake (Fauci et al., 1998). One-fourth of ulcer clients experience bleeding, which occurs more often with duodenal than with gastric ulcers. If the blood is vomited immediately after bleeding begins, it is bright red. If it stays in contact with digestive juices for a while, the vomitus is brown-black and granular, resembling coffee grounds. The medical term for this is *coffee-ground emesis*. Other symptoms of peptic ulcer are nausea, anorexia, and sometimes weight loss.

Complications of Peptic Ulcers

Hemorrhage is a complication of peptic ulcers. Scar tissue from a healed ulcer can restrict the gastric outlet, causing pyloric obstruction. If the ulcer continues to erode through the entire stomach or intestinal wall, the result is a **perforated ulcer**. Leakage of gastrointestinal contents into the sterile abdominal cavity causes **peritonitis**, an inflammation of the peritoneum (the lining of the abdominal cavity). Most perforated ulcers in clients younger than 75 years of age are attributed to smoking (Svanes, 2000).

Treatment of Peptic Ulcers

Usually a course of medical treatment is prescribed first. If *H. pylori* infection is the cause, combinations of antibiotics and other drugs are recommended (Soll, 1996). Only if such treatment prove ineffective is surgery recommended.

MEDICAL TREATMENT Before the advent of antiulcer medications, clients with peptic ulcers were usually advised to take antacids every 2 hours, alternating with milk and cream. One adverse effect of this treatment was milk alkali syndrome as discussed in Chapter 8, Minerals. New medications have revolutionized the treatment and are almost always effective without a drastic change in diet. In addition to antibiotics, commonly prescribed medications are cimetidine, ranitidine, and famotidine, which block histamine-stimulated gastric acid secretion, and omeprazole, which suppresses gastric acid production.

Diet does require some modification, however. Some experts recommend only three regular meals with no snacking between because food, including milk, stimulates gastric secretion. Other authorities recommend midmorning and midafternoon snacks. In both regimens, substances that cause gastric irritation are avoided. These include the same gastric irritants discussed in the section on gastritis. Clients should be encouraged to avoid or limit spices or foods that are not well tolerated.

Changes in an ulcer client's lifestyle improve the chances of successful treatment. Since smoking stimulates secretion of gastric acid, ulcer clients should be advised not to smoke.

SURGICAL TREATMENT When surgery is necessary, the ulcer is removed and the remaining gastrointestinal tract is sutured together. Surgical procedures designed to eliminate the diseased area include the gastroduodenostomy (stomach and duodenum anastomosed), the gastrojejunostomy (stomach and jejunum anastomosed) and the total gastrectomy (esophagus and duodenum anastomosed). **Anastomosis** is the surgical connection between tubular structures. Figure 22–4 illustrates these three procedures.

Following gastric surgery, parenteral and tube feeding are used singly or in combination. If tube feeding is used, the tube must be inserted beyond the area that was resected (removed). Once a client is advanced to an oral diet, he or she may experience the **dumping syndrome**, a complication of a surgical procedure that removes, disrupts, or bypasses the pyloric sphincter. Clinical Application 22–2 describes the dumping

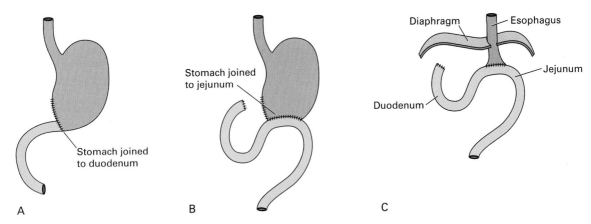

Figure 22–4:
Common gastric resection procedures. (A) Gastroduodenostomy or Billroth I procedure, (B) gastrojejunostomy or Billroth II procedure, (C) total gastrectomy. (From Williams and Hopper, p 587, with permission.)

syndrome in more detail. Table 22–4 depicts a diet to prevent or treat the dumping syndrome. Long-term nutritional consequences of reconstructive surgery for peptic ulcer include iron deficiency anemia and osteomalacia. The deficiency of iron is related to decreased gastric acidity and decreased absorptive capacity of the duodenum. The mechanism for developing osteomalacia is incompletely described, although the duodenum is a major site for calcium absorption (Stenson, 1999).

Disorders of the Intestines

Successful diagnostic studies of the bowel depend on proper preparation. It is imperative to empty the bowel for clear radiographic visualization. This is accomplished by laxatives and enemas. Often the client is advised to follow a low-residue diet for several days prior to diagnostic studies. Explaining the procedures and the necessity for them helps to gain the client's cooperation. The radiography department or the institution's diet manual lists the procedures. The nurse should ensure that the client receives maximum nourishment when tests are completed for the day. Frequently, another series of tests is scheduled for the next day.

Problems with Elimination

Several problems with frequency and consistency of bowel movements are common. These include irritable bowel syndrome, diarrhea, and constipation.

Irritable Bowel Syndrome

This condition is the most common gastrointestinal complaint seen in primary practices and accounts for 50 percent of referrals to gastroenterologists (Carlson, 1998). Signs and symptoms of **irritable bowel syndrome** are diarrhea, constipation, or alternating diarrhea and constipation; abdominal pain; and flatulence. Investigation often reveals no organic cause for the symptoms, but food intolerance is highly correlated with irritable bowel syndrome.

Treatment is symptomatic. Offending foods should be identified and avoided. The most common foods identified are lactose and gluten, each accounting for about 40 percent of the identified causes of symptoms. In one study, more than half of clients could identify between 2 and 5 foods as creating problems (Carlson, 1998), and such identification makes the condition more manageable. For all clients, stress management techniques and bowel hygiene principles should be part of the teaching plan. A high-fiber diet, designed to avoid not only constipation but also increased pressure on the walls of the intestine, often provides symptomatic relief.

CLINICAL APPLICATION 22–2

Dumping Syndrome

The pyloric sphincter normally allows only small amounts of gastric contents into the duodenum at a time. After the pyloric sphincter is surgically removed, the dumping syndrome may result. When a concentrated liquid suddenly enters the intestine, water is pulled from the bowel wall just as in osmotic diarrhea. Local effects are hyperperistalsis, diarrhea, abdominal pain, and vomiting 30 to 60 min after a meal. Systemic effects relate to fluid volume deficit: weakness, dizziness, sweating, decreased blood pressure, tachycardia, and palpitations. The dumping syndrome is most often associated with total gastrectomy or resection of two-thirds of the stomach. The same signs and symptoms can occur in a client receiving a tube feeding if the nasogastric tube is accidentally carried down into the duodenum.

Dietary treatment of the dumping syndrome attempts to delay gastric emptying and to distribute the increased osmolality in the bowel over time. This can be achieved by limiting the intake of simple sugars, consuming frequent meals, and limiting fluids with meals. Simple sugars increase the osmolality of the gastric contents and enhance the movement of food out of the stomach. Small, frequent meals will reduce the load on the intestine. Liquids should be taken between, rather than with, meals. Beverages should be low in simple carbohydrate. Very hot or cold foods will stimulate peristalsis and should be avoided. A nondietary intervention also helps to control the symptoms of the dumping syndrome. Lying down for 30 to 60 min after eating retains the meal in the stomach longer.

Table 22–4 Diet for Dumping Syndrome

Description	Indications	Adequacy
This diet consists of 6 small feedings, high in protein and low in simple sugars.	This diet and adjunct therapy, used after surgical removal of the pyloric sphincter or other treatments that speed gastric emptying, is designed to prevent rapid emptying of hypertonic gastric contents into the small intestine. Examples of such operative procedures include vagotomy, pyloroplasty, hemigastrectomy, total gastrectomy, esophagogastrectomy, Whipple's procedure, gastroenterostomy, and gastrojejunostomy. As the body adapts to its new condition, specific foods may be tolerated later in convalescence.	Deficiencies secondary to surgery or malabsorption may require supplementation. Among the nutrients likely to be needed are the vitamins B_{12}, D and folic acid, and the minerals calcium and iron.

	Choose	Decrease
Meal pattern	Six small servings Eat slowly and chew thoroughly	Fluids with meals
Adjunct therapy	Lie down for 1/2 hour after meals	
Food Group		
Milk	LactAid Aged cheese (>90 days)	Milk if lactose intolerant*
Breads and cereals	White, whole wheat, rye, Jewish, Italian, and Vienna breads* Rolls, crackers, biscuits, and muffins (milk-free)* Any cooked or dry cereal, milk-free* Rice, noodles, spaghetti, macaroni	Frosted breads Sweet rolls, doughnuts, coffeecake Bread made with milk (unless tolerated)* Sugar sweetened cereal Cereal containing milk*
Fruits	Fresh, frozen or unsweetened canned fruits, banana Juices, fresh, frozen, canned, unsweetened between meals only	Sweetened canned or frozen juices and fruits, dried fruit Raw fruits unless tolerated Juices with meals
Vegetables	Any as tolerated Juices between meals only	Those causing discomfort Juices with meals
Meat group	Any as tolerated	None
Fats and oils	Milk-free margarine if lactose intolerant* Oils Vegetable shortening	Any containing milk unless tolerated*

(Continued on next page)

Diarrhea

Diarrhea is an important cause of morbidity and mortality in the elderly and in children (see Chapter 12, Life Cycle Nutrition: Infancy, Childhood, Adolescence). A tourist has a 30–50 percent chance of contracting traveler's diarrhea in Mexico, Central and South America, the Mediterranean area, the Middle East, and Southeast Asia (Aranda-Michel and Giannella, 1999). Of special note here are foods that are perilous for travelers. Especially in primitive areas, raw vegetables, raw meat, raw seafood, tap water, ice, and unpasteurized dairy products are best avoided. If an adult is in little jeopardy from an electrolyte imbalance, self-treatment for diar-

Table 22–4 Diet for Dumping Syndrome (Continued)

	Choose	Decrease

Desserts and miscellaneous	Artificially sweetened gelatin
	Angel food and sponge cakes
	Salt, pepper, spices as tolerated
	Mustard, catsup, pickles,
	   relishes as tolerated
	Artificially sweetened beverages
	Decaffeinated tea and coffee,
	   herbal tea
	Dietetic jam and jelly
		Sugar containing cakes, pies,
		   cookies, ice cream,* sherbet*
		Seasonings that cause discomfort
		Caffeine-containing beverages
		Sugar, honey, syrup, molasses
		Jam, jelly
		Candy

Sample Menu

30 Minutes Before Breakfast	*30 Minutes Before Lunch*
Decaffeinated beverage	1 cup LactAid
Artificial sweetener	
	Lunch/Dinner
Breakfast	3 oz roast pork
1/2 banana	Barley with butter
1 egg, poached	1/2 cup squash
1 tsp milk-free margarine	1/2 cup fruit cocktail, drained
Dietetic jelly	
	1 1/2 Hours After Meal
1 1/2 Hours After Breakfast	Decaffeinated beverage
Orange juice	Artificial sweetener
Midmorning Snack	
1 slice whole-wheat toast	
Dietetic jam	

*If lactose-free restriction is necessary.

rhea following the conservative regimen listed in Table 22–5 is appropriate. Most instances of diarrhea in adults are self-limiting and resolve without treatment or the need for extensive medical work-up. On the other hand, large volumes of stool, severe abdominal pain, bloody stools, systemic symptoms such as fever, and prostration deserve investigation (Aranda-Michel and Giannella, 1999). In addition to these concerns, if the diarrhea is protracted or if a client has medical conditions for which fasting, dehydration, or infectious disease is a hazard, a physician should be consulted.

Constipation

Each person develops a usual bowel pattern, so that a bowel movement every day or every second or third day may be perfectly normal for a given individual. **Constipation** refers to a decrease in a person's normal frequency of defecation, especially if the stool is hard, dry, or difficult to expel. It is essential that changes in bowel habits be investigated thoroughly to discover or rule out other diseases. Aside from disease conditions, the causes of constipation are lack of water and fiber in the diet, lack of exercise, and voluntary retention.

Treatment for constipation involves dietary and lifestyle changes, not laxatives. Unfortunately, this message has not yet been widely heard, especially by the elderly. Up to 50 percent of adults over age 70 regularly use laxatives. Overall, Americans spend $250 million on laxatives each year.

Increasing the fiber in the diet with adequate amounts of water and exercising regularly are the keys to overcoming constipation. Even laxative habits established for years can be overcome this way.

In cases of fecal impaction, the client may experience diarrhea. Clinical Application 22–3 explains this paradox.

Problems with Absorption

Fat malabsorption may follow many diseases that damage the intestine. Celiac disease, or nontropical sprue, is a specific response to gluten-containing foods.

CLINICAL APPLICATION 22–3

Distinguishing Diarrhea from Fecal Impaction

If a client usually is constipated and then has diarrhea, the nurse should check the rectum for impacted stool. The stool will be dry and hard and the client will not be able to pass it unassisted. The diarrheal stool is passed around the impaction. This type of constipation is not treated with diet. As in many cases, prevention is preferable to diagnosis and treatment. Institutionalized clients should be monitored for elimination problems. Frequency and consistency of bowel movements should be charted.

Fat Malabsorption

Several conditions hinder fat absorption. Many of the resulting symptoms are similar, despite the differences in the underlying pathology.

When fat is not well absorbed, the fat-soluble vitamins also are poorly absorbed and the fat content of the feces is increased. These extra fatty acids bind with calcium and magnesium to form soaps in the bowel. (A chemical soap results from the union of fatty acid and alkali.) The calcium bound in the soap is thus unavailable to bind with oxalate. An increased amount of oxalate is excreted through the kidney. This is not a harmless rerouting, however, because oxalate kidney stones can form as a result.

Treatment centers on careful selection of fats in the diet and appropriate supplementation of unavailable nutrients. The later Table 22–9 compares some food choices that are low in fat to similar items that are high in fat. (Low-fat diets are discussed later in the chapter.) Because pancreatic lipase or bile is unnecessary for their absorption, medium-chain triglycerides (MCTs) are often given to increase kilocalories. MCTs as well as amino acids and monosaccharides are absorbed into the portal vein, rather than into the lymphatic system as are other lipids. Usually, MCTs are added to salad dressings, skim milk, or desserts. Because linoleic acid, an essential fatty acid, is missing from MCT, some regular fat is still needed in the diet. Supplements of the fat-soluble vitamins should be given in water-soluble form. To overcome malabsorption, the commonly used dose of supplements is twice the RDA.

Celiac Disease

An illness resembling this one was described in the first century A.D. **Celiac disease** is also called **gluten-sensitive enteropathy** or nontropical sprue. Usually diagnosed in childhood, it occasionally is not discovered until late adulthood (Scully et al., 1994) with approximately 10 percent of newly diagnosed cases occurring in persons over the age of 60 (Saltzman and Russell, 1995). Its cause is unknown, but there is a genetic predisposition. Celiac disease occurs up to 100 times more frequently in clients having a first-degree relative with the disease than in other people, but about half of these relatives are asymptomatic, leading to the conclusion that additional genetic factors or environmental conditions are needed for the disease to occur (Connon, 1999). The disease is rare in blacks, Chinese, and Japanese and varies significantly by country. For example, prevalence is 1:300 in Ireland and 1:3500 in Finland. Researchers are attempting to identify the components of gluten that cause the disease, but a single trigger seems unlikely (Saltzman and Clifford, 1994). The affected person is sensitive to gluten, a protein in wheat, oats, rye, and barley. As little as 3 grams per day may cause symptoms. Ingestion of gluten by these sensitive people causes atrophy of the intestinal villi in the jejunum. Malabsorption of all the classes of nutrients except water follows.

The outstanding sign of celiac disease is **steatorrhea**, or excessive fat in the stools, which are foul-smelling, frothy, and bulky. Clients complain of bloating, diarrhea, and cramping abdominal pain. Some of this may be temporary as the result of lactase insufficiency. Untreated, the client's anorexia leads to weight loss and malnutrition marked by anemia, muscle wasting, edema from hypoalbuminemia, bleeding due to vitamin K deficiency, and bone pain and tetany from hypocalcemia. Clients with celiac disease, especially those who are untreated or whose disease is poorly controlled, may be at increased risk of developing osteoporosis (Kemppainen et al., 1999).

The treatment is to remove gluten permanently from the diet. The disease is not outgrown, and damage to the villi continues even without symptoms. Removing gluten from the diet is easier said than done. It involves analyzing the label of every food the client ingests. See Chapter 10, Digestion, Absorption, Metabolism, and Excretion, which outlines a gluten-restricted diet. Fortunately, this treatment reverses the pathology almost completely, although it might take 3–6 months. Sometimes, a secondary lactose intolerance results from mucosal damage and requires long-term management. Also, vitamin supplementation may be needed because the vast majority of gluten-free products are not enriched (Thompson, 1999).

Inflammatory Bowel Diseases

Inflammatory bowel diseases (IBD) are a group of syndromes that share similar characteristics but have some major differences. The two most common inflammatory bowel diseases are **Crohn's disease**, also known as ileitis or regional enteritis, and **ulcerative colitis**. Although the cause of both of these conditions is unknown, autoimmunity and genetic susceptibility may be partially responsible. Occurrence of IBD in a *first-degree relative* (parent, sibling, child) is a major known risk factor

Table 22–5 Self-Treatment for Diarrhea*

Time	Oral Intake	Comments
1st 12 h	Water or oral hydration solutions at room temperature	Easily absorbed fluids to maintain hydration
2nd 12 h	Clear liquids, no caffeine or extremes of temperature	If up to 5 percent body weight lost; if more than 5 percent lost, seek medical attention. Very hot, very cold, or caffeinated beverages stimulate peristalsis
3rd 12 h	Full liquids	Experiment with milk in case lactose intolerance has developed
4th 12 h	Soft diet	Include applesauce or banana for pectin; rice, pasta, and bread without fat (digested by enzymes usually unaffected by gastroenteritis).
By 48th h	Regular diet	If diarrhea has not resolved and regular diet is not tolerated, seek medical treatment.

*Appropriate for healthy adults.

Table 22–6 Differences between Crohn's Disease and Ulcerative Colitis

	Crohn's Disease	Ulcerative Colitis
Location	Anywhere in bowel	Large intestine
	Diseased areas alternate with healthy tissue	Usually starts in rectum and spreads upward in continuous pattern
Lesions	Involves all layers of intestinal wall	Confined to mucosal and submucosal layers
Complications	Fistula, obstruction, stricture	Toxic megacolon, fistula Increased risk of colon cancer

CLINICAL APPLICATION 22–4

Short Bowel Syndrome

Because the small intestine is 16–20 ft. long in the adult, up to 50 percent can be removed, if necessary. Depending on the site of resection, the remaining bowel adjusts by becoming longer, thicker, and wider to increase its absorptive capacity. This process may take up to 6 months, however, and occurs only if the client receives food or tube feedings that stimulate gastrointestinal function. In cases in which the ileocecal valve and/or 80 percent of the small bowel is removed, the body cannot completely compensate for the loss.

Signs and symptoms of short bowel syndrome are diarrhea, weight loss, and muscle wasting. These are related to protein and fat malabsorption. Poor absorption of iron, calcium, or magnesium leads to anemia, hypocalcemia, or hypomagnesemia, respectively.

Treatment of short bowel syndrome can be intensive and requires consultation with a dietitian. Early nourishment is provided by TPN. When enteral feeding begins, elemental formulas may be chosen because they are completely absorbed in the proximal small intestine. When food is taken, it should be eaten as small low-fat meals, with medium-chain triglycerides replacing regular fats. Liquids should be taken between meals, and juices and regular soda may need to be diluted to half-strength to prevent osmotic diarrhea (Lykins and Stockwell, 1998).

In clients with intestinal failure who become intolerant to parenteral nutrition, small bowel transplantation can be a lifesaving procedure. Lengthening the small intestine by transplanting sections of a donor's small intestine has been increasingly successful, with an overall worldwide survival rate of 50 percent (Brook, 1998), and one center's survival rate for combined liver and small bowel transplantation is 80 percent (Jan et al., 1999).

(Griffiths, 1999). The most common signs and symptoms of both Crohn's disease and ulcerative colitis are diarrhea, abdominal pain, and fever. Differences between the two diseases include their location in the gastrointestinal tract, the type of lesions involved, and complications (Table 22–6). The nutritional care of clients with IBD is variable and depends on the nutritional status of the individual, the location and extent of the disease, and the nature of the surgical and medical management. Elemental diets have promoted remission in Crohn's disease of the small bowel but not of the large bowel, and not of ulcerative colitis (Sullivan and Heyman, 1995). Particularly for children with Crohn's disease, long-term enteral supplementation has extended remissions and supported growth (Griffiths, 1999).

Nutritional Therapy in Crohn's Disease

Crohn's disease may involve either the small or the large intestine, or both, as well as the stomach and esophagus in some cases. The emphasis of treatment is (1) to support the healing of tissue, (2) to avoid and/or prevent nutritional deficiencies, and (3) to prevent local trauma to inflamed areas. Parenteral and tube feedings may be used together or separately to meet nutritional goals. The diet modifications are usually based on high-kilocaloric, high-protein, low-fat, and sometimes low-fiber or low-residue intake. Small, frequent feedings may assist in promoting comfort and adequate nutrition. Seasonings and chilled foods often aggravate symptoms. Restricting lactose is appropriate only in documented cases of intolerance (Sullivan and Heyman, 1995).

Nutritional Therapy in Ulcerative Colitis

During an acute exacerbation of ulcerative colitis, tube feedings or total parenteral nutrition (TPN) are often given. A 4- to 6-week course of TPN achieves complete bowel rest. This choice may be necessary when the client has a fistula, obstruction, or abscess. Convalescent clients with ulcerative colitis must avoid irritating foods. Dietary modification is usually based on client tolerance. To maintain nutritional status, foods should not be eliminated from the diet without a fair trial. Restrictions should be limited to foods that produce gas or loose stools. Suspected foods should be tried in small amounts to determine tolerance levels. Parenteral supplements of iron and vitamin B_{12} may also be prescribed for these clients.

Surgical Treatment in Inflammatory Bowel Disease

Surgery may be recommended when inflammatory bowel disease becomes medically unmanageable. It may be curative in ulcerative colitis but is palliative in Crohn's disease (Sullivan and Heyman, 1995). The portion of the bowel that is inflamed can be surgically resected. This results in a shorter gut. Resection of the small intestine may create additional nutritional hazards for the client (Clinical Application 22–4). A **colectomy** is the surgical removal of part or all of the colon. Other surgical procedures include ileostomy and colostomy, which may be either permanent or temporary.

In an **ileostomy**, the end of the remaining portion of the small intestine (the **ileum**) is attached to a surgically established opening in the abdominal wall called a **stoma**, from which the intestinal contents are discharged. In a **colostomy**, a part of the large intestine is resected and a stoma is created in the abdominal wall. Clients who have surgery to divert

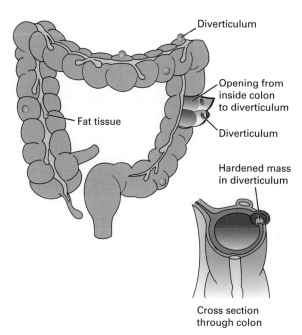

CLINICAL APPLICATION 22–5

Continent Ileostomies

Ordinarily if an ileostomy is performed, the client must wear an appliance to contain the drainage. Other procedures afford a measure of control of the drainage. Continent ileostomies sometimes can be constructed from the remaining intestine, creating an intestinal reservoir just inside the abdominal wall. The reservoir is emptied by inserting a catheter into the stoma several times a day. Sometimes an ileoanal anastomosis is done so that the anal sphincter can be used to control elimination. Even after the bowel adapts to its shorter length, the client has 7 to 10 bowel movements per day.

It is important for the nurse to know which procedure has been perormed so that the surgeon's and client's expectations can be reinforced when teaching the client.

intestinal contents through the abdominal wall often suffer psychological trauma in addition to the physical change.

ILEOSTOMY An ileostomy produces liquid drainage containing active enzymes, which irritate the skin. In addition, nutrient losses are great. A loss of as much as 2 liters of fluid per day immediately following surgery is possible. Clinical Application 22–5 discusses innovations for controlling ileostomy drainage. Over time the bowel adapts to some extent, and drainage decreases to 300–500 milliliters. This amount, however, is more than the 100–200 milliliters of water lost in the normal stool. Additional nutrient losses in ileostomy clients include sodium, potassium, and vitamin B_{12}.

COLOSTOMY In contrast to an ileostomy, a colostomy, after the convalescent period, may be so continent that a dry dressing is all that is necessary to cover the stoma. The client may do daily irrigations or not, as the surgeon suggests. Sometimes the client knows best, after the initial learning process.

DIETARY GUIDELINES FOR OSTOMY CLIENTS A soft or general diet is usually served to ostomy clients after recovery from surgery. Stringy, high-fiber foods are initially avoided until a definite tolerance has been demonstrated. Stringy, high-fiber foods include celery, coconut, corn, cabbage, coleslaw, membranes on citrus fruits, peas, popcorn, spinach, dried fruit, nuts, sauerkraut, pineapple, seeds, and fruit and vegetable skins. Some clients avoid fish, eggs, beer, and carbonated beverages because they produce excessive odor.

Clients with ostomies should be encouraged to (1) eat at regular intervals; (2) chew food well to avoid blockage at the stoma site; (3) drink adequate amounts of fluid; (4) avoid foods that produce excessive gas, loose stools, offensive odors and/or undesirable bulk; and (5) avoid excessive weight gain. Dietary restrictions are usually based on individual tolerance.

Diverticular Disease

A **diverticulum** (plural: diverticula) is an outpouching of intestinal membrane through a weakness in the intestine's muscular layer. Diverticula are present in 10 percent of the U.S. population, about 33–50 percent of the elderly, and 60 percent of those older than 80. A low-fiber diet, containing less than 15 grams of fiber per day, is believed to increase the risk for diverticula.

Figure 22–5:
Diverticula of the transverse and descending colon. (From Thomas, CL [ed]: Taber's Cyclopedic Medical Dictionary, ed 18. FA Davis, Philadelphia, 1997, p 565, by Beth Anne Willert, MS, Dictionary Illustrator, with permission.)

Diverticulosis

The presence of diverticula is called **diverticulosis**. The usual site is the sigmoid colon (Fig. 22–5). Diverticula often occur at the points at which blood vessels enter the intestinal muscle. A hypothesized cause for diverticulosis is the increased force needed to propel insufficient intestinal contents through the lumen. Often a person with diverticulosis has no signs or symptoms. Once an individual knows the diverticula are present, a high-fiber diet of 30 grams per day is advised. This should be accompanied by an adequate fluid intake.

Diverticulitis

When diverticula become inflamed, the condition is termed **diverticulitis**. Inflammation occurs in the elderly at about the same rate as in younger people with diverticulosis, 25 percent. Following the prescribed diet improves the condition of 85 percent of the clients.

Signs and symptoms of diverticulitis, with the exception of fever, occur in the abdomen. The client complains of cramps, pain in the lower left quadrant, dyspepsia, nausea and vomiting, distention and flatus, and alternating constipation and diarrhea. Some serious complications can follow diverticulitis. The inflammatory process can lead to adhesions or fistulas. A thickened intestinal wall from the scar tissue can cause an obstruction. Rupture of a diverticulum can initiate peritonitis.

The dietary treatment of diverticulitis has changed radically over the years. Whereas once a low-fiber diet was the rule, now it is only a temporary measure. While the inflammation is severe, elemental or predigested formulas or a low-fiber diet is given. After that, a high-fiber diet as for diverticulosis is prescribed. It is important that clients receive detailed

Table 22–7 Types of Viral Hepatitis

	Hepatitis A	Hepatitis B	Hepatitis C
Occurrence	Hepatitis A Worldwide, common in areas with poor sanitation Serologic evidence of prior infection in 33 percent of U.S. population	Hepatitis B Worldwide, 4 million new acute cases and 1 million deaths per year	Hepatitis C Worldwide estimates: 1.5 million persons infected in Europe, 4 million in the United States
Usual mode of transmission	Fecal-oral: contaminated water, shellfish, raw produce Rarely, blood products	Body fluids Inanimate objects contaminated with body fluids	Parenteral equipment Rarely, sexual contact
High-risk populations	Household and sexual contacts of acute cases Contacts with diapered children in day care Travelers to areas with endemic disease Men who have sex with men	Household and sexual contacts of infected persons Injecting drug users Heterosexuals with multiple partners Men who have sex with men Long-term international travelers in close contact with local people Health care and public safety workers exposed to blood in their work Hemodialysis clients	Individuals who share injecting equipment Health care workers using parenteral equipment (needlestick accidents)
Complications	Complete recovery Low fatality rate	May cause up to 80 percent of hepatocellular cancer worldwide	50–90 percent develop chronic infection 50 percent of those chronically infected will develop cirrhosis or cancer of the liver
Vaccine	Yes	Yes; believed effective for 15 years	No

Abstracted from Chin, 2000.

instructions on the incorporation of fiber back into the diet after they have followed a low-fiber diet. Fiber should be reintroduced gradually to avoid the abdominal cramping, bloating, and gas pains that can occur with drastic changes in fiber intake. Although not proven to be helpful, avoiding foods with small seeds that could get caught in a diverticulum may be recommended.

Diseases and Conditions of the Liver

The infiltration of liver cells by fat is called **fatty liver**. Many situations can cause fatty liver, including alcoholism and a low-protein or a starvation diet (because of the breakdown of adipose tissue for energy). Usually no harm occurs because of fatty liver unless it progresses. Treatment is to correct the cause. If it is alcohol consumption, abstinence reverses the pathology. More serious liver diseases are hepatitis and cirrhosis.

Hepatitis

Inflammation of the liver, or **hepatitis**, can result from viral infections, alcohol, drugs, or toxins. Two well-known viral infections are hepatitis A and hepatitis B. Hepatitis A is spread by the fecal-oral route and, rarely, by blood transfusion. It is discussed in Chapter 14, Food Management. Hepatitis B is spread by body fluids such as blood, saliva, semen, and vaginal secretions and has been associated with reusable fingerstick blood sampling devices used to monitor blood glucose levels (Centers for Disease Control, 1997b). Hepatitis C is parenterally transmitted, with the highest incidence being in drug users and hemophilia clients. From 50 to 90 percent of persons infected with hepatitis C will develop chronic hepatitis, and 50 percent of those chronically infected develop cirrhosis or cancer of the liver (Chin, 2000). Table 22–7 compares the occurrence, mode of transmission, high-risk populations, complications, and preventive vaccines for these three types of viral hepatitis.

CLINICAL APPLICATION 22–6

Nutritional Effects of Alcoholism

Alcoholism is a disease of alcohol consumption that produces tolerance, physical dependence, and characteristic organ pathology in the body. Ingestion of prodigious amounts of alcohol is not necessary for someone to become an alcoholic. The disease may be produced in some persons by 3-5 ounces per day of whiskey. The first notion to dispel is the cliché of the skid row alcoholic. There still are alcoholics on skid row, of course, but the disease is far more pervasive than that. In an affluent society, alcoholics may be obese, usually early in the disease rather than later, and may continue to function in several roles at work and in the family.

In the United States, alcoholism is the single most important factor in nutrient deficiencies. Associating the numerous functions of the liver with the fact that alcohol is toxic to all body cells, the nutritional havoc accompanying alcoholism becomes obvious. Even without liver damage, alcohol injures the intestine, thereby reducing absorption of vitamins A, D, K, thiamin, pyridoxine, folic acid, and B_{12}. Folic acid deficiency occurs in 50–80 percent of alcoholics.

The vitamin deficiency that is almost synonymous with alcoholism is that of thiamin because it is necessary to convert alcohol to energy. In the United States, thiamin deficiency is seen almost exclusively in alcoholics, affecting 30–80 percent. The neurological symptoms of thiamin deficiency, called *dry beriberi*, present a disheartening picture. Clients have atrophy of many nerves, weakness in the ankles and toes, and numbness and tingling in the feet. Even more serious is wet beriberi, in which cardiac symptoms predominate. The severe form of wet beriberi, *shoshin wet beriberi*, can rapidly lead to heart failure and carries a high mortality rate (Smith, 1998).

The behavior of an intoxicated person readily shows that alcohol penetrates the blood-brain barrier. In fact, brain damage may occur before severe liver damage. The **Wernicke-Korsakoff syndrome** is a disorder of the central nervous system that is caused by thiamin deficiency and is seen predominantly but not exclusively in alcoholics. The clients display disorientation, memory dysfunction, and **ataxia**. Weakness of the muscles that control the eyes produces double vision (*diplopia*) and abnormal movements of the eyeball (*nystagmus*).

Thiamin helps to oxidize glucose and to metabolize alcohol to energy. This is a critical piece of information for healthcare providers who care for alcoholic clients. Administering a simple solution of glucose intravenously can precipitate symptoms of Wernicke-Korsakoff syndrome if the client is thiamin-deficient. For this reason, thiamin is routinely administered parenterally to alcoholics. Because magnesium appears to be necessary for thiamin utilization, parenteral administration of this mineral is advised for shoshin wet beriberi (Smith, 1998).

Other vitamin deficiencies in alcoholics, in order of frequency after folic acid and thiamin, are of pyridoxine, niacin, vitamin C, and vitamin A. Niacin deficiency occurs in one-third of alcoholics. Scurvy in the United States is almost exclusively found in alcoholics. Vitamin C, besides being necessary for tissue repair, plays a role in folic acid metabolism and in iron absorption. Storage of vitamin A in the liver is impaired. A visual impairment, abnormal adaptation to darkness, has been reported in 50 percent of alcoholics with cirrhosis and 15 percent of those without it (Feinman and Lieber, 1999).

Other nutritional effects possible in alcoholics are bone loss and bleeding tendencies. One-half of alcoholics show bone loss. Albumin carries calcium in the bloodstream. Hypoalbuminemia, reduced stores and faulty metabolism of vitamin D, low calcium intake, and steatorrhea causing binding of calcium in the intestine may all combine to produce bone loss.

Prothrombin, normally manufactured by the liver using vitamin K, is necessary for blood clotting. Vitamin E deficiency produces neurological changes, cerebellar degeneration, and peripheral neuropathy.

Potassium, phosphorus, and magnesium are the most common major mineral deficiencies in alcoholics. Electrolyte status should be monitored during treatment. (See refeeding syndrome in Chapter 24, Stress.) Insufficient magnesium impairs central nervous system activity and increases muscular excitability and therefore is suggested to exacerbate the increased neuroirritability displayed by clients in acute alcohol withdrawal. Iron and zinc are the trace minerals most often deficient in alcoholics. Low iron stores are related to gastrointestinal bleeding, rather than poor absorption. Alcohol damages the intestinal mucosa and thereby permits increased absorption of iron. With low folic acid levels, however, red blood cell production cannot proceed normally. Anemia or bone marrow abnormalities have been found in 75 percent of clients hospitalized with alcoholism. Up to 50 percent of alcoholic clients are deficient in zinc. Zinc is needed for many enzymes that function in DNA and RNA metabolism. It plays a vital role in the growth and repair of essential organs, such as the liver. Zinc is also necessary to convert vitamin A to a functional form in the retina.

Finally, alcoholics suffer from protein-energy malnutrition. Even in early alcoholism, albumin levels are low-normal. The typical alcoholic consumes only 75 percent of required energy. The result of low-protein, low-energy intake is muscle wasting. Fat is not an adequate source of energy for alcoholics, owing to malabsorption. Steatorrhea is seen in half the clients.

Awareness of the wide range of nutritional effects of alcoholism should help the nurse to focus on early case finding. Interruption of the downward spiral in health could literally be lifesaving.

CLINICAL APPLICATION 22–7

Alcohol Contributes to Mortality

Chronic liver disease and cirrhosis ranked tenth in the causes of death in the United States in 1997. Alcohol also contributes to other causes of mortality. Accidents are the fifth leading cause of death. Alcohol is implicated in about 40 percent of motor vehicle fatalities, 45 percent of cases of accidental drowning, and 35 percent of accidental fall fatalities. Alcohol abuse has been linked to 50 percent of homicides (the thirteenth leading cause of death) and 28 percent of suicides (the eighth leading cause of death).

Alcohol can be immediately lethal if a large quantity of ethanol (or a smaller quantity of alcohols not intended for beverages) is consumed in a short period of time. Alcohol poisoning is especially heart-breaking when it kills a young person whose companions let the victim "sleep it off" through ignorance or fear of retribution. Teaching young people about the hazards of alcohol and counseling adult clients about the responsible use of alcohol are nursing functions in all settings. These interventions may be appropriate for friends and family members as well as for clients.

CLINICAL APPLICATION 22–8

CAGE Questionnaire for Identifying the Alcohol Abuser

The following instrument has been extensively validated against the psychiatric diagnostic criteria for alcoholism and alcohol abuse. Using one or more "yes" answers as indicative of alcohol abuse, the CAGE questionnaire's sensitivity was 86 percent and its specificity 93 percent in a walk-in clinic (Liskow et al., 1995). **Sensitivity** is the proportion of people correctly identified by the test as having the disease. **Specificity** is the proportion of people correctly identified by the test as not having the disease. Using two or more "yes" answers in hospitalized clients yielded a sensitivity of 76 percent and a specificity of 94 percent (Beresford et al., 1 990). The designer of the questionnaire recommended that even one "yes" answer merits further inquiry (Ewing, 1984). Since the prevalence rate of alcoholism is 20-30 percent in clinical settings, a CAGE score of 1 is recommended there (Liskow et al., 1995). The CAGE questionnaire is a screening instrument to identify a need for a diagnostic workup. Its advantages are its simplicity and its proven accuracy in clinical studies.

C—Have you ever had a need to CUT BACK on your drinking?
A—Have people ANNOYED YOU with criticism about your drinking?
G—Have you ever felt GUILTY about your drinking?
E—Have you ever needed to start the day with a drink? (an EYE-OPENER)

Signs and Symptoms of Hepatitis

Regardless of type or cause, symptoms are anorexia, nausea, epigastric discomfort, fatigue, and weakness. Signs of hepatitis are vomiting, diarrhea, and jaundice caused by the inability of the liver to convert fat-soluble bilirubin to a water-soluble (conjugated) form. The degree of jaundice gives a rough estimate of the severity of the disease. Physical examination shows an enlarged and tender liver and an enlarged spleen.

Treatment of Hepatitis

No current medications can cure hepatitis, but combinations of interferon and antiviral drugs are being tested in efforts to modify its course. Nevertheless, the cornerstones of treatment are bed rest, abstinence from alcohol, and optimum nutrition to permit the liver to heal. Convalescence may take from 3 weeks to 3 months. Clients on bed rest, especially debilitated clients, are more susceptible to pressure ulcers than the average client because of decreased synthesis of albumin and the globulins. If the client abstains from alcohol, the hepatitis is often reversible.

A high-kilocalorie, high-protein, moderate-fat diet is frequently prescribed for hepatitis clients. Energy intake should come from as much as 400 grams of carbohydrate daily. Protein in amounts up to 100 grams helps heal the liver. Many clients cannot tolerate this amount of protein, however, because the liver has sustained too much damage. Commonly dietary protein is restricted for clients with irreversible liver damage. The client may tolerate emulsified fats in dairy products and eggs better than other fats. Up to 35 percent of kilocalories in fat can provide high energy in a lower volume of food. Fluid intake should be 3–3.5 liters per day.

Coaxing a person with hepatitis to accept such a substantial meal pattern is an enormous task because of the anorexia and nausea that accompany the disease. Since the nausea is often less in the morning than later in the day, hepatitis clients should be encouraged to eat a big break-

fast. Polymeric oral feedings that are high in kilocalories and protein are widely used for between-meal feedings.

Cirrhosis of the Liver

The word cirrhosis comes from a French word for orange. In **cirrhosis** the liver becomes fibrous and contains orange-colored nodules that resemble the skin of an orange. In the United States, chronic alcohol abuse is the most common, but not the only, cause of cirrhosis. About half of the 13 million alcoholics in this country will develop cirrhosis. Cirrhosis also occurs in nondrinkers. Insults to the liver such as infection, biliary obstruction, and toxic chemicals, including medications, may precede cirrhosis. Alcohol is toxic to all body tissues, including the liver. The nutritional effects of alcoholism are summarized in Clinical Application 22–6, and its connection to mortality is described in Clinical Application 22–7.

A number of barriers interfere with alcoholism case-finding: (1) alcoholism's multiple and varied manifestations, (2) the healthcare provider's personal definition and meaning of alcoholism, and (3) denial by the client and family. The CAGE questionnaire shown in Clinical Application 22–8 is a brief, effective screening tool to identify possible alcohol abusers. In addition, morning drinking appears to indicate a current or impending alcohol problem, showing a stronger relationship in women than in men (York, 1995).

Pathophysiology

Alcohol needs no digestion. It is absorbed rapidly, 20 percent from the stomach and 80 percent from the small intestine. Immediately after absorption, the alcohol is carried throughout the body. In the liver, it is

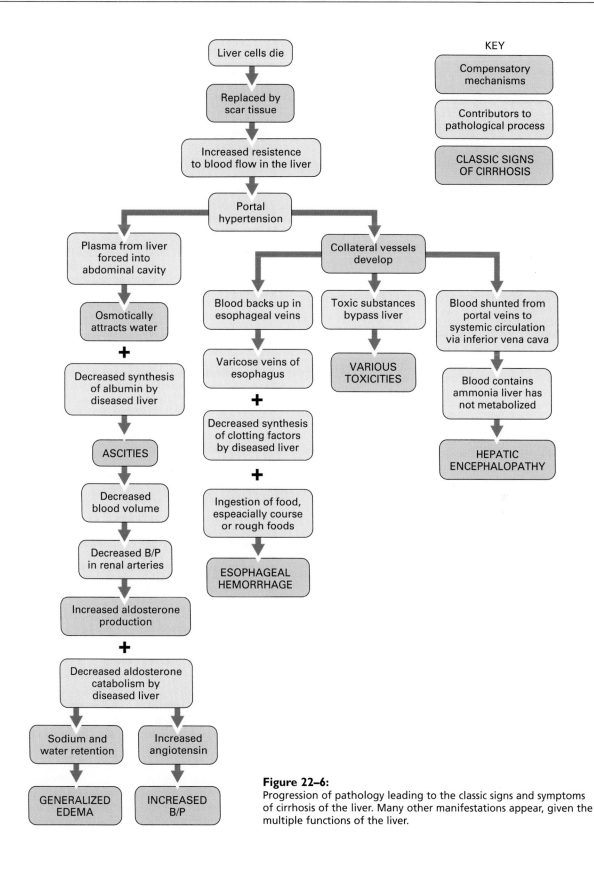

Figure 22–6:
Progression of pathology leading to the classic signs and symptoms of cirrhosis of the liver. Many other manifestations appear, given the multiple functions of the liver.

CLINICAL APPLICATION 22–9

Hepatic Encephalopathy

Hepatic encephalopathy results from liver failure, but the precise mechanism involved in the pathology is uncertain. Because hepatic encephalopathy is associated with increased serum levels of ammonia and aromatic amino acids, treatments to control one or both of these factors have been suggested. Because elevated serum ammonia levels interfere with normal mentation, the nurse should be cautious when interpreting interview data obtained from the client.

Because of its clinical similarity to hepatic encephalopathy, manganese toxicity is proposed as a mechanism that contributes to the manifestations of both these conditions, and increased manganese levels in various parts of the brain have been recorded on autopsy of clients who succumbed to hepatic encephalopathy (Layrargues et al., 1998; Rose et al., 1999). Manganese is a component of an enzyme, glutamine synthetase, that detoxifies ammonia. If manganese does prove to be a causative factor, metal-chelating agents may be added to the treatment of hepatic encephalopathy (Krieger et al., 1995).

Ammonia is produced by intestinal bacteria and by digestive enzymes breaking down protein. Even if the person consumes no protein foods, the bacteria work on the cast-off cells of the gastrointestinal tract and on the blood from gastrointestinal bleeding, which is common in alcoholic cirrhosis. Ordinarily, the liver degrades ammonia to urea, which is then excreted by the kidneys in urine. In liver failure, blood ammonia levels rise. Ammonia is toxic to all cells, including those of the liver and the brain. The laboratory values are not clearly correlated with the degree of encephalopathy, so a series of tests is necessary to monitor each client. Hypokalemia with resulting alkalosis for instance, causes ammonia retention in the brain.

The liver normally breaks down amino acids. The client with liver failure exhibits a change in the ratio of aromatic amino acids (phenylalanine, tryptophan, and tyrosine) to branched-chain amino acids (leucine, isoleucine, lysine, and valine). In the healthy client this ratio is approximately 1:1; with hepatic coma it is 3:1 or higher. The elevated levels of aromatic amino acids are thought to contribute to hepatic coma by interfering with the formation of the neurotransmitters dopamine and norepinephrine.

Some signs of hepatic encephalopathy can be observed before the onset of coma, including personality changes, irritability, weakness, apathy, confusion, and sleepiness. More specific signs are asterixis and fetor hepaticus. *Asterixis*, or liver flap, refers to involuntary jerking movements or a flapping of the hand when the arm is outstretched. *Fetor hepaticus* is a fecal odor to the breath. Finally, coma occurs.

Treatment consists of medications and dietary modifications, along with symptomatic care. Oral neomycin kills the bacteria in the intestine, thereby decreasing ammonia production. Lactulose acidifies the large intestine, causing ammonia to be converted to ammonium ions, which are not absorbed but eliminated in the feces. The diet must be carefully planned. Some foods produce higher ammonia levels than most others. These include chicken, salami, ground beef, ham, gelatin, peanut butter, potatoes, onions, and buttermilk, as well as blue, American, and cheddar cheeses (Rudman et al., 1973).

When coma is approaching, protein is limited to 40–60 grams of high-quality protein per day. Because they contain fewer aromatic amino acids, vegetable proteins may be tolerated better than animal protein. Branched-chain amino acids have been administered orally or parenterally in attempts to treat hepatic encephalopathy. This therapy is not recommended routinely but may benefit protein-intolerant clients with chronic encephalopathy (Lieber, 1999). If enteral feeding is necessary, special preparations low in aromatic amino acids are available. Two of them are Hepatic-Aid II and Travasorb-Hepatic. Aspartame (NutraSweet) contains phenylalanine, an aromatic amino acid. If the theory holds, it too should be avoided.

If the client's condition continues to deteriorate, even greater restrictions are placed on diet. Adequate kilocaloric intake, 1500–2000 kilocalories, must be maintained to prevent tissue protein from being used for energy. Dietary protein is decreased to 10–20 grams/day. As the client recovers, dietary protein is added in increments of 10 grams every 2 days. If signs of encephalopathy reappear, protein is reduced to the previous restriction.

---

metabolized at the rate of 0.5 ounce of alcohol per hour. This refers to the alcohol content, not the whole beverage. This rate cannot be rushed, and giving coffee or other stimulants to an inebriated person induces not sobriety but merely wide-awake intoxication.

If the liver is not able to repair the damage, dying liver cells are replaced by scar tissue. Figure 22–6 traces the path from cell death to several cardinal signs of cirrhosis. Because liver has multiple functions, one pathological change reinforces another. The ascites is worsened by hypoalbuminemia and is partly caused by and also worsened by sodium retention. Depressed plasma protein production, as evidenced by decreasing albumin levels, indicates a poor client outcome.

Signs and Symptoms of Cirrhosis

Cirrhosis causes anorexia, epigastric pain, and nausea that worsens as the day goes on. Signs of the disease are abdominal distention, vomiting, steatorrhea, jaundice, ascites, edema, and gastrointestinal bleeding. Of clients with advanced cirrhosis, 70 percent develop esophageal varices, which are varicose veins of the esophagus. Muscle tremors are attributed to hypomagnesemia. Laboratory tests show hypoglycemia and elevated serum triglyceride levels. The lack of enzymes for converting noncarbohydrate sources to energy causes hypoglycemia. Insufficient lipoprotein synthesis causes the elevated triglycerides and fatty liver. The end result of cirrhosis is liver failure, which leads to hepatic coma (Clinical Application 22–9).

Table 22–8 Protein-Controlled Diets for Liver Disease

Description	Indications	Adequacy
These diets are prescribed to attain and maintain normal amino acid balance, reduce blood ammonia levels, and improve clinical status. In addition to protein, fluid and sodium are often restricted.	These diets are used in severe liver disease such as acute hepatitis or advanced cirrhosis.	The diets may not meet the RDA for B complex vitamins, especially folic acid, calcium, and iron.

Meal Plan   **Sample Menu**

20-GRAM PROTEIN DIET

		40-GRAM PROTEIN DIET	
Breakfast		*Add to the Above:*	
1/2 cup milk	1/2 cup whole milk	1/2 cup milk	1 starch exchange
1 fruit	1/2 cup orange juice with 2 tbsp modular carbohydrate supplement*	2 meat exchanges	
2 starches	1/2 cup Cream of Wheat with 1 tbsp modular carbohydrate supplement and 1 slice of toast with 1 tbsp margarine and jelly	**60-GRAM PROTEIN DIET** *Add to the 20-Gram Protein Diet Meal Plan:* 2 cups milk	
Fat (as tolerated)	2 tbsp cream	1 starch exchange	1 vegetable exchange 3 meat exchanges
Beverage	As tolerated and per fluid restriction		
Lunch		2 cups milk	1 vegetable exchange
2 starches	1 cup rice with 1/4 cup unsalted tomato sauce and 1 tbsp olive oil	5 meat exchanges	4 starch exchanges
Vegetable	1/2 cup green beans with 1 tsp margarine		
Fruit	1/2 cup canned peaches with 1 tbsp modular carbohydrate supplement		
Beverage	As tolerated and per fluid restriction		
Dinner			
2 starches	1 baked potato with 2 tbsp sour cream and 1 slice of bread with 1 tsp margarine and jelly		
Vegetable	1/2 cup mushrooms (for potato topping)		
Fruit	1/2 cup strawberries with 1 tbsp modular carbohydrate supplement		
Beverage	As tolerated and per fluid restriction		

Within the sample menu area the following headings appear:

80-GRAM PROTEIN DIET
Add to the 20-Gram Diet Meal Plan:

*Polycose, Sumacal, and Moducal are all modular carbohydrate supplements.

Dietary Treatment of Cirrhosis

Treatment is ineffective if the client continues to drink. Even so, once portal hypertension has occurred, abstinence does not halt the progression of cirrhosis. A protein-restricted diet, limited to 20–40 grams per day, may be prescribed when the liver cannot process the end products of protein metabolism. Esophageal varices necessitate a soft diet. As the client improves, dietary protein can sometimes be increased to aid liver regeneration. It is necessary to monitor the client carefully for signs of excessive protein intake. Blood ammonia levels are tested frequently to assess the client's ability to metabolize dietary protein effectively. Sufficient kilocalories must be provided to prevent catabolism of tissue protein for energy. Simple carbohydrates are encouraged. Enough fat is offered for palatability. Dietary fats that are

Table 22–9 Comparison of Fat Content of Selected Foods

Low-Fat Foods	Fat (g)	High-Fat Foods	Fat (g)
		STARCH/BREADS	
Angel food cake, 1/12	<1	Pecan pie, 1/6 of pie	24
Italian bread, 1 slice	<1	Bread stuffing, 1/2 cup	13
English muffin, 1	1	Danish pastry	12
Raisin toast, 1 slice	1	Croissant, 1	12
Pancake, 4-in, 1	2	Glazed raised doughnut, 1	13
		MEATS, FISH, AND POULTRY	
Beef round, 3 oz lean roasted	9	Beef prime rib, 3 oz. lean only	24
Chicken breast, 3 oz rst., without skin	9	Chicken, deep-fried thigh, 1	14
Boiled ham, 3 oz	9	Spare ribs, 3 oz	24
Tuna, 1/2 cup water-packed	6	Tuna, 1/2 cup oil-packed, drained	24
		FRUITS AND VEGETABLES	
Banana, 8 3/4 in. long, 1	1	Avocado, 1	30
Raisins, 1 cup	1	Coconut, dried, 1 cup	50
		French fried potato, 2 x 3 1/2 in., 15	
Potato, baked 1	<1	pieces	12
Onion, raw, sliced, 1 cup	<1	French fried onion rings, 4	10
		MILK PRODUCTS	
Cottage cheese, 1 percent, 1/2 cup	1	Cottage cheese, 4 percent, 1/2 cup	5
Mozzarella, part skim, 1 oz	5	Cheddar, 1 oz	9
Skim milk, with added milk solids, 1 cup	1	Whole milk, 1 cup	8
Frozen yogurt, low-fat, 1 cup	4	Ice cream, regular, hard, vanilla, 1 cup	14
		FAST FOODS*	
Arby's			
Turkey sandwich, deluxe	6	Chicken breast sandwich	22
McDonald's			
Chicken McNuggets, 6	18	Quarter pounder with cheese	29
Taco Bell			
Chicken burrito	13	Taco salad with salsa	56
Wendy's			
Chili, 1 cup	7	Chicken club sandwich	21

*Check with the restaurant. Recipes may be revised.

already emulsified, such as those in homogenized milk and eggs, need less bile for digestion.

Fluid and electrolyte balance demands careful attention. If the client has ascites, sodium probably needs to be restricted. A limitation of 250 milligrams to 1 gram per day is common. Fluid is restricted also, often to 1.5–2 liters in 24 hours. If the serum sodium level is low, fluid may be limited to 1–1.5 liters. Monitoring the improvement or progression of ascites includes measuring abdominal girth and daily weighing. If the client has ascites without peripheral edema, a reasonable goal for weight loss is 0.5 kilogram (1.1 pounds) per day. If both ascites and peripheral edema are displayed, the goal for weight loss is 1 kilogram per day.

Table 22–8 displays various protein-controlled diets that assume the client tolerates fats. Extensive low-protein exchange lists have been developed to treat liver failure. The dietary management of these clients is complex and constantly changing, requiring the services of a dietitian. Because of the high risk of vitamin deficiencies, cirrhosis clients are given pharmaceutical supplements. Up to five times the RDA of water-soluble vitamins may be necessary.

Gallbladder Disease

On the underside of the liver is a small pouch-like organ called the **gallbladder**. Its function is to concentrate and store bile until it is needed for digestion. The liver secretes 600–800 milliliters of bile per day. The gallbladder reduces this to 60–160 milliliters.

Gallbladder disease is usually related to gallstones. The presence of gallstones is called **cholelithiasis**. One-fifth of adults over 40 years of age and one-third over 70 have gallstones. Most gallstones form when the bile is too scant or too concentrated or contains excessive cholesterol. When the gallbladder becomes inflamed from irritation by the stones, the condition is labeled **cholecystitis**.

Causative Factors

Women are three times more likely than men to have gallbladder disease. A definite nutritional link is obesity, and a tentative link is the low serum levels of ascorbic acid found in women with gallbladder disease (Sijmon and Hudes, 2000). Heredity and hypercholesterolemia are associated with gallstones, whereas cardiovascular disease and diabetes mellitus, both related to heredity and hypercholesterolemia, are associated with gallbladder disease. Other risk factors include ileal disease or resection, long-term TPN, multiple pregnancies, and oral contraceptive use. Gallstone disease is also associated with a habitual long overnight fast, with dieting, and with a low fiber intake (Sichiere, Everhart, and Rothe, 1991). A long fast between the evening meal and the first meal of the next day could be modified by a light bedtime snack and/or drinking two glasses of water on arising if breakfast will be delayed. Either practice stimulates the gallbladder to empty, thus decreasing the likelihood of very concentrated bile.

Symptoms of Gallbladder Disease

The cardinal symptom of gallbladder disease is pain after ingestion of fat. The pain is located in the right upper quadrant and often radiates to the right shoulder.

Treatment of Gallbladder Disease

Dietary modification and medical and surgical interventions are used to treat gallbladder disease. Usually, conservative medical management is tried for a time before surgery.

Dietary Modifications

During an acute attack, a full liquid diet with minimal fat is recommended. For chronic gallbladder disease, the client should limit fat and obese clients should lose weight. Some clients obtain relief with the restriction of dietary fat; others do not. A reasonable approach to fat restriction is (1) to select skim milk dairy products, (2) to limit fats or oils to 3 teaspoons per day, and (3) to consume no more than 6 ounces of very lean meat per day. Gas-forming foods also are often poorly tolerated.

Another approach is to eliminate foods that cause symptoms. Clients usually can identify foods that cause them pain. Fried foods are the worst offenders. Table 22–9 identifies some foods that are low in fat and some that are high in fat.

Medical and Surgical Interventions

New procedures have been devised to treat gallstones without surgery. One technique involves injecting solvents into the gallbladder. Another method is to break up the stones using shock waves through a procedure called *lithotripsy*. Clients and physicians still may opt for removal of the stones through an abdominal incision, a *cholecystotomy*, or for removal of the gallbladder, *cholecystectomy*, through a laparoscope or the traditional abdominal incision.

Postoperative diet routines are similar to those for other gastrointestinal surgery. When the client begins to take oral nourishment, clear liquids are given for 24 hours. The diet is progressed as tolerated. Because bile enters the duodenum continuously, balanced meals should be well tolerated. Many clients can eat a regular diet without difficulty 1 month after surgery. Clients who become nauseated and suffer pain after eating certain foods preoperatively, however, may continue to avoid them postoperatively because of the association.

Diseases and Disorders of the Pancreas

In addition to the endocrine secretions insulin, glucagon, and somatostatin, the **pancreas** secretes amylase, lipase, trypsin, and chymotrypsin. Disorders of the pancreas include pancreatitis and cystic fibrosis.

Pancreatitis

When the blood vessels of the pancreas become abnormally permeable, plasma and plasma protein leak into the interstitial spaces. The resulting edema damages the pancreatic cells. Normally, the pancreatic enzymes necessary for digestion are inactive in the pancreas and become activated only upon entering the duodenum; otherwise, the active enzymes would digest the pancreas itself. In **pancreatitis**, the retained pancreatic enzymes, especially trypsin, become activated and digest the pancreatic tissue.

Alcoholism is the most common cause of pancreatitis, generating up to 75 percent of the cases. Other conditions that can lead to pancreatitis are biliary tract disease or surgery; stomach surgery; and the administration of cancer chemotherapy, steroids, thiazides, or estrogens. In some cases, viral infection, pregnancy, or trauma has preceded pancreatitis. The characteristic symptom of pancreatitis is excruciating pain in the left upper quadrant. Nausea and vomiting accompany an attack. Laboratory tests reveal elevated levels of serum amylase and lipase.

In the treatment of pancreatitis, the client is advised to avoid alcohol. An acutely ill client is usually allowed nothing by mouth for 24–48 hours to reduce secretions. A nasogastric tube is used to suction stomach contents. Ice chips may be prescribed to lessen dryness of the mouth. Special ice chips may be made by freezing electrolyte solutions to circumvent the loss of gastric secretions that is stimulated by plain water or ice chips made with plain water. Increased secretions when administering gastric suction only escalates electrolyte losses. If necessary, the client is maintained on intravenous or TPN feedings until the acute phase subsides.

When the pain subsides and bowel sounds return, oral intake is started. Clear liquids, progressing to a low-fat, high-carbohydrate diet, are given. The use of elemental formulas may be necessary. Medium-chain triglycerides may be a better-tolerated source of fats than normal dietary fats. Six small meals per day constitute the usual pattern. The client's comfort level is monitored, and serum amylase concentrations are periodically checked. If the client's condition worsens, the acute care regimen is reinstituted.

Acute pancreatitis may or may not progress to chronic pancreatitis. For chronic pancreatitis clients, alcohol is not recommended. Fat restriction similar to that for gallbladder disease may be helpful. Pancreatic enzymes can be given orally before or with meals to aid digestion. Because pancreatitis clients do not absorb vitamin B_{12} adequately, it is given parenterally.

Cystic Fibrosis

The most common cause of pancreatic insufficiency in children and young adults is **cystic fibrosis**. It occurs in 1 of every 2500 live births. One in 20 Caucasians carries the recessive gene for this disorder. Median survival in the United States in 1995 was 30.1 years (Anthony et al., 1998).

Pathophysiology

The underlying pathology of cystic fibrosis is thick glandular mucus production. This dense mucus affects the pancreas, lungs, liver, heart, gallbladder, and small intestine. The mucus plugs the ducts through which it and other secretions are supposed to flow. The stagnant secretions then become a hospitable environment for bacteria. Fifty percent of children with cystic fibrosis have lung symptoms. Lung infection is the most common cause of death.

The pancreas is affected in 80 percent of cystic fibrosis cases. Here the thick mucus interferes with digestive secretions, leading to malabsorption of many nutrients and stunted growth (deficit in height for age). The sign of cystic fibrosis related to the gastrointestinal tract is the passage of bulky, fatty, foul-smelling feces. This is caused by the impairment of fat digestion. With increased life expectancy, more cystic fibrosis clients display hyperglycemia or diabetes mellitus.

The sweat of a cystic fibrosis client has more sodium chloride than normal. A sweat chloride level greater than 60 milliequivalents per liter is diagnostic of cystic fibrosis. The high electrolyte content of the sweat also puts the client at increased risk of imbalance during hot weather or fever.

Treatment of Cystic Fibrosis

Supportive care is the foundation of cystic fibrosis treatment. Pulmonary congestion and infections are treated as required. The client's energy needs may be double those of others the same age. When the lungs are involved, much of the client's energy is expended in respiratory effort. Because starches require amylase for digestion, carbohydrates in the form of simple sugars are a better source of energy. If the client also has diabetes mellitus, the diet will include more simple sugars than the usual diet for diabetes mellitus. Intensive therapy of the diabetes mellitus can be maintained with self-monitoring of blood glucose and multiple doses of insulin (Hayes et al., 1994).

For cystic fibrosis clients, protein needs are double those of other individuals. Fat content should be as high as possible because it is a concentrated energy source. If necessary, medium-chain triglycerides can be used to increase fat intake without overtaxing the weak

Summary

Diseases of other body systems may be more immediately life threatening, but over the long term gastrointestinal diseases can profoundly affect quality of life and life expectancy. Healthcare workers should make nutrition a priority for clients undergoing diagnostic tests or surgery. Medications have revolutionized the treatment of peptic ulcers. If the client does have a gastrectomy and develops dumping syndrome, he or she should receive frequent dry meals that are low in simple sugars and should lie down after eating. In contrast, clients with hiatal hernias may be more comfortable if they remain upright after meals.

Celiac disease and cystic fibrosis are gastrointestinal diseases found in children as well as in adults. In celiac disease, gluten destroys the intestinal villi, causing major malabsorption problems. In cystic fibrosis, thick glandular secretions plug the pancreatic ducts, causing malabsorption. The excessive mucus produced in the lungs by cystic fibrosis is life threatening, however.

Nourishing clients with Crohn's disease and ulcerative colitis poses significant challenges. Use of elemental formulas or total parenteral nutrition is often necessary to permit healing. In intractable cases, colon resection and ileostomy or colostomy may be performed. This drastic surgery presents a new set of management problems, including fluid balance, odor control, and skin integrity.

Because of its multiple functions, the liver, when diseased, produces varied and severe consequences. The different types of hepatitis can be transmitted by food, body fluids, and wastes and sometimes by inanimate objects. Complete recovery is the usual outcome of hepatitis A, but hepatitis B is thought to cause 80 percent of hepatocellular cancer. Vaccines are available to prevent these two types of hepatitis. Hepatitis C often progresses to a chronic infection that significantly increases the risk of cancer of the liver or cirrhosis. In cirrhosis, the liver becomes scarred, hard, and increasingly nonfunctional. The result is portal hypertension, absorp-

Wellness Tips 22–1

- Maximize nutrition 2–3 weeks before elective surgery. Be conscientious about consuming recommended amounts of foods high in protein, vitamins C and K, iron, and zinc.
- To avoid constipation, consume adequate fiber and fluid, obtain enough exercise, and schedule a regular time to defecate.
- Obtain appropriate hepatitis vaccinations. Implement safe food-handling practices. Wash hands thoroughly after using the toilet or changing diapers. Use universal precautions. Campaign for the adoption of safer needle systems. Report all needlestick injuries.
- Drink moderately (maximum of one drink/day for women, small men, and elderly and two drinks/day for average-size men), if at all. Teach young people the severe outcomes of acute alcohol poisoning.
- To avoid concentrated bile resulting from a long overnight fast that increases the risk of gallstones, eat breakfast or drink two glasses of water upon arising.

tion of toxins through collateral channels, esophageal varices, ascites, bleeding problems, and possible hepatic coma. Alcohol abuse underlies most, but not all, cases of cirrhosis and pancreatitis. Treatment is abstinence and supportive therapy. Diet is modified according to the client's current clinical status.

Of the major diseases discussed in this chapter, gallbladder disease is the most amenable to treatment. If a low-fat selective diet is not successful, medical and surgical techniques are available to remove the stones or the organ as necessary.

Wellness Tip 22-1 summarizes major guidelines to help maintain gastrointestinal health.

Case Study 22–1

An outpatient, Ms. C, a 40-year-old white woman, has just been evaluated for right upper quadrant pain. The pain occurs after meals and radiates to the right shoulder. Ms. C has noticed her stools have become pale gray in the past 2 months. Ms. C is 5 ft. 4 in. tall, has a medium frame, and weighs 151 lb.

Ultrasound examination of the gallbladder showed the presence of numerous stones. None is obstructing the duct system yet.

Ms. C is a single parent of four children, aged 4 to 17, and is employed as a secretary. If surgery does become necessary, she would like to delay it until the youngest child is in school. For that reason, she is electing conservative treatment.

The nurse taking a dietary history discovers that Ms. C seldom eats breakfast, substituting a doughnut and coffee during her morning coffee break. Lunch is generally a bologna sandwich with chips. Dinner at home often consists of hamburgers, pizza, or macaroni and cheese. Ms. C told the nurse she does not know much about nutrition, that she shops as her mother did, and cooks food her children will eat.

....

Nursing Care Plan

Subjective Data	Pain in right upper quadrant immediately after eating
	Pale stools for 2 months by history
	High-fat, low-fiber diet by history
	Admitted lack of knowledge about nutrition
Objective Data	Gallstones per ultrasound
	115 percent of healthy body weight
Nursing Diagnosis	NANDA: Knowledge deficit (North American Nursing Diagnosis Association, 1999, with permission.)
	Related to prescribed low-fat diet for cholecystitis as evidenced by admitted lack of knowledge about nutrition

Desired Outcomes Evaluation Criteria	Nursing Actions/ Interventions	Rationale
NOC: Knowledge (Diet) (Johnson, Maas, and Moorhead, 2000, with permission.)	NIC: Nutritional Counseling (McCloskey and Bulechek, 2000, with permission.)	
Client will verbalize foods to avoid to maintain low-fat diet by end of teaching session.	Explain low-fat diet, working in client's lifestyle. Provide written instructions for client to take home.	Having written instructions available as a teaching tool structures the session and may stimulate questions the client would not think of otherwise. Her taking the material home will reinforce the instruction.
Client will state means of modifying meals to accommodate prescribed diet by end of teaching session.	Explore Ms. C's preferences for adding fiber to her diet.	Soluble fiber will combine with cholesterol, which comprises most gallstones, and carry it out of the body. Building on the client's choices increases chances of compliance.
	Obtain client's reaction to diet and offer alternatives to her present meal pattern.	Considering the client's wishes affirms her status as an individual. Personalizing the diet for her circumstances will increase the chances of success.
	Suggest Ms. C either eat breakfast or drink 2 glasses of water first thing in the morning.	Either of these actions will stimulate the gallbladder to empty and rid itself of the concentrated bile that has accumulated overnight.
Client will return to follow-up session in 1 week with report of the week's meals and any questions she may have.	Try to obtain a commitment to return for follow-up in 1 week.	This is quite a radical change from Ms. C's usual eating habits. Follow-up in 1 week will give the nurse an opportunity to reinforce the teaching, answer questions, and counsel the client to remain committed to the therapeutic regimen.

....

Critical Thinking Questions

1. Expand this nursing care plan to a family case. What additional assessment data are needed? How might dietary interventions be modified for a 4-year-old and a 17-year-old?

2. What is your interpretation of Ms. C's financial situation? How would it impact on the implementation of the family care plan?

3. Criticize the use of knowledge deficit as a long-term evaluative criterion.

Study Aids

Subjects	Internet Sites
General Information	http://www.niddk.nih.gov/health/house/digest/digest.htm
	http://www.eatright.org
	http://www.acg.gi.org
	http://www.sgna.org
Esophagus and Stomach	http://www.gerd.com
	http://helicobacter.com
	http://www.cdc.gov/epo/mmwr/preview/mmwrhtml/00049679.htm
Bowel Diseases	http://www.girf.org
	http://www.niddk.nih.gov/health/digest/pubs/divert/divert.htm
	http://www.ccfa.org
	http://www.iffgd.org
	http://www.uoa.org
	http://207.158.234.82
	http://www.wocn.org
Celiac Disease	http://www.celiac.org
	http://csaceliacs.org
	http://www.celiac.com
Liver Diseases	http://www.cdc.gov/ncidad/diseases/hepatitis/index.htm
	http://www.hepb.org
	http://www.scn.org/health/hepatitis/index.htm
	http://www.hepfi.org
	http://www.nhtech.demon.co.uk/pbc/index.html
	http://www.liver.ca
	http://www.cdc.gov/hepatitis
	http://www.cdc.gov/epo/mmwr/preview/mmwrhtml/00046679.htm
Alcoholism	http://www.niaaa.nih/gov
	http://www.ncadd.org
	http://www.health.org/search/treatdir97.htm
	http://www.med.uc.edu/alcohol/links.htm
	http://alcoholism.miningco.com/health/alcoholism/
Cystic Fibrosis	http://www.cff.org
	http://www.ccff.ca
	http://cf-web.mit.edu
	http://vmsb.csd.mu.edu/~5418/ukasr/cystic.html
	http://www.pslgroup.com/CF.HTM
	http://www.nhlbi.nih.gov/health/public/lung/other/cystfib.htm
	http://www.nhlbi.nih.gov/health/public/lung/other/cf.htm
	http://www.phd.msu.edu/cf/art.html
Fast Food Nutrition Analysis	http://www.mcdonalds.com/countries/usa/food/nutrient_breakdown/index.html
	http://www.wendys.com/The_menu/nut_frame.html
	http://www.tacobell.com/homepage/default2.asp

Chapter Review

1. Which of the following foods is allowed for a preoperative client on a low-residue diet?
   a. 8 ounces of milk with each of the three main meals
   b. Minestrone soup containing peas and lentils
   c. Ground beef on a white bun
   d. A fresh fruit salad

2. Increased fat in the bowel due to absorption problems may lead to kidney stones because:
   a. Fatty acids form the core of kidney stones.
   b. Less calcium is available to bind with oxalate to promote its excretion.
   c. The bile supply cannot meet demand, so fats are absorbed without emulsification.
   d. Waste material moves through the intestine so fast that insufficient water is absorbed to keep the urine dilute.

3. Clients who have had resection of the ileum should be monitored for:
   a. Iron-deficiency anemia
   b. Fat-soluble vitamin deficiency
   c. Calcium and phosphorus deficiency
   d. Vitamin B_{12} deficiency

4. A client with cirrhosis of the liver should be asked if he or she experienced _____ before ordering a diet.
   a. Headache
   b. Vomiting of blood
   c. A recent course of antibiotic therapy
   d. Hives

5. Which of the following meal components is likely to lessen symptoms of the dumping syndrome?
   a. Mashed fresh strawberries
   b. Orange sherbet
   c. Salt-free tomato juice
   d. Whole-wheat toast with dietetic jelly

Clinical Analysis

Mr. W is a 55-year-old white man admitted to the acute care unit with jaundice and ascites secondary to cirrhosis of the liver. He has gained 15 pounds in the past 3 weeks. He is a diagnosed alcoholic who has been through a detoxification program several times in the past 5 years. The dietitian has instructed Mr. W on a 1000-milligram sodium diet with a fluid restriction of 1000 milliliters per day.

1. When the nurse does the beginning of shift assessment, Mr. W says he has tried "cutting down on salt" when he started gaining weight, but it didn't work. Which of the following statements best reflects the nurse's understanding of Mr. W's pathology and treatment?
   a. Just cutting out added salt is not enough, because many foods are naturally high in sodium.
   b. Fluids are always restricted with a low-sodium diet.
   c. The ascites is caused by the inability of the liver to produce water-soluble bilirubin.
   d. Besides retaining sodium, Mr. W has ascites due to decreased blood pressure in the liver.

2. Mr. W vomits immediately after his next meal. The physician then orders a hydrating solution of 5 percent dextrose in water intravenously. If thiamin is not included in that order, the nurse should inquire about it because:
   a. Thiamin is necessary to predigest the dextrose for immediate absorption.
   b. Intravenous glucose without thiamin in the cirrhosis client can precipitate the Wernicke-Korsakoff syndrome
   c. Thiamin prevents folic acid stores from being diluted by the hydrating solution.
   d. Deficiency of thiamin causes delirium tremens.

3. Mr. W 's condition worsens. He is placed on a 30-gram protein diet. Mrs. W has been told the purpose of the protein restriction. The next day, Mrs. W asks the nurse, "If protein breakdown is causing the problem, why is he getting any at all?" Which of the following responses by the nurse would be most accurate?
   a. Some protein is necessary to spare glucose for basic energy needs.
   b. If the body receives no protein, it will destroy its own tissue to obtain it.
   c. The proteins in this diet are predigested and more easily absorbed than most.
   d. Protein is needed to feed the bacterial flora in the intestine.

Bibliography

Anthony, H, et al,: Current approaches to the nutritional management of cystic fibrosis in Australia. J Paediatr Child Health 34:170, 1998.

Aranda-Michel, J, and Giannella, RA: Acute diarrhea: A practical review. Am J Med 106:670, 1999.

Beresford, TP, et al,: Comparison of CAGE questionnaire and computer-assisted laboratory profiles in screening for covert alcoholism. Lancet 336:482, 1990.

Brook, G: Quality of life issues: Parenteral nutrition to small bowel transplantation—a review. Nutrition 14:813, 1998.

Bruun, LI, et al,: Prevalence of malnutrition in surgical patients: Evaluation of nutritional support and documentation. Clin Nutr 18:141, 1999.

Carlson, E: Irritable bowel syndrome. Nurse Pract 23:82, 1998.

Centers for Disease Control: Knowledge about causes of peptic ulcer disease—United States, March-April 1997. MMWR 46:985, 1997a. Accessed 6/14/2000 at http://www.cdc.gov/epo/mmwr/preview/mmwrhtml/00049679.htm

Centers for Disease Control: Nosocomial hepatitis B virus infection associated with reusable fingerstick blood sampling devices—Ohio and New York City, 1996. MMWR 46:217, 1997b. Accessed 6/14/2000 at http://www.cdc.gov/epo/mmwr/preview/mmwrhtml/00046679.htm

Chin, J (ed): Control of Communicable Diseases Manual, ed 17. American Public Health Association, Washington, DC, 2000.

Connon, JJ: Celiac disease. In Shils, ME, et al, (eds): Modern Nutrition in Health and Disease, ed 9. Lippincott Williams and Wilkins, Philadelphia, 1999.

Dannhauser, A, Van Zyl, JM, and Nel, CJC: Preoperative nutritional status and prognostic nutritional index in patients with benign disease undergoing abdominal operations: Part I. J Am Coll Nutr 14:80, 1995.

Detsky, AS, Smalley, PS, and Chang, J: Is this patient malnourished? JAMA 271:54, 1994.

Edington, J, Kon, R, and Martyn, CN: Prevalence of malnutrition after major surgery. J Human Nutr Dietet 10:111, 1997.

Ewing, JA: Detecting alcoholism: The CAGE questionnaire. JAMA 252:1905, 1984.

Fauci, AS, et al,: Harrison's Principles of Internal Medicine Companion Handbook. McGraw-Hill, New York, 1998.

Feinman, L, and Lieber, CS: Nutrition and diet in alcoholism. In Shils, ME, et al. (eds): Modern Nutrition in Health and Disease ed 9. Lippincott Williams and Wilkins, Philadelphia, 1999.

Fraser-Moodie, et al,: Weight loss has an independent beneficial effect on symptoms of gastro-oesophageal reflux in patients who are overweight. Scan J Gastroenterol 34:337, 1999.

Gaskin, KJ: Cystic fibrosis. In Walker, WA, and Watkins, JB: Nutrition in Pediatrics, ed 2. BC Decker, Hamilton, Ontario, 1997.

Griffiths, AM: Inflammatory Bowel Disease. In Shils, ME, et al, (eds): Modern Nutrition in Health and Disease, ed 9. Lippincott Williams and Wilkins, Philadelphia, 1999.

Hayes, DR, et al,: Management dilemmas in the individual with cystic fibrosis and diabetes. J Am Diet Assoc 94:78, 1994.

Jan, D, et al,: Up-to-date evolution of small bowel transplantation in children with intestinal failure. J Pediatr Surg 34:841, 1999.

Jester, R, and Williams, S: Pre-operative fasting: Putting research into practice. Nurs Standard 13:33, 1999.

Johnson, M, Maas, M, and Moorhead, S: Nursing Outcomes Classification (NOC), ed 2. Mosby, Philadelphia, 2000.

Kemppainen, T, et al,: Osteoporosis in adult patients with celiac disease. Bone 24:249, 1999.

Krieger, D, et al,: Manganese and chronic hepatic encephalopathy. Lancet 346:270, 1995.

Layrargues, GP, et al,: Role of manganese in the pathogenesis of portal-systemic encephalopathy. Metab Brain Dis 13:311, 1998.

Lieber, CS: Nutrition in liver disorders. In Shils, ME, et al, (eds): Modern Nutrition in Health and Disease, ed 9. Lippincott Williams and Wilkins, Philadelphia, 1999.

Liskow, B, et al,: Validity of the Cage questionnaire in screening for alcohol dependence in a walk-in (triage) clinic. J Stud Alcohol 56:277, 1995.

Lykins, TC, and Stockwell, J: Comprehensive modified diet simplifies nutrition management of adults with short-bowel syndrome. J Am Diet Assoc 98:309, 1998.

McCloskey, JC, and Bulechek, GM: Nursing Interventions Classification (NIC), ed 3. Mosby, Philadelphia, 2000.

Mullen, JL: Consequences of malnutrition in the surgical patient. Surg Clin North Am 61:465, 1981.

North American Nursing Diagnosis Association: Nursing Diagnoses: Definitions and Classification 1999–2000, North American Nursing Diagnosis Association, Philadelphia, 1999.

Rose, C, et al,: Manganese deposition in basal ganglia structures results from both portal-systemic shunting and liver dysfunction. Gastroenterology 117:640, 1999.

Rosenfeld, M, et al,: Nutritional effects of long-term gastrostomy feedings in children with cystic fibrosis. J Am Diet Assoc 99:191, 1999.

Rudman, D, et al,: Ammonia content of food. Am J Clin Nutr 26:487, 1973.

Saltzman, JR, and Clifford, BD: Identification of the triggers of celiac sprue. Nutr Rev 52:317, 1994.

Saltzman, JR, and Russell, RM: Gastrointestinal function and aging. In Morley, JE, Glick, Z, and Rubenstein, LZ (eds): Geriatric Nutrition, ed 2. Raven Press, New York, 1995.

Scanlon, VT, and Sanders, T: Student Workbook for Essentials of Anatomy and Physiology. FA Davis, Philadelphia, 1995.

Scully, RE, et al,: Case records of the Massachusetts General Hospital. N Engl J Med 331:383, 1994.

Sichiere, R, Everhart, JE, and Rothe, H: A prospective study of hospitalization with gallstone disease among women: Role of dietary factors, fasting period, and dieting. Am J Public Health 81:880, 1991.

Simon, JA, and Hudes, ES: Serum ascorbic acid and gallbladder disease prevalence among US adults. Arch Intern Med 160:931, 2000.

Smith, SW: Severe acidosis and hyperdynamic circulation in a 39-year-old alcoholic. J Emerg Med 16:587, 1998.

Soll, AH: Medical treatment of peptic ulcer disease: Practice guidelines. JAMA 275:622, 1996.

Stenson, WF: The esophagus and stomach. In Shils, ME, et al, (eds): Modern Nutrition in Health and Disease, ed 9. Lippincott Williams and Wilkins, Philadelphia, 1999.

Sullivan, M, and Heyman, MB: Increasing use of nutritional therapy in pediatric inflammatory bowel disease. RD (Health Communications, Darien, CT) 15:1, 1995.

Svanes, C: Trends in perforated peptic ulcer: Incidence, etiology, treatment, and prognosis. World J Surg 24:277, 2000.

Thomas, CL, ed: Taber's Cyclopedic Medical Dictionary, ed 18. FA Davis, Philadelphia, 1997.

Thompson, T: Thiamin, riboflavin, and niacin contents of the gluten-free diet: Is there cause for concern? J Am Diet Assoc 99:858, 1999.

Williams, LS, and Hopper, PD: Understanding Medical-Surgical Nursing. FA Davis, Philadelphia, 1999.

York, JL: Progression of alcohol consumption across the drinking career in alcoholics and social drinkers. J Stud Alcohol 56:328, 1995.

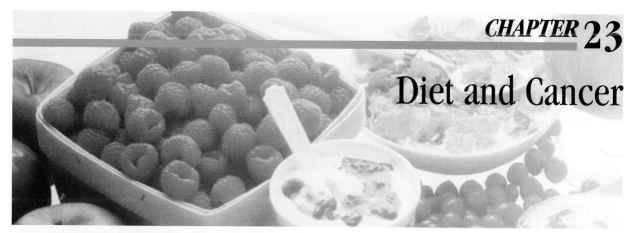

Diet and Cancer

LEARNING OBJECTIVES
After completing this chapter, the student should be able to:
1. Describe the ways in which foods are implicated in the development of cancer.
2. Identify reasons that population correlations may not apply to subgroups or to individuals.
3. List several correlations between dietary intake and cancers of specific sites.
4. Interpret dietary guidelines for the prevention of cancer.
5. Name several factors thought to contribute to loss of appetite in cancer clients.
6. Discuss measures to increase oral intake for clients with cancer.

Cancer has been known and described for thousands of years. Amazingly, one substance now linked to prevention was used as a treatment in ancient Rome, where crushed cabbage leaves were applied to cancerous ulcers (Albert-Puleo, 1983). Now cabbage is one of the cruciferous vegetables in the diet associated with reduced risk of cancers of the gastrointestinal and respiratory tracts. Cancer means "crab," for the creeping way in which it spreads.

Cancer is a general term for more than 100 types of malignant neoplastic disease. A cancer is a **neoplasm**, a new and abnormal formation of tissue (tumor) that grows at the expense of the healthy organism. Two main divisions of neoplasms are **malignant** tumors, which infiltrate surrounding tissue and spread to distant sites of the body, and **benign** tumors, which are localized. Two of the main types of cancer are sarcomas and carcinomas. **Sarcomas** arise from connective tissue, such as muscle or bone, and are more common in young people. **Carcinomas** occur in epithelial tissue and are more common in older people. Carcinomas include cancers of the lung, breast, prostate, and colon. The characteristics common to all types of cancer are uncontrolled growth and the ability to spread to distant sites (**metastasize**). Clinical Application 23–1 discusses the transformation of normal cells into cancer cells.

Cancer is the second most common cause of death in the United States after diseases of the heart. The age-adjusted death rate in 1997 was 125.6 per 100,000 standard population. Of the fifty states, Utah, Hawaii, and Colorado had the lowest age-adjusted death rates from cancer at 84.9, 95.5, and 101.4, respectively. Louisiana had the highest age-adjusted death rate at 146.6 per 100,000 standard population, followed by Kentucky with 145.7 and Delaware at 142.2 (Centers for Disease Control, 1999). The leading causes of cancer deaths in the United States for black and white men are cancers of the lung and bronchus, prostate, and colon/rectum. For white women, the most common causes of death are cancers of the lung and bronchus, breast, and colon/rectum. For black women, the top three sites are the same, but breast cancer is the leading cause of cancer death; however, it is rapidly being overtaken by cancer of the lung and bronchus (Cancer Rates, 2000). The top five sites of cancer occurrence by race or ethnicity and gender are illustrated in Figure 23–1. Figure 23–2 shows the mortality rates for all cancers in the United States. In general, the most commonly occurring cancers also cause the most deaths, except that cancer of the lung, which causes the most deaths, is second or third in frequency of occurrence (Data Evaluation and Publication Committee, 2000). Clients who are alive and without recurrence of cancer 5 years after diagnosis are considered cured. This is termed the *5-year survival rate*. The overall cancer survival rate is 55.5 percent for whites and 40.4 percent for blacks (Cancer Rates, 2000). Regardless of ethnicity, the 5-year survival rate for poor Americans is estimated to be 10–15 percent lower than that of middle-class and affluent Americans; at least half this difference in survival is a result of diagnosis late in the disease (Kagawa-Singer, 1995). Depending on the site in which the cancer occurs, the survival rates vary greatly.

This chapter considers diet and cancer. The relationship of diet to the development of cancer is explored first, followed by the nourishment of clients with cancer.

Interpreting Evidence Linking Cancer to Diet

The causes of cancer are complex and often incompletely understood. Certain cancers appear in great numbers in particular countries. Clinical Application 23–2 summarizes some of these findings. Although people in a given country may be influenced by many similar environmental factors, including diet, they also may have genes that are similar, compared to those found in people elsewhere. This chapter describes some examples

Transformation of Normal Cells into Cancer Cells

Cancer is basically uncontrolled replication of cells. Normal cells divide in the processes of growth and maintenance but stop dividing at appropriate points. Even in normal cell division, mistakes in deoxyribonucleic acid (DNA) transcription are made and corrected. Hundreds of incidents of oxidative damage to cell components, such as DNA, are estimated to occur in a cell daily but this oxidative damage has not been directly linked to cancer. Obviously, not all of these mistakes go on to turn cells cancerous. Multiple enzyme systems exist to repair or remove the damage (Poulsen, Prieme, and Loft, 1998). Several genes within a cell must be changed or **mutated** for cancer to occur.

Transformation of normal cells into cancer cells is a two-step process. The first step is **initiation**. The second step is promotion. Physical forces, chemicals, or biologic agents can damage genes. If the damage is not repairable, the gene has mutated, and if cancer develops later, the cancer cells are descendents of that mutated cell (Weinberg, 1996). The alteration may not be significant until the second step of the conversion to cancerous cells, **promotion**, takes place. The time period between initiation and promotion in some cases is 10–30 years but may be shorter if a mutated cancer-causing gene is inherited from a parent. Substances that enhance the expression of the altered gene are called promoters. They must be present at high levels for a prolonged period. Promoters are tissue specific: for instance, saccharin for cancer of the urinary bladder (in rats) and bile acids for colon cancer. In contrast to initiation, which results in permanent change, the process of promotion is reversible. Reducing exposure to high levels of promoters allows the body to repair the damaged cells.

Genes are carried in the DNA molecules of the chromosomes in the cell nucleus. Two classes of genes play major roles in the life cycle of cells: **proto-oncogenes** and **tumor suppressor genes**. In normal cells, proto-oncogenes support the growth and division of the cell, whereas tumor suppressor genes inhibit those processes. Both proto-oncogenes and tumor suppressor genes may be mutated and thus contribute to cancer development. The proto-oncogenes become carcinogenic **oncogenes** that stimulate excessive reproduction, and the tumor suppressor genes become inactivated and unable to stop the multiplication of cells. As more is learned about the molecular basis of cancer, therapies can be developed that target the aberrant cells much more accurately than the treatments currently available. Possibilities abound but might include transferring drug-resistance to healthy cells to protect them from chemotherapy agents, fortifying a client's immune system, and instilling genes into cancer cells that cause them to attract and absorb toxic drugs (Gene therapy, 1996).

of the associations that have been found and show the difficulty of pinpointing the causative links and thus the difficulty of identifying a dietary behavior to adopt or avoid to prevent cancer.

Dietary Components Associated with Cancer

It is difficult to assess the role of dietary components without also considering other factors that might contribute to the development of cancer. An estimated 50 percent of cancers may be related to diet, including 40 percent of those in men and 60 percent of those in women, despite the fact that women consume a more varied diet and less alcohol than men (Patterson et al., 1995). Diet is most strongly associated with cancers of the colon, rectum, prostate, and breast (Krebs-Smith, 1998). Much data has been compiled on breast cancer and diet. Clinical Application 23–3 gives a sample of these findings.

Excesses of Certain Substances

Some substances are associated with cancer when they are consumed in large quantities. This is the case with fat, alcohol, and pickled and smoked foods. The cooking method also may influence the development of cancer. These topics are addressed in the following section.

Fat

Some of the end products of fat metabolism are thought to be *carcinogenic*. That, plus the slow intestinal transit time, which increases the duration of exposure to the **carcinogen**, may contribute to the development of bowel cancer. Increased consumption of foods high in animal fat was linked to prostate cancer in blacks but not in whites (Hayes et al., 1999). Similarly, saturated fatty acids and animal fat from red meat were associated with a greater risk of aggressive or advanced prostate cancer (Giovannucci et al., 1993; Greco and Kulawiak, 1994). The early connection between dietary fat and breast cancer, however, is weakly present only in postmenopausal women, and the connection between colon cancer and fat intake may be a function of a component of red meat other than its fat content (Willett, 1999). Total energy, rather than the source of energy (fat, protein, or carbohydrate), was found to increase the risk for colon cancer in both men and women (Slattery et al., 1997).

Linoleic acid, an essential fatty acid found in corn oil, is classified as a promoter of cancer rather than as an initiator. Excessive intake of polyunsaturated fats has enhanced the development of breast, colon, pancreas, and prostate cancers in animals. Omega-3 fatty acids have been protective against cancer development; monounsaturated fatty acids have been neutral, neither promoting nor protecting against cancer. The current thinking is that total dietary fat is not a strong risk factor for cancer in humans but that additional information is needed regarding specific fatty acids in relation to causing or preventing cancer (Birt, Shull, and Yaktine, 1999).

Alcohol

Alcohol-induced cirrhosis, with resulting increased liver cell turnover, is associated with liver cancer. When combined with cigarettes or chewing tobacco, alcohol increases the risk of mouth, larynx, and throat cancers.

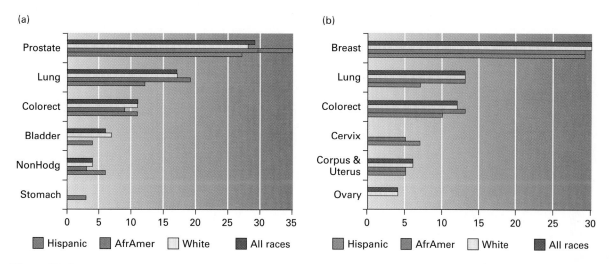

Figure 23–1:
The five most frequently occurring cancers in the United States by race/ethnic group and gender from 1993 to1997. Overall, two-thirds of the cancers developed in five sites in men and five sites in women. Shown are: (a) the five most common cancers in the United States for all races of men (prostate, lung, colon and rectum, bladder, and non-Hodgkin's lymphoma), and for white, African American, and Hispanic men; (b) the five most common cancers in the United States for all races of women (breast, lung, colon and rectum, corpus and uterus, and ovary), and for white, African American, and Hispanic women. (Data derived from Data Evaluation and Publication Committee, 2000.)

Heavy beer drinking is identified with colorectal cancer. Men who consumed more than two drinks daily had twice the risk of colon cancer as men who drank less than one-quarter of a drink daily. Inadequate folate and methionine intake increased the alcohol-associated risk for cancer of the distal colon approximately sevenfold (Giovannucci et al., 1995a). Alcohol also interferes with the availability of folic acid, which may explain its relationship to colon cancer (Willett, 1999).

Alcohol has been related to an increased risk of breast cancer. An estimated increase in risk of 40 percent was associated with each 24 grams of alcohol (about two drinks) consumed per day (Hunter and Willett, 1993). A possible pathophysiological reason for the correlation is discussed in Clinical Application 23–3.

Pickled and Smoked Foods

Cancers of the esophagus and stomach are correlated with large intakes of pickled and smoked foods. It is postulated that the process of smoking foods may result in their absorbing tar similar to that in tobacco smoke. Charcoal broiling presents the same type of danger, in that carcinogens may be deposited on the surface of the food.

Carcinogens Related to Cooking

High-temperature cooking of meat—frying, broiling, and grilling—produces substances known to cause cancer in animals when given at very high doses. Low-temperature, high-moisture cooking, such as stewing and pot-roasting, does not produce the same level of carcinogens. Even when pan frying, using lower temperatures and turning ground beef patties every minute reduced the carcinogen levels while safely inactivating bacteria (Salmon et al., 2000). In a human study, women who consumed hamburger, beef steak, and bacon that was consistently cooked to very

well done had a 4.6 times higher risk of breast cancer than women who consumed the meats cooked rare or medium done (Zheng et al., 1998). This is not as straightforward as it seems. Other researchers have demonstrated genetic differences related to an enzyme that catalyzes the formation of mutagenic products from cooked meats and fish. People who were classified as fast acetylators based on this enzyme had an 80 percent greater risk of colorectal cancer than did slow acetylators. Also, the risk increased with increasing meat consumption in the fast acetylators but not in slow acetylators (Roberts-Thomson et al., 1996).

Protective Dietary Components

Certain foods and nutrients have been associated with a decreased risk of cancer. Of particular note are fruits and vegetables and other foods containing fiber as well as vitamin E and calcium. Consumption of even relatively small amounts of fish also was found to be protective against cancers of the digestive tract (Fernandez et al., 1999).

Fruits and Vegetables

In many studies, fruits and vegetables seemed to be protective against cancer, especially of the lung and stomach (Willett, 1999). Analysis of the micronutrients contained in these fruits and vegetables shows some benefits, too, but not to the extent achieved by the whole plant foods (Hensrud and Heimburger, 1998). It is possible that all the micronutrients and phytochemicals have not been identified or that several of the components produce a synergistic effect. An Italian study found most vegetables inversely associated with cancer of the colon and rectum, high fruit intake inversely associated with rectal cancer, and only carrots and raw vegetables inversely associated with breast cancer (Franceschi et al., 1998).

Cancer mortality rates by state economic area (age-adjusted 1970 US population)

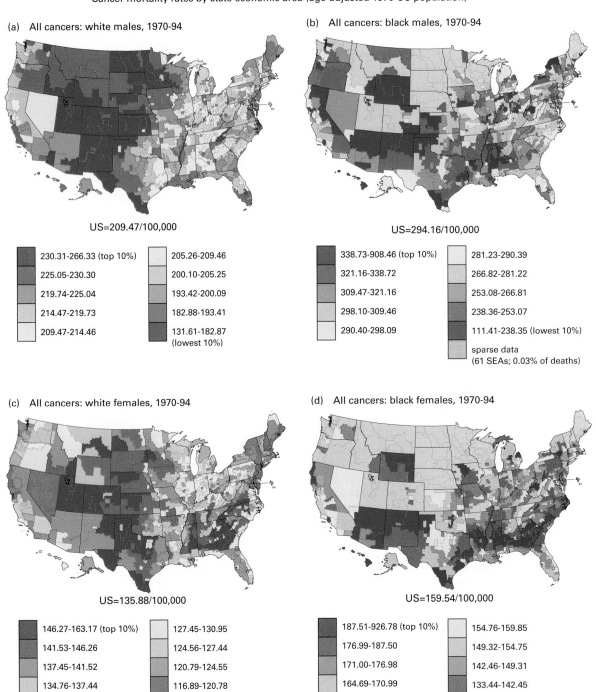

(a) All cancers: white males, 1970-94

US=209.47/100,000

230.31-266.33 (top 10%)	205.26-209.46
225.05-230.30	200.10-205.25
219.74-225.04	193.42-200.09
214.47-219.73	182.88-193.41
209.47-214.46	131.61-182.87 (lowest 10%)

(b) All cancers: black males, 1970-94

US=294.16/100,000

338.73-908.46 (top 10%)	281.23-290.39
321.16-338.72	266.82-281.22
309.47-321.16	253.08-266.81
298.10-309.46	238.36-253.07
290.40-298.09	111.41-238.35 (lowest 10%)
	sparse data (61 SEAs; 0.03% of deaths)

(c) All cancers: white females, 1970-94

US=135.88/100,000

146.27-163.17 (top 10%)	127.45-130.95
141.53-146.26	124.56-127.44
137.45-141.52	120.79-124.55
134.76-137.44	116.89-120.78
130.96-134.75	97.00-116.88 (lowest 10%)

(d) All cancers: black females, 1970-94

US=159.54/100,000

187.51-926.78 (top 10%)	154.76-159.85
176.99-187.50	149.32-154.75
171.00-176.98	142.46-149.31
164.69-170.99	133.44-142.45
159.86-164.68	54.08-133.43 (lowest 10%)
	sparse data (80 SEAs; 0.06% of deaths)

CLINICAL APPLICATION 23–2

Diet-Cancer Links in Various Populations

Particular cancers occur with greater frequency in some countries than others. When this was noted, the search began for dissimilarities in environment that could explain the differences. Because hereditary factors can confound the results when dissimilar populations are compared, the study of immigrants is especially enlightening.

In Japan there is more stomach cancer and less prostate and colon cancer than in the United States. In second-generation Japanese immigrants to the United States, however, the distribution of cancers becomes similar to that of other Americans. Similar findings are reported in Polish men for prostate cancer. Immigration, and presumed adoption of a Western diet, affects cancer development: age-adjusted breast cancer incidence rates per 100,000 Japanese women were 14 in Japan, 44 in Hawaii, and 57 in Los Angeles (Tomlinson, 1994).

Stomach and esophageal cancers are common where nitrates and nitrites are prevalent in food and water and where cured and pickled foods are popular. These areas include China, Japan, and Iceland. In Yangzhong, China, frequent intake of allium vegetables (garlic, onion, Welsh onion, and Chinese chives), raw vegetables, tomatoes, snap beans, and tea decreased the risk of stomach and esophageal cancer (Gao et al., 1999). Vitamins C and E and green tea can prevent formation of carcinogenic nitrosamines and nitrosamides (Greenwald, 1994; Ho et al., 1994; Kim et al., 1994). Residents of Linxian County, China, have one of the world's highest rates of esophageal and gastric **cardia** cancer; a 5-year trial of beta-carotene, vitamin E, and selenium reduced stomach cancer incidence by 20 percent and total mortality by 10 percent (Alberts and Garcia, 1995).

A low rate of colon cancer is seen in Africa. The diet there is high in fiber, and the Africans pass bulky stools. The theory put forth was that the fiber both dilutes the carcinogens in the feces and pushes them out of the body faster than a low-fiber diet would. New research shows that black South Africans consume less than the RDA for fiber, so the low risk for colon cancer was attributed to avoidance of excess animal protein and fat (O'Keefe et al., 1999). Avoidance is probably unintentional. The populations with high fiber intakes and low colon cancer rates also are seen in poor countries where obesity is uncommon, meat consumption is low, and physical activity is high.

VITAMIN C Foods containing vitamin C have been shown to protect against cancer of the stomach, esophagus, and oral cavity and to give moderate protection against cancers of the cervix, rectum, breast, and lung (Greenwald and McDonald, 1997). The highest intake of vitamin C from fruits and vegetables was correlated with the lowest risk for cancers of the gastrointestinal tract and lung (Birt, Shull, and Yaktine, 1999).

VITAMIN A AND CAROTENOIDS Foods high in beta-carotene have been associated with a reduced risk for stomach and lung cancers (Greenwald and McDonald, 1997). Vitamin A may control cell differentiation, influence host immune defenses, or protect against oxidation. Studies have shown that people with the overall highest cancer rates have lower serum retinol levels than other people. A clinical trial in Finland, however, when testing beta-carotene and vitamin E as cancer preventive agents for lung cancer, had the surprising finding of a 16 percent *increase* in lung cancer and an 8 percent *increase* in total mortality in the beta-carotene group. Similar results occurred, a 28 percent higher than expected incidence of lung cancer, when beta-carotene and retinol were given to men and women who had been heavy smokers and to men with extensive occupational asbestos exposure. An explanation for the increases in lung cancer awaits further study. Given the 10- to 30-year latency period for lung cancer, other variables may have contributed to the result.

Common vegetables and fruits contain approximately 50 carotenoids that possess antioxidant activity. Carotenoids other than beta-carotene (provitamin A) seem to be protective against cancer. Intake of tomatoes, tomato sauce, and pizza was found inversely associated with risk of prostate cancer (Giovannucci et al., 1995b). **Lycopene**, found in tomatoes, is the most efficient antioxidant of the carotenoids—but has no vitamin A potential—and is retained after heating (Franceschi et al., 1994). This carotenoid may explain the low rates of prostate cancer in Italy and Greece where the Mediterranean diet includes many tomato-based dishes. A high intake of raw tomatoes, more than seven servings per week, was significantly related to decreased risk for gastrointestinal cancers compared to an intake of less than two servings per week (Franceschi et al., 1994). Tomatoes have other components besides vitamin C and lycopene that may contribute to these findings, suggesting that at this stage of understanding, eating a variety of whole foods, not individual micronutrients, is the appropriate formula to decrease the risk of cancer.

FOLIC ACID Folate from dietary sources alone was related to a modest reduction in risk for colon cancer. Moreover, risk was 75 percent lower after 15 years of multivitamin use (Giovannucci et al., 1998). The women taking the most folic acid also were slightly thinner and consumed less fat and alcohol and more fiber than the other women, but after those factors were controlled, folic acid intake had the greatest impact on the reduced risk for colon cancer. Clinical Application 23–4 discusses vegetable intake, as opposed to pharmaceutical vitamin supplementation, in relation to cancer.

Figure 23–2 (Facing Page):
Mortality Rates for all cancers in the United States 1970–1994 by race and gender. Depicted here are mortality rates for all cancers for (a) white males, (b) black males, (c) white females, and (d) black females. Note that the legend colors denote different rates per 100,000 age-adjusted population for each map. The brightest red is assigned to the highest 10 percent of each group, so that it indicates rates of 230–260/100,000 population for white males but 339–908/100,000 for black males. This Web site also contains maps of mortality rates for about 40 specific cancers, maps by county, and maps for the years 1950–1969. (National Cancer Institute, 1999.)

CLINICAL APPLICATION 23–3

Breast Cancer and Diet

Early epidemiological research related high-dietary fat intake to breast cancer in many countries, but later case-control and prospective studies did not support a cause-and-effect relationship except in postmenopausal women (Howe et al., 1990; van't Veer, 1994). The type of fat also is important. Monounsaturated fats have been associated with decreased breast cancer risk (Greenwald and McDonald, 1997). Researchers in Europe did not rely on dietary data but biopsied gluteal fat, finding higher concentrations of trans fatty acids in women with postmenopausal breast cancer than in control subjects (Kohlmeier et al., 1997). The data on adult women cannot exclude the effect of fat intake in childhood or adolescence on later breast cancer (Hunter et al., 1996). Further evidence of youthful diet affecting breast cancer is the positive correlation between height and breast cancer, particularly linked to energy intake during peripubertal growth (Hunter and Willett, 1993; Vatten and Kvinnsland, 1990).

One key aspect of breast cancer involves the metabolism of estrogen. Risk of breast cancer increases 40–50 percent with estrogen replacement therapy and decreases with bilateral oophorectomy early in life (Hulka and Stark, 1995). Breast cancers with a high ability to take up estrogen, labeled estrogen receptor positive, are often treated by counteracting the hormone. Estrogen is produced not only by the ovaries but also by body fat cells. Thus, the fact that obesity increases the risk of breast cancer in postmenopausal women may be related to this source of estrogen. Of women with estrogen receptor positive breast tumors, 66 percent of the obese women had lymph node involvement compared to 32 percent of the lean women (Niwa, Swaneck, and Bradlow, 1994). Obesity at the time of diagnosis of breast cancer was associated with an increased risk of recurrence (Shils and Shike, 1999). Manipulating the fat in the diet has been shown to affect the amounts of estrogen in the blood even in the short-term. A 10- to 22-week trial to lower dietary fat intake from 37 to 20 percent of kilocalories reduced blood estradiol 17 percent (Prentice et al., 1990).

It is difficult to isolate single factors when studying the etiology of cancer. Estrogen is degraded by the liver, so impairment of liver function would increase the estrogen level in the blood. Alcohol taxes liver function and also has been associated with increased risk of breast cancer. In an analysis of six prospective studies, women who consumed 30–60 grams of alcohol per day had a 41 percent higher risk of invasive breast cancer than nondrinkers (Smith-Warner et al., 1998). In fact, data suggest the use of both alcohol and estrogen replacement therapy, considered in another context to confer cardiovascular benefits, may increase breast cancer risk more than either one used singly (Ginsburg, 1999). Enger and colleagues (1999) found that alcohol was not associated with a premenopausal risk of breast cancer, regardless of hormone receptor status, but suggested that alcohol may preferentially increase the risk of estrogen receptor positive breast cancer in postmenopausal women. In another study, however, alcohol was associated with breast cancer risk and low folate consumption. Among women who consumed at least 15 grams of alcohol (1 drink) per day, the risk of breast cancer was highest among those with low folate intake, whereas current use of multivitamin supplements was associated with lower breast cancer risk (Zhang et al., 1999).

Besides estrogen receptors, vitamin D receptors have been found on breast tumor cells. Their presence seems to be protective because clients whose tumors showed these receptors had a longer disease-free survival than those without them. These vitamin D receptors may help to explain the 55 percent higher breast cancer mortality in the Northeastern United States than in the Southeast and Southwest. Breast cancer rates are low in Japan, which is relatively far north, but the native Japanese diet contains large amounts of fish rich in vitamin D.

Attempts to correlate specific vitamins with a lower risk of breast cancer have been unsuccessful, but intake of fruits and vegetables has been shown to be protective (Hulka and Stark, 1995). Awareness that knowledge about disease etiology accrues in small increments will help to interpret the isolated and conflicting reports in the scientific and general press. Eating a balanced, varied diet in moderation, rather than supplementing with individual nutrients, is still the recommended course.

Fiber

In the United States, approximately one-third of all cancers have been attributed to the typical high-fat, low-fiber diet (Foerster, 1995). Increased intake of cereals and vegetables was related to a decreased risk of prostate cancer (Greco and Kulawick, 1994), but the relationship of fruits and vegetables to lower colon cancer rates does not seem to be caused by their fiber content, and the evidence for cereal grains contributing to low colon cancer rates is weak (Willett, 1999). Despite their relatively equal intakes of fat at 34–37 percent of kilocalories, the risk for colon cancer is lower in Finland than in either Denmark or New York and is attributed to con-

sumption of twice as much fiber in Finland (Greenwald and McDonald, 1997). It has been suggested, however, that all fiber is not of equal value and that perhaps a particular subset of fiber, as yet unspecified, confers all the protection.

Vitamin E

Vitamin E and selenium are both antioxidants that protect cells against breakdown. These two nutrients can substitute for one another, so relating one alone to cancer is a complicated process. The Finnish beta-carotene trial mentioned earlier also showed 34 percent fewer

---

The Role of Vegetables in Cancer Prevention

Low intakes of vegetables have been associated with stomach and colon cancers. In Japan, smokers who ingested yellow or green vegetables every day had 20–30 percent lower lung cancer rates than smokers who did not consume those vegetables every day.

Vegetables contain several substances that may contribute to cancer prevention. Some of these substances are carotene, indoles, and antioxidants.

Carotene, the precursor of vitamin A, is present in many green and deep-yellow vegetables. Vitamin A plays a role in cellular differentiation, a process that is faulty in the rapidly growing cancer cell. Thus, an adequate intake of carotene may be instrumental in preventing cancer. The fact that *supplementation* with beta-carotene was associated with increased morbidity and mortality from lung cancer should not deter someone from consuming vegetables rich in this nutrient.

Cruciferous vegetables, those of the cabbage family, are specifically recommended for cancer prevention. These vegetables contain phytochemicals called **indoles** that activate enzymes to destroy carcinogens (Niwa, Swaneck, and Bradlow, 1994; Stoewsand, 1995). Members of the cruciferous family include broccoli, Brussels sprouts, cabbage, cauliflower, collards, kohlrabi, and kale.

Antioxidants prevent oxidation of molecules by becoming oxidized themselves. Some molecules become very unstable when oxidized and damage nearby molecules. This reaction could modify a cell's DNA to set in motion the uncontrolled reproduction of cancer cells. Many vegetables contain carotene and vitamin C, which are antioxidants.

It is unclear which of these substances contributes the most to cancer prevention. In fact, antioxidants work together more effectively than individually (Kendler, 1995). It may be determined that another, yet-untested substance in the vegetables is more valuable for cancer prevention than those mentioned here. For these reasons, taking supplements is not recommended. Eating a variety of vegetables, including those linked to low cancer incidence, is the better method of protecting a person's health.

---

cases of prostate cancer and 16 percent fewer cases of colorectal cancer than expected in the men receiving vitamin E (Greenwald and McDonald, 1997). An adverse effect of vitamin E was seen in the increased deaths from hemorrhagic stroke in those receiving vitamin E (Alpha-Tocopherol, 1994).

Calcium

In both animals and humans, calcium seems to protect against colon cancer. Experts theorize that calcium reduces cell turnover rates and chemically interferes with bile acids and fatty acids to possibly reduce their toxicity. Increasing daily calcium intake by up to 1200 milligrams with low-fat dairy foods for 12 months in clients with prior polypectomies restored markers of normal cellular differentiation (Holt et al., 1998). In another study with an outcome of colon cancer, however, results varied according to family history, which illustrates the pitfall of focusing on diet to the exclusion of genetics. In that study, total calcium intake was inversely correlated with colon cancer among women with a negative family history for the disease but was unrelated to incidence in women with a positive family history (Sellers et al., 1998).

A component of foods recently receiving attention as having a possible role in cancer prevention is phytoestrogens or plant estrogens. These substances, found in a variety of foodstuffs, are discussed in Clinical Application 23–5.

Water

Drinking more than five glasses of water per day, compared to two glasses or less, was associated with half the risk of colon cancer in women (Shannon et al., 1996). Tap water, including coffee, tea, and cocoa, had an inverse dose-response relationship to cancer of the lower urinary tract in women, which was more pronounced in smokers (Wilkens et al., 1996). Both of these findings were part of larger investigations of food intake and cancer occurrence among men and women. The researchers did not speculate as to the lack of association of water intake in the men.

Questionable Relationships to Cancer

Studies have produced inconclusive data or conflicting reports on the relationship of certain substances to cancer. Two of these are caffeine and coffee. Total epidemiological evidence shows no substantial increase in breast cancer risk due to coffee-drinking (Hunter and Willett, 1993). Likewise, an Italian study found no appreciable association between coffee and pancreatic cancer (Soler et al., 1998).

Aflatoxins are inconclusively linked to cancer. **Aflatoxins** from molds are contaminants of improperly stored food. Aflatoxin contamination of peanuts and corn is related to primary liver cancer, especially in Africa and Asia. Interpreting this information is complicated, because hepatitis B is endemic to both continents. The cancer may be caused by the aflatoxins, by hepatitis B virus, or by both. No evidence relates aflatoxins to cancer risk in the United States. Box 23–1 outlines some of the factors to consider when confronted with research findings concerning nutrition. Even in science, there are relatively few sure things and no guarantees, even with an optimal diet, that one will not develop cancer.

Reducing the Risk of Cancer

Cancer evolves from genetic and environmental factors, of which diet is only one. Diet is likely to influence the premalignant phase of cancer development, but not frank tumor growth (Alberts and Garcia, 1995). Nevertheless, certain dietary practices are widely recommended to decrease the risk of cancer. For the most part, these practices have been incorporated into the Dietary Guidelines and the Food Guide Pyramid. Previous chapters detailed the extent to which Americans are not complying with the recommendations. Even following the rules perfectly, however, does not guarantee a disease-free life. Some advice specific to cancer prevention follows.

Phytoestrogens

These naturally occurring compounds have estrogenic or antiestrogenic activity. Phytoestrogens are present in many foods, including dried beans, broccoli, cabbage, carrots, cauliflower, chili, dark bread, grains, peas, soybeans, spinach, sprouts, and hops (Humfrey, 1998; Shoff et al., 1998). These plant estrogens are thought to balance levels of circulating hormones in both sexes. As such they are seen as playing a role in prevention of breast and prostate cancers (Stephens, 1999). Epidemiological studies suggest that phytoestrogens, especially soy and unrefined grain products, may be associated with a low risk of breast and prostate cancer (Strauss et al., 1998). A Hawaiian study showed that high consumption of soy products and other legumes was associated with a decreased risk of endometrial cancer in women who had never been pregnant or had never used unopposed estrogen medication (Goodman et al., 1997).

Some experts warn that caution is warranted. Although populations with high intakes of soy have lower prevalences of certain cancers, experimental data demonstrating a protective effect are lacking (Anderson, Smith, and Washnock, 1999). There is no direct evidence for the beneficial effects of phytoestrogens in humans, and possible adverse effects have not been evaluated (Strauss et al., 1998). For cancer of the prostate, colon, rectum, stomach, and lung, the evidence suggests a protective effect from a high intake of grains, legumes, fruits, and vegetables, but it is not possible to identify the responsible foods or components. In addition, although there is no evidence that the amount of phytoestrogens in the normal diet is harmful for adults, more research evidence is needed to recommend particular dietary practices (Humfrey, 1998). Special concern has been expressed regarding phytoestrogen exposure in infants. Infant soy formula appears to provide the highest of all phytoestrogen doses, but the effects of high doses of phytoestrogens in infants have not been documented (Humfrey, 1998; Sheehan, 1998).

Food Practices to Avoid

Persons attempting to minimize the risk of cancer should avoid excessive intakes of meat, fat, and alcohol.

Excessive Meat Consumption

Population studies link low cancer rates with low meat intake and high intake of vegetables and grains. Seventh Day Adventists and Mormons have a lower incidence of bowel cancer than other Americans, even when caffeine and alcohol differences between the study groups are equalized. Some Seventh Day Adventists eat meat, but those who did had higher rates of colon and prostate cancer than vegetarian members of the sect, and those who consumed the most beef had a higher risk of bladder cancer than those who consumed less (Fraser, 1999). A diet high in meat and fat from animal sources is associated with increased risk of non-Hodgkin's lymphoma in older women (Chiu et al., 1996).

Of particular concern is the consumption of smoked, salted, or nitrate-cured meat as indicated in Clinical Application 23-2. Consumption of bacon, sausage, and ham was associated with increased risk of lower urinary tract cancer in Hawaiian men of Japanese ancestry but not in those of Caucasian descent (Wilkens et al., 1996). These foods should be consumed infrequently. Matching these preserved foods with a good source of vitamin C to counter the effects of nitrosamines would be wise. Likewise, limiting the consumption of meats cooked at high temperatures may be desirable.

Consuming one or more servings of fish per week protected against digestive tract cancers in Italy (Fernandez, 1999). To what extent the fish-containing meals reduced meat consumption was not reported, but once again, the evidence supports the healthfulness of a varied diet.

Excessive Fat Consumption

Cancers of the uterus, colon, and prostate are linked to excessive fat consumption. Limiting fat intake to 30 percent of kilocalories is recommended. Substituting skim-milk dairy products for whole-milk products is a significant change for some people. Selecting lean meats and trimming fat is another step. Limiting fat intake without adding other foods in its place would also limit kilocalories, which seems to be beneficial.

Alcohol Consumption

When consumed by cigarette smokers, alcohol is linked to head and neck cancers. Liver cancer risk is increased by alcoholic cirrhosis. Excessive beer consumption is associated with rectal cancer, possibly due to the formation of a nitrosamine compound during direct-fire drying of barley malt. This discovery led to modification of the brewing process (Sugimura and Wakabayashi, 1999). In Italy, alcohol drinking (chiefly wine) was not correlated with colorectal cancers (Tavani et al., 1998). Evidence links alcohol consumption with breast cancer, but whether abstinence later in life reduces the risk is uncertain (Hunter, and Willett, 1993). The overall recommendation is to drink alcohol moderately, if at all.

Food Practices to Cultivate

Along with food practices to avoid, there are some food practices to cultivate to minimize cancer risk. These concern fruits, vegetables, and fiber that were addressed in a California program. Its logo is shown in Figure 23–3. The campaign used broadcast and print media and point-of-sale reminders, posters, and recipes to educate consumers (Foerster et al., 1995). Unfortunately, a survey of cancer risk behavior indicated that pressure from others (extrinsic motivation) may be less effective than beliefs (intrinsic motivation) in promoting healthful behaviors (Patterson et al., 1995).

Increase Intake of Particular Fruits and Vegetables

Even achieving an intake of two fruits and three vegetables per day would be a big improvement for many people. Regularly choosing those shown to have cancer prevention effects would be a plus.

THOSE HIGH IN VITAMIN C Ascorbic acid has both antioxidant and tissue-healing functions. It can prevent formation of carcinogenic nitrosamines and has been associated with lower rates of cancer in many populations.

THOSE HIGH IN CAROTENE These precursors of vitamin A have been associated with lower cancer rates. Because of the function of vitamin A in

Box 23–1 Research Findings: Probabilities Not Certainties

There is a natural progression in research from descriptive to experimental studies that involves an increase in the certainty that the findings reflect reality. Unfortunately, the significance and practical application of research results are often overstated and publicized in the general press before being replicated by other scientists. A single study may be interesting but should not be the basis for radical behavior changes. Peer scientists should examine all research for its strengths and weaknesses. Possible shortcomings affecting all research include:

- Inaccurate measurements. Recall data from questionnaires, although showing statistical differences in large studies, may not accurately reflect dietary intake or other behaviors. Even blood levels may be insensitive to small differences and may not correlate with cellular levels in certain organs.

- Imperfect statistical controls. Although extraneous variables are often held constant by statistical manipulation, the process is not perfect and all extraneous variables may not be considered.

- Incorrect assumptions. An underlying physiological basis for a given effect increases the credibility of research. New methods to test physiological effects often challenge earlier assumptions and conclusions. For instance, the mechanism supporting the value of cranberry juice in decreasing bladder infections was determined to be inhibition of E. coli. The earlier anecdotal evidence regarding cranberry juice was dismissed by scientists who assumed that the mechanism of action would have to be acidification of the urine, and cranberry juice did not make that much difference in pH.

The following table lists some of types of studies, their distinguishing qualities, and examples of individual studies with a nutritional focus.

TYPE OF STUDY	CHARACTERISTICS	APPLICATION TO NUTRITION	LIMITATIONS	EXAMPLE
Descriptive (Observational)	Reports naturally occurring events	Examines a population in relation to presence of risk factors, average intake of nutrients, cancer rates and mortality, utilization of health care, etc.	Diet is just one of many influences on health outcomes	In a random household survey, 70 percent of American Indian women reported they were overweight, and 12 percent reported chronic drinking. Their healthcare providers referred 30 percent of the women for breast cancer screening, 56 percent for cervical cancer screening, and only 15 percent of smokers for smoking cessation (Risendal et al., 1999).
Correlational	Compares phenomena in groups with particular outcomes	Determines the existence of systematic relationships between consumption of specific foods or supplements and cancer occurrence	Correlation does not establish causation. An untested variable may be causing the relationship.	
Case Control	Compares reported behavior by cancer patients with reported behavior by a control group of similar people without cancer		Controls may differ from cases in significant ways that were not considered and in ability to recall behavior accurately.	Total fluid intake showed a strong inverse dose-response relationship to lower urinary tract cancer among women (Wilkens et al., 1996).

(Continued on next page)

Box 23–1 Research Findings Report Probabilities Not Certainties (Continued)

TYPE OF STUDY	CHARACTERISTICS	APPLICATION TO NUTRITION	LIMITATIONS	EXAMPLE
Prospective (Cohort)	Measures phenomena of interest in a large population. Much later compares those with particular outcome to those without it in relation to the earlier determined practice.	Determines usual diet and other pertinent traits of large group of people at Point A. Waits until illness of interest develops in an adequate number of the people. Compares the groups with disease and without it in relation to the early diet.	Requires very large groups to obtain sufficient cases. May take years for illness of interest to develop.	Deaths from esophageal cancer were substantially associated with smoking, drinking alcohol, drinking very hot tea, and lower consumption of green-yellow vegetables among Japanese men and women (Kinjo et al., 1998).
Experimental	Comparing results of an intervention given to one group but not to another	Administers vitamin or specific food to one group, placebo or none to another. Measures changes in illness, symptoms, blood levels, etc.	Component selected for intervention may not be the one that gave the effect when whole foods were investigated.	
Cell and Tissue Cultures				Some omega-3 fatty acids inhibited the growth of colon, breast, and prostate cancers (Fernandez et al., 1999).
Animals			Very large doses may be used that are unrealistic to extrapolate to humans.	Caloric restriction reduced the incidence of mammary cancer in rats and prolonged the latency period to palpable mammary carcinomas in a dose-dependent manner (Zhu, Haegele, and Thompson, 1997).
Humans			Difficult to shield participant from knowing their intervention or control status. May take a long time to see an effect.	Serum levels of alpha-carotene and lutein were significantly higher in breast cancer clients encouraged to include vegetable juice in their high vegetable, low-fat diets than in breast cancer clients not instructed to drink vegetable juice (McEligot et al., 1999).

In summary, careful reading of research reports is required to make wise judgments about the applicability to health practices. Occasionally, an intervention trial is terminated early to permit an obviously effective treatment to be extended to the control group as in folic acid–neural tube defect case (MRC Vitamin Study Research Group, 1991) or to prevent harm as in the beta-carotene/vitamin A–lung cancer case (Redlich et al., 1998). Even in these rare situations, the complete reasons for the effect shown by the overwhelming evidence are not always clear. A broad perspective is necessary to guide a person's behavior toward healthy choices for a lifetime.

maintaining the integrity of epithelial tissue, carotene intake may help prevent cancers of these tissues. Preformed vitamin A as a supplement is not recommended because of possible toxicity. Supplemental beta-carotene is discouraged because of the adverse effects in smokers and lack of evidence of benefit for nonsmokers (Omenn, 1998). Consumption of foods high in beta-carotene and higher blood beta-carotene levels were found to be associated with lower rates of lung cancer, which stimulated the clinical trials of supplementation (Albanes, 1999). The association of supplemental beta-carotene and increased lung cancer occurrence in smokers and asbestos workers should not discourage people from eating foods rich in beta-carotene.

CRUCIFEROUS VEGETABLES Cancer clients have been found to eat less cabbage, broccoli, and Brussels sprouts than cancer-free persons. The other members of this vegetable family are cauliflower, collards, kale, and kohlrabi. Consuming these vegetables regularly may reduce the risk of cancer of the gastrointestinal and respiratory tracts.

Increase Fiber Intake

A diet markedly higher in fiber than the average American diet is recommended. Fiber promotes bile excretion and speeds up intestinal transit time so that carcinogens are eliminated more rapidly. Whether the increased fiber in grains and fruits and vegetables works through a mechanism of its own or by displacing meat and fat in the diet is unresolved, but the advice is still good. The Finnish people have a low colon cancer rate despite high-fat diets, but their diets are also high in fiber. International Dietary Guidelines to Prevent Cancer are shown in Box 23–2. They closely parallel the U.S. Guidelines discussed throughout the text.

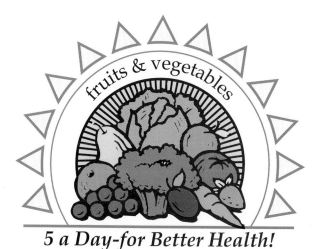

Figure 23–3:
National 5-a-Day Program logo. The program logo and slogan are registered service marks. To use them, food industry and state health authority partners sign a license agreement to follow guidelines that maintain the scientific integrity of all messages and other communications to the public. (From Foerster et al., 1995, with permission.)

Box 23–2 International Dietary Guidelines to Prevent Cancer

The American Institute for Cancer Research and the World Cancer Research Fund published these recommendations. Notice how closely they parallel the Food Guide Pyramid.
1. The diet should be based on plant products.
2. Cereals, legumes, and tubers should provide at least 50 percent of energy.
3. Sugars should provide less than 10 percent of energy.
4. 400 grams (about 14 ounces) of vegetables and fruits, to provide more than 10 percent of energy, should be consumed daily.
5. No more than 80 grams (about 2.9 ounces) of meat should be consumed, preferably fish or poultry, and limited amounts that are cured or smoked.
6. Fat intake should be limited to no more than 30 percent of energy, with a predominance of monounsaturated and polyunsaturated forms.
7. Total salt consumption should be less than 6 grams (about 1 teaspoonful of salt).
8. Perishable foods should be kept frozen or refrigerated and consumed promptly.
9. Foods should be cooked at low temperatures, and better boiled or steamed than fried or grilled.
10. Alcohol intake should not exceed two drinks a day.

(Munoz de Chavez and Chavez, 1998.)

Nutrition for Cancer Clients

Once a person has cancer, nutrition becomes part of the treatment. Despite the possible role of diet in preventing cancer, dietary manipulation has not been shown to cure cancer. The dietary goal is to maintain the client's strength to endure the treatment of the cancer. With the possible exception of those with acquired immune deficiency syndrome (AIDS), clients with cancer have the highest incidence of malnutrition among hospitalized clients (Ottery, 1995).

Cachexia

A state of malnutrition and wasting is called **cachexia**. Often associated with cancer, it is also seen in AIDS, alcoholism, malaria, tuberculosis, and pituitary disease. Cachexia affects one-third to two-thirds of cancer clients. It occurs, despite efforts to nourish the client, because of the tumor's effects on the client's metabolism. Several factors have been identified as mediators of tissue wasting in cachexia. Among them are two derived from the tumor, lipid-mobilizing factor (LMF) and protein-mobilizing factor (PMF). Of particular relevance to nutrition is that a polyunsaturated fatty acid, eicosapentaenoic acid (EPA), weakens the activity of LMF and PMF. Administration of EPA has stabilized the rate of weight loss, adipose tissue, and muscle mass in clients with inoperable pancreatic cancer (Tisdale, 1999). Figure 23–4 shows a woman with cachexia.

Cancer changes the client's carbohydrate metabolism. Insulin resistance is common. The client can no longer produce glucose efficiently from carbohydrate but instead uses tissue protein for energy. In traumatized noncancer clients, catabolism of fat for fuel gradually replaces protein breakdown. The cancer client's body does not make this adaptive change.

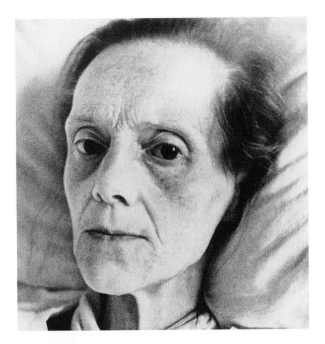

Figure 23–4:
This woman is cachectic, showing signs of malnutrition and wasting. (Reproduced from Nutrition Today, 16(3), cover, © by Williams and Wilkins, 1981, with permission.)

Special Needs

Food is therapy for cancer clients. Energy needs are one and one-half to two times the resting energy expenditure. (See Chapter 24, Nutrition During Stress.) Protein needs are 1.5–2 grams per kilogram of body weight. Optimal nutrition enhances medical treatments. During radiation therapy, good nutrition and elemental diets seem to lower the incidence of significant bowel injury (Nussbaum, Campana, and Weese, 1993).

Assessment

Unexplained weight loss is one of the seven danger signals of cancer, but it is not a universal sign. Compared to 80 percent of clients with cancers of the stomach and pancreas who experienced weight loss, just 31–40 percent of those with breast or hematologic cancers or sarcomas and 54–64 percent of those with cancers of the colon, lung, and prostate were so affected (Shils and Shike, 1999). Anorexia and changes in the sense of taste often precede the diagnosis of cancer. Because the tumor alters the person's metabolism, it is possible for weight loss to occur without a reduction in food intake. Pretreatment weight loss has been related to poor response to therapy (Ottery, 1994) and involuntary weight loss of more than 10 percent to poorer survival rates (Shils and Shike, 1999).

Cancer clients often develop ascites as well as accumulation of fluids in other body cavities. Interpreting the weight gain or loss may be difficult because of third-space sequestering of fluids. Nevertheless, weight is an important measure of progress in treating ascites

Serum proteins, particularly albumin, reflect skeletal muscle and visceral protein status. Serum protein levels were found to be lower in clients with pressure ulcers (pressure sores) if they also had cancer than

if they did not. Increased breakdown of the body's tissues and catabolism of the albumin produces low serum albumin levels. Values below 3.4 grams per deciliter are associated with increased morbidity and mortality after therapy (Daly and Shinkwin, 1991). Hypoalbuminemia also may be caused by nephrotic syndrome or loss of proteins from removal of third-space fluids. Serum transferrin is also used as a marker for protein status. Because its half-life is 8 days, compared to 20 days for albumin, serum transferrin levels reflect the client's responses to stress or to nutritional support faster than serum albumin levels.

A relatively simple summary measure of malnutrition uses three parameters: weight loss of 10 percent or more of body weight, serum albumin lower than 3.4 grams per deciliter, and serum transferrin lower than 190 milligrams per deciliter. The presence of any two of those findings indicates a need for nutritional support (Daly and Shinkwin, 1991).

Common Nutritional Problems in Cancer Clients

Some nutritional problems in cancer clients are due to the disease and others to treatment modalities. Common problems affecting the consumption of meals and nourishment of cancer clients are early satiety and anorexia, taste alterations, local effects in the mouth, nausea, vomiting and diarrhea, and altered immune response.

Early Satiety and Anorexia

Although they may look starved, cancer clients may take a few bites of food and declare that they are full. They may say that they have no appetite at all. The main source of this symptom is the cancer itself, by a mechanism that is incompletely understood (Tchekmedyian, 1993). Control of the disease improves the appetite. Sometimes, though, the physical pressure from the tumor or third-space fluid accumulation may give a feeling of fullness. Relieving that problem may improve food intake.

Some additional factors may interfere with appetite. The psychological stress of dealing with cancer may produce anxiety or depression. The person may be grappling with a body image change or may be going through the grieving process for the loss of a body function or the potential loss of life itself.

Taste Alterations

Cancer clients often have changes in taste perceptions, particularly a decreased threshold for bitterness. Accordingly, they will often say that beef and pork taste bitter or metallic. Some clients report a decreased sensation of sweet, salty, and sour tastes, and they desire increased seasonings. These taste changes are caused by the cancer and the various modes of therapy.

Local Effects in the Mouth

Clients who are being treated with radiation for head and neck cancers often experience mouth ulcers, decreased and thick saliva, and swallowing difficulty. Any of these may interfere with nutritional intake.

Nausea, Vomiting, and Diarrhea

This triad of symptoms often accompanies radiation treatment or chemotherapy, as well as certain types of tumors. Since the gastrointestinal tract cells are replaced every few days, these rapidly dividing cells are more vulnerable to the cancer treatments than are more slowly reproducing cells. Not all clients suffer these side effects to the same extent, and they generally cease when the treatment is completed.

Radiation enteritis involves injury to the intestine. Clients at greater risk of radiation enteritis are those who are thin; who have had previous abdominal surgery; who have hypertension, diabetes mellitus, or pelvic inflammatory disease; or who receive chemotherapy along with the radiation. Delays in presentation of symptoms of 20 years have been reported (Turtel and Shike, 1999).

Altered Immune Response

Sometimes, antineoplastic agents also suppress the client's immune system. Clients receiving them are at risk of overwhelming infections from organisms that would not affect other persons. Clients receiving radiation therapy or radiation as part of bone marrow transplantation also are at high risk of infections and need to be protected from all organisms, even those that are harmless to most healthy people. Clinical Application 23–6 discusses the role of the immune system in preventing cancer.

Nutritional Interventions

Based on the problem areas just discussed, dietary alterations are suggested. Parenteral therapy and tube feedings are covered in detail in Chapter 15.

For Early Satiety and Anorexia

Many nutrient-dense feedings are offered to the cancer client. For instance, adding 1 1/3 cups of instant dry skim milk powder to 1 quart of liquid milk increases the nutrient density, with little or no change in palatability.

Cancer clients should be encouraged to eat whether they are hungry or not. Appropriate exercise before meals may help to stimulate appetite. Attractively prepared food served in a pleasant environment is enticing. Very small servings, offered frequently, may increase the client's intake. For clients in the hospital, receiving favorite foods from home or sharing a meal with the family may help overcome the client's aversion to food and offer the family the opportunity to contribute to a loved one's care. Children sometimes can be coaxed to eat by decorating their food with faces or serving it in the form of designs such as cars or dolls or the child's name. Involving the child in food preparation or in choosing the menu can help to stimulate the appetite. Reorganizing a pediatric oncology unit to provide "room service" improved the children's energy intake significantly and their protein intake by 18 percent as well as their satisfaction with the hospital food service (Williams, Virtue, and Adkins, 1998).

For the severely anorexic client, offering 1 ounce of a complete nutritional supplement every hour can be effective in promoting nourishment. Clients with severe, chronic anorexia who can tolerate oral intake may benefit from drug therapy with megestrol acetate. This progesterone-like hormone with antineoplastic action has improved appetite and food intake in cancer clients, but increased survival time has not been documented (Tchekmedyian, 1993). When treating a terminally ill client, improving quality of life through some enjoyment of food and family is an appropriate goal. Nourishing the terminally ill client is the subject of Chapter 26.

To Combat Bitter or Metallic Tastes

Oral hygiene before meals freshens the mouth. Sometimes lemon-flavored beverages improve taste sensations. Cooking in a microwave oven or in glass utensils may minimize the metallic taste. As protein sources,

---

CLINICAL APPLICATION 23–6

Role of the Immune System in Preventing Cancer

Some experts believe that many cancers begin in a person's lifetime, only to be stopped by the body's defense system. The increased incidence of cancer in AIDS clients and organ transplant clients on immunosuppressive drugs offers credence to this theory.

One of the body's defenses is provided by certain white blood cells called **T-lymphocytes**. These cells have the task of recognizing foreign materials, including cancer cells, as "non-self" and acting to destroy the invaders. Some of the T-lymphocytes develop into killer cells, which bind to the foreign cell membrane and release lysosomal enzymes into the cancer cell which destroys it. The T-lymphocytes mature in the **thymus** gland in the chest, hence the name, thymic lymphocytes.

Contributing to the development of cancer in the elderly is the deterioration of the immune system. The thymus gland begins to shrink at sexual maturity. By age 50 only 10 percent of the original gland remains.

---

eggs, fish, poultry, and dairy products may be better received than beef or pork. Serving meat cold or at room temperature lessens the bitter taste. Sweet sauces and marinades added to the meat sometimes improves its palatability.

For Local Effects about the Mouth

A single canker sore can be remarkably painful. A cancer client with multiple oral ulcerations may complain of severe pain on food ingestion. In addition, some clients also have a dry mouth and difficulty swallowing. For all of these problems, good oral hygiene, before and after meals, is essential.

MOUTH ULCERATIONS Foods should be soft and mild. Sauces, gravies, and dressings may make foods easier to eat. Cream soups and milk provide much nutrition for the volume ingested. Cold foods have a somewhat numbing effect and may be better tolerated than hot food. Taking liquids with meals helps wash down the food. Drinking straws may help get the liquids past mouth ulcerations. Substances likely to irritate the mouth ulcerations should be avoided. These may include hot items, salty or spicy foods, and acidic juices.

To maintain oral intake, it may be necessary to resort to an anesthetic mouthwash. If the mouth is anesthetized, clients should be instructed to chew slowly and carefully to avoid biting their lips, tongue, or cheeks. A small study demonstrated the effectiveness of topical vitamin E oil in healing chemotherapy-induced mouth lesions (Wadleigh et al., 1992).

DRY MOUTH Adequate hydration helps keep the mouth moist. Food lubricants can be of value: gravy, butter, margarine, milk, beer, or bouillon may aid in consuming a near-adequate diet when the mouth is dry. Synthetic salivas are available also, but sips of water are often preferred. Sugarless hard candy, chewing gum, or popsicles may stimulate saliva production (Ganley, 1995).

SWALLOWING DIFFICULTY This problem may linger throughout a course of treatment. To combat it, clients should make swallowing a conscious act. They should inhale, swallow, and exhale. They should experiment with head position. Tilting the head backward or forward may help. Foods for these clients should be nonsticky and of even consistency. Lumpy gravy and mixed vegetables, for example, are hard to manage. Dunking bread products in beverages helps lubricate the passage.

For Nausea, Vomiting, and Diarrhea

Antiemetic medications should be given an appropriate number of hours before chemotherapy begins and continued on a regular schedule. These drugs are most effective if given prophylactically before the client becomes nauseated. Similarly, medications for pain and insomnia must be given liberally. Nausea and vomiting frequently accompany pain in clients without cancer, also. Controlling the pain may alleviate nausea to a great extent. A derivative of marijuana, dronabinol, has been approved by the Food and Drug Administration for prevention of serious nausea and vomiting from chemotherapy when other agents are ineffective. In addition to administering antiemetic drugs, the nurse should be alert for the need to monitor the client's hydration and electrolyte status.

As with morning sickness, eating dry crackers before arising may alleviate the nausea. Liquids taken between meals, rather than with them, reduce the volume in the stomach. Similarly, a low-fat diet is digested faster, leaving less content in the stomach to cause nausea or to be vomited. Clients should eat slowly and chew thoroughly. Resting after eating helps to control nausea. Foods the client especially likes should be saved for times when the client feels well, so that these favorite foods do not become associated with vomiting and are thereafter avoided. Food aversions develop in more than half of chemotherapy clients, usually involving two to four foods, but they may be accepted several weeks or months after the completion of therapy (Utermohlen, 1999).

As with the client who has gastrointestinal upset, clear liquids should be tried first, after vomiting ceases, and the diet progressed as tolerated. Unconventional mealtimes may be instituted to ensure that the client receives nourishment when nausea is minimal. If this means that breakfast is eaten at 2 a.m. and lunch at 6 a.m., so be it. This accommodation is truly individualized care.

Diarrhea may be countered by adding pectin-containing foods to the client's intake. Adding nutmeg to food to decrease gastric motility is suggested (Lowdermilk, 1995). A low-residue diet helps reduce intestinal stimulation. The possibility of lactose intolerance should be considered because of the destruction of the gastrointestinal mucosa. Active cultures of yogurt have been used to repopulate the intestine with bacteria when the flora normally present have been killed by the therapy or washed out by the diarrheal stools.

Pancreatic secretions and bile acids in the bowel seem to increase the susceptibility of the small bowel to radiation. Nourishing clients enterally with amino acids or partially digested protein and very little fat helped to decrease diarrhea and weight loss and to minimize interruptions to the treatment schedule. Such feedings are not recommended routinely because of the inconvenience but may be appropriate for malnourished clients or those with severe radiation toxicity (Turtel and Shike, 1999).

For Altered Immune Response

Clients may be placed in protective isolation to minimize their exposure to microorganisms. As for dietary interventions, fresh fruits and fresh vegetables may be restricted since they cannot be disinfected adequately. Yogurt also may have to be avoided because of the possibility of translocation of bacteria from the intestine to the bloodstream. Other measures are similar to those taken to protect AIDS clients and are discussed in Chapter 25, Diet in HIV and Aids.

Total Parenteral Nutrition or Tube Feedings

The principles of tube feeding and total parenteral nutrition (TPN) apply to cancer clients as well as to clients generally. Clients should be started on appropriate feeding methods before they become severely malnourished. Clients whose weight is 5 kilograms below their healthy body weight and whose serum albumin is less than 3 grams per 100 milliliters should be considered candidates for intensive nutritional support. Charting Tip 23–1 discusses documenting cancer clients' at-home treatments and diet plans.

Other Nursing Interventions

Oral hygiene before and after meals may help clients to eat better. Oral hygiene with isotonic saline alone or combined with soda bicarbonate is recommended. Alcohol and glycerine products dry the mucosa, and hydrogen peroxide damages new tissue.

Physical therapy to prevent further loss of muscle tissue due to weight loss is recommended (Ottery, 1994). Massage and relaxation exercises may assist clients in coping. Depending on the techniques used, massage can either stimulate or relax a person. Besides the local effects, the client receives the benefit of touch from another person. This can be very valuable, because cancer clients sometimes feel, rightly or wrongly, that they are being shunned. In one type of relaxation exercise, clients are coached to relax areas of the body in sequence. Others focus the client's mind on controlled breathing or mental images. These procedures have the added advantage of assisting the client to achieve some control over an oppressive situation. Clients respond differently to nursing interventions. No single technique works in every situation.

Nursing cancer clients requires creativity and patience. It also exemplifies one of the most satisfying rewards of nursing. By entering clients' lives at critical times, the nurse often shares their hopes and fears and memories. As often as not, we can learn as much from them as they can from us. Cancer clients, by confronting a potentially fatal disease, can teach themselves, their families, and their caregivers the truth of the adage that life is a journey, not a destination.

Charting Tip 23–1

- When admitting a client who provides much of his or her own care at home, try to learn all about treatments and dietary preferences and document them. If the client becomes less self-sufficient after surgery or after beginning cancer therapy, the staff will not have to ask multiple questions before providing care. Recording this information ensures that others besides the nurse who obtained it will be able to meet the client's needs.

Summary

Cancer is the second leading cause of death in the United States. Many different kinds of cancer exist, but all occur when normal cells reproduce uncontrollably both at the site of origin and in metastatic sites of the body. The two-step process of cancer development may evolve over decades, involving initiators that alter a cell's genes and promoters that then activate the altered genes to begin their unruly growth. As more is discovered about the molecular basis of cancer, more refined treatments will be possible.

Dietary guidelines to prevent cancer are similar to those discussed throughout this book. People should avoid excessive consumption of alcohol, fat, and meats, and especially meats that are cured or smoked. Positive dietary steps are to maintain generous intakes of fruits and vegetables, fiber, vitamin E, and calcium. Wellness Tips 23-1 summarizes general guidelines.

Cancer clients often present difficult nutritional challenges. Both the disease and its treatment can cause early satiety and anorexia, taste alterations, local effects in the mouth, nausea, vomiting, diarrhea, and altered immune responses. Creative interventions for these problems help make the client's life significantly more comfortable and can give a sense of accomplishment to the nurse.

Wellness Tips 23–1

- ***Do not smoke.***
- Eat a wide variety of fruits and vegetables. Eight to ten servings a day as recommended in the DASH Diet for hypertension would also be suitable in attempts to minimize cancer risk.
- Choose whole grains, cereals, and legumes to provide half the kilocalories in the daily diet.
- Select small portions (3 ounces/day) of fish, poultry, or meat and limit intake of cured or smoked products.
- Limit consumption of saturated fats in favor of monounsaturated and polyunsaturated forms.
- Confine salt intake to less than 6 grams (about 1 teaspoon) per day.
- Cook foods at low temperatures instead of by frying or grilling.
- If alcohol is consumed, restrict it to one to two standard drinks, depending on age, gender, and body size.
- If a supplemental vitamins and minerals are desired, pick a multivitamin/mineral product containing the nutrients at RDA levels rather than individual products.
- Avoid excess body weight.
- Exercise regularly.

Case Study 23–1

Ms. X is admitted to the hospital for a third course of chemotherapy. She is divorced, with no children, and lives with her mother, who is very supportive. Hopeful that this therapy will stem the cancer, Ms. X is determined to complete the prescribed treatments. Nausea and vomiting in the past two courses of chemotherapy caused her to suspend treatment before it was completed.

Ms. X is 42 years old, 5 ft, 5 in. tall, and weighs 123 lb. Her wrist measurement is 5 1/2 in. The mucous membranes of her oral cavity are intact. Her favorite foods are ice cream and steak, although for the past 2 months beef has tasted bitter to her.

Nursing Care Plan

Subjective Data	History of intolerance to chemotherapy due to excessive nausea and vomiting
	Taste alteration for beef
	Stated determination to complete treatment
Objective Data	94 percent healthy bodyy weight (131 lb)
	No breaks in mucous membranes of mouth
Nursing Diagnosis	NANDA: Altered Nutrition: Less than Body Requirements (North American Nursing Diagnosis Association, 1999, with permission.)
	Related to side effects of chemotherapy as evidenced by body weight 6 percent under healthy body weight for height

Desired Outcomes Evaluation Criteria	Nursing Actions/ Interventions	Rationale
NOC: Nutritional Status (Johnson, Maas, and Moorhead, 2000, with permission.)	NIC: Nutrition Therapy (McCloskey and Bulechek, 2000, with permission.)	
Client will maintain current weight during chemotherapy treatments.	Give antiemetics on scheduled basis for maximum effectiveness.	Antiemetics work better as preventive medicine than as curative.
	Assess daily the times nausea occurs. Schedule meals at other times.	Individualizing meal schedules for clients at high risk of malnutrition should increase dietary intake.
	Offer dry crackers whenever nausea occurs.	Some clients have received relief from nausea by eating dry crackers.
	Give gentle oral hygiene every 4 hours.	Keeping the oral cavity clean and fresh helps to maintain intake.

Continued on next page

Nursing Care Plan (Continued)

Desired Outcomes Evaluation Criteria	Nursing Actions/ Interventions	Rationale
	Encourage client to eat slowly and chew thoroughly.	Eating slowly and chewing thoroughly reduce the incidence and severity of nausea.
	Provide a back rub and quiet time after meals.	Rest after eating will lessen pressure on stomach and intestines. Appropriate massage induces relaxation.
	Teach relaxation exercises and controlled breathing to be used when nausea occurs.	These exercises give the client some control over her environment. Teaching the exercises before treatments begin will be more effective than trying to interrupt the cycle of nausea and vomiting once begun.
	If vomiting occurs, monitor weight, hydration, and electrolyte status.	Early identification and interruption of a pathological process permits easier and less invasive treatments. Loss of gastric secretions can cause fluid volume deficit and alkalosis.
	Consult with clinical dietitian and physician regarding high-protein, low-fat diet, enteral feeding, or TPN.	Although this client is not 10 percent below minimum body weight, if she loses an additional 5 lb, she will reach that benchmark. Aggressive nutritional support should begin before the client becomes severely malnourished.

Critical Thinking Question

1. What additional assessment data might impact the design of Ms. X's nursing care plan?
2. How could you involve the client's mother in her care?
3. Later, the physician's chart notes indicate Ms. X's cancer has not responded to treatment. Ms. X is aware of her situation. She tells the nurse, "If this doesn't work, I'm going to starve it out by fasting and purging." How should the nurse respond?

 # Study Aids

Subjects . . . . .Internet Sites

Cancer in General . . . . .http://www.cancer.org
http://www.cancernews.com
http://www.preventivenutrition.com
http://cancer.med.upenn.edu
http://www.nci.nih.gov/atlas

Diet and Cancer . . . . .http://rex.nih.gov
http://www.cancer.med.upenn.edu/causeprevent/diet/
http://www.aicr.org/reduce.htm
http://ificinfo.health.org/insight/dietcanc.htm

Survivors of Cancer . . . . .http://www.dianadyermsrd.com
http://wwwmother.com/~wesurviv/welcome.htm

Chapter Review

1. Excessive consumption of certain substances has been linked to increases in the occurrence of various cancers. Later research showed weaker connections than originally thought between which of the following?
   a. Alcohol and breast cancer
   b. Total dietary fat and colon cancer
   c. Red fruits and vegetables and prostate cancer
   d. Pickled and smoked foods and esophageal cancer

2. Cruciferous vegetables that are specifically thought to protect against cancer are:
   a. Corn, lima beans, and peas
   b. Carrots, green beans, and tomatoes
   c. Brussels sprouts, bean sprouts, and water chestnuts
   d. Broccoli, cauliflower, and cabbage

Continued on next page

Chapter Review (Continued)

3. Which of the following foods is likely to be well received by a cancer client with mouth ulcerations?
   a. Hot chicken noodle soup
   b. Orange juice with orange sherbet
   c. Vanilla milkshake
   d. Soda crackers with cream cheese
4. Which of the following is the best advice to increase oral intake for a chemotherapy client who suffers from nausea and vomiting?
   a. Drink plenty of fluids with the meal
   b. Eat high-fat, high-protein meals
   c. Take only foods that are well liked
   d. Eat slowly and chew thoroughly
5. If visitors brought all of the following to a client in protective isolation, which should the nurse question?
   a. Fruit basket
   b. Homemade vegetable soup
   c. Apple pie
   d. Malted milk and French fries

Clinical Analysis

Ms. P is a 38-year-old single mother of three who has returned to the clinic for follow-up after a breast biopsy. The tissue removed from her left breast was diagnosed as benign.

Ms. P is 5 feet, 6 inches tall and weighs 180 pounds. Meals at the P house are often hamburger dishes or ethnic combinations. Italian and Mexican foods are favorites of her children.

Ms. P's mother was treated for breast cancer at age 60, but is living and well. When interviewed by the nurse, Ms. P expressed interest in learning what she could do to lessen her chances of developing a malignancy of the breast.

1. Knowing that too radical a change is likely to be rejected by the client, the nurse concentrates on one improvement to be made in Ms. P's diet. Which of the following is likely to make the biggest difference in Ms. P's health?
   a. Substituting vegetable oil margarine for butter
   b. Increasing fluid intake
   c. Limiting fats to 30 percent of kilocalories
   d. Increasing protein to 20 percent of kilocalories

2. Which of the following suggestions should help Ms. P meet her new dietary goal?
   a. Avoiding gas-forming vegetables of the cabbage family
   b. Draining and rinsing cooked ground beef for one-dish meals
   c. Minimizing the use of tomato-based sauces
   d. Selecting aged cheddar rather than processed American cheese
3. Ms. P confides that her mother is a recovering alcoholic. She wonders if heavy alcohol consumption contributed to her mother's breast cancer. Which of the following answers would be best for the nurse to give?
   a. "Much evidence has shown alcohol is related to cancers of the gastrointestinal system and some evidence links it to breast cancer."
   b. "Probably not. Alcohol intake is related to liver cancer only."
   c. "Only if she also smoked. Alcohol must be potentiated by cigarettes to produce breast cancer."
   d. "Not at all. Alcohol has a sterilizing effect on the internal organs, so that any bacteria likely to translocate to the bloodstream would be eliminated."

Bibliography

Albanes, D: Beta-carotene and lung cancer: A case study. Am J Clin Nutr 69:1345S, 1999.

Albert-Puleo, M: Physiological effects of cabbage with reference to its potential as a dietary cancer-inhibitor and its use in ancient medicine. J Ethnopharmacol 9:261, 1983.

Alberts, DS, and Garcia, DJ: An overview of clinical cancer chemoprevention studies with emphasis on positive Phase III studies. J Nutr 125:692S, 1995.

Alpha-Tocopherol, Beta-carotene Cancer Prevention Study Group. Effect of vitamin E and beta-carotene on the incidence of lung cancer and other cancers in male smokers. N Engl J Med 330:1029, 1994.

Anderson, JW, Smith, BM, and Washnock, CS: Cardiovascular and renal benefits of dry bean and soybean intake. Am J Clin Nutr 70(3 suppl):464S, 1999.

Birt, DF, Shull, JD, and Yaktine, AL: Chemoprevention of cancer. In Shils, ME, et al. (eds): Modern Nutrition in Health and Disease, ed 9. Lippincott Williams and Wilkins, Philadelphia, 1999.

Cancer Rates. Accessed 01/07/2000 at http://rex.nci.nih.gov/NCI_Pub/Interface/rates30.html and http://rex.nci.nih.gov/NCI_Pub/Interface/rates/33.html.

Centers for Disease Control: Number of deaths, death rates, and age-adjusted death rates for major causes of death for the United States, each division, each state, Puerto Rico, Virgin Islands, Guam, and American Samoa, 1997. National Vital Statistics Reports. 47:82, 1999. Accessed 12/09/1999 at http://www.cdc.gov/nchs/fastats/pdf/47_19t24.pdf.

Chiu, BC-H, et al.: Diet and risk of non-Hodgkin lymphoma in older women. JAMA 275:1315, 1996.

Data Evaluation and Publication Committee: Top five most commonly diagnosed cancers diagnosed in the U.S. by race/ethnic group, 1993–1997. North American Association of Central Cancer Registries, 2000. Accessed 6/19/2000 at http://www.naaccr.org/data/cina9397/top59397.pdf.

Daly, HM, and Shinkwin, M: Nutrition and the cancer patient. In Holleb, AI, Fink, DJ, and Murphy, GP (eds): American Cancer Society Textbook of Clinical Oncology. American Cancer Society, Atlanta, 1991.

Enger, SM, et al.: Alcohol consumption and breast cancer oestrogen and progesterone receptor status. Br J Cancer 79:1308, 1999.

Fernandez, et al.: Fish consumption and cancer risk. Am J Clin Nutr 70:85, 1999.

Foerster, SB, et al.: California's "5 a Day—for Better Health" campaign: An innovative population-based effort to effect large-scale dietary change. Am J Prev Med 11:124, 1995.

Franceschi, S, et al.: Role of different types of vegetables and fruits in the prevention of cancer of the colon, rectum, and breast. Epidemiology 9:338, 1998.

Franceschi, S, et al.: Tomatoes and risk of digestive-tract cancers. Int J Cancer 59:181, 1994.

Fraser, GE: Associations between diet and cancer, ischemic heart disease, and all-cause mortality in non-Hispanic white California Seventh-day Adventists. Am J Clin Nutr 70(3Suppl):532S, 1999.

Ganley, BJ: Effective mouth care for head and neck radiation therapy patients. Medsurg Nurs 4:133, 1995.

Gao, CM, et al.: Protective effect of allium vegetables against both esophageal and stomach cancer: A simultaneous case-referent study of a high-epidemic area in Jiangsu Province, China. Jpn J Cancer Res 90:614, 1999.

Gene therapy. Cancer Smart 2:10, 1996.

Ginsburg, ES: Estrogen, alcohol and breast cancer risk. J Steroid Biochem Mol Biol 69:299, 1999.

Giovannucci, E, et al.: Alcohol, low-methionine-low-folate diets, and risk of colon cancer in men. J Natl Cancer Inst 87:265, 1995a.

Giovannucci, E, et al.: Intake of carotenoids and retinol in relation to risk of prostatic cancer. J Natl Cancer Inst 87:1767, 1995b.

Giovannucci, E, et al.: Multivitamin use, folate, and colon cancer in women in the Nurses' Health Study. Ann Intern Med 129:517, 1998.

Giovannucci, E, et al.: A prospective study of dietary fat and risk of prostate cancer. J Natl Cancer Inst 85:1571, 1993.

Greco, KE, and Kulawiak, L: Prostate cancer prevention: Risk reduction through lifestyle, diet and chemoprevention. Oncol Nurs Forum 21:1504, 1994.

Greenwald, P: Antioxidant vitamins and cancer risk. Nutrition 10:433, 1994.

Greenwald, P, and McDonald, SS: Cancer prevention: The roles of diet and chemoprevention. Cancer Control: Journal of the Moffitt Cancer Center 4:118, 1997. Accessed 01/06/2000 at http://www.medscape.com/moffitt/ CancerControl/1997/v04.n02/cc04 and at http://www.medscape.com/moffitt/CancerControl/1997v04.n02/cc0402 .03.gree.htm.

Goodman, MT, et al.: Association of soy and fiber consumption with the risk of endometrial cancer. Am J Epidemiol 146:294, 1997.

Hayes, RB, et al.: Dietary factors and risks for prostate cancer among blacks and whites in the United States. Cancer Epidemiol Biomarkers Prev 8:25, 1999.

Hensrud, DD, and Heimburger, DC: Diet, nutrients, and gastrointestinal cancer. Gastroenterol Clin North Am 27:325, 1998.

Ho, C-T, et al.: Phytochemicals in teas and rosemary and their cancer-preventive properties. In Huang, M-T, et al. (eds): Food Phytochemicals II: Teas, Spices, and Herbs. American Chemical Society, Washington, DC, 1994.

Holt, PR, et al.: Modulation of abnormal colonic epithelial cell proliferation and differentiation by low-fat dairy foods: A randomized controlled trial. JAMA 280:1074, 1998.

Howe, GR, et al.: Dietary factors and risk of breast cancer: Combined analysis of 12 case-control studies. J Natl Cancer Inst 82:561, 1990.

Hulka, BS, and Stark, A: Breast cancer: Cause and prevention. Lancet 346:883, 1995.

Humfrey, CD: Phytoestrogens and human health effects: Weighing up the current evidence. Nat Toxins 6:51, 1998.

Hunter, DJ, et al.: Cohort studies of fat intake and the risk of breast cancer—a pooled analysis. N Engl J Med 334:356, 1996.

Hunter, DJ, and Willett, WC: Diet, body size, and breast cancer. Epidemiologic Reviews 15:110, 1993.

Johnson, M, Maas, M, and Moorhead, S: Nursing Outcomes Classification (NOC), ed 2. Mosby, Philadelphia, 2000.

Kagawa-Singer, J: Socioeconomic and cultural influences on cancer care of women. Semin Oncol Nurs 11:109, 1995.

Kendler, BS: Free radicals in health and disease: Implications for primary health care providers. Nurse Pract 20:29, 1995.

Kim, M, et al.: Preventive effect of green tea polyphenols on colon carcinogenesis. In Huang, M-T, et al. (eds): Food Phytochemicals II: Teas, Spices, and Herbs. American Chemical Society, Washington, DC, 1994.

Kinjo, Y, et al.: Mortality risks of oesophageal cancer associated with hot tea, alcohol, tobacco, and diet in Japan. J Epidemiol 8:235, 1998.

Kohlmeier, L, et al.: Adipose tissue trans fatty acids and breast cancer in the European Community Multicenter Study on Antioxidants, Myocardial Infarction and Breast Cancer. Cancer Epidemiol Biomarkers Prev 6:705, 1997.

Krebs-Smith, SM: Progress in improving diet to reduce cancer risk. Cancer 83:1425, 1998.

Lowdermilk, DL: Home care of the patient with gynecologic cancer. J Obstet Gynecol Neonatal Nurs 24:157, 1995.

McCloskey, JC, and Bulechek, GM: Nursing Interventions Classification (NIC), ed 3. Mosby, Philadelphia, 2000.

McEligot, AJ, et al.: Comparison of serum carotenoid responses between women consuming vegetable juice and women consuming raw or cooked vegetables. Cancer Epidemiol Biomarkers Prev 8:227, 1999.

MRC Vitamin Study Research Group: Prevention of neural tube defects: Results of the Medical Research Council Vitamin Study. Lancet 338:131, 1991.

Munoz de Chavez, M, and Chavez, A: Diet that prevents cancer: Recommendations from the American Institute for Cancer Research. Int J Cancer Suppl 11:85, 1998.

National Cancer Institute: Atlas of Cancer Mortality in the United States, 1950–94. National Institutes of Health, 1999. Accessed 6/21/2000 at http://www.nci.nih.gov/atlas.

North American Nursing Diagnosis Association: Nursing Diagnoses: Definitions and Classification 1999–2000, North American Nursing Diagnosis Association, Philadelphia, 1999.

Niwa, T, Swaneck, G, and Bradlow, HL: Alterations in estradiol metabolism in MCF-7 cells induced by treatment with indole-3-carbinol and related compounds. Steroids 59:523, 1994.

Nussbaum, ML, Campana, TJ, and Weese, JL: Radiation-induced intestinal injury. Clin Plastic Surg 20:573, 1993.

O'Keefe, SJ, et al.: Rarity of colon cancer in Africans is associated with low animal product consumption, not fiber. Am J Gastroenterol 94:1373, 1999.

Omenn, GS: Chemoprevention of lung cancer: The rise and demise of beta-carotene. Annu Rev Public Health 19:73, 1998.

Ottery, FD: Rethinking nutritional support of the cancer patient: The new field of nutritional oncology. Semin Oncol 21:770, 1994.

Patterson, RE, et al.: Diet-cancer related beliefs, knowledge, norms, and their relationship to healthful diets. J Nutr Educ 27:86, 1995.

Poulsen, HE, Prieme, H, and Loft, S: Role of oxidative DNA damage in cancer initiation and promotion. Eur J Cancer Prev 7:9, 1998.

Prentice, R, et al.: Dietary fat reduction and plasma estradiol concentration in healthy postmenopausal women. J Natl Cancer Inst 82:129, 1990.

Redlich, CA, et al.: Effect of supplementation with beta-carotene and vitamin A on lung nutrient levels. Cancer Epidemiol Biomarkers Prev 7:211, 1998.

Risendal, B, et al.: Cancer prevention among urban southwestern American Indian women: Comparison to selected Year 2000 national health objectives. Ann Epidemiol 9:383, 1999.

Roberts-Thomson, I, et al.: Diet, acetylator phenotype, and risk of colorectal neoplasia. Lancet. 347:1372, 1996.

Salmon, CP, et al: Minimization of heterocyclic amines and thermal inactivation of *Escherichia coli* in fried ground beef. J Nat Cancer Inst 92:1773, 2000.

Sellers, TA: Diet and risk of colon cancer in a large prospective study of older women: An analysis stratified on family history (Iowa, United States). Cancer Causes Control 9:357, 1998.

Shannon, J, et al.: Relationship of food groups and water intake to colon cancer risk. Cancer Epidemiol Biomarkers Prev 5:495, 1996.

Sheehan, DM: Herbal medicines, phytoestrogens and toxicity: Risk-benefit considerations. Proc Soc Exp Biol Med 217:379, 1998.

Shils, ME, and Shike, M: Nutritional support of the cancer patient. In Shils, ME, et al. (eds): Modern Nutrition in Health and Disease, ed 9. Lippincott Williams and Wilkins, Philadelphia, 1999.

Shoff, SM, et al.: Usual consumption of plant foods containing phytoestrogens and sex hormone levels in postmenopausal women in Wisconsin. Nutr Cancer 30:207, 1998.

Slattery, ML, et al.: Dietary energy sources and colon cancer risk. Am J Epidemiol 145:199, 1997.

Smith-Warner, SA, et al.: Alcohol and breast cancer in women: A pooled analysis of cohort studies. JAMA 279:535, 1998.

Soler, M, et al.: Diet, alcohol, coffee, and pancreatic cancer: Final results from an Italian study. Eur J Cancer Prev 7:455, 1998.

Stephens, FO: The rising incidence of breast cancer in women and prostate cancer in men. Dietary influences: A possible preventive role for nature's sex hormone modifiers—the phytoestrogens (review). Oncol Rep 6:865, 1999.

Stoewsand, GS: Bioactive organosulfur phytochemicals in Brassica oleracea vegetables—a review. Food Chem Toxic 33:537, 1995.

Strauss, L, et al.: Dietary phytoestrogens and their role in hormonally dependent disease. Toxicol Lett Dec 28: 102, 1998.

Sugimura, T, and Wakabayashi, K: Carcinogens in foods. In Shils, ME, et al. (eds): Modern Nutrition in Health and Disease, ed 9. Lippincott Williams and Wilkins, Philadelphia, 1999.

Tavani, A, et al.: Alcohol intake and risk of cancers of the colon and rectum. Nutr Cancer 30:213, 1998.

Tchekmedyian, NS: Treatment of anorexia with megestrol acetate. Nutr Clin Prac 8:115, 1993.

Tisdale, MJ: Wasting in cancer. J Nutr 129(1S Suppl):243S, 1999.

Tomlinson, SS: Dietary and lifestyle factors associated with breast cancer rates. J Am Acad Phys Assist 7:622, 1994.

Turtel, PS, and Shike, M: Diseases of the small bowel. In Shils, ME, et al. (eds): Modern Nutrition in Health and Disease, ed 9. Lippincott Williams and Wilkins, Philadelphia, 1999.

Utermohlen, V: Diet, nutrition, and drug interactions. In Shils, ME, et al. (eds): Modern Nutrition in Health and Disease, ed 9. Lippincott Williams and Wilkins, Philadelphia, 1999.

van't Veer, P: Diet and breast cancer: Trial and error? Ann Med 26:453, 1994.

Vatten, LJ, and Kvinnsland, S: Body height and risk of breast cancer. A prospective study of 23,831 Norwegian women. Br J Cancer 61:881, 1990.

Wadleigh, RD, et al.: Vitamin E in the treatment of chemotherapy-induced mucositis. Am J Med 92:481, 1992.

Weinberg, RA: How cancer arises. Scientific American 275:62, 1996. Accessed 6/27/2000 at http://www.sciam.com/0996issue/0996weinberg.html.

Wilkens, LR, et al.: Risk factors for lower urinary tract cancer: The role of total fluid consumption, nitrites, and nitrosamines, and selected foods. Cancer Epidemiol Biomarkers Prev 5:161, 1996.

Willett, WC: Diet, nutrition, and the prevention of cancer. In Shils, ME, et al. (eds): Modern Nutrition in Health and Disease, ed 9. Lippincott Williams and Wilkins, Philadelphia, 1999.

Williams, R, Virtue, K, and Adkins, A: Clinical issues. Room service improves patient food intake and satisfaction with hospital food. J Pediatr Oncol Nurs 15:183, 1998.

Zhang, S, et al.: A prospective study of folate intake and the risk of breast cancer. JAMA 281:1632, 1999.

Zheng, W, et al.: Well-done meat intake and the risk of breast cancer. J Natl Cancer Inst 90:1724, 1998.

Zhu, Z, Haegele, AD, and Thompson, HJ: Effect of caloric restriction on pre-malignant and malignant stages of mammary carcinogenesis. Carcinogenesis 18:1007, 1997.

Nutrition During Stress

Stress is any stimulus or condition that threatens the body's mental or physical well-being. This chapter discusses how the body responds to four distinct types of stress and how this condition impacts nutritional needs. The chapter begins with a discussion of mental stress experienced by physically healthy persons. The body's response to mental stress differs markedly from the response to starvation, severe physical injury that invokes a hypermetabolic response, and respiratory stress. The body's response is different for each of these physical stressors. The chapter concludes with a discussion of the principles for safely refeeding nutritionally deprived clients.

Nutrition and Mental Stress

The effects of mental stress cannot be isolated easily from the effects of physical stress. The physical self and the mental self are structurally related. For example, in the presence of danger, a series of chemical reactions occurs that are associated with our feeling of fear. Hormones mediate the fight-or-flight response, discussed in Chapter 1, Evolution and the Science of Nutrition. In other words, the fear (mental factor) triggers the hormones (physical factors). Despite the relationship between mental and physical stress, no reliable evidence shows that mental stress increases the need for kilocalories or nutrients.

Not All Stress Is Negative

A balanced amount of stress maximizes health. Human beings need some stress for mental well-being. For example, boredom is stressful for many people. Mental stresses related to ambition, drive, and desire may in fact be perceived as positive. Stress, such as strain, tension, and/or anxiety, is commonly perceived as negative. Most people perceive the death of a spouse, divorce, unemployment, financial problems, and personal injury as negative. Clearly, we cannot control all the events that affect us. However, we do have some control over how we respond to such events. The relationship between nutritional status and people's response to emotional stress has not been completely researched.

Chronic Disease

Mental stress is related to the incidence of cancer, cardiovascular disease, hypertension, and some forms of gastrointestinal diseases. All of these chronic diseases are related to nutrition. Epidemiological evidence indicates that diets that contain significant amounts of fruits, vegetables, and grains are associated with a lower incidence of heart disease and certain cancers. But it is not known which, if any, specific substances in the diet are responsible or whether taking more than the RDA doses of supplements may do more harm than good (Quandt, 1999). A healthy mental state is known to be important for reducing the risk of heart disease. People who are ordinarily tense, impatient, and ambitious tend to have a high serum cholesterol level. Clients with diabetes report that emotional stress increases their blood glucose levels.

The dietary treatments for chronic diseases should focus on dietary components that are known to be related to health outcomes. For example, clients who have diabetes benefit the most from a carbohydrate-, fat-, and kilocalorie-controlled diet to normalize blood and lipid levels and maintain or lose body weight. Maintenance of body weight by both diet and exercise has been shown to help prevent cancer, diabetes, hypertension, and heart disease. Sodium-restricted diets have been shown to help control of hypertension.

Gastrointestinal Complication

Ulcers and some intestinal diseases are aggravated by perceived excessive mental stress. A client may report that he or she has specific food intolerances when under emotional stress but that the same food is easily tolerated in the absence of stress. This is partially due to impairment of gastrointestinal function during episodes of stress. Decreased motility can cause the development of anorexia, abdominal distention, gas pains, and constipation. These symptoms may contribute to food intolerances or reduced food intake. Thus, the effects of emotional stress, including food intolerances, can vary not only from person to person, but also in the same person at different times.

Food Intake

The volume of food a client consumes and the desire to prepare food are sometimes affected by emotional stress. Some people respond to stress by eating more; others respond by eating less. Mental stress can cause a person to lose interest in food preparation. Thus, mental stress can lead to either overnutrition or undernutrition. An individual's perceived stress should always be taken into consideration when formulating the nutritional component of a care plan.

The time at which food is eaten also may be important. Undernutrition is related to cognition. Extensive evidence indicates that relatively modest increases in circulating glucose concentrations enhance learning and memory processes in rats and humans. For example, students who eat breakfast score higher on examinations than those who do not (Gold, 1995).

Requirements for Nutrients

Nutrition experts believe the need for most nutrients is not increased above the RDA solely as a result of excessive mental activity. The needs for kilocalories, amino acids, and vitamins in healthy individuals have all received some attention from scientists.

Kilocalories

Mental stress alone does not increase our need for kilocalories. For example, mental effort used in studying demands few, if any, additional kilocalories. Likewise, a single person coping with financial problems, a job, and childrearing does not require extra kilocalories solely as a result of excessive mental activity. Because mental stress does not require additional kilocalories, our requirement for certain vitamins is not increased solely as a result of mental activity. Thiamin, riboflavin, and niacin requirements are based on kilocalorie or protein requirements; if the need for kilocalories (protein) is not increased, neither is the requirement for these vitamins.

A person who responds to mental stress with increased physical movement or muscle activity requires additional kilocalories to maintain his or her body weight. Mental stress may cause a person to sleep less, walk more, tremble, fidget, or otherwise increase the work of the muscles. In this situation, additional kilocalories are needed in underweight clients.

Amino Acids

Research has failed to show a relationship between amino acids and stress in healthy individuals. Recently, many health-food manufacturers have developed erogenic aids (amino acid supplements) that falsely claim to increase stamina, endurance, and muscle development by releasing growth hormone. There is no scientific evidence that these products actu-

ally release growth hormone, which is fortunate because if they did, acromegaly might result (Barrett and Herbert, 1999). Acromegaly is a disease marked by elongation and enlargement of facial and extremity bones. This condition is often associated with somnolence, moodiness, and decreased libido. The Federation of American Societies for Experimental Biology (FASEB) has criticized the widespread use of amino acids in supplements because little scientific literature exists about most amino acid supplements taken by healthy persons, because no scientific rationale has been presented to justify the use of amino acid supplements by healthy individuals, and because safety levels for amino acid supplements have not been established (Barrett and Herbert, 1999).

Vitamins and Minerals

The majority of evidence gathered thus far indicates that vitamins in excess of the RDA do not counterbalance the negative effects of mental stress. Manufacturers of nutritional supplements for "stress" have yet to produce valid scientific evidence that their products have a health benefit. In 1990, the Federal Trade Commission (FTC) barred a large manufacturer from making unsubstantiated claims that any vitamin product is needed to replace nutrients lost as a result of athletic activity or the stress of daily living (Barrett and Herbert, 1999). A healthy, well-balanced diet with adequate protein, fiber, minerals, and vitamins is the best nutritional insurance against excessive stress. Maintenance of a healthy body weight is an indication that kilocaloric intake is appropriate.

The Stress of Starvation

The physical stress of starvation does alter nutrient needs. Biologically, our bodies evolved to cope with periods of feast or famine. Our response to the stress of starvation evolved slowly over the course of millions of years. The human body's response to food deprivation differs from the body's response to other forms of stress.

Uncomplicated starvation means that the client is experiencing food deprivation without an underlying disease state. During uncomplicated starvation, clients expend about 70 percent of the kilocalories they normally need to maintain body weight. Because of the biochemical adaptation to starvation, these clients require fewer kilocalories than is normal for their height and weight.

The human body has a well-defined response to starvation. The breakdown or catabolism of nutrient stores to meet energy needs characterizes our response. Every cell within the human body needs a constant supply of energy to function. During starvation, a series of chemical reactions occurs to meet each cell's energy needs. A summary of these chemical reactions follows:

1. **Glycogenolysis** is the breakdown of glycogen (the liver's carbohydrate stores). This releases glucose into the bloodstream. However, the body's limited glycogen stores last only a few hours.
2. **Gluconeogenesis** is the production of glucose from noncarbohydrate stores (only the glycerol portion of triglycerides and amino acids derived from proteins in muscle and organ mass). The primary source of glucose in early starvation is the increased rate of gluconeogenesis.
3. **Lipolysis** is the breakdown of adipose tissue for energy. This releases free fatty acids into the bloodstream. In prolonged

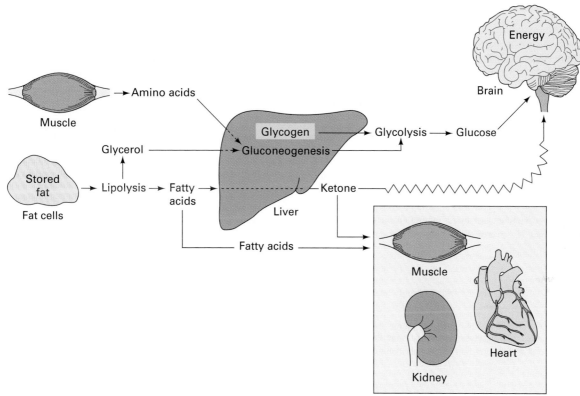

Figure 24–1:
Origin of fuel and fuel consumption during starvation. The primary source of glucose in early starvation (after the depletion of glycogen stores) is the increased rate of gluconeogensis. In prolonged starvation, adaptive mechanisms conserve protein by enabling a greater proportion of energy needs to be met by ketone bodies, with a decreased requirement for glucose.

starvation, adaptive mechanisms conserve body protein stores by enabling a greater proportion of energy needs to be met by increased fatty acids, with a decreased requirement for glucose.

4. **Ketosis** is the accumulation in the body of the ketone bodies: acetone, beta-hydroxybutyric acid, and acetoacetic acid. Ketosis results from the incomplete metabolism of fatty acids, generally from carbohydrate deficiency, and occurs commonly in starvation. The body utilizes some ketone bodies for energy during prolonged starvation to meet the central nervous system's need for glucose. This reduces, but does not eliminate, the need for glucose.

These chemical reactions are summarized in Figure 24–1.

Each body cell needs glucose, fatty acids, or the end products of fatty acids and amino acids for energy. Body cells need fuel constantly. Amino acids can be utilized for energy, but only after the liver converts them into glucose or fat. Specific organs have a preference for glucose as a fuel source. (The medical literature uses the word *preference* in this context; the word *affinity* may be substituted for preference.) The brain prefers glucose for energy. Some cells can also utilize ketone bodies for energy. The brain will use ketone bodies but prefers glucose. For the most part, the human body can use only a very small part of the fat molecule, the glycerol portion, to manufacture glucose. This means that body protein

stores must be continually broken down to supply the brain with glucose during starvation after the liver's glycogen stores are depleted.

The heart, kidney, and skeletal muscle tissues prefer fatty acids and/or ketone bodies for their fuel sources. This means that even if a starving person is fed glucose (as in intravenous feeding), some fat is still needed to prevent the breakdown of adipose tissue. A balance of the end products of fat and carbohydrate metabolism is necessary for survival.

In prolonged starvation, most body organs switch to a less preferred fuel source. Even the brain increasingly begins to utilize more ketone bodies for energy after adaptation to starvation than before. The breakdown of muscle tissue continues in prolonged starvation, but at a much lower rate than previously. The human body also becomes more efficient in reusing amino acids for protein synthesis. Thus, urea nitrogen excretion decreases during prolonged starvation. The rate of tissue breakdown in prolonged starvation also decreases because the metabolic rate and total energy expenditure decrease to conserve energy and prolong life. The catabolic or starved individual spontaneously decreases physical activity, increases sleep, and has a lower body temperature. All of these adaptations during prolonged starvation serve one purpose—to prolong life. The human body gets "more miles per gallon" as a result of individual body organs switching to a less preferred fuel source.

The Stress Response

A severe physical assault to the body invokes the stress response. The term *stress response* refers to major changes in metabolism that occur after severe injury, illness, or infection. Kilocaloric needs decrease during uncomplicated starvation and increase (sometimes markedly) as a result of bodily response to stress. The stress response is a dynamic process that has an ebb phase, a flow phase, and an anabolic phase. A client can progress or regress from one phase to another during his or her clinical course. The need for protein varies according to the client's stress level.

Ebb Phase

The **ebb phase** begins with an initial stress stimulus and typically lasts for approximately 24 hours. Blood pressure, cardiac output, body temperature, and oxygen consumption are all reduced during the ebb phase. The body does this so that it has the capacity to meet the increased demands of the environment. These clients require about 1.5 grams of protein per kilogram of body weight per day.

Flow Phase

Increased cardiac output, increased urinary nitrogen losses, altered glucose metabolism, and accelerated catabolism characterize the flow phase. In addition, the **flow phase** is marked by pronounced hormonal changes. Table 24–1 lists hormones secreted during this stage of the stress response and describes the impact these hormones have on metabolism. These hormonal conditions favor the breakdown of body protein stores to provide glucose. This leads to a rapid loss of nitrogen in the urine as lean body mass is broken down to furnish the cells with glucose. The need for protein is about 2 grams per kilogram of body weight during the flow phase but is highly dependent on the severity of the injury. The administration of elevated levels of protein may contribute to a high

TABLE 24–1 Hormonal Secretion during Phase Two of the Stress Response and the Metabolic Effect of These Hormones*

Hormonal Secretions	Effect of Metabolism
Increased epinephrine	Rate of lipolysis increased Rate of glycolysis increased Rate of gluconeogenesis increased
Decreased insulin	Storage of glucose, fatty acids, and amino acids ceases. Glucose delivery to the cells thus decreases. For this reason, hyperglycemia is commonly seen in stressed clients.
Increased glucagon	Rate of gluconeogenesis increases
Increased antidiuretic hormone	Increase in water retention
Increased aldosterone	Increase in sodium retention

*Net effect: decrease in body protein and fat stores.

Glutamine and Stress

Glutamine is a nonessential amino acid. During stress the body's requirement for glutamine appears to exceed the individual's ability to produce it in sufficient amounts. Current research is exploring the provision of supplemental glutamine to enhance the recovery of the seriously ill client. Alitraq, manufactured by Ross Laboratories, is a specialized elemental formula for medical use that is high in glutamine.

renal load, especially in infants and elderly adults, dictating routine monitoring of fluid status, blood urea nitrogen, and serum creatinine levels (Skipper, 1998).

Blood flow to the gastrointestinal tract is often diminished during this phase of the stress response. This reduced flow decreases the supply of both oxygen and nutrients to the gastrointestinal tract. The secretion of mucus is diminished, and the secretion of gastric acid is increased. Cells that line the gastrointestinal tract waste away and die as a result of these changes. The client may complain of diarrhea and bloating.

Recovery or Anabolic Phase

The third stage of the stress response, the **anabolic phase**, is also marked by changes in hormonal secretions. Insulin and growth hormone increase in the bloodstream during the anabolic phases. Secretion of most of the other hormones decreases. The building up of body tissue and nutrient stores (anabolism) characterizes this phase. Protein need during the anabolic phase is 2–3 grams per kilogram of body weight but depends on the severity of the injury.

It is obviously desirable for a client to progress to the third phase of the stress stage as rapidly as possible. Tissue building, or anabolism, is beneficial. The ability of a client to rebuild tissue after a physical stress depends on several factors. Age is one factor. The client's prior nutritional status and the severity and duration of the stress particularly influence tissue growth. Clients who have ample nutrient stores to draw on during stress are better able to tolerate the negative effects of the stress. Good nutrition is a form of insurance, because the nutrient stores are available to be used if an unexpected stress occurs. Recent research has shown that early supplementation with the amino acid glutamine may enhance the progression to the anabolic phase of the stress response (see Clinical Application 24–1).

Nutrition and Metabolic Stress from Illness, Trauma, and Infection

Cancer, major surgery, burns, infections, and trauma are the physical stressors that have the greatest impact on metabolism. The needs of clients with cancer are described in Chapter 23. This section of this chapter focuses on the nutritional needs of clients experiencing surgery, burns, infections and fevers, and trauma. Nutritional support during extreme stress is needed to decrease the length of the stress, prevent complications, and minimize human suffering.

Hypermetabolism

Hypermetabolism is an abnormal increase in the rate at which fuel or kilocalories are burned. Hypermetabolism can be identified by an increased metabolic rate, negative nitrogen balance, hyperglycemia, and increased oxygen consumption. Clients are hypermetabolic during the flow phase of the stress response.

Protein Needs

Protein needs are elevated during hypermetabolism. Injury or illness requires active protein formation. Surgical wound healing, tissue repair, replacement of red blood cells and plasma protein lost in hemorrhage, and the immune response to infection all require a constant supply of protein. For these reasons, a client who is hypermetabolic has an increased need for protein. A hypermetabolic client may lose as much as 250 grams (about 1/2 pound) of muscle tissue per day.

URINE ASSESSMENT OF PROTEIN STATUS Total urinary excretion of nitrogen increases with the client's stress level. Urinary creatinine measurements may be used to estimate muscle protein reserves. One problem common to the use of all urinary measurements is the completion of an accurate 24-hour urine collection. Nurses are typically responsible for collecting a 24-hour urine specimen from the client. If even one voiding is discarded, the measurement will be inaccurate.

Kilocalories and Hypermetabolic Stress

Clients who are hypermetabolic have an increased need for kilocalories. The negative nitrogen balance observed in hypermetabolic clients may be the result of inadequate kilocaloric intake rather than of insufficient protein intake, or of both.

EARLY FEEDING The use of early nutritional support has been studied. The use of enteral nutrition shortly after the event that precipitated the stress may be advantageous because it supplies essential nutrients, keeps the gastrointestinal tract active, and halts the elevation of levels of catabolic stress hormones. Enteral feeding has been found to directly nourish the gastrointestinal tract and may help reverse the defective gut barrier that accompanies burn shock. In contrast, intravenous nutritional support appears to lack effectiveness in burn patients and may actually increase morbidity and mortality (Hansbrough, 1998).

Although early enteral feeding offers many advantages, the introduction of nutrients into the gastrointestinal tract needs to be evaluated on an individual basis. Low mesenteric blood flow (commonly referring to the peritoneal fold that encircles the small intestine), severe tachycardia, hypotension, a volume deficit, and multi-system organ failure preclude the use of enteral feedings.

KILOCALORIE NEEDS Energy expenditure is the number of kilocalories that an individual uses to meet the body's demand for fuel. The kilocalorie need of a person is calculated by this formula:

Resting Energy Expenditure × Activity Factor = Daily Energy Allowance

The hypermetabolic client's kilocaloric need has been well researched. Major body stressors increase kilocaloric needs. The kilocaloric need of a hypermetabolic client is often calculated with this formula:

Resting Energy Expenditure × Activity Factor × Stress Factor = Estimated Energy Need

Each part of this formula is discussed in detail.

Clinical Calculation 24–1 Calculation of Kilocaloric Need for Both a Male and a Female

Male Client

Energy Need = REE
× Activity Factor × Stress Factor

Step 1: Use the following Harris-Benedict equation to calculate the male client's resting energy expenditure:

REE = 66 + (13.7 × weight in kg)
+ (5 × height in cm) − (6.8 × age)

Step 2: Multiply an activity factor by the client's REE (from Table 24-2).

Step 3: Multiply the answer obtained in step 2 by the appropriate stress factor (Table 24–3).

Female Client

Energy Need = REE
× Activity Factor × Stress Factor

Step 1: Use the following Harris-Benedict equation to calculate the female client's resting energy expenditure:

REE = 655 + (9.6 × weight in kg)
+ (1.7 × height in cm) − (4.7 x age)

Step 2: Multiply an activity factor by the client's REE (Table 24-2):

REE × Activity Factor

Step 3: Multiply the answer obtained in step 2 by the appropriate stress factor (from Table 24–3):

REE × Activity Factor × Stress Factor

Example Calculation

Assume you need to estimate the kilocalorie need of a 154-lb (70-kg) male who is 5 ft 5 in. (165 cm) tall and 25 years old. Assume he is confined to bed and has a fractured long bone.

Sample calculation for step 1:

70-kg male who is 165 cm tall and 25 years old

REE = 66 + (13.7 × 70) + (5 × 165) − (6.8 × 25)
REE = 66 + 959 + 825 − 170
REE = 680

Sample calculation for step 2:

REE × Activity Factor
1680 × 1.2
2016

Sample calculation for step 3:

Answer from step 2 × Stress Factor

2016 × 1.35
2721.6 = client's estimated energy need

RESTING ENERGY EXPENDITURE (REE) The Harris-Benedict equation is widely used to estimate REE for critically ill clients. The Harris-Benedict equation is presented in Clinical Calculation 24–1, along with an example of these calculations. Note that different equations are used for male and

Table 24–2 Activity Factors Commonly Used to Calculate a Client's Activity Kilocaloriesr

For a client confined to bed	0.2, or 20 percent
For a client out of bed	0.3, or 30 percent

female clients. The Harris-Benedict equation allows the health care provider to calculate estimated kilocalorie needs based on an individual client's height, age, and weight.

ACTIVITY FACTOR The Harris-Benedict equation calculates the patient's REE. Physical activity is not included in the REE and must be calculated. Table 24–2 shows activity factors for clients confined to bed as 0.20, or 20 percent, and for those not confined to bed as 0.30, or 30 percent.

STRESS FACTOR Research has shown that different types of stress increase kilocaloric needs differently. A **stress factor** is a number assigned to a given pathological state to predict how much a client's kilocaloric need has increased as a result of the type of stress the client is experiencing from that stress state. Table 24–3 lists various types of physical stress and the stress factor used for each disease state.

As you can see in the table, a client with burns over 50 percent of his or her body has a stress factor of 2.0. This means kilocaloric need is twice (200 percent) his or her resting energy expenditure. In contrast, the stress factor after minor surgery is 1.05. This means a client who has had minor surgery needs only 5 percent more kilocalories than his or her REE multiplied by the previously determined physical activity factor. Stress factors are convenient to use in estimating kilocaloric needs.

Kilocalorie:Nitrogen Ratios in the Hypermetabolic Client
Protein requirements cannot be totally separated from energy requirements because protein is used as an energy source in the absence of adequate kilocalories. The current practice is to calculate **kilocalorie:nitrogen ratios** for hypermetabolic clients. As a rule, the average healthy person needs 1 gram of nitrogen per 300 kilocalories (range 1:300 to 350). One gram of nitrogen is derived from 6.25 grams of protein. A hypermetabolic client needs approximately 1 gram of nitrogen per 100 to 150 kilocalories (range 100 to 200) (Souba and Wilmore,

TABLE 24–3 Stress Factors Commonly Used to Determine a Client's Need for Kilocalories

Stressor	Factor
Uncomplicated minor surgery	1.05
Starvation	0.70
For each degree F above 98.6	1.07
Cancer	1.1–1.45
Soft tissue trauma	1.14–1.37
Skeletal trauma (fracture)	1.35
Burns (10–30 percent of body surface area)	1.5
Burns (30–50 percent of body surface area)	1.75
Burns (>50 percent of body surface area)	2.0
Peritonitis	1.2–1.5
Major sepsis	1.4–1.8

1999). A hypermetabolic client needs about twice as much protein as a client not in a state of hypermetabolism. Clinical Calculation 24–2 demonstrates the calculation of kilocalorie:nitrogen ratios in a TPN solution. Most nutritional supplements have the kilocalorie:nitrogen ratio of the product listed either on the label or in a package insert.

Vitamin and Mineral Needs

The hypermetabolic client usually requires increased B vitamins, vitamin A, and zinc (Skipper, 1998). The B vitamins help release the chemical energy stored in foods. Whenever a client requires increased kilocalories, the need for the B-vitamin complex automatically increases. When anabolism or the building of body tissue is indicated, vitamin C requirements are increased. Hypermetabolic clients usually need to build up depleted tissue stores. Electrolyte (sodium, potassium, chloride, phosphorus, calcium, and magnesium) manipulation during the ebb phase is most often accomplished using the intravenous route (Skipper, 1998).

Examples of Hypermetabolic Conditions

The hypermetabolic conditions that influence nutritional needs most profoundly are major surgery, burns, infections and fevers, and trauma. All of

Clinical Calculation 24–2 Calculation of a Sample TPN Solution

Please calculate the total kilocalories, nonprotein calories, grams of nitrogen, calorie/nitrogen ratio, and percent calories from fat in the following TPN solution: 500 cc D50, 500 cc amino acids 10 percent, 250 cc lipid 20 percent.

Dextrose:

$$D50 = 0.50 \times 500 \text{ cc} = 250 \text{ g dextrose}$$
$$250 \text{ g} \times 3.4 \text{ kcal/g} = 850 \text{ kcal}$$

Amino Acids:

$$500 \text{ cc} \times 0.10 = 50 \text{ g protein}$$
$$50 \text{ g protein} \times 4 \text{ kcal/g} = 200 \text{ kcal}$$

Lipids:

$$250 \text{ cc} \times 1.1 \text{ kcal/cc} = 275 \text{ kcal}$$

Total Calories:

$$850 \text{ from dextrose} + 200 \text{ from protein} + 275 \text{ from lipid} = 1325 \text{ kcal}$$

Nonprotein Calories:

$$\text{Kcal from dextrose } 850 + \text{ kcal from lipid } 275 = 1125 \text{ nonprotein kcal}$$

Grams of Nitrogen:

$$50 \div 6.25 = 8.0 \text{ g nitrogen}$$

Calorie:Nitrogen Ratio:

$$850 \text{ (from dextrose)} + 275 \text{ (from lipid)} = 1125 \text{ nonprotein kcal}$$
$$1125 \div 8.0 \text{ g nitrogen} = 141$$
$$\text{Calorie:nitrogen ratio} = 141 \text{ to } 1$$

Percent Kilocalories from Fat:

$$\text{Total kcal} \div \text{kcal from fat}$$
$$275 \text{ total kcal} \div 1325 \text{ kcal from fat} = 21 \text{ percent}$$

these conditions increase resting energy expenditure and therefore kilocaloric requirements. The following sections discuss these conditions.

Surgery

Uncomplicated minor surgery increases the surgical client's kilocaloric requirement by only 5 percent. Surgery needed to repair soft tissue trauma requires a 14–37 percent increase in kilocalories. A surgical client with complications may require a large increase in kilocalories (Table 24–3).

Burns

Major burns are the most extreme state of stress a client can sustain. They produce a hypermetabolic state that raises kilocaloric needs higher than those of most other stress states. Kilocaloric requirements may be as high as 8000 kilocalories per day. Even a client who was well nourished before becoming burned may rapidly develop protein-kilocalorie malnutrition. As indicated in Table 24-3, the degree to which the metabolic rate increases is directly related to the body surface area burned. The percentage of body surface area burned is determined by totaling the individual percentages given in Figure 24–2. Although it is not reflected in the stress factors listed in the table, the deeper the burn, the higher is the client's kilocaloric need. Burn clients may remain in a hypermetabolic state for many weeks.

The increased load of waste products produced in some clients with burns is one reason for an increase in fluid requirements. Extra fluids help the kidneys eliminate these waste products. Capillary permeability is increased in burn clients; thus, plasma proteins, fluids, and electrolytes escape into the burn area and interstitial space. This shift reduces the volume of the plasma, so fluid volume needs to be replaced.

Physicians disagree on the best time to begin feeding burn clients. Some physicians keep the client NPO for the first 24–72 hours, and others initiate tube feedings within 4 hours following a burn injury. Here, an important consideration is that **peristalsis**, the wavelike motion that propels food through the gastrointestinal tract, ceases in some burn clients. Until peristalsis returns, the client's stomach should not be the site of choice for a tube feeding. The patient may also have an ileus caused by muscle paralysis or an obstruction. Physicians who do feed patients early insert the feeding tube into the client's intestines past the ileus and deliver a very slow, continuous-drip feeding. The slow continuous drip minimizes the likelihood of the feeding collecting in the intestines, because it is readily absorbed.

The rationale for early feeding in these patients follows. If the small intestine *maintains its digestive and absorptive properties*, enteral support is the preferred method of nutrient delivery. Several studies have shown that enteral nutrition initiated within 24 hours of injury was well tolerated and resulted in a statistically significant lower incidence of post-operative pneumonia, intra-abdominal abscess, and catheter sepsis (Souba and Wilmore, 1999). No evidence supports a delay in enteral feeding until the resuscitation period has ended (Skipper, 1998). Patients with burns of less than 20 percent of total body surface area are usually capable of orally consuming sufficient nutrients (Skipper, 1998).

Rather than beginning feedings on the day of injury, some physicians resume oral feeding of the client with the return of normal bowel activity. For most clients this is 2–4 days after the initial burn. Burn clients are

Rule of Nines

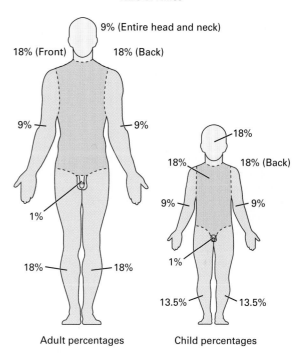

Figure 24–2:
The percentage of body surface area burned is determined by comparing the body surface area of the client's burns to the percentages given in the chart. For example, if a client has extensive burns over both legs, the total body surface area burned would be 36 percent (18 percent for the first leg plus 18 percent for the second leg). (From Thomas, CL [ed]: Taber's Cylopedic Medical Dictionary, ed 18. FA Davis, Philadelphia, 1997, p 278, by Beth Anne Willert, MS, Illustrator, with permission.)

usually allowed a clear or full liquid diet at this time. Dietary progression begins 4–10 days after the injury, as tolerated.

Burn clients are particularly susceptible to **sepsis**, the state in which disease-producing organisms are present in the blood. Major sepsis further increases a client's metabolic rate. See Table 24–3 for the stress factor to use in determining kilocaloric needs during sepsis. Clients with Foley catheters and intravenous lines are at a risk for sepsis.

Stress factors can be multiplied by each other. For example, the formula to use for a client with greater than 50 percent burns over the body surface area and major sepsis is:

Kilocalorie Need = REE × Activity Factor × Stress Factor No. 1 (2.0 for 50 percent burn) × Stress Factor No. 2 (1.5 for major sepsis)

Sepsis of course is not limited to burn clients; surgical and trauma clients may also suffer from sepsis.

For all burn clients, a nutritional assessment is essential to minimize complications and allow nutritional therapy to be effectively evaluated. The food intake of these clients should be monitored and documented. The kilocalories, grams of protein, kilocalorie:nitrogen ratio, grams of nitrogen (N), and percent of kilocalories from fat consumed or taken intravenously should be charted daily.

A high-protein, high-kilocalorie diet is ordered for most burn clients; often the diet is initially offered in six small meals. Complete nutritional oral supplements are commonly used to increase the client's kilocaloric and protein intake. The protein content of the diet can be increased by providing a between-meal feeding high in protein, a serving of two eggs at breakfast, and a large serving of meat at both lunch and supper. If the client drinks a full 8 ounces of milk with each meal, this further increases the protein content of the diet.

Infections and Fever

Malnutrition decreases resistance to infection, and infection aggravates malnutrition by depleting body nutrient stores. Fever characteristically accompanies infection but can also result from a variety of causes. The body needs extra kilocalories and fluids during fever because it takes more energy to support the higher metabolic rate. Infection often results in decreased food intake and absorption of nutrients, altered metabolism, and increased excretion of nutrients. In any hypermetabolic state, such as fever or infection, extra kilocalories are needed because the client's REE increases. Table 24–3 shows a stress factor of 1 + 0.07 for each degree Fahrenheit the client's temperature exceeds normal. For example, to determine the kilocaloric need of a client with a prolonged fever of 104.6°F, the stress factor is 1.49 (1 + 7 degrees x 0.07). Protein and fluid requirements are increased for clients with an infection. Extra protein is also needed to enable the body to produce antibodies and white blood cells to fight the infection. Perspiration entails a loss of fluids from the body, and many clients with fever have increased perspiration. Fluid may also be lost in vomiting and diarrhea, and this fluid needs to be replaced.

Trauma

Trauma may be defined as a physical injury or wound caused by an external source of violence. Stab and gunshot wounds, multiple fractures, and injuries acquired in motor vehicle accidents are examples of trauma. Victims of traumas may become hypermetabolic, depending on the severity of the injury. Vitamin supplements may be necessary. Vitamin C plays a role in wound healing, and its administration restores healing. Vitamin C functions as a cofactor in the hydroxylation of proline into collagen and enhances cellular and humoral response to stress. Doses as high as 500–1000 mg per day have been recommended (Skipper, 1998). Vitamin A, calcium, and zinc are also important in wound healing. Vitamin A enhances fibroplasia and collagen accumulation in wounds. Calcium is needed for calcium-dependent collagenases, iron for the formation of collagen, and zinc as a cofactor for enzymes responsible for cellular proliferation. These clients are at nutritional risk and may need extra kilocalories and protein.

Nutrition and Respiration

The scientific literature addresses the relationship between good nutrition and **respiration**. Respiration refers to the exchange of gases (oxygen and carbon dioxide) between a living organism and its environment. The air or oxygen inhaled and the carbon dioxide exhaled is the act of **ventilation**. Ventilation means breathing. **Pulmonary** means concerning or

involving the lungs. **Chronic obstructive pulmonary disease** (COPD) refers to a group of lung diseases with a common characteristic of chronic airflow obstruction. COPD has become the fourth leading cause of death in the United States. **Respiratory failure** is an acute or chronic disease caused by an imbalance between the amount of gases entering the lungs and the demand of body cells for gases, resulting in tissue hypoxia. Acute respiratory failure is an imbalance as a result of a disease that affects ventilation in a client who has a healthy lung and normal alveoli. Chronic respiratory failure results from a disease in the bronchial structures and/or functioning (alveoli) structures of the lung. Malnutrition is commonly seen in clients with respiratory diseases.

Effects of Impaired Nutritional Status on Respiratory Function

Poor nutrition is related to inadequate pulmonary function in five important ways. First, clients with respiratory diseases or inadequate respiratory function frequently have an inadequate food intake, which is related to anorexia, shortness of breath, and/or gastrointestinal distress. Shortness of breath during food preparation and consumption of meals may limit kilocaloric intake. Inadequate oxygen delivery to the cells causes fatigue. Impaired gastrointestinal tract motility is common in clients with respiratory diseases (see the following section).

Second, kilocaloric requirements are often increased in clients with pulmonary disease. Research has estimated that although the number of kilocalories needed to breathe ranges from 36 to 72 kilocalories per day in normal individuals, the kilocaloric cost of breathing increases to 430 to 720 kilocalories per day in clients with COPD (Brown and Light, 1983). Kilocalorie requirements can be estimated at 25 kcal/kg of body weight for maintenance therapy and 35 kcal/kg for repletion therapy (Skipper, 1998). As a result of the combined effects of decreased food intake and increased energy requirements, weight loss is commonly seen in these clients.

The third important relationship between nutrition and pulmonary function is the effect of catabolism. When kilocaloric intake is decreased, the body begins to break down muscle stores, including those of the respiratory muscles. A loss in the lean mass of any muscle affects the muscle's function. The lung's structure itself is thus affected as a result of catabolism. Malnutrition may also result in decreased lung-tissue cell replacement or growth.

Gastrointestinal distress is common in clients with pulmonary disease and is related to malnutrition. A loss of gastrointestinal structure including muscle mass may lead to hemorrhage and paralytic ileus. **Paralytic ileus** is the temporary cessation of peristalsis. This contributes to decreased food intake and the feeling of anorexia. In addition, paralytic ileus may lead to a translocation of bacteria. Decreased peristalsis in the GI tract fosters the movement (translocation) of bacteria from the GI tract into the bloodstream. This, in turn, leads to sepsis, or blood-borne infection, a sometimes fatal complication.

The fourth important relationship between nutrition and pulmonary function is that malnutrition decreases a person's resistance to infection. Lung infection is frequently the cause of death in pulmonary clients. In a state of malnutrition, the body decreases the production of antibodies, which are necessary to fight infection. Also, as a result of starvation, the lungs decrease production of pulmonary phospholipid (a fat-like substance). Phospholipids assist in keeping the lung tissue lubricated and help to protect the lungs from any disease-producing organisms that are inhaled.

The fifth important relationship between nutrition and pulmonary function is that improved nutritional status has been shown to be associated with a better ability to wean clients from ventilators. A ventilator is a machine that provides gases under pressure to clients who are unable to breathe on their own because of an insufficient number of ventilations or inspired volume amounts for cellular respiration. Clients on ventilators do not have to use their respiratory muscles to breathe. Active muscle movement stimulates muscle growth through protein stimulus. This is the same principle that applied to physical exercise increasing muscle size. To some extent, all the respiratory muscles **atrophy**, or waste away, due to inactivity while a client is artificially breathing.

Clients on ventilators are usually weaned slowly from these machines as their condition improves. Some experts have attributed clients' ability to be successfully weaned from ventilators to an increase in protein synthesis. Good nutrition stimulates respiratory muscle growth.

Nutritional Therapy

Respiratory disease can affect both food intake and nutrient utilization. Many clients with respiratory diseases also have problems with water balance.

Energy Nutrient Utilization

Many clients with COPD suffer from carbon dioxide retention and oxygen depletion. Such clients are said to be carbon dioxide retainers. The medical goal for these clients is to decrease their blood level of carbon dioxide. The following formula helps explain this concept:

$$\text{Protein (or Carbohydrate or Fat) + Oxygen =}$$
$$\text{Heat Energy + Water + Carbon Dioxide}$$

Fat kilocalories produce less carbon dioxide than carbohydrate kilocalories. For this reason, a diet high in fat is often used for carbon dioxide retainers. A high-fat diet may also assist the client with respiratory failure who must be weaned from mechanical ventilation. A high-fat diet may provide as much as 50 percent of the kilocalories in the form of fat. Figure 24–3 illustrates the relationship between nutrition and respiratory status in clients with pulmonary insufficiency and shows the influence of high-carbohydrate and high-fat diets.

Some physicians oppose the use of a high-fat diet for carbon dioxide retainers. Their opposition is based on research that has shown that a high-fat intake may be immunosuppressive in some clients (Juskelis, 1991). For this reason, fat in excess of 50 percent of total kilocalories is rarely prescribed.

Care must be taken not to overfeed clients with reduced respiratory function. Excess intake can raise the demand for oxygen and the production of carbon dioxide beyond the clients' capacity. The total number of kilocalories fed to the pulmonary client should be closely monitored. A nutritional assessment helps estimate the client's kilocaloric need and assists in therapy. Several companies market complete nutritional supplements targeted to clients who need a greater percentage of kilocalories provided from fat.

Vitamins A and C

An adequate intake of vitamins A and C is essential for helping to prevent pulmonary infections and decrease the extent of lung tissue damage. Foods high in vitamin A, such as fortified milk, dark green or yellow fruits and vegetables, some breakfast cereals (check the label), cheese, and eggs should be included in the diet. Foods high in vitamin C, such as citrus fruits and juices, strawberries, and fortified breakfast cereals (check the label) should also be included. Sources of vitamins A and C should be carefully chosen to ensure that they do not contribute to gas production.

Water, Phosphorus, and Magnesium

Water balance and serum phosphorus levels need to be closely monitored in these clients. Clients with COPD and acute respiratory failure often need fluid restriction. Fluid restriction assists in the control of pulmonary edema or a movement of fluid into interstitial lung tissue. Low serum phosphorus levels or hypophosphatemia are often seen in clients who are respirator-dependent. Phosphorus leaves the intracellular space and moves into the extracellular space during starvation. Serum phosphorus levels are in the normal or near-normal range at this point. With refeeding, phosphate moves back into the intracellular space. At this point, the serum phosphorus level may drop below normal. If this occurs, it is crucial that the client receive phosphate therapy. Because acute hypophosphatemia has been reported to cause respiratory failure, serum phosphorus levels should be monitored in all clients receiving aggressive nutritional support. A magnesium deficiency appears to cause a loss of muscle strength (American Dietetic Association, 1996).

Feeding Techniques

Many of these clients lack the energy to eat. Complaints of fatigue are common. The gastrointestinal distress experienced by these clients contributes to the anorexia. Foods from the cabbage family such as broccoli, cabbage, and Brussels sprouts may produce gas and contribute to gastrointestinal distress. Small, frequent feedings of foods with a high-nutrient density should be encouraged. Serving food items that require little or no chewing may help with difficulties chewing, breathlessness, and swallowing.

Refeeding Syndrome

Refeeding is the reintroduction of kilocalories and nutrients by oral or other routes into a patient. **Refeeding syndrome** is a detrimental state that results when a previously severely malnourished person is reintroduced to food and nutrients improperly. Complications with refeeding can occur regardless of the route by which nutrients are delivered—oral, enteral, and/or parenteral.

The term refeeding syndrome has been used to describe a series of metabolic and physiological reactions that occur in some malnourished clients when nutritional rehabilitation is begun. Improper refeeding of a chronically malnourished client can result in congestive heart failure (CHF) and respiratory failure. Clients at risk include those with alcoholism, chronic weight loss, hyperglycemia, or insulin-dependent diabetes mellitus and clients on chronic antacid or diuretic therapy. Elderly persons living alone who choose not to eat or are unable to eat because of progressive infirmity are likely candidates. Any incompetent mentally or physically challenged adult or abused child who has not

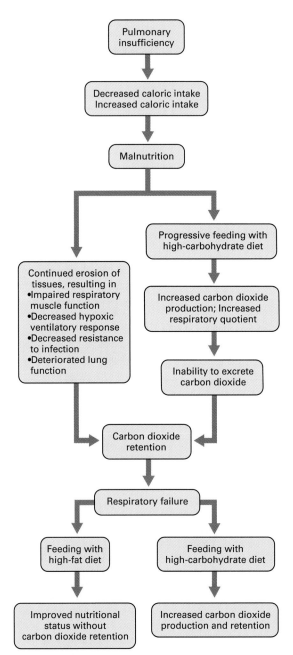

Figure 24–3:
Interrelationship between nutrition and respiratory status in clients with pulmonary insufficiency. Influence of high-carbohydrate and high-fat diets is shown. (From Specialized Nutrition for Pulmonary Patients, December 1984, p 14, Ross Laboratories, with permission.)

been eating either by choice or neglect is also likely to experience refeeding syndrome.

Starvation leads to both a loss of the lean body mass in the heart and respiratory muscles and decreased insulin secretion. When carbohydrate intake is low, the pancreas adapts by decreasing insulin secretion. With the reintroduction of carbohydrates into the diet, insulin secretion will

increase. The increased insulin secretion is associated with increased sodium and water retention. Other hormones are also activated with carbohydrate feeding. As a result of hormone action, increases in metabolic rate, oxygen consumption, and carbon dioxide production occur. The net effect of these metabolic changes is an increased workload for the cardiopulmonary system. Refeeding may increase the work of the cardiopulmonary system beyond its diminished capacity (due to the loss of lean body mass) and cause CHF and respiratory failure.

Starvation also leads to an increase in extracellular fluid and an increased loss of intracellular phosphorus, potassium, and magnesium. The degree of intracellular loss of these minerals reflects the degree of loss of lean body mass. Before refeeding, serum phosphorus and magnesium levels may remain in the lower range of normal, whereas the intracellular and total body stores of these minerals are depleted. After refeeding, these minerals are redistributed from the extracellular to the intracellular compartments. Repeated laboratory measurements taken after refeeding is started may show low serum levels of phosphorus, magnesium, and potassium. Failure to correct for these mineral deficiencies may be fatal for the client.

Principles of Safe Refeeding of the Malnourished Client

Healthcare workers need to be aware of the dangers of refeeding a severely malnourished or starved client. Starved or severely malnourished clients may be seen in outpatient settings as well as in hospital intensive care units and long-term care facilities. A high prevalence of malnutrition is common in outpatient settings. The following recommendations may help the health care worker avoid the refeeding syndrome in malnourished clients.

1. Recognize clients at risk. Refeeding syndrome occurs in clients with frank starvation, including war victims undergoing repletion, chronically ill clients who are malnourished, clients on prolonged intravenous dextrose solutions without other modes of nutritional support, hypermetabolic clients who have not received nutritional support for 1–2 weeks, clients who report prolonged fasting, obese clients who report a recent loss of a considerable amount of weight, chronic alcoholics, and clients with anorexia nervosa.

2. Healthcare workers practicing in outpatient settings not directly under the supervision of a physician need to develop a referral plan in the event they suspect a client is a likely candidate for refeeding syndrome. These clients require the expertise of a physician.

3. A physician needs to test for and correct all electrolyte abnormalities before initiating nutritional support, whether by the oral, enteral, or parenteral route. Many physicians depend on other health care workers to assist in the monitoring of serum phosphorus, magnesium, and potassium values. For nurses practicing within hospitals, this means notifying the physician on receipt of laboratory test results showing low serum levels of these minerals. It is especially important to notify the physician before implementing changes in tube feedings, oral diets, or the rate of hyperalimentation. In larger hospitals, the nutrition support service performs this service.

4. The physician needs to restore circulatory volume and to monitor pulse rate and intake and output before initiating nutritional support. Again, many physicians depend on nurses and other healthcare workers to assist in monitoring these signs.

5. The kilocaloric delivery to a previously starved client should be slow. Tube-fed and parenterally fed clients need to be closely monitored. The rate, total volume, and concentration of kilocalories delivered should be carefully monitored and documented. The concentration, volume, and rate of kilocaloric intake should be increased one at a time. Stepwise advancement to a higher kilocalorie intake should not occur unless the client is metabolically and physiologically stable.

6. Electrolytes should be monitored before nutritional support is started and at designed intervals thereafter.

Refeeding the malnourished client requires a team effort. A careful diet history taken by the dietitian can assist in the identification of clients likely to become victims of the refeeding syndrome. Changes in taste, appetite, intake, weight, or consumption of a special diet may indicate significantly altered status. Correction of electrolyte abnormalities by the physician before implementing nutritional support can prevent death. Careful observation and monitoring by the nutritional support service can identify early signs of this syndrome. Open and prompt communication among all healthcare team members may be crucial to the client's survival.

Summary

Stress is defined as any condition that threatens the body's mental or physical well-being. The best nutritional insurance against unexpected stress is good nutrient stores developed from a well-balanced diet. The use of supplemental vitamins, minerals, and amino acids in healthy individuals for excessive mental activity or stress has not been proved to provide a health benefit. However, a well-balanced diet or diet therapy for the treatment and prevention of chronic diseases exacerbated by mental stress has been shown to provide a health benefit.

The physical stress of hypermetabolism invokes the stress response and alters nutritional requirements for kilocalories, protein, and micronutrients. The stress response has three well-defined phases, which are mediated by hormones: the ebb phase, the flow phase, and the recovery (or anabolic) phase. Hypermetabolism differs from starvation in that resting energy expenditure (REE) increases during hypermetabolism and decreases during a prolonged state of starvation. Major surgery, severe infections, fever, major burns, and severe trauma are all examples of hypermetabolic states.

Respiratory status profoundly affects nutrient need and utilization as well as food intake. Nutritional support can decrease catabolism of the respiratory muscles, improve immune function, minimize carbon dioxide production, and improve the likelihood of successfully weaning clients who are on mechanical respirators.

Refeeding a previously starved client involves some risks. Refeeding may increase the work of the cardiorespiratory system beyond its diminished capacity and cause congestive heart failure and respiratory failure. Refeeding syndrome is a series of metabolic reactions seen in some malnourished clients when they are refed. All healthcare workers have a responsibility to understand this syndrome. A team approach to refeeding the malnourished client is necessary to prevent tragic complications.

Case Study 24–1

Mr. X is a 42-year-old man who was admitted to the intensive care unit (ICU) with a diagnosis of acute bronchitis. He has a known history of carbon dioxide retention and chronic obstructive pulmonary disease. Mr. X is 5 ft. 11 in. (180 cm), 140 lbs (63.6 kg), and has a medium body frame (HBW = 87.5 percent; BMI = 19.5). He reports a recent 9 lb weight loss over a 3-week period. The client is on a mechanical ventilator. The physician's goal is to wean the client from the ventilator as soon as possible. Mr. X complains of fatigue, gas pains, anorexia, dyspnea (difficulty breathing), and early satiety. The client consumed a cup of coffee and one slice of toast for breakfast before falling asleep. The physician has ordered a 50 percent fat high-kilocalorie, high-protein diet.

Nursing Care Plan

Subjective Data	Reports a 3-lb/week loss over the last 3 weeks.
	Complains of fatigue, gas pains, anorexia, dyspnea, and early satiety.
Objective Data	87.5 percent HBW; BMI = 19.5
	Observed low-food intake
	Known history of COPD with carbon dioxide retention
Nursing Diagnosis	NANDA: Nutrition: altered less than body requirements (North American Nursing Diagnosis Association, 1999)
	Related to poor food intake, recent weight loss, fatigue, gas pains, anorexia, dyspnea, and early satiety as evidenced by 87.5 percent HBW and known history of COPD and carbon dioxide retention

Desired Outcomes Evaluation Criteria	Nursing Actions/ Interventions	Rationale
NOC: Nutritional Status (Johnson, Maas, and Moorhead, 2000)	NIC: Nutrition Management (McCloskey and Bulechek, 2000)	
States that good nutrition is important to independent respiration in one day	Emphasizes the importance of the prescribed diet to independent respiration.	Successful weaning to independent respiration is enhanced by good nutrition. Good nutrition decreases respiratory muscle catabolism, fosters protein synthesis, and facilitates production of pulmonary phospholipids.
Consumes an appropriate food intake in 3 days.	Consult with the dietitian to set a nutritional goal for the client based on the client's estimated energy expenditure using the Harris-Benedict formula, total energy requirements, and protean requirements.	The pulmonary client should not be over- or underfed. Determination of the client's energy and protein requirements will provide baseline information to determine nutritional needs. Kilocalories and carbohydrates in excess will increase carbon dioxide retention. A deficiency of kilocalories and protein will increase catabolism of the respiratory muscles.
	Promote a pleasant, relaxed environment, including socialization if possible at mealtime.	Eating is both a social and biological experience. Kilocalorie intake will be greater if an attempt is made to provide a pleasant eating environment.
	Consult with the dietitian to provide a diet with modifications that meet the needs such as: • Texture and modification as necessary. • Avoidance of foods not tolerated due to questionable limited GI tract motility such as gassy vegetables, spicy foods, milk products (secondary to lactase deficiency), etc. • Between meal supplements that are acceptable to the client. • Limitation of empty kilocalories. • Meal size and volume limits. • Monitor the client's food intakes (i.e., kilocalorie count).	Clients with pulmonary disease are often too tired to eat and may have gastrointestinal complaints. Small frequent meals, easily chewed foods, and reduction of empty kilocalories may assist in helping the client to meet estimated kilocalorie and protein needs. Documentation of food intake with subsequent analysis of protein and kilocalorie content will provide an objective measure of nursing care plan effectiveness. The results of the analysis can be used to provide feedback to the client.
	Provide oral care before/after meals.	A fresh mouth increases appetite.
Maintains his weight during hospitalization.	Weigh client daily.	The best way to evaluate the effectiveness of nutritional therapy is to weigh the nonedematous client. For this client, weight gain will require a considerable effort, hence, an intermediate goal of weight maintenance is realistic.
Demonstrates progressive weight gain toward his HBW over the next 3 months.	Instruct client to weigh himself weekly.	The ultimate goal for this client is anabolism with a weight gain. A slow progressive weight gain means the approach taken is succeeding.

Critical Thinking Question

1. After 2 days of monitoring the patient's kilocalorie and protein intake and despite encouragement to eat from the nurses and the dietitian, the patient refuses to eat much food. His kilocalorie intake is less than 500 with only 12 grams of protein. What would you recommend?

2. The patient's physician has ordered a fluid restriction of 800 cc qd plus output. The patient is angry and wants more fluids. How would you handle this situation?

3. You question the client's mental competence. What should you do?

Study Aids

Subjects . . . .**Internet Sites**

Hypermetabolism http://zebu.cvm.msu.edu/courses/vm556/metabolism/sld060.htm

Starvation . . . . .www.redcross.org/news/index.html

http://www.usariem.army.mil/somalia/starve.htm

Respiration http://www2.uca.edu/biology/mobley/biology/cellresp.htm

Refeeding Syndrome http://www.medicine.uiowa.edu/pa/sresrch/Shindela/Shindelar/tsld015.htm

http://www.clinnutr.org/Jpenabs0998.htm

Chapter Review

1. Clients who complain about excessive mental stress benefit the most by counseling to:
   a. Supplement their diet with thiamin
   b. Drink extra fluids
   c. Eat a balanced diet
   d. Increase their protein intake
2. Which of these conditions does not increase a client's resting energy expenditure?
   a. Infection
   b. Chronic obstructive pulmonary disease
   c. Starvation
   d. Burn
3. A burn client's need for kilocalories is related to:
   a. The amount of protein eaten
   b. The total body surface area burned
   c. The volume of food tolerated
   d. Existing nutrient stores
4. Malnutrition is commonly seen in clients with pulmonary disease for all but one of the following reasons. Identify the exception.
   a. Many of these clients have a decreased food intake.
   b. Many of these clients expend more kilocalories to breathe.
   c. Many of these clients have impaired gastrointestinal tract function.
   d. Many of these clients have an extraordinary ability to fight infection.
5. Experts advocate the following when refeeding a malnourished client:
   a. Immediately pushing kilocalories and protein to replenish lost stores
   b. Progressing the rate, volume, and concentration of a tube feeding as rapidly as possible
   c. Full participation of all members of the health care team to manage commonly seen metabolic abnormalities
   d. Correction of the hyperphosphatemia seen during the refeeding of a malnourished client

Clinical Analysis

1. Mr. X is suffering from second- and third-degree burns over 40 percent of his body. His physician has decided to use topical agents and leave the wound open to air. In the first 30–40 days postburn, the nurse is planning nutritional support. The best supplemental feedings for the client would use:
   a. A modular feeding with a kilocalorie:nitrogen ratio of 150:1
   b. A modular feeding with a kilocalorie:nitrogen ratio of 300:1
   c. A polymeric (complete nutritional) supplement that is acceptable to the client
   d. High-kilocalorie desserts such as apple pie, cake, and ice cream
2. Mrs. J is an alcoholic who has previously reported that she has not eaten "food" for at least the last 3 months. She stated that her sole source of kilocalories had been in the form of alcohol. She was recently transferred to the unit in which you work after her treatment for alcohol withdrawal on another unit. The physician has ordered a high-kilocalorie, high-protein diet. So far, she has eaten 100 percent of the three high-kilocalorie, high-protein trays she has received while on your unit. While reviewing the client's laboratory values, you notice her serum phosphorus, magnesium, and calcium levels are decreased. Mrs. J's depressed phosphorus values may be related to:
   a. A movement of phosphorus into the extracellular space
   b. A total compartmental depletion of phosphorus
   c. A lack of phosphorus in Mrs. J's present dietary intake
   d. A movement of phosphorus into the intracellular space
3. Mr. C is a heavy smoker. He was recently admitted to your unit with carbon dioxide retention and a diagnosis of chronic obstructive pulmonary disease. He complains of gas pains. His diet should include all except the following:
   a. A high-fat complete nutritional supplement
   b. Broccoli, onions, peas, melons, and cabbage
   c. Six small meals
   d. Custard, hot cooked cereals, bananas, ground meats, and mashed potatoes

Bibliography

American Dietetic Association: Manual of Clinical Dietetics, ed 5. The American Dietetic Assoc. Chicago, 1996.

Barrett, S, and Herbert, V: Fads, frauds, and quackery. In Shils, ME, Olson, JA, Shike, M, and Ross, CA (eds): Modern Nutrition in Health and Disease, ed 9. Williams and Wilkins, Baltimore, 1999.

Bronson-Adatto, C (ed): Suggested Guidelines for Nutrition Management of the Critically Ill Patient. American Dietetic Association, Chicago, 1984.

Brown, SE, and Light, RW: What is now known about protein-energy depletion: When COPD patients are malnourished. J Respir Dis, May 1983.

Bullock, BL, and Rosendahl, PP: Pathophysiology: Adaptations and Alterations in Function, ed 3. JB Lippincott, Philadelphia, 1992.

Gold, PE: Role of glucose in regulating brain and cognition. Am J Clin Nutr. 61(suppl):9875, 1995.

Hansbrough, JF: Enteral nutritional support in burn patients. Gastrointest Endosc Clin N Am. 8(3):645, July 1998.

Johnson, M, Maas, M, and Moorhead, S: Nursing Outcomes Classification (NOC), ed 2. Mosby, Philadelphia, 2000.

Juskelis, D: Starvation in patients: Guidelines for refeeding. Registered Dietitian Clinical Interactions 11:2, 1991.

McCloskey, JC, and Bulechek, GM: Nursing Interventions Classification (NIC), ed 3. Mosby, Philadelphia, 2000.

National Research Council: Recommended Dietary Allowances, ed 10. National Academy Press, Washington DC, 1989.

North American Nursing Diagnosis Association: Nursing Diagnoses: Definitions and Classification 1999–2000, North American Nursing Diagnosis Association, Philadelphia, 1999.

Quandt, SA: Cultural influences on food consumption and nutritional status. In Shils, ME, Olson, JA, Shike, M, and Ross, CA (eds): Modern Nutrition in Health and Disease, ed 9. Williams and Wilkins, Baltimore, 1999.

Skipper, A: Dietitian's Handbook of Enteral and Parenteral Nutrition, ed 2. Aspen Publishing, Gaithersburg, MD, 1998.

Smith, MK, and Lawry, SF: The hypermetabolic state. In Shils, ME, Olson, JA, Shike, M, and Ross, CA (eds): Modern Nutrition in Health and Disease, ed 9. Williams and Wilkins, Baltimore, 1999.

Souba, WW, and Wilmore, D: Diet and nutrition in the care of the patient with surgery, trauma, and sepsis. In Shils, ME, Olson, JA, Shike, M, and Ross, CA (eds): Modern Nutrition in Health and Disease, ed 9. Williams and Wilkins, Baltimore, 1999.

Solomon, SM, and Kirby, DF: The refeeding syndrome: A review. JPEN 14:90, 1991.

Thomas, CL (ed): Taber's Cyclopedic Medical Dictionary, ed 17. FA Davis, Philadelphia, 1993.

CHAPTER 25

Diet in HIV and AIDS

LEARNING OBJECTIVES

After completing this chapter, the student should be able to:

1. Define AIDS and HIV and list transmission routes for the virus.
2. List nutrition-related complications seen in clients infected with HIV and, for each complication, describe interventions to improve nutritional status.
3. Discuss why malnutrition is commonly seen in clients with HIV or AIDS.
4. Describe why each client with AIDS needs an individualized nutritional assessment.

Acquired immune deficiency syndrome (AIDS) is a life-threatening disease and a major public health issue. The **human immunodeficiency virus** (HIV) causes AIDS. The impact of this virus on our society is and will continue to be a challenge. This chapter discusses the prevention, diagnosis, and treatment of HIV infection. The course of acquired immune deficiency syndrome is often complicated by malnutrition. For this reason, a major portion of this chapter is devoted to the nutritional care of clients infected with HIV.

Human Immunodeficiency Virus

The human immunodeficiency virus attacks both the immune system and the nervous system. **Immunity** refers to resistance to or protection against a specified disease. When the AIDS virus enters the bloodstream, it begins to attack cells with a specific protein called CD_4 on their surfaces. CD_4 is present on lymphocytes. Lymphocytes are the main source of the body's immune capability, which involves humoral immunity produced by B cells and cell-mediated immunity produced by T cells. CD_4 levels decrease as the HIV disease progresses. A healthy, uninfected person usually has 500–1500 CD_{4+} cells per cubic millimeter of blood (Ungvarski and Flaskerud, 1999).

The HIV virus enters the cell, conscripts its DNA, and reprograms it to reproduce the virus. Loss of CD_4 function leaves an individual susceptible to infections and certain cancers. Evidence shows that the AIDS virus may also attack the nervous system, causing damage to the brain.

Acquired Immune Deficiency Syndrome

AIDS is a disease complex characterized by a collapse of the body's natural immunity against disease. Every part of the human body may be affected. The disease is progressive but runs an unpredictable course with periods of remission. On the average it takes about 10 years for HIV to progress to AIDS. This disease is often diagnosed after certain indicator opportunistic diseases occur, such as infection, tumor, wasting, or dementia. The Centers for Disease Control has published a specific list of infections and cancers that are used to diagnose AIDS. This list is constantly being reviewed and revised as more information is gathered on the course of this disease. The World Health Organization defines AIDS more simply (Table 25–1).

No Known Cure

Dramatic but expensive treatment advances have changed the healthcare community's view of AIDS. The use of highly active antiretroviral therapy (HAART) has decreased mortality rates. However, findings indicate that in the vast majority of patients receiving HAART and who had undetectable levels of HIV-1 RNA in plasma, the virus has not been eradicated (Pomerantz, 1999). Also, HAART is not a treatment option for much of the world's population. Sadly, the medications are too costly.

Signs and Symptoms

The natural history of HIV infection is divided into three phases: early symptomatic phase, clinical latency, and advanced HIV disease (or AIDS).

Early Symptomatic Phase

The HIV-infected individual may develop an acute flu-like illness, with symptoms appearing about 2–6 weeks after exposure to the virus. Typically, the symptoms are not severe enough for the client to seek medical attention.

TABLE 25–1 World Health Organization's Case Definition of Adult AIDS*

Major Signs

Weight loss of greater than 10 percent of body weight

Chronic diarrhea of longer than 1 month's duration

Fever of longer than 1 month's duration, either intermittent or constant

Minor Signs

Persistent cough for greater than 1 month

General pruritic dermatitis (severe itching due to inflammation of the skin)

Recurrent herpes zoster (recurrent infectious disease caused by the varicella-zoster virus)

Oropharyngeal candidiasis (infection of the throat with any species of *Candida*)

Chronic progressive and disseminated herpes simplex infections (an acute infectious disease caused by the herpes simplex virus Type I)

Generalized lymphadenopathy (disease of the lymph nodes)

*AIDS in an adult is diagnosed if at least two major and one minor signs are present in the absence of a known cause of immunosuppression, such as cancer or severe malnutrition.

Clinical Latency

After this phase, the individual may be **asymptomatic** for years. Most HIV-infected persons have no symptoms, and many are not even aware that they are infected. The danger lies in their ability to infect other people unknowingly. Some people remain symptom-free for years after infection with the HIV virus. Even though the client is symptom-free, viral replication continues. There is a steady decline in CD_{4+} cells during this stage (about 40–80 cells per cubic millimeter of blood) for each year of infection (Ungvarski and Flasterud, 1999).

Viral load tests are also used to measure and monitor disease progression in clients who have been diagnosed. Amplicor HIV-1, better known as the PCR test, is used to determine the likelihood of disease progression. The higher the viral load, the more likely is the chance of disease progression. People who began studies with a viral load of less than 20,000 had only a 1 percent chance of experiencing disease progression during the following 60 weeks compared with 24 percent of people who started with a viral load over 200,000 (www.aidsinfonyc.org, accessed May, 2000).

Advanced HIV Disease Phase (AIDS)

After a period of 2–10 or more years, the CD_4 count drops to less than half the normal value, the viral load increases, and the immune system begins to fail, permitting opportunistic infections and other conditions characteristic of AIDS (Batterham, 1999). When the CD_{4+} cell count drops to less than 50, there is an increasing chance of treatment failure. Death becomes likely, usually within 1 year (Ungvarski and Flaskerud, 1999)

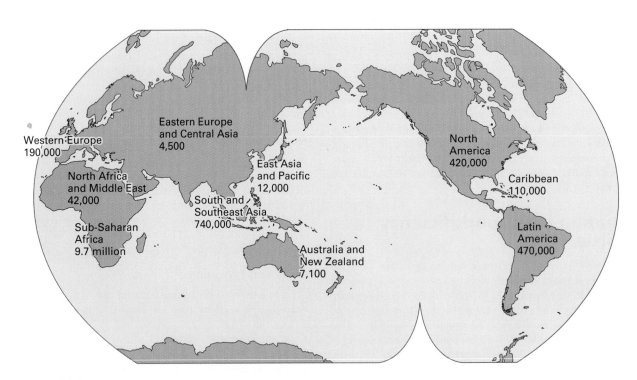

Figure 25–I:
Estimated adult and child deaths due to HIV/AIDS from the beginning of the epidemic through 1997. (WHO, 1999)

The Epidemic

Figure 25–1 illustrates the total number of people who have died from AIDS since the beginning of the epidemic. Figure 25–2 illustrates the adults and children estimated to be living with HIV/AIDS as of the end of 1997.

AIDS Worldwide

The World Health Organization (WHO) has endeavored to collect information about the number of reported cases of AIDS. This has been difficult because reporting in many countries is unreliable and the definitions used to identify AIDS vary. WHO estimates that about 30.6 million adults and children were alive with HIV/AIDS by the end of 1997.

The World Health Organization estimated adult and children deaths due to HIV/AIDS from the beginning of the epidemic to the end of 1997 as 420,000 (WHO, 1999).

AIDS in the United States

The Centers for Disease Control and Prevention cites the following figures for the United States (Centers for Disease Control, 1999):

- 16,685 deaths annually (1997)
- 227,000 hospital discharges for patients with HIV diagnosis (1996)
- 9.3 days average length of hospital stay (1995)

Transmittal Routes

The human immunodeficiency virus is not easily transmissible. Evidence indicates that the AIDS virus is spread through blood and body fluids. Direct contact of blood to blood or of virus to mucous membrane must occur for disease transmittal. In practical terms, there are three transmittal routes: blood-borne, perinatal, and sexual.

Blood-borne Route

HIV may be transmitted by exposure to contaminated blood or blood products through transfusion, sharing of drug apparatus, and injuries to healthcare workers from needles and other sharp objects. Box 25–1 outlines precautions to prevent needle-stick injuries. Intravenous drug abusers often share needles and other equipment for drug injection. This practice can result in a minute amount of blood from an infected person being injected into the bloodstream of the next user. In addition, cases of AIDS have been linked with receipt of blood products from HIV-infected donors (before donated blood was routinely tested for the HIV virus), acupuncture treatments performed with improperly sterilized needles, and receipt of transplanted organs from a person later discovered to have been HIV infected.

Perinatal Transmission

Most children with AIDS contract the virus from their infected mothers through blood-to-blood transmission before or at birth. Breast-feeding has been implicated in transmission, since HIV has been isolated from breast milk. In the United States, the Centers for Disease Control

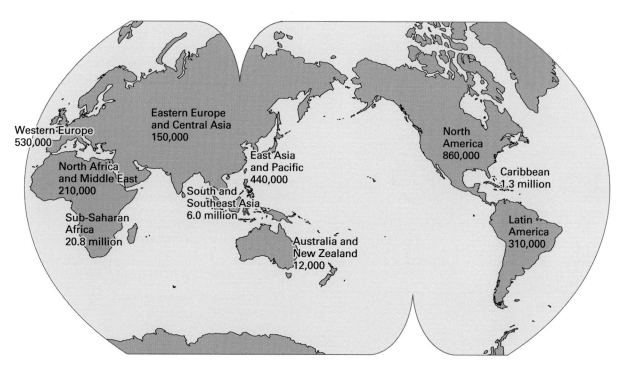

Figure 25–2:
Adults and children estimated to be living with HIV/AIDS as of the end of 1997. (WHO, 1999)

Box 25–1 Needle-Stick Injuries

To prevent needle-stick injuries, needles should not be:

- Recapped
- Purposely bent or broken by hand
- Removed from disposable syringes
- Otherwise manipulated by hand

Guidelines for disposal of syringes, needles, scalpel blades, and other sharp objects include:

- Placing them in a puncture-resistant container located as close to the area of use as is practical
- Placing large-bore reusable needles in a puncture-resistant container for transport to the processing area (Figure 25–3 illustrates a healthcare worker disposing a needle into an appropriate conatiner.)

advises HIV-positive women against breast-feeding. On the other hand, in developing countries, breast-feeding is still advocated by WHO because of the concern about infant morbidity and mortality due to poor sanitation.

Sexual Transmission

The most likely way to become infected with the HIV is to have unprotected sexual contact with an infected individual's blood, semen, and possibly vaginal secretions. The virus enters a person's bloodstream through the rectum, vagina, or penis. Small tears in the surface lining of the vagina or rectum may occur during insertion of the penis, fingers, or other objects, thus opening an avenue for entrance of the virus directly into the bloodstream. Both homosexual and heterosexual persons are at risk for AIDS. The only people not at risk of infection by this route are celibate individuals and couples who have maintained mutually faithful monogamous relationships (only one continuing sexual partner) for at least 15 years.

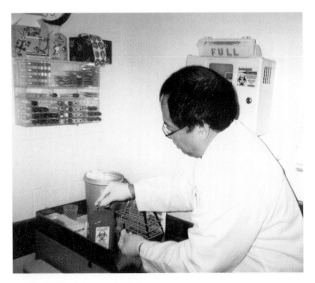

Figure 25–3:
A healthcare worker disposing of a needle in an approved "sharps" container. Note that he is wearing gloves.

AIDS: You Can Protect Yourself

The best advice for avoiding infection is to avoid direct contact with anyone's blood or body fluids. This involves practicing safer sexual behaviors and following universal precautions or body substance isolation procedures. Nurses need to advise clients to adopt safer sexual practices. Many resources are available describing precautions to prevent sexual transmission.

Universal Precautions or Body Substance Isolation

Healthcare workers need to consider all clients as potentially infected with HIV and/or other blood-borne pathogens. **Universal precautions** dictate that every client and every client's blood and certain body fluids should be considered contaminated and treated as such. **Body substance isolation** procedures are used when all body fluids should be considered contaminated and treated as such. Body substance isolation is thus more comprehensive than universal precautions. Whether universal precautions or body substance isolation procedures are followed in a given facility varies. Clinical Application 25–1 discusses the myth of transmission via casual contact.

Test Screening

Antibodies to HIV are diagnosed initially by enzyme-linked immunosorbent assays (ELISA) and agglutination assays and are confirmed by with Western Blot or more specific tests. The accuracy of existing HIV tests is limited because new strains of the virus are still being discovered that may not be identified by current tests. Negative results also can occur in infected individuals because of lack of antibody formation early in the disease and in late stages because of loss of ability to produce antibodies (Watson and Jaffe, 1995).

Complications of HIV Infection

AIDS is characterized by weakness, anorexia, diarrhea, weight loss, fever, and a decreased white blood cell count, or **leukopenia**. Common problems associated with AIDS include opportunistic infections, gastrointestinal dysfunction, tumors, AIDS dementia complex (ADC), and organ dysfunction. In the last years, several clients have developed a syndrome of "lipodystrophy" that is characterized by peripheral and facial wasting, in which all the veins in the extremities are prominent and the abdomen is enlarged (Batterham, 1999).

Opportunistic Infections

Parasitic, bacterial, viral, and fungal organisms are everywhere in our environment. The healthy person's immune system keeps these organisms in check and under control. AIDS places the client at high risk for certain infections, called **opportunistic infections**. Some of the infections these clients develop were rarely seen in the United States before the onset of the AIDS epi-

---

CLINICAL APPLICATION 25–1

No Risk of AIDS from Casual Contact

The majority of infected people contracted the virus through intimate sexual contact. No cases have been found where AIDS has been transmitted through casual (nonsexual) contact with a household member, relative, co-worker, or friend. Casual contact includes sneezing, coughing, eating or drinking from common utensils, or merely being around an infected person.

demic. Four opportunistic infections are commonly seen in AIDS clients: thrush, tuberculosis, pneumocystis pneumonia, and *cryptosporidiosis.*

THRUSH A physical assessment may show signs of **thrush**, which produces a thick whitish coating on the tongue or in the throat and may be accompanied by sore throat. Thrush is a fungal infection that can cause oral ulcers, frequent fevers, and gastrointestinal inflammation. Basic teaching for mouth care by the health educator should include:

- Keep the mouth clean by rinsing with a dilute solution of hydrogen peroxide and water at least three times a day, especially after eating. Instruct clients not to swallow the solution.
- Use a cotton swab instead of a toothbrush if brushing is painful or causes bleeding. Commercial mouthwash may cause discomfort or pain.
- Avoid hot foods.
- Try soft foods, such as scrambled eggs, cottage cheese, mashed potatoes, mashed winter squash, puddings, custards, milk, juices (not citrus), canned fruits such as peaches, pears, apricots, and bananas.
- Cut meat into small pieces or grind or blend it.
- Supplement diet with a complete oral nutritional supplement.
- Use a straw.
- Tilt head forward or backward to ease swallowing.
- Avoid any food that causes discomfort. Fried, spicy, sour, salty, and sticky foods may not be tolerated, such as chips, nuts, seeds, raw vegetables, peanut butter, pickles, citrus fruits and juices, and tomatoes

TUBERCULOSIS Tuberculosis (TB) is spread from person to person through tiny airborne particles. By sharing surroundings with a person who has active pulmonary TB, a susceptible person may inhale the disease-producing bacteria. Fortunately, most people who have inhaled these particles never become contagious or develop active TB. Even a healthy immune system cannot kill all the particles. HIV infection weakens the body's immune system and makes it more likely that the individual who has inhaled TB-related particles will develop active TB.

PNEUMOCYSTIS PNEUMONIA Pneumonia, characterized by shortness of breath, fatigue, and anorexia, is also common in AIDS clients. About 60 percent of AIDS clients are infected with one type of pneumonia-causing organism called *Pneumocystis carinii,* hence the name **pneumocystis pneumonia.** The organisms settle in the person's lungs, causing progressively worsening breathing problems and eventually leading to death.

CRYPTOSPORIDIOSIS Persons with HIV are at a high risk for food-borne illnesses. Food safety and sanitation should always be a part of client education in this population. Because of the gastrointestinal infections acquired by immunosuppressed clients, an additional safety precaution has been recommended. Because of outbreaks of *crytosporidiosis* in public drinking water, the Centers for Chronic Disease Control (CDC) has suggested that people with HIV infection and AIDS drink sterilized water and avoid tap water (American Dietetic Association, 1995).

Gastrointestinal Dysfunction

The gastrointestinal tract is a common site for expression of HIV-related symptoms. The client may feel pain in the mouth or esophagus due to the growth of opportunistic infections. The client may have difficulty swallowing because of open lesions or sores. AIDS commonly affects both the small and large intestine. The enzymes necessary for digestion and absorption in the wall of the small intestine may be lacking or present in insufficient amounts. Malabsorption may occur with diarrhea. Gut failure may follow. The medications these clients receive to control their infections also contribute to the gastrointestinal dysfunction.

AIDS Dementia Complex

AIDS dementia complex (ADC) is the most common HIV-caused central nervous system illness associated with AIDS. It is estimated that at least 40–50 percent of adults with AIDS have some neurological dysfunction. Experts believe ADC frequently is misdiagnosed as Alzheimer's disease in persons over 50 (Scharnhorst, 1992). This dysfunction is usually chronic and progressive. Early symptoms of ADC are difficulty in concentration, slowness in thinking and response, and memory impairment. Behavioral symptoms include social withdrawal, apathy, and personality changes. Such symptoms may be interpreted solely as a psychiatric disorder. Motor symptoms include clumsiness of gait, difficulty with fine motor movements, and poor balance and coordination.

Tumors

Kaposi's sarcoma is the most frequently seen malignancy among AIDS clients. The most common manifestation of Kaposi's sarcoma is single or multiple lesions appearing on the lower extremities, and especially on the feet and ankles. These open areas appear reddish, purple, or brown. Treatment consists of radiation, surgery, and/or chemotherapy.

Organ Dysfunction

AIDS affects many organs in the body, leading to organ dysfunction. Diseases of the gallbladder, liver, and kidneys are seen in some AIDS clients. **Cholecystitis**, inflammation of the gallbladder, can occur in conjunction with certain opportunistic infections seen in AIDS victims. *Hepatomegaly,* an enlarged liver, is frequently seen with pain, fever, and abnormal liver function test results, especially of the alkaline phosphatase level. **Pancreatitis**, inflammation of the pancreas, has also been noted in some infected clients. AIDS can lead to **end-stage renal failure** within weeks.

Clearly, AIDS has many complications. Ongoing research has yet to discover a cure for this terrible disease.

Lipodystrophy

Since February 1998, reports from France, Spain, Switzerland, Hong Kong, Australia, and the United States of an odd redistribution of fat, called lipodystrophy, have been received. Lipodystrophy, now preferably called fat redistribution syndrome, is characterized by increasing abdominal girth, decreasing fat mass in the extremities and face, the advent of a "buffalo hump," and breast enlargement in patients with HIV, especially those on HAART with a protease inhibitor. Also seen are increased serum triglyceride, glucose, and insulin levels and, sometimes, increased blood pressure (Kotler, 1999). It is not clear whether HAART causes fat redistribution or whether this is a natural progression of HIV infection being seen with increased longevity due to improved survival. These changes may be seen despite effective viral suppression and otherwise improved health. Although further studies to determine the clinical consequences are needed, there is

---

CLINICAL APPLICATION 25–2

Medications Used for HIV and Aids

Drug therapy for clients with HIV has increased in complexity. Clients must often take 10 or more different medications each day to treat HIV infections, suppress opportunistic infections, and control symptoms. Medications that increase blood lipid levels and promote diarrhea may require the patient to further modify his or her diet. The following table lists common mediations used in HIV/AIDS, typical dosing, and food tips.

Protease Inhibitors

Medication	Generic Name	Dosing	Food Tips
Indinavir	Crixivan	BID, every 12 hours	Take on an empty stomach to enhance absorption
		TID, every 8 hours	Take with a light snack that contains 300 kcal, 6 grams of protein, and 2 grams of fat to reduce stomach upset
			Drink at least 1 cup of water or juice (not grapefruit) with each dose
			Drink a total of 10 cups of water and/or juice every day to prevent kidney stones
Ritonavir	Norvir	BID	Take with a full meal
			Complications may include diarrhea, lipodystrophy, and elevated lipids
			Avoid alcohol
Saquinavir	Fortovase (Invirase)	BID or TID	Take within 2 hours of a high-fat meal or snack. This will increase the drug's absorption by 5–10 times. A high-fat meal should contain about 55 grams of fat
			Possible complications include lipodystrophy and elevated lipids
Nelfinavir	Viracept	TID	Take with food.
		Doses should not exceed 12 hours	Possible complications include diarrhea, lipodystrophy, and elevated lipids.

(Continued on next page)

---

little question that patients demonstrating these body composition and metabolic changes should be considered at increased risk for the development of cardiovascular disease (Kotler, 1999).

Treatment

A variety of new medications show some promise of killing or inhibiting the activity of the HIV virus. Clinical Application 25–2 discusses drug treatment for AIDS. In addition, one study has shown that progressive resistance training or weightlifting may protect lean body mass (Roubenoff, et

al, 1999). This study emphasized that progressive resistance training or weightlifting can increase lean mass without the potential side effects and expenses of pharmacologic treatments (Roubenoff, et al., 1999). Realistically, health care intervention can only suppress most infections for these clients, not cure them.

Prevention and Counseling

Notification of a positive HIV test finding creates a crisis for the individual. A person who has had pretest counseling is more prepared and likely

---

CLINICAL APPLICATION 25–2 (Continued)

NON-Nucleoside Reverse Transcriptase Inhibitor

Medication	Generic Name	Dosing	Food Tips
Didanosine (ddl)	Videx	Once per day	Take on an empty stomach
			Do not take with other medications
Lamivudine (3TC)	Epivir	BID	With or without food
Stavudine (d4T)	Zerit	BID	With or without food
Zalcitibine (ddC)	Hivid	TID	With or without food
Zidovudine (AZT)	Retrovir	BID	With food, preferably nonfat
			Take 400 IU vitamin E qd to decrease bone marrow suppression
Abacavir	1592U89	BID	With or without food
Nevirapine	Viramune	BID	No food restriction
Delavirdine	Efavirenz	Once a day at bedtime	No food restriction

How are the drugs mentioned in this table combined? Typically a protease inhibitor is combined with two non-nucleoside reverse transcriptase inhibitors. For example, Crixivan is combined with AZT and DDL. This requires following a tight schedule. Here is a sample schedule:

6:00 A.M.   Indinavir

7:00 A.M   Breakfast and AZT

9:00 A.M.   DDL on an empty stomach

11:00 A.M.   Lunch

2:00 P.M.   Indinavir

5:00 P.M.   Dinner and AZT

8:00 P.M.   Snack

10:00 P.M.   Indinavir

12:00 P.M.   DDL on an empty stomach

Other medications may be useful in reversing the nutritional decline and sequelae associated with AIDS. Marinal, dronabinal, and megace have all been shown to have significant efficacy in appetite stimulation, increased kilocalorie intake, reversing weight loss, and improving patient's sense of well-being.

---

to cope better. Counseling the individual on how best to fight the virus is important; for example, the HIV-positive individual needs to receive all current immunizations to boost his or her immunity. Behaviors that interfere with wellness and reduce immunity, such as drinking alcohol, smoking, and illegal drug use, should be discouraged. Adequate rest, good nutrition, and exercise all can improve general good health and should be encouraged.

Nutrition and HIV Infection

Nutritional management is both a preventive and a therapeutic treatment in HIV infection. Malnutrition is a major mediator and predictor of death from AIDS (Solomons, 1999). A malnourished client has a limited ability to fight infection. Well-nourished individuals infected with the HIV virus are better able to offer some resistance to opportunistic infections and tolerate the side effects of treatment. Good nutritional status may influence response to medications by decreasing the incidence of adverse drug reactions, providing available raw materials for reactions evoked by medications, and supporting organ functions. Because these patients take multiple prescribed medications, almost all need extensive counseling on food and medication interactions.

Some experts believe that the most effective medical intervention involves the prevention, early identification, and early treatment of enteric infections and malabsorption. Keeping AIDS clients well nourished is often a challenge because of their numerous medical complications. Dietary modifications are frequently indicated for many of them.

Nutrition and Immunity

The function of the immune system is to protect the body against foreign invasion. Foreign invaders include viruses, bacteria, tumor cells, fungi, and transplant material. Studies have shown that a deficiency of almost any nutrient affects a cell's ability to fight infection and handle foreign invaders. Therefore, malnutrition itself can result in an immune deficiency. Many experts believe that malnutrition aggravates AIDS and may suppress any residual immune function. Deficiencies of iron, zinc, pyridoxine, folic acid, and vitamins B_{12}, C, and A are associated with immunologic changes. Malnourished clients with AIDS have minimal internal resources to fight opportunistic infections.

Malnutrition in AIDS Clients

Malnutrition causes a number of physiological alterations that may lead to decreased resistance to infection. For example, malnutrition can cause increased gut permeability, which allows more alien material to be absorbed into the body. Malnutrition may also result in decreased intestinal secretions. Some of these secretions are necessary for the proper digestion and absorption of food. Malnutrition may also cause a change in intestinal flora. This may affect the utilization of nutrients. Malnutrition may lead to hormonal imbalances and a decreased ability to repair tissue. The body ceases to replace and repair tissue because it lacks the raw materials to do so. A well-balanced diet is essential to optimal immune function.

Some HIV-positive clients need an additional 400 kilocalories per day to maintain their weight and prevent wasting. Wasting is a loss of both body fat and lean body mass and always accompanies an inadequate intake of kilocalories and protein. Wasting has been shown to increase mortality and shorten life.

Cachexia is a loss of lean body mass without a weight loss. Weight can be rising while lean body mass is decreasing. This happens because cachexia occurs when the body's immune response is turned on and certain catabolic cytokines, such as interleukin-1 and tumor necrosis factor, are also turned on. These cytokines alter metabolism in such a way that protein is utilized excessively and fat is utilized insufficiently. Thus, the protein compartment of the body declines and the fat compartment is relatively spared (Mason and Roubenoff, 1999). Cachexia is a slower process than wasting, and life can be sustained for quite a period of time during the process. Death results when approximately 40 percent of baseline lean body mass is lost. Clients with HIV should be alerted to this phenomenon and have their body composition monitored. Nutrition education is indicated (Box 25–2). Also, exercise has been shown to help conserve lean body mass.

Malabsorption

Diarrhea and malabsorption are probably the major nutrition-related problems for AIDS clients. Mucosal atrophy and decreased digestive enzyme activity contribute to the malabsorption seen in persons with AIDS. Carbohydrate malabsorption and steatorrhea are frequently seen in AIDS clients with diarrhea. Gastrointestinal problems such as diarrhea may occur in children with HIV infection due to disaccharide intolerance rather than to enteric infection with known pathogens. Malabsorption of

---

Box 25–2 Counseling the Client with HIV and AIDS

1. Offer nutrition education soon after the initial diagnosis. Even if the client has not lost weight or seems to be eating a balanced diet, teach the client the basics of good nutrition.
2. Decreased fat and cholesterol levels have been linked to adverse clinical outcomes (Chlebowski et al., 1995). Closely monitor blood lipids and cholesterol levels.
3. Evaluate the client's diet which should contain at least 100 percent of the RDA for all vitamins and minerals. A multivitamin/mineral supplement may or may not be indicated.
4. Recommend the HIV-infected person consume a few hundred more kilocalories per day than usual. Discourage weight loss as many HIV clients lose lean body mass and fat second.
5. Encourage more and frequent meals to increase energy intake. Snacks, complete nutritional supplements, and intravenous feedings may be necessary.

---

fat, simple sugars, and vitamin B_{12} is known to occur in clients with intestinal infections. AIDS clients who have diarrhea or malabsorption clearly have additional vitamin and mineral needs. Clinicians measure 25-hydroxy–vitamin D levels (as an indicator of fat-soluble vitamin absorption) and folate or zinc (as an indicator of water-soluble vitamin status) (Mason and Roubenoff, 1999).

Other factors may contribute to the diarrhea seen in these clients. Malnutrition can cause a decrease in pancreatic secretions, decreased levels of the enzymes found in the walls of the small intestine (lactase, sucrase, maltase), villous atrophy, and decreased absorptive surfaces. Side effects of medication therapy may be related to malabsorption. For example, bacterial overgrowth of organisms that are not susceptible to the chosen antibiotic may occur with long-term anti-infective therapy. The colon contains colonies of bacteria that aid in food digestion. Whenever an individual takes an antibiotic, these helpful bacterial colonies are disrupted and may permit overgrowth of other relatively resistant bacteria that promote diarrhea.

Initially, dietary treatment involves identification of the cause of the diarrhea and a determination of which nutrients the client cannot absorb. The concentration of hydrogen in the breath can be measured after oral lactose or sucrose administration to determine whether the client is intolerant to either of these sugars. An elevated breath hydrogen level implies intolerance, because the hydrogen is primarily a product of metabolism of these sugars by colon bacteria. Fecal microbiologic evaluations and intestinal biopsies are used to determine absorptive capability. In some clients infected with HIV, malabsorption of sucrose, maltose, lactose, and fat has been documented, even in the absence of diarrhea.

Clients with a form of carbohydrate intolerance may benefit from either a lactose-restricted or a disaccharide-free diet. A disaccharide-free diet is indicated for severe intolerance to sugar. Sucrose needs to be broken down into glucose and fructose (lactose into glucose and galactose; maltose into glucose and glucose) before absorption is possible. A disaccharide-free diet excludes most fruits and vegetables and many starches and is nutritionally inadequate. Vitamin C is deficient, and daily supplementation is recommended. Some of these clients may tolerate a small

---

CLINICAL APPLICATION 25-3

Incorporating Medium-Chain Triglyceride Oil into Table Foods

Medium-chain triglyceride (MCT) oil can replace vegetable oil in most recipes with satisfactory results. The easiest ways to introduce MCT oil in food preparation are in salad dressings, blended with milk (pretreated with lactase enzyme if necessary) or fruit juices, and in sauteed foods MCT oil can be used to make cookies, bread, pancakes, French toast, muffins, and pie crusts. MCT oil is made by Mead-Johnson and can usually be purchased from a pharmacy.

amount of sugar, but they usually need assistance in understanding their tolerance level. A lactose-free diet may be sufficient for clients who are deficient only in lactase.

A low-fat diet may be necessary to control steatorrhea. In cases of severe fat intolerance, medium-chain triglycerides are more readily absorbed. Clinical Application 25–3 discusses several ways in which medium-chain triglycerides can be incorporated into table foods. Usually the physician prescribes this diet as needed.

Several additional meal-planning tips are suggested to promote the client's well-being and to control the malabsorption:

1. Fluids should be encouraged to maintain hydration when large fluid volume is lost in stools.
2. Yogurt and other foods that contain the *Lactobacillus acidophilus* culture may be helpful if bacteria overgrowth is a problem secondary to long-term anti-infective use.
3. Small, frequent meals make the best use of a limited absorptive capacity of the gut.
4. A multivitamin supplement is indicated to increase the amount of vitamin available for absorption.
5. An elemental formula for medical use or parenteral nutrition may be necessary during severe bouts of malabsorption. An elemental formula for medical use contains partially digested nutrients. Promising studies have shown that clients experienced increased weight gain and good tolerance when this type of formula was given at home (Trujillo et al., 1992).
6. Avoidance of sorbital, which is used as a sweetening agent in both sugar-free candies and some medications, has been shown to cause diarrhea and should be avoided.

In some situations, the malabsorption is highly resistant to any treatment. Nutritional therapy goals should maximize client comfort. Fiber-containing supplements or foods high in fiber may be beneficial for decreasing diarrhea; eliminating caffeine intake also may help control it. The benefits of overly restricting the client's diet may not suffice to offset the resulting loss in client comfort in an incurable situation.

Increased Nutritional Requirements

Several studies suggest that the resting energy expenditure (REE) is elevated in patients with early HIV infection and increases with subsequent AIDS (Smith and Lowry, 1999). Fever and infection increase kilocaloric, protein, and certain mineral and vitamin requirements.

Dietitians frequently use the **Harris-Benedict equation** and multiply by appropriate stress and activity factors to determine kilocaloric requirements. Protein requirements should reflect a 150:1 kilocalorie:nitrogen ratio (McCorkindale, 1990) if the client shows signs of hypermetabolism. Chapter 24, Nutrition During Stress, discusses hypermetabolism in more detail.

Not all patients with AIDS become hypermetabolic. Studies have indicated that a small percentage of the AIDS population without secondary infection may be hypometabolic and demonstrate a response similar to that seen in starvation (Smith and Lowry, 1999). Hypometabolic patients need a gradual increase in kilocalories and a lower kilocalorie:nitrogen ratio. These patients should also be monitored for refeeding syndrome.

Decreased Food Intake

Anorexia can be a major problem for many clients with AIDS. A poor food intake may be the result of fever, respiratory infections, drug side effects, gastrointestinal complications, oral and esophageal pain, and emotional stress. Clients with ADC may experience mechanical problems with eating. Some drugs used in these clients, such as bactrim and pentamine, may cause nausea, vomiting, and taste changes that decrease the client's desire to eat. Interaction with the client to encourage food intake is particularly important when the person is feeling relatively well.

Nutritional Care in AIDS

Manifestations of the HIV virus vary greatly from one client to another. Therefore, nutritional care must be tailored to each client's unique set of symptoms. Quality nutritional care starts with screening.

Screening

Screening HIV-infected clients for nutritional problems is a crucial component of quality client care. Early indicators of decreased nutritional status include decreases in body weight, percent body fat, and body mass index (BMI) (McCorkindale, 1990). The recent food intake of all clients infected with the HIV virus should be assessed. An effort should be made to correct all nutritional deficiencies as soon as possible. This intervention will help support response to treatment of opportunistic infections and improve client strength and comfort. A baseline measure of percent body fat and lean body mass helps monitor disease progression.

Planning Nutrient Delivery

In keeping with the general principle, "if the gut works, use it," every effort should be made to feed the client orally. The anorexia commonly seen in AIDS clients can sometimes be resolved by changing the meal plan. Try offering smaller, frequent feedings. Serving food cold or at room temperature may help some clients consume more kilocalories. Modification of seasonings and kilocaloric density may also improve intake. Modification of texture may assist the client with poor chewing ability or oral lesions.

The Centers for Disease Control recommends the use of regular dishware for clients with blood-borne diseases. Because AIDS is not transmitted through food, food handling, or dishes, regular dishes and utensils may be used without risk. This means an isolation setup is not necessary. Historically, an isolation setup included only disposable dishware, a cardboard tray, and plastic utensils. Disposable dishware compounds the client's feelings of social isolation. Regular dishware provides better quality food at appropriate temperatures and allows the food to appear more appetizing. However, many healthcare institutions require all workers to wear protective gloves when handling soiled dishes to protect them from infection with opportunistic organisms.

If the client is unable to consume sufficient nutrients from table foods, supplemental feedings and/or other enteral feedings should be considered. The type of malnutrition should influence the food and supplements offered, which the dietitian usually determines. For example, if the client's protein status is adequate but the client has an energy deficit, a carbohydrate and/or fat supplement may be the best choice. In such a situation, the client's serum albumin level is normal but the client still may be losing weight. On the other hand, if the client's albumin is low but his or her body weight is stable, a protein supplement would be preferable. Of course, water balance also influences body weight, so this example is necessarily an oversimplification. The point is that not all supplemental feedings are equally desirable at any given stage of illness. Clients are encouraged to consume particular nutrients based on individual assessment data.

If the client is unable to consume sufficient nutrients orally and the gut is working, a tube feeding may be considered. If the gut is not functioning properly, PPN or TPN may be considered. The goal with these clients should always be to prolong living, not to prolong dying. A client has the right to refuse any alternative-feeding route offered.

Monitoring

To ensure that adequate nutrients are being consumed, the client must be evaluated periodically. Body weight and nutritional intake should be monitored frequently. BMI and percent body fat should be monitored every few weeks. Throughout this process, healthcare workers should maintain a supportive, nonjudgmental approach, which is the key to establishing a trusting relationship.

Client Teaching

Nutritional education is an important part of total client care. All AIDS clients need instruction on food safety because low immune system functioning makes them much more susceptible to food-borne illnesses. This will minimize the likelihood of opportunistic infection. Instructions on dietary modifications and the use of supplemental feedings are also indicated. Many of these clients need instruction on the importance of good nutrition and how to prepare nutrient-dense meals. An assessment of the client's knowledge level and understanding of the individualized meal plan is appropriate. Food tips for travelers with HIV are discussed in Table 25–2.

FOOD FADDISM AND QUACKERY Some clients with AIDS are vulnerable to both food faddism and quackery because they become desperate enough to try anything that arouses hope. **Food faddism** is an unusual pattern of food behavior enthusiastically adapted by its adherents. **Food quackery**

TABLE 24–2 Food Tips for Travelers with HIV Infection

Travel, particularly to third world countries, may carry a significant risk for the exposure of HIV-infected persons to opportunistic pathogens. For this reason, HIV-infected travelers should be counseled on the following prior to departure from home:

- Raw or undercooked seafood, eggs (Caesar dressings), and poultry should be avoided.
- Unpasteurized milk and dairy products should be avoided.
- Items purchased from street vendors should be avoided.
- Tap water and ice made from tap water should be avoided. Hot coffee or tea, beer, wine, or water brought to a rolling boil for 1 minute is preferable. Treatment of water with iodine or chlorine may not be as effective as boiling but can be used, perhaps in conjunction with filtration, when boiling is not practical.
- Items generally considered safe include: steaming hot foods served, fruits peeled by the traveler, and bottled (especially carbonated) beverages.
- Accidental ingestion of lake or river water while swimming or engaging in other recreational activities may carry a risk. In the severely immunocompromised client, an additional restriction may be necessary. Some soft cheese and ready-to-eat foods (e.g., hot dogs and cold cuts from delicatessen counters) have been known to cause listeriosis. These foods should be reheated until they are steaming hot before ingestlon.

---

is the promotion for profit of a medical scheme or remedy that is unproved or known to be false (Barrett and Herbet, 1999).

Healthcare educators need to carefully balance and consider the danger of unusual food behaviors versus taking away any hope the client may have. Clients may tune out educators if they perceive that their beliefs and feelings are discounted without sensitivity. Some unusual food behaviors are not harmful, and some food behaviors can result in negative health consequences. The client with limited resources who spends all his or her money on dietary supplements and herbal products with limited health benefits and very little or no money on food will develop malnutrition. A reliable desktop reference and carefully chosen Internet sites can help the health educator determine what is inappropriate. Care must be taken not to use Internet sites that sell questionable products.

Follow-up Care

The nutritional status of a client often depends on appropriate follow-up care. A referral to a community agency, a home health care program, an outpatient clinic, or a dietitian should be made to provide continuity of care.

Summary

The AIDS epidemic is worldwide. Although HAART and protease inhibitors have reduced mortality rates, no cure has been found for AIDS. Known transmittal routes include blood-to-blood, perinatal, and sexual contact. As healthcare professionals, we can all protect ourselves from AIDS by using extreme care when handling blood and equipment that has been in contact with blood and as private individuals by practicing safe sexual

behaviors. HIV attacks the immune system and leaves its victims defenseless against opportunistic infections. AIDS is a disease with many clinical complications. Nutritional management is both a preventive and a therapeutic treatment in clients infected with HIV. Increased nutrient needs, decreased food intake, and impaired nutrient absorption contribute to the malnutrition seen in AIDS clients.

Case Study 25–1

Ms. S is a 30-year-old woman who acquired HIV from her drug-abusing husband and subsequently infected their son in utero. She could not believe the test results when she was first told. Now she is seeking nutritional information to allow her to increase her chance for a quality life and her son's chance to survive infancy. Her knowledge of basic nutrition is good.

Nursing Care Plan

Subjective Data	Lack of information on relationship of nutrition to AIDS
	Concrete goals established
Objective Data	HIV-positive tests, both mother and infant
	Percent body fat, 25
Nursing Diagnosis	NANDA: Knowledge deficit (North American Nursing Diagnosis Association, 1999)
	Related to AIDS progression and verbal statements

Desired Outcomes Evaluation Criteria	Nursing Actions/ Interventions	Rationale
NOC: Knowledge: disease (Johnson, Maas, and Moorhead, 2000, with permission.)	NIC: Teaching: Disease Process (McCloskey and Bulechek, 2000)	
Client will verbalize areas in which nutrition could affect AIDS development.	Reinforce need for regular, balanced meals. Emphasize adequate kilocalories.	The stress of receiving this diagnosis may impede use of previously learned information.
	Instruct Ms. S to keep home environment clean, especially kitchen, bathroom, and basements where molds and fungi could thrive.	Organisms that are harmless to persons with normal immune systems can cause opportunistic infections in HIV-infected persons.
	Teach client to monitor herself and her son for changes in health related to food intake or digestion.	Discovering beginning malabsorption problems would permit treatment before malnutrition becomes apparent.
Client will monitor her % body fat	Explain the relationships among percent body fat, percent lean body mass, and exercise.	Exercise can prevent a loss of lean body mass.
		Weight can be stable, but body fat content can increase.

Critical Thinking Question

1. The client has developed mouth sores from thrush and would like you to arrange for her to have TPN. She claims it is just too painful to eat. What would you recommend?
2. The client's child has been diagnosed HIV positive. During a home visit, you notice the kitchen is filthy. You instruct the client on food safety and sanitation. On a return visit, despite prior instruction on food safety, you notice that the client's kitchen is still not clean. The client claims she is too tired to clean. What do you do?
3. The client went to a health food store and purchased several bottles of vitamin pills and herbal supplements. She believes she can take these in lieu of eating. What should you do?

 # Study Aids

Subjects . . . . .Internet Sites	
Center for Chronic Disease Control . . . . .http://www.cdc.gov/ncnswww/fastata/aids-hiv.htm, accessed December 1999 Statistical information by disease	
HIV/AIDS and STD surveillance . . . . .http://www.who, accessed December 1999	
HIV/AIDS continuing education . . . . .http://cyberounds.com/conferences/nutrition/conferences/0499/ conference.html, accessed December 1999	
An HIV/AIDS information resource . . . . .www.thebody.com, accessed May 2000	
AIDS Treatment Data Network . . . . .www.aidsinfonyc.org, accessed May 2000	
HIV/AIDS information site . . . . .www.aegis.com, accessed May 2000	

Chapter Review

1. The healthcare worker's best insurance against HIV transmission on the job is:
   a. Frequent hand washing
   b. Universal precautions
   c. Body substance isolation
   d. Adherence to all food safety policies and procedures
2. A client on HAART can partially compensate for fat redistribution syndrome by:
   a. Taking medications as prescribed
   b. Taking supplemental vitamins and minerals
   c. Consuming a low-fat diet
   d. Exercising
3. Compared to wasting, cachexia is:
   a. A slower process
   b. The result of both a protein and kilocalorie deficit
   c. Always the result of a poor food intake
   d. Best treated by the inclusion of 400 additional kilocalories per day
4. Clinicians measure _____ as an indicator of fat-soluble vitamin absorption.
   a. Folate
   b. Zinc
   c. 25-hyroxy–vitamin D
   d. Glucose
5. Educating an AIDS client about food safety is important because:
   a. AIDS clients are less likely to develop rare tumors
   b. AIDS clients are less likely to have body fat redistribution
   c. AIDS clients are less likely to have renal complications
   d. AIDS clients are less likely to develop opportunistic infections

Clinical Analysis

1. Mr. Y, a 45-year-old black male, was diagnosed as HIV positive 1 month ago. His height is 6 feet 0 inches, and his weight is 178 pounds and stable. He reports no signs or symptoms and has not seen a physician yet. He wants to know what he should eat. As the nurse during this first visit, it may be appropriate to discuss:
   a. The many benefits of HAART
   b. Food safety, exercise, good nutrition, and the importance of follow-up with a physician
   c. The expected outcome and potential complications
   d. Vitamin-mineral supplementation, increased kilocalorie needs, and the treatment for malabsorption
2. Carlos, a 25-year-old Hispanic male, presents with severe diarrhea. He was diagnosed with HIV about 8 years ago. He has five to six watery stools each day that do not appear to be related to his medications. His height is 5 feet 10 inches, and his weight is 140 pounds (usual weight is 175 pounds). He is an inpatient, and the physician has ordered a stool culture but the results are not back. You recommend:
   a. Extra fluids with meals to prevent dehydration
   b. A clear liquid, complete nutritional supplement
   c. A high-fat and high-fiber diet to provide both kilocalories and bulk to his diet
   d. Six small meals with a milkshake between meals to push kilocalories and protein
3. Dave, a 36-year-old white male, complains of fatigue. He is often too tired to cook and has little interest in food. He lives alone and is on disability. His CD_4 cell count is 400, and his viral load is 100,000. You recommend:
   a. A tube feeding
   b. Referral to a social service agency for a friendly visitor
   c. Meals-on-Wheels
   d. Six small meals daily

Bibliography

American Dietetic Association: Manual of Clinical Dietetics, ed 5. The American Dietetic Association, Chicago, 1995.

Barrett, S, and Herbet, V: Fads, frauds, and quackery. In Shils, ME, Olson, JE, Shikes, M, and Ross, CA (eds): Modern Nutrition in Health and Disease, ed 9. Williams and Wilkins, Baltimore, 1999.

Bartletti, JG (ed): New Trials Reach Same Conclusion: Two Drugs Are Better Than AZT Alone. AIDS Alert 10:133, 1995.

Batterham, M: Lipodystrophy—a side effect of protease inhibitor therapy. Positive Communications: A publication of the HIV/AIDS dietetic practice group. The American Dietetic Association, Chicago, IL 2(2), Summer 1998

Centers for Disease Control: AIDS Information Hotline (404/332-4565). Document No. 320210, 1994.

Centers for Disease Control: www.cdc.gov/ncnswww/fastats/aids-hiv.htm accessed August 1999.

Chlebowski, RT, et al.: Diet intake and counseling, weight maintenance, and the course of HIV infection. J Am Diet Assoc 95:428, 1995.

Coffin, J: Current understanding of HIV disease: A summary. Positive Communications: A publication of the HIV/AIDS dietetic practice group. The American Dietetic Association, Chicago, IL, Vol 2, No 4, Summer 1998.

Collier, AC, et al.: Treatment of human immunodeficiency virus infection with saquinavir, zidovudine, and zalcitabine. New Engl J Med 334:1011, 1996.

Garrett, L: The Coming Plague, p 477. Penguin Books, New York, 1994.

Greene, WC: Denying HIV safe haven. New Engl J Med 334:1264, 1996.

Heckt, FM, et al..: Optimizing care for patients with HIV infection. Ann Intern Med 131:136, 1999.

HIV InSite, www.hivinsite.ucsf.edu, accessed May 2000.

Johnson, M, Maas, M, and Moorhead, S: Nursing Outcomes Classification (NOC), ed 2. Mosby, Philadelphia, 2000.

Kotler, D: Metabolism, Wasting/Nutrition, HIV/AIDS Course. The American Dietetic Association Eighty-first Annual Meeting and Exhibition Workshop, Kansas City, Missouri, October 18, 1998.

Mandell, GL, Bennett, JE, and Dolin, R: Principles and Practice of Infectious Diseases, ed 4. Churchill Livingstone, New York, 1995.

Mason, J, and Roubenoff, R: Nutritional issues of clinical concern in HIV patients. http://www.cyberounds.com/conferences/0499/conference.html accessed July 28, 1999.

Maurice, J: Hypertriglyceremia in HIV patients?possible solutions. Positive Communications: A publication of the HIV/AIDS dietetic practice group. The American Dietetic Association, Chicago, IL 2(2), Summer 1998.

McCloskey, JC, and Bulechek, GM: Nursing Interventions Classification (NIC), 3 ed. Mosby, Philadelphia, 2000.

McCorkindale, C: Nutrition status of HIV-infected patients during early disease stages. J Am Diet Assoc 90:1236, 1990.

North American Nursing Diagnosis Association: Nursing Diagnoses: Definitions and Classification 1999–2000, North American Nursing Diagnosis Association, Philadelphia, 1999.

Pomerantz, R: Residual HIV-1 disease in the era of highly active anti-retroviral therapy. N Engl J Med 340:1672. 1999.

Position Paper of the American and Canadian Dietetic Association: Nutrition intervention in the care of persons with human immunodeficiency virus infection. J Am Diet Assoc 94:1042, 1994.

Roubenoff, R, et al.: Short-term progressive resistance training increases strength and lean body mass in adults infected with human immunodeficiency virus, 1999. http://www.cyberounds.com. Accessed July 1999.

Scharnhorst, S: AIDS dementia complex in the elderly. Nurse Pract 17(8):41, 1992.

Smith, MK, and Lowry, SF: The hypermetabolic state. In Shils, ME, Olson, JE, Shikes, M, and Ross, CA (eds): Modern Nutrition in Health and Disease, ed 9. Williams and Wilkins, Baltimore, 1999.

Solomons, NE: International priorities for clinical and therapeutic nutrition in the context of public relations. In Shils, ME, Olson, JE, Shikes, M, and Ross, CA (eds): Modern Nutrition in Health and Disease, ed 9. Williams and Wilkins, Baltimore, 1999.

Trujillo, EB, et al.: Assessment of nutritional status, nutrient intake, and nutrition support in AIDS patients. J Am Diet Assoc 92:477, 1992.

Ungvarski, PJ, and Flaskerud, JH: HIV/AIDS: A Guide to Primary Care Management. WB Saunders, Philadelphia, 1999.

US Public Health Service: Guidelines for the prevention of opportunistic infections in persons infected with human immunodeficiency virus: A summary. Ann Intern Med 124:349, 1996.

Viral load tests, www.aidsinfonyc.org accessed, May 2000

Volberding, PA: Improving the outcomes of care for patients with human immunodeficiency virus infection. New Engl J Med 334:729, 1996.

Watson, J, and Jaffe, MS: Nurse's Manual of Laboratory and Diagnostic Tests, ed 2. FA Davis, Philadelphia, 1995.

Woods, SE: Nutrition beliefs of men with human immunodeficiency virus disease in a self-selected population. The American Dietetic Association Seventy-eighth Annual Meeting and Exhibition (abstracts). J Am Diet Assoc 95:A-88, 1995.

World Health Organization: http://www.who, accessed July 22, 1999.

CHAPTER 26

Nutritional Care of the Terminally Ill

LEARNING OBJECTIVES

After completing this chapter, the student should be able to:

1. Differentiate between palliative and curative nutritional care.
2. State appropriate nutritional screening questions for the terminally ill client.
3. List at least two appropriate dietary management techniques for symptom control for each of the following: anemia, anorexia, bowel obstruction, cachexia, constipation, cough, dehydration, diarrhea, dysgeusia, esophageal reflux, fever, fluid accumulation, hiccups, incontinence, jaundice and hepatic encephalopathy, migraine headache, nausea and vomiting, pruritus, stomatitis, weakness, wounds and pressure sores, and **xerostomia**.
4. State appropriate assessment questions for a terminally ill client.
5. Discuss the ethical and legal considerations for feeding a terminally ill client.

This chapter discusses clients who have been certified by physicians to be terminally ill. An individual is considered terminally ill if he or she has a medical prognosis of 6 months or less based on the usual disease progression. Although a physician can estimate life expectancy based on disease progression, this is not an exact science. A client diagnosed with a terminal disease may live longer or less long than predicted because the disease may not follow its usual progression. Individuals who have been certified by a physician as terminally ill can elect the Hospice benefit under federal guidelines (www.ncfa.gov/medicaid). Hospice is the major health care program for the terminally ill in the United States.

Dealing with Death

Our culture emphasizes the enjoyment of life. At the beginning of this century, most people died at home, and many died young. Death was a part of everyday life. In the past 50 years, most people have died in hospitals or long-term care facilities. Often an ambulance is called if a person is dying. Although healthcare workers have received much training on how to reverse the effects of disease, we have received much less training on how to assist our clients with dying. With changes in the healthcare system bringing decreased lengths of hospital stays, an increasing number of clients will again be cared for in their homes. Training healthcare workers to provide homecare for terminally ill clients is becoming essential.

To help the dying, healthcare workers must first contemplate and then accept their own mortality. Nurses, physicians, and other health care workers tend to deny death as much as lay people do. One study showed that basic interventions to maintain comfort were often not provided in hospitals, including the following: oral hygiene was often poor; thirst remained unquenched; little assistance was given to encourage eating; contact between nurses and dying patients was minimal; and distancing between nurses and dying patients was evident; and this isolation increased as death approached (Mills, Davis, and Micrea, 1994). Health care providers may also become attached to particular clients and become overwhelmed by feelings, thereby becoming ineffective as helping caregivers. Nutritional and dietary issues are at the center of some ethical questions concerning the care of these clients. Becoming an advocate for clients' best interests is a priority when providing quality care to the dying.

The Dying Process

Death is an unavoidable part of the life cycle. Both physiological and psychological changes occur as part of the dying process. The client's age, diagnosis, and physical condition influence physiological changes. Regardless of the underlying disease, cardiopulmonary failure is the final cause of death. Pulmonary and circulatory failure may be gradual or sudden. The major signs and symptoms in the final days and hours of life include cessation of eating and drinking, oliguria and incontinence, muscle weakness, difficulty in breathing, cyanosis, decreased mental alertness, and changes in vital signs.

Hospice team members may describe clients with a terminal diagnosis as actively dying. An actively dying client has a life expectancy of a few hours or a few days. The reason for the actively dying designation is to determine staff needs. The following sections discuss the criteria team members use to determine the actively dying status.

Cessation of Eating and Drinking

Life will soon cease when a client's eating and drinking diminishes critically. One study reported that 8 percent of clients with cancer completely cease to eat and/or drink (Feuz and Rapin, 1994). Oral intake dwindles because a client has no desire to eat or because disease prevents digestion. This greatly decreased oral intake is often worrisome to family members. Healthcare workers need to counsel family members that dehydration at this time is believed to have a euphoric effect and is not painful. Clinical Application 26–1 discusses the physiological responses to fluid restriction. Oral dryness can be alleviated by good oral care, the use of ice chips, giving sips of fluids, and applying oil to the lips. It is unkind to force food or fluids on a client who is actively dying.

Oliguria and Incontinence

Because oral intake is usually decreased for several days before death, urine output is often diminished and may cease. The color of the urine may become very dark. A period of incontinence often precedes the oliguria, and anuria occurs. General fatigue, muscle weakness, and decreased mental acuity are among the reasons for the incontinence. Bedding should be changed as quickly as possible to avoid skin irritation. Death usually occurs within 48–72 hours after urine output stops.

Difficulty in Breathing

Most clients have some difficulty breathing before death. Caregivers may become alarmed when they hear a loud, hoarse, and bubbling sound. This sound is caused by the passage of breath through pharyngeal and pulmonary secretions that lodge at the back of the client's throat. Atropine is often administered to decrease the secretions. Elevating the head of the bed, gentle suctioning, and positioning the client on his or her side help maintain a clear airway. All terminally ill clients do not have these sounds with respiration. Some clients experience apnea (a temporary cessation of breathing). A change such as these in breathing is an indicator that life will soon cease.

Cyanosis

Slightly bluish, grayish, or dark purple discoloration of the skin caused by poor oxygenation is called **cyanosis**. The client's feet, legs, hands, and groin feel cold. Many healthcare workers believe this is one of the most useful indicators that the end of life is approaching. Slowed circulation and decreased tissue perfusion cause these signs.

Decreased Mental Alertness

The amount of blood reaching the brain, lungs, liver, and kidneys decreases as general circulation slows. Sleepiness, apathy, disorientation, confusion, restlessness, and finally a decreased level of consciousness that frequently progresses to a sleep-like state are among the signs that death is imminent.

Changes in Vital Signs

A decrease in body temperature, an increase in pulse rate, a rise and then a decrease in respirations, and a fall in blood pressure are signs

---

CLINICAL APPLICATION 26–1

Physiological Response to Fluid Restriction

Young, healthy, active individuals who are derived of water develop thirst, dry mouth, and headache, followed by fatigue; cognitive impairment occurs as dehydration progresses and becomes severe with abnormal electrolytes, rising blood urea nitrogen, and hemoconcentration (Shils, 1999). If water is not taken, renal failure is likely.

Hospice workers taking care of terminally ill clients report the following (Junkerman and Schiedermayer, 1998):

- Actively dying clients often voluntarily stop eating and drinking and do not tolerate a substantial amount of tube feedings.
- Actively dying clients who are given normal fluid replacement commonly show signs of fluid overload, including pulmonary edema.
- Actively dying clients almost never report feelings of hunger or thirst.
- Dehydration results in less vomiting and diarrhea, less need to suction secretions, less dyspnea, and peripheral edema.

Hospice discourages the use of tube feedings and orally administered fluids for dying patients. However, fluids should be offered to clients and given if requested by clients

---

of impending death. Death occurs when there is no pulse and respiration ceases.

Family members and caregivers of terminally ill clients often express fear at the thought of being alone with an actively dying client. For this reason, healthcare workers often remain with the client and their loved ones during this time. Some nurses resist working with the terminally ill because they think that they cannot cope with this experience. However, death is not always a painful experience. Death can provide an opportunity for personal growth, joyous affirmation of life, and meaningful attachments. Healthcare workers who share the death experience with a client and the client's family often describe the experience as rewarding and profound.

Palliative Versus Curative Care

The goal of curative care is arresting the disease. The goal of palliative care is the relief of symptoms to alleviate or ease pain and discomfort. Emphasis in palliative care is placed on addressing the problems of pain, loneliness, and loss of control that are common in dying clients. Palliative care programs address and/or include the client and family members in the plan of care.

Hospice is a concept that dates back to medieval times. During the crusades, travelers needed a place to stop for comfort. The Knights of Hospitallers of the Order of St. John of Jerusalem in the twelfth century sheltered sick and religious pilgrims. They established hospices in England, Germany, Italy, Cyprus, and Rhodes. The soul, the mind, and the spirit were considered as much in need of help as the body. Around the fifteenth century, anatomic and surgical practices developed. Physicians moved into hospitals that emphasized curative treatments. Monks and nuns remained in cloisters and cared for the people the physicians could not heal, including the disabled, the chronically ill, and the terminally ill. During the eighteenth and nineteenth centuries, great advances in curative treatments occurred, and hospitals became highly specialized in acute life-threatening situations. Hospitals were less able to offer shelter to people nearing life's end. At the same time, caring for the terminally ill became less a private or religious function and more a public and governmental one.

The modern hospice has its roots in the late nineteenth century, when a place of shelter for the incurable ill was founded in Dublin. The British physician Dr. Cicely Saunders inspired the hospice movement in the United States. Dr. Saunders is noted for her work in pain control and for the founding of St. Christopher's Hospice in London in 1967. The first operational hospice program in the United States was established in New Haven, Connecticut, in the early 1970s.

Hospice philosophy includes the belief that death is a natural aspect of life. Hospice is committed to the philosophy that persons have the right to die in the setting of their choice and to be as comfortable as possible. Central to the hospice philosophy is the idea that palliative care is appropriate when treatment of the client's disease becomes ineffective and irrelevant.

Nutrition Screening

The goal of palliative nutritional care is to assist the client and/or caregiver(s) with any food-related concerns. These difficulties may be related to uncomfortable symptoms and/or attitudes and beliefs held about food. Screening the client with a terminal illness for food-related concerns is the first step. There are major differences between screening a client who is undergoing curative and/or preventive treatment and screening a terminally ill client who is receiving palliative care. First, the healthcare worker needs to ascertain if the client has any symptoms that may be diminished by nutritional intervention. Second, the attitudes and beliefs of the client and/or caregiver(s) about food need to be examined. Some clients and their caregivers have difficulty accepting that the

terminally ill client frequently eats much less than is needed to sustain life. Table 26–1 is an example of a nutrition screening form for the client with a terminal condition.

Assessment

During the nutritional assessment, it is important that every question posed to the client and/or caregiver has a purpose. Healthcare workers generally need to know the results of laboratory tests, diagnostic procedures, physical examinations, and anthropometric measures as well as the level of immune function and food intake information to determine a client's nutritional status. These nutritional parameters may have no value in the provision of nutritional care for a terminally ill client, however. For example, why ask if a client drinks milk? Is it to estimate if the client is meeting the calcium, riboflavin, and vitamin D allowances? If it is determined that the client's milk intake is suboptimal, however, would anything be done about the inadequacy? If the client has diarrhea with severe abdominal cramping after the ingestion of milk, however, a recommendation to drink lactose-free milk would be appropriate. Unless the client will experience relief from bothersome symptoms, it is best not to recommend behavioral changes that may be difficult for the client to make.

Intervention and Symptom Control

Table 26–2 describes appropriate dietary management for symptom control for a client with a terminal illness. If a nurse feels uncomfortable discussing these issues with the client or lacks the time to counsel the client, a referral to the dietitian is indicated.

Ethical and Legal Considerations

Many of the legal and ethical issues concerning healthcare delivery and healthcare provider–client relations involve the provision of nutrition and hydration. In the past, before the development of tube feedings and intra-

---

Table 26–1 A Sample Nutrition Screening Form for the Client with a Terminal Condition

Name _____ Caregiver's Name _____
Date _____ Diagnosis _____
1. Have you had any concerns about weight changes or food intake?
   _____ No _____ Yes Describe _____
2. (For clients on tube feedings or parenteral feedings only): Have your feedings created or increased discomfort, diarrhea, distension, etc.?
   Type: _____ Amt. _____ Infusion rate _____
3. Do you feel your symptoms could be decreased/controlled through dietary change?
   _____ No _____ Yes Describe _____
4. Do you feel diet or nutritional supplement would benefit you or your disease process?
   _____ No _____ Yes Type _____
5. Do you believe that your diet caused your disease or will slow the progression of your disease?
   _____ No _____ Yes Describe _____
6. Do you find eating enhances comfort? _____ No _____ Yes
7. What concerns do your have regarding your diet intake? _____
8. Would you (client or caregiver) like to discuss food-related concerns with the dietitian? _____ No _____ Yes

TABLE 26–2 Dietary Management for Symptom Control

Anemia
1. Recommend vitamin C source with red meats and iron fortified foods.
2. Discourage use of coffee, tea, and chocolate if the client has gastrointestinal bleeding.
3. Recommend multivitamin supplement if client desires, but avoid megadose vitamins.

Anorexia
1. Discuss practical issues with client and/or caregiver such as food attitudes, social aspects of eating, and unpredictable food preferences (Dietitians Assoc of Australia Position Paper, 1992).
2. Evaluate client's desire for a sense of well-being.
3. Suggest use of small frequent feedings.
4. Educate caregiver to recognize early signs of malnutrition and provide protein supplements, make food accessible, and encourage eating as desired by the client and/or caregiver, if the client's prognosis is more than a few weeks.
5. Evaluate client acceptance of a liquid diet and recommend complete oral nutritional supplements.
6. Teach caregiver that the client has the right to self-determination and may refuse to eat and/or drink when actively dying. The caregiver should continue to offer nourishment as a sign of love and caring but not harass the client to eat or drink.

Bowel Obstruction
1. Recommend limiting intake to sips of fluids if the client has a complete obstruction.
2. Encourage small meals low in fiber and residue if oral intake is not contraindicated.
3. Encourage the client to eat slowly, chew food well, and rest after each meal if oral intake is not contraindicated.
4. Recommend dry feedings if oral intake is not contraindicated.
5. Recommend avoidance of sugary fatty foods, alcohol, and foods with a strong odor.

Cachexia
I. Teach relaxation techniques and encourage use before mealtime.
2. Encourage client and/or caregiver to concentrate on the sensual pleasures of eating such as setting an attractive table and plate, the use of food garnishes, and the importance of an appetizing eating environment (remove bedpans and emesis basin, etc. before serving the food).
3. Evaluate client for dysgeusia and dysphagia, and xerostomia. Refer to symptoms and definitions of terms on this table.

Constipation
1. Encourage high-fiber foods (bran, whole grains, fruits, vegetables, nuts, and legumes) if an adequate fluid intake can be maintained.
2. Instruct the client to avoid high-fiber foods if dehydration or an obstruction is suspected or anticipated.
3. Assess the client's fluid intake and recommend an increased intake if needed.
4. Recommend taking 1–2 oz with the evening meal of a special recipe: 2 cups applesauce, 2 cups unprocessed bran (All-bran), and 1 cup of 100 percent prune juice. (Gallagher-Allred, 1989). Refrigerate this mixture between uses and discard after 5 days if not used.
5. Suggest limiting cheese and high-fat, sugary foods (doughnuts, cakes, pies, cookies) that may be constipating.
6. Discontinue calcium and iron supplements if contributing to constipation.
7. Review the client's medications. If the client is taking bulking agents (milk of magnesia, magnesium citrate, Metamucil, or Golytely), a large fluid intake is essential. Suggest the client and/or caregiver mask the taste of these medications in applesauce, mashed potatoes, gravy, orange juice, and nectars.

Cough
1. Encourage fluids and ice chips.
2. Recommend hard candy including sour balls.
3. Have the client try tea and coffee to dilate pulmonary vessels.

Dehydration
1. Encourage fluids such as juices, ice cream, gelatin, custards, puddings, soups, and juices, if the client's life expectancy is more than a few days.
2. Encourage the client to try creative beverages such as orange sherbet and milk shake.
3. Consider a nasogastric tube feeding for fluid delivery only after a discussion with other team members, client, and caregivers. Plain water and foods high in electrolytes can be delivered via a tube feeding.
4. Consider a parenteral line only after a tube feeding is considered and rejected and after an in depth discussion with the team members, client, and family. Client goals, expectations, and quality of life issues should all be very carefully considered. Parenteral lines for the delivery of nutrients and water are rarely indicated in terminally ill clients.
5. Be prepared to accept that dehydration is still considered by some health professionals to be painful or uncomfortable. The impression that starvation and dehydration are terrible ways to die is especially prominent among nonhospice physicians. Generally, the impression of hospice clinicians is that starvation and dehydration do not contribute to suffering among the dying and might contribute to a comfortable passage from life (Byock, 1995). Evidence for the potential benefits of not rehydrating and for the withdrawal of intravenous fluids for terminally ill clients is increasing but is still not conclusive (Malone, 1994). This is an area of active research. *(Continued on next page)*

TABLE 26–2 Dietary Management for Symptom Control (Continued)

Diarrhea
1. Consider modification of diet to omit lactose, gluten, or fat if related to diarrhea.
2. Suggest a decrease in dietary fiber content.
3. Consider the omission of gas-forming vegetables if an association between the consumption of these foods and diarrhea can be ascertained.
4. Consider the use of a low-residue diet.
5. Encourage high-potassium foods (bananas, tomato juice, orange juice, potatoes, etc.) if the client is dehydrated.
6. Recommend dry feedings (drink fluids 1 hour before or 30–60 min after meals).
7. Encourage intake of medium-chain triglycerides and a diet high in protein and carbohydrates for steatorrhea due to pancreatic insufficiency.
8. Consider the use of a complete oral nutritional supplement to provide adequate nutrient composition while helping the client overcome mild-to-moderate malabsorption.
9. For copious diarrhea and/or diarrhea combined with a decubitus on the coccyx, consider use of a clear liquid complete nutritional supplement or a predigested oral nutritional supplement.

Disgeusia (abnormal taste)
1. Encourage oral care before mealtime.
2. Evaluate whether client experiences a bitter, sweet, or no taste after food consumption.

If foods taste bitter encourage consumption of poultry, fish, milk and milk products, and legumes. Recommend the use of marinated meats and poultry in juices or wine. Sour and salty foods are generally not liked when a client experiences a bitter taste. Cook food in a glass or porcelain container to improve taste. Recommend a decreased use of red meats, sour juices, coffee, tea, tomatoes, and chocolate. The use of a modular protein supplement may be helpful if the client's protein intake is suboptimal.

If food has no taste, recommend foods served at room temperature, highly seasoned foods, and sugary foods.

If foods have a sweet taste, recommend sour juices, tart foods, lemon juice, vinegar, pickles, spices, herbs, and the use of a modular carbohydrate supplement.

Dyspnea (difficulty breathing)
1. Encourage coffee, tea, carbonated beverages, and chocolate. These foods are bronchodilators that increase blood pressure, dilate pulmonary vessels, increase glomerular filtration rate, and thereby break up and expel pulmonary secretions and fluids (Gallagher-Allred, 1989).
2. Encourage use of a soft diet. Liquids are usually better tolerated than solids. Cold foods are often better accepted than hot foods.
3. Recommend small frequent feedings.
4. Encourage ice chips, frozen fruit juices, and popsicles; these are often well accepted.
5. Consider the use of a complete high-fat, low-carbohydrate nutritional supplement. This decreases carbon dioxide retention and assists in breathing.

Esophageal Reflux
1. Recommend small feedings.
2. Discourage foods that lower esophageal sphincter pressure such as high-fat foods, chocolate, peppermint, spearmint, and alcohol.
3. Encourage client to sit up while eating and for 1 hour afterward.
4. Recommend avoidance of food within 3 hours before bedtime.
5. Teach relaxation techniques.

Fever
1. Recommend a high-fluid intake.
2. Consider a tube feeding for severe dehydration to maintain hydration after a discussion with team members. This is not recommended if death is imminent (hours/days).
3. Recommend high-protein, high-caloric foods.

Fluid Accumulation
1. Recommend a mild sodium restriction (3–4 g/day). Recommend a lower sodium restriction only if this is the wish of the client.
2. Discourage a fluid restriction unless the client has significant hyponatremia.
3. Provide a list of foods high in protein and potassium.

Hiccups
1. Recommend smaller meals and slow eating.
2. Discourage the use of a straw.
3. Add peppermint to food to decrease gastric distention (Gallagher-Allred, 1989).
4. Recommend client swallow a large teaspoon of granulated sugar.

(Continued on next page)

TABLE 26–2 Dietary Management for Symptom Control (Continued)

Hypoglycemia
1. Assess the client's and/or caregiver's knowledge about diabetes and hypoglycemia.
2. Determine if the client is truly insulin dependent as part of the admission assessment process. The following suggest true insulin-dependence (Tatling, Houston, and Hill, 1985): a. The introduction of insulin soon after the diagnosis b. A history of previous ketoacidosis c. Use of more than one daily dose of insulin for years
3. Evaluate the client's expressed desire for extent of medical care. The primary guide for determining the level of nutritional intervention is the wish of the client.
4. Determine the last time the client experienced the signs of a hypoglycemic episode. Many of these clients have deficiencies in the counterregulatory hormones, especially epinephrine, and may lapse into a coma without any warning signs. Caregivers need to be informed of this potential complication. Educate the client and/or caregiver on the treatment of hypoglycemia (15–15 rule, "Diet in Diabetes Mellitus and Hypoglycemia").
5. Monitor client's blood glucose level. A suitable range for blood sugars would be 127-309 mg/dL in the hospice population (Boyd, 1993).
6. Encourage 30-50 g of carbohydrate every 3 hours to prevent starvation ketosis. Each of the following is equal to 30-50 g of carbohydrate:
   3/4 cup Carnation Instant Breakfast
   1 cup regular gelatin
   1 cup vanilla ice cream
   1 1/2 cups gingerale
   1 cup orange Juice
   1 cup apple juice

Incontinence
1. Discourage intake of coffee, tea, carbonated beverages containing caffeine, especially before bedtime.
2. Continue to encourage adequate fluid intake.

Jaundice and Hepatic Encephalopathy
1. Encourage a high-carbohydrate diet.
2. Encourage a protein-restricted diet only if the client desires.
3. Specialized oral nutritional supplements for clients with liver disease are often ineffective for the terminally ill but may be beneficial when the client desires to "live long enough to _____

Nausea and Vomiting
1. Discuss practical issues with client and/or caregiver such as food attitudes, social aspects of eating, and unpredictable food preferences (Dietitians Association of Australia, 1992).
2. Recommend client restrict fluids to 1 hour before or after meals to prevent early satiety.
3. Assess if sweet, fried, or fatty foods are poorly tolerated; recommend avoidance if necessary.
4. Evaluate if starchy foods such as crackers, breads, potatoes, rice, and pasta are better tolerated. Encourage increased consumption if helpful.
5. Encourage the client to eat slowly, chew feed well, and rest after each meal as these behaviors may increase food intake.
6. Recommend the client avoid offensive odors during food preparation.
7. Recommend that the person who has recently experienced severe nausea and vomiting try 1-2 bites of food per hour.
8. Emphasize the sensual aspects of food including: appearance (serve garnished food on attractive tableware); odor of environment (remove bedpans and emesis basins from room); taste (cater to the client's likes and dislikes); and the importance of companionship during mealtime.
9. Recommend the avoidance of food if nausea and vomiting becomes severe and food makes the client feel worse. Feeding may not be desirable if death is expected within hours or a few days and the effects of partial dehydration or the withdrawal of nutrition support will not adversely alter client comfort (American Dietetic Association, 1987).

Migraine Headaches
1. Recommend that the client eat at regular intervals. Hunger or missed meals can trigger a migraine headache.
2. Recommend that the highly motivated client keep a food diary and record the onset of any headaches. Migraine headaches can be triggered by one or many foods. Common food offenders include: many common food additives, processed meats, peanuts and peanut products, soybeans, yeast, chocolate, aged cheeses, seasonings, caffeine, some types of alcohol, and flavorings.

Pruritus (severe itching)
1. Recommend avoidance of known allergy foods.
2. Encourage fluid intake for clients receiving antihistamines.
3. Recommend avoidance of coffee, tea, carbonated beverages containing caffeine, alcohol, and cocoa that can cause vasodilation and itching.

(Continued on next page)

TABLE 26–2 Dietary Management for Symptom Control (Continued)

Stomatitis (Inflammation of the mouth)
1. Consider multivitamin supplement with folic acid and vitamin B12.
2. Recommend avoidance of spicy, acidic, rough, hot, and salty foods.
3. Recommend a consistency modification such as pureed, soft, or liquid.
4. Consider the use of a complete nutritional supplement.
5. Recommend creamy foods, whites sauces, and gravies.
6. Consider between meal supplements such as milkshakes, eggnogs, and puddings.
7. Recommend caregiver add sugar to acid or salty foods to alter the food's taste.
8. Recommend meals be served when the client's pain is under control.
9. Recommend good oral care before and after meals.

Weakness
1. Recommend multivitamin-mineral supplement with folic acid, vitamin B_{12}, and iron.
2. Encourage high-potassium foods (bananas, cantaloupe, milk, baked winter squash, etc.) if client vomits easily.
3. Recommend a modification in the food's consistency (mechanical soft or full liquid) to decrease the energy cost of eating

Wounds and Pressure Sores
1. Recommend caregiver cater to the client's food preferences.
2. Use of aggressive nutritional support is rarely effective, but may be appropriate if the client and family desire quantity. For example, "I want to live and see my _____."
3. Correct elevated glucose levels to decrease risk of infection.
4. Evaluate the use of a multiple vitamin and mineral supplement which contains zinc and vitamin C. As excess dietary zinc impedes healing, do not routinely recommend a zinc supplement without assessment information.
5. Encourage protein and caloric intake equal to estimated needs only if the client desires and is able.

Xerostomia (dry mouth)
1. Encourage frequent sips of water, fruit juices, ice chips, popsicles, ice cream, and sherbet.
2. Recommend the use of hard candy.
3. Consider a modification of food consistency such as soft, mechanical soft, or full liquids.
4. Recommend avoidance of extremely hot or cold foods. Foods served at room temperature are generally better tolerated.
5. Recommend creamy foods, white sauces, and gravies.
6. Encourage the client to dip foods in gravy, margarine, butter, olive oil, coffee, and broth.
7. Consider the need for a complete liquid nutritional supplement between meals.

---

venous feedings, the inability to eat and drink by mouth meant death from progressive body wasting. Now a decision needs to be made whether or not to feed a client. A client may experience a more comfortable death if he or she is slightly dehydrated. On the other hand, efforts to hydrate some clients (not those actively dying) may offer a benefit. This is controversial. Sometimes a client, significant other, or physician thinks that artificial hydration may promote client comfort and prolong life in a given situation. Perhaps a client's vital signs had been fluctuating and are now stable. Ethicists use rational processes for determining the most morally desirable course of action in the face of conflicting value choices. The process of choosing an ethical course of action involves medical goals and proportionality, client preferences, quality of life, and contextual features. Contextual features are the characteristics of a given situation.

Medical Care Goals and Proportionality

The medical care goals that apply to the client with a terminal illness include:

- Relieving symptoms, pain, and suffering
- Preventing untimely death ("I want to live long enough to . . .")
- Improving functional status or maintaining compromised status
- Educating and counseling the client and his or her significant others regarding the client's condition and prognosis
- Avoiding harming the client in the course of care

- Promoting health and preventing disease not related to the terminal disease

The physician is responsible for the initial education and counseling of clients regarding their condition and prognosis.

The principle of proportionality is an important ethical consideration in the treatment of terminally ill clients. **Proportionality** means a medical treatment is ethically mandatory to the extent that it is likely to confer greater benefits than burdens to the client. For example, many experts believe that a client who is actively dying and is slightly dehydrated has a more comfortable death. Dehydration has been reported to reduce a client's secretions and excretions, thus decreasing breathing problems, emesis, and incontinence. Dehydration can sedate the brain just before death. Greatly diminished oral intake or its cessation is one of the signs that death is imminent. In another context, a client who is terminally ill but whose condition is stable and enjoys many activities of daily living may appreciate or request education on how to maintain hydration. A nutritional intervention is appropriate if the client would receive greater benefits than burdens.

Client Preference

The most important ethical principle to consider is the client's right to self-determination. Some individuals may perceive suffering as an important means of personal growth or a religious experience. Other individuals may hope a miracle cure will be discovered for his or her disease. Others may be ready for and accepting of death. Healthcare workers have a responsibility to provide a combination of emotional support and technical nutritional advice on how best to achieve each client's goals.

Quality of Life

The most fundamental goal of medical care is an improvement in the quality of life for those who seek care. If improvement is not possible, a goal of medical care is maintenance of the same quality of life or slowing a decline in quality of life. Oral feeding is part of being human and associated with human dignity. One study found that 92 percent of all cancer clients could eat and/or drink until the day they died (Feuz and Rapin, 1994). These clients derived some pleasure from the sensual aspect of food and the socialization that accompanies meals. Food conveys emotional, spiritual, sociological, and biologic meanings. If food remains enjoyable for a client with a terminal illness, the healthcare worker should encourage mealtimes to be shared with loved ones. If eating is not a pleasant experience, however, it should not be overemphasized.

Contextual

Every terminally ill client has his or her own story, with both a history and a future. A client's decision to eat or not to eat is part of his or her narrative. Two examples can illustrate why eating issues should always be given consideration when formulating a care plan. Client 1 lives in a rooming house without air conditioning; his family doesn't want to get involved; he does not have cooking facilities; he refuses to eat the meals delivered to him from the Senior Nutrition Center; and he insists he wants to die at home. Client 2 lives with his male companion in a beach house; his friend carries him every day to the beach to watch the sunset; meals are prepared for him by his boyfriend and many other neighbors and friends. Client 1 refuses to eat. Client 2 tries to eat a small amount at least six times a day. The willingness to eat is part of each man's story.

The contextual features in a patient's situation often relate to food acceptance. In Client 1's situation, the healthcare worker may offer a valuable service by reassuring the client that he will not be abandoned because he refuses to eat. The fear of abandonment is among the most frequently cited apprehensions of dying (American Dietetic Association, 1987). Even if a client refuses to eat, healthcare workers should remain supportive. The client may change his or her mind. The healthcare worker should not consider the rejection of food as a sign of personal or professional failure.

A consideration of a client's medical goals, preferences, quality of life, and contextual features may provide a framework for resolution of ethical dietary issues. Hospice programs have interdisciplinary care teams, and the interdisciplinary team conference is the best arena in which to discuss ethical feeding conflicts.

Legal Issues

The issue of whether to discontinue food and fluid to a client with a terminal illness first emerged in the 1960s. Clients have the legal right to refuse treatment, including artificial feedings. This right is based on the Fourteenth Amendment to the Constitution, which refers to the right to liberty, including the right to be left alone and not invaded or treated against one's will. Courts have recognized that competent adults have the right to refuse treatment, including artificial feeding. The state may exert its authority to expand the individual's right to liberty, however, based on other concepts. The preservation of life, the prevention of suicide, the protection of innocent third parties (such as minor children), and the protection of the ethical integrity and professional discretion of the medical profession are among these concepts. Healthcare workers need to be familiar with the laws in their individual states and the policies and procedures of the organization for which they work. They should also know their professional organization's standards of practice. In some states, a charge of battery can be made if a client is fed artificially against his or her wishes. In some states, a charge of negligence can be made if clients are allowed to intentionally starve themselves to death. Situations such as these should be discussed at the interdisciplinary team meeting or brought to the risk manager's attention. (The risk manager is hired by a health care organization to identify, evaluate, and correct potential risks of injuring clients, staff, visitors, or property.)

With incompetent adult clients, caretakers and family should try to ascertain the client's wishes from past written and oral statements and actions. State laws differ as to whether nutrition and hydration are medically obligatory or medically optional. Some clients may wish for the withdrawal of antibiotics and ventilators but wish to continue nutritional support. This situation may occur when an individual has a permanent feeding tube in place because of an inability to swallow, such as may occur with cancer of the esophagus. What can the nurse legally do if the client is incompetent and the family wants the feeding tube removed? What can the nurse legally do if family members disagree about whether to have the feeding tube removed? When in doubt, the best advice is to continue to feed the client until the healthcare team, the institution's ethics committee, or the facility's risk manager reviews the case. The artificial feeding can be stopped at a future time if the decision is changed, but a deceased person cannot be brought back to life.

Individuals may make their wishes known in writing through advanced directives, such as a living will or durable power of attorney. Although such legal documents are technically different, the common element is that trust is given to another party to make decisions for an individual if he or she becomes incompetent. In the event that a client does not have a written directive, the next of kin or guardian should be consulted about probable preference for the level of nutritional intervention (American Dietetic Association, 1987).

General Considerations

Oral feedings should be advocated over tube and intravenous feedings for terminally ill clients. Food and control of food intake can be one of life's last pleasures. The client's decision to eat or not to eat is his or her right. An effort should be made to enhance the individual's enjoyment of food. A pleasant dining environment that includes a cheerful attitude by caregivers may encourage food intake. The use of complete oral nutrition supplements may provide some relief from symptoms associated with hunger, thirst, and malnutrition. Previously prescribed dietary restrictions should be reevaluated and liberalized. The client's right to self-determination should guide the health care worker in determining whether to allow foods that are not permitted within the diet prescription.

Palliative care does not automatically preclude aggressive nutritional support. The client's informed preference for the level of nutrition intervention is important. If the client wants maximal nutrition support and the policy of the organization is not to provide hyperalimentation or tube feedings for terminally ill clients, the client has the right to be informed of the name of a facility that will provide this service. Artificial feeding is generally not desirable if death is expected within hours or a few days. The effects of partial dehydration and the withdrawal of nutritional support will not adversely alter the client's comfort. Enteral or parenteral feeding would probably worsen the client's condition, symptoms, or discomfort when shock, pulmonary edema, diarrhea, or aspiration is a potential or actual complication. The client or surrogate needs to be informed of these facts when he or she requests maximal support.

Summary

Death is an aspect of life. If we want to help the dying, we must examine our own attitudes toward death. Treatment for terminally ill clients is palliative. The goal of care is symptomatic relief to reduce or alleviate pain. Nutritional intervention can frequently alleviate or reduce the pain and suffering of a terminally ill client. The use of oral feedings should always be given preferential consideration over tube and parenteral feedings. Oral feeding is ordinary care, whereas tube feedings and hyperalimentation are considered by some to be extraordinary care.

In the United States, the client's expressed desire is the primary guide for determining the extent of nutritional and hydration therapy. Our Constitution guarantees clients the right to self-determination. Ethical and legal dilemmas should be brought to the attention of the interdisciplinary team, the risk manager, or the facility's ethics committee promptly. Artificial feeding should never be stopped unless one of these parties has investigated the situation and made a legal and ethical determination that the feeding should cease.

Case Study 26–1

Ms. Z is a 60-year-old woman who has a diagnosis of amyotrophic lateral sclerosis (ALS), also called Lou Gehrig's Disease, with a prognosis of less than 6 months. The client has at least two swallowing impediments. She is unable to dislodge food that collects under her tongue, in cheeks, and on her hard palate. She does not have adequate swallow control (the bolus goes down before she wants it to). Because of these impediments, Ms. Z is unable to tolerate thin liquids and the maintenance of hydration and aspiration are of concern to the caregiver. Ms. Z is alert, oriented, and highly educated. She saw a television program that led her to believe that a high-protein diet would delay the progression of ALS. She would like instruction on a high-protein diet.

Nursing Care Plan

Subjective Data	Client believes a high-protein diet will delay the progression of her ALS
	The caregiver is concerned about the danger of aspiration and the maintenance of hydration.
Objective Data	Diagnosis ALS with a prognosis of less than 6 months
	Lack of swallowing control
Nursing Diagnosis	Knowledge deficit related to lack of desired information about foods high in protein as evidenced by verbal statements. Knowledge deficit related to a lack of understanding of how to increase and/or maintain hydration with the client's swallowing impediments as evidenced by the caregiver's verbal statements.

Desired Outcomes Evaluation Criteria	Nursing Actions/ Interventions	Rationale
NOC: Knowledge: Diet (Johnson, Maas, and Moorhead, 2000, with permission.)	NIC: Diet (McCloskey and Bulechek, 2000, with permission.)	
The client will indicate how she can incorporate foods high in protein and of semisolid or pureed consistency into her diet.	Plan a 70–80 g protein semiliquid/pureed diet (2 cups thickened milk, 6 oz meat or equivalent, 2 vegetables, and 6 starches) for the client or refer the client to the dietitian to plan and instruct the client and/or caregiver on the diet.	Because a 70–80 g protein diet would most likely not harm the client and would make her feel in control, instruction on the diet is appropriate.

(Continued on next page)

Nursing Care Plan (Continued)

Desired Outcomes Evaluation Criteria	Nursing Actions/ Interventions	Rationale
The caregiver will verbalize how to reduce the likelihood of aspiration by following safety precautions for clients with dysphagia.	Discuss feeding issues with the caregiver such as the correct body positioning and eating conditions (American Dietetic Association, 1992).	The risk of aspiration is high in clients with dysphagia.
	Eliminate distractions	
	Position individual in an upright position (90degrees at the hip) with feet flat on floor.	
	Give semiliquids in very small amounts (syringe) and only after food has been cleared from the mouth.	
	Feed the client very small bites. Encourage several dry swallows between bites of food.	
	If the Adam's apple rises, it is likely the food is being swallowed and not deposited in the cheeks. A wet sounding voice with a gurgle may mean food is resting on the vocal cords.	

Critical Thinking Question

1. The client's swallowing disorders are becoming more severe. Ms. Z is capable of eating only very small bites of food very slowly. The client's daughter is her caregiver and she states, "It has been taking me 2 hours to feed my mother each meal. If I go any faster, she chokes. My husband is becoming very resentful and has asked me to make a decision. He says I can't continue to spend all day with my mother and ignore him." What would you say to this caregiver?

2. The caregiver believes the client is still mentally alert and oriented, although the client cannot communicate. The client has progressed to the point where she has lost all motor function. She cannot talk or walk and has lost the use of her hands. The client's physician now believes Ms. Z has an ileus (paralysis of the bowel). Why does this mean the patient cannot be fed orally? What are the treatment options? Who needs to be informed of the treatment options?

 Study Aids

Subjects .Internet Sites

Hospice . . . . .http://www.nho.org/general.htm

. . . . .http://www.teleport.com/~hospice/index.htm

Cachexia . . . . .http://cahn.mankato.msus.edu/cancerupdate/_disc9/00000022.htm

. . . . .http://orthopedics.medscape.com/adis/DTP/1998/v12.n12/dtp1212.02/dtp1212.02-01.html

Migraine Headaches . . . . .http://www.imitrex.com/what/triggers/index.html

. . . . .http://www.eatright.org/nfs/nfs48.html

. . . . .http://www.hivdent.org/oralm/oralm.htm

Xerostomia . . . . .http://www.cdha.org/articles/drymouth.htm

. . . . .http://www.umanitoba.ca/outreach/wisdomtooth/drymouth.htm

Chapter Review

1. A diet prescription consistent with palliative care goals is:
   a. 40 grams of protein for liver failure
   b. Low-cholesterol, low-saturated fat diet for hyperlipoproteinemia
   c. Gluten-free diet for diarrhea and celiac disease
   d. High-calorie, high-protein diet for anorexia in an actively dying client

2. An appropriate nutritional screening question for a client with a terminal illness is:
   a. "How many times a day do you eat?"
   b. "How much weight have you lost in the past month?"
   c. "Do you look forward to meals?"
   d. "Do you include a green or yellow vegetable in your diet each day?"

3. The most important ethical principle to consider when a decision must be made about whether or not to feed a client is:
   a. The client's right to self-determination
   b. Proportionality
   c. Medical goals
   d. The client's quality of life
4. Which recommendation would be appropriate for a client with end-stage congestive heart failure who requests dietary advice?
   a. Recommend a low-potassium diet
   b. Recommend a 1000 cc fluid restriction
   c. Monitor the client's fluid intake and output
   d. Recommend a 3- or 4-gram sodium diet
5. The intervention appropriate for a terminally ill client with dyspnea who requests dietary treatment is:
   a. Encourage a high-fiber diet
   b. Consider a high-fat, low-carbohydrate diet
   c. Recommend fresh fruits, whole grains, and vegetables
   d. Encourage avoidance of caffeine

Clinical Analysis

1. Mr. O is actively dying. Mr. O's wife is concerned because her husband adamantly refuses all food and fluids. The nurse should:
   a. Call the doctor and request an order for a tube feeding
   b. Call the doctor and request an order for an intravenous feeding
   c. Instruct the caregiver to be more creative in the type of food and fluids she gives the client
   d. Counsel the caregiver that oral intake often ceases near the end of life
2. Mrs. P has diagnoses of brain cancer and insulin-dependent diabetes mellitus and a prognosis of a few days. She and her caregiver have been self-monitoring her blood glucose levels. The caregiver is quite concerned because Mrs. P's blood glucose levels are running between 400 to 500 milligrams per deciliter. Historically, the client claims to have followed her 1200-calorie diet faithfully. Recently, her appetite is markedly reduced and her blood glucose levels are elevated (hypermetabolism). The physician has been contacted and refuses to increase the client's insulin further but recommends to Mrs. P's caregiver to stop monitoring the client's blood glucose levels. The nurse should:
   a. Encourage the caregiver to offer Mrs. P frequent sips of clear liquid fruit juices (about 30 grams of carbohydrate every 3 hours)
   b. Encourage the caregiver to continue to offer the client the 1200-calorie diet to avoid a hypoglycemic episode
   c. Recommend the caregiver look for a new doctor because obviously the doctor does not know how to treat clients with insulin-dependent diabetes
   d. Contact the hospice medical director and ask for an order to increase the client's insulin
3. Mr. J has a partial bowel obstruction and shows signs of dehydration. He has an order for Metamucil prn. The nurse should immediately recommend:
   a. High-fiber foods such as bran, whole grains, fruits, vegetables, etc.
   b. Discontinuation of the Metamucil
   c. Increasing the dose of Metamucil
   d. Encourage the use of cheese, cakes, pies, cookies, and doughnuts

Bibliography

Albert, SM: Do family caregivers recognize malnutrition in frail elderly? J Am Geriatr Soc 93:617, 1993.

American Dietetic Association: Manual of Clinical Dietetics. American Dietetic Association, Chicago, 1995.

American Dietetic Association: Migraine headaches and food. The "trigger" factor. J Am Diet Assoc 95:1240, 1995.

American Dietetic Association: Position of the American Dietetic Association: Issues in feeding the terminally ill adult. J Am Diet Assoc 87:76, 1987.

American Dietetic Association: Position of the American Dietetic Association: Legal and ethical issues in feeding permanently unconscious patients. J Am Diet Assoc 95:231, 1995.

Boyd, K: Diabetes mellitus in hospice patients: Some guidelines. Palliative Med 7:163, 1993.

Byock, I: Patient refusal of nutrition and hydration: Walking the ever-fine line. Am J Hospice Palliative Care 12:8, 1995.

Dietitians Association of Australia: Position Paper: Nutrition priorities in palliative care of oncology patients. Dietitians Association of Australia 92–93, 1992.

Feuz, A, and Rapin, C: An observational study of the role of pain management and food adaptation of elderly patients with terminal cancer. J Am Diet Assoc 94:767, 1994.

Finucane, TE, Christmas, C, and Travis, K: Tube feeding in patients with advanced dementia. JAMA 14:282, 1999.

Gallagher-Allred, CR: Nutritional Care of the Terminally Ill. Aspen Publishers, Gaithersburg, MD, 1989.

Johnson, M, Maas, M, and Moorhead, S: Nursing Outcomes Classification (NOC), ed 2. Mosby, Philadelphia, 2000.

Junkerman, C, and Schiedermayer, D: Practical Ethics for Student, Interns, and Residents, ed 2. University Publishing Group, Fredrick, MD, 1998.

Malone, N: Hydration in the terminally ill patient. Clin Palliative Care 8:20, 1994.

McCloskey, JC, and Bulechek, GM: Nursing Interventions Classification (NIC), ed 3. Mosby, Philadelphia, 2000.

McKinley, MJ, et al.: Improved body weight as a result of nutrition intervention in adult, HIV-positive outpatients. J Am Diet Assoc 94:1014, 1994.

Mills, M, Davies, HTO, and Macrae, WA: Care of dying patients in hospital. Br Med J: 583, 1994.

Morley, JE, and Kraenzle, D: Causes of weight loss in a community nursing home. J Am Geriatr Soc 94:583, 1994.

North American Nursing Diagnosis Association: Nursing Diagnoses: Definitions and Classification 1999–2000, North American Nursing Diagnosis Association, Philadelphia, 1999.

Shils, ME: Nutrition and medical ethics: The interplay of medical decisions, patients rights, and the judicial system. In Shils, ME, Olson, JA, Shike, M, and Ross, CA (eds): Modern Nutrition in Health and Disease, ed 9. Williams and Wilkins, Baltimore, 1999.

Tatling, W, Houston, DC, and Hill, RD: The prevalence of diabetes mellitus in a typical English community. Jr Coll Phys Lond 19:248, 1985.

Towers, AL, et al.: Constipation in the elderly: Influence of dietary, psychological, and physical factors. J Am Geriatr Soc 94:701, 1994.

Appendices

APPENDIX A

Exchange Lists of the American Dietetic and American Diabetes Associations

STARCH LIST

One starch exchange equals 15 g carbohydrate, 3 g protein, 0–1 g fat, and 80 cal.

Bread

Bagel	1/2 (1 oz)
Bread, reduced-calorie	2 slices (1 1/2 oz)
Bread, white, whole-wheat, pumpernickel, rye	1 slice (1 oz)
Bread sticks, crisp, 4 in long 3 1/2 in	2 (2/3 oz)
English muffin	1/2
Hot dog or hamburger bun	1/2 (1 oz)
Pita, 6 in across	1/2
Roll, plain, small	1 (1 oz)
Raisin bread, unfrosted	1 slice (1 oz)
Tortilla, corn, 6 in across	1
Tortilla, flour, 7–8 in across	1
Waffle, 4 1/2 in square, reduced-fat	1

Cereals and Grains

Bran cereals	1/2 cup
Bulgur	1/2 cup
Cereals	1/2 cup
Cereals, unsweetened, ready-to-eat	3/4 cup
Cornmeal (dry)	3 tbsp
Couscous	1/3 cup
Flour (dry)	3 tbsp
Granola, low-fat	1/4 cup
Grape-Nuts	1/4 cup
Grits	1/2 cup
Kasha	1/2 cup
Millet	1/4 cup
Muesli	1/4 cup

Oats	1/2 cup
Pasta	1/2 cup
Puffed cereal	1 1/2 cups
Rice milk	1/2 cup
Rice, white or brown	1/3 cup
Shredded Wheat	1/2 cup
Sugar-frosted cereal	1/2 cup
Wheat germ	3 tbsp

Starchy Vegetables

Baked beans	1/3 cup
Corn	1/2 cup
Corn on cob, medium	1 (5 oz)
Mixed vegetables with corn, peas, or pasta	1 cup
Peas, green	1/2 cup
Plantain	1/2 cup
Potato, baked or boiled	1 small (3 oz)
Potato, mashed	1/2 cup
Squash, winter (acorn, butternut)	1 cup
Yam, sweet potato, plain	1/2 cup

Crackers and Snacks

Animal crackers	8
Graham crackers, 2 1/2 in square	3
Matzoh	3/4 oz
Melba toast	4 slices
Oyster crackers	24
Popcorn (popped, no fat added or low-fat microwave)	3 cups
Pretzels	3/4 oz
Rice cakes, 4 in across	2

Saltine-type crackers	6
Snack chips, fat-free (tortilla, potato)	15–20 (3/4 oz)
Whole-wheat crackers, no fat added	2–5 (3/4 oz)

Dried Beans, Peas, and Lentils
(Count as 1 starch exchange, plus 1 very lean meat exchange.)

Beans and peas (garbanzo, pinto, kidney, white, split, black-eyed)	1/2 cup
Lima beans	2/3 cup
Lentils	1/2 cup
Misc*	3 tbsp

Starchy Foods Prepared with Fat
(Count as 1 starch exchange, plus 1 fat exchange.)

| Biscuit, 2 1/2 in across | 1 |

*= 5 400 mg or more of sodium per serving.

Chow mein noodles	1/2 cup
Corn bread, 2 in cube	1 (2 oz)
Crackers, round butter type	6
Croutons	1 cup
French-fried potatoes	16–25 (3 oz)
Granola	1/4 cup
Muffin, small	1 (1 1/2 oz)
Pancake, 4 in across	2
Popcorn, microwave	3 cups
Sandwich crackers, cheese or peanut butter filling	3
Stuffing, bread (prepared)	1/3 cup
Taco shell, 6 in across	2
Waffle, 4 1/2 in square	1
Whole-wheat crackers, fat added	4–6 (1 oz)

FRUIT LIST

One fruit exchange equals 15 g carbohydrate and 60 cal. The weight includes skin, core, seeds, and rind.

Fruit

Apple, unpeeled, small	1 (4 oz)
Applesauce, unsweetened	1/2 cup
Apples, dried	4 rings
Apricots, fresh	4 whole (5 1/2 oz)
Apricots, dried	8 halves
Apricots, canned	1/2 cup
Banana, small	1 (4 oz)
Blackberries	3/4 cup
Blueberries	3/4 cup
Cantaloupe, small	1/3 melon (11 oz) or 1 cup cubes
Cherries, sweet, fresh	12 (3 oz)
Cherries, sweet, canned	1/2 cup
Dates	3
Figs, fresh	1 1/2 large or 2 medium (3 1/2 oz)
Figs, dried	1 1/2
Fruit cocktail	1/2 cup
Grapefruit, lg	1/2 (11 oz)
Grapefruit sections, canned	3/4 cup
Grapes, small	17 (3 oz)
Honeydew melon	1 slice (10 oz) or 1 cup cubes
Kiwi	1 (3 1/2 oz)
Mandarin oranges, canned	3/4 cup
Mango, small	1/2 fruit (5 1/2 oz) or 1/2 cup
Nectarine, small	1 (5 oz)
Orange, small	1 (6 1/2 oz)
Papaya	1/2 fruit (8 oz) or 1 cup cubes
Peach, medium, fresh	1 (6 oz)
Peaches, canned	1/2 cup
Pear, lg, fresh	1/2 (4 oz)
Pears, canned	1/2 cup
Pineapple, fresh	3/4 cup
Pineapple, canned	1/2 cup
Plums, small	2 (5 oz)
Plums, canned	1/2 cup
Prunes, dried	3
Raisins	2 tbsp
Raspberries	1 cup
Strawberries	1 1/4 cup whole berries
Tangerines, small	2 (8 oz)
Watermelon	1 slice (13 1/2 oz) or 1 1/4 cup cubes

Fruit Juice

Apple juice/cider	1/2 cup
Cranberry juice cocktail	1/3 cup
Cranberry juice cocktail reduced-calorie	1 cup
Fruit juice blends, 100 percent juice	1/3 cup
Grape juice	1/3 cup
Grapefruit juice	1/2 cup
Orange juice	1/2 cup
Pineapple juice	1/2 cup
Prune juice	1/3 cup

MILK LIST

One milk exchange equals 12 g carbohydrate and 8 g protein.

Skim and Very Low-Fat Milk
(0–3 g fat per serving)

Skim milk	1 cup
1/2 percent milk	1 cup
1 percent milk	1 cup
Nonfat or low-fat buttermilk	1 cup
Evaporated skim milk	1/2 cup
Nonfat dry milk	1/3 cup dry
Plain nonfat yogurt	3/4 cup
Nonfat or low-fat fruit-flavored yogurt sweetened with aspartame or with a nonnutritive sweetener	1 cup

Low-Fat
(5 g fat per serving)

2 percent milk	1 cup
Plain low-fat yogurt	3/4 cup
Sweet acidophilus milk	1 cup

Whole Milk
(8 g fat per serving)

Whole milk	1 cup
Evaporated whole milk	1/2 cup
Goat's milk	1 cup
Kefir	1 cup

OTHER CARBOHYDRATES LIST

One exchange equals 15 g carbohydrate, or 1 starch, or 1 fruit, or 1 milk.

Food	Serving Size	Exchanges Per Serving
Angel food cake, unfrosted	1/12th cake	2 carbohydrates
Brownie, small, unfrosted	2 in square	1 carbohydrate, 1 fat
Cake, unfrosted	2 in square	1 carbohydrate, 1 fat
Cake, frosted	2 in square	2 carbohydrates, 1 fat
Cookie, fat-free	2 small	1 carbohydrate
Cookie or sandwich cookie with creme filling	2 small	1 carbohydrate, 1 fat
Cupcake, frosted	1 small	2 carbohydrates, 1 fat
Cranberry sauce, jellied	1/4 cup	2 carbohydrates
Doughnut, plain cake	1 medium (1 1/2 oz)	1 1/2 carbohydrates, 2 fats
Doughnut, glazed	3 3/4 in across (2 oz)	2 carbohydrates, 2 fats
Fruit juice bars, frozen, 100 percent juice	1 bar (3 oz)	1 carbohydrate
Fruit snacks, chewy (pureed fruit concentrate)	1 roll (3/4 oz)	1 carbohydrate
Fruit spreads, 100 percent fruit	1 tbsp	1 carbohydrate
Gelatin, regular	1/2 cup	1 carbohydrate
Gingersnaps	3	1 carbohydrate
Granola bar	1 bar	1 carbohydrate, 1 fat
Granola bar, fat-free	1 bar	2 carbohydrates
Hummus	1/3 cup	1 carbohydrate, 1 fat
Ice cream	1/2 cup	1 carbohydrate, 2 fats
Ice cream, light	1/2 cup	1 carbohydrate, 1 fat
Ice cream, fat-free, no sugar added	1/2 cup	1 carbohydrate
Jam or jelly, regular	1 tbsp	1 carbohydrate
Milk, chocolate, whole	1 cup	2 carbohydrates, 1 fat
Pie, fruit, 2 crusts	1/6 pie	3 carbohydrates, 2 fats
Pie, pumpkin or custard	1/8 pie	1 carbohydrate, 2 fats
Potato chips	12–18 (1 oz)	1 carbohydrate, 2 fats
Pudding, regular (made with low-fat milk)	1/2 cup	2 carbohydrates
Pudding, sugar-free (made with low-fat milk)	1/2 cup	1 carbohydrate
Salad dressing, fat-free*	1/4 cup	1 carbohydrate
Sherbet, sorbet	1/2 cup	2 carbohydrates
Spaghetti or pasta sauce, canned*	1/2 cup	1 carbohydrate, 1 fat
Sweet roll or Danish	1 (2 1/2 oz)	2 1/2 carbohydrates, 2 fats
Syrup, light	2 tbsp	1 carbohydrate

Food	Serving Size	Exchanges Per Serving
Syrup, regular	1 tbsp	1 carbohydrate
Syrup, regular	1/4 cup	4 carbohydrates
Tortilla chips	6–12 (1 oz)	1 carbohydrate, 2 fats
Yogurt, frozen, low-fat, fat-free	1/3 cup	1 carbohydrate, 0–1 fat
Yogurt, frozen, fat-free, no sugar added	1/2 cup	1 carbohydrate
Yogurt, low-fat with fruit	1 cup	3 carbohydrates, 0–1 fat
Vanilla wafers	5	1 carbohydrate, 1 fat

* 5 400 mg or more sodium per exchange.

VEGETABLE LIST

In general, one vegetable exchange is 1/2 cup cooked vegetable or juice or 1 cup raw vegetable.
One vegetable exchange equals 5 g carbohydrate, 2 g protein, 0 g fat, and 25 cal.

Artichoke	Mushrooms
Artichoke hearts	Okra
Asparagus	Onions
Beans (green, wax, Italian)	Pea pods
Bean sprouts	Peppers (all varieties)
Beets	Radishes
Broccoli	Salad greens (endive, escarole, lettuce, romaine, spinach)
Brussels sprouts	
Cabbage	Sauerkraut*
Carrots	Spinach
Cauliflower	Summer squash
Celery	Tomato
Cucumber	Tomatoes, canned
Eggplant	Tomato sauce*
Green onions or scallions	Tomato/vegetable juice*
Greens (collard, kale, mustard, turnip)	Turnips
Kohlrabi	Water chestnuts
Leeks	Watercress
Mixed vegetables (without corn, peas, or pasta)	Zucchini

* 5 400 mg or more sodium per exchange.

MEAT AND MEAT SUBSTITUTES LIST

Very Lean Meat and Substitutes List

One exchange equals 0 g carbohydrate, 7 g protein, 0–1 g fat, and 35 cal. One very lean meat exchange is equal to any one of the following items.

Poultry: Chicken or turkey (white meat, no skin), Cornish hen (no skin)	1 oz
Fish: Fresh or frozen cod, flounder, haddock, halibut, trout; tuna fresh or canned in water	1 oz
Shellfish: Clams, crab, lobster, scallops, shrimp, imitation shellfish	1 oz
Game: Duck or pheasant (no skin), venison, buffalo, ostrich	1 oz
Cheese with 1 g or less fat per ounce:	
Nonfat or low-fat cottage cheese	3/4 cup
Fat-free cheese	1 oz
Other: Processed sandwich meats with 1 g or less fat per ounce, such as deli thin, shaved meats, chipped beef,* turkey ham	1 oz

Egg whites	2
Egg substitutes, plain	1/4 cup
Hot dogs with 1 g or less fat per ounce*	1 oz
Kidney (high in cholesterol)	1 oz
Sausage with 1 g or less fat per ounce	1 oz

Count as one very lean meat and one starch exchange.

Dried beans, peas, lentils (cooked)	1/2 cup

Lean Meat and Substitutes List

One exchange equals 0 g carbohydrate, 7 g protein, 3 g fat, and 55 cal. One lean meat exchange is equal to any one of the following items.

Beef: USDA Select or Choice grades of lean beef trimmed of fat, such as round, sirloin, and flank steak; tenderloin; roast (rib, chuck, rump); steak (T-bone, porterhouse, cubed), ground round	1 oz

Pork: Lean pork, such as fresh ham; canned, cured, or boiled ham; Canadian bacon*; tenderloin, center loin chop — 1 oz

Lamb: Roast, chop, leg — 1 oz

Veal: Lean chop, roast — 1 oz

Poultry: Chicken, turkey (dark meat, no skin), chicken white meat (with skin), domestic duck or goose (well drained of fat, no skin) — 1 oz

Fish:

Herring (uncreamed or smoked)	1 oz
Oysters	6 medium
Salmon (fresh or canned), catfish	1 oz
Sardines (canned)	2 medium
Tuna (canned in oil, drained)	1 oz

Game: Goose (no skin), rabbit — 1 oz

Cheese:

4.5 percent fat cottage cheese	1/2 cup
Grated Parmesan	2 tbsp
Cheeses with 3 g or less fat per ounce	1 oz

Other:

Hot dogs with 3 g or less fat per ounce*	1 1/2 oz
Processed sandwich meat with 3 g or less fat per ounce, such as turkey pastrami or kielbasa	1 oz
Liver, heart (high in cholesterol)	1 oz

Medium-Fat Meat and Substitutes List

One exchange equals 0 g carbohydrate, 7 g protein, 5 g fat, and 75 cal. One medium-fat meat exchange is equal to any one of the following items.

Beef: Most beef products fall into this category (ground beef, meatloaf, corned beef, short ribs, Prime grades of meat trimmed of fat, such as prime rib) — 1 oz

Pork: Top loin, chop, Boston butt, cutlet — 1 oz

Lamb: Rib roast, ground — 1 oz

Veal: Cutlet (ground or cubed, unbreaded) — 1 oz

FAT LIST

Poultry: Chicken dark meat (with skin), ground turkey or ground chicken, fried chicken (with skin) — 1 oz

Fish: Any fried fish product — 1 oz

Cheese: With 5 g or less fat per ounce

Feta	1 oz
Mozzarella	1 oz
Ricotta	1/4 cup (2 oz)

Other:

Egg (high in cholesterol, limit to 3 per week)	1
Sausage with 5 g or less fat per ounce	1 oz
Soy milk	1 cup
Tempeh	1/4 cup
Tofu	4 oz or 1/2 cup

High-Fat Meat and Substitutes List

One exchange equals 0 g carbohydrate, 7 g protein, 8 g fat, and 100 cal.

Remember these items are high in saturated fat, cholesterol, and calories and may raise blood cholesterol levels if eaten on a regular basis. One high-fat meat exchange is equal to any one of the following items.

Pork: Spareribs, ground pork, pork sausage — 1 oz

Cheese: All regular cheeses, such as American*, cheddar, Monterey Jack, Swiss — 1 oz

Other: Processed sandwich meats with 8 g or less fat per ounce, such as bologna, pimento loaf, salami — 1 oz

Sausage, such as bratwurst, Italian, knockwurst, Polish, smoked — 1 oz

Hot dog (turkey or chicken)*	1 (10/lb)
Bacon	3 slices (20 slices/lb)

Count as one high-fat meat plus one fat exchange.

Hot dog (beef, pork, or combination)*	1 (10/lb)
Peanut butter (contains unsaturated fat)	2 tbsp

* 5 400 mg or more sodium per exchange.

Monounsaturated Fats List

One fat exchange equals 5 g fat and 45 cal.

Avocado, medium	1/8 (1 oz)
Oil (canola, olive, peanut)	1 tsp
Olives: ripe (black)	8 large
green, stuffed*	10 large
Nuts	
almonds, cashews	6 nuts
mixed (50% peanuts)	6 nuts
peanuts	10 nuts
pecans	4 halves
Peanut butter, smooth or crunchy	2 tsp
Sesame seeds	1 tbsp
Tahini paste	2 tsp

Polyunsaturated Fats List

One fat exchange equals 5 g fat and 45 cal.

Margarine: stick, tub, or squeeze	1 tsp
lower-fat (30 percent to 50 percent vegetable oil)	1 tbsp
Mayo: regular	1 tsp
reduced-fat	1 tbsp
Nuts, walnuts, English	4 halves
Oil (corn, safflower, soybean)	1 tsp
Salad dressing: regular*	1 tbsp
reduced-fat	2 tbsp
Miracle Whip Salad Dressing®:	
regular	2 tsp
reduced-fat	1 tbsp
Seeds: pumpkin, sunflower	1 tbsp

Saturated Fats List†
One fat exchange equals 5 g of fat and 45 cal.

Bacon, cooked	1 slice (20 slices/lb)
Bacon, grease	1 tsp
Butter: stick	1 tsp
whipped	2 tsp
reduced-fat	1 tbsp
Chitterlings, boiled	2 tbsp (1/2 oz)

Coconut, sweetened, shredded	2 tbsp
Cream, half and half	2 tbsp
Cream cheese: regular	1 tbsp (1/2 oz)
reduced-fat	2 tbsp (1 oz)
Fatback or salt pork, see below‡	
Shortening or lard	1 tsp
Sour cream: regular	2 tbsp
reduced-fat	3 tbsp

* 5 400 mg or more sodium per exchange.
† Saturated fats can raise blood cholesterol levels.
‡ Use a piece 1 in 3 1 in 3 1/4 in if you plan to eat the fatback cooked with vegetables. Use a piece 2 in 3 1 in 3 1/2 in when eating only the vegetables with the fatback removed.

FREE FOODS LIST

A *free food* is any food or drink that contains less than 20 cal or less than 5 g of carbohydrate per serving. Foods with a serving size listed should be limited to three servings per day. Be sure to spread them out throughout the day. If you eat all three servings at one time, it could affect your blood glucose level. Foods listed without a serving size can be eaten as often as you like.

Fat-Free Or Reduced-Fat Foods

Cream cheese, fat-free	1 tbsp
Creamers, nondairy, liquid	1 tbsp
Creamers, nondairy, powdered	2 tsp
Mayo, fat-free	1 tbsp
Mayo, reduced-fat	1 tsp
Margarine, fat-free	4 tbsp
Margarine, reduced-fat	1 tsp
Miracle Whip®, nonfat	1 tbsp
Miracle Whip®, reduced-fat	1 tsp
Nonstick cooking spray	
Salad dressing, fat-free	1 tbsp
Salad dressing, fat-free, Italian	2 tbsp
Salsa	1/4 cup
Sour cream, fat-free, reduced-fat	1 tbsp
Whipped topping, regular or light	2 tbsp

Sugar-Free or Low-Sugar Foods

Candy, hard, sugar-free	1 candy
Gelatin dessert, sugar-free	2 tsp
Gelatin, unflavored	
Gum, sugar-free	
Jam or jelly, low-sugar or light	
Sugar substitutes*	
Syrup, sugar-free	2 tbsp

Drinks

Bouillon, broth, consommé†	1 tbsp
Bouillon or broth, low-sodium	
Carbonated or mineral water	
Cocoa powder, unsweetened	

Coffee
Club soda
Diet soft drinks, sugar-free
Drink mixes, sugar-free
Tea
Tonic water, sugar-free

Condiments

Catsup	1 tbsp
Horseradish	
Lemon juice	
Lime juice	
Mustard	
Pickles, dill†	1 1/2 large
Soy sauce, regular or light†	
Taco sauce	1 tbsp
Vinegar	

Seasonings

Be careful with seasonings that contain sodium or are salts, such as garlic or celery salt, and lemon pepper.

Flavoring extracts
Garlic
Herbs, fresh or dried
Pimento
Spices
Tabasco® or hot pepper sauce
Wine, used in cooking
Worcestershire sauce

* Sugar substitutes, alternatives, or replacements that are approved by the Food and Drug Administration (FDA) are safe to use. Common brand names include: Equal® (aspartame), Sprinkle Sweet® (saccharin), Sweet One® (acesulfame K), Sweet-10® (saccharin), Sugar Twin® (saccharin), Sweet 'n Low® (saccharin).

† 5 400 mg or more of sodium per choice.

COMBINATION FOODS LIST

Many of the foods we eat are mixed together in various combinations. These combination foods do not fit into any one exchange list. Often it is hard to tell what is in a casserole dish or prepared food item. This is a list of exchanges for some typical combination foods. This list will help you fit these foods into your meal plan. Ask your dietitian for information about any other combination foods you would like to eat.

Food	Serving Size	Exchanges Per Serving
Entrees		
Tuna noodle casserole, lasagna, spaghetti with meatballs, chili with beans, macaroni and cheese*	1 cup (8 oz)	2 carbohydrates, 2 medium-fat meats
Chow mein (without noodles or rice)	2 cups (16 oz)	1 carbohydrate, 2 lean meats
Pizza, cheese, thin crust*	1/4 of 10 in (5 oz)	2 carbohydrates, 2 medium-fat meats, 1 fat
Pizza, meat topping, thin crust*	1/4 of 10 in (5 oz)	2 carbohydrates, 2 medium-fat meats, 2 fats
Pot pie*	1 (7 oz)	2 carbohydrates, 1 medium-fat meat, 4 fats
Frozen entrees		
Salisbury steak with gravy, mashed potato*	1 (11 oz)	2 carbohydrates, 3 medium-fat meats, 3–4 fats
Turkey with gravy, mashed potato, dressing*	1 (11 oz)	2 carbohydrates, 2 medium-fat meats, 2 fats
Entree with less than 300 cal*	1 (8 oz)	2 carbohydrates, 3 lean meats
Soups		
Bean*	1 cup	1 carbohydrate, 1 very lean meat
Cream (made with water)*	1 cup (8 oz)	1 carbohydrate, 1 fat
Split pea (made with water)*	1/2 cup (4 oz)	1 carbohydrate
Tomato (made with water)*	1 cup (8 oz)	1 carbohydrate
Vegetable beef, chicken noodle, or other broth-type*	1 cup (8 oz)	1 carbohydrate

* 5 400 mg or more of sodium per choice.

FAST FOODS*

Food	Serving Size	Exchanges Per Serving
Burritos with beef†	2	4 carbohydrates, 2 medium-fat meats, 2 fats
Chicken nuggets†	6	1 carbohydrate, 2 medium-fat meats, 1 fat
Chicken breast and wing, breaded and fried†	1 ea.	1 carbohydrate, 4 medium-fat meats, 2 fats
Fish sandwich/tartar sauce†	1	3 carbohydrates, 1 medium-fat meat, 3 fats
French fries, thin	20–25	2 carbohydrates, 2 fats
Hamburger, regular	1	2 carbohydrates, 2 medium-fat meats
Hamburger, large†	1	2 carbohydrates, 3 medium-fat meats, 1 fat
Hot dog with bun†	1	1 carbohydrate, 1 high-fat meat, 1 fat
Individual pan pizza†	1	5 carbohydrates, 3 medium-fat meats, 3 fats
Soft-serve cone	1 medium	2 carbohydrates, 1 fat
Submarine sandwich†	1 sub (6 in)	3 carbohydrates, 1 vegetable, 2 medium-fat meats, 1 fat
Taco, hard shell†	1 (6 oz)	2 carbohydrates, 2 medium-fat meats, 2 fats
Taco, soft shell†	1 (3 oz)	1 carbohydrate, 1 medium-fat meat, 1 fat

* 5 400 mg or more sodium per exchange.

† Ask at your fast-food restaurant for nutrition information about your favorite fast foods.

USING FOOD LABELS

Nutrition Facts on food labels can help you with food choices. These labels are required by law for most foods and are based on standard serving sizes. However, these serving sizes may not always be the same as the serving sizes in this booklet.

- Check the serving size on the label. Is it nearly the same size as the food exchange? You may need to adjust the size of the serving to fit your meal plan.
- Look at the grams of carbohydrate in the serving size. (One starch, fruit, milk, or other carbohydrate has about 15 grams of carbohydrate.) So, if 1 cup of cereal has 30 grams of carbohydrate, it will count as 2 starch choices in your meal plan. You may need to adjust the size of the serving so it contains the number of carbohydrate choices you have for a meal or a snack.
- Look at the grams of protein in the serving size. (One meat choice has 7 grams of protein.) If the food has more than 7 grams of protein in a serving, you can figure out the number of meat choices by dividing the grams of protein by 7. Meats generally contain fat, too.
- Look at the grams of fat in the serving size. (One fat choice has 5 grams of fat.) If one waffle has 15 grams of carbohydrate and 5 grams of fat, it counts as 1 starch choice and 1 fat choice.
- Look at the number of calories in the serving size. If there are less than 20 calories per serving, it is a free food. However, if it has more than 20 calories, follow the steps listed above to count the food choices.

Ask your dietitian for help using information on food labels. Some food labels may also give exchanges. These are based on information in this appendix.

Chili With Beans
Nutrition Facts

Serving Size 1 cup (253 g)
Servings Per Container 2

Amount Per Serving
Calories 260   Calories from Fat 72

	% Daily Value
Total Fat 8 g	13%
Saturated Fat 3 g	17%
Cholesterol 130 mg	44%
Sodium 1010 mg	42%
Total Carbohydrate 22 g	7%
Dietary Fiber 9 g	36%
Sugars 4 g	
Protein 25 g	

The Exchange Lists are the basis of a meal-planning system designed by a committee of the American Diabetes Association and the American Dietetic Association. While designed primarily for people with diabetes and others who must follow special diets, the Exchange Lists are based on principles of good nutrition that apply to everyone. Copied with permission.

Source: Adapted from Exchange Lists for Meal Planning © 1995, American Diabetes Association, The American Dietetic Association.

Nutritive Values of Foods

Foods, approximate measures, units, and weight (weight of edible portion only)			Water	Food energy	Pro-tein	Fat	Fatty Acids		
							Satu-rated	Mono-unsatu-rated	Poly-unsatu-rated
			Per-cent	Cal-ories					
		Grams			Grams	Grams	Grams	Grams	Grams
BEVERAGES									
Alcoholic:									
Beer:									
Regular- - - - - - - - - - - -	12 fl oz- - - - - - - -	360	92	150	1	0	0.0	0.0	0
Light- - - - - - - - - - - -	12 fl oz- - - - - - - -	355	95	95	1	0	0.0	0.0	0.0
Gin, rum, vodka, whiskey:									
86-proof- - - - - - - - - -	1½ fl oz- - - - - - - -	42	64	105	0	0	0.0	0.0	0.0
Wines:									
Dessert- - - - - - - - - - -	3½ fl oz- - - - - - - -	103	77	140	Tr	0	0.0	0.0	0.0
Table:									
Red- - - - - - - - - - - -	3½ fl oz- - - - - - - -	102	88	75	Tr	0	0.0	0.0	0.0
White- - - - - - - - - -	3½ fl oz- - - - - - - -	102	87	80	Tr	0	0.0	0.0	0.0
Carbonated:[2]									
Club soda- - - - - - - - - -	12 fl oz- - - - - - - -	355	100	0	0	0	0.0	0.0	0.0
Cola type:									
Regular- - - - - - - - - - -	12 fl oz- - - - - - - -	369	89	160	0	0	0.0	0.0	0.0
Diet, artificially sweet-ened- - - - - - - - - - - -	12 fl oz- - - - - - - -	355	100	Tr	0	0	0.0	0.0	0.0
Ginger ale- - - - - - - - - - -	12 fl oz- - - - - - - -	366	91	125	0	0	0.0	0.0	0.0
Root beer- - - - - - - - - - -	12 fl oz- - - - - - - -	370	89	165	0	0	0.0	0.0	0.0
Coffee:									
Brewed- - - - - - - - - - - -	6 fl oz- - - - - - - -	180	100	Tr	Tr	Tr	Tr	Tr	Tr
Instant, prepared (2 tsp powder plus 6 fl oz water)- - - - - - - - - - - -	6 fl oz- - - - - - - -	182	99	Tr	Tr	Tr	Tr	Tr	Tr
Fruit drinks, noncarbonated:									
Canned:									
Fruit punch drink- - - - -	6 fl oz- - - - - - - -	190	88	85	Tr	0	0.0	0.0	0.0
Grape drink- - - - - - - -	6 fl oz- - - - - - - -	187	86	100	Tr	0	0.0	0.0	0.0
Pineapple-grapefruit juice drink- - - - - - - -	6 fl oz- - - - - - - -	187	87	90	Tr	Tr	Tr	Tr	Tr
Fruit juices. See type under Fruits and Fruit Juices.									
Milk beverages. See Dairy Products									
Tea:									
Brewed- - - - - - - - - - - -	8 fl oz- - - - - - - -	240	100	Tr	Tr	Tr	Tr	Tr	Tr
Instant, powder, prepared:									
Unsweetened (1 tsp powder plus 8 fl oz water)- - - - - - - - - - -	8 fl oz- - - - - - - -	241	100	Tr	Tr	Tr	Tr	Tr	Tr
Sweetened (3 tsp powder plus 8 fl oz water)- - -	8 fl oz- - - - - - - -	262	91	85	Tr	Tr	Tr	Tr	Tr
DAIRY PRODUCTS									
Cheese:									
Natural:									
Blue- - - - - - - - - - - -	1 oz- - - - - - - - -	28	42	100	6	8	5.3	2.2	0.2

(Tr indicates nutrient present in trace amounts.)

Nutrients in Indicated Quantity

Cho-les-terol	Carbo-hydrate	Calcium	Phos-phorus	Iron	Potas-sium	Sodium	Vitamin A value (IU)	Vitamin A value (RE)	Thiamin	Ribo-flavin	Niacin	Ascorbic acid
Milli-grams	Grams	Milli-grams	Milli-grams	Milli-grams	Milli-grams	Milli-grams	Inter-national units	Retinol equiva-lents	Milli-grams	Milli-grams	Milli-grams	Milli-grams
0	13	14	50	0.1	115	18	0	0	0.02	0.09	1.8	0
0	5	14	43	0.1	64	11	0	0	0.03	0.11	1.4	0
0	Tr	Tr	Tr	Tr	1	Tr	0	0	Tr	Tr	Tr	0
0	8	8	9	0.2	95	9	(1)	(1)	0.01	0.02	0.2	0
0	3	8	18	0.4	113	5	(1)	(1)	0.00	0.03	0.1	0
0	3	9	14	0.3	83	5	(1)	(1)	0.00	0.01	0.1	0
0	0	18	0	Tr	0	78	0	0	0.00	0.00	0.0	0
0	41	11	52	0.2	7	18	0	0	0.00	0.00	0.0	0
0	Tr	14	39	0.2	7	[3]32	0	0	0.00	0.00	0.0	0
0	32	11	0	0.1	4	29	0	0	0.00	0.00	0.0	0
0	42	15	0	0.2	4	48	0	0	0.00	0.00	0.0	0
0	Tr	4	2	Tr	124	2	0	0	0.00	0.02	0.4	0
0	1	2	6	0.1	71	Tr	0	0	0.00	0.03	0.6	0
0	22	15	2	0.4	48	15	20	2	0.03	0.04	Tr	[4]61
0	26	2	2	0.3	9	11	Tr	Tr	0.01	0.01	Tr	[4]64
0	23	13	7	0.9	97	24	60	6	0.06	0.04	0.5	[4]110
0	Tr	0	2	Tr	36	1	0	0	0.00	0.03	Tr	0
0	1	1	4	Tr	61	1	0	0	0.00	0.02	0.1	0
0	22	1	3	Tr	49	Tr	0	0	0.00	0.04	0.1	0
21	1	150	110	0.1	73	396	200	65	0.01	0.11	0.3	0

Nutritive Value of Foods *(Continued)*

Foods, approximate measures, units, and weight (weight of edible portion only)		Water	Food energy	Pro-tein	Fat	Satu-rated	Mono-unsatu-rated	Poly-unsatu-rated
							Fatty Acids	
		Grams	Per-cent	Cal-ories	Grams	Grams	Grams	Grams	Grams

Foods, approximate measures, units, and weight (weight of edible portion only)		Grams	Per-cent	Cal-ories	Grams	Grams	Grams	Grams	Grams
DAIRY PRODUCTS—Con.									
Camembert (3 wedges per 4-oz container)- - - - -	1 wedge- - - - - - - -	38	52	115	8	9	5.8	2.7	0.3
Cheddar:									
Cut pieces- - - - - - - -	1 oz- - - - - - - - - -	28	37	115	7	9	6.0	2.7	0.3
	1 in³- - - - - - - - -	17	37	70	4	6	3.6	1.6	0.2
Shredded- - - - - - - -	1 cup- - - - - - - - -	113	37	455	28	37	23.8	10.6	1.1
Cottage (curd not pressed down):									
Lowfat (2%)- - - - - - -	1 cup- - - - - - - - -	226	79	205	31	4	2.8	1.2	0.1
Uncreamed (cottage cheese dry curd, less than ½% fat)- - - - -	1 cup- - - - - - - - -	145	80	125	25	1	0.4	0.2	Tr
Cream- - - - - - - - - - - - -	1 oz- - - - - - - - - -	28	54	100	2	10	6.2	2.8	0.4
Feta- - - - - - - - - - - - - -	1 oz- - - - - - - - - -	28	55	75	4	6	4.2	1.3	0.2
Mozzarella, made with:									
Whole milk- - - - - - - -	1 oz- - - - - - - - - - -	28	54	80	6	6	3.7	1.9	0.2
Parmesan, grated:									
Tablespoon- - - - - - - -	1 tbsp- - - - - - - - -	5	18	25	2	2	1.0	0.4	Tr
Ounce- - - - - - - - - - -	1 oz- - - - - - - - - -	28	18	130	12	9	5.4	2.5	0.2
Provolone- - - - - - - - - -	1 oz- - - - - - - - - -	28	41	100	7	8	4.8	2.1	0.2
Ricotta, made with:									
Whole milk- - - - - - - -	1 cup- - - - - - - - -	246	72	430	28	32	20.4	8.9	0.9
Part skim milk- - - - -	1 cup- - - - - - - - -	246	74	340	28	19	12.1	5.7	0.6
Swiss- - - - - - - - - - - - -	1 oz- - - - - - - - - -	28	37	105	8	8	5.0	2.1	0.3
Pasteurized process cheese:									
American- - - - - - - - - -	1 oz- - - - - - - - - -	28	39	105	6	9	5.6	2.5	0.3
Swiss- - - - - - - - - - - - -	1 oz- - - - - - - - - -	28	42	95	7	7	4.5	2.0	0.2
Pasteurized process cheese food, American- - - - -	1 oz- - - - - - - - - -	28	43	95	6	7	4.4	2.0	0.2
Cream, sweet:									
Half-and-half (cream and milk)- - - - - - - - - - - -	1 cup- - - - - - - - -	242	81	315	7	28	17.3	8.0	1.0
	1 tbsp- - - - - - - - -	15	81	20	Tr	2	1.1	0.5	0.1
Light, coffee, or table- - - -	1 cup- - - - - - - - -	240	74	470	6	46	28.8	13.4	1.7
	1 tbsp- - - - - - - - -	15	74	30	Tr	3	1.8	0.8	0.1
Whipping, unwhipped (volume about double when whipped):									
Light- - - - - - - - - - - - -	1 tbsp- - - - - - - - -	15	64	45	Tr	5	2.9	1.4	0.1
Heavy- - - - - - - - - - - - -	1 tbsp- - - - - - - - -	15	58	50	Tr	6	3.5	1.6	0.2
Whipped topping, (pressurized)- - - - - - - - - - - - -	1 tbsp- - - - - - - - -	3	61	10	Tr	1	0.4	0.2	Tr
Cream, sour- - - - - - - - - - -	1 tbsp- - - - - - - - -	12	71	25	Tr	3	1.6	0.7	0.1
Cream products, imitation (made with vegetable fat):									

(Tr indicates nutrient present in trace amounts.)

Nutrients in Indicated Quantity

Cho-les-terol	Carbo-hydrate	Calcium	Phos-phorus	Iron	Potas-sium	Sodium	Vitamin A value (IU)	Vitamin A value (RE)	Thiamin	Ribo-flavin	Niacin	Ascorbic acid
Milli-grams	Grams	Milli-grams	Milli-grams	Milli-grams	Milli-grams	Milli-grams	Inter-national units	Retinol equiva-lents	Milli-grams	Milli-grams	Milli-grams	Milli-grams
27	Tr	147	132	0.1	71	320	350	96	0.01	0.19	0.2	0
30	Tr	204	145	0.2	28	176	300	86	0.01	0.11	Tr	0
18	Tr	123	87	0.1	17	105	180	52	Tr	0.06	Tr	0
119	1	815	579	0.8	111	701	1,200	342	0.03	0.42	0.1	0
19	8	155	340	0.4	217	918	160	45	0.05	0.42	0.3	Tr
10	3	46	151	0.3	47	19	40	12	0.04	0.21	0.2	0
31	1	23	30	0.3	34	84	400	124	Tr	0.06	Tr	0
25	1	140	96	0.2	18	316	130	36	0.04	0.24	0.3	0
22	1	147	105	0.1	19	106	220	68	Tr	0.07	Tr	0
4	Tr	69	40	Tr	5	93	40	9	Tr	0.02	Tr	0
22	1	390	229	0.3	30	528	200	49	0.01	0.11	0.1	0
20	1	214	141	0.1	39	248	230	75	0.01	0.09	Tr	0
124	7	509	389	0.9	257	207	1,210	330	0.03	0.48	0.3	0
76	13	669	449	1.1	307	307	1,060	278	0.05	0.46	0.2	0
26	1	272	171	Tr	31	74	240	72	0.01	0.10	Tr	0
27	Tr	174	211	0.1	46	406	340	82	0.01	0.10	Tr	0
24	1	219	216	0.2	61	388	230	65	Tr	0.08	Tr	0
18	2	163	130	0.2	79	337	260	62	0.01	0.13	Tr	0
89	10	254	230	0.2	314	98	1,050	259	0.08	0.36	0.2	2
6	1	16	14	Tr	19	6	70	16	0.01	0.02	Tr	Tr
159	9	231	192	0.1	292	95	1,730	437	0.08	0.36	0.1	2
10	1	14	12	Tr	18	6	110	27	Tr	0.02	Tr	Tr
17	Tr	10	9	Tr	15	5	170	44	Tr	0.02	Tr	Tr
21	Tr	10	9	Tr	11	6	220	63	Tr	0.02	Tr	Tr
2	Tr	3	3	Tr	4	4	30	6	Tr	Tr	Tr	0
5	1	14	10	Tr	17	6	90	23	Tr	0.02	Tr	Tr

Nutritive Value of Foods *(Continued)*

Foods, approximate measures, units, and weight (weight of edible portion only)		Water	Food energy	Pro-tein	Fat	Fatty Acids		
						Satu-rated	Mono-unsatu-rated	Poly-unsatu-rated
		Grams	Per-cent	Cal-ories	Grams	Grams	Grams	Grams	Grams

		Grams	Per-cent	Cal-ories	Grams	Grams	Grams	Grams	Grams
DAIRY PRODUCTS—Con.									
Sweet:									
Creamers:									
Powdered- - - - - - - - -	1 tsp- - - - - - - - - -	2	2	10	Tr	1	0.7	Tr	Tr
Whipped topping:									
Frozen- - - - - - - - - -	1 cup- - - - - - - - -	75	50	240	1	19	16.3	1.2	0.4
	1 tbsp- - - - - - - - -	4	50	15	Tr	1	0.9	0.1	Tr
	1 tbsp- - - - - - - - -	12	75	20	Tr	2	1.6	0.2	0.1
Ice cream. See Milk desserts, frozen.									
Ice milk. See Milk desserts, frozen.									
Milk:									
Fluid:									
Whole (3.3% fat)- - - - -	1 cup- - - - - - - - -	244	88	150	8	8	5.1	2.4	0.3
Lowfat (2%):									
No milk solids added-	1 cup- - - - - - - - -	244	89	120	8	5	2.9	1.4	0.2
Lowfat (1%):									
No milk solids added-	1 cup- - - - - - - - -	244	90	100	8	3	1.6	0.7	0.1
Nonfat (skim):									
No milk solids added-	1 cup- - - - - - - - -	245	91	85	8	Tr	0.3	0.1	Tr
Buttermilk- - - - - - - - -	1 cup- - - - - - - - -	245	90	100	8	2	1.3	0.6	0.1
Canned:									
Evaporated:									
Whole milk- - - - - - -	1 cup- - - - - - - - -	252	74	340	17	19	11.6	5.9	0.6
Skim milk- - - - - - -	1 cup- - - - - - - - -	255	79	200	19	1	0.3	0.2	Tr
Dried:									
Nonfat, instantized:									
Envelope, 3.2 oz, net wt.[6]- - - - - - - - - -	1 envelope- - - - - -	91	4	325	32	1	0.4	0.2	Tr
Milk beverages:									
Chocolate milk (commer-cial):									
Regular- - - - - - - - - - -	1 cup- - - - - - - - -	250	82	210	8	8	5.3	2.5	0.3
Lowfat (2%)- - - - - - -	1 cup- - - - - - - - -	250	84	180	8	5	3.1	1.5	0.2
Cocoa and chocolate-flavored beverages:									
Eggnog (commercial)- - - -	1 cup- - - - - - - - -	254	74	340	10	19	11.3	5.7	0.9
Malted milk:									
Chocolate:									
Powder									
Prepared (8 oz whole milk plus ¾ powder)- - - - - - -	1 serving- - - - - - -	265	81	235	9	9	5.5	2.7	0.4
Shakes, thick:									
Chocolate- - - - - - - - - -	10-oz container- -	283	72	335	9	8	4.8	2.2	0.3
Vanilla- - - - - - - - - - - -	10-oz container- -	283	74	315	11	9	5.3	2.5	0.3

(Tr indicates nutrient present in trace amounts.)

Nutrients in Indicated Quantity

Cholesterol	Carbohydrate	Calcium	Phosphorus	Iron	Potassium	Sodium	Vitamin A value (IU)	Vitamin A value (RE)	Thiamin	Riboflavin	Niacin	Ascorbic acid
Milligrams	Grams	Milligrams	Milligrams	Milligrams	Milligrams	Milligrams	International units	Retinol equivalents	Milligrams	Milligrams	Milligrams	Milligrams
0	1	Tr	8	Tr	16	4	Tr	Tr	0.00	Tr	0.0	0
0	17	5	6	0.1	14	19	[5]650	[5]65	0.00	0.00	0.0	0
0	1	Tr	Tr	Tr	1	1	[5]30	[5]3	0.00	0.00	0.0	0
1	1	14	10	Tr	19	6	Tr	Tr	Tr	0.02	Tr	Tr
33	11	291	228	0.1	370	120	310	76	0.09	0.40	0.2	2
18	12	297	232	0.1	377	122	500	139	0.10	0.40	0.2	2
10	12	300	235	0.1	381	123	500	144	0.10	0.41	0.2	2
4	12	302	247	0.1	406	126	500	149	0.09	0.34	0.2	2
9	12	285	219	0.1	371	257	80	20	0.08	0.38	0.1	2
74	25	657	510	0.5	764	267	610	136	0.12	0.80	0.5	5
9	29	738	497	0.7	845	293	1,000	298	0.11	0.79	0.4	3
17	47	1,120	896	0.3	1,552	499	[7]2,160	[7]646	0.38	1.59	0.8	5
31	26	280	251	0.6	417	149	300	73	0.09	0.41	0.3	2
17	26	284	254	0.6	422	151	500	143	0.09	0.41	0.3	2
149	34	330	278	0.5	420	138	890	203	0.09	0.48	0.3	4
34	29	304	265	0.5	500	168	330	80	0.14	0.43	0.7	2
30	60	374	357	0.9	634	314	240	59	0.13	0.63	0.4	0
33	50	413	326	0.3	517	270	320	79	0.08	0.55	0.4	0

Nutritive Value of Foods *(Continued)*

Foods, approximate measures, units, and weight (weight of edible portion only)			Water	Food energy	Pro-tein	Fat	Fatty Acids		
							Satu-rated	Mono-unsatu-rated	Poly-unsatu-rated
		Grams	*Per-cent*	*Cal-ories*	*Grams*	*Grams*	*Grams*	*Grams*	*Grams*
DAIRY PRODUCTS—Con.									
Milk desserts, frozen:									
Ice cream, vanilla:									
Regular (about 11% fat):									
Hardened---------	1 cup---------	133	61	270	5	14	8.9	4.1	0.5
	3 fl oz---------	50	61	100	2	5	3.4	1.6	0.2
Soft serve (frozen cus-									
tard)-----------	1 cup---------	173	60	375	7	23	13.5	6.7	1.0
Rich (about 16% fat),									
hardened--------	1 cup---------	148	59	350	4	24	14.7	6.8	0.9
Ice milk, vanilla:									
Hardened (about									
4% fat)---------	1 cup---------	131	69	185	5	6	3.5	1.6	0.2
Soft serve (about									
3% fat)---------	1 cup---------	175	70	225	8	5	2.9	1.3	0.2
Sherbert (about 2% fat)--	1 cup---------	193	66	270	2	4	2.4	1.1	0.1
Yogurt:									
With added milk solids:									
Made with lowfat milk:									
Fruit-flavored⁸----	8-oz container---	227	74	230	10	2	1.6	0.7	0.1
Plain-----------	8-oz container---	227	85	145	12	4	2.3	1.0	0.1
Made with nonfat milk-	8-oz container---	227	85	125	13	Tr	0.3	0.1	Tr
EGGS									
Eggs, large (24 oz per dozen):									
Raw:									
Whole, without shell---	1 egg---------	50	75	80	6	6	1.7	2.2	0.7
White------------	1 white--------	33	88	15	3	Tr	0.0	0.0	0.0
Yolk-------------	1 yolk--------	17	49	65	3	6	1.7	2.2	0.7
Cooked:									
Fried in butter-------	1 egg---------	46	68	95	6	7	2.7	2.7	0.8
Hard-cooked, shell									
removed---------	1 egg---------	50	75	80	6	6	1.7	2.2	0.7
Poached----------	1 egg---------	50	74	80	6	6	1.7	2.2	0.7
Scrambled (milk added)									
in butter. Also omelet-	1 egg---------	64	73	110	7	8	3.2	2.9	0.8
FATS AND OILS									
Butter (4 sticks per lb):									
Tablespoon (⅛ stick)----	1 tbsp---------	14	16	100	Tr	11	7.1	3.3	0.4
Pat (1 in square, ⅓ in high;									
90 per lb)-----------	1 pat---------	5	16	35	Tr	4	2.5	1.2	0.2
Fats, cooking (vegetable									
shortenings)---------	1 tbsp---------	13	0	115	0	13	3.3	5.8	3.4
Lard-----------------	1 tbsp---------	13	0	115	0	13	5.1	5.9	1.5
Margarine:									
Imitation (about 40% fat),									
soft-----------	1 tbsp---------	14	58	50	Tr	5	1.1	2.2	1.9

(Tr indicates nutrient present in trace amounts.)

Nutrients in Indicated Quantity

Cholesterol	Carbohydrate	Calcium	Phosphorus	Iron	Potassium	Sodium	Vitamin A value		Thiamin	Riboflavin	Niacin	Ascorbic acid
							(IU)	(RE)				
Milligrams	Grams	Milligrams	Milligrams	Milligrams	Milligrams	Milligrams	International units	Retinol equivalents	Milligrams	Milligrams	Milligrams	Milligrams
59	32	176	134	0.1	257	116	540	133	0.05	0.33	0.1	1
22	12	66	51	Tr	96	44	200	50	0.02	0.12	0.1	Tr
153	38	236	199	0.4	338	153	790	199	0.08	0.45	0.2	1
88	32	151	115	0.1	221	108	900	219	0.04	0.28	0.1	1
18	29	176	129	0.2	265	105	210	52	0.08	0.35	0.1	1
13	38	274	202	0.3	412	163	175	44	0.12	0.54	0.2	1
14	59	103	74	0.3	198	88	190	39	0.03	0.09	0.1	4
10	43	345	271	0.2	442	133	100	25	0.08	0.40	0.2	1
14	16	415	326	0.2	531	159	150	36	0.10	0.49	0.3	2
4	17	452	355	0.2	579	174	20	5	0.11	0.53	0.3	2
274	1	28	90	1.0	65	69	260	78	0.04	0.15	Tr	0
0	Tr	4	4	Tr	45	50	0	0	Tr	0.09	Tr	0
272	Tr	26	86	0.9	15	8	310	94	0.04	0.07	Tr	0
278	1	29	91	1.1	66	162	320	94	0.04	0.14	Tr	0
274	1	28	90	1.0	65	69	260	78	0.04	0.14	Tr	0
273	1	28	90	1.0	65	146	260	78	0.03	0.13	Tr	0
282	2	54	109	1.0	97	176	350	102	0.04	0.18	Tr	Tr
31	Tr	3	3	Tr	4	[9]116	[10]430	[10]106	Tr	Tr	Tr	0
11	Tr	1	1	Tr	1	[9]41	[10]150	[10]38	Tr	Tr	Tr	0
0	0	0	0	0.0	0	0	0	0	0.00	0.00	0.0	0
12	0	0	0	0.0	0	0	0	0	0.00	0.00	0.0	0
0	Tr	2	2	0.0	4	[11]134	[12]460	[12]139	Tr	Tr	Tr	Tr

Nutritive Value of Foods *(Continued)*

Foods, approximate measures, units, and weight (weight of edible portion only)		Water	Food energy	Pro-tein	Fat	Fatty Acids Satu-rated	Mono-unsatu-rated	Poly-unsatu-rated
		Per-cent	*Cal-ories*					
FATS AND OILS—Con.	*Grams*			*Grams*	*Grams*	*Grams*	*Grams*	*Grams*
Regular (about 80% fat):								
Hard (4 sticks per lb):								
Tablespoon (⅛ stick)-	1 tbsp- - - - - - - - -	14	16	100	Tr	11	2.2	5.0	3.6
Pat (1 in square, ⅓ in								
high; 90 per lb)- - - -	1 pat- - - - - - - - -	5	16	35	Tr	4	0.8	1.8	1.3
Soft- - - - - - - - - - - - -	1 tbsp- - - - - - - - -	14	16	100	Tr	11	1.9	4.0	4.8
Spread (about 60% fat):								
Hard (4 sticks per lb):								
Tablespoon (⅛ stick)-	1 tbsp- - - - - - - - -	14	37	75	Tr	9	2.0	3.6	2.5
Pat (1 in square, ⅓ in								
high; 90 per lb)- - - -	1 pat- - - - - - - - -	5	37	25	Tr	3	0.7	1.3	0.9
Soft- - - - - - - - - - - - -	8-oz container- - -	227	37	1,225	1	138	29.1	71.5	31.3
	1 tbsp- - - - - - - - -	14	37	75	Tr	9	1.8	4.4	1.9
Oils, salad or cooking:								
Corn- - - - - - - - - - - - -	1 tbsp- - - - - - - - -	14	0	125	0	14	1.8	3.4	8.2
Olive- - - - - - - - - - - - -	1 tbsp- - - - - - - - -	14	0	125	0	14	1.9	10.3	1.2
Peanut- - - - - - - - - - - -	1 tbsp- - - - - - - - -	14	0	125	0	14	2.4	6.5	4.5
Safflower- - - - - - - - - - -	1 tbsp- - - - - - - - -	14	0	125	0	14	1.3	1.7	10.4
Soybean oil, hydrogenated								
(partially hardened)- - -	1 tbsp- - - - - - - - -	14	0	125	0	14	2.1	6.0	5.3
Soybean-cottonseed oil								
blend, hydrogenated- - -	1 tbsp- - - - - - - - -	14	0	125	0	14	2.5	4.1	6.7
Sunflower- - - - - - - - - - -	1 tbsp- - - - - - - - -	14	0	125	0	14	1.4	2.7	9.2
Salad dressings:								
Commercial:								
Blue cheese- - - - - - - -	1 tbsp- - - - - - - - -	15	32	75	1	8	1.5	1.8	4.2
French:								
Regular- - - - - - - - -	1 tbsp- - - - - - - - -	16	35	85	Tr	9	1.4	4.0	3.5
Low calorie- - - - - - -	1 tbsp- - - - - - - - -	16	75	25	Tr	2	0.2	0.3	1.0
Italian:								
Regular- - - - - - - - -	1 tbsp- - - - - - - - -	15	34	80	Tr	9	1.3	3.7	3.2
Low calorie- - - - - - -	1 tbsp- - - - - - - - -	15	86	5	Tr	Tr	Tr	Tr	Tr
Mayonnaise:								
Regular- - - - - - - - -	1 tbsp- - - - - - - - -	14	15	100	Tr	11	1.7	3.2	5.8
Imitation- - - - - - - -	1 tbsp- - - - - - - - -	15	63	35	Tr	3	0.5	0.7	1.6
Mayonnaise type- - - - -	1 tbsp- - - - - - - - -	15	40	60	Tr	5	0.7	1.4	2.7
Tartar sauce- - - - - - - -	1 tbsp- - - - - - - - -	14	34	75	Tr	8	1.2	2.6	3.9
Thousand island:								
Regular- - - - - - - - -	1 tbsp- - - - - - - - -	16	46	60	Tr	6	1.0	1.3	3.2
Low calorie- - - - - - -	1 tbsp- - - - - - - - -	15	69	25	Tr	2	0.2	0.4	0.9
Prepared from home recipe:								
Cooked type[13]- - - - - - -	1 tbsp- - - - - - - - -	16	69	25	1	2	0.5	0.6	0.3
FISH AND SHELLFISH								
Clams:								
Raw, meat only- - - - - - -	3 oz- - - - - - - - - -	85	82	65	11	1	0.3	0.3	0.3
Canned, drained solids- - -	3 oz- - - - - - - - - -	85	77	85	13	2	0.5	0.5	0.4
Crabmeat, canned- - - - - - -	1 cup- - - - - - - - -	135	77	135	23	3	0.5	0.8	1.4

(Tr indicates nutrient present in trace amounts.)

Nutrients in Indicated Quantity

Cho-les-terol	Carbo-hydrate	Calcium	Phos-phorus	Iron	Potas-sium	Sodium	Vitamin A value (IU)	(RE)	Thiamin	Ribo-flavin	Niacin	Ascorbic acid
Milli-grams	Grams	Milli-grams	Milli-grams	Milli-grams	Milli-grams	Milli-grams	Inter-national units	Retinol equiva-lents	Milli-grams	Milli-grams	Milli-grams	Milli-grams
0	Tr	4	3	Tr	6	[11]132	[12]460	[12]139	Tr	0.01	Tr	Tr
0	Tr	1	1	Tr	2	[11]47	[12]170	[12]50	Tr	Tr	Tr	Tr
0	Tr	4	3	0.0	5	[11]151	[12]460	[12]139	Tr	Tr	Tr	Tr
0	0	3	2	0.0	4	[11]139	[12]460	[12]139	Tr	Tr	Tr	Tr
0	0	1	1	0.0	1	[11]50	[12]170	[12]50	Tr	Tr	Tr	Tr
0	0	47	37	0.0	68	[11]2,256	[12]7,510	[12]2,254	0.02	0.06	Tr	Tr
0	0	3	2	0.0	4	[11]139	[12]460	[12]139	Tr	Tr	Tr	Tr
0	0	0	0	0.0	0	0	0	0	0.00	0.00	0.0	0
0	0	0	0	0.0	0	0	0	0	0.00	0.00	0.0	0
0	0	0	0	0.0	0	0	0	0	0.00	0.00	0.0	0
0	0	0	0	0.0	0	0	0	0	0.00	0.00	0.0	0
0	0	0	0	0.0	0	0	0	0	0.00	0.00	0.0	0
0	0	0	0	0.0	0	0	0	0	0.00	0.00	0.0	0
0	0	0	0	0.0	0	0	0	0	0.00	0.00	0.0	0
3	1	12	11	Tr	6	164	30	10	Tr	0.02	Tr	Tr
0	1	2	1	Tr	2	188	Tr	Tr	Tr	Tr	Tr	Tr
0	2	6	5	Tr	3	306	Tr	Tr	Tr	Tr	Tr	Tr
0	1	1	1	Tr	5	162	30	3	Tr	Tr	Tr	Tr
0	2	1	1	Tr	4	136	Tr	Tr	Tr	Tr	Tr	Tr
8	Tr	3	4	0.1	5	80	40	12	0.00	0.00	Tr	0
4	2	Tr	Tr	0.0	2	75	0	0	0.00	0.00	0.0	0
4	4	2	4	Tr	1	107	30	13	Tr	Tr	Tr	0
4	1	3	4	0.1	11	182	30	9	Tr	Tr	0.0	Tr
4	2	2	3	0.1	18	112	50	15	Tr	Tr	Tr	0
2	2	2	3	0.1	17	150	50	14	Tr	Tr	Tr	0
9	2	13	14	0.1	19	117	70	20	0.01	0.02	Tr	Tr
43	2	59	138	2.6	154	102	90	26	0.09	0.15	1.1	9
54	2	47	116	3.5	119	102	90	26	0.01	0.09	0.9	3
135	1	61	246	1.1	149	1,350	50	14	0.11	0.11	2.6	0

Nutritive Value of Foods *(Continued)*

Foods, approximate measures, units, and weight (weight of edible portion only)		Water	Food energy	Pro-tein	Fat	Fatty Acids Satu-rated	Mono-unsatu-rated	Poly-unsatu-rated
		Per-cent	Cal-ories					
FISH AND SHELLFISH—Con.	Grams			Grams	Grams	Grams	Grams	Grams
Fish sticks, frozen, reheated, (stick, 4 by 1 by ½ in)- -	1 fish stick- - - - -	28	52	70	6	3	0.8	1.4	0.8
Flounder or Sole, baked, with lemon juice:									
With butter- - - - - - - - -	3 oz- - - - - - - - -	85	73	120	16	6	3.2	1.5	0.5
With margarine- - - - - - -	3 oz- - - - - - - - -	85	73	120	16	6	1.2	2.3	1.9
Without added fat- - - - - -	3 oz- - - - - - - - -	85	78	80	17	1	0.3	0.2	0.4
Haddock, breaded, fried[14]- - -	3 oz- - - - - - - - -	85	61	175	17	9	2.4	3.9	2.4
Halibut, broiled, with butter and lemon juice- - - - - -	3 oz- - - - - - - - -	85	67	140	20	6	3.3	1.6	0.7
Herring, pickled- - - - - - - -	3 oz- - - - - - - - -	85	59	190	17	13	4.3	4.6	3.1
Ocean perch, breaded, fried[14]	1 fillet- - - - - - -	85	59	185	16	11	2.6	4.6	2.8
Oysters:									
Raw, meat only (13–19 medium Selects)- - - - - - -	1 cup- - - - - - - -	240	85	160	20	4	1.4	0.5	1.4
Breaded, fried[14]- - - - - - -	1 oyster- - - - - - -	45	65	90	5	5	1.4	2.1	1.4
Salmon:									
Canned (pink), solids and liquid- - - - - - - - - - - - -	3 oz- - - - - - - - -	85	71	120	17	5	0.9	1.5	2.1
Baked (red)- - - - - - - - - -	3 oz- - - - - - - - -	85	67	140	21	5	1.2	2.4	1.4
Smoked- - - - - - - - - - - -	3 oz- - - - - - - - -	85	59	150	18	8	2.6	3.9	0.7
Sardines, Atlantic, canned in oil, drained solids- - - - -	3 oz- - - - - - - - -	85	62	175	20	9	2.1	3.7	2.9
Scallops, breaded, frozen, re-heated- - - - - - - - - - - -	6 scallops- - - - - -	90	59	195	15	10	2.5	4.1	2.5
Shrimp:									
Canned, drained solids- - -	3 oz- - - - - - - - -	85	70	100	21	1	0.2	0.2	0.4
French fried (7 medium)[16]-	3 oz- - - - - - - - -	85	55	200	16	10	2.5	4.1	2.6
Trout, broiled, with butter and lemon juice- - - - - - - -	3 oz- - - - - - - - -	85	63	175	21	9	4.1	2.9	1.6
Tuna, canned, drained solids:									
Oil pack, chunk light- - - -	3 oz- - - - - - - - -	85	61	165	24	7	1.4	1.9	3.1
Water pack, solid white- -	3 oz- - - - - - - - -	85	63	135	30	1	0.3	0.2	0.3
Tuna salad[17]- - - - - - - - - -	1 cup- - - - - - - -	205	63	375	33	19	3.3	4.9	9.2
FRUITS AND FRUIT JUICES									
Apples:									
Raw:									
Unpeeled, without cores:									
2¾-in diam. (about 3 per lb with cores)- -	1 apple- - - - - - -	138	84	80	Tr	Tr	0.1	Tr	0.1
3¼-in diam. (about 2 per lb with cores)- -	1 apple- - - - - - -	212	84	125	Tr	1	0.1	Tr	0.2
Dried, sulfured- - - - - - -	10 rings- - - - - - -	64	32	155	1	Tr	Tr	Tr	0.1
Apple juice, bottled or canned[19]- - - - - - - - - - -	1 cup- - - - - - - -	248	88	115	Tr	Tr	Tr	Tr	0.1
Applesauce, canned:									
Sweetened- - - - - - - - - -	1 cup- - - - - - - -	255	80	195	Tr	Tr	0.1	Tr	0.1

(Tr indicates nutrient present in trace amounts.)

Nutrients in Indicated Quantity

Cholesterol	Carbohydrate	Calcium	Phosphorus	Iron	Potassium	Sodium	Vitamin A value		Thiamin	Riboflavin	Niacin	Ascorbic acid
							(IU)	(RE)				
Milligrams	Grams	Milligrams	Milligrams	Milligrams	Milligrams	Milligrams	International units	Retinol equivalents	Milligrams	Milligrams	Milligrams	Milligrams
26	4	11	58	0.3	94	53	20	5	0.03	0.05	0.6	0
68	Tr	13	187	0.3	272	145	210	54	0.05	0.08	1.6	1
55	Tr	14	187	0.3	273	151	230	69	0.05	0.08	1.6	1
59	Tr	13	197	0.3	286	101	30	10	0.05	0.08	1.7	1
75	7	34	183	1.0	270	123	70	20	0.06	0.10	2.9	0
62	Tr	14	206	0.7	441	103	610	174	0.06	0.07	7.7	1
85	0	29	128	0.9	85	850	110	33	0.04	0.18	2.8	0
66	7	31	191	1.2	241	138	70	20	0.10	0.11	2.0	0
120	8	226	343	15.6	290	175	740	223	0.34	0.43	6.0	24
35	5	49	73	3.0	64	70	150	44	0.07	0.10	1.3	4
34	0	[15]167	243	0.7	307	443	60	18	0.03	0.15	6.8	0
60	0	26	269	0.5	305	55	290	87	0.18	0.14	5.5	0
51	0	12	208	0.8	327	1,700	260	77	0.17	0.17	6.8	0
85	0	[15]371	424	2.6	349	425	190	56	0.03	0.17	4.6	0
70	10	39	203	2.0	369	298	70	21	0.11	0.11	1.6	0
128	1	98	224	1.4	104	1,955	50	15	0.01	0.03	1.5	0
168	11	61	154	2.0	189	384	90	26	0.06	0.09	2.8	0
71	Tr	26	259	1.0	297	122	230	60	0.07	0.07	2.3	1
55	0	7	199	1.6	298	303	70	20	0.04	0.09	10.1	0
48	0	17	202	0.6	255	468	110	32	0.03	0.10	13.4	0
80	19	31	281	2.5	531	877	230	53	0.06	0.14	13.3	6
0	21	10	10	0.2	159	Tr	70	7	0.02	0.02	0.1	8
0	32	15	15	0.4	244	Tr	110	11	0.04	0.03	0.2	12
0	42	9	24	0.9	288	[18]56	0	0	0.00	0.10	0.6	2
0	29	17	17	0.9	295	7	Tr	Tr	0.05	0.04	0.2	[20]2
0	51	10	18	0.9	156	8	30	3	0.03	0.07	0.5	[20]4

Nutritive Value of Foods *(Continued)*

Foods, approximate measures, units, and weight (weight of edible portion only)			Water	Food energy	Protein	Fat	Fatty Acids: Saturated	Fatty Acids: Monounsaturated	Fatty Acids: Polyunsaturated
FRUITS AND FRUIT JUICES—Con.		*Grams*	*Percent*	*Calories*	*Grams*	*Grams*	*Grams*	*Grams*	*Grams*
Unsweetened	1 cup	244	88	105	Tr	Tr	Tr	Tr	Tr
Apricots:									
Raw, without pits (about 12 per lb with pits)	3 apricots	106	86	50	1	Tr	Tr	0.2	0.1
Canned (fruit and liquid):									
Heavy syrup pack	3 halves	85	78	70	Tr	Tr	Tr	Tr	Tr
Juice pack	3 halves	84	87	40	1	Tr	Tr	Tr	Tr
Dried:									
Uncooked (28 large or 37 medium halves per cup)	1 cup	130	31	310	5	1	Tr	0.3	0.1
Cooked, unsweetened, fruit and liquid	1 cup	250	76	210	3	Tr	Tr	0.2	0.1
Apricot nectar, canned	1 cup	251	85	140	1	Tr	Tr	0.1	Tr
Avocados, raw, whole, without skin and seed:									
California (about 2 per lb with skin and seed)	1 avocado	173	73	305	4	30	4.5	19.4	3.5
Florida (about 1 per lb with skin and seed)	1 avocado	304	80	340	5	27	5.3	14.8	4.5
Bananas, raw, without peel:									
Whole (about 2½ per lb with peel)	1 banana	114	74	105	1	1	0.2	Tr	0.1
Sliced	1 cup	150	74	140	2	1	0.3	0.1	0.1
Blackberries, raw	1 cup	144	86	75	1	1	0.2	0.1	0.1
Blueberries:									
Raw	1 cup	145	85	80	1	1	Tr	0.1	0.3
Frozen, sweetened	10-oz container	284	77	230	1	Tr	Tr	0.1	0.2
	1 cup	230	77	185	1	Tr	Tr	Tr	0.1
Cantaloup. See Melons.									
Cherries:									
Sour, red, pitted, canned, water pack	1 cup	244	90	90	2	Tr	0.1	0.1	0.1
Sweet, raw, without pits and stems	10 cherries	68	81	50	1	1	0.1	0.2	0.2
Cranberry juice cocktail, bottled, sweetened	1 cup	253	85	145	Tr	Tr	Tr	Tr	0.1
Cranberry sauce, sweetened, canned, strained	1 cup	277	61	420	1	Tr	Tr	0.1	0.2
Dates:									
Whole, without pits	10 dates	83	23	230	2	Tr	0.1	0.1	Tr
Figs, dried	10 figs	187	28	475	6	2	0.4	0.5	1.0
Fruit cocktail, canned, fruit and liquid:									
Heavy syrup pack	1 cup	255	80	185	1	Tr	Tr	Tr	0.1
Juice pack	1 cup	248	87	115	1	Tr	Tr	Tr	Tr

(Tr indicates nutrient present in trace amounts.)

Nutrients in Indicated Quantity

Cholesterol	Carbohydrate	Calcium	Phosphorus	Iron	Potassium	Sodium	Vitamin A value (IU)	Vitamin A value (RE)	Thiamin	Riboflavin	Niacin	Ascorbic acid
Milligrams	Grams	Milligrams	Milligrams	Milligrams	Milligrams	Milligrams	International units	Retinol equivalents	Milligrams	Milligrams	Milligrams	Milligrams
0	28	7	17	0.3	183	5	70	7	0.03	0.06	0.5	[20]3
0	12	15	20	0.6	314	1	2,770	277	0.03	0.04	0.6	11
0	18	8	10	0.3	119	3	1,050	105	0.02	0.02	0.3	3
0	10	10	17	0.3	139	3	1,420	142	0.02	0.02	0.3	4
0	80	59	152	6.1	1,791	13	9,410	941	0.01	0.20	3.9	3
0	55	40	103	4.2	1,222	8	5,910	591	0.02	0.08	2.4	4
0	36	18	23	1.0	286	8	3,300	330	0.02	0.04	0.7	[20]2
0	12	19	73	2.0	1,097	21	1,060	106	0.19	0.21	3.3	14
0	27	33	119	1.6	1,484	15	1,860	186	0.33	0.37	5.8	24
0	27	7	23	0.4	451	1	90	9	0.05	0.11	0.6	10
0	35	9	30	0.5	594	2	120	12	0.07	0.15	0.8	14
0	18	46	30	0.8	282	Tr	240	24	0.04	0.06	0.6	30
0	20	9	15	0.2	129	9	150	15	0.07	0.07	0.5	19
0	62	17	20	1.1	170	3	120	12	0.06	0.15	0.7	3
0	50	14	16	0.9	138	2	100	10	0.05	0.12	0.6	2
0	22	27	24	3.3	239	17	1,840	184	0.04	0.10	0.4	5
0	11	10	13	0.3	152	Tr	150	15	0.03	0.04	0.3	5
0	38	8	3	0.4	61	10	10	1	0.01	0.04	0.1	[21]108
0	108	11	17	0.6	72	80	60	6	0.04	0.06	0.3	6
0	61	27	33	1.0	541	2	40	4	0.07	0.08	1.8	0
0	122	269	127	4.2	1,331	21	250	25	0.13	0.16	1.3	1
0	48	15	28	0.7	224	15	520	52	0.05	0.05	1.0	5
0	29	20	35	0.5	236	10	760	76	0.03	0.04	1.0	7

Nutritive Value of Foods *(Continued)*

Foods, approximate measures, units, and weight (weight of edible portion only)		Water	Food energy	Pro-tein	Fat	Satu-rated	Mono-unsatu-rated	Poly-unsatu-rated
							Fatty Acids	
	Grams	Per-cent	Cal-ories	Grams	Grams	Grams	Grams	Grams
FRUITS AND FRUIT JUICES—Con.								
Grapefruit:								
Raw, without peel, membrane and seeds (3¾-in diam., 1 lb 1 oz, whole, with refuse)-------- ½ grapefruit----	120	91	40	1	Tr	Tr	Tr	Tr
Canned, sections with syrup)------------ 1 cup--------	254	84	150	1	Tr	Tr	Tr	0.1
Grapefruit juice:								
Raw---------------- 1 cup--------	247	90	95	1	Tr	Tr	Tr	0.1
Canned:								
Unsweetened-------- 1 cup--------	247	90	95	1	Tr	Tr	Tr	0.1
Frozen concentrate, unsweetened								
Diluted with 3 parts water by volume-------- 1 cup--------	247	89	100	1	Tr	Tr	Tr	0.1
Grapes, European type (adherent skin), raw:								
Thompson Seedless----- 10 grapes------	50	81	35	Tr	Tr	0.1	Tr	0.1
Tokay and Emperor, seeded types------------- 10 grapes------	57	81	40	Tr	Tr	0.1	Tr	0.1
Grape juice:								
Canned or bottled------ 1 cup--------	253	84	155	1	Tr	0.1	Tr	0.1
Kiwifruit, raw, without skin (about 5 per lb with skin)- 1 kiwifruit------	76	83	45	1	Tr	Tr	0.1	0.1
Lemons, raw, without peel and seeds (about 4 per lb with peel and seeds)-------- 1 lemon------	58	89	15	1	Tr	Tr	Tr	0.1
Lemon juice:								
Raw---------------- 1 cup--------	244	91	60	1	Tr	Tr	Tr	Tr
Canned or bottled, unsweetened------------- 1 cup--------	244	92	50	1	1	0.1	Tr	0.2
1 tbsp--------	15	92	5	Tr	Tr	Tr	Tr	Tr
Lime juice:								
Raw---------------- 1 cup--------	246	90	65	1	Tr	Tr	Tr	0.1
Canned, unsweetened---- 1 cup--------	246	93	50	1	1	0.1	0.1	0.2
Mangos, raw, without skin and seed (about 1½ per lb with skin and seed)---- 1 mango------	207	82	135	1	1	0.1	0.2	0.1
Melons, raw, without rind and cavity contents:								
Cantaloup, orange-fleshed (5-in diam., 2⅓ lb, whole, with rind and cavity contents)------------ ½ melon------	267	90	95	2	1	0.1	0.1	0.3
Honeydew (6½-in diam., 5¼ lb, whole, with rind and cavity contents)------ ⅒ melon------	129	90	45	1	Tr	Tr	Tr	0.1

(Tr indicates nutrient present in trace amounts.)

Nutrients in Indicated Quantity

Cho-les-terol	Carbo-hydrate	Calcium	Phos-phorus	Iron	Potas-sium	Sodium	Vitamin A value		Thiamin	Ribo-flavin	Niacin	Ascorbic acid
							(IU)	(RE)				
Milli-grams	Grams	Milli-grams	Milli-grams	Milli-grams	Milli-grams	Milli-grams	Inter-national units	Retinol equiva-lents	Milli-grams	Milli-grams	Milli-grams	Milli-grams
0	10	14	10	0.1	167	Tr	[22]10	[22]1	0.04	0.02	0.3	41
0	39	36	25	1.0	328	5	Tr	Tr	0.10	0.05	0.6	54
0	23	22	37	0.5	400	2	20	2	0.10	0.05	0.5	94
0	22	17	27	0.5	378	2	20	2	0.10	0.05	0.6	72
0	24	20	35	0.3	336	2	20	2	0.10	0.05	0.5	83
0	9	6	7	0.1	93	1	40	4	0.05	0.03	0.2	5
0	10	6	7	0.1	105	1	40	4	0.05	0.03	0.2	6
0	38	23	28	0.6	334	8	20	2	0.07	0.09	0.7	[20]Tr
0	11	20	30	0.3	252	4	130	13	0.02	0.04	).4	74
0	5	15	9	0.3	80	1	20	2	0.02	0.01	0.1	31
0	21	17	15	0.1	303	2	50	5	0.07	0.02	0.2	112
0	16	27	22	0.3	249	[23]51	40	4	0.10	0.02	0.5	61
0	1	2	1	Tr	15	[23]3	Tr	Tr	0.01	Tr	Tr	4
0	22	22	17	0.1	268	2	20	2	0.05	0.02	0.2	72
0	16	30	25	0.6	185	[23]39	40	4	0.08	0.01	0.4	16
0	35	21	23	0.3	323	4	8,060	806	0.12	0.12	1.2	57
0	22	29	45	0.6	825	24	8,610	861	0.10	0.06	1.5	113
0	12	8	13	0.1	350	13	50	5	0.10	0.02	0.8	32

Nutritive Value of Foods *(Continued)*

Foods, approximate measures, units, and weight (weight of edible portion only)		Water	Food energy	Pro-tein	Fat	Fatty Acids Satu-rated	Mono-unsatu-rated	Poly-unsatu-rated
		Grams	Per-cent	Cal-ories	Grams	Grams	Grams	Grams Grams
FRUITS AND FRUIT JUICES—Con.								
Nectarines, raw, without pits (about 3 per lb with pits)	1 nectarine	136	86	65	1	1	0.1	0.2	0.3
Oranges, raw:									
Whole, without peel and seeds (2⅝-in diam., about 2½ per lb, with peel and seeds)	1 orange	131	87	60	1	Tr	Tr	Tr	Tr
Orange juice:									
Raw, all varieties	1 cup	248	88	110	2	Tr	0.1	0.1	0.1
Canned, unsweetened	1 cup	249	89	105	1	Tr	Tr	0.1	0.1
Chilled	1 cup	249	88	110	2	1	0.1	0.1	0.2
Frozen concentrate:									
Diluted with 3 parts water by volume	1 cup	249	88	110	2	Tr	Tr	Tr	Tr
Orange and grapefruit juice, canned	1 cup	247	89	105	1	Tr	Tr	Tr	Tr
Papayas, raw, ½-in cubes	1 cup	140	86	65	1	Tr	0.1	0.1	Tr
Peaches:									
Raw: Whole, 2½-in diam., peeled, pitted (about 4 per lb with peels and pits)	1 peach	87	88	35	1	Tr	Tr	Tr	Tr
Canned, fruit and liquid:									
Heavy syrup pack	1 half	81	79	60	Tr	Tr	Tr	Tr	Tr
Juice pack	1 half	77	87	35	Tr	Tr	Tr	Tr	Tr
Dried:									
Uncooked	1 cup	160	32	380	6	1	0.1	0.4	0.6
Cooked, unsweetened, fruit and liquid	1 cup	258	78	200	3	1	0.1	0.2	0.3
Frozen, sliced, sweetened	10-oz container	284	75	265	2	Tr	Tr	0.1	0.2
	1 cup	250	75	235	2	Tr	Tr	0.1	0.2
Pears:									
Raw, with skin, cored:									
Bartlett, 2½-in diam. (about 2½ per lb with cores and stems)	1 pear	166	84	100	1	1	Tr	0.1	0.2
Bosc, 2½-in diam. (about 3 per lb with cores and stems)	1 pear	141	84	85	1	1	Tr	0.1	0.1
D'Anjou, 3-in diam. (about 2 per lb with cores and stems)	1 pear	200	84	120	1	1	Tr	0.2	0.2
Canned, fruit and liquid:									
Heavy syrup pack	1 half	79	80	60	Tr	Tr	Tr	Tr	Tr
Juice pack	1 half	77	86	40	Tr	Tr	Tr	Tr	Tr
Pineapple:									
Raw, diced	1 cup	155	87	75	1	1	Tr	0.1	0.2

(Tr indicates nutrient present in trace amounts.)

Nutrients in Indicated Quantity

| Cho-les-terol | Carbo-hydrate | Calcium | Phos-phorus | Iron | Potas-sium | Sodium | Vitamin A value | | Thiamin | Ribo-flavin | Niacin | Ascorbic acid |
| | | | | | | | (IU) | (RE) | | | | |
Milli-grams	Grams	Milli-grams	Milli-grams	Milli-grams	Milli-grams	Milli-grams	Inter-national units	Retinol equiva-lents	Milli-grams	Milli-grams	Milli-grams	Milli-grams
0	16	7	22	0.2	288	Tr	1,000	100	0.02	0.06	1.3	7
0	15	52	18	0.1	237	Tr	270	27	0.11	0.05	0.4	70
0	26	27	42	0.5	496	2	500	50	0.22	0.07	1.0	124
0	25	20	35	1.1	436	5	440	44	0.15	0.07	0.8	86
0	25	25	27	0.4	473	2	190	19	0.28	0.05	0.7	82
0	27	22	40	0.2	473	2	190	19	0.20	0.04	0.5	97
0	25	20	35	1.1	390	7	290	29	0.14	0.07	0.8	72
0	17	35	12	0.3	247	9	400	40	0.04	0.04	0.5	92
0	10	4	10	0.1	171	Tr	470	47	0.01	0.04	0.9	6
0	16	2	9	0.2	75	5	270	27	0.01	0.02	0.5	2
0	9	5	13	0.2	99	3	290	29	0.01	0.01	0.4	3
0	98	45	190	6.5	1,594	11	3,460	346	Tr	0.34	7.0	8
0	51	23	98	3.4	826	5	510	51	0.01	0.05	3.9	10
0	68	9	31	1.1	369	17	810	81	0.04	0.10	1.9	[21]268
0	60	8	28	0.9	325	15	710	71	0.03	0.09	1.6	[21]236
0	25	18	18	0.4	208	Tr	30	3	0.03	0.07	0.2	7
0	21	16	16	0.4	176	Tr	30	3	0.03	0.06	0.1	6
0	30	22	22	0.5	250	Tr	40	4	0.04	0.08	0.2	8
0	15	4	6	0.2	51	4	Tr	Tr	0.01	0.02	0.2	1
0	10	7	9	0.2	74	3	Tr	Tr	0.01	0.01	0.2	1
0	19	11	11	0.6	175	2	40	4	0.14	0.06	0.7	24

Nutritive Value of Foods *(Continued)*

Foods, approximate measures, units, and weight (weight of edible portion only)		Water	Food energy	Pro-tein	Fat	Satu-rated	Mono-unsatu-rated	Poly-unsatu-rated
							Fatty Acids	
		Grams	Per-cent	Cal-ories	Grams	Grams	Grams	Grams	Grams

Foods, approximate measures, units, and weight (weight of edible portion only)		Grams	Per-cent	Cal-ories	Grams	Grams	Grams	Grams	Grams
FRUITS AND FRUIT JUICES—Con.									
Canned, fruit and liquid:									
Heavy syrup pack:									
Slices	1 slice	58	79	45	Tr	Tr	Tr	Tr	Tr
Juice pack:									
Slices	1 slice	58	84	35	Tr	Tr	Tr	Tr	Tr
Pineapple juice, unsweetened, canned	1 cup	250	86	140	1	Tr	Tr	Tr	0.1
Plantains, without peel:									
Cooked, boiled, sliced	1 cup	154	67	180	1	Tr	0.1	Tr	0.1
Plums, without pits:									
Raw:									
2⅛-in diam. (about 6½ per lb with pits)	1 plum	66	85	35	1	Tr	Tr	0.3	0.1
1½-in diam. (about 15 per lb with pits)	1 plum	28	85	15	Tr	Tr	Tr	0.1	Tr
Canned, purple, fruit and liquid:									
Heavy syrup pack	3 plums	133	76	120	Tr	Tr	Tr	0.1	Tr
Juice pack	3 plums	95	84	55	Tr	Tr	Tr	Tr	Tr
Prunes, dried:									
Uncooked	4 extra large or 5 large prunes	49	32	115	1	Tr	Tr	0.2	0.1
Cooked, unsweetened, fruit and liquid	1 cup	212	70	225	2	Tr	Tr	0.3	0.1
Prune juice, canned or bottled	1 cup	256	81	180	2	Tr	Tr	0.1	Tr
Raisins, seedless:									
Cup, not pressed down	1 cup	145	15	435	5	1	0.2	Tr	0.2
Packet, ½ oz (1½ tbsp)	1 packet	14	15	40	Tr	Tr	Tr	Tr	Tr
Raspberries:									
Raw	1 cup	123	87	60	1	1	Tr	0.1	0.4
Frozen, sweetened	10-oz container	284	73	295	2	Tr	Tr	Tr	0.3
Rhubarb, cooked, added sugar	1 cup	240	68	280	1	Tr	Tr	Tr	0.1
Strawberries:									
Raw, capped, whole	1 cup	149	92	45	1	1	Tr	0.1	0.3
Frozen, sweetened, sliced	10-oz container	284	73	275	2	Tr	Tr	0.1	0.2
	1 cup	255	73	245	1	Tr	Tr	Tr	0.2
Tangerines:									
Raw, without peel and seeds (2⅜-in diam., (about 4 per lb, with peel and seeds)	1 tangerine	84	88	35	1	Tr	Tr	Tr	Tr
Watermelon, raw, without rind and seeds:									
Piece (4 by 8 in wedge with rind and seeds; 1/16 of 32⅔-lb melon, 10 by 16 in)	1 piece	482	92	155	3	2	0.3	0.2	1.0

(Tr indicates nutrient present in trace amounts.)

Nutrients in Indicated Quantity

Cholesterol	Carbohydrate	Calcium	Phosphorus	Iron	Potassium	Sodium	Vitamin A value		Thiamin	Riboflavin	Niacin	Ascorbic acid
							(IU)	(RE)				
Milligrams	Grams	Milligrams	Milligrams	Milligrams	Milligrams	Milligrams	International units	Retinol equivalents	Milligrams	Milligrams	Milligrams	Milligrams
0	12	8	4	0.2	60	1	10	1	0.05	0.01	0.2	4
0	9	8	3	0.2	71	1	20	2	0.06	0.01	0.2	6
0	34	43	20	0.7	335	3	10	1	0.14	0.06	0.6	27
0	48	3	43	0.9	716	8	1,400	140	0.07	0.08	1.2	17
0	9	3	7	0.1	114	Tr	210	21	0.03	0.06	0.3	6
0	4	1	3	Tr	48	Tr	90	9	0.01	0.03	0.1	3
0	31	12	17	1.1	121	25	340	34	0.02	0.05	0.4	1
0	14	10	14	0.3	146	1	960	96	0.02	0.06	0.4	3
0	31	25	39	1.2	365	2	970	97	0.04	0.08	1.0	2
0	60	49	74	2.4	708	4	650	65	0.05	0.21	1.5	6
0	45	31	64	3.0	707	10	10	1	0.04	0.18	2.0	10
0	115	71	141	3.0	1,089	17	10	1	0.23	0.13	1.2	5
0	11	7	14	0.3	105	2	Tr	Tr	0.02	0.01	0.1	Tr
0	14	27	15	0.7	187	Tr	160	16	0.04	0.11	1.1	31
0	74	43	48	1.8	324	3	170	17	0.05	0.13	0.7	47
0	75	348	19	0.5	230	2	170	17	0.04	0.06	0.5	8
0	10	21	28	0.6	247	1	40	4	0.03	0.10	0.3	84
0	74	31	37	1.7	278	9	70	7	0.05	0.14	1.1	118
0	66	28	33	1.5	250	8	60	6	0.04	0.13	1.0	106
0	9	12	8	0.1	132	1	770	77	0.09	0.02	0.1	26
0	35	39	43	0.8	559	10	1,760	176	0.39	0.10	1.0	46

Nutritive Value of Foods *(Continued)*

Foods, approximate measures, units, and weight (weight of edible portion only)		Water	Food energy	Pro-tein	Fat	Fatty Acids		
						Satu-rated	Mono-unsatu-rated	Poly-unsatu-rated
		Per-cent	Cal-ories	Grams	Grams	Grams	Grams	Grams
GRAIN PRODUCTS	Grams							
Bagels, plain or water, enriched, 3½-in diam.[24]	1 bagel	68	29	200	7	2	0.3	0.5	0.7
Barley, pearled, light, uncooked	1 cup	200	11	700	16	2	0.3	0.2	0.9
Biscuits, baking powder, 2-in diam. (enriched flour, vegetable shortening):								
From home recipe	1 biscuit	28	28	100	2	5	1.2	2.0	1.3
Breadcrumbs, enriched:								
Soft. See White bread.								
Breads:								
Boston brown bread, canned, slice, 3¼ in by ½ in[25]	1 slice	45	45	95	2	1	0.3	0.1	0.1
Cracked-wheat bread (¾ enriched wheat flour, ¼ cracked wheat flour):[25]								
Slice (18 per loaf)	1 slice	25	35	65	2	1	0.2	0.2	0.3
French or vienna bread, enriched:[25]								
Slice:								
French, 5 by 2½ by 1 in	1 slice	35	34	100	3	1	0.3	0.4	0.5
Vienna, 4¾ by 4 by ½ in	1 slice	25	34	70	2	1	0.2	0.3	0.3
Italian bread, enriched:								
Slice, 4½ by 3¼ by ¾ in	1 slice	30	32	85	3	Tr	Tr	Tr	0.1
Mixed grain bread, enriched:[25]								
Slice (18 per loaf)	1 slice	25	37	65	2	1	0.2	0.2	0.4
Oatmeal bread, enriched:[25]								
Slice (18 per loaf)	1 slice	25	37	65	2	1	0.2	0.4	0.5
Pita bread, enriched, white, 6½-in diam.	1 pita	60	31	165	6	1	0.1	0.1	0.4
Pumpernickel (⅔ rye flour, ⅓ enriched wheat flour):[25]								
Slice, 5 by 4 by ⅜ in	1 slice	32	37	80	3	1	0.2	0.3	0.5
Raisin bread, enriched:[25]								
Slice (18 per loaf)	1 slice	25	33	65	2	1	0.2	0.3	0.4
Rye bread, light (⅔ enriched wheat flour, ⅓ rye flour):[25]								
Slice, 4¾ by 3¾ by 7/16 in	1 slice	25	37	65	2	1	0.2	0.3	0.3
Wheat bread, enriched:[25]								
Slice (18 per loaf)	1 slice	25	37	65	2	1	0.2	0.4	0.3

(Tr indicates nutrient present in trace amounts.)

Nutrients in Indicated Quantity

Cholesterol	Carbohydrate	Calcium	Phosphorus	Iron	Potassium	Sodium	Vitamin A value (IU)	Vitamin A value (RE)	Thiamin	Riboflavin	Niacin	Ascorbic acid
Milligrams	Grams	Milligrams	Milligrams	Milligrams	Milligrams	Milligrams	International units	Retinol equivalents	Milligrams	Milligrams	Milligrams	Milligrams
0	38	29	46	1.8	50	245	0	0	0.26	0.20	2.4	0
0	158	32	378	4.2	320	6	0	0	0.24	0.10	6.2	0
Tr	13	47	36	0.7	32	195	10	3	0.08	0.08	0.8	Tr
3	21	41	72	0.9	131	113	[26]0	[26]0	0.06	0.04	0.7	0
0	12	16	32	0.7	34	106	Tr	Tr	0.10	0.09	0.8	Tr
0	18	39	30	1.1	32	203	Tr	Tr	0.16	0.12	1.4	Tr
0	13	28	21	0.8	23	145	Tr	Tr	0.12	0.09	1.0	Tr
0	17	5	23	0.8	22	176	0	0	0.12	0.07	1.0	0
0	12	27	55	0.8	56	106	Tr	Tr	0.10	0.10	1.1	Tr
0	12	15	31	0.7	39	124	0	0	0.12	0.07	0.9	0
0	33	49	60	1.4	71	339	0	0	0.27	0.12	2.2	0
0	16	23	71	0.9	141	177	0	0	0.11	0.17	1.1	0
0	13	25	22	0.8	59	92	Tr	Tr	0.08	0.15	1.0	Tr
0	12	20	36	0.7	51	175	0	0	0.10	0.08	0.8	0
0	12	32	47	0.9	35	138	Tr	Tr	0.12	0.08	1.2	Tr

Nutritive Value of Foods *(Continued)*

Foods, approximate measures, units, and weight (weight of edible portion only)		Water	Food energy	Pro-tein	Fat	Fatty Acids		
						Satu-rated	Mono-unsatu-rated	Poly-unsatu-rated
		Per-cent	*Cal-ories*	*Grams*	*Grams*	*Grams*	*Grams*	*Grams*
GRAIN PRODUCTS—Con.	*Grams*							
Wheat bread, enriched:[25]								
Slice (18 per loaf)- - - - - 1 slice- - - - - - - - -	25	37	65	2	1	0.3	0.4	0.2
Whole-wheat bread:[25]								
Slice (16 per loaf)- - - - - 1 slice- - - - - - - - -	28	38	70	3	1	0.4	0.4	0.3
Breakfast cereals:								
Hot type, cooked:								
Corn, (hominy) grits:								
Regular and quick, enriched- - - - - - - - 1 cup- - - - - - - - -	242	85	145	3	Tr	Tr	0.1	0.2
Instant, plain- - - - - - 1 pkt- - - - - - - - -	137	85	80	2	Tr	Tr	Tr	0.1
Cream of Wheat®:								
Regular, quick, instant- - - - - - - - 1 cup- - - - - - - - -	244	86	140	4	Tr	0.1	Tr	0.2
Mix'n Eat, plain- - - - 1 pkt- - - - - - - - -	142	82	100	3	Tr	Tr	Tr	0.1
Malt-O-Meal®- - - - - - - 1 cup- - - - - - - - -	240	88	120	4	Tr	Tr	Tr	0.1
Oatmeal or rolled oats:								
Regular, quick, instant, nonfortified- - - - - 1 cup- - - - - - - - -	234	85	145	6	2	0.4	0.8	1.0
Ready to eat:								
All-Bran® (about ⅓ cup)- - - - - - - - 1 oz- - - - - - - - - -	28	3	70	4	1	0.1	0.1	0.3
Cap'n Crunch® (about ¾ cup)- - - - - - - - - - 1 oz- - - - - - - - - -	28	3	120	1	3	1.7	0.3	0.4
Cheerios® (about 1¼ cup)- - - - - - - - - - 1 oz- - - - - - - - - -	28	5	110	4	2	0.3	0.6	0.7
Corn Flakes (about 1¼ cup):								
Kellogg's®- - - - - - - 1 oz- - - - - - - - - -	28	3	110	2	Tr	Tr	Tr	Tr
40% Bran Flakes:								
Kellogg's® (about ¾ cup)- - - - - - - - - - 1 oz- - - - - - - - - -	28	3	90	4	1	0.1	0.1	0.3
Post® (about ⅔ cup)- 1 oz- - - - - - - - - -	28	3	90	3	Tr	0.1	0.1	0.2
Froot Loops® (about 1 cup)- - - - - - - - - - 1 oz- - - - - - - - - -	28	3	110	2	1	0.2	0.1	0.1
Golden Grahams® (about ¾ cup)- - - - - 1 oz- - - - - - - - - -	28	2	110	2	1	0.7	0.1	0.2
Grape-Nuts® (about ¼ cup)- - - - - - - - - - 1 oz- - - - - - - - - -	28	3	100	3	Tr	Tr	Tr	0.1
Honey Nut Cheerios® (about ¾ cup)- - - - - 1 oz- - - - - - - - - -	28	3	105	3	1	0.1	0.3	0.3
Lucky Charms® (about 1 cup)- - - - - - - - - - 1 oz- - - - - - - - - -	28	3	110	3	1	0.2	0.4	0.4
Nature Valley® Granola (about ⅓ cup)- - - - - 1 oz- - - - - - - - - -	28	4	125	3	5	3.3	0.7	0.7
100% Natural Cereal (about ¼ cup)- - - - - 1 oz- - - - - - - - - -	28	2	135	3	6	4.1	1.2	0.5

(Tr indicates nutrient present in trace amounts.)

Nutrients in Indicated Quantity

Cholesterol	Carbohydrate	Calcium	Phosphorus	Iron	Potassium	Sodium	Vitamin A value (IU) International units	Vitamin A value (RE) Retinol equivalents	Thiamin	Riboflavin	Niacin	Ascorbic acid
Milligrams	Grams	Milligrams	Milligrams	Milligrams	Milligrams	Milligrams			Milligrams	Milligrams	Milligrams	Milligrams
0	12	32	27	0.7	28	129	Tr	Tr	0.12	0.08	0.9	Tr
0	13	20	74	1.0	50	180	Tr	Tr	0.10	0.06	1.1	Tr
0	31	0	29	[27]1.5	53	[28]0	[29]0	[29]0	[27]0.24	[27]0.15	[27]2.0	0
0	18	7	16	[27]1.0	29	343	0	0	[27]0.18	[27]0.08	[27]1.3	0
0	29	[30]54	[31]43	[30]10.9	46	[31,32]5	0	0	[30]0.24	[30]0.07	[30]1.5	0
0	21	[30]20	[30]20	[30]8.1	38	241	[30]1,250	[30]376	[30]0.43	[30]0.28	[30]5.0	0
0	26	5	[30]24	[30]9.6	31	[33]2	0	0	[30]0.48	[30]0.24	[30]5.8	0
0	19	178		1.6	131	[34]2	40	4	0.26	0.05	0.3	0
0	21	23	264	[30]4.5	350	320	[30]1,250	[30]375	[30]0.37	[30]0.43	[30]5.0	[30]15
0	23	5	36	[27]7.5	37	213	40	4	[27]0.50	[27]0.55	[27]6.6	0
0	20	48	134	[30]4.5	101	307	[30]1,250	[30]375	[30]0.37	[30]0.43	[30]5.0	[30]15
0	24	1	18	[30]1.8	26	351	[30]1,250	[30]375	[30]0.37	[30]0.43	[30]5.0	[30]15
0	22	14	139	[30]8.1	180	264	[30]1,250	[30]375	[30]0.37	[30]0.43	[30]5.0	0
0	22	12	179	[30]4.5	151	260	[30]1,250	[30]375	[30]0.37	[30]0.43	[30]5.0	0
0	25	3	24	[30]4.5	26	145	[30]1,250	[30]375	[30]0.37	[30]0.43	[30]5.0	[30]15
Tr	24	17	41	[30]4.5	63	346	[30]1,250	[30]375	[30]0.37	[30]0.43	[30]5.0	[30]15
0	23	11	71	1.2	95	197	[30]1,250	[30]375	[30]0.37	[30]0.43	[30]5.0	0
0	23	20	105	[30]4.5	99	257	[30]1,250	[30]375	[30]0.37	[30]0.43	[30]5.0	[30]15
0	23	32	79	[30]4.5	59	201	[30]1,250	[30]375	[30]0.37	[30]0.43	[30]5.0	[30]15
0	19	18	89	0.9	98	58	20	2	0.10	0.05	0.2	0
Tr	18	49	104	0.8	140	12	20	2	0.09	0.15	0.6	0

Nutritive Value of Foods *(Continued)*

Foods, approximate measures, units, and weight (weight of edible portion only)		Water	Food energy	Pro-tein	Fat	Fatty Acids		
						Satu-rated	Mono-unsatu-rated	Poly-unsatu-rated
		Grams	Per-cent	Cal-ories	Grams	Grams	Grams	Grams	Grams

Foods, approximate measures, units, and weight (weight of edible portion only)		Grams	Per-cent	Cal-ories	Grams	Grams	Grams	Grams	Grams
GRAIN PRODUCTS—Con.									
Product 19® (about ¾ cup)	1 oz	28	3	110	3	Tr	Tr	Tr	0.1
Raisin Bran:									
Kellogg's® (about ¾ cup)	1 oz	28	8	90	3	1	0.1	0.1	0.3
Post® (about ½ cup)	1 oz	28	9	85	3	1	0.1	0.1	0.3
Rice Krispies® (about 1 cup)	1 oz	28	2	110	2	Tr	Tr	Tr	0.1
Shredded Wheat (about ⅔ cup)	1 oz	28	5	100	3	1	0.1	0.1	0.3
Special K® (about 1⅓ cup)	1 oz	28	2	110	6	Tr	Tr	Tr	Tr
Super Sugar Crisp® (about ⅞ cup)	1 oz	28	2	105	2	Tr	Tr	Tr	0.1
Sugar Frosted Flakes, Kellogg's® (about ¾ cup)	1 oz	28	3	110	1	Tr	Tr	Tr	Tr
Sugar Smacks® (about ¾ cup)	1 oz	28	3	105	2	1	0.1	0.1	0.2
Total® (about 1 cup)	1 oz	28	4	100	3	1	0.1	0.1	0.3
Trix® (about 1 cup)	1 oz	28	3	110	2	Tr	0.2	0.1	0.1
Wheaties® (about 1 cup)	1 oz	28	5	100	3	Tr	0.1	Tr	0.2
Buckwheat flour, light, sifted	1 cup	98	12	340	6	1	0.2	0.4	0.4
Bulgur, uncooked	1 cup	170	10	600	19	3	1.2	0.3	1.2
Cakes prepared from cake mixes with enriched flour:[35]									
Angelfood:									
Piece, 1/12 of cake	1 piece	53	38	125	3	Tr	Tr	Tr	0.1
Coffeecake, crumb:									
Piece, ⅙ of cake	1 piece	72	30	230	5	7	2.0	2.8	1.6
Devil's food with chocolate frosting:									
Piece, 1/16 of cake	1 piece	69	24	235	3	8	3.5	3.2	1.2
Cupcake, 2½-in diam.	1 cupcake	35	24	120	2	4	1.8	1.6	0.6
Gingerbread:									
Piece, ⅑ of cake	1 piece	63	37	175	2	4	1.1	1.8	1.2
Yellow with chocolate frosting:									
Piece, 1/16 of cake	1 piece	69	26	235	3	8	3.0	3.0	1.4
Cakes prepared from home recipes using enriched flour:									
Carrot, with cream cheese frosting:[36]									
Piece, 1/16 of cake	1 piece	96	23	385	4	21	4.1	8.4	6.7

(Tr indicates nutrient present in trace amounts.)

Nutrients in Indicated Quantity

Cho-les-terol	Carbo-hydrate	Calcium	Phos-phorus	Iron	Potas-sium	Sodium	Vitamin A value		Thiamin	Ribo-flavin	Niacin	Ascorbic acid
							(IU)	(RE)				
Milli-grams	Grams	Milli-grams	Milli-grams	Milli-grams	Milli-grams	Milli-grams	Inter-national units	Retinol equiva-lents	Milli-grams	Milli-grams	Milli-grams	Milli-grams
0	24	3	40	[30]18.0	44	325	[30]5,000	[30]1,501	[30]1.50	[30]1.70	[30]20.0	[30]60
0	21	10	105	[30]3.5	147	207	[30]960	[30]288	[30]0.28	[30]0.34	[30]3.9	0
0	21	13	119	[30]4.5	175	185	[30]1,250	[30]375	[30]0.37	[30]0.43	[30]5.0	0
0	25	4	34	[30]1.8	29	340	[30]1,250	[30]375	[30]0.37	[30]0.43	[30]5.0	[30]15
0	23	11	100	1.2	102	3	0	0	0.07	0.08	1.5	0
Tr	21	8	55	[30]4.5	49	265	[30]1,250	[30]375	[30]0.37	[30]0.43	[30]5.0	[30]15
0	26	6	52	[30]1.8	105	25	[30]1,250	[30]375	[30]0.37	[30]0.43	[30]5.0	0
0	26	1	21	[30]1.8	18	230	[30]1,250	[30]375	[30]0.37	[30]0.43	[30]5.0	[30]15
0	25	3	31	[30]1.8	42	75	[30]1,250	[30]375	[30]0.37	[30]0.43	[30]5.0	[30]15
0	22	48	118	[30]18.0	106	352	[30]5,000	[30]1,501	[30]1.50	[30]1.70	[30]20.0	[30]60
0	25	6	19	[30]4.5	27	181	[30]1,250	[30]375	[30]0.37	[30]0.43	[30]5.0	[30]15
0	23	43	98	[30]4.5	106	354	[30]1,250	[30]375	[30]0.37	[30]0.43	[30]5.0	[30]15
0	78	11	86	1.0	314	2	0	0	0.08	0.04	0.4	0
0	129	49	575	9.5	389	7	0	0	0.48	0.24	7.7	0
0	29	44	91	0.2	71	269	0	0	0.03	0.11	0.1	0
47	38	44	125	1.2	78	310	120	32	0.14	0.15	1.3	Tr
37	40	41	72	1.4	90	181	100	31	0.07	0.10	0.6	Tr
19	20	21	37	0.7	46	92	50	16	0.04	0.05	0.3	Tr
1	32	57	63	1.2	173	192	0	0	0.09	0.11	0.8	Tr
36	40	63	126	1.0	75	157	100	29	0.08	0.10	0.7	Tr
74	48	44	62	1.3	108	279	140	15	0.11	0.12	0.9	1

Nutritive Value of Foods *(Continued)*

Foods, approximate measures, units, and weight (weight of edible portion only)			*Water*	*Food energy*	*Protein*	*Fat*	*Fatty Acids: Saturated*	*Fatty Acids: Monounsaturated*	*Fatty Acids: Polyunsaturated*
GRAIN PRODUCTS—Con.		*Grams*	*Percent*	*Calories*	*Grams*	*Grams*	*Grams*	*Grams*	*Grams*
Fruitcake, dark:[36]									
Piece, 1/32 of cake, 2/3-in arc	1 piece	43	18	165	2	7	1.5	3.6	1.6
Plain sheet cake:[37]									
Without frosting:									
Piece, 1/9 of cake	1 piece	86	25	315	4	12	3.3	5.0	2.8
With uncooked white frosting:									
Piece, 1/9 of cake	1 piece	121	21	445	4	14	4.6	5.6	2.9
Pound:[38]									
Slice, 1/17 of loaf	1 slice	30	22	120	2	5	1.2	2.4	1.6
Cakes, commercial, made with enriched flour:									
Pound:									
Slice, 1/17 of loaf	1 slice	29	24	110	2	5	3.0	1.7	0.2
Snack cakes:									
Devil's food with creme filling (2 small cakes per pkg)	1 small cake	28	20	105	1	4	1.7	1.5	0.6
Sponge with creme filling (2 small cakes per pkg)	1 small cake	42	19	155	1	5	2.3	2.1	0.5
White with white frosting:									
Piece, 1/16 of cake	1 piece	71	24	260	3	9	2.1	3.8	2.6
Yellow with chocolate frosting:									
Piece, 1/16 of cake	1 piece	69	23	245	2	11	5.7	3.7	0.6
Cheesecake:									
Piece, 1/12 of cake	1 piece	92	46	280	5	18	9.9	5.4	1.2
Cookies made with enriched flour:									
Brownies with nuts:									
Commercial, with frosting, 1½ by 1¾ by ⅞ in	1 brownie	25	13	100	1	4	1.6	2.0	0.6
From home recipe, 1¾ by 1¾ by ⅞ in[36]	1 brownie	20	10	95	1	6	1.4	2.8	1.2
Chocolate chip:									
Commercial, 2¼-in diam., ⅜ in thick	4 cookies	42	4	180	2	9	2.9	3.1	2.6
From home recipe, 2⅓-in diam.[25]	4 cookies	40	3	185	2	11	3.9	4.3	2.0
From refrigerated dough, 2¼-in diam., ⅜ in thick	4 cookies	48	5	225	2	11	4.0	4.4	2.0
Oatmeal with raisins, 2⅝-in diam., ¼ in thick	4 cookies	52	4	245	3	10	2.5	4.5	2.8
Peanut butter cookie, from home recipe, 2⅝-in diam.[25]	4 cookies	48	3	245	4	14	4.0	5.8	2.8

(Tr indicates nutrient present in trace amounts.)

Nutrients in Indicated Quantity

Cholesterol	Carbohydrate	Calcium	Phosphorus	Iron	Potassium	Sodium	Vitamin A value (IU)	Vitamin A value (RE)	Thiamin	Riboflavin	Niacin	Ascorbic acid
Milligrams	Grams	Milligrams	Milligrams	Milligrams	Milligrams	Milligrams	International units	Retinol equivalents	Milligrams	Milligrams	Milligrams	Milligrams
20	25	41	50	1.2	194	67	50	13	0.08	0.08	0.5	16
61	48	55	88	1.3	68	258	150	41	0.14	0.15	1.1	Tr
70	77	61	91	1.2	74	275	240	71	0.13	0.16	1.1	Tr
32	15	20	28	0.5	28	96	200	60	0.05	0.06	0.5	Tr
64	15	8	30	0.5	26	108	160	41	0.06	0.06	0.5	0
15	17	21	26	1.0	34	105	20	4	0.06	0.09	0.7	0
7	27	14	44	0.6	37	155	30	9	0.07	0.06	0.6	0
3	42	33	99	1.0	52	176	40	12	0.20	0.13	1.7	0
38	39	23	117	1.2	123	192	120	30	0.05	0.14	0.6	0
170	26	52	81	0.4	90	204	230	69	0.03	0.12	0.4	5
14	16	13	26	0.6	50	59	70	18	0.08	0.07	0.3	Tr
18	11	9	26	0.4	35	51	20	6	0.05	0.05	0.3	Tr
5	28	13	41	0.8	68	140	50	15	0.10	0.23	1.0	Tr
18	26	13	34	1.0	82	82	20	5	0.06	0.06	0.6	0
22	32	13	34	1.0	62	173	30	8	0.06	0.10	0.9	0
2	36	18	58	1.1	90	148	40	12	0.09	0.08	1.0	0
22	28	21	60	1.1	110	142	20	5	0.07	0.07	1.9	0

Nutritive Value of Foods *(Continued)*

Foods, approximate measures, units, and weight (weight of edible portion only)		Water	Food energy	Pro-tein	Fat	Fatty Acids		
						Satu-rated	Mono-unsatu-rated	Poly-unsatu-rated
		Per-cent	*Cal-ories*	*Grams*	*Grams*	*Grams*	*Grams*	*Grams*
GRAIN PRODUCTS—Con.	*Grams*							
Sandwich type (chocolate or vanilla), 1¾-in diam., ⅜ in thick - - - - 4 cookies - - - - - - -	40	2	195	2	8	2.0	3.6	2.2
Shortbread:								
Commercial - - - - - - - - - 4 small cookies - - -	32	6	155	2	8	2.9	3.0	1.1
Sugar cookie, from refriger-ated dough, 2½-in diam., ¼ in thick - - - - 4 cookies - - - - - - -	48	4	235	2	12	2.3	5.0	3.6
Vanilla wafers, 1¾-in diam., ¼ in thick - - - - - - - - 10 cookies - - - - - -	40	4	185	2	7	1.8	3.0	1.8
Corn chips - - - - - - - - - - - - 1-oz package - - - -	28	1	155	2	9	1.4	2.4	3.7
Cornmeal:								
Whole-ground, unbolted, dry form - - - - - - - - - - 1 cup - - - - - - - -	122	12	435	11	5	0.5	1.1	2.5
Bolted (nearly whole-grain), dry form - - - - - 1 cup - - - - - - - -	122	12	440	11	4	0.5	0.9	2.2
Degermed, enriched:								
Dry form - - - - - - - - - - - 1 cup - - - - - - - -	138	12	500	11	2	0.2	0.4	0.9
Crackers:[39]								
Cheese:								
Plain, 1 in square - - - - - 10 crackers - - - - -	10	4	50	1	3	0.9	1.2	0.3
Sandwich type (peanut butter) - - - - - - - - - - - 1 sandwich - - - - -	8	3	40	1	2	0.4	0.8	0.3
Graham, plain, 2½ in square - - - - - - - 2 crackers - - - - - -	14	5	60	1	1	0.4	0.6	0.4
Melba toast, plain - - - - - - 1 piece - - - - - - - -	5	4	20	1	Tr	0.1	0.1	0.1
Rye wafers, whole-grain, 1⅞ by 3½ in - - - - - - - - - - 2 wafers - - - - - - -	14	5	55	1	1	0.3	0.4	0.3
Saltines[40] - - - - - - - - - - - 4 crackers - - - - - -	12	4	50	1	1	0.5	0.4	0.2
Snack-type, standard - - - - 1 round cracker - -	3	3	15	Tr	1	0.2	0.4	0.1
Wheat, thin - - - - - - - - - 4 crackers - - - - - -	8	3	35	1	1	0.5	0.5	0.4
Whole-wheat wafers - - - - 2 crackers - - - - - -	8	4	35	1	2	0.5	0.6	0.4
Croissants, made with enriched flour, 4½ by 4 by 1¾ in - - - - - - - - - - - - - - 1 croissant - - - - -	57	22	235	5	12	3.5	6.7	1.4
Danish pastry, made with enriched flour:								
Plain without fruit or nuts:								
Round piece, about 4¼-in diam., 1 in high - - - - - 1 pastry - - - - - - -	57	27	220	4	12	3.6	4.8	2.6
Fruit, round piece - - - - - - 1 pastry - - - - - - -	65	30	235	4	13	3.9	5.2	2.9
Doughnuts, made with enriched flour:								
Cake type, plain, 3¼-in diam., 1 in high - - - - - - 1 doughnut - - - - -	50	21	210	3	12	2.8	5.0	3.0
Yeast-leavened, glazed, 3¾-in diam., 1¼ in high - - 1 doughnut - - - - -	60	27	235	4	13	5.2	5.5	0.9

(Tr indicates nutrient present in trace amounts.)

Nutrients in Indicated Quantity

Cho-les-terol	Carbo-hydrate	Calcium	Phos-phorus	Iron	Potas-sium	Sodium	Vitamin A value		Thiamin	Ribo-flavin	Niacin	Ascorbic acid
							(IU)	(RE)				
Milli-grams	Grams	Milli-grams	Milli-grams	Milli-grams	Milli-grams	Milli-grams	Inter-national units	Retinol equiva-lents	Milli-grams	Milli-grams	Milli-grams	Milli-grams
0	29	12	40	1.4	66	189	0	0	0.09	0.07	0.8	0
27	20	13	39	0.8	38	123	30	8	0.10	0.09	0.9	0
29	31	50	91	0.9	33	261	40	11	0.09	0.06	1.1	0
25	29	16	36	0.8	50	150	50	14	0.07	0.10	1.0	0
0	16	35	52	0.5	52	233	110	11	0.04	0.05	0.4	1
0	90	24	312	2.2	346	1	620	62	0.46	0.13	2.4	0
0	91	21	272	2.2	303	1	590	59	0.37	0.10	2.3	0
0	108	8	137	5.9	166	1	610	61	0.61	0.36	4.8	0
6	6	11	17	0.3	17	112	20	5	0.05	0.04	0.4	0
1	5	7	25	0.3	17	90	Tr	Tr	0.04	0.03	0.6	0
0	11	6	20	0.4	36	86	0	0	0.02	0.03	0.6	0
0	4	6	10	0.1	11	44	0	0	0.01	0.01	0.1	0
0	10	7	44	0.5	65	115	0	0	0.06	0.03	0.5	0
4	9	3	12	0.5	17	165	0	0	0.06	0.05	0.6	0
0	2	3	6	0.1	4	30	Tr	Tr	0.01	0.01	0.1	0
0	5	3	15	0.3	17	69	Tr	Tr	0.04	0.03	0.4	0
0	5	3	22	0.2	31	59	0	0	0.02	0.03	0.4	0
13	27	20	64	2.1	68	452	50	13	0.17	0.13	1.3	0
49	26	60	58	1.1	53	218	60	17	0.16	0.17	1.4	Tr
56	28	17	80	1.3	57	233	40	11	0.16	0.14	1.4	Tr
20	24	22	111	1.0	58	192	20	5	0.12	0.12	1.1	Tr
21	26	17	55	1.4	64	222	Tr	Tr	0.28	0.12	1.8	0

Nutritive Value of Foods *(Continued)*

Foods, approximate measures, units, and weight (weight of edible portion only)		Water	Food energy	Pro-tein	Fat	Fatty Acids		
						Satu-rated	Mono-unsatu-rated	Poly-unsatu-rated
GRAIN PRODUCTS—Con.		Grams	Per-cent	Cal-ories	Grams	Grams	Grams	Grams
English muffins, plain,								
enriched- - - - - - - - - - -	1 muffin- - - - - - -	57	42	140	5	1	0.3	0.2	0.3
Toasted- - - - - - - - - - - -	1 muffin- - - - - - -	50	29	140	5	1	0.3	0.2	0.3
French toast, from home								
recipe- - - - - - - - - - - - - -	1 slice - - - - - - - - -	65	53	155	6	7	1.6	2.0	1.6
Macaroni, enriched, cooked (cut lengths, elbows, shells):								
Firm stage (hot)- - - - - -	1 cup- - - - - - - - -	130	64	190	7	1	0.1	0.1	0.3
Tender stage:								
Cold- - - - - - - - - - - - -	1 cup- - - - - - - - -	105	72	115	4	Tr	0.1	0.1	0.2
Hot- - - - - - - - - - - - - -	1 cup- - - - - - - - -	140	72	155	5	1	0.1	0.1	0.2
Muffins made with enriched flour, 2½-in diam., 1½ in high:								
From home recipe:								
Blueberry[25]- - - - - - - - -	1 muffin- - - - - - -	45	37	135	3	5	1.5	2.1	1.2
Bran[36]- - - - - - - - - - - -	1 muffin- - - - - - -	45	35	125	3	6	1.4	1.6	2.3
Corn (enriched, de-germed cornmeal and flour)[25]- - - - - - - - - - -	1 muffin- - - - - - -	45	33	145	3	5	1.5	2.2	1.4
From commercial mix (egg and water added):								
Blueberry- - - - - - - - - -	1 muffin- - - - - - -	45	33	140	3	5	1.4	2.0	1.2
Bran- - - - - - - - - - - - - -	1 muffin- - - - - - -	45	28	140	3	4	1.3	1.6	1.0
Corn- - - - - - - - - - - - -	1 muffin- - - - - - -	45	30	145	3	6	1.7	2.3	1.4
Noodles (egg noodles), enriched, cooked- - - - - -	1 cup- - - - - - - - -	160	70	200	7	2	0.5	0.6	0.6
Noodles, chow mein, canned	1 cup- - - - - - - - -	45	11	220	6	11	2.1	7.3	0.4
Pancakes, 4-in diam.:								
Buckwheat, from mix (with buckwheat and enriched flours), egg and milk added- - - - -	1 pancake- - - - - -	27	58	55	2	2	0.9	0.9	0.5
Plain:								
From home recipe using enriched flour- - - - - -	1 pancake- - - - - -	27	50	60	2	2	0.5	0.8	0.5
From mix (with enriched flour), egg, milk, and oil added- - - - - - - - - - - -	1 pancake- - - - - -	27	54	60	2	2	0.5	0.9	0.5
Piecrust, made with enriched flour and vegetable short-ening, baked:								
From home recipe, 9-in diam.- - - - - - - - - - - - -	1 pie shell- - - - - -	180	15	900	11	60	14.8	25.9	15.7
From mix, 9-in diam.- - - -	Piecrust for 2-crust pie- - - - - - - -	320	19	1,485	20	93	22.7	41.0	25.0

(Tr indicates nutrient present in trace amounts.)

Nutrients in Indicated Quantity

Cho-les-terol	Carbo-hydrate	Calcium	Phos-phorus	Iron	Potas-sium	Sodium	Vitamin A value		Thiamin	Ribo-flavin	Niacin	Ascorbic acid
							(IU)	(RE)				
Milli-grams	Grams	Milli-grams	Milli-grams	Milli-grams	Milli-grams	Milli-grams	Inter-national units	Retinol equiva-lents	Milli-grams	Milli-grams	Milli-grams	Milli-grams
0	27	96	67	1.7	331	378	0	0	0.26	0.19	2.2	0
0	27	96	67	1.7	331	378	0	0	0.23	0.19	2.2	0
112	17	72	85	1.3	86	257	110	32	0.12	0.16	1.0	Tr
0	39	14	85	2.1	103	1	0	0	0.23	0.13	1.8	0
0	24	8	53	1.3	64	1	0	0	0.15	0.08	1.2	0
0	32	11	70	1.7	85	1	0	0	0.20	0.11	1.5	0
19	20	54	46	0.9	47	198	40	9	0.10	0.11	0.9	1
24	19	60	125	1.4	99	189	230	30	0.11	0.13	1.3	3
23	21	66	59	0.9	57	169	80	15	0.11	0.11	0.9	Tr
45	22	15	90	0.9	54	225	50	11	0.10	0.17	1.1	Tr
28	24	27	182	1.7	50	385	100	14	0.08	0.12	1.9	0
42	22	30	128	1.3	31	291	90	16	0.09	0.09	0.8	Tr
50	37	16	94	2.6	70	3	110	34	0.22	0.13	1.9	0
5	26	14	41	0.4	33	450	0	0	0.05	0.03	0.6	0
20	6	59	91	0.4	66	125	60	17	0.04	0.05	0.2	Tr
16	9	27	38	0.5	33	115	30	10	0.06	0.07	0.5	Tr
16	8	36	71	0.7	43	160	30	7	0.09	0.12	0.8	Tr
0	79	25	90	4.5	90	1,100	0	0	0.54	0.40	5.0	0
0	141	131	272	9.3	179	2,602	0	0	1.06	0.80	9.9	0

Nutritive Value of Foods *(Continued)*

Foods, approximate measures, units, and weight (weight of edible portion only)		Water	Food energy	Pro-tein	Fat	Fatty Acids		
						Satu-rated	Mono-unsatu-rated	Poly-unsatu-rated
		Grams	Per-cent	Cal-ories	Grams	Grams	Grams	Grams	Grams

		Grams	Per-cent	Cal-ories	Grams	Grams	Grams	Grams	Grams
GRAIN PRODUCTS—Con.									
Pies, piecrust made with enriched flour, vegetable shortening, 9-in diam.:									
Apple:									
Piece, ⅙ of pie- - - - - - -	1 piece- - - - - - - -	158	48	405	3	18	4.6	7.4	4.4
Blueberry:									
Piece, ⅙ of pie- - - - - - -	1 piece- - - - - - - -	158	51	380	4	17	4.3	7.4	4.6
Cherry:									
Piece, ⅙ of pie- - - - - - -	1 piece- - - - - - - -	158	47	410	4	18	4.7	7.7	4.6
Creme:									
Piece, ⅙ of pie- - - - - - -	1 piece- - - - - - - -	152	43	455	3	23	15.0	4.0	1.1
Custard:									
Piece, ⅙ of pie- - - - - - -	1 piece- - - - - - - -	152	58	330	9	17	5.6	6.7	3.2
Lemon meringue:									
Piece, ⅙ of pie- - - - - - -	1 piece- - - - - - - -	140	47	355	5	14	4.3	5.7	2.9
Peach:									
Piece, ⅙ of pie- - - - - - -	1 piece- - - - - - - -	158	48	405	4	17	4.1	7.3	4.4
Pecan:									
Piece, ⅙ of pie- - - - - - -	1 piece- - - - - - - -	138	20	575	7	32	4.7	17.0	7.9
Pumpkin:									
Piece, ⅙ of pie- - - - - - -	1 piece- - - - - - - -	152	59	320	6	17	6.4	6.7	3.0
Pies, fried:									
Apple- - - - - - - - - - - - - -	1 pie- - - - - - - - - -	85	43	255	2	14	5.8	6.6	0.6
Cherry- - - - - - - - - - - - - -	1 pie- - - - - - - - - -	85	42	250	2	14	5.8	6.7	0.6
Popcorn, popped:									
Air-popped, unsalted- - - -	1 cup- - - - - - - - -	8	4	30	1	Tr	Tr	0.1	0.2
Popped in vegetable oil, salted- - - - - - - - - - - -	1 cup- - - - - - - - -	11	3	55	1	3	0.5	1.4	1.2
Sugar syrup coated- - - - - -	1 cup- - - - - - - - -	35	4	135	2	1	0.1	0.3	0.6
Pretzels, made with enriched flour:									
Stick 2¼ in long- - - - - - -	10 pretzels- - - - - -	3	3	10	Tr	Tr	Tr	Tr	Tr
Twisted, dutch 2¾ by 2⅝ in- - - - - - - - -	1 pretzel- - - - - - -	16	3	65	2	1	0.1	0.2	0.2
Twisted, thin, 3¼ by 2¼ by ¼ in- - - - - - - - - - - -	10 pretzels- - - - - -	60	3	240	6	2	0.4	0.8	0.6
Rice:									
Brown, cooked, served hot-	1 cup- - - - - - - - -	195	70	230	5	1	0.3	0.3	0.4
White enriched:									
Commercial varieties, all types:									
Cooked, served hot- - -	1 cup- - - - - - - - -	205	73	225	4	Tr	0.1	0.1	0.1
Instant, ready-to-serve, hot- - - - - - - - - - - -	1 cup- - - - - - - - -	165	73	180	4	0	0.1	0.1	0.1
Parboiled:									
Cooked, served hot- - -	1 cup- - - - - - - - -	175	73	185	4	Tr	Tr	Tr	0.1

(Tr indicates nutrient present in trace amounts.)

Nutrients in Indicated Quantity

| Cholesterol | Carbohydrate | Calcium | Phosphorus | Iron | Potassium | Sodium | Vitamin A value | | Thiamin | Riboflavin | Niacin | Ascorbic acid |
| | | | | | | | (IU) | (RE) | | | | |
Milligrams	Grams	Milligrams	Milligrams	Milligrams	Milligrams	Milligrams	International units	Retinol equivalents	Milligrams	Milligrams	Milligrams	Milligrams
0	60	13	35	1.6	126	476	50	5	0.17	0.13	1.6	2
0	55	17	36	2.1	158	423	140	14	0.17	0.14	1.7	6
0	61	22	40	1.6	166	480	700	70	0.19	0.14	1.6	0
8	59	46	154	1.1	133	369	210	65	0.06	0.15	1.1	0
169	36	146	172	1.5	208	436	350	96	0.14	0.32	Œ0.9	0
143	53	20	69	1.4	70	395	240	66	0.10	0.14	0.8	4
0	60	16	46	1.9	235	423	1,150	115	0.17	0.16	2.4	5
95	71	65	142	4.6	170	305	220	54	0.30	0.17	1.1	0
109	37	78	105	1.4	243	325	3,750	416	0.14	0.21	1.2	0
14	31	12	34	0.9	42	326	30	3	0.09	0.06	1.0	1
13	32	11	41	0.7	61	371	190	19	0.06	0.06	0.6	1
0	6	1	22	0.2	20	Tr	10	1	0.03	0.01	0.2	0
0	6	3	31	0.3	19	86	20	2	0.01	0.02	0.1	0
0	30	2	47	0.5	90	Tr	30	3	0.13	0.02	0.4	0
0	2	1	3	0.1	3	48	0	0	0.01	0.01	0.1	0
0	13	4	15	0.3	16	258	0	0	0.05	0.04	0.7	0
0	48	16	55	1.2	61	966	0	0	0.19	0.15	2.6	0
0	50	23	142	1.0	137	0	0	0	0.18	0.04	2.7	0
0	50	21	57	1.8	57	0	0	0	0.23	0.02	2.1	0
0	40	5	31	1.3	0	0	0	0	0.21	0.02	1.7	0
0	41	33	100	1.4	75	0	0	0	0.19	0.02	2.1	0

Nutritive Value of Foods *(Continued)*

Foods, approximate measures, units, and weight (weight of edible portion only)		Water	Food energy	Pro- tein	Fat	Fatty Acids		
						Satu- rated	Mono- unsatu- rated	Poly- unsatu- rated
		Grams	Per- cent	Cal- ories	Grams	Grams	Grams	Grams
GRAIN PRODUCTS—Con.								
Rolls, enriched:								
Commercial:								
Dinner, 2½-in diam., 2 in high	1 roll	28	32	85	2	2	0.5	0.8	0.6
Frankfurter and ham- burger (8 per 11½-oz pkg.)	1 roll	40	34	115	3	2	0.5	0.8	0.6
Hard, 3¾-in diam., 2 in high	1 roll	50	25	155	5	2	0.4	0.5	0.6
Hoagie or submarine, 11½ by 3 by 2½ in	1 roll	135	31	400	11	8	1.8	3.0	2.2
From home recipe:								
Dinner, 2½-in diam., 2 in high	1 roll	35	26	120	3	3	0.8	1.2	0.9
Spaghetti, enriched, cooked:								
Firm stage, "al dente," served hot	1 cup	130	64	190	7	1	0.1	0.1	0.3
Tortillas, corn	1 tortilla	30	45	65	2	1	0.1	0.3	0.6
Waffles, made with enriched flour, 7-in diam.:								
From home recipe	1 waffle	75	37	245	7	13	4.0	4.9	2.6
From mix, egg and milk added	1 waffle	75	42	205	7	8	2.7	2.9	1.5
Wheat flours:								
All-purpose or family flour, enriched:								
Sifted, spooned	1 cup	115	12	420	12	1	0.2	0.1	0.5
Cake or pastry flour, enriched, sifted, spooned	1 cup	96	12	350	7	1	0.1	0.1	0.3
Self-rising, enriched, unsifted, spooned	1 cup	125	12	440	12	1	0.2	0.1	0.5
Whole-wheat, from hard wheats, stirred	1 cup	120	12	400	16	2	0.3	0.3	1.1
LEGUMES, NUTS, AND SEEDS								
Almonds, shelled:								
Slivered, packed	1 cup	135	4	795	27	70	6.7	45.8	14.8
Whole	1 oz	28	4	165	6	15	1.4	9.6	3.1
Beans, dry:								
Cooked, drained:								
Black	1 cup	171	66	225	15	1	0.1	0.1	0.5
Great Northern	1 cup	180	69	210	14	1	0.1	0.1	0.6
Lima	1 cup	190	64	260	16	1	0.2	0.1	0.5
Pea (navy)	1 cup	190	69	225	15	1	0.1	0.1	0.7
Pinto	1 cup	180	65	265	15	1	0.1	0.1	0.5

(Tr indicates nutrient present in trace amounts.)

Nutrients in Indicated Quantity

Cho-les-terol	Carbo-hydrate	Calcium	Phos-phorus	Iron	Potas-sium	Sodium	Vitamin A value (IU)	Vitamin A value (RE)	Thiamin	Ribo-flavin	Niacin	Ascorbic acid
Milli-grams	Grams	Milli-grams	Milli-grams	Milli-grams	Milli-grams	Milli-grams	Inter-national units	Retinol equiva-lents	Milli-grams	Milli-grams	Milli-grams	Milli-grams
Tr	14	33	44	0.8	36	155	Tr	Tr	0.14	0.09	1.1	Tr
Tr	20	54	44	1.2	56	241	Tr	Tr	0.20	0.13	1.6	Tr
Tr	30	24	46	1.4	49	313	0	0	0.20	0.12	1.7	0
Tr	72	100	115	3.8	128	683	0	0	0.54	0.33	4.5	0
12	20	16	36	1.1	41	98	30	8	0.12	0.12	1.2	0
0	39	14	85	2.0	103	1	0	0	0.23	0.13	1.8	0
0	13	42	55	0.6	43	1	80	8	0.05	0.03	0.4	0
102	26	154	135	1.5	129	445	140	39	0.18	0.24	1.5	Tr
59	27	179	257	1.2	146	515	170	49	0.14	0.23	0.9	Tr
0	88	18	100	5.1	109	2	0	0	0.73	0.46	6.1	0
0	76	16	70	4.2	91	2	0	0	0.58	0.38	5.1	0
0	93	331	583	5.5	113	1,349	0	0	0.80	0.50	6.6	0
0	85	49	446	5.2	444	4	0	0	0.66	0.14	5.2	0
0	28	359	702	4.9	988	15	0	0	0.28	1.05	4.5	1
0	6	75	147	1.0	208	3	0	0	0.06	0.22	1.0	Tr
0	41	47	239	2.9	608	1	Tr	Tr	0.43	0.05	0.9	0
0	38	90	266	4.9	749	13	0	0	0.25	0.13	1.3	0
0	49	55	293	5.9	1,163	4	0	0	0.25	0.11	1.3	0
0	40	95	281	5.1	790	13	0	0	0.27	0.13	1.3	0
0	49	86	296	5.4	882	3	Tr	Tr	0.33	0.16	0.7	0

Nutritive Value of Foods *(Continued)*

Foods, approximate measures, units, and weight (weight of edible portion only)		Water	Food energy	Pro-tein	Fat	Fatty Acids		
						Satu-rated	Mono-unsatu-rated	Poly-unsatu-rated
		Grams	Per-cent	Cal-ories	Grams	Grams	Grams	Grams	Grams

Foods, approximate measures, units, and weight (weight of edible portion only)		Grams	Per-cent	Cal-ories	Grams	Grams	Grams	Grams	Grams
LEGUMES, NUTS, AND SEEDS—Con.									
Canned, solids and liquid:									
White with:									
Frankfurters (sliced)-	1 cup- - - - - - - - -	255	71	365	19	18	7.4	8.8	0.7
Pork and tomato									
sauce- - - - - - - - -	1 cup- - - - - - - - -	255	71	310	16	7	2.4	2.7	0.7
Pork and sweet sauce-	1 cup- - - - - - - - -	255	66	385	16	12	4.3	4.9	1.2
Red kidney- - - - - - - -	1 cup- - - - - - - - -	255	76	230	15	1	0.1	0.1	0.6
Black-eyed peas, dry, cooked (with residual cooking liquid)- - - - - - - - - - - - -	1 cup- - - - - - - - -	250	80	190	13	1	0.2	Tr	0.3
Brazil nuts, shelled- - - - - -	1 oz- - - - - - - - -	28	3	185	4	19	4.6	6.5	6.8
Carob flour- - - - - - - - - - -	1 cup- - - - - - - - -	140	3	255	6	Tr	Tr	0.1	0.1
Cashew nuts, salted:									
Dry roasted- - - - - - - - - -	1 oz- - - - - - - - -	28	2	165	4	13	2.6	7.7	2.2
Roasted in oil- - - - - - - -	1 oz- - - - - - - - -	28	4	165	5	14	2.7	8.1	2.3
Chestnuts, European (Italian), roasted, shelled- - - - - - - - - - - - -	1 cup- - - - - - - - -	143	40	350	5	3	0.6	1.1	1.2
Chickpeas, cooked, drained-	1 cup- - - - - - - - -	163	60	270	15	4	0.4	0.9	1.9
Coconut:									
Raw:									
Piece, about 2 by 2 by ½ in- - - - - - - -	1 piece- - - - - - -	45	47	160	1	15	13.4	0.6	0.2
Dried, sweetened, shredded- - - - - - - -	1 cup- - - - - - - - -	93	13	470	3	33	29.3	1.4	0.4
Filberts (hazelnuts), chopped- - - - - - - - - - - -	1 oz- - - - - - - - -	28	5	180	4	18	1.3	13.9	1.7
Lentils, dry, cooked- - - - - -	1 cup- - - - - - - - -	200	72	215	16	1	0.1	0.2	0.5
Macadamia nuts, roasted in oil, salted- - - - - - - - - - -	1 oz- - - - - - - - -	28	2	205	2	22	3.2	17.1	0.4
Mixed nuts, with peanuts, salted:									
Dry roasted- - - - - - - - - -	1 oz- - - - - - - - -	28	2	170	5	15	2.0	8.9	3.1
Roasted in oil- - - - - - - -	1 oz- - - - - - - - -	28	2	175	5	16	2.5	9.0	3.8
Peanuts, roasted in oil, salted- - - - - - - - - - - - - -	1 oz- - - - - - - - -	28	2	165	8	14	1.9	6.9	4.4
Peanut butter- - - - - - - - - -	1 tbsp- - - - - - - -	16	1	95	5	8	1.4	4.0	2.5
Peas, split, dry, cooked- - - -	1 cup- - - - - - - - -	200	70	230	16	1	0.1	0.1	0.3
Pecans, halves- - - - - - - - -	1 oz- - - - - - - - -	28	5	190	2	19	1.5	12.0	4.7
Pine nuts (pinyons), shelled-	1 oz- - - - - - - - -	28	6	160	3	17	2.7	6.5	7.3
Pistachio nuts, dried, shelled	1 oz- - - - - - - - -	28	4	165	6	14	1.7	9.3	2.1
Pumpkin and squash kernels, dry, hulled- - - - - - - - - - -	1 oz- - - - - - - - -	28	7	155	7	13	2.5	4.0	5.9
Refried beans, canned- - - - -	1 cup- - - - - - - - -	290	72	295	18	3	0.4	0.6	1.4
Sesame seeds, dry, hulled- - -	1 tbsp- - - - - - - -	8	5	45	2	4	0.6	1.7	1.9
Soybeans, dry, cooked, drained- - - - - - - - - - - - -	1 cup- - - - - - - - -	180	71	235	20	10	1.3	1.9	5.3

(Tr indicates nutrient present in trace amounts.)

Nutrients in Indicated Quantity

Cholesterol	Carbohydrate	Calcium	Phosphorus	Iron	Potassium	Sodium	Vitamin A value		Thiamin	Riboflavin	Niacin	Ascorbic acid
							(IU)	(RE)				
Milligrams	Grams	Milligrams	Milligrams	Milligrams	Milligrams	Milligrams	International units	Retinol equivalents	Milligrams	Milligrams	Milligrams	Milligrams
30	32	94	303	4.8	668	1,374	330	33	0.18	0.15	3.3	Tr
10	48	138	235	4.6	536	1,181	330	33	0.20	0.08	1.5	5
10	54	161	291	5.9	536	969	330	33	0.15	0.10	1.3	5
0	42	74	278	4.6	673	968	10	1	0.13	0.10	1.5	0
0	35	43	238	3.3	573	20	30	3	0.40	0.10	1.0	0
0	4	50	170	1.0	170	1	Tr	Tr	0.28	0.03	0.5	Tr
0	126	390	102	5.7	1,275	24	Tr	Tr	0.07	0.07	2.2	Tr
0	9	13	139	1.7	160	[41]181	0	0	0.06	0.06	0.4	0
0	8	12	121	1.2	150	[42]177	0	0	0.12	0.05	0.5	0
0	76	41	153	1.3	847	3	30	3	0.35	0.25	1.9	37
0	45	80	273	4.9	475	11	Tr	Tr	0.18	0.09	0.9	0
0	7	6	51	1.1	160	9	0	0	0.03	0.01	0.2	1
0	44	14	99	1.8	313	244	0	0	0.03	0.02	0.4	1
0	4	53	88	0.9	126	1	20	2	0.14	0.03	0.3	Tr
0	38	50	238	4.2	498	26	40	4	0.14	0.12	1.2	0
0	4	13	57	0.5	93	[43]74	Tr	Tr	0.06	0.03	0.6	0
0	7	20	123	1.0	169	[44]190	Tr	Tr	0.06	0.06	1.3	0
0	6	31	131	0.9	165	[44]185	10	1	0.14	0.06	1.4	Tr
0	5	24	143	0.5	199	[45]122	0	0	0.08	0.03	4.2	0
0	3	5	60	0.3	110	75	0	0	0.02	0.02	2.2	0
0	42	22	178	3.4	592	26	80	8	0.30	0.18	1.8	0
0	5	10	83	0.6	111	Tr	40	4	0.24	0.04	0.3	1
0	5	2	10	0.9	178	20	10	1	0.35	0.06	1.2	1
0	7	38	143	1.9	310	2	70	7	0.23	0.05	0.3	Tr
0	5	12	333	4.2	229	5	110	11	0.06	0.09	0.5	Tr
0	51	141	245	5.1	1,141	1,228	0	0	0.14	0.16	1.4	17
0	1	11	62	0.6	33	3	10	1	0.06	0.01	0.4	0
0	19	131	322	4.9	972	4	50	5	0.38	0.16	1.1	0

Nutritive Value of Foods *(Continued)*

Foods, approximate measures, units, and weight (weight of edible portion only)		Water	Food energy	Pro-tein	Fat	Fatty Acids		
						Satu-rated	Mono-unsatu-rated	Poly-unsatu-rated
		Grams	Per-cent	Cal-ories	Grams	Grams	Grams	Grams	Grams

		Grams	Per-cent	Cal-ories	Grams	Grams	Grams	Grams	Grams
LEGUMES, NUTS, AND SEEDS—Con.								
Soy products:								
Miso- - - - - - - - - - - - -	1 cup- - - - - - - -	276	53	470	29	13	1.8	2.6	7.3
Tofu, piece 2½ by 2¾								
by 1 in- - - - - - - - - - -	1 piece- - - - - - -	120	85	85	9	5	0.7	1.0	2.9
Sunflower seeds, dry, hulled-	1 oz- - - - - - - -	28	5	160	6	14	1.5	2.7	9.3
Tahini- - - - - - - - - - - - -	1 tbsp- - - - - - - -	15	3	90	3	8	1.1	3.0	3.5
Walnuts:								
Black, chopped- - - - - - -	1 oz- - - - - - - - -	28	4	170	7	16	1.0	3.6	10.6
English or Persian, pieces								
or chips- - - - - - - - - - -	1 oz- - - - - - - - -	28	4	180	4	18	1.6	4.0	11.1
MEAT AND MEAT PRODUCTS								
Beef, cooked:[46]								
Cuts braised, simmered, or pot roasted:								
Relatively fat such as chuck blade:								
Lean and fat, piece, 2½ by 2½ by ¾ in- - - - -	3 oz- - - - - - - - -	85	43	325	22	26	10.8	11.7	0.9
Lean only- - - - - - - - -	2.2 oz- - - - - - - -	62	53	170	19	9	3.9	4.2	0.3
Relatively lean, such as bottom round:								
Lean and fat, piece, 4⅛ by 2¼ by ½ in- - - -	3 oz- - - - - - - - -	85	54	220	25	13	4.8	5.7	0.5
Lean only- - - - - - - - -	2.8 oz- - - - - - - -	78	57	175	25	8	2.7	3.4	0.3
Ground beef, broiled, patty, 3 by ⅝ in:								
Lean- - - - - - - - - - - - -	3 oz- - - - - - - - -	85	56	230	21	16	6.2	6.9	0.6
Regular- - - - - - - - - - -	3 oz- - - - - - - - -	85	54	245	20	18	6.9	7.7	0.7
Liver, fried, slice, 6½ by 2⅜ by ⅜ in[47]- - - - - - -	3 oz- - - - - - - - -	85	56	185	23	7	2.5	3.6	1.3
Roast, oven cooked, no liquid added:								
Relatively fat, such as rib:								
Lean and fat, 2 pieces, 4⅛ by 2¼ by ¼ in- -	3 oz- - - - - - - - -	85	46	315	19	26	10.8	11.4	0.9
Lean only- - - - - - - - -	2.2 oz- - - - - - - -	61	57	150	17	9	3.6	3.7	0.3
Relatively lean, such as eye of round:								
Lean and fat, 2 pieces, 2½ by 2½ by ⅜ in- -	3 oz- - - - - - - - -	85	57	205	23	12	4.9	5.4	0.5
Lean only- - - - - - - - -	2.6 oz- - - - - - - -	75	63	135	22	5	1.9	2.1	0.2
Steak:								
Sirloin, broiled:								
Lean and fat, piece, 2½ by 2½ by ¾ in- - - - -	3 oz- - - - - - - - -	85	53	240	23	15	6.4	6.9	0.6
Lean only- - - - - - - - -	2.5 oz- - - - - - - -	72	59	150	22	6	2.6	2.8	0.3
Beef, canned, corned- - - - -	3 oz- - - - - - - - -	85	59	185	22	10	4.2	4.9	0.4

(Tr indicates nutrient present in trace amounts.)

Nutrients in Indicated Quantity

Cholesterol	Carbohydrate	Calcium	Phosphorus	Iron	Potassium	Sodium	Vitamin A value		Thiamin	Riboflavin	Niacin	Ascorbic acid
							(IU)	(RE)				
Milligrams	Grams	Milligrams	Milligrams	Milligrams	Milligrams	Milligrams	International units	Retinol equivalents	Milligrams	Milligrams	Milligrams	Milligrams
0	65	188	853	4.7	922	8,142	110	11	0.17	0.28	0.8	0
0	3	108	151	2.3	50	8	0	0	0.07	0.04	0.1	0
0	5	33	200	1.9	195	1	10	1	0.65	0.07	1.3	Tr
0	3	21	119	0.7	69	5	10	1	0.24	0.02	0.8	1
0	3	16	132	0.9	149	Tr	80	8	0.06	0.03	0.2	Tr
0	5	27	90	0.7	142	3	40	4	0.11	0.04	0.3	1
87	0	11	163	2.5	163	53	Tr	Tr	0.06	0.19	2.0	0
66	0	8	146	2.3	163	44	Tr	Tr	0.05	0.17	1.7	0
81	0	5	217	2.8	248	43	Tr	Tr	0.06	0.21	3.3	0
75	0	4	212	2.7	240	40	Tr	Tr	0.06	0.20	3.0	0
74	0	9	134	1.8	256	65	Tr	Tr	0.04	0.18	4.4	0
76	0	9	144	2.1	248	70	Tr	Tr	0.03	0.16	4.9	0
410	7	9	392	5.3	309	90	[48]30,690	[48]9,120	0.18	3.52	12.3	23
72	0	8	145	2.0	246	54	Tr	Tr	0.06	0.16	3.1	0
49	0	5	127	1.7	218	45	Tr	Tr	0.05	0.13	2.7	0
62	0	5	177	1.6	308	50	Tr	Tr	0.07	0.14	3.0	0
52	0	3	170	1.5	297	46	Tr	Tr	0.07	0.13	2.8	0
77	0	9	186	2.6	306	53	Tr	Tr	0.10	0.23	3.3	0
64	0	8	176	2.4	290	48	Tr	Tr	0.09	0.22	3.1	0
80	0	17	90	3.7	51	802	Tr	Tr	0.02	0.20	2.9	0

Nutritive Value of Foods *(Continued)*

Foods, approximate measures, units, and weight (weight of edible portion only)		Water	Food energy	Pro-tein	Fat	*Fatty Acids*		
						Satu-rated	Mono-unsatu-rated	Poly-unsatu-rated
	Grams	Per-cent	Cal-ories	Grams	Grams	Grams	Grams	Grams
MEAT AND MEAT PRODUCTS—Con.								
Beef, dried, chipped- - - - - - - 2.5 oz- - - - - - - - -	72	48	145	24	4	1.8	2.0	0.2
Lamb, cooked:								
Chops, (3 per lb with bone):								
Arm, braised:								
Lean and fat- - - - - - - 2.2 oz- - - - - - - - -	63	44	220	20	15	6.9	6.0	0.9
Lean only- - - - - - - - - 1.7 oz- - - - - - - - -	48	49	135	17	7	2.9	2.6	0.4
Loin, broiled:								
Lean and fat- - - - - - - 2.8 oz- - - - - - - - -	80	54	235	22	16	7.3	6.4	1.0
Lean only- - - - - - - - - 2.3 oz- - - - - - - - -	64	61	140	19	6	2.6	2.4	0.4
Leg, roasted:								
Lean and fat, 2 pieces, 4⅛								
by 2¼ by ¼ in- - - - - 3 oz- - - - - - - - - -	85	59	205	22	13	5.6	4.9	0.8
Lean only- - - - - - - - - 2.6 oz- - - - - - - - -	73	64	140	20	6	2.4	2.2	0.4
Rib, roasted:								
Lean and fat, 3 pieces, 2½								
by 2½ by ¼ in- - - - - 3 oz- - - - - - - - - -	85	47	315	18	26	12.1	10.6	1.5
Lean only- - - - - - - - - 2 oz- - - - - - - - - -	57	60	130	15	7	3.2	3.0	0.5
Pork, cured, cooked:								
Bacon:								
Regular- - - - - - - - - - - 3 medium slices- -	19	13	110	6	9	3.3	4.5	1.1
Canadian-style- - - - - - - 2 slices- - - - - - - -	46	62	85	11	4	1.3	1.9	0.4
Ham, light cure, roasted:								
Lean and fat, 2 pieces, 4⅛								
by 2¼ by ¼ in- - - - - - 3 oz- - - - - - - - - -	85	58	205	18	14	5.1	6.7	1.5
Lean only- - - - - - - - - 2.4 oz- - - - - - - - -	68	66	105	17	4	1.3	1.7	0.4
Luncheon meat:								
Canned, spiced or un-spiced, slice, 3 by 2 by ½								
in- - - - - - - - - - - - - - 2 slices- - - - - - - -	42	52	140	5	13	4.5	6.0	1.5
Cooked ham (8 slices per 8-oz pkg):								
Regular- - - - - - - - - - 2 slices- - - - - - - -	57	65	105	10	6	1.9	2.8	0.7
Extra lean- - - - - - - - 2 slices- - - - - - - -	57	71	75	11	3	0.9	1.3	0.3
Pork, fresh, cooked:								
Chop, loin (cut 3 per lb with bone):								
Broiled:								
Lean and fat- - - - - - - 3.1 oz- - - - - - - - -	87	50	275	24	19	7.0	8.8	2.2
Lean only- - - - - - - - - 2.5 oz- - - - - - - - -	72	57	165	23	8	2.6	3.4	0.9
Pan fried:								
Lean and fat- - - - - - - 3.1 oz- - - - - - - - -	89	45	335	21	27	9.8	12.5	3.1
Lean only- - - - - - - - - 2.4 oz- - - - - - - - -	67	54	180	19	11	3.7	4.8	1.3
Ham (leg), roasted:								
Lean and fat, piece, 2½ by								
2½ by ¾ in- - - - - - - 3 oz- - - - - - - - - -	85	53	250	21	18	6.4	8.1	2.0
Lean only- - - - - - - - - 2.5 oz- - - - - - - - -	72	60	160	20	8	2.7	3.6	1.0

(Tr indicates nutrient present in trace amounts.)

Nutrients in Indicated Quantity

Cholesterol	Carbohydrate	Calcium	Phosphorus	Iron	Potassium	Sodium	Vitamin A Value (IU)	Vitamin A Value (RE)	Thiamin	Riboflavin	Niacin	Ascorbic acid
Milligrams	Grams	Milligrams	Milligrams	Milligrams	Milligrams	Milligrams	International units	Retinol equivalents	Milligrams	Milligrams	Milligrams	Milligrams
46	0	14	287	2.3	142	3,053	Tr	Tr	0.05	0.23	2.7	0
77	0	16	132	1.5	195	46	Tr	Tr	0.04	0.16	4.4	0
59	0	12	111	1.3	162	36	Tr	Tr	0.03	0.13	3.0	0
78	0	16	162	1.4	272	62	Tr	Tr	0.09	0.21	5.5	0
60	0	12	145	1.3	241	54	Tr	Tr	0.08	0.18	4.4	0
78	0	8	162	1.7	273	57	Tr	Tr	0.09	0.24	5.5	0
65	0	6	150	1.5	247	50	Tr	Tr	0.08	0.20	4.6	0
77	0	19	139	1.4	224	60	Tr	Tr	0.08	0.18	5.5	0
50	0	12	111	1.0	179	46	Tr	Tr	0.05	0.13	3.5	0
16	Tr	2	64	0.3	92	303	0	0	0.13	0.05	1.4	6
27	1	5	136	0.4	179	711	0	0	0.38	0.09	3.2	10
53	0	6	182	0.7	243	1,009	0	0	0.51	0.19	3.8	0
37	0	5	154	0.6	215	902	0	0	0.46	0.17	3.4	0
26	1	3	34	0.3	90	541	0	0	0.15	0.08	1.3	Tr
32	2	4	141	0.6	189	751	0	0	0.49	0.14	3.0	[49]16
27	1	4	124	0.4	200	815	0	0	0.53	0.13	2.8	[49]15
84	0	3	184	0.7	312	61	10	3	0.87	0.24	4.3	Tr
71	0	4	176	0.7	302	56	10	1	0.83	0.22	4.0	Tr
92	0	4	190	0.7	323	64	10	3	0.91	0.24	4.6	Tr
72	0	3	178	0.7	305	57	10	1	0.84	0.22	4.0	Tr
79	0	5	210	0.9	280	50	10	2	0.54	0.27	3.9	Tr
68	0	5	202	0.8	269	46	10	1	0.50	0.25	3.6	Tr

Nutritive Value of Foods *(Continued)*

Foods, approximate measures, units, and weight (weight of edible portion only)		Water	Food energy	Pro-tein	Fat	Fatty Acids		
						Satu-rated	Mono-unsatu-rated	Poly-unsatu-rated
		Per-cent	*Cal-ories*	*Grams*	*Grams*	*Grams*	*Grams*	*Grams*
MEAT AND MEAT PRODUCTS—Con.	*Grams*							
Rib, roasted:								
Lean and fat, piece, 2½ by								
¾ in- - - - - - - - - - 3 oz- - - - - - - - -	85	51	270	21	20	7.2	9.2	2.3
Lean only- - - - - - - - - 2.5 oz- - - - - - - -	71	57	175	20	10	3.4	4.4	1.2
Shoulder cut, braised:								
Lean and fat, 3 pieces, 2½								
by 2½ by ¼ in- - - - 3 oz- - - - - - - - -	85	47	295	23	22	7.9	10.0	2.4
Lean only- - - - - - - - - 2.4 oz- - - - - - - -	67	54	165	22	8	2.8	3.7	1.0
Sausages (See also Luncheon meats):								
Bologna, slice (8 per 8-oz pkg)- - - - - - - - - - - - 2 slices- - - - - - - -	57	54	180	7	16	6.1	7.6	1.4
Braunschweiger, slice (6 per 6-oz pkg)- - - - - - - - 2 slices- - - - - - - -	57	48	205	8	18	6.2	8.5	2.1
Brown and serve (10–11 per 8-oz pkg), browned- - - 1 link- - - - - - - - -	13	45	50	2	5	1.7	2.2	0.5
Frankfurter (10 per 1-lb pkg), cooked (reheated)- - - - - - - - - 1 frankfurter- - - -	45	54	145	5	13	4.8	6.2	1.2
Pork link (16 per 1-lb pkg), cooked[60]- - - - - - - - - 1 link- - - - - - - - -	13	45	50	3	4	1.4	1.8	0.5
Salami:								
Cooked type, slice (8 per 8-oz pkg)- - - - - - - - 2 slices- - - - - - - -	57	60	145	8	11	4.6	5.2	1.2
Dry type, slice (12 per 4-oz pkg)- - - - - - - - 2 slices- - - - - - - -	20	35	85	5	7	2.4	3.4	0.6
Sandwich spread (pork, beef)- - - - - - - - - - - 1 tbsp- - - - - - - - -	15	60	35	1	3	0.9	1.1	0.4
Vienna sausage (7 per 4-oz can)- - - - - - - - - - - 1 sausage- - - - - -	16	60	45	2	4	1.5	2.0	0.3
Veal, medium fat, cooked, bone removed:								
Cutlet, 4⅛ by 2¼ by ½ in, braised or broiled- - - - 3 oz- - - - - - - - -	85	60	185	23	9	4.1	4.1	0.6
Rib, 2 pieces, 4⅛ by 2¼ by ¼ in, roasted- - - - - - - - - 3 oz- - - - - - - - -	85	55	230	23	14	6.0	6.0	1.0
MIXED DISHES AND FAST FOODS								
Mixed dishes:								
Chicken potpie, from home recipe, baked, piece, ⅓ of 9-in diam. pie[51]- - - 1 piece- - - - - - - -	232	57	545	23	31	10.3	15.5	6.6
Chili con carne with beans, canned- - - - - - - - - - - 1 cup- - - - - - - - -	255	72	340	19	16	5.8	7.2	1.0
Chop suey with beef and pork, from home recipe- - - - - - - - - - - 1 cup- - - - - - - - -	250	75	300	26	17	4.3	7.4	4.2

(Tr indicates nutrient present in trace amounts.)

Nutrients in Indicated Quantity

Cho-les-terol	Carbo-hydrate	Calcium	Phos-phorus	Iron	Potas-sium	Sodium	Vitamin A value		Thiamin	Ribo-flavin	Niacin	Ascorbic acid
							(IU)	(RE)				
Milli-grams	Grams	Milli-grams	Milli-grams	Milli-grams	Milli-grams	Milli-grams	Inter-national units	Retinol equiva-lents	Milli-grams	Milli-grams	Milli-grams	Milli-grams
69	0	9	190	0.8	313	37	10	3	0.50	0.24	4.2	Tr
56	0	8	182	0.7	300	33	10	2	0.45	0.22	3.8	Tr
93	0	6	162	1.4	286	75	10	3	0.46	0.26	4.4	Tr
76	0	5	151	1.3	271	68	10	1	0.40	0.24	4.0	Tr
31	2	7	52	0.9	103	581	0	0	0.10	0.08	1.5	[48]12
89	2	5	96	5.3	113	652	8,010	2,405	0.14	0.87	4.8	[49]6
9	Tr	1	14	0.1	25	105	0	0	0.05	0.02	0.4	0
23	1	5	39	0.5	75	504	0	0	0.09	0.05	1.2	[48]12
11	Tr	4	24	0.2	47	168	0	0	0.10	0.03	0.6	Tr
37	1	7	66	1.5	113	607	0	0	0.14	0.21	2.0	[49]7
16	1	2	28	0.3	76	372	0	0	0.12	0.06	1.0	[49]5
6	2	2	9	0.1	17	152	10	1	0.03	0.02	0.3	0
8	Tr	2	8	0.1	16	152	0	0	0.01	0.02	0.3	0
109	0	9	196	0.8	258	56	Tr	Tr	0.06	0.21	4.6	0
109	0	10	211	0.7	259	57	Tr	Tr	0.11	0.26	6.6	0
56	42	70	232	3.0	343	594	7,220	735	0.32	0.32	4.9	5
28	31	82	321	4.3	594	1,354	150	15	0.08	0.18	3.3	8
68	13	60	248	4.8	425	1,053	600	60	0.28	0.38	5.0	33

Nutritive Value of Foods *(Continued)*

Foods, approximate measures, units, and weight (weight of edible portion only)			Water	Food energy	Pro-tein	Fat	Fatty Acids		
							Satu-rated	Mono-unsatu-rated	Poly-unsatu-rated
		Grams	Per-cent	Cal-ories	Grams	Grams	Grams	Grams	Grams
MIXED DISHES AND FAST FOODS—Con.									
Macaroni (enriched) and cheese:									
Canned[52]	1 cup	240	80	230	9	10	4.7	2.9	1.3
Quiche Lorraine, ⅛ of 8-in diam. quiche[51]	1 slice	176	47	600	13	48	23.2	17.8	4.1
Spaghetti (enriched) in to-mato sauce with cheese:									
Canned	1 cup	250	80	190	6	2	0.4	0.4	0.5
From home recipe	1 cup	250	77	260	9	9	3.0	3.6	1.2
Spaghetti (enriched) with meatballs and tomato sauce:									
From home recipe	1 cup	248	70	330	19	12	3.9	4.4	2.2
Fast food entrees:									
Cheeseburger:									
Regular	1 sandwich	112	46	300	15	15	7.3	5.6	1.0
4 oz patty	1 sandwich	194	46	525	30	31	15.1	12.2	1.4
Chicken, fried. See Poultry and Poultry Products.									
Enchilada	1 enchilada	230	72	235	20	16	7.7	6.7	0.6
English muffin, egg, cheese, and bacon	1 sandwich	138	49	360	18	18	8.0	8.0	0.7
Fish sandwich:									
Regular, with cheese	1 sandwich	140	43	420	16	23	6.3	6.9	7.7
Large, without cheese	1 sandwich	170	48	470	18	27	6.3	8.7	9.5
Hamburger:									
Regular	1 sandwich	98	46	245	12	11	4.4	5.3	0.5
4 oz patty	1 sandwich	174	50	445	25	21	7.1	11.7	0.6
Pizza, cheese, ⅛ of 15-in diam. pizza[51]	1 slice	120	46	290	15	9	4.1	2.6	1.3
Roast beef sandwich	1 sandwich	150	52	345	22	13	3.5	6.9	1.8
Taco	1 taco	81	55	195	9	11	4.1	5.5	0.8
POULTRY AND POULTRY PRODUCTS									
Chicken:									
Fried, flesh, with skin:[53]									
Batter dipped:									
Breast, ½ breast (5.6 oz with bones)	4.9 oz	140	52	365	35	18	4.9	7.6	4.3
Drumstick (3.4 oz with bones)	2.5 oz	72	53	195	16	11	3.0	4.6	2.7
Flour coated:									
Breast, ½ breast (4.2 oz with bones)	3.5 oz	98	57	220	31	9	2.4	3.4	1.9
Drumstick (2.6 oz with bones)	1.7 oz	49	57	120	13	7	1.8	2.7	1.6

(Tr indicates nutrient present in trace amounts.)

Nutrients in Indicated Quantity

| Cho-les-terol | Carbo-hydrate | Calcium | Phos-phorus | Iron | Potas-sium | Sodium | Vitamin A value | | Thiamin | Ribo-flavin | Niacin | Ascorbic acid |
| | | | | | | | (IU) | (RE) | | | | |
Milli-grams	Grams	Milli-grams	Milli-grams	Milli-grams	Milli-grams	Milli-grams	Inter-national units	Retinol equiva-lents	Milli-grams	Milli-grams	Milli-grams	Milli-grams
24	26	199	182	1.0	139	730	260	72	0.12	0.24	1.0	Tr
285	29	211	276	1.0	283	653	1,640	454	0.11	0.32	Tr	Tr
3	39	40	88	2.8	303	955	930	120	0.35	0.28	4.5	10
8	37	80	135	2.3	408	955	1,080	140	0.25	0.18	2.3	13
89	39	124	236	3.7	665	1,009	1,590	159	0.25	0.30	4.0	22
44	28	135	174	2.3	219	672	340	65	0.26	0.24	3.7	1
104	40	236	320	4.5	407	1,224	670	128	0.33	0.48	7.4	3
19	24	97	198	3.3	653	1,332	2,720	352	0.18	0.26	Tr	Tr
213	31	197	290	3.1	201	832	650	160	0.46	0.50	3.7	1
56	39	132	223	1.8	274	667	160	25	0.32	0.26	3.3	2
91	41	61	246	2.2	375	621	110	15	0.35	0.23	3.5	1
32	28	56	107	2.2	202	463	80	14	0.23	0.24	3.8	1
71	38	75	225	4.8	404	763	160	28	0.38	0.38	7.8	1
56	39	220	216	1.6	230	699	750	106	0.34	0.29	4.2	2
55	34	60	222	4.0	338	757	240	32	0.40	0.33	6.0	2
21	15	109	134	1.2	263	456	420	57	0.09	0.07	1.4	1
119	13	28	259	1.8	281	385	90	28	0.16	0.20	14.7	0
62	6	12	106	1.0	134	194	60	19	0.08	0.15	3.7	0
87	2	16	228	1.2	254	74	50	15	0.08	0.13	13.5	0
44	1	6	86	0.7	112	44	40	12	0.04	0.11	3.0	0

Nutritive Value of Foods *(Continued)*

Foods, approximate measures, units, and weight (weight of edible portion only)		Water	Food energy	Pro-tein	Fat	Satu-rated	Mono-unsatu-rated	Poly-unsatu-rated
							Fatty Acids	
POULTRY AND POULTRY PRODUCTS—Con.	*Grams*	*Per-cent*	*Cal-ories*	*Grams*	*Grams*	*Grams*	*Grams*	*Grams*
Roasted, flesh only:								
Breast, ½ breast (4.2 oz with bones and skin)- - - - - - - 3.0 oz- - - - - - - -	86	65	140	27	3	0.9	1.1	0.7
Drumstick, (2.9 oz with bones and skin)- - - 1.6 oz- - - - - - - -	44	67	75	12	2	0.7	0.8	0.6
Stewed, flesh only, light and dark meat, chopped or diced- - - - - - - - 1 cup- - - - - - - -	140	67	250	38	9	2.6	3.3	2.2
Chicken liver, cooked- - - - - 1 liver- - - - - - - -	20	68	30	5	1	0.4	0.3	0.2
Duck, roasted, flesh only- - - ½ duck- - - - - - -	221	64	445	52	25	9.2	8.2	3.2
Turkey, roasted, flesh only:								
Dark meat, piece, 2½ by 1⅝ by ¼ in - - - - - - - - - - 4 pieces- - - - - - -	85	63	160	24	6	2.1	1.4	1.8
Light meat, piece, 4 by 2 by ¼ in - - - - - - - - - - - 2 pieces- - - - - - -	85	66	135	25	3	0.9	0.5	0.7
Poultry food products:								
Turkey:								
Loaf, breast meat (8 slices per 6-oz pkg)- - - - - - 2 slices- - - - - - -	42	72	45	10	1	0.2	0.2	0.1
Roast, boneless, frozen, seasoned, light and dark meat, cooked- - - 3 oz- - - - - - - - - -	85	68	130	18	5	1.6	1.0	1.4
SOUPS, SAUCES, AND GRAVIES								
Soups:								
Canned, condensed:								
Prepared with equal volume of milk:								
Clam chowder, New England- - - - - - - 1 cup- - - - - - - -	248	85	165	9	7	3.0	2.3	1.1
Cream of chicken- - - - 1 cup- - - - - - - -	248	85	190	7	11	4.6	4.5	1.6
Cream of mushroom- - 1 cup- - - - - - - -	248	85	205	6	14	5.1	3.0	4.6
Tomato- - - - - - - - - - 1 cup- - - - - - - -	248	85	160	6	6	2.9	1.6	1.1
Prepared with equal volume of water:								
Bean with bacon- - - - 1 cup- - - - - - - -	253	84	170	8	6	1.5	2.2	1.8
Beef broth, bouillon, consomme- - - - - - - 1 cup- - - - - - - -	240	98	15	3	1	0.3	0.2	Tr
Beef noodle- - - - - - - 1 cup- - - - - - - -	244	92	85	5	3	1.1	1.2	0.5
Chicken noodle- - - - - 1 cup- - - - - - - -	241	92	75	4	2	0.7	1.1	0.6
Chicken rice- - - - - - - 1 cup- - - - - - - -	241	94	60	4	2	0.5	0.9	0.4
Clam chowder, Manhattan- - - - - - - - 1 cup- - - - - - - -	244	90	80	4	2	0.4	0.4	1.3
Cream of chicken- - - - 1 cup- - - - - - - -	244	91	115	3	7	2.1	3.3	1.5
Cream of mushroom- - 1 cup- - - - - - - -	244	90	130	2	9	2.4	1.7	4.2
Minestrone- - - - - - - 1 cup- - - - - - - -	241	91	80	4	3	0.6	0.7	1.1
Pea, green- - - - - - - - 1 cup- - - - - - - -	250	83	165	9	3	1.4	1.0	0.4

(Tr indicates nutrient present in trace amounts.)

Nutrients in Indicated Quantity

Cho-les-terol	Carbo-hydrate	Calcium	Phos-phorus	Iron	Potas-sium	Sodium	Vitamin A value (IU)	Vitamin A value (RE)	Thiamin	Ribo-flavin	Niacin	Ascorbic acid
Milli-grams	Grams	Milli-grams	Milli-grams	Milli-grams	Milli-grams	Milli-grams	Inter-national units	Retinol equiva-lents	Milli-grams	Milli-grams	Milli-grams	Milli-grams
73	0	13	196	0.9	220	64	20	5	0.06	0.10	11.8	0
41	0	5	81	0.6	108	42	30	8	0.03	0.10	2.7	0
116	0	20	210	1.6	252	98	70	21	0.07	0.23	8.6	0
126	Tr	3	62	1.7	28	10	3,270	983	0.03	0.35	0.9	3
197	0	27	449	6.0	557	144	170	51	0.57	1.04	11.3	0
72	0	27	173	2.0	246	67	0	0	0.05	0.21	3.1	0
59	0	16	186	1.1	259	54	0	0	0.05	0.11	5.8	0
17	0	3	97	0.2	118	608	0	0	0.02	0.05	3.5	54 0
45	3	4	207	1.4	253	578	0	0	0.04	0.14	5.3	0
22	17	186	156	1.5	300	992	160	40	0.07	0.24	1.0	3
27	15	181	151	0.7	273	1,047	710	94	0.07	0.26	0.9	1
20	15	179	156	0.6	270	1,076	150	37	0.08	0.28	0.9	2
17	22	159	149	1.8	449	932	850	109	0.13	0.25	1.5	68
3	23	81	132	2.0	402	951	890	89	0.09	0.03	0.6	2
Tr	Tr	14	31	0.4	130	782	0	0	Tr	0.05	1.9	0
5	9	15	46	1.1	100	952	630	63	0.07	0.06	1.1	Tr
7	9	17	36	0.8	55	1,106	710	71	0.05	0.06	1.4	Tr
7	7	17	22	0.7	101	815	660	66	0.02	0.02	1.1	Tr
2	12	34	59	1.9	261	1,808	920	92	0.06	0.05	1.3	3
10	9	34	37	0.6	88	986	560	56	0.03	0.06	0.8	Tr
2	9	46	49	0.5	100	1,032	0	0	0.05	0.09	0.7	1
2	11	34	55	0.9	313	911	2,340	234	0.05	0.04	0.9	1
0	27	28	125	2.0	190	988	200	20	0.11	0.07	1.2	2

Nutritive Value of Foods *(Continued)*

Foods, approximate measures, units, and weight (weight of edible portion only)		Water	Food energy	Pro-tein	Fat	Fatty Acids Satu-rated	Mono-unsatu-rated	Poly-unsatu-rated
		Per-cent	Cal-ories					
SOUPS, SAUCES, AND GRAVIES—Con.	Grams			Grams	Grams	Grams	Grams	Grams
Tomato- - - - - - - - - 1 cup- - - - - - - -	244	90	85	2	2	0.4	0.4	1.0
Vegetable beef- - - - - 1 cup- - - - - - - -	244	92	80	6	2	0.9	0.8	0.1
Vegetarian- - - - - - - - 1 cup- - - - - - - -	241	92	70	2	2	0.3	0.8	0.7
Dehydrated:								
Prepared with water:								
Chicken noodle- - - - - 1 pkt (6-fl-oz)- - -	188	94	40	2	1	0.2	0.4	0.3
Onion- - - - - - - - - - - 1 pkt (6-fl-oz)- - -	184	96	20	1	Tr	0.1	0.2	0.1
Tomato vegetable- - - 1 pkt (6-fl-oz)- - -	189	94	40	1	1	0.3	0.2	0.1
Sauces:								
From dry mix:								
Hollandaise, prepared								
with water- - - - - - - 1 cup- - - - - - - -	259	84	240	5	20	11.6	5.9	0.9
White sauce, prepared								
with milk- - - - - - - - 1 cup- - - - - - - -	264	81	240	10	13	6.4	4.7	1.7
From home recipe:								
White sauce, medium[55]- 1 cup- - - - - - - -	250	73	395	10	30	9.1	11.9	7.2
Ready to serve:								
Barbecue- - - - - - - - - - 1 tbsp- - - - - - - -	16	81	10	Tr	Tr	Tr	0.1	0.1
Soy- - - - - - - - - - - - - - 1 tbsp- - - - - - - -	18	68	10	2	0	0.0	0.0	0.0
SUGARS AND SWEETS								
Candy:								
Caramels, plain or choco-								
late- - - - - - - - - - - - - 1 oz- - - - - - - - -	28	8	115	1	3	2.2	0.3	0.1
Chocolate:								
Milk, plain- - - - - - - - 1 oz- - - - - - - - -	28	1	145	2	9	5.4	3.0	0.3
Milk, with almonds- - - - 1 oz- - - - - - - - -	28	2	150	3	10	4.8	4.1	0.7
Milk, with peanuts- - - - 1 oz- - - - - - - - -	28	1	155	4	11	4.2	3.5	1.5
Milk, with rice cereal- - 1 oz- - - - - - - - -	28	2	140	2	7	4.4	2.5	0.2
Semisweet, small pieces								
(60 per oz)- - - - - - - - 1 cup or 6 oz- - - -	170	1	860	7	61	36.2	19.9	1.9
Sweet (dark)- - - - - - - 1 oz- - - - - - - - -	28	1	150	1	10	5.9	3.3	0.3
Fudge, chocolate, plain- - - 1 oz- - - - - - - - -	28	8	115	1	3	2.1	1.0	0.1
Gum drops- - - - - - - - - - 1 oz- - - - - - - - -	28	12	100	Tr	Tr	Tr	Tr	0.1
Hard- - - - - - - - - - - - - - 1 oz- - - - - - - - -	28	1	110	0	0	0.0	0.0	0.0
Jelly beans- - - - - - - - - - 1 oz- - - - - - - - -	28	6	105	Tr	Tr	Tr	Tr	0.1
Marshmallows- - - - - - - - 1 oz- - - - - - - - -	28	17	90	1	0	0.0	0.0	0.0
Custard, baked- - - - - - - - 1 cup- - - - - - - -	265	77	305	14	15	6.8	5.4	0.7
Gelatin dessert prepared with								
gelatin dessert powder and								
water- - - - - - - - - - - - - ½ cup- - - - - - - -	120	84	70	2	0	0.0	0.0	0.0
Honey, strained or extracted 1 cup- - - - - - - -	339	17	1,030	1	0	0.0	0.0	0.0
1 tbsp- - - - - - - -	21	17	65	Tr	0	0.0	0.0	0.0
Jams and preserves- - - - - - 1 tbsp- - - - - - - -	20	29	55	Tr	Tr	0.0	Tr	Tr
1 packet- - - - - - -	14	29	40	Tr	Tr	0.0	Tr	Tr
Jellies- - - - - - - - - - - - - - 1 tbsp- - - - - - - -	18	28	50	Tr	Tr	Tr	Tr	Tr
1 packet- - - - - - -	14	28	40	Tr	Tr	Tr	Tr	Tr
Popsicle, 3-fl-oz size- - - - - 1 popsicle- - - - - -	95	80	70	0	0	0.0	0.0	0.0

(Tr indicates nutrient present in trace amounts.)

Nutrients in Indicated Quantity

Cho-les-terol	Carbo-hydrate	Calcium	Phos-phorus	Iron	Potas-sium	Sodium	Vitamin A value (IU)	Vitamin A value (RE)	Thiamin	Ribo-flavin	Niacin	Ascorbic acid
Milli-grams	Grams	Milli-grams	Milli-grams	Milli-grams	Milli-grams	Milli-grams	Inter-national units	Retinol equiva-lents	Milli-grams	Milli-grams	Milli-grams	Milli-grams
0	17	12	34	1.8	264	871	690	69	0.09	0.05	1.4	66
5	10	17	41	1.1	173	956	1,890	189	0.04	0.05	1.0	2
0	12	22	34	1.1	210	822	3,010	301	0.05	0.05	0.9	1
2	6	24	24	0.4	23	957	50	5	0.05	0.04	0.7	Tr
0	4	9	22	0.1	48	635	Tr	Tr	0.02	0.04	0.4	Tr
0	8	6	23	0.5	78	856	140	14	0.04	0.03	0.6	5
52	14	124	127	0.9	124	1,564	730	220	0.05	0.18	0.1	Tr
34	21	425	256	0.3	444	797	310	92	0.08	0.45	0.5	3
32	24	292	238	0.9	381	888	1,190	340	0.15	0.43	0.8	2
0	2	3	3	0.1	28	130	140	14	Tr	Tr	0.1	1
0	2	3	38	0.5	64	1,029	0	0	0.01	0.02	0.6	0
1	22	42	35	0.4	54	64	Tr	Tr	0.01	0.05	0.1	Tr
6	16	50	61	0.4	96	23	30	10	0.02	0.10	0.1	Tr
5	15	65	77	0.5	125	23	30	8	0.02	0.12	0.2	Tr
5	13	49	83	0.4	138	19	30	8	0.07	0.07	1.4	Tr
6	18	48	57	0.2	100	46	30	8	0.01	0.08	0.1	Tr
0	97	51	178	5.8	593	24	30	3	0.10	0.14	0.9	Tr
0	16	7	41	0.6	86	5	10	1	0.01	0.04	0.1	Tr
1	21	22	24	0.3	42	54	Tr	Tr	0.01	0.03	0.1	Tr
0	25	2	Tr	0.1	1	10	0	0	0.00	Tr	Tr	0
0	28	Tr	2	0.1	1	7	0	0	0.10	0.00	0.0	0
0	26	1	1	0.3	11	7	0	0	0.00	Tr	Tr	0
0	23	1	2	0.5	2	25	0	0	0.00	Tr	Tr	0
278	29	297	310	1.1	387	209	530	146	0.11	0.50	0.3	1
0	17	2	23	Tr	Tr	55	0	0	0.00	0.00	0.0	0
0	279	17	20	1.7	173	17	0	0	0.02	0.14	1.0	3
0	17	1	1	0.1	11	1	0	0	Tr	0.01	0.1	Tr
0	14	4	2	0.2	18	2	Tr	Tr	Tr	0.01	Tr	Tr
0	10	3	1	0.1	12	2	Tr	Tr	Tr	Tr	Tr	Tr
0	13	2	Tr	0.1	16	5	Tr	Tr	Tr	0.01	Tr	1
0	10	1	Tr	Tr	13	4	Tr	Tr	Tr	Tr	Tr	1
0	18	0	0	Tr	4	11	0	0	0.00	0.00	0.0	0

Nutritive Value of Foods *(Continued)*

Foods, approximate measures, units, and weight (weight of edible portion only)		Water	Food energy	Pro-tein	Fat	Satu-rated	Mono-unsatu-rated	Poly-unsatu-rated
							Fatty Acids	
		Grams	Per-cent	Cal-ories	Grams	Grams	Grams	Grams	Grams

SUGARS AND SWEETS—Con.								
Puddings:								
Canned:								
Vanilla- - - - - - - - - - -	5-oz can- - - - - -	142	69	220	2	10	9.5	0.2	0.1
Dry mix, prepared with whole milk:								
Chocolate:								
Instant- - - - - - - - - -	½ cup- - - - - - - -	130	71	155	4	4	2.3	1.1	0.2
Regular (cooked)- - - -	½ cup- - - - - - - -	130	73	150	4	4	2.4	1.1	0.1
Rice- - - - - - - - - - - -	½ cup- - - - - - - -	132	73	155	4	4	2.3	1.1	0.1
Tapioca- - - - - - - - - - -	½ cup- - - - - - - -	130	75	145	4	4	2.3	1.1	0.1
Vanilla:								
Instant- - - - - - - - - -	½ cup- - - - - - - -	130	73	150	4	4	2.2	1.1	0.2
Sugars:								
Brown, pressed down- - - -	1 cup- - - - - - - -	220	2	820	0	0	0.0	0.0	0.0
White:								
Granulated- - - - - - - -	1 cup- - - - - - - -	200	1	770	0	0	0.0	0.0	0.0
	1 tbsp- - - - - - - -	12	1	45	0	0	0.0	0.0	0.0
	1 packet- - - - - - -	6	1	25	0	0	0.0	0.0	0.0
Powdered, sifted, spooned into cup- - - -	1 cup- - - - - - - -	100	1	385	0	0	0.0	0.0	0.0
Syrups:								
Chocolate-flavored syrup or topping:								
Thin type- - - - - - - - -	2 tbsp- - - - - - - -	38	37	85	1	Tr	0.2	0.1	0.1
Fudge type- - - - - - - - -	2 tbsp- - - - - - - -	38	25	125	2	5	3.1	1.7	0.2
Molasses, cane, blackstrap	2 tbsp- - - - - - - -	40	24	85	0	0	0.0	0.0	0.0
Table syrup (corn and maple)- - - - - - - - - - -	2 tbsp- - - - - - - -	42	25	122	0	0	0.0	0.0	0.0
VEGETABLES AND VEGETABLE PRODUCTS								
Alfalfa seeds, sprouted, raw-	1 cup- - - - - - - -	33	91	10	1	Tr	Tr	Tr	0.1
Artichokes, globe or French, cooked, drained- - - - - - -	1 artichoke- - - - -	120	87	55	3	Tr	Tr	Tr	0.1
Asparagus, green:								
Cooked, drained:								
From raw:								
Cuts and tips- - - - - -	1 cup- - - - - - - -	180	92	45	5	1	0.1	Tr	0.2
Spears, ½-in diam. at base- - - - - - - - - -	4 spears- - - - - - -	60	92	15	2	Tr	Tr	Tr	0.1
From frozen:								
Cuts and tips- - - - - -	1 cup- - - - - - - -	180	91	50	5	1	0.2	Tr	0.3
Spears, ½-in diam. at base- - - - - - - - - -	4 spears- - - - - - -	60	91	15	2	Tr	0.1	Tr	0.1
Canned, spears, ½-in diam. at base- - - - - - - -	4 spears- - - - - - -	80	95	10	1	Tr	Tr	Tr	0.1
Bamboo shoots, canned, drained- - - - - - - - - - - -	1 cup- - - - - - - -	131	94	25	2	1	0.1	Tr	0.2

(Tr indicates nutrient present in trace amounts.)

Nutrients in Indicated Quantity

Cho-les-terol	Carbo-hydrate	Calcium	Phos-phorus	Iron	Potas-sium	Sodium	Vitamin A value		Thiamin	Ribo-flavin	Niacin	Ascorbic acid
							(IU)	(RE)				
Milli-grams	Grams	Milli-grams	Milli-grams	Milli-grams	Milli-grams	Milli-grams	Inter-national units	Retinol equiva-lents	Milli-grams	Milli-grams	Milli-grams	Milli-grams
1	33	79	94	0.2	155	305	Tr	Tr	0.03	0.12	0.6	Tr
14	27	130	329	0.3	176	440	130	33	0.04	0.18	0.1	1
15	25	146	120	0.2	190	167	140	34	0.05	0.20	0.1	1
15	27	133	110	0.5	165	140	140	33	0.10	0.18	0.6	1
15	25	131	103	0.1	167	152	140	34	0.04	0.18	0.1	1
15	27	129	273	0.1	164	375	140	33	0.04	0.17	0.1	1
0	212	187	56	4.8	757	97	0	0	0.02	0.07	0.2	0
0	199	3	Tr	0.1	7	5	0	0	0.00	0.00	0.0	0
0	12	Tr	Tr	Tr	Tr	Tr	0	0	0.00	0.00	0.0	0
0	6	Tr	Tr	Tr	Tr	Tr	0	0	0.00	0.00	0.0	0
0	100	1	Tr	Tr	4	2	0	0	0.00	0.00	0.0	0
0	22	6	49	0.8	85	36	Tr	Tr	Tr	0.02	0.1	0
0	21	38	60	0.5	82	42	40	13	0.02	0.08	0.1	0
0	22	274	34	10.1	1,171	38	0	0	0.04	0.08	0.8	0
0	32	1	4	Tr	7	19	0	0	0.00	0.00	0.0	0
0	1	11	23	0.3	26	2	50	5	0.03	0.04	0.2	3
0	12	47	72	1.6	316	79	170	17	0.07	0.06	0.7	9
0	8	43	110	1.2	558	7	1,490	149	0.18	0.22	1.9	49
0	3	14	37	0.4	186	2	500	50	0.06	0.07	0.6	16
0	9	41	99	1.2	392	7	1,470	147	0.12	0.19	1.9	44
0	3	14	33	0.4	131	2	490	49	0.04	0.06	0.6	15
0	2	11	30	0.5	122	[56]278	380	38	0.04	0.07	0.7	13
0	4	10	33	0.4	105	9	10	1	0.03	0.03	0.2	1

Nutritive Value of Foods *(Continued)*

Foods, approximate measures, units, and weight (weight of edible portion only)		Water	Food energy	Pro-tein	Fat	Fatty Acids		
						Satu-rated	Mono-unsatu-rated	Poly-unsatu-rated
		Per-cent	*Cal-ories*	*Grams*	*Grams*	*Grams*	*Grams*	*Grams*

Foods, approximate measures, units, and weight (weight of edible portion only)		Grams	Water *Per-cent*	Food energy *Cal-ories*	Pro-tein *Grams*	Fat *Grams*	Satu-rated *Grams*	Mono-unsatu-rated *Grams*	Poly-unsatu-rated *Grams*
VEGETABLES AND VEGETABLE PRODUCTS—Con.									
Beans:									
Lima, immature seeds, frozen, cooked, drained:									
Thick-seeded types (Fordhooks)	1 cup	170	74	170	10	1	0.1	Tr	0.3
Thin-seeded types (baby limas)	1 cup	180	72	190	12	1	0.1	Tr	0.3
Snap:									
Cooked, drained:									
From raw (cut and French style)	1 cup	125	89	45	2	Tr	0.1	Tr	0.2
From frozen (cut)	1 cup	135	92	35	2	Tr	Tr	Tr	0.1
Canned, drained solids (cut)	1 cup	135	93	25	2	Tr	Tr	Tr	0.1
Beans, mature. See Beans, dry and Black-eyed peas, dry.									
Bean sprouts (mung):									
Raw	1 cup	104	90	30	3	Tr	Tr	Tr	0.1
Beets:									
Cooked, drained:									
Diced or sliced	1 cup	170	91	55	2	Tr	Tr	Tr	Tr
Canned, drained solids, diced or sliced	1 cup	170	91	55	2	Tr	Tr	Tr	0.1
Beet greens, leaves and stems, cooked, drained	1 cup	144	89	40	4	Tr	Tr	0.1	0.1
Black-eyed peas, immature seeds, cooked and drained:									
From raw	1 cup	165	72	180	13	1	0.3	0.1	0.6
From frozen	1 cup	170	66	225	14	1	0.3	0.1	0.5
Broccoli:									
Raw	1 spear	151	91	40	4	1	0.1	Tr	0.3
Cooked, drained:									
From raw:									
Spear, medium	1 spear	180	90	50	5	1	0.1	Tr	0.2
Spears, cut into ½-in pieces	1 cup	155	90	45	5	Tr	0.1	Tr	0.2
Brussels sprouts, cooked, drained:									
From frozen	1 cup	155	87	65	6	1	0.1	Tr	0.3
Cabbage, common varieties:									
Raw, coarsely shredded or sliced	1 cup	70	93	15	1	Tr	Tr	Tr	0.1
Cooked, drained	1 cup	150	94	30	1	Tr	Tr	Tr	0.2
Cabbage, Chinese:									
Pak-choi, cooked, drained	1 cup	170	96	20	3	Tr	Tr	Tr	0.1
Pe-tsai, raw, 1-in pieces	1 cup	76	94	10	1	Tr	Tr	Tr	0.1

(Tr indicates nutrient present in trace amounts.)

Nutrients in Indicated Quantity

Cholesterol	Carbohydrate	Calcium	Phosphorus	Iron	Potassium	Sodium	Vitamin A value		Thiamin	Riboflavin	Niacin	Ascorbic acid
							(IU)	(RE)				
Milligrams	Grams	Milligrams	Milligrams	Milligrams	Milligrams	Milligrams	International units	Retinol equivalents	Milligrams	Milligrams	Milligrams	Milligrams
0	32	37	107	2.3	694	90	320	32	0.13	0.10	1.8	22
0	35	50	202	3.5	740	52	300	30	0.13	0.10	1.4	10
0	10	58	49	1.6	374	4	[57]830	[57]83	0.09	0.12	0.8	12
0	8	61	32	1.1	151	18	[58]710	[58]71	0.06	0.10	0.6	11
0	6	35	26	1.2	147	[59]339	[60]470	[60]47	0.02	0.08	0.3	6
0	6	14	56	0.9	155	6	20	2	0.09	0.13	0.8	14
0	11	19	53	1.1	530	83	20	2	0.05	0.02	0.5	9
0	12	26	29	3.1	252	[61]466	20	2	0.02	0.07	0.3	7
0	8	164	59	2.7	1,309	347	7,340	734	0.17	0.42	0.7	36
0	30	46	196	2.4	693	7	1,050	105	0.11	0.18	1.8	3
0	40	39	207	3.6	638	9	130	13	0.44	0.11	1.2	4
0	8	72	100	1.3	491	41	2,330	233	0.10	0.18	1.0	141
0	10	205	86	2.1	293	20	2,540	254	0.15	0.37	1.4	113
0	9	177	74	1.8	253	17	2,180	218	0.13	0.32	1.2	97
0	13	37	84	1.1	504	36	910	91	0.16	0.18	0.8	71
0	4	33	16	0.4	172	13	90	9	0.04	0.02	0.2	33
0	7	50	38	0.6	308	29	130	13	0.09	0.08	0.3	36
0	3	158	49	1.8	631	58	4,370	437	0.05	0.11	0.7	44
0	2	59	22	0.2	181	7	910	91	0.03	0.04	0.3	21

Nutritive Value of Foods *(Continued)*

Foods, approximate measures, units, and weight (weight of edible portion only)		Water	Food energy	Pro-tein	Fat	Fatty Acids		
						Satu-rated	Mono-unsatu-rated	Poly-unsatu-rated
VEGETABLES AND VEGETABLE PRODUCTS—Con.		Grams	Per-cent	Cal-ories	Grams	Grams	Grams	Grams
Cabbage, red, raw, coarsely shredded or sliced- - - - - -	1 cup- - - - - - - -	70	92	20	1	Tr	Tr	Tr	0.1
Cabbage, savoy, raw, coarsely shredded or sliced- - - - - -	1 cup- - - - - - - -	70	91	20	1	Tr	Tr	Tr	Tr
Carrots:								
Raw, without crowns and tips, scraped:								
Whole, 7½ by 1⅛ in, or strips, 2½ to 3 in long-	1 carrot or 18 strips- - - - - - - -	72	88	30	1	Tr	Tr	Tr	0.1
Cooked, sliced, drained:								
From frozen- - - - - - - -	1 cup- - - - - - - -	146	90	55	2	Tr	Tr	Tr	0.1
Canned, sliced, drained solids- - - - - - - - - - -	1 cup- - - - - - - -	146	93	35	1	Tr	0.1	Tr	0.1
Cauliflower:								
Cooked, drained:								
From raw (flowerets)- - -	1 cup- - - - - - - -	125	93	30	2	Tr	Tr	Tr	0.1
From frozen (flowerets)-	1 cup- - - - - - - -	180	94	35	3	Tr	0.1	Tr	0.2
Celery, pascal type, raw:								
Stalk, large outer, 8 by 1½ in (at root end)- - - - - - - -	1 stalk- - - - - - - -	40	95	5	Tr	Tr	Tr	Tr	Tr
Collards, cooked, drained:								
From raw (leaves without stems)- - - - - - - - - - - - -	1 cup- - - - - - - -	190	96	25	2	Tr	0.1	Tr	0.2
Corn, sweet:								
Cooked, drained:								
From raw, ear 5 by 1¾ in - - - - - - - - -	1 ear- - - - - - - -	77	70	85	3	1	0.2	0.3	0.5
From frozen:								
Kernels- - - - - - - - -	1 cup- - - - - - - -	165	76	135	5	Tr	Tr	Tr	0.1
Canned:								
Cream style- - - - - - - -	1 cup- - - - - - - -	256	79	185	4	1	0.2	0.3	0.5
Whole kernel, vacuum pack- - - - - - - - - - -	1 cup- - - - - - - -	210	77	165	5	1	0.2	0.3	0.5
Cowpeas. See Black-eyed peas.								
Cucumber, with peel, slices, ⅛ in thick (large, 2⅛-in diam.; small, 1¾-in diam.)- - - - -	6 large or 8 small slices- - - - - - - -	28	96	5	Tr	Tr	Tr	Tr	Tr
Dandelion greens, cooked, drained- - - - - - - - - - - - -	1 cup- - - - - - - -	105	90	35	2	1	0.1	Tr	0.3
Eggplant, cooked, steamed- -	1 cup- - - - - - - -	96	92	25	1	Tr	Tr	Tr	0.1
Endive, curly (including escarole), raw, small pieces- - - - - - - - - - - - - -	1 cup- - - - - - - -	50	94	10	1	Tr	Tr	Tr	Tr
Jerusalem-artichoke, raw, sliced- - - - - - - - - - - - - -	1 cup- - - - - - - -	150	78	115	3	Tr	0.0	Tr	Tr

(Tr indicates nutrient present in trace amounts.)

Nutrients in Indicated Quantity

Cholesterol	Carbohydrate	Calcium	Phosphorus	Iron	Potassium	Sodium	Vitamin A value (IU)	Vitamin A value (RE)	Thiamin	Riboflavin	Niacin	Ascorbic acid
Milligrams	Grams	Milligrams	Milligrams	Milligrams	Milligrams	Milligrams	International units	Retinol equivalents	Milligrams	Milligrams	Milligrams	Milligrams
0	4	36	29	0.3	144	8	30	3	0.04	0.02	0.2	40
0	4	25	29	0.3	161	20	700	70	0.05	0.02	0.2	22
0	7	19	32	0.4	233	25	20,250	2,025	0.07	0.04	0.7	7
0	12	41	38	0.7	231	86	25,850	2,585	0.04	0.05	0.6	4
0	8	37	35	0.9	261	[62]352	20,110	2,011	0.03	0.04	0.8	4
0	6	34	44	0.5	404	8	20	2	0.08	0.07	0.7	69
0	7	31	43	0.7	250	32	40	4	0.07	0.10	0.6	56
0	1	14	10	0.2	114	35	50	5	0.01	0.01	0.1	3
0	5	148	19	0.8	177	36	4,220	422	0.03	0.08	0.4	19
0	19	2	79	0.5	192	13	[63]170	[63]17	0.17	0.06	1.2	5
0	34	3	78	0.5	229	8	[63]410	[63]41	0.11	0.12	2.1	4
0	46	8	131	1.0	343	[64]730	[63]250	[63]25	0.06	0.14	2.5	12
0	41	11	134	0.9	391	[65]571	[63]510	[63]51	0.09	0.15	2.5	17
0	1	4	5	0.1	42	1	10	1	0.01	0.01	0.1	1
0	7	147	44	1.9	244	46	12,290	1,229	0.14	0.18	0.5	19
0	6	6	21	0.3	238	3	60	6	0.07	0.02	0.6	1
0	2	26	14	0.4	157	11	1,030	103	0.04	0.04	0.2	3
0	26	21	117	5.1	644	6	30	3	0.30	0.09	2.0	6

Nutritive Value of Foods *(Continued)*

Foods, approximate measures, units, and weight (weight of edible portion only)		Water	Food energy	Pro-tein	Fat	Satu-rated	Mono-unsatu-rated	Poly-unsatu-rated
							Fatty Acids	
		Per-cent	*Cal-ories*	*Grams*	*Grams*	*Grams*	*Grams*	*Grams*
VEGETABLES AND VEGETABLE PRODUCTS—Con.	*Grams*							
Kale, cooked, drained:								
From raw, chopped- - - - - 1 cup- - - - - - - - -	130	91	40	2	1	0.1	Tr	0.3
From frozen, chopped- - - - 1 cup- - - - - - - - -	130	91	40	4	1	0.1	Tr	0.3
Kohlrabi, thickened bulb-like stems, cooked, drained, diced- - - - - - - - - - - - - - 1 cup- - - - - - - - -	165	90	50	3	Tr	Tr	Tr	0.1
Lettuce, raw:								
Butterhead, as Boston types:								
Head, 5-in diam- - - - - 1 head- - - - - - - -	163	96	20	2	Tr	Tr	Tr	0.2
Leaves- - - - - - - - - - - 1 outer or 2 inner leaves- - - - - - -	15	96	Tr	Tr	Tr	Tr	Tr	Tr
Crisphead, as iceberg:								
Head, 6-in diam- - - - - 1 head- - - - - - - -	539	96	70	5	1	0.1	Tr	0.5
Looseleaf (bunching varie-ties including romaine or cos), chopped or shredded pieces- - - - - 1 cup- - - - - - - - -	56	94	10	1	Tr	Tr	Tr	0.1
Mushrooms:								
Raw, sliced or chopped- - - 1 cup- - - - - - - - -	70	92	20	1	Tr	Tr	Tr	0.1
Cooked, drained- - - - - - - 1 cup- - - - - - - - -	156	91	40	3	1	0.1	Tr	0.3
Canned, drained solids- - - 1 cup- - - - - - - - -	156	91	35	3	Tr	0.1	Tr	0.2
Mustard greens, without stems and midribs, cooked, drained- - - - - - - - - - - - - 1 cup- - - - - - - - -	140	94	20	3	Tr	Tr	0.2	0.1
Okra pods, 3 by ⅝ in, cooked 8 pods- - - - - - - - -	85	90	25	2	Tr	Tr	Tr	Tr
Onions:								
Raw:								
Sliced- - - - - - - - - - - - - 1 cup- - - - - - - - -	115	91	40	1	Tr	0.1	Tr	0.1
Cooked (whole or sliced), drained- - - - - - - - - - 1 cup- - - - - - - - -	210	92	60	2	Tr	0.1	Tr	0.1
Onions, spring, raw, bulb (⅜-in diam.) and white portion of top- - - - - - - - - - - - - - 6 onions- - - - - - -	30	92	10	1	Tr	Tr	Tr	Tr
Onion rings, breaded, par-fried, frozen, prepared- - - 2 rings- - - - - - - -	20	29	80	1	5	1.7	2.2	1.0
Parsley:								
Raw- - - - - - - - - - - - - - - 10 sprigs- - - - - - -	10	88	5	Tr	Tr	Tr	Tr	Tr
Parsnips, cooked (diced or 2 in lengths), drained- - - - - - - 1 cup- - - - - - - - -	156	78	125	2	Tr	0.1	0.2	0.1
Peas, edible pod, cooked, drained- - - - - - - - - - - - - 1 cup- - - - - - - - -	160	89	65	5	Tr	0.1	Tr	0.2
Peas, green:								
Canned, drained solids- - - 1 cup- - - - - - - - -	170	82	115	8	1	0.1	0.1	0.3
Frozen, cooked, drained- - 1 cup- - - - - - - - -	160	80	125	8	Tr	0.1	Tr	0.2
Peppers:								
Hot chili, raw- - - - - - - - - 1 pepper- - - - - - -	45	88	20	1	Tr	Tr	Tr	Tr

(Tr indicates nutrient present in trace amounts.)

Nutrients in Indicated Quantity

Cholesterol	Carbohydrate	Calcium	Phosphorus	Iron	Potassium	Sodium	Vitamin A value (IU)	Vitamin A value (RE)	Thiamin	Riboflavin	Niacin	Ascorbic acid
Milligrams	Grams	Milligrams	Milligrams	Milligrams	Milligrams	Milligrams	International units	Retinol equivalents	Milligrams	Milligrams	Milligrams	Milligrams
0	7	94	36	1.2	296	30	9,620	962	0.07	0.09	0.7	53
0	7	179	36	1.2	417	20	8,260	826	0.06	0.15	0.9	33
0	11	41	74	0.7	561	35	60	6	0.07	0.03	0.6	89
0	4	52	38	0.5	419	8	1,580	158	0.10	0.10	0.5	13
0	Tr	5	3	Tr	39	1	150	15	0.01	0.01	Tr	1
0	11	102	108	2.7	852	49	1,780	178	0.25	0.16	1.0	21
0	2	38	14	0.8	148	5	1,060	106	0.03	0.04	0.2	10
0	3	4	73	0.9	259	3	0	0	0.07	0.31	2.9	2
0	8	9	136	2.7	555	3	0	0	0.11	0.47	7.0	6
0	8	17	103	1.2	201	663	0	0	0.13	0.03	2.5	0
0	3	104	57	1.0	283	22	4,240	424	0.06	0.09	0.6	35
0	6	54	48	0.4	274	4	490	49	0.11	0.05	0.7	14
0	8	29	33	0.4	178	2	0	0	0.07	0.01	0.1	10
0	13	57	48	0.4	319	17	0	0	0.09	0.02	0.2	12
0	2	18	10	0.6	77	1	1,500	150	0.02	0.04	0.1	14
0	8	6	16	0.3	26	75	50	5	0.06	0.03	0.7	Tr
0	1	13	4	0.6	54	4	520	52	0.01	0.01	0.1	9
0	30	58	108	0.9	573	16	0	0	0.13	0.08	1.1	20
0	11	67	88	3.2	384	6	210	21	0.20	0.12	0.9	77
0	21	34	114	1.6	294	[66]372	1,310	131	0.21	0.13	1.2	16
0	23	38	144	2.5	269	139	1,070	107	0.45	0.16	2.4	16
0	4	8	21	0.5	153	3	[67]4,840	[67]484	0.04	0.04	0.4	109

Nutritive Value of Foods *(Continued)*

Foods, approximate measures, units, and weight (weight of edible portion only)		Water	Food energy	Pro-tein	Fat	Fatty Acids		
						Satu-rated	Mono-unsatu-rated	Poly-unsatu-rated
		Grams	Per-cent	Cal-ories	Grams	Grams	Grams	Grams	Grams

		Grams	Per-cent	Cal-ories	Grams	Grams	Grams	Grams	Grams
VEGETABLES AND VEGETABLE PRODUCTS—Con.									
Sweet (about 5 per lb, whole), stem and seeds removed:									
Raw	1 pepper	74	93	20	1	Tr	Tr	Tr	0.2
Cooked, drained	1 pepper	73	95	15	Tr	Tr	Tr	Tr	0.1
Potatoes, cooked:									
Baked (about 2 per lb, raw):									
With skin	1 potato	202	71	220	5	Tr	0.1	Tr	0.1
Flesh only	1 potato	156	75	145	3	Tr	Tr	Tr	0.1
Boiled (about 3 per lb, raw):									
Peeled after boiling	1 potato	136	77	120	3	Tr	Tr	Tr	0.1
Peeled before boiling	1 potato	135	77	115	2	Tr	Tr	Tr	0.1
French fried, strip, 2 to 3½ in long, frozen:									
Oven heated	10 strips	50	53	110	2	4	2.1	1.8	0.3
Fried in vegetable oil	10 strips	50	38	160	2	8	2.5	1.6	3.8
Potato products, prepared:									
Hashed brown, from frozen	1 cup	156	56	340	5	18	7.0	8.0	2.1
Mashed:									
From home recipe:									
Milk added	1 cup	210	78	160	4	1	0.7	0.3	0.1
Milk and margarine added	1 cup	210	76	225	4	9	2.2	3.7	2.5
Potato salad, made with mayonnaise	1 cup	250	76	360	7	21	3.6	6.2	9.3
Scalloped:									
From dry mix	1 cup	245	79	230	5	11	6.5	3.0	0.5
Potato chips	10 chips	20	3	105	1	7	1.8	1.2	3.6
Pumpkin:									
Cooked from raw, mashed	1 cup	245	94	50	2	Tr	0.1	Tr	Tr
Canned	1 cup	245	90	85	3	1	0.4	0.1	Tr
Radishes, raw, stem ends, rootlets cut off	4 radishes	18	95	5	Tr	Tr	Tr	Tr	Tr
Sauerkraut, canned, solids and liquid	1 cup	236	93	45	2	Tr	0.1	Tr	0.1
Seaweed:									
Kelp, raw	1 oz	28	82	10	Tr	Tr	0.1	Tr	Tr
Southern peas. See Black-eyed peas.									
Spinach:									
Raw, chopped	1 cup	55	92	10	2	Tr	Tr	Tr	0.1
Cooked, drained:									
From raw	1 cup	180	91	40	5	Tr	0.1	Tr	0.2
Canned, drained solids	1 cup	214	92	50	6	1	0.2	Tr	0.4
Squash, cooked:									
Summer (all varieties), sliced, drained	1 cup	180	94	35	2	1	0.1	Tr	0.2

(Tr indicates nutrient present in trace amounts.)

Nutrients in Indicated Quantity

Cholesterol	Carbohydrate	Calcium	Phosphorus	Iron	Potassium	Sodium	Vitamin A value		Thiamin	Riboflavin	Niacin	Ascorbic acid
							(IU)	(RE)				
Milligrams	Grams	Milligrams	Milligrams	Milligrams	Milligrams	Milligrams	International units	Retinol equivalents	Milligrams	Milligrams	Milligrams	Milligrams
0	4	4	16	0.9	144	2	[68]390	[68]39	0.06	0.04	0.4	[69]95
0	3	3	11	0.6	94	1	[70]280	[70]28	0.04	0.03	0.3	[71]81
0	51	20	115	2.7	844	16	0	0	0.22	0.07	3.3	26
0	34	8	78	0.5	610	8	0	0	0.16	0.03	2.2	20
0	27	7	60	0.4	515	5	0	0	0.14	0.03	2.0	18
0	27	11	54	0.4	443	7	0	0	0.13	0.03	1.8	10
0	17	5	43	0.7	229	16	0	0	0.06	0.02	1.2	5
0	20	10	47	0.4	366	108	0	0	0.09	0.01	1.6	5
0	44	23	112	2.4	680	53	0	0	0.17	0.03	3.8	10
4	37	55	101	0.6	628	636	40	12	0.18	0.08	2.3	14
4	35	55	97	0.5	607	620	360	42	0.18	0.08	2.3	13
170	28	48	130	1.6	635	1,323	520	83	0.19	0.15	2.2	25
27	31	88	137	0.9	497	835	360	51	0.05	0.14	2.5	8
0	10	5	31	0.2	260	94	0	0	0.03	Tr	0.8	8
0	12	37	74	1.4	564	2	2,650	265	0.08	0.19	1.0	12
0	20	64	86	3.4	505	12	54,040	5,404	0.06	0.13	0.9	10
0	1	4	3	0.1	42	4	Tr	Tr	Tr	0.01	0.1	4
0	10	71	47	3.5	401	1,560	40	4	0.05	0.05	0.3	35
0	3	48	12	0.8	25	66	30	3	0.01	0.04	0.1	(1)
0	2	54	27	1.5	307	43	3,690	369	0.04	0.10	0.4	15
0	7	245	101	6.4	839	126	14,740	1,474	0.17	0.42	0.9	18
0	7	272	94	4.9	740	[72]683	18,780	1,878	0.03	0.30	0.8	31
0	8	49	70	0.6	346	2	520	52	0.08	0.07	0.9	10

Nutritive Value of Foods *(Continued)*

Foods, approximate measures, units, and weight (weight of edible portion only)		Water	Food energy	Pro-tein	Fat	Satu-rated	Mono-unsatu-rated	Poly-unsatu-rated
							Fatty Acids	
		Grams	Per-cent	Cal-ories	Grams	Grams	Grams	Grams	Grams
VEGETABLES AND VEGETABLE PRODUCTS—Con.									
Winter (all varieties), baked, cubes	1 cup	205	89	80	2	1	0.3	0.1	0.5
Sunchoke. See Jerusalem-artichoke.									
Sweet potatoes:									
Cooked (raw, 5 by 2 in; about 2½ per lb):									
Baked in skin, peeled	1 potato	114	73	115	2	Tr	Tr	Tr	0.1
Boiled, without skin	1 potato	151	73	160	2	Tr	0.1	Tr	0.2
Candied, 2½ by 2-in piece	1 piece	105	67	145	1	3	1.4	0.7	0.2
Canned:									
Solid pack (mashed)	1 cup	255	74	260	5	1	0.1	Tr	0.2
Vacuum pack, piece 2¾ by 1 in	1 piece	40	76	35	1	Tr	Tr	Tr	Tr
Tomatoes:									
Raw, 2⅗-in diam. (3 per 12 oz pkg.)	1 tomato	123	94	25	1	Tr	Tr	Tr	0.1
Canned, solids and liquid	1 cup	240	94	50	2	1	0.1	0.1	0.2
Tomato juice, canned	1 cup	244	94	40	2	Tr	Tr	Tr	0.1
Tomato products, canned:									
Paste	1 cup	262	74	220	10	2	0.3	0.4	0.9
Puree	1 cup	250	87	105	4	Tr	Tr	Tr	0.1
Sauce	1 cup	245	89	75	3	Tr	0.1	0.1	0.2
Turnips, cooked, diced	1 cup	156	94	30	1	Tr	Tr	Tr	0.1
Turnip greens, cooked, drained:									
From raw (leaves and stems)	1 cup	144	93	30	2	Tr	0.1	Tr	0.1
From frozen (chopped)	1 cup	164	90	50	5	1	0.2	Tr	0.3
Vegetable juice cocktail, canned	1 cup	242	94	45	2	Tr	Tr	Tr	0.1
Vegetables, mixed:									
Frozen, cooked, drained	1 cup	182	83	105	5	Tr	0.1	Tr	0.1
Water chestnuts, canned	1 cup	140	86	70	1	Tr	Tr	Tr	Tr
MISCELLANEOUS ITEMS									
Baking powders for home use:									
Sodium aluminum sulfate:									
With monocalcium phos-phate monohydrate	1 tsp	3	2	5	Tr	0	0.0	0.0	0.0
Catsup	1 cup	273	69	290	5	1	0.2	0.2	0.4
	1 tbsp	15	69	15	Tr	Tr	Tr	Tr	Tr
Chili powder	1 tsp	2.6	8	10	Tr	Tr	0.1	0.1	0.2
Chocolate:									
Bitter or baking	1 oz	28	2	145	3	15	9.0	4.9	0.5
Semisweet, see Candy									
Cinnamon	1 tsp	2.3	10	5	Tr	Tr	Tr	Tr	Tr
Curry powder	1 tsp	2	10	5	Tr	Tr	(1)	(1)	(1)

(Tr indicates nutrient present in trace amounts.)

Nutrients in Indicated Quantity

Cholesterol	Carbohydrate	Calcium	Phosphorus	Iron	Potassium	Sodium	Vitamin A value		Thiamin	Riboflavin	Niacin	Ascorbic acid
							(IU)	(RE)				
Milligrams	Grams	Milligrams	Milligrams	Milligrams	Milligrams	Milligrams	International units	Retinol equivalents	Milligrams	Milligrams	Milligrams	Milligrams
0	18	29	41	0.7	896	2	7,290	729	0.17	0.05	1.4	20
0	28	32	63	0.5	397	11	24,880	2,488	0.08	0.14	0.7	28
0	37	32	41	0.8	278	20	25,750	2,575	0.08	0.21	1.0	26
8	29	27	27	1.2	198	74	4,400	440	0.02	0.04	0.4	7
0	59	77	133	3.4	536	191	38,570	3,857	0.07	0.23	2.4	13
0	8	9	20	0.4	125	21	3,190	319	0.01	0.02	0.3	11
0	5	9	28	0.6	255	10	1,390	139	0.07	0.06	0.7	22
0	10	62	46	1.5	530	[73]391	1,450	145	0.11	0.07	1.8	36
0	10	22	46	1.4	537	[74]881	1,360	136	0.11	0.08	1.6	45
0	49	92	207	7.8	2,442	[75]170	6,470	647	0.41	0.50	8.4	111
0	25	38	100	2.3	1,050	[76]50	3,400	340	0.18	0.14	4.3	88
0	18	34	78	1.9	909	[77]1,482	2,400	240	0.16	0.14	2.8	32
0	8	34	30	0.3	211	78	0	0	0.04	0.04	0.5	18
0	6	197	42	1.2	292	42	7,920	792	0.06	0.10	0.6	39
0	8	249	56	3.2	367	25	13,080	1,308	0.09	0.12	0.8	36
0	11	27	41	1.0	467	883	2,830	283	0.10	0.07	1.8	67
0	24	46	93	1.5	308	64	7,780	778	0.13	0.22	1.5	6
0	17	6	27	1.2	165	11	10	1	0.02	0.03	0.5	2
0	1	58	87	0.0	5	329	0	0	0.00	0.00	0.0	0
0	69	60	137	2.2	991	2,845	3,820	382	0.25	0.19	4.4	41
0	4	3	8	0.1	54	156	210	21	0.01	0.01	0.2	2
0	1	7	8	0.4	50	26	910	91	0.01	0.02	0.2	2
0	8	22	109	1.9	235	1	10	1	0.01	0.07	0.4	0
0	2	28	1	0.9	12	1	10	1	Tr	Tr	Tr	1
0	1	10	7	0.6	31	1	20	2	0.01	0.01	0.1	Tr

Nutritive Value of Foods *(Continued)*

Foods, approximate measures, units, and weight (weight of edible portion only)		Grams	Water Per-cent	Food energy Cal-ories	Pro-tein Grams	Fat Grams	Satu-rated Grams	Mono-unsatu-rated Grams	Poly-unsatu-rated Grams
								Fatty Acids	
MISCELLANEOUS ITEMS—Con.									
Garlic powder	1 tsp	2.8	6	10	Tr	Tr	Tr	Tr	Tr
Gelatin, dry	1 envelope	7	13	25	6	Tr	Tr	Tr	Tr
Mustard, prepared, yellow	1 tsp or individual packet	5	80	5	Tr	Tr	Tr	0.2	Tr
Olives, canned:									
Green	4 medium or 3 extra large	13	78	15	Tr	2	0.2	1.2	0.1
Ripe, Mission, pitted	3 small or 2 large	9	73	15	Tr	2	0.3	1.3	0.2
Oregano	1 tsp	1.5	7	5	Tr	Tr	Tr	Tr	0.1
Paprika	1 tsp	2.1	10	5	Tr	Tr	Tr	Tr	0.2
Pepper, black	1 tsp	2.1	11	5	Tr	Tr	Tr	Tr	Tr
Pickles, cucumber:									
Dill, medium, whole, 3¾ in long, 1¼-in diam.	1 pickle	65	93	5	Tr	Tr	Tr	Tr	0.1
Fresh-pack, slices 1½-in diam., ¼ in thick	2 slices	15	79	10	Tr	Tr	Tr	Tr	Tr
Sweet, gherkin, small, whole, about 2½ in long, ¾-in diam.	1 pickle	15	61	20	Tr	Tr	Tr	Tr	Tr
Popcorn. See Grain Products									
Salt	1 tsp	5.5	0	0	0	0	0.0	0.0	0.0
Vinegar, cider	1 tbsp	15	94	Tr	Tr	0	0.0	0.0	0.0
Yeast:									
Baker's, dry, active	1 pkg	7	5	20	3	Tr	Tr	0.1	Tr

(Tr indicates nutrient present in trace amounts.)

[1] Value not determined.

[2] Mineral content varies depending on water source.

[3] Blend of aspartame and saccharin; if only sodium saccharin is used, sodium is 75 mg; if only aspartame is used, sodium is 23 mg.

[4] With added ascorbic acid.

[5] Vitamin A value is largely from beta-carotene used for coloring.

[6] Yields 1 qt of fluid milk when reconstituted according to package directions.

[7] With added vitamin A.

[8] Carbohydrate content varies widely because of amount of sugar added and amount and solids content of added flavoring. Consult the label if more precise values for carbohydrate and calories are needed.

[9] For salted butter; unsalted butter contains 12 mg sodium per stick, 2 mg per tbsp, or 1 mg per pat.

[10] Values for vitamin are year-round average.

[11] For salted margarine.

[12] Based on average vitamin A content of fortified margarine. Federal specifications for fortified margarine require a minimum of 15,000 IU per pound.

[13] Fatty acid values apply to product made with regular margarine.

[14] Dipped in egg, milk, and breadcrumbs; fried in vegetable shortening.

[15] If bones are discarded, value for calcium will be greatly reduced.

[16] Dipped in egg, breadcrumbs, and flour; fried in vegetable shortening.

[17] Made with drained chunk light tuna, celery, onion, pickle relish, and mayonnaise-type salad dressing.

Nutrients in Indicated Quantity

| Cho-les-terol | Carbo-hydrate | Calcium | Phos-phorus | Iron | Potas-sium | Sodium | Vitamin A value | | Thiamin | Ribo-flavin | Niacin | Ascorbic acid |
| | | | | | | | (IU) | (RE) | | | | |
Milli-grams	Grams	Milli-grams	Milli-grams	Milli-grams	Milli-grams	Milli-grams	Inter-national units	Retinol equiva-lents	Milli-grams	Milli-grams	Milli-grams	Milli-grams
0	2	2	12	0.1	31	1	0	0	0.01	Tr	Tr	Tr
0	0	1	0	0.0	2	6	0	0	0.00	0.00	0.0	0
0	Tr	4	4	0.1	7	63	0	0	Tr	0.01	Tr	Tr
0	Tr	8	2	0.2	7	312	40	4	Tr	Tr	Tr	0
0	Tr	10	2	0.2	2	68	10	1	Tr	Tr	Tr	0
0	1	24	3	0.7	25	Tr	100	10	0.01	Tr	0.1	1
0	1	4	7	0.5	49	1	1,270	127	0.01	0.04	0.3	1
0	1	9	4	0.6	26	1	Tr	Tr	Tr	0.01	Tr	0
0	1	17	14	0.7	130	928	70	7	Tr	0.01	Tr	4
0	3	5	4	0.3	30	101	20	2	Tr	Tr	Tr	1
0	5	2	2	0.2	30	107	10	1	Tr	Tr	Tr	1
0	0	14	3	Tr	Tr	2,132	0	0	0.00	0.00	0.0	0
0	1	1	1	0.1	15	Tr	0	0	0.00	0.00	0.0	0
0	3	3	90	1.1	140	4	Tr	Tr	0.16	0.38	2.6	Tr

[18] Sodium bisulfite used to preserve color; unsulfited product would contain less sodium.
[19] Also applies to pasteurized apple cider.
[20] Without added ascorbic acid. For value with added ascorbic acid, refer to label.
[21] With added ascorbic acid.
[22] For white grapefruit; pink grapefruit have about 310 IU or 31 RE.
[23] Sodium benzoate and sodium bisulfite added as preservatives.
[24] Egg bagels have 44 mg cholesterol and 22 IU or 7 RE vitamin A per bagel.
[25] Made with vegetable shortening.
[26] Made with white cornmeal. If made with yellow cornmeal, value is 32 IU or 3 RE.
[27] Nutrient added.
[28] Cooked without salt. If salt is added according to label recommendations, sodium content is 540 mg.
[29] For white corn grits. Cooked yellow grits contain 145 IU or 14 RE.
[30] Value based on label declaration for added nutrients.
[31] For regular and instant cereal. For quick cereal, phosphorus is 102 mg and sodium is 142 mg.
[32] Cooked without salt. If salt is added according to label recommendations, sodium content is 390 mg.
[33] Cooked without salt. If salt is added according to label recommendations, sodium content is 324 mg.
[34] Cooked without salt. If salt is added according to label recommendations, sodium content is 374 mg.
[35] Excepting angelfood cake, cakes were made from mixes containing vegetable shortening and frostings were made with margarine.
[36] Made with vegetable oil.

(Footnotes continue on next page.)

[37] Cake made with vegetable shortening; frosting with margarine.

[38] Made with margarine.

[39] Crackers made with enriched flour except for rye wafers and whole-wheat wafers.

[40] Made with lard.

[41] Cashews without salt contain 21 mg sodium per cup or 4 mg per oz.

[42] Cashews without salt contain 22 mg sodium per cup or 5 mg per oz.

[43] Macadamia nuts without salt contain 9 mg sodium per cup or 2 mg per oz.

[44] Mixed nuts without salt contain 3 mg sodium per oz.

[45] Peanuts without salt contain 22 mg sodium per cup or 4 mg per oz.

[46] Outer layer of fat was removed to within approximately ½ inch of the lean. Deposits of fat within the cut were not removed.

[47] Fried in vegetable shortening.

[48] Value varies widely.

[49] Contains added sodium ascorbate. If sodium ascorbate is not added, ascorbic acid content is negligible.

[50] One patty (8 per pound) of bulk sausage is equivalent to 2 links.

[51] Crust made with vegetable shortening and enriched flour.

[52] Made with corn oil.

[53] Fried in vegetable shortening.

[54] If sodium ascorbate is added, product contains 11 mg ascorbic acid.

[55] Made with enriched flour, margarine, and whole milk.

[56] For regular pack; special dietary pack contains 3 mg sodium.

[57] For green varieties; yellow varieties contain 101 IU or 10 RE.

[58] For green varieties; yellow varieties contain 151 IU or 15 RE.

[59] For regular pack; special dietary pack contains 3 mg sodium.

[60] For green varieties; yellow varieties contain 142 IU or 14 RE.

[61] For regular pack; special dietary pack contains 78 mg sodium.

[62] For regular pack; special dietary pack contains 61 mg sodium.

[63] For yellow varieties; white varieties contain only a trace of vitamin A.

[64] For regular pack; special dietary pack contains 8 mg sodium.

[65] For regular pack; special dietary pack contains 6 mg sodium.

[66] For regular pack; special dietary pack contains 3 mg sodium.

[67] For red peppers; green peppers contain 350 IU or 35 RE.

[68] For green peppers; red peppers contain 4220 IU or 422 RE.

[69] For green peppers; red peppers contain 141 mg ascorbic acid.

[70] For green peppers; red peppers contain 2740 IU or 274 RE.

[71] For green peppers; red peppers contain 121 mg ascorbic acid.

[72] With added salt; if none is added, sodium content is 58 mg.

[73] For regular pack; special dietary pack contains 31 mg sodium.

[74] With added salt; if none is added, sodium content is 24 mg.

[75] With no added salt; if salt is added, sodium content is 2070 mg.

[76] With no added salt; if salt is added, sodium content is 998 mg.

[77] With salt added.

Adapted from Nutritive Value of Foods, Home and Garden Bulletin, No. 72, U.S. Dept. of Agriculture.

Nutritional Assessment Tools

The Warning Signs of poor nutritional health are often overlooked. Use this checklist to find out if you or someone you know is at nutritional risk.

Read the statements below. Circle the number in the yes column for those that apply to you or someone you know. For each yes answer, score the number in the box. Total your nutritional score.

DETERMINE YOUR NUTRITIONAL HEALTH

		YES
*D	I have an illness or condition that made me change the kind and/or amount of food I eat.	**2**
E	I eat fewer than 2 meals per day.	**3**
	I eat few fruits or vegetables, or milk products.	**2**
T	I have 3 or more drinks of beer, liquor or wine almost every day.	**2**
E	I have tooth or mouth problems that make it hard for me to eat.	**2**
R	I don't always have enough money to buy the food I need.	**4**
	I eat alone most of the time.	**1**
M	I take 3 or more different prescribed or over-the-counter drugs a day.	**1**
I	Without wanting to, I have lost or gained 10 pounds in the last 6 months.	**2**
N	I am not always physically able to shop, cook and/or feed myself.	**2**
E	Age_____ Today's Date_____	**TOTAL**

NAME _____ SEX _____ PHONE # _____

ADDRESS _____ CITY _____ STATE ____ ZIP CODE ____

Total Your Nutritional Score. If it's...

0-2 **Good!** Recheck your nutritional score in 6 months.

3-5 **You are at moderate nutritional risk.** See what can be done to improve your eating habits and lifestyle. Your office of aging, senior nutrition program, senior citizens center or health department can help. Recheck your nutritional score in 3 months.

6 or more **You are at high nutritional risk.** Bring this checklist the next time you see your doctor, dietitian or other qualified health or social service professional. Talk with them about any problems you may have. Ask for help to improve your nutritional health.

These materials developed and distributed by the Nutrition Screening Initiative, a project of:

AMERICAN ACADEMY OF FAMILY PHYSICIANS
THE AMERICAN DIETETIC ASSOCIATION
NATIONAL COUNCIL ON THE AGING, INC.

FOR OFFICE USE ONLY

INTERVENTION RECOMMENDED
☐ Social Service   ☐ Medication Use
☐ Nutrition Education/   ☐ Oral Health
   Counseling   ☐ Nutrition Support
☐ MentalHealth

Continued on following page

Remember that warning signs suggest risk, but do not represent diagnosis of any condition.
See below to learn more about the warning signs of poor nutritional health.

Disease

Any disease, illness or chronic condition which causes you to change the way you eat, or makes it hard for you to eat, puts your nutritional health at risk. Four out of five adults have chronic diseases that are affected by diet. Confusion or memory loss that keeps getting worse is estimated to affect one out of five or more of older adults. This can make it hard to remember what, when or if you've eaten. Feeling sad or depressed, which happens to about one in eight older adults, can cause big changes in appetite, digestion, energy level, weight and well-being.

Eating Poorly

Eating too little and eating too much both lead to poor health. Eating the same foods day after day or not eating fruit, vegetables, and milk products daily will also cause poor nutritional health. One in five adults skip meals daily. Only 13% of adults eat the minimum amount of fruit and vegetables needed. One in four older adults drink too much alcohol. Many health problems become worse if you drink more than one or two alcoholic beverages per day.

Tooth Loss/Mouth Pain

A healthy mouth, teeth and gums are needed to eat. Missing, loose or rotten teeth or dentures which don't fit well or cause mouth sores make it hard to eat.

Economic Hardship

As many as 40% of older Americans have incomes of less than $6,000 per year. Having less–or choosing to spend less–than $25-30 per week for food makes it very hard to get the foods you need to stay healthy.

Reduced Social Contact

One-third of all older people live alone. Being with people daily has a positive effect on morale, well-being and eating.

Multiple Medicines

Many older Americans must take medicines for health problems. Almost half of older Americans take multiple medicines daily. Growing old may change the way we respond to drugs. The more medicines you take, the greater the chance for side effects such as increased or decreased appetite, change in taste, constipation, weakness, drowsiness, diarrhea, nausea, and others. Vitamins or minerals when taken in large doses act like drugs and can cause harm. Alert your doctor to everything you take.

Involuntry Weight Loss/Gain

Losing or gaining a lot of weight when you are not trying to do so is an important warning sign that must not be ignored. Being overweight or underweight also increases your chance of poor health.

Needs Assistance in Self Care

Although most older people are able to eat, one of every five have trouble walking, shopping, buying and cooking food, especially as they get older.

Elder Years Above Age 80

Most older people lead full and productive lives. But as age increases, risk of frailty and health problems increase. Checking your nutritional health regularly makes good sense.

SOURCE: Reprinted with permission by the Nutrition Screening Initiative, a project of the American Academy of Family Physicians, the American Dietetic Association, and the National Council on the Aging, Inc., and funded in part by a grant from Ross Products Division, Abbott Laboratories.

Level 1 Screen

Body Weight

Measure height to the nearest inch and weight to the nearest pound. Record the values below and mark them on the Body Mass Index (BMI) scale to the right. Then use a straight edge (ruler) to connect the two points and circle the spot where the straight line crosses the center line (body mass index). Record the number below.

Healthy older adults should have a BMI between 24 and 27.

Height (in): _____
Weight (lbs): _____
Body Mass Index: _____
(number from center column)

Check any boxes that are true for the individual:

❑ Has lost or gained 10 pounds (or more) in the past 6 months.

❑ Body mass index <24

❑ Body mass index >27

For the remaining sections, please ask the individual which of the statements (if any) is true for him or her and place a check by each that applies.

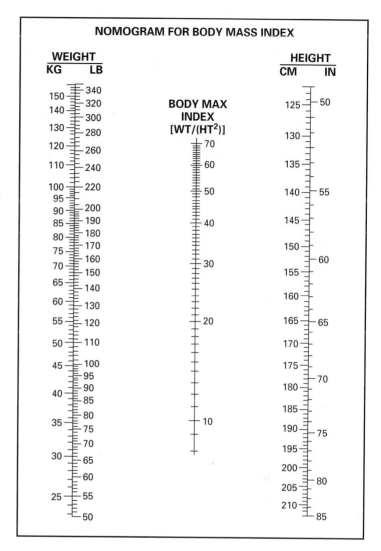

Eating Habits

❑ Does not have enough food to eat each day

❑ Usually eats alone

❑ Does not eat anything on one or more days each month

❑ Has poor appetite

❑ Is on a special diet

❑ Eats vegetables two or fewer times a day

❑ Eats milk or milk products once or not at all daily

❑ Eats fruit or drinks fruit juice once or not at all daily

❑ Eats breads, cereals, pasta, rice, or other grains five or fewer times daily

❑ Has difficulty chewing or swallowing

❑ Has more than one alcoholic drink per day (if woman); more than two drinks per day (if man)

❑ Has pain in mouth, teeth, or gums

A physician should be contacted if the individual has gained or lost 10 pounds unexpectedly or without intending to during the past 6 months. A physician should also be notified if the individual's body mass index is above 27 or below 22.

Living Environment

☐ Lives on an income of less than $6,000 per year (per individual in the household)

☐ Lives alone

☐ Is housebound

☐ Is concerned about home security

☐ Lives in a home with inadequate heating or cooling

☐ Does not have a stove and/or refrigerator

☐ Is unable or prefers not to spend money on food (<$25-30 per person spent on food each week)

Functional Status

Usually or always needs assistance with (check each that applies):

☐ Bathing

☐ Dressing

☐ Grooming

☐ Toileting

☐ Eating

☐ Walking or moving about

☐ Traveling (outside the home)

☐ Preparing food

☐ Shopping for food or other necessities

If you have checked one or more statements on this screen, the individual you have interviewed may be at risk for poor nutritional status. Please refer this individual to the appropriate health care or social service professional in your area. For example, a dietitian should be contacted for problems with selecting, preparing, or eating a healthy diet, or a dentist if the individual experiences pain or difficulty when chewing or swallowing. Those individuals whose income, lifestyle, or functional status may endanger their nutritional and overall health should be referred to available community services: home-delivered meals, congregate meal programs, transportation services, counseling services (alcohol abuse, depression, bereavement, etc.) home health care agencies, day care programs, etc.

Please repeat this screen at least once each year—sooner if the individual has a major change in his or her health, income, immediate family (e.g., spouse dies), or functional status.

Figure 2. Level I Screen. (From the Nutrition Screening Initiative: A project of the American Academy of Family Physicians, The American Dietetic Association, and the National Council on the Aging, Inc. and funded in part by a grant from Ross Laboratories, a division of Abbott laboratories, with permission.)

FEATURES OF SUBJECTIVE GLOBAL ASSESSMENT (SGA)

Select appropriate category with a check mark, or enter numerical value where indicated by "#".

A. History
1. Weight change
   —Overall loss in past 6 months: amount 5 = _____ kg; % loss 5 = _____
   —Change in past 2 weeks: _____ increase
                                 _____ no change
                                 _____ decrease
2. Dietary intake change (relative to normal)
   _____ No change
   _____ Change _____ duration 5 = _____ weeks
                    _____ type: _____ suboptimal solid diet   _____ full liquid diet
                                       _____ hypocaloric liquids   _____ starvation
3. Gastrointestinal symptoms (that persisted for > 2 weeks)
   _____ none   _____ nausea   _____ vomiting   _____ diarrhea   _____ anorexia
4. Functional capacity
   _____ No dysfunction (eg, full capacity)
   _____ Dysfunction   _____ duration 5 = _____ weeks
                                   _____ type: _____ working suboptimally
                                         _____ ambulatory
                                         _____ bedridden
5. Disease and its relation to nutritional requirements
   Primary diagnosis (specify):
   Metabolic demand (stress): _____ no stress   _____ low stress
                                    _____ moderate stress   _____ high stress

B. Physical (for each trait specify: 0 = normal, 1+ = mild, 2+ = moderate, 3+ = severe)
   # _____ loss of subcutaneous fat (triceps, chest)
   # _____ muscle wasting (quadriceps, deltoids)
   # _____ ankle edema
   # _____ sacral edema
   # _____ ascites

C. SGA rating (select one):
   _____ A = Well nourished
   _____ B = Moderately (suspected of being) malnourished
   _____ C = Severely malnourished

SOURCE: Detsky, et al: What is subjective global assessment? JPEN 11:8, 1987, with permission.

Nutritional Screening Form

Name _____ Date _____ Adm. Date _____

Sex _____ Birthdate _____ Physician's Name _____

Adm. Dx. _____

Diet	Diet order_____ Date prescribed_____
Information	Accepts all major groups _____
	Feeds self _____ Type of assistance needed _____

Physical Height _____ Weight _____ Healthy body weight % _____
Weight change in last 3 months _____ Chewing ability _____
Weight history _____ Swallowing ability _____
Hearing _____ Vision _____ Bowel function _____
Bladder function _____ Edema _____ Nausea _____
Pressure ulcer _____ Stage _____ Allergies _____

Laboratory Blood glucose _____ Albumin _____ Potassium_____
Lymphocytes _____ Hemoglobin _____ Hematocrit_____
Cholesterol _____

Medications Insulin _____ Diuretics _____ Laxatives _____ Vit/min supp _____
Antibiotics _____ Thyroid _____ Anticoagulants _____
Antidepressants (MAO) _____ Antabuse _____ Flagyl _____
Lithium _____

If the above identifies a problem, continue with in-depth assessment.

_____ (Signature) _____ (Date)

Growth Charts for Boys and Girls Birth to 20 Years

Growth charts, such as the eight that follow, are used to evaluate growth in infants, children and adolescents. The charts are a valuable tool in nutritional assessment. This expanded file of charts, just released in 2000, permits use of weight, length or stature, age, head circumference, body mass index (BMI), and gender to document an individual's status. The charts, and other versions showing different percentiles, can be downloaded from http://cdc.gov/growthcharts.

To use a chart, select the appropriate one for the characteristics you wish to plot. For example, for a male infant weighing 28 lb at 15 months of age, the correct chart is labeled "Weight-for-age percentiles: Boys, birth to 36 months." By following the lines for 28 lb at the left and 15 months on the bottom, you see that the two lines intersect about at the curved line marked "90th." This indicates the boy is heavier than 90% of 15-month-old males. The heavy dark line marked "50th" is the point at which half the 15-month old boys are heavier and half are lighter than 24.5 lb.

A child's progress can be plotted on a chart to immdiately see if there have been drastic changes in the growth pattern. The physician will probably want to know about a child above the 95th percentile or below the 5th percentile, or one with rapid changes above the 75th or below the 25th percentiles.

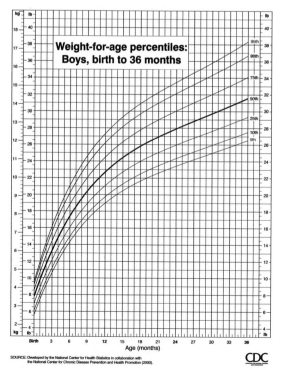

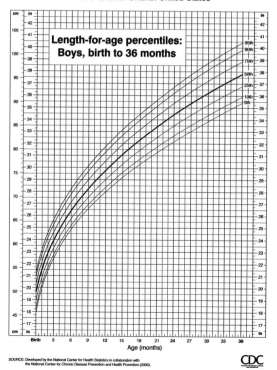

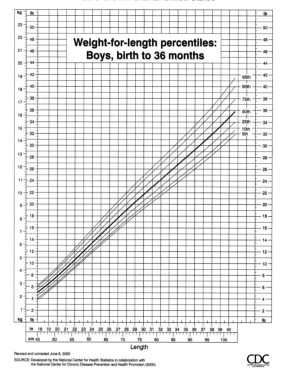

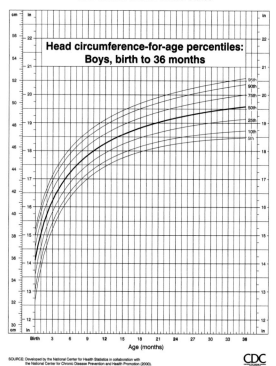

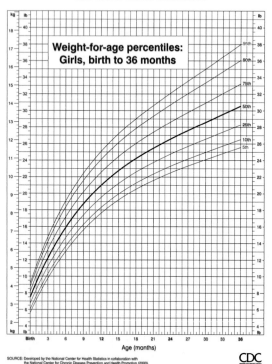

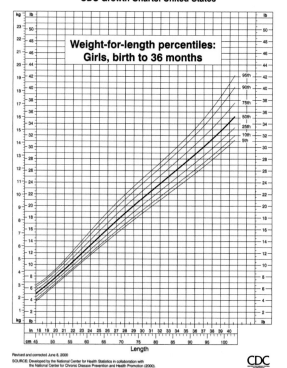

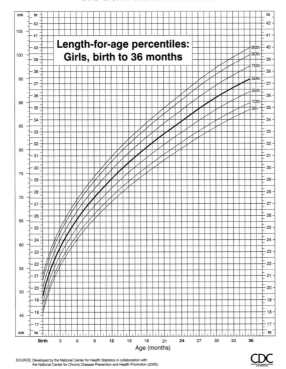

CDC Growth Charts: United States

Length-for-age percentiles:
Girls, birth to 36 months

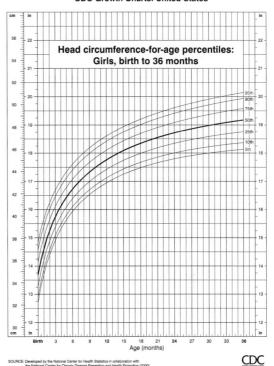

CDC Growth Charts: United States

Head circumference-for-age percentiles:
Girls, birth to 36 months

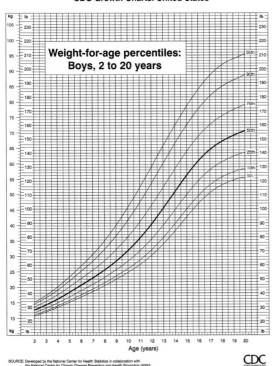

CDC Growth Charts: United States

Weight-for-age percentiles:
Boys, 2 to 20 years

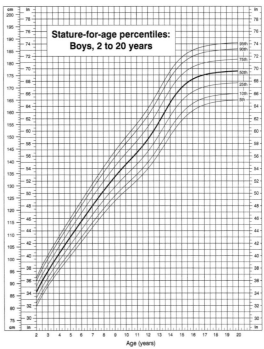

CDC Growth Charts: United States

Stature-for-age percentiles:
Boys, 2 to 20 years

CDC Growth Charts: United States

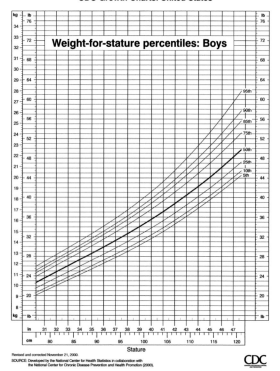

Weight-for-stature percentiles: Boys

Revised and corrected November 21, 2000.
SOURCE: Developed by the National Center for Health Statistics in collaboration with
the National Center for Chronic Disease Prevention and Health Promotion (2000).

CDC Growth Charts: United States

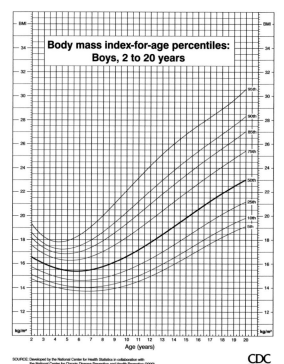

Body mass index-for-age percentiles: Boys, 2 to 20 years

SOURCE: Developed by the National Center for Health Statistics in collaboration with
the National Center for Chronic Disease Prevention and Health Promotion (2000).

CDC Growth Charts: United States

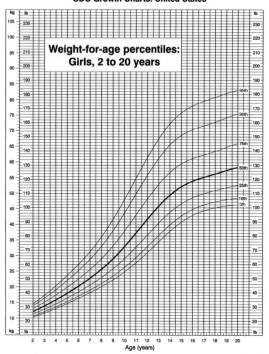

Weight-for-age percentiles: Girls, 2 to 20 years

SOURCE: Developed by the National Center for Health Statistics in collaboration with
the National Center for Chronic Disease Prevention and Health Promotion (2000).

CDC Growth Charts: United States

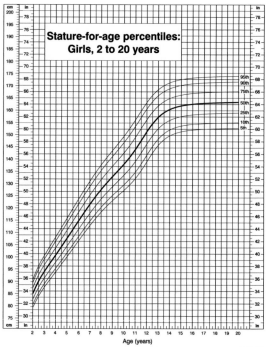

Stature-for-age percentiles: Girls, 2 to 20 years

SOURCE: Developed by the National Center for Health Statistics in collaboration with
the National Center for Chronic Disease Prevention and Health Promotion (2000).

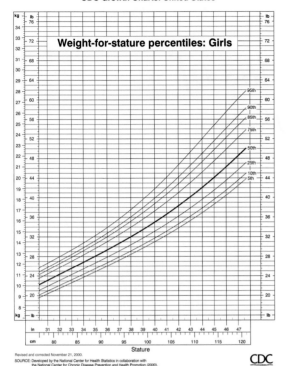

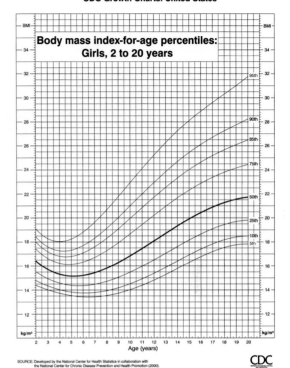

Body Fat and Skinfolds of Adults and Children

| TABLE A | *Body Fat and Skinfolds of Men* | | | |

Skinfolds (mm)	Ages			
	17–29	30–39	40–49	50+
15	4.8	—	—	—
20	8.1	12.2	12.2	12.6
25	10.5	14.2	15.0	15.6
30	12.9	16.2	17.7	18.6
35	14.7	17.7	19.6	20.8
40	16.4	19.2	21.4	22.9
45	17.7	20.4	23.0	24.7
50	19.0	21.5	24.6	26.5
55	20.1	22.5	25.9	27.9
60	21.2	23.5	27.1	29.2
65	22.2	24.3	28.2	30.4
70	23.1	25.1	29.3	31.6
75	24.0	25.9	30.3	32.7
80	24.8	26.6	31.2	33.8
85	25.5	27.2	32.1	34.8
90	26.2	27.8	33.0	35.8
95	26.9	28.4	33.7	36.6
100	27.6	29.0	34.4	37.4
105	28.2	29.6	35.1	38.2
110	28.8	30.1	35.8	39.0
115	29.4	30.6	36.4	39.7
120	30.0	31.1	37.0	40.4
125	30.5	31.5	37.6	41.1
130	31.0	31.9	38.2	41.8
135	31.5	32.3	38.7	42.4
140	32.0	32.7	39.2	43.0
145	32.5	33.1	39.7	43.6
150	32.9	33.5	40.2	44.1

TABLE A   *Body Fat and Skinfolds of Men (Continued)*

Skinfolds (mm)	Ages			
	17–29	30–39	40–49	50+
155	33.3	33.9	40.7	44.6
160	33.7	34.3	41.2	45.1
165	34.1	34.6	41.6	45.6
170	34.5	34.8	42.0	46.1
175	34.9	—	—	—
180	35.3	—	—	—
185	35.6	—	—	—
190	35.9	—	—	—
195	—	—	—	—
200	—	—	—	—
205	—	—	—	—
210	—	—	—	—

TABLE B   *Body Fat and Skinfolds of Women*

Skinfolds (mm)	Ages			
	16–29	30–39	40–49	50+
15	10.5	—	—	—
20	14.1	17.0	19.8	21.4
25	16.8	19.4	22.2	24.0
30	19.5	21.8	24.5	26.6
35	21.5	23.7	26.4	28.5
40	23.4	25.5	28.2	30.3
45	25.0	26.9	29.6	31.9
50	26.5	28.2	31.0	33.4
55	27.8	29.4	32.1	34.6
60	29.1	30.6	33.2	35.7
65	30.2	31.6	34.1	36.7
70	31.2	32.5	35.0	37.7
75	32.2	33.4	35.9	38.7
80	33.1	34.3	36.7	39.6
85	34.0	35.1	37.5	40.4
90	34.8	35.8	38.3	41.2
95	35.6	36.5	39.0	41.9
100	36.4	37.2	39.7	42.6
105	37.1	37.9	40.4	43.3
110	37.8	38.6	41.0	43.9
115	38.4	39.1	41.5	44.5
120	39.0	39.6	42.0	45.1
125	39.6	40.1	42.5	45.7
130	40.2	40.6	43.0	46.2
135	40.8	41.1	43.5	46.7
140	41.3	41.6	44.0	47.2
145	41.8	42.1	44.5	47.7
150	42.3	42.6	45.0	48.2

TABLE B   *Body Fat and Skinfolds of Women (Continued)*

Skinfolds (mm)	Ages			
	16–29	30–39	40–49	50+
155	42.8	43.1	45.4	48.7
160	43.3	43.6	45.8	49.2
165	43.7	44.0	46.2	49.6
170	44.1	44.4	46.6	50.0
175	—	44.8	47.0	50.4
180	—	45.2	47.4	50.8
185	—	45.6	47.8	51.2
190	—	45.9	48.2	51.6
195	—	46.2	48.5	52.0
200	—	46.5	48.8	52.4
205	—	—	49.1	52.7
210	—	—	49.4	53.0

In two thirds of the instances, the error was within +3.5% of the body-weight as fat for the women and ±5% for the men.

The relationship of skinfold thickness to body fat in children and individuals under 17 is addressed by The American Alliance for Health, Physical Education, Recreation and Dance in the publication *Lifetime Health Related Physical Fitness Test Manual.* They suggest that national percentile norms provide the best reference. They further suggest that the ideal is at the 50th percentile. Those below the 25th percentile should be encouraged to reduce amount of body fat, while those above the 90th percentile should not be encouraged to lose body fat.

TABLE C *Percentile Norms. Ages 6–18* for Sum of Triceps plus Subscapular Skinfolds (mm) for Boys*

Age	6	7	8	9	10	11	12	13	14	15	16	17
Percentile												
99	7	7	7	7	7	8	8	7	7	8	8	8
95	8	9	9	9	9	9	9	9	9	9	9	9
90	9	9	9	10	10	10	10	10	9	10	10	10
85	10	10	10	10	11	11	10	10	10	11	11	11
80	10	10	10	11	11	12	11	11	11	11	11	12
75	11	11	11	11	12	12	11	12	11	12	12	12
70	11	11	11	12	12	12	12	12	12	12	12	13
65	11	11	12	12	13	13	13	12	12	13	13	13
60	12	12	12	13	13	14	13	13	13	13	13	14
55	12	12	13	13	14	15	14	14	13	14	14	14
50	12	12	13	14	14	16	15	15	14	14	14	15
45	13	13	14	14	15	16	15	16	14	15	15	16
40	13	13	14	15	16	17	16	17	15	16	16	16
35	13	14	15	16	17	19	17	18	16	18	17	17
30	14	14	16	17	18	20	19	19	18	18	18	19

TABLE C *Percentile Norms. Ages 6–18* for Sum of Triceps plus Subscapular Skinfolds (mm) for Boys (Continued)*

Age	6	7	8	9	10	11	12	13	14	15	16	17
Percentile												
25	14	15	17	18	19	22	21	22	20	20	20	21
20	15	16	18	20	21	24	24	25	23	22	22	24
15	16	17	19	23	24	28	27	29	27	25	24	26
10	18	18	21	26	28	33	33	36	31	30	29	30
5	20	24	28	34	33	38	44	46	37	40	37	38

*The norms for age 17 may be used for age 18.

Source: Based on data from Johnston, F.E., Hamill, D.V., and Lemeshow, S.: (1) *Skinfold Thickness of Children 6–11 Years* (Series II, No. 120, 1972), and (2) *Skinfold Thickness of Youths 12–17 Years* (Series II, No. 132, 1974). US National Center for Health Statistics, US Department of HEW, Washington, DC.

TABLE D *Percentile Norms Ages 6–18* for Sum of Triceps plus Subscapular Skinfolds (mm) for Girls*

Age	6	7	8	9	10	11	12	13	14	15	16	17
Percentile												
99	8	8	8	9	9	8	9	10	10	11	11	12
95	9	10	10	10	10	11	11	12	13	14	14	15
90	10	11	11	12	12	12	12	13	15	16	16	16
85	11	12	12	12	13	13	13	14	16	17	18	18
80	12	12	12	13	13	14	14	15	17	18	19	19
75	12	12	13	14	14	15	15	16	18	20	20	20
70	12	13	14	15	15	16	16	17	19	21	21	22
65	13	13	14	15	16	16	17	18	20	22	22	23
60	13	14	15	16	17	17	17	19	21	23	23	24
55	14	15	16	16	18	18	19	20	22	24	24	26
50	14	15	16	17	18	19	19	20	24	25	25	27
45	15	16	17	18	20	20	21	22	25	26	27	28
40	15	16	18	19	20	21	22	23	26	28	29	30
35	16	17	19	20	22	22	24	25	27	29	30	32
30	16	18	20	22	24	23	25	27	30	32	32	34
25	17	19	21	24	25	25	27	30	32	34	34	36
20	18	20	23	26	28	28	31	33	35	37	37	40
15	19	22	25	29	31	31	35	39	39	42	42	42
10	22	25	30	34	35	36	40	43	42	48	46	46
5	26	28	36	40	41	42	48	51	52	56	57	58

*The norms for age 17 may be used for age 18.

Source: Based on data from Johnston, F.E., Hamill, D.V. and Lemeshow, S: (1) *Skinfold Thickness of Children 6–11 Years* (Series II, No. 120, 1972), and (2) *Skinfold Thickness of Youths 12–17 Years* (Series II, No. 132, 1974). US National Center for Health Statistics, US Department of HEW, Washington, DC.

Tables from Lifetime Health Related Physical Fitness Test Manual, ADHPERD, Reston, VA., 1980. With permission of the American Alliance for Health, Physical Education, Recreation and Dance.

Dietary Reference Intakes: RDAs and AIs

Food and Nutrition Board, Institute of Medicine-National Academy of Sciences—Dietary Reference Intakes: Recommended levels for individual intake[a]

Life-stage group	Calcium (mg/d)	Phosphorus (mg/d)	Magnesium (mg/d)	Vitamin D[b,c] (µg/d)	Fluoride (mg/d)	Thiamin (mg/d)	Riboflavin (mg/d)	Niacin[d] (mg/d)	Vitamin B-6 (mg/d)	Folate[e] (µg/d)	Vitamin B-12 (µg/d)	Pantothenic Acid (mg/d)	Biotin (µg/d)	Choline[f] (mg/d)
Infants														
0-6 mo	210*	100*	30*	5*	0.01*	0.2*	0.3*	2*	0.1*	65*	0.4*	1.7*	5*	125*
7-12 mo	270*	275*	75*	5*	0.5*	0.3*	0.4*	4*	0.3*	80*	0.5*	1.8*	6*	150*
Children														
1-3 y	500*	460	80	5*	0.7*	0.5	0.5	6	0.5	150	0.9	2*	8*	200*
4-8 y	800*	500	130	5*	1*	0.6	0.6	8	0.6	200	1.2	3*	12*	250*
Males														
9-13 y	1,300*	1,250*	240	5*	2*	0.9	0.9	12	1.0	300	1.8	4*	20*	375*
14-18 y	1,300*	1,250*	410	5*	3*	1.2	1.3	16	1.3	400	2.4	5*	25*	550*
19-30 y	1,000*	700	400	5*	4*	1.2	1.3	16	1.3	400	2.4	5*	30*	550*
31-50 y	1,000*	700	420	5*	4*	1.2	1.3	16	1.3	400	2.4	5*	30*	550*
51-70 y	1,200*	700	420	10*	5*	1.2	1.3	16	1.7	400	2.4[g]	5*	30*	550*
>70 y	1,200*	700	420	15*	4*	1.2	1.3	16	1.7	400	2.4[g]	5*	30*	550*
Females														
9-13 y	1,300*	1,250*	240	5*	2*	0.9	0.9	12	1.0	300	1.8	4*	20*	375*
14-18 y	1,300*	1,250*	360	5*	3*	1.0	1.0	14	1.2	400[h]	2.4	5*	25*	400*
19-30 y	1,000*	700	310	5*	3*	1.1	1.1	14	1.3	400[h]	2.4	5*	30*	425*
31-50 y	1,000*	700	320	5*	3*	1.1	1.1	14	1.3	400[h]	2.4	5*	30*	425*
51-70 y	1,200*	700	320	10*	3*	1.1	1.1	14	1.5	400	2.4[g]	5*	20*	425*
>70 y	1,200*	700	320	15*	3*	1.1	1.1	14	1.5	400	2.4[g]	5*	30*	425*
Pregnancy														
≤18 y	1,300*	1,250*	400	5*	3*	1.4	1.4	18	1.9	600[i]	2.6	6*	30*	450*
19-30 y	1,000*	700	350	5*	3*	1.4	1.4	18	1.9	600[i]	2.6	6*	30*	450*
31-50 y	1,000*	700	360	5*	3*	1.4	1.4	18	1.9	600[i]	2.6	6*	30*	450*
Lactation														
≤18 y	1,300*	1,250*	360	5*	3*	1.5	1.6	17	2.0	500	2.8	7*	35*	550*
19-30 y	1,000*	700	310	5*	3*	1.5	1.6	17	2.0	500	2.8	7*	35*	550*
31-50 y	1,000*	700	320	5*	3*	1.5	1.6	17	2.0	500	2.8	7*	35*	550*

[a]Recommended Dietary Allowances (RDAs) are presented in bold type and Adequate intakes (AIs) in ordinary type followed by an asterisk (*). RDAs and AIs may both be used as goals for individual intake. RDAs are set to meet the needs of most all (97% to 98%) individuals in a group. For healthy breast-fed infants, the AI is the mean intake. The AI for other life-stage and gender groups is believed to cover needs of all individuals in the group, but lack of data or uncertainty in the data prevent being able to specify with confidence the percentage of persons covered by this intake.

[b]As cholecalciferol. 1 µg cholecalciferol = 40 IU vitamin D.

[c]In the absence of adequate exposure to sunlight.

[d]As niacin equivalents (NE). 1 mg niacin=60 mg tryptophan; 0 to 6 mo = performed niacin (not NE).

[e]As dietary folate equivalent (DFE). 1 DFE = 1 µg food folate = 0.6 µg folic acid (from fortified food or supplement) consumed with food = 0.5 µg synthetic (supplemental) folic acid taken on an empty stomach.

[f]Although AIs have been set for choline, there are few data to assess whether a dietary supply of choline is needed at all stages of the life cycle, and it may be that the choline requirement can be met by endogenous synthesis at some of these stages.

[g]Because 10% to 30% of older people may malabsorb food-bound vitamin B-12, it is advisable for those older than 50 years to meet their RDA mainly by consuming foods fortified with vitamin B-12 or a supplement containing vitamin B-12.

[h]In view of evidence linking folate intake with neural tube defects in the fetus, it is recommended that all women capable of becoming pregnant consume 400 µg synthetic folic acid from fortified foods and/or supplements in addition to intake of food folate from a varied diet,

[i]It is assumed that women will continue consuming 400 µg folic acid until their pregnancy is confirmed and they enter prenatal care, which ordinarily occurs after the end of the periconceptional period—the critical time for formation of the neural tube.

Source: From Dietary Reference Intakes, copyright © 1998, by the National Academy of Sciences, National Academy Press, Washington, DC, with permission.

Dietary Reference Intake Values for Vitamin C by Life Stage and Gender Group

Life Stage Group	RDA (mg/d)[b]		AI (mg/d)[c]	
	Male	Female	Male	Female
0 through 6 mo			40	40
7 through 12 mo			50	50
1 through 3 y	15	15		
4 through 8 y	25	25		
9 through 13 y	45	45		
14 through 18 y	75	65		
19 through 30 y	90	75		
31 through 50 y	90	75		
51 through 70 y	90	75		
>70 y	90	75		
Pregnancy				
−18 y		80		
19 through 50 y		85		
Lactation				
−18 y		115		
19 through 50 y		120		

[b]RDA = Recommended Dietary Allowance. The intake that meets the nutrient needs of almost all (97-98 percent) individuals in a group.

[c]AI = Adequate Intake. The observed average or experimentally set intake by a defined population or subgroup that appears to sustain a defined nutritional status, such as a growth rate, normal circulating nutrient values, or other functional indicators of health. An AI is used if sufficient scientific evidence is not available to derive an EAR. For healthy human milk-fed infants, the AI is the mean intake. **The AI is not equivalent to an RDA.**

Dietary Reference Intake Values for α-Tocopherol[a] by Life Stage Group

Life Stage Group[b]	RDA (mg/d)[d]	AI (mg/d)[e]
0 through 6 mo		4
7 through 12 mo		6
1 through 3 y	6	
4 through 8 y	7	
9 through 13 y	11	
14 through 18 y	15	
19 through 30 y	15	
31 through 50 y	15	
51 through 70 y	15	
>70 y	15	
Pregnancy		
−18 y	15	
19 through 50 y	15	
Lactation		
−18 y	19	
19 through 50 y	19	

[a]α-Tocopherol includes *RRR*-α-tocopherol, the only form of α-tocopherol that occurs naturally in foods, and the 2*R*-stereoisomeric forms of α-tocopherol (*RRR*-, *RSR*-, *RRS*-, and *RSS*-α-tocopherol) that occur in fortified foods and supplements. Does not include the 2*S*-stereoisomeric forms of α-tocopherol (*SRR*-, *SSR*-, *SRS*-, and *SSS*-α-tocopherol), also found in fortified foods and supplements.

[b]All groups except Pregnancy and Lactation are males and females.

[d]RDA = Recommended Dietary Allowance. The intake that meets the nutrient needs of almost all (97-98 percent) individuals in a group.

[e]AI = Adequate Intake. The observed average or experimentally set intake by a defined population or subgroup that appears to sustain a defined nutritional status, such as growth rate, normal circulating nutrient values, or other functional indicators of health. An AI is used if sufficient scientific evidence is not available to derived an EAR. For healthy human milk-fed infants, the AI is the mean intake. **The AI is not equivalent to an RDA.**

Source: From Dietary Reference Intakes for Vitamin C, Vitamin E, Selenium, and Carotenoids, © 2000, by the National Academy of Sciences, National Academy Press, Washington, DC, with permission.

Dietary Reference Intake Values for Selenium by Life Stage Group

Life Stage Group[a]	RDA (µg/d)[c]	AI (µg/d)[d]
0 through 6 mo		15
7 through 12 mo		20
1 through 3 y	20	
4 through 8 y	30	
9 through 13 y	40	
14 through 18 y	55	
19 through 30 y	55	
31 through 50 y	55	
51 through 70 y	55	
> 70 y	55	
Pregnancy		
− 18 y	60	
19 through 50 y	60	
Lactation		
− 18 y	70	
19 through 50 y	70	

[a]All groups except Pregnancy and Lactation are males and females.

[c]RDA = Recommended Dietary Allowance. The intake that meets the nutrient needs of almost all (97-98 percent) individuals in a group.

[d]AI = Adequate Intake. The observed average or experimentally set intake by a defined population or subgroup that appears to sustain a defined nutritional status, such as growth rate, normal circulating nutrient values, or other functional indicators of health. An AI is used if sufficient scientific evidence is not available to derived an EAR. For healthy human milk-fed infants, the AI is the mean intake. **The AI is not equivalent to an RDA.**

Source: From Dietary Reference Intakes for Vitamin C, Vitamin E, Selenium, and Carotenoids, © 2000, by the National Academy of Sciences, National Academy Press, Washington, DC, with permission.

Dietary Reference Intakes: ULs

Tolerable Upper Intake Levels[a] (ULs) for certain nutrients[b]

Life-stage group	Calcium (g/d)	Phosphorus (g/d)	Magnesium[c] (mg/d)	Vitamin D (µg/d)	Fluoride (mg/d)	Niacin[d] (mg/d)	Vitamin B-6 (mg/d)	Synthetic folic acid[d] (µg/d)	Choline (g/d)
0-6 mo	ND[e]	ND	ND	25	0.7	ND	ND	ND	ND
7-12 mo	ND	ND	ND	25	0.9	ND	ND	ND	ND
1-3 y	2.5	3	65	50	1.3	01	30	300	1.0
4-8 y	2.5	3	110	50	2.2	15	40	400	1.0
9-13 y	2.5	4	350	50	10	20	60	600	2.0
14-18 y	2.5	4	350	50	10	30	80	800	3.0
19-17 y	2.5	4	350	50	10	35	100	1,000	3.5
>70 y	2.5	3	350	50	10	35	100	1,000	3.5
Pregnancy									
≤ 18 y	2.5	3.5	350	50	10	30	80	800	3.0
19-50 y	2.5	3.5	350	50	10	35	100	1,000	3.5
Lactation									
≤ 18 y	2.5	4	350	50	10	30	80	800	3.0
19-50 y	2.5	4	350	50	10	35	100	1,000	3.5

[a]UL = the maximum level of daily intake that is likely to pose no risk of adverse effects. Unless otherwise specified, the UL represents total intake from food, water, and supplements. Due to lack of suitable data, ULs could not be established for thiamin, riboflavin, vitamin B-12, pantothenic acid, or biotin. In the absence of ULs, extra caution may be warranted in consuming levels above recommended intake.

[b]Source: references 1 and 5.

[c]The UL for magnesium represents intake from a pharmacological agent only and does not include intake from food and water.

[d]The ULs for niacin and synthetic folic acid apply to forms obtained from supplements, fortified foods, or a combination of the two.

[e]ND: Not determinable due to lack of data of adverse effects in this age group and concern with regard to lack of ability to handle excess amounts. Source of intake should be from food only to prevent high levels of intake.

Tolerable Upper Intake Levels (UL[a]) by Life Stage Group

Life Stage Group	Vitamin C (mg/d)	α-Tocopherol (mg/d)[b]	Selenium (µg/d)
0 through 6 mo	ND[c]	ND	45
7 through 12 mo	ND	ND	60
1 through 3 y	400	200	90
4 through 8 y	650	300	150
9 through 13 y	1,200	600	280
14 through 18 y	1,800	800	400
19 through 70 y	2,000	1,000	400
>70 y	2,000	1,000	400
Pregnancy			
−18 y	1,800	800	400
19 through 50 y	2,000	1,000	400
Lactation			
−18 y	1,800	800	400
19 through 50 y	2,000	1,000	400

[a]The UL is the highest level of daily nutrient intake that is likely to pose no risk of adverse health effects to almost all individuals in the general population. As intake increases above the UL, the risk of adverse effects increases. Unless specified otherwise, the UL represents total nutrient intake from food, water, and supplements.
[b]The UL for α-tocopherol applies to any form of supplemental α-tocopherol.
[c]ND. Not determinable due to lack of data of adverse effects in this age group and concern with regard to lack of ability to handle excess amounts. Source of intake should be from food and formula in order to prevent high levels of intake.

Source: From Dietary Reference Intakes for Vitamin E. Selenium, and Carotenoids, © 2000, by the National Academy of Sciences, National Academy Press, Washington, DC, with permission.

Recommended Dietary Allowances, 1989

Recommended Dietary Allowances (RDA), Revised 1989[a]

Age (Years)	Weight[b] (kg)	Weight[b] (lb)	Height[b] (cm)	Height[b] (inches)	Fat-Soluble Vitamins (g) Protein)	Fat-Soluble Vitamins (µg RE)[c] Vitamin A	Fat-Soluble Vitamins (µg) Vitamin K	Minerals (mg) Iron	Minerals (mg) Zinc	Minerals (µg) Iodine
Infants										
0.0-0.5	6	13	60	24	13	375	5	6	5	40
0.5-1.0	9	20	7	28	14	375	10	10	5	50
Children										
1-3	13	29	90	35	16	400	15	10	10	70
4-6	20	44	112	44	24	500	20	10	10	90
7-10	28	62	132	52	28	700	30	10	10	120
Males										
11-14	45	99	107	62	45	1000	45	12	15	150
15-18	66	145	176	69	59	1000	65	12	15	150
19-24	72	160	177	70	58	1000	70	10	15	150
25-50	79	174	176	70	63	1000	80	10	15	150
51+	77	170	173	68	63	1000	80	10	15	150
Females										
11-14	46	101	157	62	46	800	45	15	12	150
15-18	55	120	163	64	44	800	55	15	12	150
19-24	58	128	164	65	46	800	60	15	12	150
25-50	63	138	163	64	50	800	65	15	12	150
51+	65	143	160	63	50	800	65	10	12	150
Pregnant					60	800	65	30	15	175
Lactating										
1st 6 months					65	1300	65	15	19	200
2nd 6 months					62	1200	65	15	16	200

[a]The allowances, expressed as average daily intakes over time, are intended to provide for individual variations among most normal persons as they live in the United States under usual environmental stresses. Diets should be based on a variety of common foods in order to provide other nutrients for which human requirements have been less well defined.

[b]Weights and heights of Reference Adults are actual medians for the U.S. population of the designated age, as reported by NHANES II. The use of these figures does not imply that the height-to-weight ratios are ideal.

[c]Retinol equivalents. 1 retinol equivalent = 1 µg retinol or 6 µg β-carotene. See Clinical Calculation 6–1 to convert IU of vitamin A to retinol equivalents.

Note: The Committee on Dietary Allowances has published a separate table showing energy allowances which appears as Table 8–4.

Source: From Recommended Dietary Allowances, © 1989, by the National Academy of Sciences, National Academy Press, Washington, DC, with permission.

APPENDIX I

Estimated Safe and Adequate Daily Dietary Intakes of Selected Minerals, 1989[a]

	Age (Years)	Trace Elements[b]			
		Copper (mg)	Manganese (mg)	Chromium (µg)	Molybdenum (µg)
Infants	0–0.5	0.4–0.6	0.3–0.6	10–40	15–30
	0.5–1	0.6–0.7	0.6–1.0	20–60	20–40
Children and adolescents	1–3	0.7–1.0	1.0–1.5	20–80	25–50
	4–6	1.0–1.5	1.5–2.0	30–120	30–75
	7–10	1.0–2.0	2.0–3.0	50–200	50–150
	11+	1.5–2.5	2.0–5.0	50–200	75–250
Adults		1.5–3.0	2.0–5.0	50–200	75–250

[a]Because there is less information on which to base allowances, these figures are not given in the main table of RDA and are provided here in the form of ranges of recommended intakes.

[b]Since the toxic levels for many trace elements may be only several times usual intakes, the upper levels for the trace elements given in this table should not be habitually exceeded.

Source: From Recommended Dietary Allowances, © 1989, by the National Academy of Sciences, National Academy Press, Washington, DC, with permission.

Estimated Sodium, Chloride, and Potassium Minimum Requirements of Healthy Persons[a]

Age	Weight (kg)[d]	Sodium (mg)[a,b]	Chloride (mg)[a,b]	Potassium (mg)[c]
Months				
0–5	4.5	120	180	500
6–11	8.9	200	300	700
Years				
1	11.0	225	350	1,000
2–5	16.0	300	500	1,400
6–9	25.0	400	600	1,600
10–18	50.0	500	750	2,000
>18[d]	70.0	500	750	2,000

[a]No allowance has been included for large, prolonged losses from the skin through sweat.

[b]There is no evidence that higher intakes confer any health benefit.

[c]Desirable intakes of potassium may considerably exceed these values (~3,500 mg for adults—see text).

[d]No allowance included for growth. Values for those below 18 years assume a growth rate at the 50th percentile reported by the National Center for Health Statistics (Hamill et al., 1979) and averaged for males and females. See text for information on pregnancy and lactation.

Source: From Recommended Dietary Allowances, © 1989, by the National Academy of Sciences, National Academy Press, Washington, DC, with permission.

Medical Nutritional Formulas

MODULAR FORMULAS

A modular formula contains only one nutrient and can be used to supplement the diet orally or as an additional component of a tube feeding.

Nutrient	Formula	Comments
Protein	*Casec* *ProMod* *Propac* *Pro-Mix*	Orally best used as an additive to soups, beverages, cooked cereals, canned fruits, and gravies. Used when protein intake is inadequate to meet need.
Carbohydrate	*Polycose* *Moducal* *Sumacal* *Nutrisource*	Orally best added to fruits and fruit juices. Frequently used for protein-fat-electrolyte-restricted diets to boost kilocalories.
Fat	*MCT oil*	Orally best used in milkshakes and hot cereals and as an oil. Contains medium-chain triglycerides and is used for lipid malabsorption.

Selected Elemental Formulas

Elemental formulas are designed for metabolically stressed patients with impaired GI function. Most of the nutrients are predigested.

Formula	Description	Comments
Sandosource Peptide *Tolerex* *Vivonex Plus* *Vivonex TEN* *Crucial* *Peptamen* *Peptamen VHP* *Reabilian* *Criticare HN* *Vivionex Pediatric* *Vital HN*	Complete nutritional supplements that meet 100% of the U.S. RDA for Vit/Min in a specified volume.	Expensive—should be used only if indicated. May be given orally or as a tube feeding. Not acceptable orally to many patients.

Complete Nutritional Supplements

Complete nutritional supplements (CNS) contain all the essential nutrients in a specified volume. There are dozens of these products. Some of them are designed for oral use and some are designed for tube feedings. Most healthcare facilities select only one or two of these formulas to use as the standard in-house formula.

Product	Manufacturer	Description	Volume for 100% U.S. RDA	MOsm/kg water	Kcal/ml	Protein grams/1000 kcal
Sustacal Basic	Mead Johnson	Oral Supplement Intact Protein	1890	500	1.06	33
Sustacal Plus	Mead Johnson	Oral Supplement Intact Protein	1180	630–670	1.52	40.1
Resource Standard	Novartis	Oral Supplement Intact Protein	1890	430	1.06	34.9
Ensure	Ross Products, Abbott Laboratories	Oral Supplement Intact Protein	948	555	1.06	35.1
Ensure Plus	Ross Products, Abbott Laboratories	Oral Supplement Intact Protein	1420	690	1.5	36.6
Ensure Plan High Nitrogen	Ross Products, Abbott Laboratories	Oral Supplement Intact Protein	947	650	1.5	41.7
Sustacal Liquid	Mead Johnson	High Protein Intact Protein Oral Supplement	1080	650–690	1.0	61
Ensure High Protein	Ross Products, Abbott Laboratories	High Protein Intact Protein Oral Supplement	948	610	0.95	53.3
Jevity	Ross Products, Abbott Laboratories	Tube Feeding Intact Protein Fiber Containing	1321	300	1.06	41.8
Jevity Plus	Ross Products, Abbott Laboratories	Tube Feeding Intact Protein Fiber Containing	1000	450	1.2	46.3
FiberSource HN	Novaritis	Tube Feeding Intact Protein Fiber Containing	1500	390	1.2	44.2

Specilized Formulas

Product	Manufacturer	Description	Volume for 100% U.S. RDA	MOsm/kg water	Kcal/ml	Protein grams/1000 kcal
Nepro	Ross Products, Abbott Laboratories	Renal Dialysis	960	665	2.0	70
Suplena	Ross Products, Abbott Laboratories	Renal Insufficiency	960	600	2.0	30
Impact	Novartis	Critical Care Healing Support	1500	375	1.0	56
Replete	Nestle Clinical Nutrition	Critical Care Healing Support Diets	1000	300–350	1.0	62.5
TraumaCal	Mead Johnson	Critical Care Healing Support	2000	560	1.5	54.7
Promote with Fiber	Ross Products, Abbott Laboratories	Critical Care Healing Support	1000	370	1.0	62.5
Glucerna	Ross Products, Abbott Laboratories	Glucose Intolerance	1422	355	1.0	41.8
Hepatic-Aid II	McGaw	Hepatic	N/A	560	1.2	36.8
PediaSure	Ross Products, Abbott Laboratories	Pediatric	1000 (children 1–6) 1300 (children 7–10)	345	1.0	30
Amin-Aid	R & D Laboratories	Renal	N/A	700	2.0	9.7
Pulmocare	Ross Products Abbott Laboratories	Pulmonary	947	475	1.5	16.7

Client Teaching Aids

1200-Calorie Simplified Meal Plan

Breakfast:
1/2 cup orange juice or 1/2 banana or 1 fresh orange
1 small bagel or 2 slices of toast or 1 slice of toast and 1/2 cup cooked cereal
1 egg or 1 oz or low-fat cheese
1 cup of skim milk

Lunch and Dinner:
2 oz. of processed lunch meat with 3 grams of fat or less per oz or 1/2 cup water pack tuna or
    1/2 cup of cottage cheese or 2 oz. of any lean meat
1 slice of bread or 6 small crackers or 1/2 cup of cooked pasta or 3/4 oz matzoh or 1/3 cup couscous
    or 1/2 cup of rice
1/2 to 1 cup of vegetables
1 small piece of fresh fruit or 1/2 cup of 100% fruit juice or 1-1/4 cup of fresh berries or melon
1 teaspoon of margarine or 1 tbsp. of salad dressing or 2 Tbsp. of reduced-fat salad dressing or 1 tsp. olive or
canola oil or 5 large olives or 2 whole walnuts

Snack:
1 cup of skim milk
1 small piece of fresh fruit or 1/2 cup of 100% fruit juice or 1-1/4 cup of fresh berries or melon

1500-Calorie Simplified Meal Plan

Breakfast:
1 cup orange juice or 1 banana or 1/4 cup of raisins
1/2 of a small bagel or 1 slice of toast or 1/2 cup cooked cereal
1 cup of skim milk
2 tsp. of margarine or 2 tbsp. of cream cheese

Lunch and Dinner:
3 oz. of processed lunch meat with 3 grams of fat or less per oz or 3/4 cup water pack tuna or
    3/4 cup of cottage cheese or 3 oz of any lean meat or 1 cup of tofu
2 slices of bread or 12 small crackers or 1 cup of cooked pasta or 1-1/2 oz matzoh or 2/3 cup couscous or
    2/3 cup of rice or 1 small baked potato
1/2 to 1 cup of vegetables
1 small piece of fresh fruit or 1/2 cup of 100% fruit juice or 1-1/4 cup of fresh berries or melon
1 tsp. of margarine or 1 tbsp. of salad dressing or 2 tbsp. of reduced-fat salad dressing or 1 tsp. olive or canola
    oil or 5 large olives or 2 whole walnuts

Snack:
1 cup of skim milk or 1 cup of plain unsweetened yogurt
1 slice of bread or 5 small crackers or 3/4 cup of unsweetened cold cereal or 1-1/2 cup of fat-free popcorn
1 small piece of fresh fruit or 1/2 cup of 100% fruit juice or 1-1/4 cup of fresh berries or melon

Sodium-Restricted Diet

Description

A sodium-restricted diet is often recommended to assist in the control of blood pressure and/or prevent water retention. The level of restriction (measured in grams or milligrams of sodium) depends on individual tolerance for sodium.

Sodium is in table salt, foods, medications, and water. Approximately one-half of salt is sodium. A sodium-restricted diet restricts the use of table salt and many foods processed with salt and sodium. Food naturally contains sodium. Sometimes a recommendation is made to restrict the intake of milk, regular salted breads, cereal, meat, and salted fats. If this is your situation, please consult a registered dietitian to prevent a nutritional deficiency. Local water supplies and water that has been chemically softened may contain considerable sodium. Sometimes a recommendation is made to drink bottled sodium-free water. Read food and medication labels and avoids those products that contain excessive amounts of sodium.

Nutritional Adequacy

The suggested meal plan provides foods in amounts that meet the recommended standards for all nutrients (except iron for females) for the average adult.

Food Group from Food Pyramid Model/ Recommended Intake	Foods Recommended	Foods Not Recommended	Hints
Grain Group/ 6–11 servings per day	Bread products without salted tops Cooked cereals Cold cereals without excessive added sodium (check label or speak with a dietitian) Puffed Wheat, Puffed Rice, and Shredded Wheat Homemade bread products without excessive added salt Rice and pasta To lower sodium further purchase bread products made without any salt, soda, and baking powder (this isn't necessary for all individuals on sodium-restricted diets)	Bread products that look salty Instant hot cereals Seasoned pasta and rice mixes	Choose whole grains whenever possible The first ingredient on the food label after the word *ingredient* should be whole wheat or whole grain
Vegetable Group/ 3-5 servings per day	Vegetables are naturally low in sodium Fresh, frozen, or unsalted canned vegetables	Most canned vegetables, unless labeled unsalted, are higher in sodium than those recommended Sauerkraut Vegetables juices can contain excessive sodium Frozen convenience vegetable casseroles frequency contain excessive sodium	Try to eat at least 3 servings per day—most people do not eat enough vegetables Try to include a green or yellow vegetable each day
Fruits/ 2 to 4 servings per day	Fruits are naturally low in sodium	Some dried fruits contain sodium preservatives and should be avoided	Remember to include a source of vitamin C each day (citrus, cantaloupe, strawberries)

Food Group from Food Pyramid Model/ Recommended Intake	Foods Recommended	Foods Not Recommended	Hints
Milk / 2–3 servings	Most	Buttermilk is higher in sodium than other milk products Malted milk and other milk mixes may contain appreciable amounts of sodium	Many individual's diets lack sufficient calcium, which is essential for healthy bones, because they do not drink milk
Meat and Meat Substitute Group/ 2–3 servings	Unprocessed meat, fish, and poultry Eggs Low-sodium peanut butter Dried peas and beans Tofu	Processed meats: canned, salted, smoked, and cured including lunch meats, bacon, ham, sausage, hot dogs Many convenience meat products—check labels Salted nuts	Frozen convenience meat products that contain more than 500 mg of sodium per serving should be used infrequently Many low- and reduced-sodium meat products are available, such as reduced-sodium hot dogs
Others/ Oils, sweets, and desserts	Lemons, limes, cornstarch, flour, unsalted popcorn, vinegar, low-sodium catsup, low-sodium mustard, cocoa powder, cream of tartar, homemade unsalted gravies, unsalted broth and bouillon Avoid seasonings with the word *salt* such as celery salt. Use celery powder instead	Olives, salted condiments such as catsup, mustard, mayonnaise, relishes, steak sauces, barbecue sauce, soy sauce, monosodium glutamate (MSG), Worcestershire sauce, bacon bits, prepared horseradish sauce, dill pickles	There are many salt-free seasoning mixes in the grocery store Salted snack foods such as potato chips and salted pretzels are very high in sodium Remember sodium is an acquired taste and most people can adjust to a lower sodium intake in time. Many people find the use of highly salted foods objectionable especially after they have followed a sodium-restricted diet for some time.

Meal Plan – approximately 1250 mg of sodium

Breakfast
1 cup skim milk
1/2 cup unsalted oatmeal
1 slice of whole grain bread
1 teaspoon of margarine and jelly
1/2 cup of orange juice
Coffee, if desired

Lunch and Dinner
2–3 oz of unsalted unprocessed meat or meat substitute
1/2 cup of low-sodium and unsalted whole grain pasta or rice
1/2 cup of an unsalted vegetable
Fresh fruit
Whole-grain dinner roll
1 teaspoon of margarine
Green leafy salad at one meal with an unsalted salad dressing or vinegar and monounsaturated oil
1 cup of skim milk at one meal
Coffee or tea, if desired
To decrease sodium further, encourage the use of unsalted bread and margarine.
To increase sodium further, increase the servings of whole grains from 3 to 6 per day and margarine from 3 tsp. to 5 tsp.

WHAT TO CONSIDER BEFORE TAKING DIETARY SUPPLEMENTS

Items sold as dietary supplements in the United States do not receive the same oversight from the Food and Drug Administration as that given to food and prescription or over-the-counter drugs. Nevertheless, many supplements have effects equal in power to those of drugs.

Some people have experienced problems because of the lack of product standardization, poor quality control, and contamination with harmful substances.

If you decide to take dietary supplements:
- Discuss your desires and plans with your primary healthcare provider.
- Treat the supplement as medicine. You are expecting medicinal results.
- Store the supplements in childproof containers.
- Take the product as directed.
- Add just one supplement at a time. Observe for desired actions and for side effects.
- Discontinue use and report to your primary healthcare provider if desired effects do not occur or if new symptoms appear.
- Use the supplements for short periods of time only.
- Inform surgeons and anesthesiologists of your intake. They may want you to stop taking supplements 2–3 weeks before scheduled surgery.
- Purchase the products from a reputable supplier. Use the same brand consistently. European sources are preferable to Asian ones. Some suppliers that have been recommended in the scientific literature are:

N.S.D. Products, P.O. Box 880, Brandon, MS 39043
Phone 601-825-6831   Fax 601-825-5575
Physiologics, 6565 Odell Place, Boulder, CO 80301-3330
Phone 800-765-6775   Fax 303-530-2592
PhytoPharmica, 825 Challenger Dr., Green Bay, WI 54311
Phone 800-553-2370   Fax 920-469-4418

DO NOT:
- Do not give supplements or medicinal teas to infants or children.
- Do not consume supplements if you are pregnant, planning to become pregnant, or are breast-feeding.
- Do not take supplements if you are elderly.
- Do not use supplements if you are subject to allergies, except with careful investigation and extreme caution.
- Do not add to your treatment plan any products with the same effects as other drugs you are taking, particularly blood thinners or aspirin and other nonsteroidal anti-inflammatory drugs (NSAIDS).

It is best to avoid the following botanicals: borage, chaparral, comfrey, ephedra, germander, kombucha, lobelia, pennyroyal, sassafras, and wormwood.

Monitor for side effects and report them to your primary healthcare provider or to the **FDA's MEDWATCH at 1-800-FDA-1088** or on the Internet at http://www.fda.gov/medwatch/report/consumer/consumer.htm

SURVIVAL SKILLS FOR PATIENTS WITH DIABETES ON MEDICATION

ACCEPTABLE BLOOD GLUCOSE LEVELS

A normal blood glucose level is between 60 and 120 mg/dL before a meal and less than 140 mg/dL 2 hours after a meal. Glycosylated hemoglobin is a test that measures the average blood glucose for the past 60 days. The physician typically determines acceptable blood glucose and glycosylated hemoglobin for clients with diabetes. Here are some guidelines:

- *Intensive Treatment*: 70–140 mg/dL before meals; less than 180 mg/dL 2 hours after meals; glycosylated hemoglobin within 1 percent of normal.
- *Average Treatment:* 80–160 mg/dL before meals; less than 200 mg/dL 2 hours after meals; glycosylated hemoglobin within 2 percent of normal

HYPERGLYCEMIA (BLOOD GLUCOSE GREATER THAN 250 mg/dL)

Controlling your diabetes means dealing with your blood glucose when it is too high. This condition can occur rapidly or gradually. Usually, you will be able to lower your own blood glucose. There are times, however, when emergency care is needed.

Causes

- Too little insulin or oral medication
- Too much food
- Less activity or exercise than usual
- More stress than usual
- Illness, infection, or injury

Symptoms

- Fatigue
- Increased thirst
- Unexplained weight loss
- Blurry vision
- Increased hunger
- Dry mouth and skin
- Increased urination

Treatment

- Check your blood glucose more frequently.
- **Take your insulin or oral medication as prescribed (adjust dosage only if told to do so by your doctor).**
- Follow your meal plan, adding more calorie-free liquids.
- Follow the 4 sick day rules listed below.

HYPOGLYCEMIA (BLOOD GLUCOSE LESS THAN 60 mg/dL)

Controlling blood glucose means dealing with your blood glucose when it drops too low. This condition is called hypoglycemia.

Causes of Hypoglycemia

- Too much insulin or oral medication
- More exercise or activity than usual
- Skipping or delaying meals or snacks or eating less food than usual

Signs

- Slurred speech
- Headache
- Tingling of lips
- Coma
- Weakness
- Nervousness

- Sweating
- Tremors
- Hunger
- Rapid heart beat
- Confusion/disorientation

Treatment

1. Test your blood glucose immediately.
2. Quickly take 15 grams of carbohydrate; 15 grams of carbohydrate is equal to any of the foods listed in the Food Substitutions When Ill section or:

3 glucose tabs (from pharmacy)	6 hard candies
1 tube of glucose gel (from pharmacy)	1 fruit exchange
8 oz. of skim milk (no fat)	1 starch exchange
4 oz. juice or regular cola	

3. Test your blood glucose again 15 minutes later.
4. If your blood glucose has not risen, take another glucose dose as above.
5. Treatment of low blood glucose should not take the place of a meal or snack.
6. Eat a meal.

EXERCISE GUIDELINES

Before beginning any exercise program, consult your doctor, especially if you are over age 40 or have had diabetes for 10 years or longer.

General Recommendations

1. Type of Exercise: Aerobic, high repetitions, low weight-bearing
2. Frequency: Daily exercise aids blood glucose control
3. Duration: 40–60 minutes; longer than 40 minutes is required to begin breakdown of body fat
4. Timing: 60–90 minutes after meals when the blood glucose level is highest; consistency in time of day will assist in the regulation of blood glucose levels

Benefits of Exercise

- Helps your body use insulin more effectively
- Can lower blood glucose levels
- Strengthens heart and lungs
- Reduces body fat and increases muscle
- Assists with weight control
- Helps you cope with stress
- Helps improve body image
- Lowers blood pressure

Risks of Exercise

- Certain types of exercise may worsen eye, kidney, or nerve problems.
- Blood pressure may rise higher during exercise in people with diabetes than in those without diabetes.

- People with diabetes are at increased risk for heart problems. **Stop exercising and consult your doctor if you have any of the following symptoms: chest pain, unusual fatigue, dizziness, visual disturbances, or nausea.**
- Know how to prevent hypoglycemia if you take insulin or diabetes pills.
- Wear your diabetes ID during exercise.

Special Considerations for Patients with Type 2 Diabetes
- Food intake must be regulated and maintained, not increased, despite increased appetite.
- Check your blood glucose level before and after exercise.
- Exercise is most beneficial when the blood glucose level is below 200 mg/dL.
- Exercise in the evening may benefit blood glucose levels the next morning.
- Regular exercise is more beneficial than sporadic exercise.
- Exercise is best done 60–90 minutes after eating.

SICK DAY GUIDELINES
Illness, such as a cold or flu, can cause serious problems with diabetes control. The four main rules for sick day management are:
1. Continue to take the insulin or diabetes pill prescribed.
2. Test blood glucose frequently (every 2–4 hours); record results.
3. Frequent fluid intake is recommended (8–12 oz/hour).
4. Try to eat the usual amount of carbohydrate (milk, fruit, and starch exchanges), divided into smaller meals and snacks if necessary; if blood glucose is 250 mg/dL or higher, all of the usual amount of carbohydrate is not necessary. **Call your doctor if your blood glucose is higher than 250 mg/dL for more than two tests in a row.**

Food Substitutions When Ill
Each of the following may be substituted for a fruit or starch exchange on sick days:

1/2 cup regular gelatin	1/2 cup ice cream
1/4 cup sherbet	1/4 cup plain pudding
4 oz. cola	1 cup cream soup
6 oz. ginger ale	1 cup yogurt
1 Tbs. honey	1 Tbs. corn syrup
1 Tbs. brown sugar	

MEAL PLAN
What and when you eat influences your blood glucose levels. For this reason, it is necessary that you follow some type of meal plan. Many different types of meal plans are available for you to choose from including:
1. American Dietetic Association Food Exchange Lists
2. *Month of Meals*—menus for one month
3. Food Pyramid and Healthy Food Choices
4. Carbohydrate counting

The dietitian will assist you in the selection of an appropriate meal-planning system. The effectiveness of any diet is objectively evaluated by consistently monitoring lipid, glycosylated hemoglobin, and blood glucose levels as well as body weight.

Dietary Guidelines

The *Dietary Guidelines for Healthy Americans* was written with the intent to help reduce the risks associated with chronic disease in the general population (http://www.usda.gov). Almost all the risk factors for heart and circulatory diseases for the general population are more common in the diabetic population. For this reason, it is important to know and follow the dietary guidelines to reduce the risk of developing the chronic complications of diabetes.

1. Aim for fitness
   - Aim for a healthy body weight
   - Be physically active each day
2. Build a healthy base
   - Let the Pyramid guide your food choices
   - Choose a variety of whole grains each day
   - Choose a variety of fruits and vegetables
   - Keep food safe to eat
3. Choose sensibly
   - Choose a diet low in saturated fat and cholesterol and moderate in fat
   - Choose beverages and foods to moderate your intake of sugars
   - Choose and prepare foods with less salt
   - If you drink alcoholic beverages, do so in moderation

Eating Out

With the help of a meal plan, the person with diabetes can enjoy eating in restaurants. Care must be taken not to consume more fat and calories than usual. Some patients save their daily fat calories and use them at the meal that they plan to eat in the restaurant. Here is a list of suggestions for reducing fat and calories:
- Order salad dressings on the side
- Ask that broiled, grilled, or baked entrees be prepared without added oil, butter, or margarine.
- Request that vegetables, rice, potatoes, and pasta be prepared without fat.
- Select raw vegetables, fresh fruit, crackers, and diet dressing from salad bars.
- The key to reducing fat in a fast-food restaurant is to buy a small, plain hamburger, side salad, fruit juice, and skimmed milk.

Snacking

For persons with Type 2 diabetes, snacking is discouraged. Snacking prevents normalization of glucose levels during the day. Also, most persons with Type 2 diabetes are overweight, and weight reduction assists in the control of blood glucose levels. Some overweight people are unable to stop eating once they start.

Some people with Type 2 diabetes have a long history of snacking and are not willing to change their usual pattern of eating. For these individuals, snacks that contain less than 20 calories per serving may be the most feasible approach to weight control. Following is a list of low-calorie snacks:

Raw vegetables

1 cup air-popped popcorn

1/2 cup unsweetened rhubarb

7 pretzel sticks

2 gingersnaps

3 mini rice cakes

1/2 cup unsweetened cranberries

1 dill pickle (high in sodium)

2 vanilla wafers

ADDITIONAL TIPS

1. Drink alcohol in moderation only when your blood glucose has been in good control. Do *not* drink alcohol on an empty stomach if you take insulin or oral diabetes medication. It may cause a low blood sugar reaction.
2. Have an annual exam with a board-certified ophthalmologist (a doctor specializing in eye care).
3. Over the long term, diabetes can lead to foot problems, including infection and amputation. Check your feet (and legs) daily. Look between toes and on bottoms for sores, redness, infection, drainage, swelling, or bruises. Report problems to your doctor early. Keep your feet clean and wear clean, dry socks. Never go barefoot. Protect any area where sensation is lost.
4. Communicate with your family doctor. Maintain good daily records of your food intake, medication schedule, and blood glucose levels. Share these with your doctor.
5. Join the local chapter of the American Diabetes Association.
6. Eliminating smoking and controlling blood pressure and elevated blood cholesterol levels is important for reducing the risk of heart and circulatory problems. Controlling high blood pressure reduces the chance of having heart attacks, strokes, and kidney disease. Have your blood pressure checked at least once a year, and take blood pressure medication as prescribed.
7. A physician should promptly treat urinary tract infections. Contact your physician if you experience pain, burning, or urgency on urination. Frequent urination is also a symptom of a urinary tract infection.
8. Keep up-to-date on immunizations.

SURVIVAL SKILLS FOR PATIENTS WITH TYPE 2 DIABETES DIET CONTROLLED

ACCEPTABLE BLOOD GLUCOSE LEVELS
A normal blood glucose level is 60–120 mg/dL before a meal and less than 140 mg/dL after a meal. A glycosylated hemoglobin measures your average blood glucose for the past 60 days.   Acceptable blood glucose and glycosylated hemoglobin levels for patients with diabetes are typically within 1 percent of normal.

EXERCISE GUIDELINES
Before beginning any exercise program, consult your doctor, especially if you are over age 40 or have had diabetes for 10 years or longer.

General Recommendations
Type of Exercise: Aerobic, high repetitions, low weight-bearing
Frequency: Daily frequency aids blood glucose control
Duration: 40–60 minutes; longer than 40 minutes is required to begin breakdown of body fat
Timing: 60–90 minutes after meals when the blood glucose level is highest
Consistency in time of day will assist in the regulation of blood glucose levels

Benefits of Exercise
- Helps your body use insulin more effectively
- Can lower blood glucose levels
- Strengthens heart and lungs
- Reduces body fat and increases muscle
- Assists with weight control
- Helps you to cope with stress
- Helps improve body image
- Lowers blood pressure

Risks of exercise
Certain types of exercise may worsen eye, kidney, or nerve problems. Blood pressure may rise higher during exercise in people with diabetes than in those without diabetes.
People with diabetes are at increased risk for heart problems. **Stop exercising and consult your doctor if you have any of the following symptoms: chest pain, unusual fatigue, dizziness, visual disturbances or nausea.**
Wear your diabetes ID during exercise.

Special Considerations for patients with Type 2 Diabetes
- Food intake must be regulated and maintained, not increased despite increased appetite.
- Check your blood glucose level before and after exercise.
- Exercise is the most beneficial if your blood glucose is below 200 mg/dL.
- Exercise in the evening may benefit blood glucose levels the next morning.
- Regular exercise is more beneficial than sporadic exercise.
- Exercise is best done 60–90 minutes after eating.

HYPERGLYCEMIA (BLOOD GLUCOSE GREATER THAN 250 mg/dL)

Controlling your diabetes means dealing with your blood glucose when it is too high. This condition can occur rapidly or gradually. Usually, you will be able to lower your own blood glucose. There are times, however, when emergency care is needed.

Causes
- Too much food
- Less activity or exercise than usual
- More stress than usual
- Illness, infection, or injury

Symptoms
- Fatigue
- Blurry vision
- Dry mouth & skin
- Increased thirst
- Increased hunger
- Increased urination
- Unexplained weight loss

Treatment
- Check your blood glucose more frequently
- Follow your meal plan, adding more calorie free liquids
- Follow your exercise plan only if blood glucose level is less than 250 mg/dL

Meal Plan

Nutrition is an essential component of management for all persons with diabetes as diabetes is directly related to how the body uses food. Patients report improved health, better control over body weight and improved control of blood glucose and lipid levels when they adhere to dietary recommendations.

For all of these reasons, it is necessary to follow some type of meal plan. Many different types of meal plans are available for you to choose from including:
1. American Dietetic Association Food Exchange Lists
2. *Month of Meals* - menus for one month
3. Food Pyramid and "Healthy Food Choices"

The patient needs to select and follow an appropriate meal planning system. The effectiveness of any diet can be objectively evaluated by consistently monitoring lipid, glycosylated hemoglobin, and blood glucose levels and body weight. All meal-planning systems are based on the *Dietary Guidelines for Healthy Americans.*

Dietary Guidelines

The *Dietary Guidelines for Healthy Americans* was written with the intent to help reduce the risks associated with chronic disease in the general population (US Department of Agriculture and US Department of Health Education and Welfare). Almost all the risk factors for heart and circulatory diseases for the general population are more common in the diabetic population. For this reason, it is important to know the dietary guidelines and follow them to reduce the risk of developing the chronic complications of diabetes.

1. Aim for Fitness
   - Aim for a healthy body weight
   - Be physically active each day

2. Build a Healthy Base
   - Let the pyramid guide your food choices
   - Choose a variety of whole grains each day
   - Choose a variety of fruits and vegetables
   - Keep food safe to eat

3. Choose Sensibly
   - Choose a diet low in saturated fat and cholesterol and moderate in fat
   - Choose beverages and foods to moderate your intake of sugars
   - Choose and prepare foods with less salt
   - If you drink alcoholic beverages, do so in moderation

Eating Out

With the help of a meal plan, the person with diabetes can enjoy eating in restaurants. Care must be taken not to consume more fat and calories than usual. Some patients save their daily fat calories and use them at the meal that they plan to eat in the restaurant. Here is a list of suggestions for reducing fat and calories:
- Order salad dressings on the side
- Ask that broiled, grilled, or baked entrees be prepared without additional oil, butter, and margarine
- Request that vegetables, rice, potatoes, and pasta is prepared without fat
- Select raw vegetables, fresh fruit, crackers, and diet dressing from salad bars
   The key to reducing fat in a fast food restaurant is to buy small a plain hamburger, side salad, fruit juice, and skimmed milk.

Snacking

For persons with Type 2 diabetes, snacking is discouraged. Snacking prevents normalization of glucose levels during the day. Also, most persons with Type 2 diabetes are overweight and weight reduction assists in the control of blood glucose levels. Some overweight people are unable to stop eating once they start.

   Some people with Type 2 diabetes have a long history of snacking and are not willing to change their usual pattern of eating. For these individuals, snacks, which contain less than 20 calories per serving, may be the most feasible approach to weight control. Following is a list of low calorie snacks:

Raw vegetables	3 mini rice cakes
1-cup air-popped popcorn	1/2 cup unsweetened cranberries
1/2 cup unsweetened rhubarb	1 dill pickle (high in sodium)
7 pretzel sticks	2 vanilla wafers
	2 gingersnaps

ADDITIONAL TIPS

1. Drink alcohol in moderation only when your blood glucose has been in good control. Do **not** drink alcohol on an empty stomach as it may cause a low blood sugar reaction. Visible medical identification should be carried or worn when drinking away from home.
2. Have an annual exam with a board-certified ophthalmologist (a doctor specializing in eye care)
3. Over the long term, diabetes can lead to foot problems, including infection and amputation. Check your feet (and legs) daily. Look between toes and on bottoms for sores, redness, infection, drainage, swelling or bruises. Report problems to your doctor early. Keep your feet clean and wear clean dry socks. Never go barefoot. Protect any area where sensation is lost.
4. Eliminating smoking and controlling blood pressure and elevated blood cholesterol levels are important for reducing the risk or heart and circulatory problems. Controlling high blood pressure reduces the chance of having heart attacks, strokes, and kidney disease. Have your blood pressure checked at least once a year and take blood pressure medication as prescribed.
5. Urinary tract infections should be promptly treated by a physician. Contact your physician if you experience pain, burning, or urgency on urination. Frequent urination is also a symptom of a urinary tract infection.
6. Keep up-to-date on immunizations.

Answers to Questions

Chapter 1

Chapter Review
1. b   2. c   3. a   4. b   5. d

Clinical Analysis
1. d   2. a   3. d

Chapter 2

Chapter Review
1. b   2. b   3. c   4. a   5. c

Clinical Analysis
1. d   2. b   3. a

Chapter 3

Chapter Review
1. b   2. c   3. c   4. d   5. a

Clinical Analysis
1. c   2. d   3. a

Chapter 4
Chapter Review
1. c   2. b   3. c   4. b   5. c
Clinical Analysis
1. d   2. a   3. c

Chapter 5

Chapter Review
1. a   2. c   3. b   4. b   5. d

Clinical Analysis
1. d   2. c   3. a

Chapter 6

Chapter Review
1. c   2. a   3. c   4. b   5. d

Clinical Analysis
1. d   2. d   3. b

Chapter 7

Chapter Review
1. c   2. d   3. a   4. a   5. b

Clinical Analysis
1. d   2. c   3. b

Chapter 8

Chapter Review
1. b   2. b   3. c   4. a   5. c
Clinical Analysis
1. b   2. a   3. b

Chapter 9

Chapter Review
1. c.   2. d   3. b   4. a   5. d

Clinical Analysis
1. a   2. d   3. c

Chapter 10

Chapter Review
1. d   2. a   3. c   4. b   5. b

Clinical Analysis
1. a   2. d   3. a

Chapter 11

Chapter Review
1. b   2. a   3. c   4. a   5. d

Clinical Analysis
1. c   2. b.   3. d

Chapter 12

Chapter Review
1. c   2. b   3. c   4. b   5. d

Clinical Analysis
1. d   2. c   3. a

Chapter 13

Chapter Review
1. b   2. d   3. b   4. a   5. d

Clinical Analysis
1. b   2. b   3. c

Chapter 14

Chapter Review
1. c   2. a   3. d   4. b   5. a

Clinical Analysis
1. b   2. a   3. c

Chapter 15

Chapter Review
1. c   2. a   3. c   4. b   5. a

Clinical Analysis
1. c   2. c   3. a

Chapter 16

Chapter Review
1. c   2. a   3. b   4. b   5. a

Clinical Analysis
1. c   2. d   3. d

Chapter 17

Chapter Review
1. b   2. e   3. c   4. d   5. a

Clinical Analysis
1. c   2. c   3. a

Chapter 18

Chapter Review
1. a   2. b   3. d   4. b   5. b

Clinical Analysis
1. a   2. b   3. c

Chapter 19

Chapter Review
1. a   2. b   3. d   4. b   5. a

Clinical Analysis
1. c   2. a   3. b

Chapter 20

Chapter Review
1. a   2. c   3. d   4. b   5. d

Clinical Analysis
1. b   2. d   3. c

Chapter 21

Chapter Review
1. b   2. b   3. d   4. a   5. d

Clinical Analysis
1. c   2. b   3. a

Chapter 22

Chapter Review
1. c   2. b   3. d   4. b   5. d

Clinical Analysis
1. a   2. b   3. b

Chapter 23

Chapter Review
1. b   2. d   3. c   4. d   5. a

Clinical Analysis
1. c   2. b   3. a

Chapter 24

Chapter Review
1. c   2. c   3. b   4. d   5. c

Clinical Analysis
1. c   2. d   3. b

Chapter 25

Chapter Review
1. b   2. d   3. a   4. c   5. d

Clinical Analysis
1. b   2. b   3. b

Chapter 26

Chapter Review
1. c   2. c   3. a   4. d   5. b

Clinical Analysis
1. d   2. a   3. b

Glossary

Commonly used terms and terms that appear in **boldface** in the chapters can be found in this glossary. After each definition, the chapter or chapters in which the term is either introduced or discussed extensively are identified numerically in parentheses.

Abdominal circumference (girth)—Distance around the trunk at the umbilicus. (2)

Abdominal obesity—Excess body fat located between the chest and pelvis. (18)

Abortifacient—Anything used to cause or induce an abortion (16)

Absorption—The movement of the end products of digestion from the gastrointestinal tract into the blood and/or lymphatic system. (10)

Accreditation—Process by which a nongovernmental agency recognizes an institution for meeting established criteria of quality. (2)

Acculturation—Process of adopting the values, attitudes, and behaviors of another culture. (2)

Acetone—A ketone body found in urine, which can be due to the excessive breakdown of stored body fat. (3)

Acetonemia (Ketonemia)—Large amounts of acetone in the blood. (17)

Acetylcholine—A chemical necessary for the transmission of nervous impulses. (7)

Acetyl CoA—Important intermediate by-product in metabolism formed from the breakdown of glucose, fatty acids, and certain amino acids. (10)

Achalasia—Failure of the gastrointestinal muscle fibers to relax where one part joins another. (22)

Achlorhydria—Absence of free hydrochloric acid in the stomach. (13)

Acidosis—Condition that results when the pH of the blood falls below 7.35; may be caused by diarrhea, uremia, diabetes mellitus, respiratory depression, and certain drug therapies. (9)

Acquired immune deficiency syndrome (AIDS)—A disease complex caused by a virus that attacks the immune system and causes neurological disease and permits opportunistic infections and malignancies. (25)

Acrodermatitis enteropathica—Rare autosomal recessive disease that causes zinc deficiency through an unknown mechanism of absorptive failure; fatal if untreated. (8)

Acute illness—A sickness characterized by rapid onset, severe symptoms, and a short course. (15)

Acute renal failure—Condition that occurs suddenly, in which the kidneys are unable to perform essential functions; usually temporary. (21)

Adaptive thermogenesis—The adjustment in energy expenditure the body makes to a large increase or decrease in kilocalorie intake of several days' duration. (6)

Additive—A substance added to food to increase its flavor, shelf life, and/or characteristics such as texture, color, and aroma. (14)

Adequate Intake (AI)—The average observed or experimentally defined intake by a defined population or subgroup that appears to sustain a defined nutritional state; incorporates information on the reduction of disease risk; may be used as a goal for an individual's nutrient intake if an EAR or RDA cannot be set. (2)

Adipose cells—Cells in the human body that store fat. (4)

Adipose tissue—Tissue containing masses of fat cells. (4)

Adipose tissue mass—Fat plus its supporting cellular and extracellular structures consisting of protein and water. (2)

Adolescence—Time from the onset of puberty until full growth is reached. (12)

ADP (adenosine diphosphate)—A substance present in all cells involved in energy metabolism. Energy is released when molecules of ATP, another compound in cells, release a phosphoric acid chain and become ADP. The opposite chemical reaction of adding the third phosphoric acid group to ADP requires much energy. (8)

Adrenal glands—Small organs on the superior surface of the kidneys that secrete many hormones, including epinephrine (adrenalin) and aldosterone. (7)

Aerobic exercise—Training methods such as running or swimming that require continuous inspired oxygen. (6)

Afferent—Proceeding toward a center, as arteries, veins, lymphatic vessels, and nerves. (18)

Afferent arteriole—Small blood vessel by which blood enters the glomerulus (functional unit of the kidney). (21)

Aflatoxin—A naturally occurring food contaminant produced by some strains of *Aspergillus* molds found especially on peanuts and peanut products. (14, 23)

AIDS dementia complex (ADC)—A central nervous system disorder caused by the human immunodeficiency virus. (25)

Albumin—A plasma protein responsible for much of the colloidal osmotic pressure of the blood. (9)

Aldosterone—An adrenocorticoid hormone that increases sodium and water retention by the kidneys. (9)

Alimentary canal—The digestive tube extending from the mouth to the anus. (10)

Alkaline phosphatase—An enzyme found in highest concentration in the liver, biliary tract epithelium, and bones; enzyme levels are elevated in liver, bone, and biliary disease. (14)

Alkalosis—Condition that results when the pH of the blood rises above 7.45; may be caused by vomiting, nasogastric suctioning, or hyperventilation. (8)

Allele—One of two or more different genes containing specific inheritable characteristics that occupy corresponding positions (loci) on paired chromosomes; an individual possessing a pair of identical alleles, either dominant or recessive, is homozygous for this gene. (11)

Allergen—Substance that provokes an abnormal, individual hypersensitivity. (12)

Allergy—State of abnormal, individual hypersensitivity to a substance. (10)

Alopecia—Hair loss, especially of the head; baldness. (8)

Alpha-tocopherol equivalent (α-TE)—The measure of vitamin E; 1 milligram of alpha-tocopherol equivalent equals 1.5 of the older measure, International Units. (7)

Amenorrhea—Absence of menstruation; normally occurs before puberty, after menopause, and during pregnancy and lactation. (12)

Amino acids—Organic compounds that are the building blocks of protein; also the end products of protein digestion. (5)

Amniotic fluid—Albuminous liquid that surrounds and protects the fetus throughout pregnancy. (11)

Amylase—A class of enzymes that splits starches; for example, salivary amylase, pancreatic amylase. (10)

Anabolic phase—The third and last phase of stress; characterized by the building up of body tissue and nutrient stores; also called recovery phase. (24)

Anabolism—The building up of body compounds or tissues by the synthesis of more complex substances from simpler ones; the constructive phase of metabolism. (5, 8)

Anaerobic exercise—A form of physical activity such as weight lifting or sprinting that does not rely on continuous inspired oxygen. (6)

Anaphylaxis—Exaggerated, life-threatening hypersensitivity response to a previously encountered antigen; in severe cases, produces bronchospasm, vascular collapse, and shock. (12)

Anastomosis—The surgical connection between tubular structures. (22)

Anemia—Condition of less-than-normal values for red blood cells or hemoglobin, or both; result is decreased effectiveness in oxygen transport. (7, 8)

Anencephaly—Congenital absence of the brain; cerebral hemispheres missing or reduced to small masses; fatal within a few weeks. (11)

Angina pectoris—Severe pain and a sense of constriction about the heart caused by lack of oxygen to the heart muscle. (20)

Angiogram—A radiographic record of the heart and blood vessels taken after injection of a contrast material. (20)

Angiotensin II—End product of complex reaction in response to low blood pressure; effect is vasoconstriction and aldosterone secretion. (9)

Anorexia—Loss of appetite. (13)

Anorexia of aging—Loss of appetite in an elderly individual related to physiologic, social, psychological, or medical causes. (13)

Anion—An ion with a negative charge. (9)

Antagonist—A substance that counteracts the action of another substance. (7)

Anthropometry—The science of measuring the human body. (2)

Anti-insulin antibodies (AIAs)—A protein found to be elevated in persons with insulin-dependent diabetes mellitus. (19)

Anorexia nervosa—A mental disorder characterized by a 25 percent loss of usual body weight, an intense fear of becoming obese, and self-starvation. (18)

Anorexigenic—Causing loss of appetite. (18)

Anthropometric measurements—Physical measurements of the human body such as height, weight, and skinfold thickness; used to determine body composition and growth. (2)

Anthropometry—Science of measuring the body. (2)

Antibody—A specific protein developed in the body in response to a substance that the body senses to be foreign. (5)

Anticholinergic—An agent that blocks parasympathetic nerve impulses, thereby causing dry mouth, blurred vision due to dilated pupils, and decreased gastrointestinal and bronchial secretions. (16)

Antidiuretic hormone (ADH)—Hormone formed in the hypothalamus and released from the posterior pituitary in response to blood that is too concentrated; effect is return of water to the bloodstream by the kidney. (9, 19)

Antineoplastic Drug—A drug that combats tumors. (17)

Antioxidant—A substance that prevents or inhibits the uptake of oxygen; in the body, antioxidants prevent tissue damage; in foods, antioxidants prevent deterioration. (1)

Anuria—A total lack of urine output. (21)

Apgar Score—a system for evaluating an infant's physical condition at birth; heart rate, respiration, muscle tone, response to stimuli, and color are rated 0 to 2 at 1 minute and 5 minutes after birth; scores of 7 to 10 are good to excellent.

Apoferritin—A protein found in intestinal mucosal cells that combines with iron to form ferritin; it is always found attached to iron in the body. (8)

Appetite—A strong desire for food or for a pleasant sensation, based on previous experience, that causes one to seek food for the purpose of tasting and enjoying. (6)

Aquaporin—Water transport proteins, found in many cell membranes, that serve as water-selective channels and explain the speed at which water moves across cell membranes (9)

Arachidonic acid—an omega-6 polyunsaturated fatty acid present in peanuts; precursor of prostaglandins (12)

Ariboflavinosis—Condition arising from a deficiency of riboflavin in the diet. (7)

Arrhythmia—Irregular heartbeat. (20)

Arteriosclerosis—Common arterial disorder characterized by thickening, hardening, and loss of elasticity of the arterial walls; also called "hardening of the arteries." (20)

Arthritis—Inflammatory condition of the joints, usually accompanied by pain and swelling. (13)

Ascites—Accumulation of serous fluid in the peritoneal (abdominal) cavity. (9, 22)

Ascorbic acid—Vitamin C; *ascorbic* literally means "without scurvy." (7)

Ash—The residue that remains after an item is burned; usually refers to the mineral content of the human body. (1)

Aspartame—Artificial sweetener composed of aspartic acid and phenylalanine; 180 times sweeter than sucrose; brand names: Equal, Nutrasweet. (5)

Aspergillus—Genus of molds that produce aflatoxins. (14)

Aspiration—The state whereby a substance has been drawn into the nose, throat, or lungs. (15)

Assessment—An organized procedure to gather pertinent facts. (2)

Asymptomatic—Without symptoms. (25)

Ataxia—Defective muscular coordination, especially seen in voluntary movement attempts. (22)

Atherosclerosis—A form of arteriosclerosis characterized by the deposit of fatty material inside the arteries; major factor contributing to heart disease. (20)

Atom—Smallest particle of an element that has all the properties of the element. An atom consists of the nucleus, which contains protons (positively charged particles), neutrons (particles with no electrical charge), and surrounding electrons (negatively charged particles). (3, 9)

Atopic—Pertaining to a hereditary tendency to develop allergy; the tendency is inherited but the specific clinical form (hay fever, asthma, dermatitis) is not. (12)

ATP (adenosine triphosphate)—Compound in cells, especially muscle cells, that stores energy; when needed, enzymes break off one phosphoric acid group, which releases energy for muscle contraction. (8)

Atrophy—Decrease in size of a normally developed organ or tissue. (24)

Autoimmune disease—A disorder in which the body produces an immunologic response against itself. (19)

Autonomy—Achieving independence; the psychosocial developmental task of the toddler. (12)

Autosomal recessive inheritance—Nonsex-linked pattern of inheritance in which an affected gene must be received from both parents for the individual to be affected; examples: cystic fibrosis, PKU, galactosemia, sickle cell disease. (20)

Avidin—Protein in raw egg white that inhibits the B vitamin biotin. (7)

Bacteria—Single-celled microorganisms that lack a true nucleus; may be either harmless to humans or disease producing. (3)

Balanced diet—One that contains all the essential nutrients in required amounts. (2)

Barium enema—Series of x-ray studies of the colon used to demonstrate the presence and location of polyps, tumors, diverticula, or positional abnormalities. The client is first administered an enema containing a radioopaque substance (barium) that enhances visualization when the film is exposed. (15)

Barium swallow—The primary diagnostic tool for direct visualization of the swallowing mechanism is called the "cookie swallow" or "modified barium swallow." During this procedure, the client consumes three items of different viscosities. Each item contains a dye called barium. The dye in the food or beverage allows all phases of the swallowing mechanism to be visualized in x-rays. A physician is always present during this procedure. (10)

Basal ganglia—Four masses of gray matter located in the cerebrum; contribute to the subconscious aspects of voluntary movement; inhibit tremors. (8)

Benign—Tumor that is localized; does not infiltrate surrounding tissue or metastasize; may be life-threatening in crucial tissue such as the brain. (23)

Beriberi—Disease caused by deficiency of vitamin B_1 (thiamin). (7)

Beta-endorphin—Chemical released in the brain during exercise that produces a state of relaxation. (6)

Bicarbonate—Any salt containing the HCO_3 anion; blood bicarbonate is a measure of alkali (base) reserve of the body; bicarbonate of soda is sodium bicarbonate ($NaHCO_3$). (9)

Bile—Yellow secretion of the liver that alkalinizes the intestine and breaks large fat globules into smaller ones to facilitate enzyme digestive action. (10)

Binging—Eating to excess; eating from 5,000 to 20,000 kilocalories per day. (18)

Bioavailability—The rate and extent to which an active drug or nutrient or metabolite enters the general circulation permitting access to the site of action. (14)

Bioelectric impedance—Indirect measure of body fatness based on differences in electrical conductivity of fat, muscle, and bone. (2)

Biologic value—Measure of how well food proteins can be converted into body protein. (5)

Biotin—B-complex vitamin widely available in foods. (7)

Bladder—A body organ, also called the urinary bladder, that receives urine from the kidneys and discharges it through the urethra. (10)

Blood pressure—Force exerted against the walls of blood vessels by the pumping action of the heart. (20)

Blood urea nitrogen (BUN)—The amount of nitrogen present in the blood as urea, often elevated in renal disorders; may be referred to as serum urea nitrogen (SUN). (13, 21)

Body frame size—Designation of a person's skeletal structure as small, medium, or large; used to determine healthy body weight (HBW). (2)

Body image—The mental image a person has of himself or herself. (18)

Body mass index (BMI)—Weight in kilograms divided by height in meters squared; BMIs of 20.8 to 27.7 for men and 19.2 to 27.2 for women are considered normal. (2)

Body substance isolation—A situation in which all body fluids should be considered contaminated and treated as such by all healthcare workers. (25)

Bolus—A mass of food that is ready to be swallowed; or a single dose of feeding or medication. (10, 15)

Bolus feeding—Giving a 4- to 6-hour volume of a tube feeding within a few minutes. (15)

Bomb calorimeter—A device used to measure the energy content of food. (6)

Botulism—An often fatal form of food intoxication caused by the ingestion of food containing poisonous toxins produced by the microorganism *Clostridium botulinum*. (14)

Bowman's capsule—The cuplike top of an individual nephron; functions as a filter in the formation of urine. (21)

Brewer's yeast—Unicellular fungus used in brewing beer and baking bread; good source of vitamin B complex. (7)

Buffer—A substance that can react to offset excess acid or excess alkali (base) in a solution; blood buffers include carbonic acid, bicarbonate, phosphates, and proteins, including hemoglobin. (9)

Bulimia—Excessive food intake followed by extreme methods, such as self-induced vomiting and the use of laxatives, to rid the body of the foods eaten. (18)

Cachexia—State of malnutrition and wasting seen in chronic conditions such as cancer, AIDS, malaria, tuberculosis, and pituitary disease. (23)

Calcidiol—Inactive form of vitamin D produced by the liver. (7)

Calcification—Process in which tissue becomes hardened with calcium deposits. (7)

Calcitonin—Hormone produced by the C cells of the thyroid gland that slows bone resorption when serum calcium levels are high. (8)

Calcitriol—The activated form of vitamin D, 1,25-dihydroxycholecalciferol. (7, 21)

Calorie—A measurement unit of energy; unit equaling the amount of heat required to raise the temperature of 1 gram of water 1 degree Celsius; laypersons' term for kilocalorie. (6)

Campylobacter—Flagellated, gram-negative bacteria; important cause of diarrheal illnesses. (14)

Candida albicans—Microscopic fungal organism normally present on skin and mucous membranes of healthy people; cause of thrush, vaginitis, opportunistic infections. (25)

Capillary—Minute vessel connecting arteriole and venule; wall acts as semipermeable membrane to exchange substances between blood and lymph and interstitial fluid. (10)

Carbohydrate—Any of a group of organic compounds, including sugar, starch, and cellulose, that contains only carbon, oxygen, and hydrogen. (3)

Carbonic acid—Aqueous solution of carbon dioxide; carbon dioxide in solution or in blood is carbonic acid. (9)

Carcinogen—Any substance or agent that causes the development of or increases the risk of cancer. (23)

Carcinoma—A malignant neoplasm that occurs in epithelial tissue. (23)

Cardia—Upper orifice of the stomach connecting with the esophagus. (23)

Cardiac arrhythmia—Irregular heartbeat. (18)

Cardiac output—The amount of blood discharged per minute from the left or right ventricle of the heart. (20)

Cardiac sphincter—Smooth muscle band at the lower end of the esophagus; prevents reflux of stomach contents. (10, 22)

Cardiomyopathy—Disease of heart muscle; may be primary due to unknown cause or secondary to another cardiac disorder or systemic disease. (8)

Carotene—Yellow pigment in vegetables; the form with greatest vitamin A activity is beta-carotene (provitamin A). (7)

Carotenemia—Excess carotene in the blood, producing yellow skin but not discoloring the whites of the eyes. (7)

Carotenoid—Group of red, orange, or yellow pigments found in carrots, sweet potatoes, and green, leafy vegetables; includes carotene, a precursor of vitamin A, and lycopene which is not. (20)

Casein—Principal protein in cow's milk

Catabolism—The breaking down of body compounds or tissues into simpler substances; the destructive phase of metabolism. (5)

Catalyst—A substance that speeds up a chemical reaction without entering into or being changed by the reaction. (5)

Cataract—Clouding of the lens of the eye. (13)

Cation—An ion with a positive charge. (9)

Cecum—The first portion of the large intestine between the ileum and the ascending colon. (10)

Celiac disease (gluten-sensitive enteropathy)—An intolerance to dietary gluten, which damages the intestine and produces diarrhea and malabsorption. (10, 22)

Cell—The smallest functional unit of structure in all plants and animals. (10)

Cellular immunity—Delayed immune response produced by T-lymphocytes, which mature in the thymus gland; examples of this type of response are rejection of transplanted organs and some autoimmune diseases. (23)

Cerebrovascular accident (CVA)—An abnormal condition in which the brain's blood vessels are occluded by a thrombus, an embolus, or hemorrhage, resulting in damaged brain tissue; stroke. (20)

Chelating agent—A chemical compound that binds metallic ions into a ring structure, inactivating them; used to remove poisonous metals from the body. (8)

Chemical digestion—Digestive process that involves the splitting of complex molecules into simpler forms. (10)

Chemical reaction—The process of combining or breaking down substances to obtain different substances. (10)

Chlorophyll—The green plant pigment necessary for the manufacture of carbohydrates. (3)

Cholecalciferol—Vitamin D_3, formed when the skin is exposed to sunlight; further processed by the liver and kidneys. (7)

Cholecystitis—Inflammation of the gallbladder. (22, 25)

Cholecystokinin—A hormone secreted by the duodenum; stimulates contraction of the gallbladder (releases bile) and the secretion of pancreatic juice. (10)

Cholelithiasis—The presence of gallstones. (22)

Cholestasis—Blockage of the flow of bile; due to liver disease or obstructions in the duct system. (8)

Cholesterol—A fat-like substance made in the human body and found in foods of animal origin; associated with an increased risk of heart disease. (4, 20)

Chronic illness—A sickness persisting for a long period that shows little change or a slow progression over time. (15)

Chronic obstructive pulmonary disease (COPD)—A group of chronic diseases with a common characteristic of chronic airflow obstruction. (24)

Chronic renal failure—An irreversible condition in which the kidneys cannot perform vital functions. (21)

Chvostek's sign—Spasm of facial muscles following a tap over the facial nerve in front of the ear; indication of tetany. (8)

Chylomicron—A lipoprotein that carries triglycerides in the bloodstream after meals. (10, 20)

Chyme—The mixture of partly digested food and digestive secretions found in the stomach and small intestine during digestion of a meal. (10)

Chymotrypsin—A protein-splitting enzyme produced by the pancreas; active in the intestine. (10)

Cirrhosis—Chronic disease of the liver in which functioning cells degenerate and are replaced by fibrosed connective tissue. (22)

Client care conference—A meeting that includes all health care team members and may include the client or a significant other to review and update the client's nursing care plan. (15)

Clostridium botulinum—An anaerobic (grows without air) organism that produces a poisonous toxin; the cause of botulism. (14)

Clostridium perfringens—A bacterium that produces a poisonous toxin that causes a food intoxication; the symptoms are generally mild and of short duration and include intestinal disorders. (14)

Coenzyme—A substance that combines with an enzyme to activate it. (7)

Cognitive—Referring to or associated with the act of knowing. (18)

Colectomy—Surgical removal of part or all of the colon. (22)

Collagen—Fibrous insoluble protein found in connective tissue. (7)

Collecting tubule—The last segment of the renal tubule; follows the distal convoluted tubule. Several nephrons usually share a single collecting tubule. (21)

Colloidal osmotic pressure—Pressure produced by plasma and cellular proteins. (9)

Colon—The large intestine from the end of the small intestine to the rectum. (10)

Colostomy—Surgical procedure in which an opening to the large intestine is constructed on the abdomen. (22)

Co-morbidity—A disease co-existing with the primary disease. (18)

Complementation—Principle of meal planning advocating combining plant foods within a meal so that it contains all the essential amino acids; now applied to daily intake rather than to single meals. (5)

Complete protein—A protein containing all essential amino acids that humans need; usually found in animal sources such as milk, meat, eggs, and fish. (5)

Complex carbohydrate—A carbohydrate composed of many molecules of $C_6H_{12}O_6$ joined together; polysaccharide; includes starch, glycogen, and fiber. (3)

Compound—Two or more elements united chemically in specific proportions. (9)

Compound fat—Substance obtained when one of the fatty acids joined to the glycerol molecule is replaced by another molecule, such as a protein. (4)

Congestive heart failure (CHF)—Condition resulting from the failure of the heart to maintain adequate blood circulation; due to complex reactive mechanisms, fluid is retained in the body's tissues. (20)

Constipation—Decrease in a person's normal frequency of defecation; stool often hard, dry, or difficult to expel. (22)

Contamination iron—Iron that leaches from cookware into the food; in special circumstances, can become hazardous. (8)

Continuous ambulatory peritoneal dialysis (CAPD)—A form of self-dialysis in which the dialysate is allowed to remain in the abdominal cavity for 4–6 hours before replacement. (21)

Continuous feeding—Nutritional support on an ongoing basis. (15)

Contraindication—Any circumstance under which treatment should not be given. (15)

Coronary heart disease (CHD)—Disease resulting from the decreased flow of blood through the coronary arteries to the heart muscle. (20)

Coronary occlusion—Blockage of one or more branches of the coronary arteries, which supply the heart muscle with oxygen and nutrients. (20)

Creatine—Nonprotein substance synthesized in the body from arginine, glycine, and methionine; combines with phosphate to form creatine phosphate, which is stored in muscle tissue as an energy source.

Creatinine—Nonprotein nitrogenous end product of creatine metabolism; because creatinine is excreted by the kidneys, serum creatinine levels are used to detect and monitor renal disease and to estimate muscle protein reserves. (21)

Cretinism—A congenital condition resulting from a lack of thyroid secretions characterized by a stunted and malformed body and arrested mental development. (8)

Crohn's disease—Inflammatory disease appearing in any area of the bowel in which diseased areas can be found alternating with healthy tissue. (22)

Cross-contamination—The spreading of a disease-producing organism from one food, person, or object to another food, person, or object. (14)

Cruciferous—Belonging to a botanical mustard family; includes broccoli, Brussels sprouts, cabbage, cauliflower, kale, kohlrabi, and swiss chard. (23)

Crystalluria—The presence of crystals in the urine; may be caused by the administration of sulfonamides. (17)

Culture—The learned, shared, and transmitted values, beliefs, and norms of a particular group that guides their thinking, decisions, and actions in patterned ways. (2)

Cyanocobalamin—Vitamin B$_{12}$; essential for proper blood formation. (7)

Cyclical variation—A recurring series of events during a specified period. (1)

Cystic fibrosis—Hereditary disease often affecting the lungs and pancreas in which glandular secretions are abnormally thick. (22)

Cystitis—Inflammation of the bladder. (21)

Cytochrome P450 enzyme—Group of genetically determined enzymes that help to metabolize fat-soluble vitamins, steroids, fatty acids, and other substances and to detoxify drugs and environmental pollutants. (17)

Daily food guide—Tool used to assist consumers in making informed food choices. (2)

Deamination—Metabolic process whereby nitrogen is removed from an amino acid. (10)

Deciliter (dL)—100 milliliters or 100 cubic centimeters. (19)

Decubitus ulcer—A pressure sore on the lower back, such as a bedsore. (13, 15)

Degenerative Joint Disease (DJD)—Osteoarthritis. (13)

Dehiscence—Separation of the edges of a surgical incision. (5)

Delusion—False belief that is firmly maintained despite obvious proof to the contrary. (7)

Dementia—The impairment of intellectual function that usually is progressive and interferes with normal social and occupational activities. (1)

Dental caries—The gradual decay and disintegration of the teeth; a dental cavity is a hole in a tooth caused by dental caries. (3)

Dental plaque—Colorless and transparent gummy mass of microorganisms that grows on the teeth, predisposing them to decay. (3)

Deoxyribonucleic acid (DNA)—Protein substance in the cell nucleus that directs all the cell's activities, including reproduction. (5)

Desirable body weight—A person's body weight as compared with the 1959 Desirable Height/Weight Table. (18)

Desired outcome—The behavioral or physical change in a client that indicates the achievement of a nursing goal. (2)

Development—Gradual process of changing from a simple to a more complex organism; involves psychosocial and physical changes, not only an increase in size. (12)

Dextrose—Another name for the simple sugar glucose. (3)

Diabetes incipidus—Increased water intake and increased urine output resulting from inadequate secretion of antidiuretic hormone (ADH) by the posterior pituitary or by failure of the kidney tubules to respond to ADH; underlying causes can be tumor, surgery, trauma, infection, radiation injury, or congenital anomaly. (9)

Diabetes mellitus—Disease caused by insufficient insulin secretion by the pancreas or insulin resistance by body tissues causing excess glucose in the blood and deranged carbohydrate, fat, and protein metabolism. (19)

Diabetic neuropathy—Degeneration of peripheral nerves occurring in diabetes; possible causes are microscopic changes in blood vessels or metabolic defects in nerve tissue. (19)

Diacetic acid—A ketone body found in the urine, which can be due to the excessive breakdown of stored body fat. (3)

Diagnostic—Relating to scientific and skillful methods to establish the cause and nature of a sick person's illness. (15)

Dialysate—In renal failure, the fluid used to remove or deliver compounds or electrolytes that the failing kidney cannot excrete or retain in proper concentrations. (21)

Dialysis—The process of diffusing blood across a semipermeable membrane to remove toxic materials and to maintain fluid, electrolyte, and acid-base balances in cases of impaired kidney function or absence of the kidneys. (21)

Dialysis dementia—A neurological disturbance seen in clients who have been on dialysis for a number of years. (21)

Diastolic pressure—Pressure exerted against the arteries between heart beats; the lower number of a blood pressure reading. (9, 20)

Dietary fiber—Material in foods, mostly from plants, that the human body cannot break down or digest. (3)

Dietary recall, 24-hour—Description of what a person has eaten for the previous 24 hours. (2)

Dietary Reference Intake (DRI)—Four nutrient-based reference values that can be used for assessing and planning diets for the healthy general population; refer to average daily intakes for one or more weeks; include Estimated Average Requirements (EARs), Recommended Dietary Allowances (RDAs), Adequate Intakes (AIs), and Tolerable Upper Intake Levels (ULs). (2)

Dietary status—Description of what a person has been eating; his or her usual intake. (2)

Digestion—The process by which food is broken down mechanically and chemically in the gastrointestinal tract into forms simple enough for intestinal absorption. (10)

Diglyceride—Two fatty acids joined to a glycerol molecule. (4)

Dilutional hyponatremia—Serum sodium that is low, not because of an absolute lack of sodium, but because of an excess of water. (8)

Disaccharide—A simple sugar composed of two units of $C_6H_{12}O_6$ joined together; examples include sucrose, lactose, and maltose. (3)

Disulfide linkage—Specific chemical bond joining amino acids; in hair, skin, and nails, holds amino acids in their distinct shapes. (8)

Diverticulitis—Inflammation of a diverticulum. (22)

Diverticulosis—Presence of one or more diverticula. (22)

Diverticulum—A sac or pouch in the walls of a tubular organ; pl., diverticula. (22)

Docosahexaenoic acid (DHA)—Omega-3 polyunsaturated fatty acid found in fish oils. (4)

Dopamine—Catecholamine synthesized by the adrenals; immediate precursor in the synthesis of norepinephrine. (17)

Double-blind—Technique of scientific investigation in which neither the investigator nor the subject knows what treatment, if any, the subject is receiving. (16)

Double bond—A type of chemical connection in which, for example, a fatty acid has two neighboring carbon atoms, each lacking one hydrogen atom. (4)

Drink—An alcoholic beverage; one drink is usually 12 ounces of beer, 4 ounces of wine, or 1.5 ounces of liquor. (20)

Dual-energy x-ray absorptiometry (DEXA)—Diagnostic test using two x-ray beams to determine body composition; used to measure bone mineral density as an indicator of osteopenia and osteoporosis. (2)

Duct—A structural tube designed to allow secretions to move from one body part to another body part. (10, 19)

Dumping syndrome—A condition in which the contents of the stomach empty too rapidly into the duodenum; mostly occurs in patients who have had gastric resections. (22)

Duodenum—The first part of the small intestine between the stomach and the jejunum. (10)

Dysphoria—A speech disorder characterized by hoarseness. (18)

Dyspnea—Difficulty breathing. (24)

Ebb phase—The first phase in the stress response; the body reduces blood pressure, cardiac output, body temperature, and oxygen consumption to meet increased demands. (24)

Eclampsia—An obstetrical emergency involving hypertension, edema, proteinuria, and convulsions appearing after the twentieth week of pregnancy. (11)

Eczema—Skin inflammation, acute or chronic; cause by external (chemical irritation or microbial invasion) or internal (genetic or psychological) factors. (12)

Edema—The accumulation of excessive amounts of fluid in interstitial spaces. (9)

Edentulous—The state of having no teeth. (13)

Efferent—Directed away from a center; used to describe arteries, veins, lymphatic vessels, and nerves. (18)

Efferent arteriole—Small blood vessel by which blood leaves the nephron. (21)

Efficacy—Ability of a drug to achieve the desired effect. (16)

Electrocardiogram (ECG)—A graphic record produced by an electrocardiograph that shows the electrical activity of the heart. (9)

Electroencephalogram (EEG)—The record obtained from an electroencephalograph that shows the electrical activity of the brain. (9)

Electrolyte—An element or compound that when dissolved in water separates (dissociates) into ions that are capable of conducting an electrical current; acids, bases, and salts are common electrolytes. (9)

Element—A substance that cannot be separated into simpler parts by ordinary means. (3)

Elemental or "predigested" formula—Formula that contains either partially or totally predigested nutrients. (15)

Embolus—A circulating mass of undissolved matter in a blood or lymphatic vessel; may be composed of tissues, fat globules, air bubbles, clumps of bacteria, or foreign bodies, including pieces of medical devices. (20)

Embryo—A developing infant in the prenatal period between the second and eighth weeks inclusive. (11)

Empty kilocalories—Refers to a food that contains kilocalories and almost no other nutrients. (6)

Emulsification—The physical breaking up of fat into tiny droplets. (10)

Emulsifier—A molecule that attracts both water- and fat-soluble molecules. (14)

Emulsion—One liquid evenly distributed in a second liquid with which it usually does not mix. (4)

Endemic—The constant presence of a disease or infectious agent within a given geographic area; the usual prevalence of a given disease within such an area. (8)

Endogenous—Produced within or caused by factors within the organism. (16)

Endoscope—A device consisting of a tube and an optical system for observing the inside of a hollow organ or cavity. (15)

End-stage renal failure—A state in which the kidneys have lost most or all of their ability to maintain internal homeostasis and produce urine. (21, 25)

Energy—The capacity to do work. (1)

Energy balance—A situation in which kilocaloric intake equals kilocaloric output. (6)

Energy expenditure—The amount of fuel the body uses for a specified period. (6)

Energy imbalance—Situation in which kilocalories eaten do not equal the number of kilocalories used for energy. (18)

Energy nutrients—The chemical substances in food that are able to supply fuel; refers collectively to carbohydrate, fat, and protein. (1)

Enrichment—The addition of nutrients previously present in a food but removed during food processing or lost during storage. (3)

Enteral tube feeding—The feeding of a formula by tube into the gastrointestinal tract. (15)

Enteric-coated—A type of drug preparation designed to dissolve in the intestine rather than in the stomach. (17)

Enteritis—Inflammation of the intestines, particularly the small intestine. (12)

Enzyme—Complex protein produced by living cells that acts as a catalyst. (5, 6)

Epidemic—Occurrence in a region of more than the expected number of cases of a communicable disease. (25)

Epinephrine—Hormone of the adrenal gland; produces the fight-or-flight response. (24)

Epithelial tissue—A type of tissue that forms the outer layer of skin and lines body surfaces opening to the outside; functions include protection, absorption, and secretion. (7)

Ergocalciferol—Vitamin D_2 formed by the action of sunlight on plants. (7)

Ergot poisoning—Poisoning resulting from excessive use of the drug ergot or from the ingestion of grain or grain products infected with the *Claviceps purpurea* fungus. (14)

Erikson, Erik—Psychologist who devised a theory of human development consisting of eight stages of life, each with a psychosocial developmental task to be mastered. (12)

Erosion—Destruction of the surface of a tissue, either on the external surface of the body or internally. (22)

Erythropoietin—Hormone released by the kidney to stimulate red blood cell production. (21)

Esophagostomy—A surgical opening in the esophagus. (15)

Esophagus—A muscular canal extending from the mouth to the stomach. (10, 22)

Essential amino acid—One of the amino acids that cannot be manufactured by the human body; must be obtained from food or artificial feeding. (5)

Essential (primary) hypertension—Elevated blood pressure that develops without apparent cause. (20)

Essential nutrient—A substance found in food that must be present in the diet because the human body lacks the ability to manufacture it in sufficient amounts for optimal health. (1)

Estimated Average Requirement—Intake that meets the estimated nutrient need of 50% of the individuals in a life-stage and gender group; used to set the RDA and to assess or plan the intake of groups. (2)

Estimated Safe and Adequate Daily Dietary Intake (ESADDI)—Intake of four minerals for which insufficient information is available to establish a Recommended Dietary Allowance (RDA). (2)

Ethanol—Grain alcohol; ounces of ethanol in beverages can be estimated with the conversion factors of 0.045 for beer, 0.121 for wine, and 0.409 for liquor. (20)

Ethnocentrism—Belief that one's own view of the world is superior to anyone else's. (2)

Evaluation—The final step in the nursing process in which the actual outcome is compared to the desired outcome. (2)

Evaporative water loss—Insensible water loss through the skin. (9)

Exchange—A defined quantity of food on the American Dietetic and Diabetes associations' food exchange list or on another, similar exchange list. (2)

Exchange list—A food guide developed by the American Dietetic and Diabetes associations; often used in clinical practice to aid in meal planning. (2)

Excretion—The elimination of waste products from the body in feces, urine, exhaled air, and perspiration. (10)

Exogenous—Outside the body. (19)

External muscle layer—Muscle layer of the alimentary canal. (6)

External water loss—Water lost to the outside of the body. (9)

Extracellular fluid—Fluid found between the cells and within the blood and lymph vessels. (9)

Extrinsic factor—Vitamin B_{12}, necessary for proper red blood cell development. (7)

Failure to thrive (FTT)—Medical diagnosis for infants who fail to gain weight appropriately or who lose weight. (12)

Fasting—The state of having had no food or fluid enterally or no parenteral nutrition. (15)

Fasting blood sugar (FBS)—Blood glucose measured in the fasting state; normal values are 70–110 mg per deciliter. (3, 19)

Fat-free mass—Lean body mass plus nonfat components of adipose tissue. (2)

Fatty acid—Part of the structure of a fat. (4)

Fatty liver—Accumulation of lipids in the liver cells; may be reversible if the cause, of which there are many, is removed. (22)

Ferric iron—Oxidized iron, which is less absorbable from the gastrointestinal tract than ferrous iron; abbreviated Fe^{3+}. (8)

Ferritin—An iron-phosphorus-protein complex formed in the intestinal mucosa by the union of ferric iron with apoferritin; the form in which iron is stored in the tissues, mainly in liver, spleen, and bone marrow cells. (8, 21)

Ferrous iron—The more absorbable form of iron for humans; abbreviated Fe^{2+}. (8)

Fetal alcohol syndrome (FAS)—A condition characterized by mental and physical abnormalities in an infant caused by the mother's consumption of alcohol during pregnancy. (11)

Fetus—The human child in utero from the third month until birth; also applicable to the later stages of gestation of other animals. (11)

Fiber, dietary—Material in foods, mostly from plants, that the human body cannot break down or digest. (3)

Fibrin—Insoluble protein formed from fibrinogen by the action of thrombin; forms the meshwork of a blood clot. (8)

Fibrinogen—Protein in blood essential to the clotting process; also called Factor I; see fibrin. (8)

Filtration—The process of removing particles from a solution by allowing the liquid to pass through a membrane or other partial barrier. (21)

First pass effect—Process whereby drugs are extensively metabolized by the liver immediately after absorption into the portal circulation from the intestinal tract; result is that less drug reaches the systemic circulation. (17)

Flatus—Gas in the digestive tract, averaging 400 to 1200 milliliters per day. (22)

Flavonoids—Nonnutritive antioxidant compounds that occur naturally in certain foods such as onions, apples, tea, and red wine; inhibit oxidation of LDL in laboratory experiments. (20)

Flow phase—The second phase in the stress response; marked by pronounced hormonal changes. (24)

Fluorosis—Condition due to excessive prolonged intake of fluoride; tissues affected are teeth and bones. (8)

Folate conjugase—Enzyme needed to separate folic acid from the amino acids that usually bind to it in foods; found in salivary, gastric, pancreatic, and jejunal secretions. (7)

Folic acid—B-complex vitamin necessary for DNA formation and proper red blood cell formation. (7)

Food acceptance record—A checklist that indicates food items accepted or rejected by the client. (15)

Food allergy—Sensitivity to a food that does not cause a negative reaction in most people. (10)

Food faddism—An unusual pattern of food behavior enthusiastically adapted by its adherents. (25)

Food frequency—A usual food intake or a description of what an individual usually eats during a typical day. (2)

Food quackery—The promotion for profit of a medical scheme or remedy that is unproven or known to be false. (25)

Food infection—Infection acquired through contact with food or water contaminated with disease-producing microorganisms. (14)

Food intoxication—An illness caused by the consumption of a food in which bacteria have produced a poisonous toxin. (14)

Food Pyramid—Food guide commonly used to evaluate a person's dietary status and to educate clients about food choices; food is divided into six groups: each contains foods of similar nutritional content. (2)

Food record—A diary of a person's self-reported food intake. (2)

Fortification—Process of adding nutritive substances not naturally occurring in the given food to increase its nutritional value; for example, milk fortified with vitamins A and D. (7)

Free-living—Following a way of life in which one freely indulges one's appetites and desires. (7)

Free radicals—Atoms or molecules that have lost an electron and vigorously pursue its replacement; in doing so, free radicals can damage normal cell constituents. (7)

Fructose—A monosaccharide found in fruits and honey; a simple sugar. (3)

Fundus—Larger part of a hollow organ; the part of the stomach above its attachment to the esophagus. (22)

Galactose—A monosaccharide derived mainly from the breakdown of the sugar in milk, lactose; a simple sugar. (3)

Galactosemia—Lack of an enzyme needed to metabolize galactose. (12)

Gallbladder—A pear-shaped organ on the underside of the liver that concentrates and stores bile. (10, 22)

Gastric bypass—A surgical procedure that routes food around the stomach. (18)

Gastric lipase—An enzyme in the stomach that aids in the digestion of fats. (10)

Gastric stapling—A surgical procedure on the stomach to induce weight loss by reducing the size of the stomach; also known as gastroplasty. (18)

Gastrin—A hormone secreted by the gastric mucosa; stimulates the secretion of gastric juice. (10)

Gastritis—Inflammation of the stomach. (22)

Gastroesophageal reflux (acid-reflux disorder) abbr. GERD—Regurgitation of stomach contents into the esophagus. (22)

Gastroparesis—Partial paralysis of the stomach. (19)

Gastrostomy—A surgical opening in the stomach. (15)

Gene—Basic unit of heredity; linear segment of deoxyribonucleic acid (DNA) that occupies a specific location on a specific chromosome; provides the instructions for protein synthesis. (5, 23)

Generativity—The seventh of Erikson's developmental stages, in which the middle-aged adult guides the next generation. (13)

Generic name—The name given to a drug by its original developer; usually the same as the official name given to it by the Food and Drug Administration. (17)

Genetic susceptibility—The likelihood of an individual developing a given trait as determined by heredity. (3)

Geriatrics—The branch of medicine involved in the study and treatment of diseases of the elderly. (13)

Gestation—The time from fertilization of the ovum until birth; in humans the length of gestation is usually 38–42 weeks. (11)

Gestational diabetes (GDM)—Hyperglycemia and altered carbohydrate, protein, and fat metabolism related to the increased demands of pregnancy. (11, 19)

Globin—The simple protein portion of hemoglobin. (5)

Glomerular filtrate—The fluid that has been passed through the glomerulus. (21)

Glomerular filtration rate (GFR)—An index of kidney function; the amount of filtrate formed each minute in all the nephrons of both kidneys. (21)

Glomerulonephritis—Inflammation of the glomeruli. (21)

Glomerulus—The network of capillaries inside Bowman's capsule. (21)

Glucagon—A hormone secreted by the alpha cells of the pancreas; increases the concentration of glucose in the blood. (5, 19)

Gluconeogenesis—The production of glucose from noncarbohydrate sources such as amino acids and glycerol. (24)

Glucose—A monosaccharide (simple sugar) commonly called the blood sugar; the same as dextrose. (3)

Glucose tolerance factor (GTF)—Organic compound containing chromium, which enhances the action of insulin, facilitating the uptake of glucose by the body's cells. (8)

Glucose tolerance test—A test of blood and urine after the patient receives a concentrated dose of glucose; used to diagnose abnormalities of glucose metabolism. (19)

Gluteal-femoral obesity—Excess body fat centered around an individual's buttocks, hips, and thighs. (18, 20)

Gluten—A type of protein found in wheat, rye, oats, and barley. (10)

Gluten-sensitive enteropathy (celiac disease)—An intestinal disorder caused by an abnormal response following the consumption of gluten. (10, 22)

Glycemic index—A measure of how much the blood glucose level increases following consumption of a particular food that contains a given amount of carbohydrate. (19)

Glycerol—The backbone of a fat molecule; pharmaceutical preparation is glycerin. (4)

Glycogen—The form in which carbohydrate is stored in liver and muscle. (3)

Glycogenolysis—The breakdown of glycogen. (24)

Glycosuria—Glucose in the urine. (19)

Glycosylated hemoglobin—Hemoglobin to which a glucose group is attached; in diabetes mellitus, if the blood glucose level has not been controlled over the previous 120 days, the glycosylated hemoglobin level is elevated. (19)

Goiter—Enlargement of the thyroid gland characterized by pronounced swelling in the neck. (8)

Goitrogens—Substances that block the absorption of iodine, thereby causing goiter; found in cabbage, rutabaga, and turnips, but only related to goiter in cassava. (8)

Gout—A hereditary metabolic disease that is a form of acute arthritis and is marked by inflammation of the joints. (21)

Growth—Progressive increase in size of a living thing that entails the synthesis of new protoplasm and multiplication of cells. (12)

"Gut failure"—Impaired absorption due to structural damage to the small intestine; symptoms include diarrhea, malabsorption, and unsuccessful absorption of oral food. (10)

Harris-Benedict equation—A formula commonly used to estimate resting energy expenditure in a stressed client. (24, 25)

Health—The state of complete physical, mental, and social well-being, not just the absence of disease or infirmity. (1)

Healthy body weight (HBW)—Estimate of a weight suitable for an individual based on frame size and height and weight tables. (2)

Healthy Eating Index—Measure of diet quality devised by the United States Department of Agriculture Center for Nutrition Policy and Promotion; sections include Food Guide Pyramid, fat consumption, sodium, and variety (12)

Helminthiasis—Infestation with intestinal parasites or worms. (8)

Hematocrit—Percent of total blood volume that is red blood cells; normals are 40–54 percent for men; 37–47 percent for women. (8)

Hematuria—Blood in the urine. (21)

Heme—The iron-containing portion of the hemoglobin molecule. (8)

Heme iron—Iron bound to hemoglobin and myoglobin in meat, fish, and poultry; 10–30 percent of the iron in these foods is absorbed. (8)

Hemochromatosis—A disease of iron metabolism in which iron accumulates in the tissues. (8)

Hemodialysis—A method for cleansing the blood of wastes by circulating blood through a machine that contains tubes made of synthetic semipermeable membranes. (21)

Hemoglobin—The iron-carrying pigment of the red blood cells; carries oxygen from the lungs to the tissues. (5, 8)

Hemolysis—Rupture of red blood cells releasing hemoglobin into the plasma; causes include bacterial toxins, chemicals, inappropriate medications, vitamin E deficiency. (7)

Hemolytic anemia—An abnormal reduction in the number of red blood cells due to hemolysis. (8)

Hemosiderin—An iron oxide-protein compound derived from hemoglobin; a secondary storage form of iron. (8)

Hemosiderosis—Condition resulting from excess deposits of hemosiderin, especially in the liver and spleen; caused by destruction of red blood cells, which occurs in diseases such as hemolytic anemia, pernicious anemia, and chronic infection. (8)

Heparin—A chemical, found naturally in many tissues, that inhibits blood clotting by preventing the conversion of prothrombin to thrombin; also given as an anticoagulant medication. (7)

Hepatic portal circulation—A subdivision of the vascular system in which blood from the digestive organs and spleen circulates through the liver before returning to the heart. (10)

Hepatitis—Inflammation of the liver, caused by viruses, drugs, alcohol, or toxic substances. (22)

Heterozygous—Having two different genes, one from each parent, governing a particular trait; the dominant gene will produce the given trait in the individual. (11)

Hiatal hernia—A protrusion of part of the stomach into the chest cavity. (22)

High-density lipoprotein (HDL)—A plasma protein that carries fat in the bloodstream to the tissues or to the liver to be excreted; elevated blood levels are associated with a decreased risk of heart disease. (20)

High-fructose corn syrup (HFCS)—A common food additive used as a sweetener; made from fructose. (3)

Hives (urticaria)—Sudden swelling and itching of skin or mucous membranes, often caused by allergies; if the respiratory tract is involved, may be life-threatening. (12)

Homeostasis—Tendency toward balance in the internal environment of the body, achieved by automatic monitoring and regulating mechanisms. (6)

Homozygous—Having two identical genes, one from each parent, governing a particular trait; necessary condition to produce a disease caused by a recessive gene, such as sickle cell anemia. (11)

Hormone—A substance produced by cells of the body that is released into the bloodstream and carried to target sites to regulate the activity of other cells and organs. (4, 5)

Human immunodeficiency virus (HIV)—The virus that causes AIDS. (25)

Humoral immunity—Development of antibodies to specific antigens by the B-lymphocytes, some of which retain the ability to recognize the antigen if it is encountered again; basis of immunizations. (23)

Humulin—Exact duplicate of human insulin manufactured by altering bacterial DNA. (19)

Hunger—The sensation resulting from a lack of food, characterized by dull or acute pain around the lower part of the chest. (18)

Hydrochloric acid (HCl)—Strong acid secreted by the stomach that aids in protein digestion. (10)

Hydrogenation—The process of adding hydrogen to a fat to make it more highly saturated. (4)

Hydrolysis—A chemical reaction that splits a substance into simpler compounds by the addition of water. (10)

Hydrostatic pressure—The pressure created by the pumping action of the heart on the fluid in the blood vessels. (9)

Hyperalimentation—Another name for total parenteral nutrition. (15)

Hyperbilirubinemia—Excessive bilirubin in the blood; bilirubin is produced by the breakdown of red blood cells. (8)

Hypercalcemia—A serum calcium level that is too high; in adults, more than 5.5 milliequivalents per liter. (8)

Hypercholesterolemia—Excessive cholesterol in the blood. (20)

Hyperemesis gravidarum—Severe nausea and vomiting persisting after the fourteenth week of pregnancy. (11)

Hyperglycemia—An elevated level of glucose in the blood; fasting value above 110 or 120 milligrams per deciliter, depending on measuring technique used. (19)

Hyperglycemic hyperosmolar nonketotic syndrome (HHNS)—Life-threatening complication of NIDDM characterized by blood glucose levels greater than 600 milligrams per deciliter, absence of or slight ketosis, profound cellular dehydration, and electrolyte imbalances. (19)

Hyperkalemia—Excessive potassium in the blood; greater than 5.0 milliequivalents per liter of serum in adults. (8)

Hyperlipoproteinemia—Increased lipoproteins and lipids in the blood. (20)

Hypermetabolism—An abnormal increase in the rate at which fuel or kilocalories are burned. (24)

Hypernatremia—An excess of sodium in the blood; greater than 145 milliequivalents per liter of serum in adults. (8)

Hyperparathyroidism—Excessive secretion of parathyroid hormone, causing changes in the bones, kidney, and gastrointestinal tract. (8)

Hyperphosphatemia—Excessive amount of phosphates in the blood; in adults, greater than 4.7 milligrams per 100 milliliters of serum. (8)

Hypertension—Condition of elevated blood pressure; diagnosed if B/P is greater than 140/90 on three successive occasions or if person is receiving antihypertensive medication (20)

Hypertensive kidney disease—A condition in which vascular or glomerular lesions cause hypertension but not total renal failure. (21)

Hyperthyroidism—Oversecretion of thyroid hormones, which increases the metabolic rate above normal. (8)

Hypertonic—A solution that contains more particles and exerts more osmotic pressure than the plasma. (9)

Hypervitaminosis—Condition caused by excessive intake of vitamins. (7)

Hypocalcemia—A depressed level of calcium in the blood; less than 4.5 milliequivalents per liter of serum in adults. (8)

Hypoglycemia—A depressed level of glucose in the blood; less than 70 milligrams per deciliter. (19)

Hypokalemia—Potassium depletion in the circulating blood; less than 3.5 milliequivalents per liter of serum in adults. (8, 17, 21)

Hyponatremia—Too little sodium per volume of blood; less than 135 milliequivalents per liter of serum in adults. (8)

Hypophosphatemia—Too little phosphate per volume of blood; in adults, less than 2.4 milligrams per 100 milliliters of serum. (8)

Hypothalamus—A portion of the brain that helps to regulate water balance, thirst, body temperature, carbohydrate and fat metabolism, and sleep. (9)

Hypothyroidism—Undersecretion of thyroid hormones; reduces the metabolic rate. (8)

Hypotonic—A solution that contains fewer particles and exerts less osmotic pressure than the plasma does. (9)

Iatrogenic malnutrition—Excessive or deficit intake of one or more nutrients induced by the oversight or omissions of healthcare workers. (15)

Ideal body weight—A person's weight as compared with the 1943 Height/Weight Tables. (18)

Identity—The fifth developmental task in Erikson's theory, in which the adolescent decides on an appropriate role. (12)

Ileocecal valve—The valve between the ileum and cecum. (10)

Ileostomy—Surgical procedure in which an opening to the small intestine (ileum) is constructed on the abdomen. (22)

Ileum—The lower portion of the small intestine. (10, 22)

Immune—Produced by, involved in, or concerned with resistance or protection against a specified disease. (23)

Immune system—The organs in the body responsible for fighting off substances interpreted as foreign. (23)

Immunity—The state of being protected from a particular disease, especially an infectious disease. (5, 25)

Immunoglobulin—Blood proteins with known antibody activity; five classes of immunoglobulins have been identified. (5)

Immunosuppressive agent—Medication that interferes with the body's ability to fight infection. (14)

Impaired glucose tolerance (IGT)—A type of classification for hyperglycemia; for persons who have a glucose intolerance but do not meet the criteria for classification as having diabetes. (19)

Implantation—Embedding of the fertilized egg in the lining of the uterus 6 or 7 days after fertilization. (11)

Incidence—The frequency of occurrence of any event or condition over a given time and in relation to the population in which it occurs. (18)

Incomplete protein—Protein lacking one or more of the essential amino acids that humans need; found primarily in plant sources such as grains and vegetables; gelatin is an animal product but is an incomplete protein. (5)

Incubation period—The time it takes to show disease symptoms after exposure to the causative organism. (14)

Indication—A circumstance that indicates when a treatment should or can be used. (15)

Indoles—Compounds found in vegetables of the cruciferous family that activate enzymes to destroy carcinogens. (23)

Industry—The fourth stage of development in Erikson's theory in which the school-age child learns to work effectively. (12)

Infection—Entry and development of parasites or entry and multiplication of microorganisms in the bodies of persons or animals; may or may not cause signs and symptoms. (25)

Initiation—The first step in the cell's becoming cancerous, when physical forces, chemicals, or biologic agents permanently alter the cell's DNA. (23)

Initiative—The third stage of development in Erikson's theory, in which the preschooler learns to set and achieve goals. (12)

Insensible water loss—Water that is lost invisibly through the lungs and skin. (9)

Insoluble—Incapable of being dissolved. (3)

Insulin—Hormone secreted by the beta cells of the pancreas in response to an elevated blood glucose level. (5)

Insulin-dependent diabetes mellitus (IDDM)—Type 2 diabetes; persons with this disorder must take insulin to survive. (18)

Insulin resistance—A disorder characterized by elevated levels of both glucose and insulin; thought to be related to a lack of insulin receptors. (19)

Intact feeding—A feeding consisting of nutrients that have not been predigested. (15)

Intact nutrients—Nutrients that have not been predigested. (15)

Intact or "polymeric" formula—An oral or enteral feeding that contains all the essential nutrients in a specified volume. (15)

Integrity—The final stage of Erikson's theory of psychosocial development, in which the older adult learns to look back on his or her life as worthwhile. (13)

Intermittent feeding—Giving a 4- to 6-hour volume of a tube feeding over 20–30 minutes. (15)

Intermittent peritoneal dialysis—Method of dialysis treatment in which the dialysate remains in a patient's abdominal cavity for about 30 minutes and then drains from the body by gravity. (21)

International Unit (IU)—Individually scaled measure of vitamins A, D, and E agreed to by a committee of scientists; largely replaced by finer measures. (7)

Interstitial fluid—Extracellular fluid located between the cells. (9)

Intimacy—The sixth stage of development in Erikson's theory, in which the young adult builds reciprocal, caring relationships. (13)

Intracellular fluid—Fluid located within the cells. (9)

Intravascular fluid—Fluid found in the blood and lymph vessels. (9)

Intravenous—Through a vein. (3)

Intrinsic factor—Specific protein-binding factor secreted by the stomach, necessary for the absorption of vitamin B_{12}. (7)

Invisible fat—Dietary fats that cannot be seen easily; hidden fats in foods such as baked goods, peanut butter, emulsified milk, and so forth. (4)

Involution—Diminishing of an organ in vital power or in size. (13)

Ion—An atom or group of atoms carrying an electrical charge; an ion with a positive charge is called a cation; an ion with a negative charge is called an anion. (9)

Ionic bond—A chemical bond formed between atoms by the loss and gain of electrons. (9)

Iron-deficiency anemia—Anemia due to a greater demand on the stored iron than can be supplied; causes include inadequate iron intake, malabsorption, and chronic or acute blood loss. (8, 11)

Irrigation—Flushing a prescribed solution through a tube or cavity. (15)

Irritable bowel syndrome—Diarrhea or alternating constipation-diarrhea with no discernible organic cause. (22)

Islet cell antibody—A protein found to be elevated in a person with insulin-dependent diabetes mellitus. (19)

Islets of Langerhans—Clusters of cells in the pancreas including alpha, beta, and delta cells; alpha cells produce glucagon, beta cells produce insulin, and delta cells produce somatostatin. (19)

Isotonic—A solution that has the same osmotic pressure as blood plasma. (9, 15)

Jaundice—Yellowing of skin, whites of eyes, and mucous membranes due to excessive bilirubin in the blood; causes may be obstructed bile duct, liver disease, or hemolysis of red blood cells. (7)

Jejunoileal bypass—A surgical procedure that removes a portion of the small intestine, bypassing about 90 percent of it. (18)

Jejunostomy—A surgical opening in the jejunum. (15)

Jejunum—The second portion of the small intestine. (8, 10)

Kaposi's sarcoma—A type of cancer often related to the immunocompromised state that accompanies AIDS; characterized by multiple areas of cell proliferation, initially in the skin and eventually in other body sites. (25)

Keshan disease—Deterioration of the heart due to selenium deficiency but heart failure not reversible by supplementation; named for the province of Keshan, China; fatality rate as high as 80%; in mice, linked to a mutation of an avirulent virus to a virulent one producing myocardial disease; virulent strain then caused heart disease in mice not selenium-deficient. (8)

Keto acid—Amino acid residue left after deamination. (5)

Ketoacidosis—Acidosis due to an excess of ketone bodies. (19)

Ketone bodies—Compounds such as acetone and diacetic acid that are formed when fat is metabolized incompletely. (4)

Ketonuria—The presence of ketone bodies in the urine. (19)

Ketosis—The physical state of the human body with ketones elevated in the blood and present in the urine; one example is diabetic ketoacidosis. (3, 24)

Kilocaloric density—The kilocalories contained in a given volume of a food. (6)

Kilocalorie—A measurement unit of energy; the amount of heat required to raise 1 kilogram of water 1 degree Celsius; often referred to as calories by the general public. (6)

Kilocalori: nitrogen ratios—A mathematical relationship expressed as the number of kilocalories per gram of nitrogen provided in a feeding. (24)

Kilojoule—A measurement unit of energy; one kilocalorie equals 4.184 kilojoules. (6)

Korsakoff's psychosis—Amnesia, often seen in chronic alcoholism, caused by degeneration of the thalamus due to thiamin deficiency; characterized by loss of short-term memory and inability to learn new skills. (7)

Krebs cycle—A complicated series of reactions that results in the release of energy from carbohydrates, fats, and proteins, also known as the TCA (tricarboxylic acid) cycle. (10)

Kussmaul respirations—Pattern of rapid and deep breathing due to the body's attempt to correct metabolic acidosis by eliminating carbon dioxide through the lungs. (19)

Kwashiorkor—Severe protein deficiency in child after weaning; symptoms include edema, pigmentation changes, impaired growth and development, and liver pathology. (5, 9)

Lactalbumin—Simple soluble protein found in greater concentration in human breast milk than in cow's milk; easily absorbed by the infant. (12)

Lactase—An intestinal enzyme that converts lactose into glucose and galactose. (10)

Lacteal—The central lymph vessel in each villus. (10)

Lactose—A disaccharide found mainly in milk and milk products. (3)

Large intestine—The part of the alimentary canal that extends from the small intestine to the anus. (10)

LCAT deficiency—A lack of LCAT, an enzyme that transports cholesterol from the tissues to the liver for removal from the body. (21)

Legumes—Plants that have nitrogen-fixing bacteria in their roots; a good alternative to meat as a protein source; examples are dried beans, lentils. (5)

Lesion—Area of diseased or injured tissue. (21)

Leukopenia—Abnormal decrease in the number of white blood corpuscles; usually below 5000 per cubic millimeter. (25)

Life expectancy—The probable number of years that persons of a given age may be expected to live. (13)

Limiting amino acid—Particular essential amino acid lacking or undersupplied in a food that classifies the food as an incomplete protein. (5)

Linoleic acid—An essential fatty acid. (4)

Lipectomy—Surgical removal of adipose tissue. (18)

Lipid—Any one of a group of fats or fat-like substances that are insoluble in water; includes true fats (fatty acids and glycerol), lipoids, and sterols. (4)

Lipoid—Substances resembling fats, but containing groups other than glycerol and fatty acids that make up true fats; example: phospholipids. (4)

Lipolysis—The breakdown of adipose tissue for energy. (19, 24)

Lipoprotein—Combination of a protein with lipid components such as cholesterol, phospholipids, and triglycerides. (4)

Lipoprotein (a)—Genetic variant of LDL cholesterol; independent risk factor for coronary artery disease. (20)

Lipoprotein lipase—An enzyme that breaks down chylomicrons. (20)

Liposuction—Surgical removal of adipose tissue through a vacuum hose. (18)

Listeriosis—Bacterial infection caused by *Listeria monocytogenes* that is particularly virulent for fetuses; transmitted from the mother to the fetus in utero or through the birth canal; outbreaks associated with raw or contaminated milk, soft cheeses, contaminated vegetables, and ready-to-eat meats. (11)

Liver—A digestive organ that aids in the metabolism of all the energy nutrients, screens toxic substances from the blood, manufactures blood proteins, and performs many other important functions. (10)

Loop of Henle—The segment of the renal tubule that follows the proximal convoluted tubule. (21)

Low-birth-weight (LBW)—Characterizing an infant that weighs less than 2500 g (5.5 lb) at birth. (11)

Low-density lipoprotein (LDL)—A plasma protein containing more cholesterol and triglycerides than protein; elevated blood levels are associated with increased risk of heart disease. (20)

Luminal effect—Drug-induced changes within the intestine that affect the absorption of nutrients and drugs without altering the intestine. (17)

Lycopene—A red pigmented carotenoid with powerful antioxidant functions but no provitamin A activity; found in tomatoes and various berries and fruits. (23)

Lymph—A body fluid collected from the interstitial fluid all over the body and returned to the bloodstream via the lymphatic vessels. (10)

Lymphatic system—All the structures involved in the transportation of lymph from the tissues to the bloodstream. (10)

Lysine—Amino acid often lacking in grains. (4)

Macrocytic anemia—Anemia in which the red blood cells are larger than normal; also found in folic acid deficiency; one characteristic of pernicious anemia. (7)

Major minerals—Those present in the body in quantities greater than 5 grams (approximately 1 teaspoonful); human's daily need at least 100 milligrams (approximately 1/50 teaspoonful); also called macrominerals. (8)

Malabsorption—Inadequate movement of digested food from the small intestine into the blood or lymphatic system. (10)

Malignant—Tumor that infiltrates surrounding tissue and spreads to distant sites of the body. (23)

Malnutrition—Poor nutrition; results when the body's cells receive either an excess or a deficiency of one or more nutrients. (1)

Maltase—An intestinal enzyme that converts maltose into glucose. (10)

Maltose—A disaccharide produced when starches are broken down by the body into simpler units; two units of glucose joined together. (3)

Marasmus—Malnutrition due to a protein and kilocalorie deficit. (5)

Mastication—The process of chewing. (10)

Mechanical digestion—The digestive process that involves the physical breaking down of food into smaller pieces. (10)

Megadose—Dose providing 10 times or more the recommended dietary allowance. (7)

Megaloblastic anemia—Anemia characterized by the formation of large immature red blood cells that cannot carry oxygen properly; caused by folic acid deficiency. (7)

Menaquinone—Vitamin K that is synthesized by intestinal bacteria; also called vitamin K_2. (7)

Meninges—Three membranes covering the brain and spinal cord; from the outside named the dura, arachnoid, and pia maters. (11)

Meningocele— Congenital protrusion of the meninges through a defect in the skull or the spinal column. (11)

Meningoencephalocele—Protrusion of the brain and its coverings through a defect in the skull. (11)

Menkes' disease—Metabolic defect blocking the absorption of copper in the gastrointestinal tract. (8)

Meta-analysis—Statistical procedure for combining data from a number of studies to analyze therapeutic effectiveness. (16)

Metabolism—The sum of all physical and chemical changes that take place in the body; the two fundamental processes involved are anabolism and catabolism. (1, 6, 10)

Metastasis—The "seeding" of cancer cells to distant sites of the body; spread via blood or lymph vessels or by spilling into a body cavity. (23)

Methionine—Amino acid often lacking in legumes. (5)

Microalbuminuria—Small amounts of protein in the urine. Detected by a laboratory using methods more sensitive than traditional urinalysis. (19)

Microgram—One-millionth of a gram or one-thousandth of a milligram; abbreviated mcg or µg. (7)

Micronize—To pulverize a substance into very tiny particles. (17)

Microvilli—Microscopic, hairlike rodlets (resembling bristles on a brush) covering the edge of each villus. (10)

Midarm circumference—Measure of the distance around the middle of the upper arm; used to assess body protein stores. (2)

Mildly obese—Twenty to 40 percent overweight; 120–140 percent healthy body weight. (18)

Milk-alkali syndrome—Condition characterized by high blood calcium and a more alkaline urine that predisposes to the precipitation of calcium in the kidney; caused by ingestion of excessive absorbable alkali and milk; associated with the milk and cream and antacid treatment of peptic ulcers used years ago. (8)

Milliequivalent—Unit of measure used for determining the concentration of electrolytes in solution; expressed as milliequivalents per liter. (9)

Milling—The process of grinding grain into flour. (3)

Milliosmole—Unit of measure for osmotic activity. (9)

Mineral—An inorganic element or compound occurring in nature; in the body, minerals help regulate bodily functions and are essential to good health. (8)

Mixed malnutrition—The result of a deficiency or excess of more than one nutrient. (15)

Moderately obese—Forty-one to 100 percent overweight; 141 to 200 percent healthy body weight. (18)

Modified diet—A term used in healthcare institutions to mean the food served to a client has been altered or changed from that served to clients on regular diets, usually by physician order. (1)

Modular supplement—A nutritional supplement that contains a limited number of nutrients, usually only one. (15)

Mold—Any of a group of parasitic or other organisms living on decaying matter; fungi. (14)

Molecule—The smallest quantity into which a substance may be divided without loss of its characteristics. (3)

Monoamine oxidase inhibitor (MAO inhibitor)—A class of antidepressant drugs that may have critical interactions with foods. (17)

Monoglyceride—One fatty acid joined to a glycerol molecule. (4)

Monosaccharide—A simple sugar composed of one unit of $C_6H_{12}O_6$; examples include glucose, fructose, and galactose. (3)

Monounsaturated fat—A lipid in which the majority of fatty acids contain one carbon-to-carbon double bond. (4)

Morbidity—The state of being diseased; number of cases of disease in relation to population. (15)

Mortality—The death rate; number of deaths per unit of population. (13)

Motility—Power to move spontaneously. (13)

Mucosa—A mucous membrane that lines body cavities. (10)

Mucosal effect—Drug-induced changes within the intestine that affect the absorption of drugs or nutrients by damaging the tissues. (17)

Mucus—A thick fluid secreted by the mucous membranes and glands. (10)

Multiparous— Having borne more than one child. (11)

Muscular dystrophy—A disease characterized by wasting away of skeletal muscle with replacement of muscle cells by fat and connective tissue; most forms are genetic, but one form is associated with a vitamin E deficiency. (7)

Mutation—Permanent transmissible change in a gene; *natural* mutation produces evolutionary change in organisms; *induced* mutation results from exposure to environmental influences such as physical forces, chemicals, or biologic agents. (23)

Mycotoxin—A substance produced by mold growing in food that can cause illness or death when ingested by humans or animals. (14)

Myelin sheath—Fatty covering surrounding the long appendages of some nerves; serves to increase the transmission speed of impulses. (7)

Myocardial infarction (MI)—Area of dead heart muscle; usually the result of coronary occlusion. (20)

Myocardium—The heart muscle. (20)

Myoglobin—A protein located in muscle tissue that contains and stores oxygen. (8)

Myxedema—A condition that occurs in older children and adults, resulting from hypofunction of the thyroid gland characterized by a drying and thickening of the skin and slowing of physical and mental activity. (8)

Narcolepsy—A chronic condition consisting of recurrent attacks of drowsiness and sleep. (18)

Nasoduodenal tube (ND tube)—A tube inserted via the nose into the duodenum. (15)

Nasogastric tube (NG tube)—A tube inserted via the nose into the stomach. (15)

Nasojejunal tube (NJ tube)—A tube inserted via the nose into the jejunum. (15)

Neoplasm—A new and abnormal formation of tissue (tumor) that grows at the expense of the healthy organism. (23)

Nephritis—General term for inflammation of the kidneys. (21)

Nephron—The structural and functional unit of the kidney. (20)

Nephropathy—A kidney disease characterized by inflammation and degenerative lesions. (19)

Nephrosclerosis—A hardening of the renal arteries; may be caused by arteriosclerosis of the kidney arteries. (21)

Nephrotic syndrome—The end result of a variety of diseases that cause the abnormal passage of plasma proteins into the urine. (21)

Neuropathy—Any disease of the nerves. (19)

Niacin—A B-vitamin that functions as a coenzyme in the production of energy from glucose; obtained from meat or produced from the amino acid tryptophan, present in milk, eggs, and meat; also called nicotinic acid. (7)

Niacin equivalent (NE)—Measure of niacin activity; equal to 1 milligram of preformed niacin or 60 milligrams of tryptophan. (7)

Night blindness—Vision that is slow to adapt to dim light; caused by vitamin A deficiency or hereditary factors, or, in the elderly, by poor circulation. (7)

Nitrogen—Colorless, odorless, tasteless gas forming about 80 percent of the earth's air. (5)

Nitrogen balance—The difference between the amount of nitrogen ingested and that excreted each day; when intake is greater, a positive balance exists; when intake is less, a negative balance exists. (5)

Nitrogen-fixing bacteria—Organisms that absorb nitrogen from the air, which, upon the death of the bacteria, is released for legume plants to use in the anabolism of protein. (5)

Nomogram—A chart that shows a relationship between numerical values. (18)

Nonessential—In nutrition, refers to a chemical substance or nutrient the body can manufacture. (1)

Nonessential amino acid—Any amino acid that can be synthesized by the body in sufficient quantities. (5)

Nonheme iron—Iron that is not bound to hemoglobin or myoglobin; all the iron in plant sources. (8)

Noninsulin-dependent diabetes mellitus (NIDDM)—Type 2 diabetes; insulin resistance commonly occurs; although some persons with this disorder take insulin, it is not necessary for their long-term survival. (19, 20)

North American Nursing Diagnosis Association—An organization of nurses, established in 1973, that fosters the use of standard terminology in describing client problems. (2)

Norwalk virus—A causative organism that is responsible for more than 50% of the reported cases of epidemic viral gastroenteropathy. The incubation period ranges from 18 to 72 hours, and the outbreaks are usually self-limiting. Flu-like intestinal symptoms last for 24–48 hours. (14)

Nulliparous—Never having borne a child. (11)

Nursing action (intervention)—Specific care to be administered, including physical and psychological care, teaching, counseling, and referring. (2)

Nursing-bottle syndrome—A condition in which an infant has many dental caries caused by drinking milk or other sweet liquids during sleep. (3)

Nursing diagnosis—Statement of a client's nursing problem that the nurse is licensed to treat. (2)

Nursing process—Systematic and orderly method of delivering nursing care, composed of five steps: assessment, nursing diagnosis, planning, implementation, and evaluation. (2)

Nutrient—Chemical substance supplied by food that the body needs for growth, maintenance, and/or repair. (1)

Nutrient density—The concentration of nutrients in a given volume of food compared with the food's kilocalorie content. (6)

Nutrition—The science of food and its relationship to living beings. (1)

Nutrition support service—A team service for clients on enteral and parenteral feedings that assesses, monitors, and counsels these clients. (15)

Nutritional assessment—The evaluation of a client's nutritional status based on a physical examination, anthropometric measurements, laboratory data, and food intake information. (2)

Nutritional status—Refers to the condition of the body as it relates to the intake and use of nutrients. (1)

Obese—Body fat content greater than 24 percent in males or 33 percent in females. (18)

Obesity—Excessive amount of fat on the body; obesity for women is a fat content greater than 33 percent; obesity for men is a fat content greater than 24 percent. (18)

Objective data—Findings verifiable by another through physical assessment or diagnostic tests, also termed signs. (2)

Obligatory excretion—Minimum amount of urine production necessary to keep waste products in solution, amounting to 400 to 600 milliliters per day. (9)

Oliguria—A decreased output of urine. (21)

Odds ratio—A measure of disease occurrence in epidemiological, case-control studies; the odds in favor of a particular event occurring in an exposed group are divided by the odds in favor of the disease occurring in an unexposed group. If the condition under study is rare, the odds ratio is a close approximation to the relative risk. (20)

Oncogene—Carcinogenic gene that stimulates excessive reproduction of the cell. (23)

Opportunistic infection—Infection caused by normally nonpathogenic organisms in a host with decreased resistance. (25)

Opsin—A protein that combines with vitamin A to form rhodopsin, a chemical in the retina necessary for vision. (7)

Optic nerve—The second cranial nerve, which transmits impulses for the sense of sight. (7)

Oral cavity—The cavity in the skull bounded by the mouth, palate, cheeks, and tongue. (10)

Organ—Somewhat independent body part having specific functions. Examples: stomach, liver. (10)

Orthostatic hypotension—A drop in blood pressure producing dizziness, fainting, or blurred vision when arising from a lying or sitting position or when standing motionless in a fixed position. (9)

Osmolality—Measure of osmotic pressure exerted by the number of dissolved particles per weight of liquid; clinically usually reported as mOsm/kg. (9)

Osmolarity—Measure of osmotic pressure exerted by the number of dissolved particles per volume of liquid; clinically usually reported as mOsm/L. (9)

Osmosis—The movement of water across a semipermeable cell membrane from an area with fewer particles to one with more particles. (9)

Osmotic pressure—The pressure that develops when a concentrated solution is separated from a less concentrated solution by a semipermeable membrane; only water crosses the membrane. (9)

Osteoarthritis—Progressive deterioration of the cartilage in the joints; risk factors are aging, obesity, occupational or athletic abuse of joints, and trauma. (13)

Osteoblasts—Bone cells that build bone. (8)

Osteocalcin—Hormonally regulated calcium-binding protein made almost exclusively by the bone-building cells called osteoblasts; vitamin K facilitates synthesis of osteocalcin. (7)

Osteoclasts—Bone cells that break down bone. (8)

Osteodystrophy—Defective bone formation. (21)

Osteomalacia—Adult form of rickets. (7)

Osteopenia—Bone mineral density 1 to 2.5 standard deviations below the mean of healthy young adults. (8)

Osteoporosis—Bone mineral density more than 2.5 standard deviations below the mean of young adults. (8)

Ostomy—A surgically formed opening to permit passage of urine or bowel contents to the outside. (15)

Overnutrition—The result of an excess of one or more nutrients in the diet. (1)

Overweight—Ten to 20 percent above healthy body weight; 110–120 percent healthy body weight. (18)

Ovum—The egg cell that, after fertilization by a sperm cell, develops into a new individual. (11)

Oxalates—Salts of oxalic acid found in some plant foods; bind with the calcium in the plant, making it unavailable to the body. (8)

Oxidation—The process in which a substance is combined with oxygen. (7, 10)

Oxytocin—A hormone produced by the posterior pituitary gland in the brain; effects are uterine contractions and release of milk. (11)

Pancreas—An abdominal gland that secretes enzymes important in the digestion of carbohydrates, fats, and proteins; also secretes the hormones insulin and glucagon. (10, 22)

Pancreatic lipase—An enzyme produced by the pancreas; used in fat digestion. (10)

Pancreatitis—Inflammation of the pancreas. (22, 25)

Pantothenic acid—A B-complex vitamin found in almost all foods; deficiencies from lack of food have not been documented. (7)

Paralytic ileus—A temporary cessation of peristalsis that causes an intestinal obstruction. (24)

Paralytic shellfish poisoning—Disease caused by the consumption of poisonous clams, oysters, mussels, or scallops. (14)

Parasite—An organism that lives within, upon, or at the expense of a living host. (14)

Parathyroid hormone (PTH)—Hormone secreted by the parathyroid glands; regulates calcium and phosphorus metabolism in the body. (7, 8, 21)

Parenteral feeding—A feeding administered by any route other than the gastrointestinal tract. (15)

Parietal—Two bones that form the sides and roof of the skull; also two lobes of the cerebrum lying roughly under those bones. (16)

Parotid glands—One of the salivary glands of the mouth, located just below and in front of the ears; the mumps virus causes infectious parotitis. (10)

Pectin—Purified carbohydrate obtained from peel of citrus fruits or apple pulp; gels when cooked with sugar at correct pH to thicken jelly and jam; contained in mashed raw apple, applesauce, firm banana prescribed for diarrhea to contribute firmness to stools. (22)

Pellagra—Deficiency disease due to lack of niacin and tryptophan; characterized by the so-called three Ds: dermatitis, diarrhea, and dementia. (7)

Pepsin—An enzyme secreted in the stomach that begins protein digestion. (10)

Pepsinogen—The antecedent of pepsin; activated by hydrochloric acid, a component of gastric juice. (10)

Peptidases—Enzymes that assist in the digestion of protein by reducing the smaller molecules to single amino acids. (10)

Peptide bond—Chemical bond that links two amino acids in a protein molecule. (5, 10)

Percutaneously—Affected through the skin. (15)

Perforated ulcer—Condition in which an ulcer penetrates completely through the stomach or intestinal wall, spilling the organ's contents into the peritoneal cavity. (22)

Periodontal disease—Any disorder of the supporting structures of the teeth. (13)

Peripheral parenteral nutrition (PPN)—An intravenous feeding via a vein away from the center of the body. (15)

Peristalsis—A wave-like movement that propels food along the alimentary canal. (10, 24)

Peritoneal dialysis—Method of removing waste products from the blood by injecting the flushing solution into a client's abdomen and using the client's peritoneum as the semipermeable membrane. (21)

Peritoneum—The membrane that covers the internal abdominal organs and lines the abdominal cavity. (21)

Peritonitis—Inflammation of the peritoneal cavity. (22)

Pernicious anemia—Inadequate red blood cell formation due to lack of intrinsic factor from the stomach, which is required for the absorption of vitamin B_{12}; leads to neural deterioration. (7)

Pesticides—A chemical used to kill insects or rodents. (14)

Petechiae—Pinpoint, flat, round, red lesions caused by intradermal or submucosal hemorrhage. (7)

pH—A scale representing the relative acidity or alkalinity of a solution; a value of 7 is neutral, less than 7 is acidic, and greater than 7 is alkaline. (9)

Pharynx—The muscular passage between the oral cavity and the esophagus. (10)

Phenylalanine—Essential amino acid, which is indigestible if a person lacks a particular enzyme. Accumulation of phenylalanine in the blood can lead to mental retardation. (5)

Phenylketonuria (PKU)—Hereditary disease caused by the body's failure to convert phenylalanine to tyrosine because of a defective enzyme. (5)

Phospholipid—An organic compound in the lipid group composed of one glycerol, two fatty acids, and one phosphate molecule; examples include lecithin and myelin. (8)

Photosynthesis—Process by which plants containing chlorophyll are able to manufacture carbohydrates from carbon dioxide and water using the sun's energy. (3)

Phylloquinone—Vitamin K_1, found in foods. (7)

Phytic acid—A substance found in grains that forms an insoluble complex with calcium; phytates. (8)

Phytochemicals—Nonnutritive food components that provide medical or health benefits including the prevention or treatment of a disease. (1)

Phytonadione—Synthetic, water-soluble pharmaceutical form of Vitamin K_1; can be administered orally or by injection. (7)

Pica—The craving to eat nonfood substances such as clay and starch. (11)

Placenta—The organ in the uterus through which the unborn child exchanges carbon dioxide for oxygen and wastes for nourishment; lay term is afterbirth. (11)

Plasma—The liquid portion of the blood including the clotting elements. (9)

Plasma transferrin receptor—Measure of iron status; increases even in mild deficiency; unaffected by inflammation. (8)

Plumbism—Lead poisoning. (8)

Pneumocystis pneumonia—A type of lung infection frequently seen in AIDS patients; caused by the organism *Pneumocystis carinii*. (25)

Polydipsia—Excessive thirst. (19)

Polymer—A natural or synthetic substance formed by combining two or more molecules of the same substance. (3)

Polypeptide—A chain of amino acids linked by peptide bonds that form proteins. (5, 10)

Polyphagia—Excessive appetite. (19)

Polysaccharide—Complex carbohydrates composed of many units of $C_6H_{12}O_6$ joined together; examples important in nutrition include starch, glycogen, and fiber. (3)

Polyunsaturated fat—A fat in which the majority of fatty acids contain more than one carbon-to-carbon double bond; intake is associated with a decreased risk of heart disease. (4)

Polyuria—Excessive urination. (19)

Positive feedback cycle—Situation in which a condition provokes a response that worsens the condition. Example: low blood pressure due to a failing heart stimulates the kidney to save sodium and water. (20)

Potassium pump—Proteins located in cell membranes that provide an active transport mechanism to move potassium ions across a membrane to their area of greater concentration; moves potassium ions into the cells. (9)

Precursor—A substance from which another substance is derived. (7)

Preeclampsia—Hypertension, edema, and proteinuria, appearing after the twentieth week of pregnancy. (11)

Preformed vitamin—A vitamin already in a complete state in ingested foods, as opposed to a provitamin, which requires conversion in the body to be in a complete state. (7)

Pregnancy-induced hypertension (PIH)—A potentially life-threatening disorder that may develop after the twentieth week of pregnancy; includes preeclampsia and eclampsia. (11)

Pressure ulcer—Tissue breakdown from external force impairing circulation. (13, 15)

Prevalence—The likelihood of an occurrence taking place within a population group. (18)

Primary malnutrition—A nutrient deficiency due to poor food choices or a lack of nutritious food to eat. (15)

Principle of complementarity—Combining incomplete-protein foods so that each supplies the amino acids lacking in the other. (5)

Prion—A proteinaceous infectious agent, extremely difficult to destroy; resistant to heat, pressure cooking, ultraviolet light, irradiation, bleach, formaldehyde, and weak acids; even autoclaving at 135° for 18 minutes does not eliminate infectivity. (14)

Prognosis—Probable outcome of an illness based on client's condition and natural course of the disease. (25)

Promotion—The second step in a cell turning cancerous, through the action of environmental substances on the altered, initiated gene. (23)

Prostaglandins—Long-chain, unsaturated fatty acids mostly synthesized in the body from arachidonic acid; have hormone-like effects. (4)

Protein—Nutrient necessary for building body tissue; composed of carbon, hydrogen, oxygen, and nitrogen (and sometimes with sulfur, phosphorus, or iron); amino acids represent the basic structure of proteins. (5)

Protein binding sites—Various sites in the body tissues to which drugs may become attached, rendering the drug temporarily inactive. (17)

Proteinuria—Protein in the urine. (21)

Protein-calorie malnutrition (PCM)—Condition in which the person's diet lacks both protein and kilocalories. (5)

Prothrombin—A protein essential to the blood-clotting process; manufactured by the liver using vitamin K. (7)

Protocol—A description of steps to be followed when performing a procedure or providing care for a particular condition. (15)

Proto-oncogene—Gene that in the normal cell stimulates growth and maintenance; when mutated, becomes an oncogene. (23)

Provitamin—Inactive substance that the body converts to an active vitamin. (7)

Provitamin A—Carotene. (7)

Proximal convoluted tubule—The first segment of the renal tubule. (21)

Psychology—The science of mental processes and their effects on behavior. (18)

Psychosis—Severe mental disturbance with personality derangement and loss of contact with reality. (7)

Psychosocial development—The maturing of an individual in relationships with others and within himself or herself. (12)

Ptyalin—A salivary enzyme that breaks down starch and glycogen to maltose and a small amount of glucose; also known as salivary amylase. (10)

Puberty—The period of life at which the physical ability to reproduce is attained. (12)

Pulmonary—Concerning or involving the lungs. (24)

Pulmonary edema—The accumulation of fluid in the lungs. (20)

Pulse pressure—The difference between systolic and diastolic blood pressure; normally 30–40 mmHg; narrows in fluid volume deficit and widens in fluid volume excess. (9)

Purging—The intentional clearing of food out of the human body by vomiting and/or using enemas, laxatives, and/or diuretics. (18)

Purines—One of the end products of the digestion of some nitrogen-containing compounds. (21)

Pyelonephritis—An inflammation of the central portion of the kidney. (21)

Pyloric sphincter—The sphincter muscle guarding the opening between the stomach and small intestine. (10)

Pyridoxine—Coenzyme in the synthesis and catabolism of amino acids; also called vitamin B_6. (7)

Pyruvate—An intermediate in the metabolism of energy nutrients. (10)

Quality assurance—A planned and systematic program for evaluating the quality and appropriateness of services rendered. (15)

Quetelet's Index—Body Mass Index. (2)

Radiologist—Physician with special training in diagnostic imaging and radiation treatments. (14)

Rancid—Having the rank smell and sour taste of stale fat or oil from decomposition. (1)

Rate—The speed or frequency of an event per unit of time. (18)

Rationale—Reason certain actions are likely to achieve a desired outcome; in nursing, ideally based on research indicating a nursing action was effective in similar circumstances. (2)

Rebound scurvy—Vitamin C deficiency produced in a person following cessation of megadosing due to a habitually lessened rate of absorption. (7)

Recessive trait—One that requires two recessive genes for the trait, one from each parent, for the trait to be expressed (to be manifested) in the individual. (22)

Recommended Dietary Allowance—Intake that meets the needs of 97–98% of the individuals in a life-stage and gender group; intended as a goal for daily intake by individuals, not for assessing adequacy of an individual's nutrient intake. (2)

Rectum—The lower part of the large intestine. (10)

Refeeding—The reintroduction of kilocalories and nutrients into a patient either orally or parenterally. (24)

Refeeding syndrome—A detrimental state that results when a previously severely malnourished person is reintroduced to food and/or nutrients and kilocalories improperly. (24)

Regurgitate—To cause to flow backward, as with an infant "spitting up." (15)

Relative risk—In epidemiological studies, the ratio of the frequency of a certain disorder in groups exposed and groups not exposed to a particular hereditary or environmental factor. (19)

Renal—Pertaining to the kidney. (9, 21)

Renal corpuscle—Refers collectively to both Bowman's capsule and the glomerulus. (21)

Renal exchange lists—A specialized type of exchange list for clients with kidney disease who require restriction of one or more of the following: protein, sodium, phosphorus, and potassium. (21)

Renal osteodystrophy—Defective bone development caused by phosphorus retention, a low or normal serum calcium level, and increased parathyroid activity. (21)

Renal pelvis—A structure inside the kidney that receives urine from the collecting tubules. (21)

Renal threshold—The blood glucose level at which glucose begins to spill into the urine. (19)

Renal tubule—The second major portion of the nephron; appears rope-like. (21)

Renin—An enzyme produced by the kidney that catalyzes the conversion of angiotensinogen to angiotensin I. (9)

Rennin—An enzyme that coagulates milk. (10)

Reservoir—Place that an infectious agent normally lives and multiplies so that it can be transmitted to a susceptible host. (14)

Residue—Trace amount of any substance in a product at the time of sale; substance remaining in the bowel after absorption. (14, 22)

Respiration—The exchange of oxygen and carbon dioxide between a living organism and the environment. (24)

Respirator—A machine used to assist respiration. (24)

Respiratory acidosis—Blood pH less than 7.35 caused by pulmonary disease, characterized by a retention of carbon dioxide. (24)

Respiratory alkalosis—Blood pH greater than 7.45 caused by pulmonary disease, characterized by a loss of carbon dioxide. (24)

Resting energy expenditure (REE)—The amount of fuel the human body uses at rest for a specified period of time; often used interchangeably with basal metabolic rate (BMR). (6)

Retina—Inner lining of eyeball that contains light-sensitive nerve cells; corresponds to film in camera. (7)

Retinol—The chemical name for preformed vitamin A. (7)

Retinol equivalents (RE)—A measure of vitamin A activity that considers both preformed vitamin A (retinol) and its precursor (carotene); 1 RE equals 3.3 International Units from animal foods and 10 International Units from plant foods; 1 RE corresponds to 1 microgram of retinol. (7)

Retinopathy—Any disorder of the retina. (19)

Retrolental fibroplasia (RLF)—A disease of the vessels of the retina present in premature infants; often caused by exposure to high postnatal oxygen concentration. (12)

Rhodopsin—Light-sensitive protein in the retina that contains vitamin A; also called visual purple. (7)

Riboflavin—Coenzyme in the metabolism of protein; also called vitamin B_2. (7)

Ribonucleic acid (RNA)—A substance in the cell nucleus that controls protein synthesis in all living cells. (5)

Rickets—Disease caused by a deficiency of vitamin D that affects the young during the period of skeletal growth, resulting in bones that are abnormally shaped and weak. (7)

Ritter syndrome—An inflammatory skin disease seen in newborns, characterized by pustules that fill with a straw-colored fluid and become encrusted. (14)

Rooting reflex—The infant's natural response to a stroke on its cheek, which turns the head toward that side to nurse. (12)

Rotavirus—Most common cause of infectious enteritis in human infants; associated with about one-third of the cases of diarrhea requiring hospitalization in children younger than 5 years old. (12)

Roux-en-Y—a surgical connection between the distal end of the small bowel and another organ such as the stomach. (18)

Rugae—Folds of mucosa of organs such as the stomach. (10)

Salivary amylase—An enzyme that initiates the breakdown of starch in the mouth. (10)

Salivary glands—The glands that secrete saliva into the mouth. (10)

Salmonella—A genus of bacteria responsible for many cases of foodborne illness. (14)

Salmonellosis—A bacterial infection manifested by the sudden onset of headache, abdominal pain, diarrhea, nausea, and vomiting. Fever is almost always present. Contaminated food is the predominant method of transmission. (14)

Sarcoma—A malignant neoplasm that occurs in connective tissue such as muscle or bone. (23)

Satiety—The feeling after consuming food that enough has been eaten; the sensation of satisfaction. (3)

Saturated fat—A fat in which the majority of fatty acids contain no carbon-to-carbon double bonds. (4)

Scurvy—Disease due to deficiency of vitamin C marked by bleeding problems and, later, by bony skeleton changes. (7)

Seasonal variation—Refers to differences during spring, summer, fall, and winter. (1)

Sebaceous gland—Oil-secreting gland of the skin; most sebaceous glands have a hair follicle associated with them. (4)

Secondary diabetes—A World Health Organization (WHO) classification for diabetes when the hyperglycemia occurs as a result of a second disorder. (19)

Secondary hypertension—High blood pressure that develops as the result of another condition. (20)

Secondary malnutrition—A nutrient deficiency due to improper absorption and distribution of nutrients. (15)

Secretin—A hormone that stimulates the production of bile by the liver and the secretion of sodium bicarbonate juice by the pancreas. (10)

Self-monitoring of blood glucose (SMBG)—A procedure that persons with diabetes follow to test their own blood glucose levels. (19)

Sensible water loss—Visible water loss through perspiration, urine, and feces. (9)

Sensitivity—Characteristic of diagnostic test; the proportion of people correctly identified as having the condition in question; a score of 100% would indicate that all the affected persons were identified by the test. (22)

Sepsis—A condition in which disease-producing organisms are present in the blood. (24)

Serosa—A serous membrane that covers internal organs and lines body cavities. (6)

Serotonin—A body chemical that assists the transmission of nerve impulses; it produces constriction of blood vessels and is thought to be related to sleep. (7, 18)

Serum—The liquid portion of the blood minus the clotting elements. (9)

Serum transferrin—Globulin in the blood that binds and transports iron; level increases in early iron deficiency, before hemoglobin and hematocrit readings drop. (8)

Severely obese—Greater than 100 percent overweight; also expressed as greater than 201 percent healthy body weight. (18)

Shelf life—The duration of time a product can remain in storage without deterioration. (4)

Shigella—Organisms causing intestinal disease; spread by fecal-oral transmission from a client or carrier via direct contact or indirectly by contaminated food. (14)

Shock—Acute peripheral circulatory failure due to loss of circulatory fluid or derangement of circulatory control producing decreased blood pressure, increased pulse rate, skin becomes cool and clammy from perspiration; urine output decreased. (9)

Signs—See objective data. (2)

Simple carbohydrate—Composed of one or two units of $C_6H_{12}O_6$; includes the monosaccharides (glucose, fructose, and galactose) and the disaccharides (sucrose, lactose, and maltose). (3)

Simple fat—Lipids that consist of fatty acids or a simple filler such as a hydroxyl (OH) molecule joined to glycerol. (4)

Small for gestational age (SGA)—Infant weighing less at birth than considered normal for the calculated length of the pregnancy. (12)

Small intestine—The part of the alimentary canal between the stomach and the large intestine, where most absorption of nutrients occurs. (10)

Sodium pump—Proteins located in cell membranes that provide an active transport mechanism to move sodium ions across a membrane to their area of greater concentration; moves sodium ions out of the cells and water follows. (9)

Solubility—The ability of one substance to dissolve into another in solution. (3)

Soluble—Able to be dissolved. (3)

Solute—The substance that is dissolved in a solvent. (9)

Solvent—A liquid holding another substance in solution. (9)

Somatostatin—A hormone produced by the delta cells of the islets of Langerhans that inhibits both the release of insulin and the production of glucagon. (19)

Specific gravity—The weight of a substance compared to an equal volume of a standard substance; usual standard for liquids is water, its specific gravity set at 1.000. (17)

Specificity—Characteristic of diagnostic test; the proportion of people correctly identified as not having the condition in question; a score of 100% would indicate that all the unaffected persons were identified by the test. (22)

Sphincter—A circular band of muscles that constricts a passage. (10)

Spina bifida—Congenital defect in spinal column whereby the vertebrae fail to close; clinical manifestations may or may not include protrusion of the meninges outside the spinal canal. (11)

Spore—A form assumed by some bacteria that is highly resistant to heat, drying, and chemicals. (12)

Sprue—Chronic form of malabsorption syndrome affecting the small intestine; subcategories: tropical and nontropical. (10, 22)

Staphylococcus aureus—One of the most common species of bacteria, which produces a poisonous toxin. The main reservoir is nose and throat discharge. Food can act as a vehicle for transmission, so proper hand washing is an essential means of control. (14)

Starches—Polysaccharides; many units of $C_6H_{12}O_6$ joined together; complex carbohydrates. (3)

Steatorrhea—The presence of greater than normal amounts of fat in the stool, producing foul-smelling, bulky excrement. (10, 22)

Sterol—Substance related to fats and belonging to the lipoids; for example, cholesterol. (4)

Stimulus control—The identification of cues that precede a behavior and rearranging daily activities to avoid such cues. (18)

Stoma—A surgically created opening in the abdominal wall. (22)

Stomach—The portion of the alimentary canal between the esophagus and small intestine. (10)

Stomatitis—An inflammation of the mouth. (17, 21)

Stress—Any threat to a person's mental or physical well-being. (24)

Stress factor—A number used to predict how much a client's kilocalorie need has increased as a result of a disease state. (24)

Subcutaneously—Beneath the skin. (19)

Subdural hematoma—Collection of blood under the outermost membrane covering the brain and spinal cord; usually resulting from head injury. (16)

Subjective data—Experiences the client reports, also termed symptoms. (2)

Submucosa—Structural layer of the alimentary canal below the mucosa; contains tissues and blood vessels. (10)

Sucrase—An enzyme in the intestinal mucosa that splits sucrose into glucose and fructose. (10)

Sucrose—A disaccharide; one unit of glucose and one unit of fructose joined together; ordinary white table sugar. (3)

Superior vena cava—One of the largest diameter veins in the human body; used to deliver total parenteral nutrition. (15)

Symptoms—See subjective data. (2)

System—An organized grouping of related structures or parts. (10)

Systemic circulation—Refers to the blood flow from the left part of the heart through the aorta and all branches (arteries) to the capillaries of the tissues. Systemic circulation also includes the blood's return to the heart through the veins and lymph vessels. (23)

Systolic pressure—Pressure exerted against the arteries when the heart contracts; the upper number of the blood pressure reading. (9, 20)

T-lymphocytes (T-cells)—White blood cells that recognize and fight foreign cells such as cancer; thymic lymphocytes. (23)

Tapeworm—A parasitic intestinal worm that is acquired by humans through the ingestion of raw seafood or undercooked beef or pork. (14)

Target heart rate—Seventy percent of maximum heart rate (number of heartbeats per minute); a person's target heart rate can be objectively determined by a stress test. Individuals can estimate their target heart rate by subtracting their age from 220 and multiplying the difference by 70 percent. A person's target heart rate is the rate at which the pulse should be maintained for at least 20 minutes during aerobic exercise. (6)

Teratogenic—Capable of causing abnormal development of the embryo; results in a malformed fetus. (11)

Term infant—One born between the beginning of the 38th week through the 41st week of gestation. (12)

Tetany—Muscle contractions, especially of the wrists and ankles, resulting from a disorder characterized by low levels of ionized calcium in the blood; causes include parathyroid deficiency, vitamin D deficiency, and alkalosis. (7)

Thermic effect of exercise (TEE)—The number of kilocalories used above resting energy expenditure as a result of physical activity. (6)

Thermic effect of foods (diet-induced thermogenesis, specific-dynamic action)—The energy cost to extract and utilize the kilocalories and nutrients in foods; the heat produced after eating a meal. (6)

Thiamin—Coenzyme in the metabolism of carbohydrates and fats; vitamin B_1. (7)

Thiaminase—An enzyme in raw fish that destroys thiamin. (7)

Third-space losses—Sequestering of fluid in body cavities such as the chest and abdomen; in the abdominal cavity, it produces ascites. (9)

Thoracic—Pertaining to the chest, or thorax. (10)

Thoracic duct—Major lymphatic vessel draining all except the right upper half of the body; empties into left internal jugular and left subclavian veins. (9)

Threonine—Essential amino acid often lacking in grains. (5)

Thrombus—A blood clot that obstructs a blood vessel; obstruction of a vessel of the brain or heart is among the most serious effects. (20)

Thrush—An infection caused by the organism *Candida albicans;* characterized by the formation of white patches and ulcers in the mouth and throat. (25)

Thymus—Gland in the chest, above and in front of the heart, which contributes to the immune response, including the maturation of T-lymphocytes. (23)

Thyroid-stimulating hormone (TSH)—A hormone secreted by the pituitary gland that stimulates the thyroid gland to secrete thyroxine and triiodothyronine; thyrotropin. (8)

Thyrotropin-releasing factor (TRF)—Stimulates the secretion of thyroid-stimulating hormone; produced in the hypothalamus. (8)

Thyroxine (T_4)—A hormone secreted by the thyroid gland; increases the rate of metabolism and energy production. (8)

Tissue—A group or collection of similar cells and their similar intercellular substance that acts together in the performance of a particular function. (11)

Tolerable Upper Intake Level (UL)—Maximum intake by an individual that is unlikely to pose risks of adverse health effects in 97–98% of individuals in specified life-stage and gender group; ordinarily refers to intake from food, fortified food, water, and supplements. (2)

Tolerance level—The highest dose at which a residue causes no ill effects in laboratory animals. (14)

Total parenteral nutrition (TPN)—An intravenous feeding that provides all nutrients known to be required. (15)

Trace minerals—Those present in the body in amounts less than 5 grams; daily intake of less than 100 milligrams needed; also called microminerals or trace elements. (8)

Traction—The process of using weights to draw a part of the body into alignment. (15)

Transcellular fluid—Located in body cavities and spaces; constantly being secreted and absorbed; examples: cerebrospinal fluid, pericardial fluid, pleural fluid. (9)

Transferrin—Protein in the blood that binds and transports iron. (8)

Trauma—A physical injury or wound caused by an external force; an emotional or psychological shock that usually results in disordered behavior. (24)

Triceps skinfold—Measure of skin and subcutaneous tissue over the triceps muscle in the upper arm; used in body fat assessment. (2)

Trichinella spiralis—A worm-like parasite that becomes embedded in the muscle tissue of pork. (14)

Trichinosis—The infestation of _Trichinella spiralis;_ a parasitic roundworm, transmitted by eating raw or insufficiently cooked pork. (14)

Triglyceride—Three fatty acids joined to a glycerol molecule. (4)

Triiodothyronine (T_3)—A hormone secreted by the thyroid gland that increases the rate of metabolism and energy production. (8)

Trousseau's sign—Spasms of the forearm and hand upon inflation of the blood pressure cuff; sign of tetany or lack of ionized calcium in the blood. (8)

Trust—First stage of Erikson's theory of psychosocial development, in which the infant learns to rely on those caring for it. (12)

Trypsin—An enzyme formed in the intestine that assists in protein digestion. (10)

Tryptophan—An essential amino acid, often lacking in legumes. (7)

Tubular reabsorption—The movement of fluid back into the blood from the renal tubule. (19)

Tubule—A small tube or canal. (21)

Tumor suppressor gene—Gene that inhibits growth and division of the cell. (23)

Turgor—Resilience of skin; when pinched, quickly returns to original shape in well-hydrated young person; test for fluid volume deficit that is not reliable for elderly clients. (9)

Type 1 diabetes—Persons with this disorder must take insulin to survive and are prone to ketoacidosis; also called insulin-dependent diabetes mellitus (IDDM), type II diabetes, and juvenile diabetes. (19)

Type 2 diabetes—Although some persons with this disorder take insulin, it is not necessary for their survival; also called noninsulin-dependent diabetes (NIDDM) and adult-onset diabetes mellitus. (19)

Tyramine—A monoamine present in various foods that will provoke a hypertensive crisis in persons taking monoamine oxidase (MAO) inhibitors. (17)

Ulcer—An open sore or lesion of the skin or mucous membrane. (22)

Ulcerative colitis—Inflammatory disease of the large intestine that usually begins in the rectum and spreads upward in a continuous pattern. (22)

Ultrasound bone densitometer—Machine that uses sound waves to estimate bone density as a screening test. (2)

Uncomplicated starvation—A food deprivation without an underlying stress state. (24)

Undernutrition—The state that results from a deficiency of one or more nutrients. (1)

Underwater weighing—Most accurate measure of body fatness. (2)

Universal precautions—A list of procedures developed by the Centers for Disease Control for when blood and certain other body fluids should be considered contaminated and treated as such. (25)

Unsaturated fat—A fat in which the majority of fatty acids contain one or more carbon-to-carbon double bonds. (9)

Urea—The chief nitrogenous constituent of urine; the final product, along with CO_2, of protein metabolism. (10)

Uremia—A toxic condition produced by the retention of nitrogen-containing substances normally excreted by the kidneys. (21)

Ureter—The tube that carries urine from the kidney to the bladder. (21)

Urinary calculus—A kidney stone, or deposit of mineral salts. (21)

Urinary tract infection (UTI)—The condition in which disease-producing microorganisms invade a client's bladder, ureter, or urethra. (21)

USDA Dietary Guidelines—Ten guidelines for health promotion issued by the U.S. Departments of Agriculture and Health and Human Services; revised in 2000. (2)

Usual food intake—A description of what a person habitually eats. (2)

Vaginitis—Inflammation of the vagina, most often caused by an infectious agent. (19)

Vasopressin—Antidiuretic hormone; abbreviated ADH. (9)

Ventilation—Process by which gases are moved into and out of the lungs; two aspects of ventilation are inhalation and exhalation. (24)

Very-low-calorie diet (VLCD)—Diet that contains less than 800 kilocalories per day. (18)

Very low-density lipoprotein (VLDL)—A plasma protein containing mostly triglycerides with small amounts of cholesterol, phospholipid, and protein; transports triglycerides from the liver to tissues. (20)

Villi—Multiple minute projections on the surface of the folds of the small intestine that absorb fluid and nutrients; plural of villus. (10)

Virus—Very small noncellular parasite that is entirely dependent on the nutrients inside host cells for its metabolic and reproductive needs. (14)

Visible fat—Dietary fat that can be easily seen, such as the fat on meat or in oil. (4)

Vitamin—Organic substance needed by the body in very small amounts; yields no energy and does not become part of the body's structure. (7)

Waist-to-Hip Ratio (WHR)—Waist measurement divided by hip measurement; if >0.85 in women or >1.0 in men, indicates increased risk of health problems related to obesity. (2)

Warfarin sodium—Anticoagulant that interferes with the liver's synthesis of vitamin K-dependent clotting factors II, VII, IX, and X. (7)

Water intoxication—Excess intake or abnormal retention of water. (9)

Weight cycling—The repeated gain and loss of body weight. (18)

Wernicke-Korsakoff syndrome—A disorder of the central nervous system seen in chronic alcoholism and resulting thiamin depletion; signs and symptoms include motor, sensory, and memory deficits. (7, 22)

Wernicke's encephalopathy—Inflammatory, hemorrhagic, degenerative lesions in several areas of the brain resulting in double vision, involuntary eye movements, lack of muscle cordination, and mental deficits; caused by thiamin deficiency often in chronic alcoholism but also in gastrointestinal tract disease and hyperemesis gravidarum. (7)

Whey—Component of milk; in human milk, contains soluble proteins that are easily digested; major whey protein in breast milk is alpha-lactalbumin, with an amino acid pattern much like that of the body tissues. (12)

Wilson's disease—Rare genetic defect of copper metabolism. (8, 17)

Women, Infants, and Children (WIC)—Federal program providing nutrition education and supplemental food to low-income pregnant or breast-feeding women and children up to 5 years of age. (12)

Xerophthalmia—Drying and thickening of the epithelial tissues of the eye; can be caused by vitamin A deficiency. (7)

Xerostomia—Dry mouth caused by decreased salivary secretions. (13)

Yo-yo effect—The repeated loss and gain of body weight. (18)

Index

INDEX

Abdominal circumference, 16
Abdominal obesity, 335
Abdominal quadrants, 428
Absorption, 169–175
    of alcohol, 438
    of drugs, effects of food on, 316, 318, 319
    factors decreasing, 171
    food allergies and, 172–175
    inadequate, 171. See also Malabsorption
    interfering factors in, 171–172, 316, 318
    intestinal disorders and, 432–433
    in large intestine, 171
    of minerals. See specific mineral
    of nutrients, drug effects on, 313–314
    in small intestine, 169–171
    unabsorbed materials, excretion of, 171
    of vitamins. See specific vitamin
    of water, 143–144
Acculturation, 26–27
ACE (angiotensin converting enzyme) inhibitors, 322
Acetylcholine, 101, 112
Acetylsalicylic acid, 313, 315, 316, 318
Achalasia, 424–425
Achlorhydria, 238
Acid-base balance, 148–150
    drug excretion and, 322
    renal function in, 403
Acidity control agents, 266
Acidosis, 149, 355
Acid urine, 322
Acquired immune deficiency syndrome. See AIDS
Acrodermatitis enteropathica, 129
Acromegaly, 470
Activity Pyramid for Children, 81
Acute, 277
Acute renal failure, 406
ADA Exchange Lists, 24–25, 42. See also Exchange lists
Adaptive response to exercise, 79
Adaptive thermogenesis, 75
ADC (AIDS dementia complex), 487
Additives, 266–267
Adenosine diphosphate (ADP), 117
Adenosine triphosphate (ATP), 117, 175, 177
Adequate intakes (AIs), 24
    of biotin, 101
    of calcium, 112
    of choline, 102
    of pantothenic acid, 101
ADH (antidiuretic hormone), 148, 149
Adolescence
    definition of, 224
    growth and development in, 225
    identity in, 224–225
    nutrition in, 224–227
    pregnancy in, 184, 189, 190
    weight in, 225–227
    young adulthood and, 235–236
ADP (adenosine diphosphate), 117
Adrenal glands, 95
Adulthood, 235–253
    definition of, 235
    intimacy in, 235, 236
    middle years in, 236–237
    nutrition education for, 248–249
    obesity and inactivity in, 236

older years in. See Older adulthood
    younger years in, 235–236
Adult onset diabetes, 350–351, 378, 381. See also
    Diabetes mellitus
Aerobic exercise, 79–80
Aflatoxins, 455
African Americans
    cancer in, 451
    diet in, 27, 28
    hypertension in, 377, 379
    stroke in, 373
Age
    body water and, 142
    cardiovascular disease and, 377, 382
    food-borne disease and, 259
    food guide compliance by, 236–237
    Healthy Eating Index and, 219
    mortality rates and, 373, 374
    overweight and obesity prevalence and, 331
    resting energy expenditure and, 77
    weight and, 227
Aging. See also Growth and development; Older
    adulthood
    anorexia of, 245
Agriculture, 3, 4
AIDS (acquired immune deficiency syndrome),
    483–495
    avoidance of, 486
    complications of, 486–488
    definition of, 483, 484
    epidemiology of, 485–486
    food safety and, 256, 492
    nutrition and, 489–492
    signs and symptoms of, 484
    test screening for, 486, 491
    treatment of, 483, 488–489
AIDS dementia complex (ADC), 487
AIs (adequate intakes). See Adequate intakes
Albumin, 60, 66
Alcohol consumption
    CAGE questionnaire for, 438
    cancer and, 450–451, 454, 456
    cardiovascular disease and, 381, 382, 383, 384
    cirrhosis and, 438, 440
    diabetes mellitus and, 366
    fetal alcohol syndrome and, 189
    hepatitis and, 436
    hypertension and, 381, 386
    iron and, 123, 126
    magnesium deficiency and, 119
    nutrition effects of, 311, 314, 315, 316, 317,
        318, 437
    osteoporosis and, 116
    pancreatitis and, 443
    pregnancy and, 189–190
    water loss and, 151
    Wernicke-Korsakoff syndrome and, 97
Alcoholism, 437, 438
Aldosterone, 148, 149
Alertness, death and, 498
Alimentary canal, 163, 164–166, 168–169, 171
Alkaline urine, 322
Alkalosis, 116–117
Allele, 184
Allergen, 214

Allergies. See Food allergies
Allergy I and II diets, 175, 176
Allium sativum, 297, 299
Alpha-tocopherol equivalents (a-TE), 92
Amenorrhea, 226, 343
American Diabetes Association, 24, 360
American Dietetic Association, 24, 360
Amino acids, 59–63
    absorption of, 318
    catabolic reactions of, 175
    digestion and, 168–169
    as ergogenic aids, 301–302
    hepatic encephalopathy and, 440
    protein food classifications and, 66
    stress and, 470
Ammonia levels, 440
Amniotic fluid, 184
Anabolic phase, 472
Anabolic steroids, 302–303
Anabolism, 62, 63, 177
Anaerobic exercise, 80
Analgesics. See Acetylsalicylic acid
Analysis
    of botanical remedies, 301
    nursing process and, 11, 12, 17–21, 22–23
Anaphylaxis, 214, 215
Anastomosis, 429
Androgenic anabolic steroids, 302–303
Anemia, megaloblastic, 100. See also Iron-deficiency
    anemia; Pernicious anemia
Anesthesia, 422–423
Angina pectoris, 314, 377
Angiograms, 379
Angiotensin converting enzyme (ACE) inhibitors, 322
Angiotensin I, 148, 149, 322
Angiotensin II, 148, 149, 322
Angiotensinogen, 149
Animal production, hormones in, 267
Anionic bond, 142
Anions, 142
Anorexia
    of aging, 245
    cancer and, 460, 461
    drug interaction causing, 312–313
    HIV/AIDS and, 491
    terminally ill and, 500
Anorexia nervosa, 343
Antacids, 317
Antagonist, 98
Anthropometric data, 14, 16–17
Antibacterial soap, 259
Antibiotics, 259
Antibodies, 65
Anticholinergic poisoning, 295
Anticoagulants, 297, 299
Anticoagulant therapy, oral, 315
Anticonvulsants, 318
Antidepressants, 313, 317
Antidiuretic hormone (ADH), 148, 149
Antiepileptics, 318
Antigout agents, 317
Antihistamines, 317
Antihypertensives, 317
Anti-infectives, 317, 318
Anti-inflammatories, 318

Antimanics, 317
Antineoplastics, 312–313, 317, 318
Antioxidants, 266
    cancer and, 455
    cardiovascular disease and, 380, 384
    as ergogenic aids, 302
    eye disease and, 93
    vitamins as, 92, 93, 95
Antiparkinson agents, 315, 318
Antitubercular agents, 315, 318
Anuria, 406, 415
Apgar score, 206
Apoferritin, 123
Appearance, 14, 16
Appetite, 79, 312–313
Aquaporins, 142
Ariboflavinosis, 98
Arrhythmias, 393
Arteriosclerosis, 373. *See also* Atherosclerosis
Arthritis, 244–245
Artificial feeding, 97, 504
Artificial sweeteners, 37
Ascites, 155, 460
Ascorbic acid. *See* Vitamin C
Asian ginseng, 296, 299
Aspartame, 37
Aspergillus molds, 261
Aspiration, 282, 283
Aspirin. *See* Acetylsalicylic acid
Assessment, 11, 14–17
    of botanical remedies, 300, 301
    of cancer client, 460
    of dementia client, 240
    D-E-N-T-A-L Screening Survey Form, 239
    of drug-nutrient interaction risk, 312
    of fluid volume deficit and excess, 155–156, 157
    of HIV/AIDS client, 486, 491
    of nutritional care, 273–274
    of older adults, 246
    PEACH survey, 222
    of preschoolers, 221, 222
    SCALES screen, 245
    of terminally ill client, 499
    of water loss, 152
    for weight loss programs, 327, 343
Assisted feeding, 279
Asymptomatic, 484
Ataxia, 437
a-TE (alpha-tocopherol equivalents), 92
Atherosclerosis, 373–374, 375–377, 380
Athletes, 300–304
Atoms, 35, 141–142
Atopic disease, 208, 215
ATP (adenosine triphosphate), 117, 175, 177
Atrophy, 477
Autoimmune diseases, 354
    autoimmune thyroid disease, 127
Autonomy, 217–218

Bacteria
    breast-feeding and, 205, 208
    dental caries and, 39
    food-borne disease and, 255–260
    intestinal, 94, 314
Barium enema, 277, 278
B-Complex vitamins. *See* Vitamin B

Beef, 52–54
    insulin molecule of, 60
Beer, 456
Behavior modification
    diabetes client and, 360
    weight control and, 339–340
Benign tumors, 449
Beriberi, 97, 437
Beta-adrenergic blockers, 318
Beta-carotene
    atherosclerosis and, 380
    cancer and, 453
Beverages
    consistency modifications of, 277
    gluten in, 173
    heart attack and, 393
    oxalic acid in, 416
    sodium content of, 392
    water in, 151
Bicarbonate, 145, 302
Bile, 163
Billroth procedures, 430
Binding sites, 315, 316, 320
Binging, 344
Bioelectrical impedance tests, 16
Biotin, 94, 97, 101, 104
Birth, premature, 211
Birth weight, 204, 211
Bladder cancer, 451, 456
Blood
    albumin in, 60, 66
    cholesterol levels in, 50
    clotting of, 93, 437
    composition of, 144
    HIV transmission via, 485
    lead levels in, 122
    proteins in, 66
    serum electrolytes in, 146
Blood glucose. *See* Glucose
Blood pressure
    alcohol intake and, 381
    DASH Diet and, 383–384, 386
    exercise and, 381
    hypertension and, 374, 376
    orthostatic hypotension and, 155, 156
    renal control of, 403
    smoking and, 381, 383
Blood sugar. *See* Glucose
Blood transfusions, 157
Blood urea nitrogen (BUN), 239
    renal disease and, 406, 415
Blue cohosh, 300
BMI. *See* Body mass index
Body. *See* Human body
Body fat
    brown fat in, 336
    fat cells in, 336
    function of, 50
    health and, 52
    ketosis and, 38–39
    loss of, 332–333
    percent of, 328–329
    storage of, 331–332
Body image disturbances, 334
Body mass index (BMI), 18–19
    child and adolescent weight and, 227

    reduced, 342–344
    weight control and, 329–330, 338
Body substance isolation, 486
Bolus, 164
Bolus feeding, 282
Bomb calorimeter, 76
Bonding, chemical, 141–142, 315
Bone
    calcium and, 112, 113
    fluoride in, 127
    phosphorus in, 117
    vitamin A and, 89
    vitamin K and, 93–94
Bone loss
    alcoholism and, 437
    fracture risk and, 245
    osteoporosis causing, 115, 116
    vitamin A and, 242
Bone mineral density, 115, 116, 245
Botanical remedies, 293–300
    commerce in, 294–295
    contamination of, 295–296
    errors associated with, 298–300
    health care providers and, 300
    nursing process and, 301
    potentially safe products, 296–298
    regulation of, 294
    standardization of, 295
Bottle-feeding, 208–209, 210, 216
Botulism, 258–259, 260
Bovine spongiform encephalopathy (BSE), 260
Bowel. *See also* Intestinal disorders
    cancer of, 456
    obstruction of, 500
    radiation and, 462
    surgery, nutrition and, 423–424
Bowman's capsule, 403
Brain function
    glucose and, 39
    iron and, 120
    in older adulthood, 239
    undernutrition and, 8
Branch-chain amino acids, 302
Breads
    childhood and, 217
    diet specifications for. *See specific diet*
    exchanges for, 41, 66, 67
    lactose intolerance and, 167–168
    older adulthood and, 243
    oxalic acid in, 416
Breast cancer, 449, 451
    alcohol consumption and, 456
    breast-feeding and, 194
    diet and, 450, 453, 454, 456
    weight loss in, 460
Breast-feeding, 193–196, 206–208
    benefits of, 194, 206–208
    botanicals and, 297, 299
    contraindications to, 195
    food guide for, 189
    genetic abnormalities and, 297
    HIV transmission and, 485–486
    infant cognition and, 205
    infantile colic and, 216
    infantile diarrhea and, 216
    nutritional needs in, 68, 82, 83, 193–194

premature delivery and, 211
techniques for, 194
Breast milk
composition of, 207
contamination of, 195
HIV in, 485–486
nutritional components in, 194, 204–206
premature delivery and, 211
storage of, 207
Breathing, in terminally ill, 498, 501
Bronchial cancer, 449
Brown fat, 336
BSE (bovine spongiform encephalopathy), 260
Buddhism, 29
Bulimia, 343–344
BUN. *See* Blood urea nitrogen
Burns
in infancy, 213
metabolic stress in, 474, 475–476

Cachexia
cancer and, 459
HIV/AIDS and, 490
terminally ill and, 500
CAD (coronary artery disease), 377, 384
Caffeine
arrhythmia and, 393
calcium absorption and, 115
drug metabolism and, 321
as ergogenic aid, 303
heart attack and, 393
pregnancy and, 190
water loss and, 151
CAGE questionnaire, 438
Calcidiol, 90
Calcitonin, 112, 113
Calcitriol, 90, 403, 406
Calcium, 111–117, 121
absorption and excretion of, 113–115
breast-feeding and, 193
cancer and, 455
in cereals, 125
control mechanisms for, 112
deficiencies of, 115–117
dietary reference intakes for, 112
function of, 112, 145
hypermetabolism and, 476
hypertension and, 378–379
infancy and, 211, 214
iron absorption and, 123
kidney stones and, 414
older adulthood and, 243
pregnancy and, 186–187
renal disease and, 409–410, 411
renal function and, 403, 406
sources of, 112–113
supplements, 122
toxicity of, 117
Calories, 76. *See also* Kilocalories
Calorimeter, bomb, 76
Campylobacter jejuni, 257, 258
Cancer, 449–462
cell changes in, 450
diet and, 449–451, 453–455
mortality rates from, 449, 452
nursing interventions in, 462

nutrition in, 456, 459–462
prevalence of, 451
prevention of, 459, 461
research findings and, 455, 457–458
risk reduction for, 455–456, 459
terminology, 449
vitamin A and, 89, 453
Canning, 259
Canola oil, 390
CAPD (continuous ambulatory peritoneal dialysis), 408, 415
Carbohydrate counting, 362, 364–365, 366
Carbohydrates, 35–42
in breast milk, 205
cholesterol and, 47
classification of, 35–38
composition of, 35, 37, 47
consumption patterns of, 39
definition of, 35
dental health and, 39
diabetes mellitus and, 361–363, 364–365, 366, 367, 368
dietary recommendations for, 42
digestion of, 166, 169
as ergogenic aids, 301
exchange list values for, 41–42
fat replacers, 55
food sources, 39–41
function of, 38–39
indigestible, 171
infancy and, 205, 211
intolerance of, 167
pulmonary disease and, 478
renal disease and, 408–409, 412
thermic effect of, 78
Carbon dioxide retention, 477, 478
Carbonic, 149
Carbonic acid, 149
Carcinogenic, 450
Carcinogens, 450, 451
Carcinomas, 449
Cardia, 453
Cardiac output, 403
Cardiac sphincter, 424–425
Cardiopulmonary system, 478–479
Cardiospasm, 424–425
Cardiovascular disease, 373–395
dietary modifications in, 387–395
mortality rates, 373, 374
occurrence of, 373
pathology underlying, 373–377
prevention of, 383–387
risk factors in, 377–383
Cardiovascular system
dehydration indicators, 244
in older adulthood, 241
water imbalances and, 155, 157
Carotene, 88, 89
cancer and, 453, 456, 459
Carotenemia, 89–90
Carotenoids, 453
Casual contact, AIDS and, 486
Catabolism
cancer and, 459
of nutrients, 175, 177
of protein, 62, 63

pulmonary function and, 476
renal disease and, 406
Cataracts, 93
Catheter, 285
Catholicism, 29
Caulophyllum thalictroides, 300
Cavities. *See* Dental caries
CD_4 protein, 483, 484
Celiac disease, 172, 433
Cells
energy production and release in, 175
fat cells, 336
membrane of, fat and, 50
transformations, in cancer, 450
Centers for Disease Control and Prevention, 485, 491
Central nervous system, 119–120
food intake and, 335
HIV and, 483, 487
in infancy, 204
in older adulthood, 239
Cereals
childhood and, 217
diet specifications for. *See specific diet*
iron and calcium in, 125
lactose intolerance and, 167–168
older adulthood and, 243
soyfood guide, 385
Cerebrovascular disease, 373, 374, 375
Cervical cancer, 451, 453
Chaparral ingestion, 298–299
CHD. *See* Coronary heart disease
Cheese, 39
Chelating agents, 128, 317, 318
Chemical bonding, 141–142, 315
Chemical digestion, 164
Chemical toxins, 195, 265–266
Chemotherapy, 460–461, 462
Childcare programs, 221
Childhood, 217–224. *See also* Adolescence; Growth and development; Infancy
activity pyramid for, 81
cholesterol in, 379
definition of, 217
diabetes mellitus in, 368
fluorosis in, 128
food allergies in, 175
Food Guide Pyramid for, 217, 218
iron deficiency and toxicity in, 125, 126
kwashiorkor in, 64, 147
lead poisoning in, 122
nutritional needs in, 217–224
nutrition screening in, 221, 222
preschoolers, 220–222
renal disease in, 413, 415
school-aged children, 222–224
toddlers, 217–220
urine output in, 152
vitamin deficiencies in, 89, 91, 100
weight in, 226–227, 332
Chinese
diet of, 28
herbal contaminants and, 296
Chinese American diet, 30
Chloride, 120, 121, 145
Choking, 212
Cholecalciferol, 90

Cholecystitis, 442
  HIV/AIDS and, 487
Cholecystokinin, 166
Cholelithiasis, 442
Cholestasis, 131
Cholesterol, 50, 379–381
  carbohydrates and, 47
  cardiovascular disease and, 382, 384, 387
  lowering of, diets for, 387–392
  population studies and, 384
  renal disease and, 410–411
  soy products and, 383
  zinc and, 129
Cholestyramine, 313, 317
Choline, 101–102
Chromium, 130–131, 133
  diabetes mellitus and, 365–366
Chronic, 277
Chronic disease, stress and, 469–470
Chronic obstructive pulmonary disease (COPD), 476
Chronic renal failure, 406–407, 410, 413–415
Chvostek's sign, 117
Chylomicrons, 380
Chyme, 166, 171
Cigarette smoke. *See* Smoking
Ciguatera poisoning, 261
Circulatory system, 66
Cirrhosis, 438–442, 450, 456
Cis configuration double bond, 51, 52
Clear liquid diet, 275
Client care. *See* Assessment; Nursing process; *specific condition/disease*
Climate, 78
Clinical pharmacist (RPh), 5
Clostridium botulinum, 258–259, 262
Clostridium perfringens, 258, 262
Clotting, 93, 437
Cobalt, 131, 134
Cocaine use, 191
Coenzymes, 87, 97
Coffee, 380. *See also* Caffeine
Coffee-ground emesis, 429
Cognition
  behavior modification strategies, 339, 340
  breast-feeding and, 205
Colchicine, 314, 317
Colds, 128
Colectomy, 434
Colic, 216
Collagen, 95
Collecting tubule, 403
Colloidal osmotic pressure, 147
Colon. *See also* Colorectal cancer
  absorption and, 171
  diverticula of, 435
  x-ray studies of, 277, 278
Colorectal cancer, 449, 451, 456
  alcohol consumption and, 456
  diet and, 450, 452, 455, 456
  epidemiology of, 453
  weight loss in, 460
Colostomy, 434
Colostrum, 207
Combination feedings, 287, 289
Co-morbidity factors, 335
Complementary medicines, 293–307

Complementation, 66
Complete proteins, 66
Complex carbohydrates, 37–38
Compound, 141
Compound fats, 49
Computerized diet programs, 21
Conditionally (acquired) essential amino acids, 61, 63
Congestive heart failure, 377, 393
Consistency modifications, 277
Constipation, 431–432
  in infancy, 213
  in older adulthood, 244
  in pregnancy, 191
  in terminally ill, 500
Contamination
  of botanicals, 295–296
  of feeding tubes, 282
  of supplements, 114
Contamination iron, 125
Continent ileostomy, 435
Continuous ambulatory peritoneal dialysis (CAPD), 408, 415
Continuous feeding, 282
Contraceptives, 195
Contraindication, 275
Cooking
  cancer and, 451
  food safety in, 257, 259
  water-soluble vitamins and, 94
Cooling, of food, 268, 269
COPD (chronic obstructive pulmonary disease), 476
Copper, 129–130, 133
Coronary artery disease (CAD), 377, 384
Coronary heart disease (CHD), 373, 374, 377
  alcohol intake and, 381
  antioxidants and, 380
  genetics and, 378
  occurrence and mortality rates in, 373, 374
  population studies of, 384
  soyfoods and, 383
Coronary occlusion, 377
Corticosteroids, 314
Cough, 500
Counseling
  of diabetic client, 352, 360, 361, 367
  of HIV/AIDS client, 488–489, 490
  on nutritional care, 273, 274
  of terminally ill client, 503
Cow's milk, 204–206, 209, 215–216
Cow's milk protein-induced intestinal injury, 215–216
Cramps, 153, 191
Cranberry juice, 416
Creatine, 302, 415
Cretinism, 127
Crohn's disease, 101, 433–435
Cross-contamination, 267, 268
Cruciferous vegetables, 455, 459
Cryptosporidiosis, 487
Crystalluria, 322
Cuban diet, 28
Culture
  food preferences and, 27–30
  nutrition and, 25–30
  obesity and, 333–334
  undernutrition and, 63–64

  weight control and, 342
Curative care, 498–499
Cyanocobalamin. *See* Vitamin B_{12}
Cyanosis, 498
Cyclospora outbreak, 256
Cystic fibrosis, 443–444
Cystitis, 416
Cytochrome P450 enzymes, 315

Dairy products. *See* Milk and dairy products
DASH Diet, 383–384, 386, 387
Data
  analysis in nursing process, 12, 17–21, 22–23
  anthropometric, 14, 16–17
Death. *See also* Terminal illness
  AIDS-related, 483, 484
  alcohol-related, 438
  cancer-related, 449, 452
  cardiovascular disease and, 373, 374
  dealing with, 497
  heat-related, 154
  height-weight tables and, 327–328
  hospice and, 499
  infant mortality, 203, 352
  obesity and, 334
  process of, 497–498
Dehydration. *See also* Fluid volume deficit
  enteral tube feeding and, 283
  ketoacidosis and, 355
  in older adulthood, 244
  terminally ill and, 500, 503
Delayed gastric emptying, 428–429
Dementia
  AIDS dementia complex, 487
  assessment and care in, 240
Dental caries
  carbohydrate intake and, 39–40
  fluoride and, 127–128
  in preschoolers, 221
  surgical client with, 422
D-E-N-T-A-L Screening Survey Form, 239
Dentition
  calcium and, 112
  cavities in. *See* Dental caries
  dentures, 238, 248
  evaluation of, 264
  fluoride and, 127
  in older adulthood, 238–239
  phosphorus and, 117
  screening form, 239
Dentures, 238, 248
Deoxyribonucleic acid (DNA), 65, 450
Desirable body weight, 327
Desired outcomes, 24
Desserts
  consistency modifications of, 277
  diet specifications for. *See specific diet*
  gluten in, 174
  lactose intolerance and, 167–168
Development. *See* Growth and development
DEXA (dual-energy x-ray absorptiometry), 16
Dexfenfluramine, 340
Diabetes insipidus, 148
Diabetes mellitus, 349–368
  acute illness episodes in, 366–367
  alcohol consumption in, 366

cardiovascular disease and, 381, 382
causes of, 353–354
in childhood, 368
complications of, 355–356
coronary heart disease and, 378
definition and classification of, 349–351
diet in, 358–367, 368
fetal nutrition and, 381
gestational, 193, 351, 352
hypoglycemia and, 349, 355, 356, 367
nutrient metabolism in, 351–353
Ojibway mythology and, 27
renal disease and, 406, 408–409
self-care in, 356–357, 367
signs and symptoms of, 354–355
supplements and, 365–366
treatment of, 356–365
type 1, 349–350, 351
type 2, 350–351, 378, 381
Diabetic ketoacidosis, 355
Diabetic neuropathy, 406
Diagnostic procedures, diet and, 276–277
Dialysate, 407
Dialysis, 407–408, 409, 411–415
Diarrhea, 430–431
cancer client and, 460–461, 462
versus fecal impaction, 432
HIV/AIDS client and, 490
infantile, 216–217
self-treatment for, 433
terminally ill and, 501
Diastolic pressure, 147
DASH Diet and, 383–384, 386
hypertension and, 374, 376
Diazepam, 316
Diet. *See also* Diet therapy; Exchange lists; Food;
    Food Guide Pyramid; *specific type of diet*
in adulthood, 235–237, 241–244, 248–249
analysis Web page, 22–23
breast-feeding and, 193–194, 208
in childhood, 219–222, 224
computerized analysis of, 21
disease-related. *See specific disease*
ethnic preferences in, 27–30
guidelines for, 19, 21
human evolution and, 3–4
in pregnancy, 189–191, 192, 208
as risk factor, 172, 175, 378–379
Dietary Approaches to Stop Hypertension (DASH)
    Diet, 383–384, 386, 387
Dietary fiber. *See* Fiber
Dietary Guidelines for Americans, 19, 20
diabetes mellitus and, 362
Dietary reference intakes (DRIs), 23–24
calcium, 112
vitamin C, 96
Dietary status, 263–264
Dietary Supplement Health Education Act (DSHEA),
    294
Dietary supplements. *See* Supplements
Dietetic technician (DT), 5
Dietitian, 5
Diet manuals, 274
Diet orders, 274–276
in cardiovascular disease, 392
Diet therapy, 8–9, 338. *See also* Menus; *specific diet*

in allergies, 175, 176
for burn client, 475–476
in cancer, 461–462
in cardiovascular disease, 383–395
in chronic disease, 469–470
in diabetes mellitus, 358–367, 368
in diagnostic procedures, 276–277
in diverticulitis, 435
in dumping syndrome, 431–432
in gallbladder disease, 443
in gastroesophageal reflux disease, 426–427
in gastrointestinal disease, 421–424, 425
in gluten-sensitive enteropathy, 172, 173–174,
    433
in gout, 414
in hepatic disease, 440–442
in hepatitis, 436, 438
in hiatal hernia, 426–427
in HIV/AIDS, 490–492
in hypoglycemia, 367, 368, 369
in inflammatory bowel disease, 433–434, 435
in lactose intolerance, 167–168
MAO inhibitors and, 319–320
in myocardial infarction, 393
in oral anticoagulant therapy, 315
in peptic ulcers, 429
in renal disease, 408–415
in terminal illness, 499, 500–503
in thrush, 487
Digestion, 163–169
accessory organs and, 163–164
alimentary canal and, 163
digestive action, 164, 314
food pathway in, 164, 166, 168–169
in infancy, 204–205, 211
Digestive enzymes, 164, 314
Diglycerides, 45, 46
Dilutional hyponatremia, 118
Disabled client, 279
Disaccharides, 35, 36–37
Disease. *See also specific disease or condition*
breast-feeding and, 207–208
decreased absorption and, 171–172
dietary fat and, 51–52
food-borne, 255–262, 492
formulas specifically for, 281
germ theory and, 30
obesity and, 334–335
phytochemicals and, 7
stress and, 469–470, 472
tube feeding indications in, 281
undernutrition causing, 64
vitamin supplements for, 89, 102
Disease-specific formulas, 281
Disulfide linkages, 120
Diuretics, 157, 316, 318
Diverticulitis, 435
Diverticulosis, 435
Diverticulum, 435
DNA (deoxyribonucleic acid), 65, 450
Dolomite, 114
Dopamine, 99
Double-blind trials, 294
Double bonds, 51, 52
Drinking (of fluids), in terminal illness, 498
DRIs. *See* Dietary reference intakes

Drug use, 191, 195. *See also* Medications; *specific
    drug*
Dry beriberi, 437
Dry mouth, 461
DSHEA (Dietary Supplement Health Education Act), 294
DT (dietetic technician), 5
Dual-energy x-ray absorptiometry (DEXA), 16
Dumping syndrome, 429, 430, 431–432
Dysgeusia, 501
Dysphagia, 165
Dysphoria, 334
Dyspnea, 498, 501

EARs (estimated average requirements), 24
Eating behavior. *See also* Nutrient delivery
behavior scale for, 240
death and, 498
disorders of, 343–344
environment and, 279
GERD and, 427
pulmonary disease and, 477
slowed-down, 339, 340
stress and, 470
terminal illness and, 504
in thrush client, 487
weight control and. *See* Diet therapy; Weight
    control; Weight loss
Eating Behavior Scale, 240
Ebb phase, 472
ECG (electrocardiogram), 142
Echinacea, 297, 299
Echinacea sp., 297, 299
Eclampsia, 192–193
Eczema, 208, 214, 215
Edema
definition of, 144
fluid volume excess and, 157
heat-related, 153
nutrient control in, 415
postoperative, 421
Education
on botanicals, 300
of diabetic client, 360, 361, 366, 367
of HIV/AIDS client, 492
on nutrition, 248–249, 341–342, 492
of terminally ill client, 503
EEG (electroencephalogram), 142
Efficacy, of botanicals, 294
Eggs
in cholesterol-lowering diet, 390
handling guidelines for, 259
Salmonella outbreak from, 256
Elderly clients. *See* Older adulthood
Electrocardiogram (ECG), 142
Electroencephalogram (EEG), 142
Electrolytes, 145
definition of, 142
diagnostic uses and hazards of, 142
drug excretion and, 322
fluid balance and, 144–145, 322
imbalances in, 146–147, 156, 355
measurement of, 145
serum, 146
Electrolyte therapy, 216, 317
Elemental formulas, 281
Elements, 35, 141

Embolus, 377
Embryo, 183
Emulsified fats, 48–49
Emulsifiers, 266
Encephalopathy, Wernicke's, 97
Endemic cretinism, 127
Endocrine system, 239, 241
End-stage renal failure, 406–407
  in HIV/AIDS client, 487
Enema, barium, 277, 278
Energy, 75–83. *See also* Energy nutrients
  adolescence and, 225
  allowances for, 82
  breast-feeding and, 193
  cancer and, 459, 460
  carbohydrates as source of, 38
  composition in exchange lists, 25
  dietary recommendations for, 82–83
  expenditure of, 75, 76–80
  fats as source of, 49, 50
  homeostasis and, 75
  imbalance in, 331–333
  infancy and, 204–205
  intake of, 75, 80, 82
  measurement of, 76
  older adulthood and, 241–242
  pregnancy and, 183
  production, in cells, 175
  protein as source of, 66
  starvation and, 471
  vitamin A and, 89
Energy imbalance, 331–333
Energy nutrients, 6, 314
  diabetes mellitus and, 352, 360–365
  older adulthood and, 241–242
  renal disease and, 411–412
  respiratory disease and, 477
  values of, 76
Enrichment, 40–41
Enteral tube feeding, 278, 281–285
  in hypermetabolism, 473
Enteric-coated medication, 297, 316, 319
Enteritis, 216
Environment
  for eating, 279
  obesity and, 337
  pollutants in, 265–266
Enzymes
  cytochrome P450, 315
  digestive, 164, 314
  obesity and, 336
  regulatory function of, 65
Ephedrine, 303
Epithelial tissue, 88, 89
Ergocalciferol, 90
Ergogenic aids, 300–304
  judgment and, 303–304
  nonnutrient, 302–303
  nutrient, 301–302
  stress and, 470
Erikson, Erik, 203, 217, 220, 223, 224, 235, 236, 237
Erosion, 429
Erythropoietin, 406
ESADDI. *See* Estimated Safe and Adequate Dietary Intakes

Escherichia coli, 205, 208, 256, 258
Esophageal cancer, 451, 453
Esophageal hiatus, 427
Esophageal reflux, 501. *See also* Gastroesophageal reflux disease
Esophagostomy, 281
Esophagus
  cancer of, 451, 453
  digestive function of, 166, 169
  disorders of, 424–427, 428
  reflux in, 501
Essential amino acids, 61, 63
Essential fatty acids, 49–50
Essential hypertension, 376
Essential nutrients, 6
Estimated average requirements (EARs), 24
Estimated Safe and Adequate Dietary Intakes (ESADDI), 23
  of minerals, 120, 130, 131
Estrogen
  breast cancer and, 454
  breast-feeding and, 195
  calcium and, 112
  nutrients and, 318
  phytoestrogens, 456
Ethics, terminal illness and, 499, 503–504
Ethnicity/race
  cancer rates by, 449, 451, 456
  cardiovascular disease and, 377, 382
  celiac disease and, 433
  diabetes mellitus in, 350–351
  ethnocentrism and, 26
  food preferences by, 27–30
  iron deficiencies and toxicity and, 125, 126
  obesity and inactivity and, 236
  teenage pregnancy and, 190
  U.S. infant mortality and, 203
  weight and, 227
Ethnocentrism, 26
Evaluation, 11, 12, 25
  of dentition, 264
  of dietary status, 263–264
  of use of botanical remedies, 301
Evaporative water loss, 151, 152
Evolution, 3–4
Exchange lists, 24–25, 26, 362. *See also specific food group*
  for diabetic client, 360, 364, 365, 369
Exchange Lists of the American Dietetic and the American Diabetes Associations, 362
Excretion, 177
  of drugs, homeostasis and, 321–322
  intestinal disorders and, 431–432
  of minerals. *See specific mineral*
  of nutrients, drug effects on, 315–316, 318
  obligatory, 151
  renal function and, 403
  of unabsorbed material, 171
  of vitamins. *See specific vitamin*
  of waste products, 177
  of water, regulation, 147, 148
Exercise
  Activity Pyramid for Children, 81
  blood pressure and, 381
  cardiovascular disease and, 382
  diabetes mellitus and, 357–358

energy expenditure and, 78–80
  hypermetabolism and, 474
  obesity and, 227, 338–339, 342
  older adulthood and, 241, 247
  osteoporosis and, 116
  school-aged children and, 224
Exhaustion, heat, 153
External fluid losses, 155
Extracellular fluid, 142, 143, 149–150
Extrinsic factor, 100
Eye disease, 93

Fad diets, 337
Failure to thrive (FTT), 204
Famine, 3–4
FAS (fetal alcohol syndrome), 189
Fasting, 277
Fasting blood sugar, 350
Fat, bodily. *See* Body fat
Fat cells, 336
Fat redistribution syndrome, 487–488
Fat replacers, 55
Fats, dietary, 45–56, 442
  absorption of, 170
  American diet and, 50–51
  avoidance of, 342
  breast cancer and, 454
  cancer and, 451, 454, 456
  carbon dioxide retention and, 477
  as carcinogens, 450
  cardiovascular disease and, 383
  childhood and, 218, 220
  cholesterol in. *See* Cholesterol
  classification of, 48–49
  composition of, 45–46
  consistency modifications of, 277
  diabetes mellitus and, 363–364
  dietary recommendations for, 51. *See also specific diet*
  digestion of, 166, 168, 169
  exchanges for, 25–26, 52–54, 55
  food sources for, 46–48, 54–55
  function of, 49–50
  gallbladder disease and, 442–443
  gluten in, 173
  health and, 51–52
  infancy and, 205, 211
  malabsorption of, 172, 432–433
  in meat, 52–54, 388, 390, 391
  older adulthood and, 243
  properties of, 46–48
  pulmonary disease and, 477, 478
  renal disease and, 408, 412, 414
  replacers, 55
  soyfood guide, 385
  thermic effect of, 78
Fat soluble vitamins, 49, 87–94. *See also specific vitamin*
  deficiencies of, conditions mimicking, 96
  older adulthood and, 242–243
  pregnancy and, 184, 186
  renal disease and, 411
Fatty acids
  catabolic reactions of, 175
  chain length of, 45–46
  cholesterol and, 379–380, 390–391

definition of, 45
digestion and, 169
double bond configuration of, 51, 52
essential, 49–50
in fish, 383
glyceride formation, 45, 46
saturation of, 46
starvation and, 471
Fatty liver, 435–436
FDA. *See* Food and Drug Administration
Fe^{3+} (ferric iron), 123
Feast-famine conditions, 3–4
Fecal impaction, 432
Feces, 171, 432
Feeding tubes, 281–282, 284. *See also* Enteral tube
    feeding; Tube feeding
    medications via, 284
    terminally ill and, 504
Fenfluramine, 340
Ferric iron (Fe3+), 123
Ferritin, 121, 123, 411, 415
Ferrous, 95
Ferrous iron, 123
Fetal alcohol syndrome (FAS), 189
Fetus, 89, 183
    cardiovascular disease and, 381
    development of, 183, 184, 187
    diabetes mellitus and, 381
    fetal alcohol syndrome in, 189
    HIV and, 485–486
    listeriosis and, 190–191
    maternal drug use and, 191
    maternal nutrition and, 183–193
    neural tube defects in, 184, 185
Fever, 78
    metabolic stress and, 472, 476
    terminally ill and, 501
    water loss from, 152
Feverfew, 297, 299
Fiber, 38
    adolescence and, 225
    cancer and, 453, 454, 459
    in cholesterol-lowering diet, 391
    content, estimating, 41
    exchanges for, 42
    food processing and, 40–41
    foods high in, 192
    obesity and, 342
Fibrin, 112
Fibrinogen, 112
First-pass effect, 320
The First Step in Diabetes Meal Planning, 362
Fish, 52–53
    cancer and, 451, 456
    cardiovascular disease and, 383
    diet specifications for. *See specific diet*
    poisoning from, 261
    soyfood guide, 385
FIT (failure to thrive), 204
5 a Day program, 459
Five-hundred rule, 331
5-year survival rate, 449
Flatus, 423
Flavonoids, 380, 384
Flavors, 266
Flow phase, 472

Fluid accumulation, 501
Fluid balance, 144–148
    drug excretion and, 322
Fluid compartments, 142–143
Fluid intake and output
    drug excretion and, 322
    monitoring, 154–155
    renal diet and, 412
    renal disease and, 410, 411
Fluid-restriction, 410, 498
Fluid volume deficit, 155–156, 157, 244
Fluid volume excess, 156–157
Fluoride, 127–128, 133
    infancy and, 214
    pregnancy and, 187
Fluorosis, 128
Folate deficiency, 100
Folic acid, 94, 97, 99–100, 103, 104
    alcoholism and, 437
    atherosclerosis and, 375
    colon cancer and, 453
    displacement and excretion of, 315, 316
    infancy and, 214
    neural tube defects and, 185
    pregnancy and, 184
    vitamin C and, 95
Food, 255–268. *See also* Diet; Digestion; Nutrition;
    Recommended Dietary Allowances; *specific*
    food or food groups
    additives in, 266–267
    adolescence and, 225–227
    allergies to. *See* Food allergies
    composition tables, 20–21
    consistency modifications of, 277
    density considerations for, 82
    drug interactions with, 311–323
    fortification of. *See* Fortification, of food
    glycemia index for, 365
    handling guidelines for, 256, 259, 262, 267–269
    human evolution and, 3–4
    illness caused by, 255–262, 265–266, 492
    infancy and, 210, 212
    intake assessment, 14, 15
    intake regulation, 335–336
    intoxicants in, 258–259, 266
    labeling of, 53, 55, 262–264
    pollutants in, 265–266
    processing and enrichment of, 40–41, 97, 127
    safety of, 4, 256, 259, 492
    selection of, 69, 388, 390–391
    stress and, 470
    as therapy. *See* Diet therapy
    thermic effect of, 78, 79
Food allergies, 172–175, 214–216
    breast-feeding and, 208
    diets for, 175, 176
    in infancy, 208, 214–216
    latex allergies and, 216
Food and Drug Administration (FDA)
    fat replacers, approval of, 55
    regulatory function of, 294
Food faddism, 492
Food Guide Pyramid, 19–20
    for adolescents, 225
    adult compliance with, 236–237
    for breast-feeding, 189

    diabetes mellitus and, 362, 366
    for older adults, 241, 243
    for pregnancy, 187, 189
    for soyfoods, 385
    for 2- to 6- year-olds, 217, 218
    for vegetarians, 70
Food infections, 256, 257–258, 262
Food insufficiency, 245
Food intoxication, 258–259, 262, 266
Food pathway, 164, 166, 168–169, 335–336
Food quackery, 492
Food service, institutional, 273
Food Stamps Program, 189
Formulas
    disease-specific, 281
    elemental or predigested, 281
    infant, 206, 208–210, 211, 227
    intact or polymeric, 279–280
    osmolality of, 282, 284
Fortification, of food, 91, 92
    calcium in, 113
    infant formula, 210, 211
    iron in, 125
    neural tube defects and, 185
Fractures, 116, 245
Fructose, 35, 36
Fruits
    cancer and, 451, 453, 456, 459
    cardiovascular disease and, 380, 383
    childhood and, 217, 218
    consistency modifications of, 277
    diet specifications for. *See specific diet*
    exchanges for, 25–26, 41, 364
    food-borne illness from, 256
    gluten in, 174
    lactose intolerance and, 167–168
    latex allergies and, 216
    minerals in, 121, 132
    older adulthood and, 243
    oxalic acid in, 416
    recommendations, compliance with, 242
    soyfood guide, 385
    vitamins in, 104–105
Fuel reserve, 50
Fuel supply, 50
Full liquid diet, 276

Galactose, 35, 36
Galactosemia, 208
Gallbladder, 442
    digestive function of, 163
    disease of, 442–443
Garlic, 297, 299
Gasoline, 122
Gastrectomy, 429, 430
Gastric acid, 123, 125
Gastric acid-pump inhibitor, 317
Gastric bypass, 340, 341
Gastric cardia cancer, 453
Gastric emptying, delayed, 428–429
Gastric irritation, 313
Gastric stapling, 340, 341
Gastrin, 166
Gastritis, 427–428
Gastroduodenostomy, 429, 430

Gastroesophageal reflux disease (GERD), 425–427, 428
Gastrointestinal disease, 421–444. *See also specific disease or disorder*
  esophageal, 424–427, 428
  gallbladder disease, 442–443
  hepatic, 421–422, 435–442
  intestinal, 429–435
  mouth and throat disorders, 424
  pancreatic, 443–444
  stomach disorders, 427–429, 430
  stress and, 469, 470
  surgical client, diet in, 421–424, 425
Gastrointestinal system
  in burn client, 475
  enteral tube feeding and, 281, 283, 285
  HIV and, 487
  in infancy, 204
  mucosal effects in, 314
  nutrient utilization and, 319
  in older adulthood, 238
  pulmonary disease and, 476
  secretions of, 151–152
  total parental nutrition and, 289
  water imbalances and, 155, 156, 157
Gastrojejunostomy, 429, 430
Gastroparesis, 356
Gastroplasty, 341
Gastrostomy, 281
Gender. *See* Sex
General diet, 276
Generativity, 236
Genes, 65
Genetics
  breast-feeding and, 208
  cardiovascular disease and, 382
  coronary heart disease and, 378
  diabetes mellitus and, 353–354
  energy expenditure and, 78
  obesity and, 337
  susceptibility and, 39
Genetic susceptibility, 39
GERD (gastroesophageal reflux disease), 425–427, 428
German Commission E, 294, 297, 298
Germ theory, 30
Gestation, 183
Gestational diabetes, 193, 351, 352
GFR (glomerular filtration rate), 403, 407
Ginger, 297, 299
Ginkgo, 297–298, 299
Ginkgo biloba, 297–298, 299
Ginseng, 296, 299
Girth, 16
Glomerular filtrate, 406
Glomerular filtration, 403, 405
Glomerular filtration rate (GFR), 403, 407
Glomerulonephritis, 406
Glomerulus, 403
Glucagon, 351, 352, 353
Glucocorticoids, 318
Gluconeogenesis, 470, 471
Glucose, 35–36
  blood glucose curve, 353
  brain function and, 39
  catabolic reactions of, 175

diabetes mellitus and, 349–351
  protein stores and, 38
  self-monitoring of, 356–357
  sources of, 353
  starvation and, 470, 471
Glucose tolerance factor (GTF), 130
Glucose tolerance test, 350
Glutamine
  as ergogenic aid, 301–302
  stress and, 472
Gluteal-femoral obesity, 335
Gluten-restricted diet, 172, 173–174
Gluten-sensitive enteropathy, 172, 433
Glycemia index, 365
Glycerides, 45–46, 168, 169
Glycerol
  catabolic reactions of, 175
  digestion and, 169
  as ergogenic aid, 303
Glycogen, 37–38, 470, 471
Glycogenolysis, 314, 470, 471
Glycosuria, 354–355
Glycosylated hemoglobin (HbAic), 350
Goiter, 127
Goitrogens, 127
Gout, 414, 416
Grains
  cancer and, 504
  childhood and, 218
  diet specifications for. *See specific diet*
  gluten in, 173
  gluten sensitivity and, 172
  minerals in, 121, 132–134
  oxalic acid in, 416
  recommendations, compliance with, 242
  soyfood guide, 385
  vitamins in, 104–105
Grapefruit juice, 320
Grape juice, 384
Gravity. *See* Specific gravity
Griseofulvin, 319
Growth and development, 8. *See also* Mental development; Psychosocial development
  in adolescence, 225
  definitions in, 204
  energy balance and, 77–78
  failure, 413, 415
  fetal, 183, 184, 187
  folate deficiency and, 100
  in infancy, 204, 211
  in preschoolers, 220
  protein and, 61, 63–64
  resting energy expenditure and, 77–78
  in school-aged children, 223
  in toddlers, 218
  vitamin A and, 89
Growth spurt, 225
GTF (glucose tolerance factor), 130
Gut failure, 171–172

HAART (highly active antiretroviral therapy), 483, 487
Hair growth, 60
Hand washing, 259, 262, 267, 268
Harris-Benedict equation, 473–474, 491
Hawaiian native diet, 27, 30

HDL (high-density lipoproteins), 379–381, 383
Headaches
  magnesium and, 119
  terminally ill and, 502
Head and neck cancers, 456
Health
  human evolution and, 3–4
  nutrition and, 8–9
Health care
  attitudes toward, 4
  culturally competent, 27
Health care professionals
  botanical remedies and, 300
  changing roles of, 4–5
  death and, 497
  medications, responsibility for, 322–323
Healthy Eating Index (HEI), 217, 219
Hearing, 238
Heart attack. *See* Myocardial infarction
Heartburn, 191
Heart disease. *See* Cardiovascular disease; *specific disease*
Heart rate, 80
Heat cramps, 153
Heating, of food, 267, 268, 269
Heat-related illness and death, 153, 154
Heavy metals, 265, 296
HEI (Healthy Eating Index), 217, 219
Height
  height-weight tables, 18, 327–328
  measurement of, 14
  zinc and, 129
Helicobacter pylori, 429
Helminthiasis, 125
Hematocrit, 126, 157
Hematuria, 406, 414
Heme iron, 123
Hemochromatosis, 126
Hemodialysis
  dietary recommendations in, 411–415
  malnutrition in, 409
  process of, 407
Hemoglobin, 60, 120, 125, 126
Hemorrhage
  parietal, 297
  peptic ulcers and, 429
Hemosiderin, 121, 126
Hemosiderosis, 126
Hepatic disease, 421–422, 435–442
Hepatic encephalopathy, 440, 502
Hepatic portal circulation, 170
Hepatitis, 436, 438
Hepatitis A, 256, 261, 436
Hepatitis B, 436
Hepatitis C, 436
Hepatomegaly, in AIDS client, 487
Herbal medicine, 293. *See also* Botanical remedies; Ergogenic aids
Hernia, hiatal, 425, 426–427
Heterozygous, 184
HHNS (hyperglycemic hyperosmolar nonketotic syndrome), 356
Hiatal hernia, 425, 426–427
Hiccoughs/hiccups
  in infancy, 213
  in terminally ill, 501

High-density lipoproteins (HDL), 379–381, 383
Highly active antiretroviral therapy (HAART), 483, 487
Hinduism, 29
Hip
    fractures of, 116, 245
    measurement of, 16, 19
Hispanic Americans
    cancer in, 451
    diet of, 27, 28
Histamine H$_2$ receptor antagonist, 317
HIV (human immunodeficiency virus), 483–492.
        See also AIDS
    avoidance of, 486
    complications of, 486–488
    epidemiology of, 484, 485–486
    nutrition and, 489–492
    signs and symptoms of, 483–484
    test screening for, 486, 491
    treatment of, 483, 488–489
Hives, 214
Home enteral nutrition, 285
Homeostasis
    drug excretion and, 321–322
    energy and, 75
Home parenteral nutrition, 289
Homocysteine, 374, 375–376
Homocysteinemia, 374
Homocystinuria, 375
Homozygous, 184
Honey, infancy and, 205
Hormones, 317, 318
    animal production and, 267
    bone tissue and, 112
    diabetes mellitus and, 351–352
    digestion and, 164, 166
    refeeding syndrome and, 478
    regulatory function of, 65
    stress response and, 472
    water balance and, 148, 149
Hormone therapy, 116
Hospice, 497, 498–499
Hospitalization
    linoleic acid deficiency during, 50
    of malnourished client, 277–278, 421
    Nutrition Support Decision Tree, 288
    of older adults, 249
Human body
    anthropometric data for, 14, 16–17
    body fat. *See* Body fat
    composition of, 8, 16, 332–333
    evolution of, 3–4
    growth of. *See* Growth and development
    image disturbances of, 334
    processes, regulation of, 6, 65–66
    protein in, 60
    size, energy needs and, 78
    temperature regulation in, 143
    water in. *See* Water, bodily
Human immunodeficiency virus. *See* AIDS; HIV
Human milk fortifiers, 210, 211
Hydrodensitometry, 16
Hydrogenation, 47–48
Hydrolysis, 164, 166
Hydrostatic pressure, 147
Hydroxocobalamin, 101

Hygiene, personal, 267, 268
Hyperactivity, 122
Hyperalimentation, 285, 286–289
Hypercalcemia, 117
Hypercapnia, enteral tube feeding and, 283
Hyperemesis gravidarum, 192
Hyperglycemia, 349. *See also* Diabetes mellitus, enteral tube feeding and, 283
Hyperglycemic hyperosmolar nonketotic syndrome (HHNS), 356
Hyperhomocysteinemia, 375, 376
Hypericum perforatum, 298, 299
Hyperinsulinism, 368
Hyperkalemia, 119
    blood transfusion and, 157
    enteral tube feeding and, 283
    nutrient control in, 415
    salt substitutes and, 322
Hyperlipoproteinemia, 378
    diets for, 387–388, 389, 391–392
    renal disease and, 410–411
Hypermetabolism, 473–476, 491
Hypernatremia, 118, 283
Hyperparathyroidism, 117
Hyperphosphatemia, 118
    nutrient control in, 415
Hypertension, 373, 374, 376–377, 378–379
    alcohol intake and, 381, 386
    cardiovascular disease and, 382
    pregnancy-induced, 192–193
    renal disease and, 406
    sodium intake and, 378, 387, 392–393
Hyperthyroidism, 127
Hypertonic, 146
Hypertriglyceridemia, 411
Hypervitaminosis A, 89, 90
Hypervitaminosis D, 92
Hypoalbuminemia, 421
Hypocalcemia, 115
Hypochromic, 125
Hypodermoclysis, 156
Hypoglycemia, 368
    alcohol consumption in, 440
    diabetes mellitus and, 349, 355, 356, 367
    meal plan for, 369
    oral agents for, 358–359
    pregnancy and, 352
    terminally ill and, 502
Hypokalemia, 119
    enteral tube feeding and, 283
    renal disease and, 409
Hyponatremia, 118, 148
    enteral tube feeding and, 283
Hypophosphatemia, 118
    enteral tube feeding and, 283
Hypotension, orthostatic, 155, 156
Hypothalamus
    food intake and, 335
    thirst and, 147–148
    weight gain and, 336
Hypothyroidism, 127
Hypotonic, 146

Iatrogenic malnutrition, 278
IBD (inflammatory bowel disease), 101, 433–435

IDDM (insulin-dependent diabetes mellitus),
        349–350, 351. *See also* Diabetes mellitus
Ideal body weight, 327
Identity, 224–225
IFG (impaired fasting glucose), 351
IGT (impaired glucose tolerance), 351
Ileostomy, 434, 435
Ileum, 434
Illness. *See also* Disease; Terminal illness
    food-borne, 255–262, 265–266, 492
    heat-related, 153
Image disturbances, 334
Immune system
    cancer and, 461, 462
    food safety and, 256
    function of, nutrition and, 490
    HIV and, 483
Immunity, 65, 483, 490
Immunoglobulins, 65
Immunosuppressive agents, 256
Impaired fasting glucose (IFG), 351
Impaired glucose tolerance (IGT), 351
Implantation, 183
Implementation, 11, 12, 24–25
    botanical remedies and, 301
    older adult nourishment and, 246–247
Inactivity in adulthood, 236
Incidence, 330
Incomplete proteins, 66
Incontinence, 498, 502
Incubation period, 261
Indication, 275
Indoles, 455
Industry, 223
Infancy, 203–217. *See also* Fetus
    allergies in, 208, 214–216
    anemia in, 125, 126, 213
    breast-feeding and. *See* Breast-feeding
    energy expenditure in, 77–78
    formula-feeding and, 206, 208–209, 210, 211, 227
    GERD in, 425
    growth and development in, 204, 211
    HIV and, 485–486
    linoleic acid deficiency in, 50
    mineral deficiencies in. *See specific mineral*
    mortality rates in, 203, 352
    nutritional needs in, 204–206
    nutritional problems in, 213–217
    phenylketonuria in, 65, 184, 208
    phosphorus toxicity in, 118
    premature birth and, 211
    protein requirements in, 68, 204–205
    semisolid foods and, 210, 212
    supplements in, 205, 206, 214
    vitamin deficiencies in. *See specific vitamin*
    water balance in, 151, 154, 156, 206, 211
    weaning in, 212–213
Infant formulas, 206, 208–209, 210, 211, 227
Infection
    cancer and, 461
    food infections, 256, 257–258, 262
    metabolic stress and, 472, 476
    opportunistic, HIV and, 486–487
    parasitic, 256, 260–261
    stress response to, 472
    viral, 256, 259, 261, 354. *See also* HIV

Inflammation, in atherosclerosis, 374
Inflammatory bowel disease (IBD), 101, 433–435
Initiation, of cancer cells, 450
Initiative, 220
Injury. *See also* Burns; Trauma
    cow's milk protein-induced intestinal injury,
        215–216
    needle-stick, 486
Insensible water loss, 151, 152
Insoluble fiber, 38
Institutional food service, 273
Insulation, fat as, 50
Insulin, 358. *See also* Diabetes mellitus
    beef molecule of, 60
    function of, 351–352, 353, 381
Insulin-dependent diabetes mellitus (IDDM),
        349–350, 351. *See also* Diabetes mellitus
Insulin resistance, 354
Intact formulas, 279–280
Integrity, 236, 237–238
Integumentary system
    dehydration indicators, 244
    drug effects on, 320–321
    in older adulthood, 238
    perspiration and, 151, 152
    water imbalances and, 155, 157
Intense sweeteners, 37
Interactions, food and drug, 311–323. *See also*
        Medications
Intermittent feeding, 282
Intermittent peritoneal dialysis, 408
International Units, 87–88
Internet. *See* Web sites
Interstitial fluid, 142, 143
Intestinal disorders, 429–435
    absorption-related, 432–433
    elimination-related, 431–432
    inflammatory bowel diseases, 433–435
    stress and, 470
Intimacy, 235, 236
Intoxicants, food, 258–259, 262, 266
Intracellular fluid, 142–143
    acid-base balance and, 150
Intradialytic parenteral nutrition, 408
Intravascular fluid, 143
Intravenous feeding, 285–289
    postoperative, 423
Intrinsic factor, 100–101
Invisible fats, 48–49
Iodine, 126–127, 133
    pregnancy and, 187
Ions, 141, 142
Iron, 120–121, 123–126, 133
    absorption of, 95, 121, 123
    excretion of, 123
    function of, 120–121
    infancy and, 214
    pregnancy and, 186
    supplements, 122
    toxicity of, 126
    zinc and, 128
Iron-deficiency anemia, 95, 125–126
    in infancy, 125, 126, 213
    in preschoolers, 221
    renal disease and, 411
Irritable bowel syndrome, 430

Islam, 29
Islets of Langerhans, 351, 353
Isotonic feeding, 284
Isotretinoin, 184
Italian diet, 28
Itching, 502
IV. *See* Intravenous feeding

Japanese
    cancer in, 453
    diet of, 29
Japanese Americans
    cancer in, 453
    diet of, 29
Jaundice, 502
Jejunoileal bypass, 340
Joules, 76
Judaism, 29, 30
Juices, 320, 384, 416
Juniper tree, calcium and, 113
Juvenile onset diabetes, 349–350, 351. *See also*
        Diabetes mellitus

Kaposi's sarcoma, 487
Keshan disease, 130
Ketoacidosis, 349, 355
Ketonuria, 350
Ketosis
    carbohydrate intake and, 38–39
    in pregnancy, 352
    in starvation, 471
Kidneys. *See* Renal disease; Renal system
Kidney stones, 413–414, 416
Kidney transplant, 408
Kilocaloric density, 82
Kilocalorie:nitrogen ratios, 474
Kilocalories, 76
    adolescence and, 225
    breast-feeding and, 193
    diabetic client and, 360–365, 368
    energy expenditure of, 76–80
    energy intake of, 80, 82, 83
    fat as source of, 51
    hypermetabolism and, 473–476
    infancy and, 205
    in IV solutions, 286
    kilocaloric density, 82
    older adulthood and, 241
    in oral supplements, 280
    pulmonary disease and, 476
    renal disease and, 408–409, 412, 414
    in Step diets, 388
    stress and, 470
Korsakoff's psychosis, 97
Kussmaul respirations, 355
Kwashiorkor, 64, 147

Labeling
    of dietary supplements, 294
    of food, 53, 55, 262–264
    of sodium content, 393
Laboratory tests, 17
Lactation. *See* Breast-feeding
Lactobacillus, 215
Lactobacillus acidophilus, 491
Lactobacillus bifidus, 208

Lactose, 36
Lactose intolerance, 166, 167–168
Large intestine. *See* Colon
Larrea tridentata, 298–299
Latex allergies, 216
Latino diet, 28
Laxatives, 313, 317
LBW (low-birth-weight), 183, 211
LCAT deficiency, 410
LDL (low-density lipoproteins), 378, 379–380,
        383
Lead poisoning, 122, 265, 295–296
Learning, 39
Leavening agents, 266
Lecithin-cholesterol acyltransferase (LCAT)
        deficiency, 410
Legal issues, terminally ill and, 499, 503, 504
Leg cramps, 153, 191
Legumes, 67
Leptin, 336
Leukopenia, 486
Levodopa, 318
Licensed practical nurse (LPN), 5
Licensed vocational nurse (LVN), 5
Licorice, 322
Life expectancy, obesity and, 334
Light, conserving rhodopsin, 88
Limiting amino acids, 66
Linoleic acid, 49–50
    cancer and, 450
Lipectomy, 340
Lipid-lowering agents, 317
Lipids, 45. *See also* Fats, dietary
    cardiovascular disease and, 374
    lowering agents, 317
Lipodystrophy, 487–488
Lipolysis, 314, 356
    in starvation, 470–471
Lipoprotein (a), 383
Lipoprotein lipase, 381
Lipoproteins, 378, 379, 380, 381, 383
Liposuction, 340
Liquid diets, 275, 276
    postoperative, 423–424
    supplemental, 279
Listeria, 257–258
Listeria monocytogenes, 191
Listeriosis, 190–191, 256
Lithium carbonate, 313, 317, 322
Lithotripsy, 443
Liver
    absorption and, 170
    bile production in, 163
    disease of. *See* Hepatic disease; *specific
        disease*
    metabolic modifications in, 170
Liver cancer, 450
    alcohol consumption and, 456
Low-birth-weight (LBW), 183, 211
Low-density lipoproteins (LDL), 378, 379–380, 383
Low-fat diets, 387–392
Low-fat foods, 54–55, 386–387
Low-residue diet, 423
LPN (licensed practical nurse), 5
Lubrication, of body tissue, 50
Luminal effects, of medications, 313–314

Lung cancer, 449, 451
  diet and, 453, 459
  weight loss in, 460
Lungs
  cystic fibrosis and, 443–444
  pulmonary disease, 476–477, 478
  respiratory function of, 476–477
LVN (licensed vocational nurse), 5
Lycopene, 453
Lymph fluid, 143
Lymphoma, non-Hodgkin's, 451, 456

Macrominerals, 111–120, 121
Macular degeneration, 93
Mad cow disease, 260
Magnesium, 119–120, 121, 145
  diabetes mellitus and, 365, 366
  hypertension and, 378–379
  pregnancy and, 187
  pulmonary disease and, 477
  starvation and, 479
Ma-huang, 321
Major minerals, 111–120, 121
Malabsorption, 171–172
  of fats, 172, 432–433
  gastrointestinal surgery and, 424, 425
  HIV/AIDS and, 490–491
Malignant tumors, 449
Malnutrition, 6–7. See also Cachexia
  alcoholic client and, 437
  cancer and, 460
  congestive heart failure and, 393
  hemodialysis client and, 408
  HIV/AIDS and, 489, 490
  hospitalized client and, 277–278, 421
  iatrogenic, 278
  in older adulthood, 245–246
  pulmonary function and, 476–477, 478
  refeeding guidelines in, 479
Malonyl-CoA, 335
Maltose, 36
Manganese, 131, 134
  hepatic encephalopathy and, 440
MAO inhibitors. See Monoamine oxidase inhibitors
Marasmus, 64
Massage, 462
Mature milk, 207
MCT (medium-chain triglycerides), 491
Meal management. See also Menus
  in diabetes mellitus, 358–367
  in HIV/AIDS, 491
  in older adulthood, 248
  in oral nutrient delivery, 278–279
  in pregnancy, 187–188
  service patterns in, 273
Measles, 89
Meats
  cancer and, 456
  cardiovascular disease and, 383
  childhood and, 217, 218
  consistency modifications of, 277
  diet specifications for. See specific diet
  exchanges for, 25–26, 52–54, 66, 364
  fat content in, 52–54, 390, 391
  food-borne illness from, 256
  gluten in, 173

iron absorption and, 123
lactose intolerance and, 167–168
minerals in, 121, 132–134
older adulthood and, 243
pregnancy and, 190
recommendations for compliance with, 242
selection of, 69
soyfood guide, 385
steroids in, 267
storage of, 257
vitamins in, 104–105
Mechanical digestion, 164
Medications
  absorption of, 316, 318, 319
  botanical, 293–300
  breast-feeding and, 195
  chemotherapy and, 462
  complementary, 293–307
  decreased absorption and, 171, 316, 318
  for diabetes mellitus, 358–359
  ergogenic, 300–303
  excretion of, 321–322
  feeding tube administration of, 284
  food interactions with, 311–323
  health care professionals and, 322–323
  for hepatic encephalopathy, 440
  for HIV/AIDS, 488–489
  metabolism of, 319–322
  nutritional status and, 311–312
  regulation of, 294
  standards for, 296
  vitamins as, 102
  for weight loss, 340
Medium-chain triglycerides (MCT), 491
Megadoses, 102
Megaloblastic anemia, 100
Memory, 39
Menaquinone, 93
Menkes' disease, 130
Menopause, 115, 116
Mental alertness, death and, 498
Mental development, 8
  fetal alcohol syndrome and, 189
  iodine and, 127
Mental stress, 469–470
Menus
  for Allergy I and II diets, 176
  for cholesterol-lowering diet, 390
  for diabetic diet, 364, 368
  for dumping syndrome, 431–432
  for gastroesophageal reflux, 426–427
  for gluten-restricted diet, 174
  for hiatal hernia, 426–427
  for hypoglycemic diet, 369
  for lactose-restricted diet, 168
  for liquid diet, 275–276
  for liver disease, 441
  for renal disease diet, 415
  for sodium-controlled diet, 395
Mercury poisoning, 265
Metabolic stress, 472–476
Metabolism, 6, 175, 177. See also Hypermetabolism;
    Nutrient metabolism; specific mineral or
    vitamin
  anabolic reactions in, 177
  catabolic reactions in, 175, 177

of drugs, effects of food on, 319–322
liver in, 170
minerals and, 111
obesity and, 336
stress in, 472–476
TPN feeding complications, 287
tube feeding complications, 283
vitamins and, 87, 314–315
water, 143–144
Metals, toxicity of, 265, 296
Metastasize, 449
Methotrexate, 315, 317, 318
Metropolitan Life Insurance Company, 18, 327–328
Mexican diet, 28
Microcytic, 125
Microgram, 89
Microminerals, 120–134
Micronized form of drugs, 319
Microorganisms
  as alternative protein source, 69
  food-borne disease from, 255–262
Midarm circumference, 14, 16
Middle adulthood, 236–237
Middle Eastern European diet, 29
Migraine headaches
  magnesium and, 119
  terminally ill and, 502
Milk-alkali syndrome, 117
Milk and dairy products
  calcium in, 112–114
  cancer and, 456
  childhood and, 217, 218, 220
  consistency modifications of, 277
  diet specifications for. See specific diet
  exchanges for, 25–26, 41, 52, 67, 364
  gluten in, 173
  infancy and, 204–206
  lactose intolerance and, 167–168
  milk-alkali syndrome, 117
  milk nutrients, 114
  minerals in, 121, 132–134
  older adulthood and, 243
  pregnancy and, 190
  recommendations for, compliance with, 242
  soyfoods guide, 385
  vitamins in, 104–105
Milliequivalents, 119, 145, 146
Milligrams, 146
Milliosmole, 146
Mineral deficiencies, 121, 133–134
  in infancy, 206, 210, 211, 214
Minerals, 111–134
  adolescence and, 225
  breast-feeding and, 193
  classification of, 111
  diabetes mellitus and, 365–366
  function of, 111
  hypermetabolism and, 474
  infancy and, 206, 210, 211, 214
  major minerals, 111–120, 121, 132
  metabolism and, 111
  older adulthood and, 244
  pregnancy and, 186–187
  renal disease and, 411
  starvation and, 479
  stress and, 470

Minerals *(cont'd.)*
supplements, 131
trace minerals, 120–134
Misdiagnosis, 277
Modular supplements, 279
Molds, 261–262
Molecule, 35
of beef insulin, 60
food intake and, 335–336
Molybdenum, 131, 134
Monitoring
of HIV/AIDS client, 492
of nutritional care, 273, 274
of TPN client, 286–287
of tube-fed client, 284–285
Monoamine oxidase (MAO) inhibitors, 319–320
hypertension and, 376
Monoglycerides, 45, 46
digestion and, 169
Monosaccharides, 35–36, 37
digestion and, 166, 169
Monounsaturated fats, 48, 52
cholesterol and, 388, 390
exchanges for, 55
Month-O-Meals, 362
Morbidity, 94, 278
Morning sickness, 191
Mortality, 94, 278. *See also* Death
Mouth
cancer and, 453, 460, 461
digestion and, 164, 169
function in older adulthood, 248
HIV/AIDS and, 487
terminally ill and, 502
throat disorders and, 424
Mucous membranes
cystic fibrosis and, 443
medications and, 314
nutrient absorption and, 314
water imbalances and, 155, 157
Multiparous, 193
Musculoskeletal system, 239, 244
Mutation, 450
Myelin sheaths, 97
Myocardial infarction, 374, 377
dietary effects and, 388, 390
diet following, 393
renal system and, 406
Myoglobin, 120
Myxedema, 127

NANDA (North American Nursing Diagnosis
Association), 11
Narcolepsy, 93
Nasoduodenal tube, 281
Nasogastric tube, 281
Nasojejunal tube, 281
National 5 a Day program, 459
National Health and Nutrition Examination Surveys
(NHANES), 39
National Institutes of Health, overweight and obesity
guidelines, 327, 330, 338–342
National Renal Diet, 411–415
Native American mythology, 27

Nausea
cancer client and, 460–461, 462
terminally ill and, 502
NE (niacin equivalents), 98
Neck cancers, 456
Needle-stick injuries, 486
Negative nitrogen balance, 63–64
Neomycin, 314, 317
Neoplasm, 449
Nephritis, 406
Nephron, 403, 404
Nephropathy, 356
Nephrosclerosis, 406
Nephrotic syndrome, 406
Nervous system. *See* Central nervous system
Neural tube defects (NTDs), 184, 185
Neurological system, dehydration indicators, 244
Neuropathy, peripheral, 92, 97
NHANES (National Health and Nutrition Examination
Surveys), 39
Niacin (vitamin B$_3$), 94, 97, 98–99, 103–105
Niacin equivalents (NE), 98
NIC (Nursing Interventions Classification), 11, 24
NIDDM. *See* Noninsulin-dependent diabetes mellitus
Night blindness, 88, 89, 186
Nines, Rule of, 475
Nitrates, cancer and, 453
Nitrites, cancer and, 453
Nitrogen, 62, 63–64
food intake and, 335
hypermetabolism and, 474
renal disease and, 409
NOC (Nursing Outcomes Classification), 11, 13
Nonemulsified fats, 48–49
Nonessential amino acids, 61, 63
Nonheme iron, 123
Non-Hodgkin's lymphoma, 451, 456
Noninsulin-dependent diabetes mellitus (NIDDM),
350–351, 378, 381. *See also* Diabetes mellitus
Non-nucleoside reverse transcriptase inhibitors, 489
Nonsteroidal-antiinflammatory drugs (NSAIDs), 429
Nontropical sprue, 172
North American Nursing Diagnosis Association
(NANDA), 11
Norwalk virus, 256, 258, 259
NSAIDs (nonsteroidal-antiinflammatory drugs), 429
NTDs (neural tube defects), 184, 185
Nucleoproteins, 65
Nurses
cancer client and, 462
classifications of, 4–5
food selection for client, 69
Nursing-bottle syndrome, 39, 213
Nursing Interventions Classification (NIC), 11, 24
Nursing Outcomes Classification (NOC), 11, 13
Nursing process, 11
assessment in, 14–17. *See also* Assessment
botanical remedies and, 301
data analysis in, 12, 17–21, 22–23
dementia client and, 240
evaluation in, 12, 25
fluid intake and output, monitoring of, 154–155
for iatrogenically malnourished, 278
implementation in, 12, 24–25, 246–247
nutritional responsibilities in, 4–5

older adulthood and, 246–248
planning in, 12, 21–24
pregnancy-related visitation in, 196
terminology, 11, 13–14
Nut allergies, 208, 214, 215, 216
Nutrient delivery, 273–289
enteral tube feeding, 278, 281–285
institutional food service, 273
malnutrition and, 277–278
nutritional care service, 273–278
oral, 278–281
parenteral, 285–289
Nutrient density, 82
Nutrient metabolism, 175, 177
in diabetes mellitus, 351–353
drug effects on, 314, 318
Nutrients. *See also* Nutrient delivery; Nutrient
metabolism
absorption of, 169–175, 313–314, 317–318
classification and function of, 6
density in food, 82
digestion of, 163–169
drug interactions and, 311–325
as ergogenic aids, 301–302
excess, storage of, 177
excretion of, drug effects on, 315–316, 318
nutrition levels of, 6–7
renal disease guidelines for, 413, 414
stress and, 470
Nutrition
in adolescence, 224–227
alcohol consumption and, 311, 314, 315, 316,
317, 318, 437
breast-feeding and, 68, 82, 83, 193–194
in childhood, 217–224
definition of, 5
disease-related. *See specific disease*
gastrointestinal surgery and, 421–424, 425
hazards in, avoidance of, 262–264
health and, 8–9
immunity and, 490
in infancy, 203–217
in middle adulthood, 236–237
nursing care. *See* Nursing process
in older adulthood, 237–249
in pregnancy, 183–193, 352
respiration and, 476–477, 478
as a science, 5–7
terminology, 13–14
therapeutic. *See* Diet therapy
in young adulthood, 235–236
Nutritional care services, 273–278
assessment, monitoring, and counseling in,
273–274
diet for diagnostic procedures and, 276–277
diet manuals and, 274
diet orders and, 274–276
iatrogenic malnutrition and, 278
importance of, 277–278
Nutritional status
appearance and, 14, 16
assessment of. *See* Assessment
drug effects on, 311–312
Nutrition education, 248–249, 341–342, 492
Nutrition screening. *See* Assessment
Nutrition Support Decision Tree, 288

Nutrition support service, 285
Nuts
    allergies to, 208, 214, 215, 216
    in DASH Diet, 386, 387
    soy, 385

Obesity
    in adulthood, 236
    breast cancer and, 454
    breast-feeding and, 208
    cardiovascular disease and, 381, 382
    in childhood and adolescence, 226–227
    consequences of, 333–335
    evaluation and treatment of, 338–342
    identification of, 337–338
    in pregnancy, 187
    prevalence of, 330, 331
    prevention of, 341–342, 342
    renal disease and, 406
    theories on, 336–337
    weight loss and, 333, 337
Objective data, 14, 16–17
Obligatory excretion, 151
Obstruction, of bowel, 500
Oil, dietary
    canola, 390
    diet specifications for. See specific diet
    gluten in, 173
    older adulthood and, 243
    soyfood guide, 385
Ojibway mythology, 27
Older adulthood, 237–249
    body systems in, 239, 241
    cancer in, 461
    distinctions among, 237
    energy balance in, 241–244
    food and drug interactions in, 311
    hospitalization in, 249
    integrity and, 237–238
    nourishment in, increasing, 246–247
    nursing process and, 246–248
    nutrition education in, 248–249
    nutrition in, 241–244
    nutrition-related problems in, 244–246
    pathogenic bacterial effects in, 259
    physical changes in, 238–241
    psychosocial development in, 237–238
    weight control in, 342
Olestra, 55
Oliguria, 406, 498
Oncogenes, 450
Opportunistic infections, HIV and, 486–487
Opsin, vitamin A and, 88
Oral anticoagulant therapy, dietary restrictions in, 315
Oral cavity, 164. See also Dentition; Mouth; Taste
Oral contraceptives, 195
Oral feeding, 278–281
    postoperative, 423–424
    terminal illness and, 504
Oral hygiene, in cancer client, 462
Oral hypoglycemic agents, 358–359
Oral supplements, 279–281
Oral ulcerations, 461
Orders, diet, 274–276
Organ protection, 50

Orlistat, 340
Orthodox Judaism, 29
Orthostatic hypotension, 155, 156
Osmolality, 146
    of feeding solutions, 282, 284
Osmolarity, 145–146
Osmosis, 145, 146
Osmotic pressure, 145–146, 156, 157
    infant formula and, 206
Osteoarthritis, 244
Osteoblasts, 93, 112
Osteocalcin, 93
Osteoclasts, 112
Osteomalacia, 91
Osteopenia, 115
Osteoporosis, 115, 116
    fracture risk in, 245
    in pregnancy, 186
Ostomy, 281, 434–435
Ovarian cancer, 451
Overeating, 227
Overhydration, enteral tube feeding and, 283
Overweight, 226–227
    evaluation and treatment of, 338–342
    identification of, 337–338
    prevalence of, 330–331
    prevention of, 341–342
Ovum, 183
Oxalates
    calcium absorption and, 114
    kidney stones and, 414
Oxalic acid
    foods high in, 416
    poisoning from, 115
Oxidation, 92
Oxytocin, 194

Pain control, in cancer client, 462
Paint, leaded, 122
Palliative care, 498–499
Panax ginseng, 296, 299
Pancreas, 351, 353
    diseases and disorders of, 443–444
    function of, 164, 443
Pancreatic cancer
    diet and, 455
    weight loss in, 460
Pancreatic lipase, 112
Pancreatitis, 443
    in AIDS client, 487
Pantothenic acid, 94, 97, 101, 104
Paralytic ileus, 423–424, 476
Paralytic shellfish poisoning, 261
Parasites
    decreased absorption and, 171
    illness related to, 256, 260–261
Parathyroid hormone (PTH), 90
    calcium and, 112, 113
    deficiency of, 115–116
    renal disease and, 409–410
Parenteral nutrition, 278, 285–289
    intradialytic, 408
Parietal hemorrhage, 297
Pathogens, food-borne, 255–262. See also specific pathogen
PCM (protein-calorie malnutrition), 63–64

PDR® for Herbal Medicines, 300
PEACH survey, 222
Peanut allergies, 208, 214, 215, 216
Pedialyte, 156
Pellagra, 98
Penicillamine, 313, 317, 318
Pepsin, 166
Peptic ulcers, 429, 430
Peptides, 168–169
Percent body fat, 328–329
Percent reasonable body weight, 328
Perforated ulcer, 429
Periodontal disease, 238
Peripherally placed central catheter, 285
Peripheral neuropathy, 92, 97
Peripheral parenteral nutrition (PPN), 285–286
Peripheral vascular disease (PVD), 377
Peristalsis, 164, 166
    in burn client, 475
    drugs and, 313
Peritoneal dialysis, 407–408, 411
Peritoneum, 407
Peritonitis, peptic ulcers and, 429
Pernicious anemia, 101
    terminally ill and, 500
Personal hygiene, 267, 268
Perspiration, 151, 152
pH, 148–150
    cooking and, 97
    nutrient absorption and, 313–314
    urinary, drugs and, 322
Pharmacist (RPh), 5
Pharmacotherapy. See Medications
Pharynx, 166
Phenylketonuria (PKU), 65, 184, 208
Phosphate, 145
Phospholipids, 117
Phosphorus, 117–118, 121
    calcium balance and, 117
    infancy and, 211, 214
    pregnancy and, 187
    pulmonary disease and, 477
    renal disease and, 409–410, 411, 412
    renal function and, 403, 406
    starvation and, 479
Phylloquinone, 93
Physical activity. See Exercise
Physical growth. See Growth and development
Physician, 5
Physician's Desk Reference® for Herbal Medicines, 300
Phytic acid
    calcium absorption and, 114
    iron absorption and, 123
Phytochemicals, 7
Phytoestrogens, 456
Phytonadione, 93
Pica, 192
Pickled foods, 451
PKU (phenylketonuria), 65, 184, 208
Placenta, 183
Planning, 11, 12, 21–24
    botanical remedies and, 301
    of meals. See Meal management; Menus
Plants, toxicity, 298–300
Plasma, 143

Plasma proteins
  binding sites on, 315, 316
  water balance and, 147
Plasma transferrin receptor, 126
Plumbism. *See* Lead poisoning
Pneumocystis carinii, 487
Pneumocystis pneumonia, 487
PNI (prognostic nutritional index), 421
Poisoning
  botanical, 295–296
  chemical, 265–266
  food, 258–259, 261
  iron, 126
  lead, 122, 265, 295–296
  mercury, 265
  oxalic acid, 115
Polish Americans, cancer in, 453
Pollutants, environmental, 265–266
Polydipsia, 354–355
Polymeric formulas, 279–280
Polyphagia, 354–355
Polysaccharides, 37–38
Polyunsaturated fats, 48, 52
  exchanges for, 55
Polyuria, 354–355
Population studies
  of cancer, 451, 452, 453, 456
  of cardiovascular disease, 384
Pork, 52–54
Positive feedback cycle, 376
Positive nitrogen balance, 63
Postmenopausal women, breast cancer in, 454
Potassium, 119, 121, 145, 317
  food sources for, 409–410
  hypertension and, 378–379
  renal disease and, 409, 411, 412
  sodium-controlled diet and, 392–393
  starvation and, 479
Potassium pumps, 145
Poultry, 52–53. *See also specific diets*
PPN (peripheral parenteral nutrition), 285–286
Precursor, 88
Predigested formulas, 281
Preeclampsia-eclampsia syndrome, 192–193
Pregnancy, 183–193
  botanicals and, 297–298, 299
  complications and problems in, 183, 191–193
  diabetes in, 193, 351, 352
  diet in, 189–191, 192, 208
  drug use and, 191
  energy in, 183
  folate deficiency in, 100
  HIV transmission in, 485–486
  hypertension in, 192–193
  hypothyroidism in, 127
  kilocaloric intake in, 82–83
  meal pattern in, 187–188, 189
  minerals in, 186–187
  nurse visitation in, 196
  protein in, 68, 184
  teenage, 184, 189, 190
  vitamins in, 184–186
  water and weight gain in, 187, 188
Pregnancy-induced hypertension, 192–193
Prejudice, against obese persons, 333–334
Premature birth, 211

Preschoolers, 220–222. *See also* Childhood
  food guide pyramid, 217, 218
Preservation
  of vitamin A, 89
  of vitamin C, 96–97
  of vitamin E, 92
Preservatives, 266
Pressure sores, 502
Pressure ulcers, 247
Primary hypertension, 376
Prognostic nutritional index (PNI), 421
Promotion, of cancer cells, 450
Proportionality, 503
Prostate cancer, 449, 451, 453, 456
  diet and, 450, 453, 455, 456
  weight loss in, 460
Protease inhibitors, 487, 488
Protein(s), 59–70
  calcium absorption and, 113–115
  cancer and, 460
  carbohydrate intake and, 38
  CD_4, 483, 484
  cirrhosis and, 440, 441
  classification of foods containing, 66–68, 70
  composition of, 59–61
  deficiency of, 96
  definition of, 59
  diabetes mellitus and, 363, 364
  digestion of, 168–169
  as ergogenic aids, 301–302
  fat replacers, 55
  function of, 60, 61, 63–66
  hepatic encephalopathy and, 440
  hydrolysis, 166
  hypermetabolism and, 473, 474
  infancy and, 68, 204–205
  loss of, 332–333
  plasma proteins, 147, 315, 316
  postoperative healing and, 421
  pregnancy and, 184
  RDAs for, 68
  renal disease and, 409, 411, 412
  selection of foods containing, 69
  soy protein formulas, 209
  thermic effect of, 78
  ulcers and, 247
Protein binding sites, 315, 316, 320
Protein-calorie malnutrition (PCM), 63–64
Protein-energy malnutrition, 63, 245–246
Proteinuria, 406, 415
Prothrombin, 93
Protocols, 286–287
Proto-oncogenes, 450
Provitamin A, 88
Pruritus, 502
Psychosis
  Korsakoff's, 97
  vitamin B_{12} deficiency and, 101
Psychosocial development, 203
  in adolescence, 224–225
  in adulthood, 235, 236, 237–238
  in childhood, 217–218, 220, 223
PTH. *See* Parathyroid hormone
Puerto Rican diet, 28
Pulmonary, 476
Pulmonary disease, 476–477, 478. *See also* Lung cancer

Pulse pressure, 155
Purging, 344
Purines, 101, 414, 416
PVD (peripheral vascular disease), 377
Pyelonephritis, 409
Pylorus, water loss and, 151–152
Pyridoxine. *See* Vitamin B_6

Quality of life, 504
Quetelet's Index, 18

Race. *See* Ethnicity/race
Radiation, 460–461, 462
Radiation enteritis, 461
Rate, 343
RD (registered dietitian), 5
RDAs. *See* Recommended Dietary Allowances
RE (retinol equivalents), 89
Reabsorption
  renal, 403, 405
  of sodium, 316
Rebound scurvy, 97
Recommended Dietary Allowances (RDA)
  of carbohydrates, 42
  of energy, 82–83
  Estimated Safe and Adequate Dietary Intakes and, 23
  of fat intake, 51
  food composition tables and, 21
  megadoses of, 102
  of mineral intake, 111, 121, 133–134
  in pregnancy, 184–187
  of protein intake, 68, 69
  of vitamins, 87, 96, 103
  of water, 150
Rectal cancer. *See* Colorectal cancer
Red light, 88
Reduced body mass, 342–344
REE. *See* Resting energy expenditure
Refeeding, 477
Refeeding syndrome, 118, 477–479
Registered dietitian (RD), 5
Registered nurse (RN), 4–5
Regular diet, 276
Regurgitation, 282, 283
  in infancy, 213
Reheating, of food, 268, 269
Rehydration, 156
Relaxation exercise, 462
Religious customs, diet and, 29
Renal disease, 403–416
  causes of, 406
  nutritional care in, 408–415
  treatment of, 407–408
  types of, 406–407, 487
  urinary tract infections, 416
Renal osteodystrophy, 410
Renal pelvis, 413
Renal system
  acid-base balance and, 149–150
  function of, 403, 405–406
  infant formula and, 206
  internal structure of, 403, 404
  kidney stones in, 413–414, 416
  sodium reabsorption in, 316
Renal threshold, 350

Renal tubule, 403, 405
Renin, 149
Replacers, fat, 55
Residues, chemical, 265
Respiration
    acid-base balance and, 149
    Kussmaul respirations, 355
    nutrition and, 476–477, 478
    water loss in, 152
Respiratory failure, 476, 478
Respiratory gas analyzer, 77
Resting energy expenditure (REE), 76–79
    HIV/AIDS and, 491
    hypermetabolism and, 473–474, 475, 476
    in older adulthood, 239
Retina, 88
Retinol, 88
Retinol equivalents (RE), 89
Retinopathy, 356
Reward system, weight and, 339, 340
Rheumatoid arthritis, 244–245
Rhodopsin, 88, 89
Riboflavin (vitamin B_2), 97, 98, 103–105
Ribonucleic acid (RNA), 65
Rickets, 91
Risk factors
    for bone fractures, 245
    in cardiovascular disease, 377–383
    diet as, 172, 175, 378–379
    for food and drug interactions, 311, 312
    obesity as, 334–335
RN (registered nurse), 4–5
RNA (ribonucleic acid), 65
Rooting reflex, 204
Rotavirus, 216
Roux-en-Y, 340
RPh (registered pharmacist), 5
Rule of Nines, 475

Saccharin, 37
Safety, of food, 4, 256, 259
Saliva, dental caries and, 39
Salmonella sp., 256, 257, 258, 259, 262
Salmonella typhimurium, 257
Salmonellosis, 257
Salt. *See* Sodium
Salt substitutes, 322, 392, 393
Sanitation, 267, 268
Sarcomas, 449, 487
Satiety
    cancer and, 460, 461
    fats and, 49–50
Saturated fats, 46–47
    exchanges for, 55
    renal disease and, 410–411
Saturation, of fatty acids, 46
Saw palmetto, 298, 299
SCALES screen, 245
Scar tissue, 60
School-aged children, 222–224
School Breakfast Program, 223
Screening. *See* Assessment
Scromboid fish poisoning, 261
Scurvy, 96, 97
SDA (specific dynamic action), 78
Seafood, toxicity of, 261

Seasonings, in sodium-controlled diets, 395
Secondary diabetes, 351
Secondary hypertension, 376
Secretin, 166
Secretions, digestive, 164
Seeds, in DASH Diet, 386, 387
Selenium, 130, 133
    cancer and, 454–455
Self-care
    in diabetes mellitus, 356–357, 367
    dialysis via, 408
    for diarrhea, 433
Self-determination, terminal illness and, 503–504
Self-feeding, 279
Self-monitoring of blood glucose (SMBG), 356–357, 358
Self-monitoring, of weight control, 339
Semisolid foods, infancy and, 210, 212
Sensible water loss, 151–152
Sensitivity, 438
Sensory system, in older adulthood, 238
Sepsis, in burn client, 475
Serenoa repens, 298, 299
Serotonin, 99
Serum, 143
Serum electrolytes, 146
Serum transferrin, 126
Set point theory, 336
Seventh-Day Adventists, 29
Sex
    cancer rates and, 451, 452
    cardiovascular disease and, 377, 382
    food guide compliance and, 236–237
    gallbladder disease and, 442
    Healthy Eating Index and, 227
    obesity and inactivity and, 236
    resting energy expenditure and, 77
    weight and, 227
Sexual activity, HIV and, 486
SGA (small-for-gestational-age), 183
Shellfish poisoning, 261
Shigella sonnei, 256
Shock, fluid volume deficit and, 156
Shopping considerations, 267, 268
Short bowel syndrome, 434
SIADH (syndrome of inappropriate secretion of antidiuretic hormone), 148
Sibutramine, 340
Sickle cell disease, 61
Simple carbohydrates, 35–37
Simple fats, 49
Skin. *See* Integumentary system
Slowed-down eating, 339, 340
Small-for-gestational-age (SGA), 183
Small intestine
    absorption in, 169–171
    digestion in, 166, 168–169
    nontropical sprue and, 172
SMBG (self-monitoring of blood glucose), 356–357, 358
Smell
    medications and, 313
    in older adulthood, 238
Smoked food, cancer and, 451, 456
Smoking
    cancer and, 456, 459
    cardiovascular disease and, 380, 381, 382, 383

osteoporosis and, 116
    weight control and, 342
Snacks
    fat content in, 54
    fat replacers in, 55
Soap, antibacterial, 259
Sodium, 118, 121, 145
    beverage content of, 392
    calcium absorption and, 115
    composition of, 141–142
    diets controlling, 392–393, 394
    drug excretion and, 322
    food labeling and, 393
    hypertension and, 378, 387, 392–393
    infancy and, 211
    iodine deficiency and, 127
    reabsorption of, 316
    renal disease and, 409, 411, 412
    substitutes for, 322, 392, 393
Sodium pumps, 145
Soft diets, 275–276
Software, diet analysis, 21
Solubility, 38
Soluble fiber, 38
Solute, 143
Solvent, water as, 143
Somatostatin, 351, 352, 353
Soup
    consistency modifications of, 277
    gluten in, 174
Soyfoods
    cancer and, 456
    cardiovascular disease and, 383, 385
    in cholesterol-lowering diet, 391
    food guide pyramid for, 385
    infant formula, 209, 214
Specialty foods, 386–387
Specific dynamic action (SDA), 78
Specific gravity, 155
    of urine, 322
Specificity, 438
Sprue, nontropical, 172
Stability, of vitamins. *See specific vitamin*
Stabilizers, 266
Staphylococcus aureus, 258, 262
Starch(es), 35, 37–38
    consistency modifications of, 277
    consumption patterns of, 39
    exchanges for, 25–26, 41, 66, 67, 364
    processing and enrichment of, 40–41
    in renal diet, 412, 413
    sources of, 37
Starvation, 470–471, 477–479. *See also* Malnutrition
Steatorrhea, 172, 433
Step I and Step II diets, 387–388, 389–390
Steroids, 267
    as ergogenic aids, 302–303
Stevia, 37
Stimulants, appetite and, 312
Stimulus-control strategies, weight control and, 339
St. John's wort, 298, 299
Stoma, 434
Stomach
    digestive function of, 166, 169
    disorders of, 427–429, 430
    drug absorption and, 316

Stomach cancer, 451, 453
    diet and, 453
    weight loss in, 460
Stomatitis, 312–313, 407, 503
Stool softener, 317
Storage
    of body fat, 331–332
    of breast milk, 207
    of excess nutrients, 177
    of food, 257, 267, 268
    of water, 143–144
Streptococcus, 205, 207
Streptococcus mutans, 208
Stress, 469–479
    mental, 469–470
    metabolic, 472–476
    refeeding syndrome and, 477–479
    respiratory, 476–477
    response to, 472
    of starvation, 470–471
Stress factor, 474, 475
Stress response, 472
Stroke
    cerebrovascular, 373, 374, 375
    eating following, 393
    heat-induced, 153
Subcutaneous injection, 358
Subdural hematoma, 297
Subjective data, 14
Substitutes
    salt, 322, 392, 393
    wheat flour, 175
Sucralose, 37
Sucrose, 36
Sugar(s), 35–37. *See also* Glucose
    in cholesterol-lowering diet, 391
    consumption patterns of, 39
    cystic fibrosis and, 444
    dental caries and, 39
    intake, estimations of, 40
Sugar alcohols, 36–37
Sulfur, 120, 121
Sunlight
    cardiovascular disease and, 384
    vitamin D from, 91
Superior vena cava, 285
    intravenous feeding and, 286–289
Supplemental Feeding Program for Women, Infants,
    and Children (WIC), 189
Supplemental feedings, 279–281
Supplements. *See also specific supplement*
    atherosclerosis and, 375
    botanical, 293–300
    in childhood, 221–222, 224
    contamination of, 114
    diabetes mellitus and, 365–366
    ergogenic, 300–303
    excessive intake, 131
    infancy and, 205, 206, 214
    intake levels for, 131
    labeling of, 294
    lead poisoning and, 122
    Ma-huang in, 321
    neural tube defects and, 185
    in older adulthood, 242–244, 248–249
    osteoporosis and, 116

    regulation of, 294
    renal disease and, 410, 411
    ulcers and, 247
    zinc and, 128
Surgery
    decreased absorption and, 171
    dental caries and, 422
    gastrointestinal, 423–424, 425
    for inflammatory bowel disease, 434–435
    for kidney stones, 416
    metabolic stress and, 472, 473, 475
    for peptic ulcers, 429, 430
    for weight loss, 340, 341
Survival skills, for diabetic client, 360, 361
Swallowing disorders, 165
    cancer and, 461–462
Sweets/sweeteners
    artificial/intense, 37
    childhood and, 218
    consistency modifications of, 277
    gluten in, 174
    older adulthood and, 243
    in sodium-controlled diets, 395
    soyfood guide, 385
Syncope, heat, 153
Syndrome of inappropriate secretion of antidiuretic
    hormone (SIADH), 148
Systolic pressure, 147, 374, 376
    DASH Diet and, 383–384

Tanacetum parthenium, 297, 299
Tannates, 123
Tapeworms, 261
Target heart rate, 80
Taste
    cancer and, 460, 461
    medications and, 313
    in older adulthood, 238, 248
    terminally ill and, 501
Teenage pregnancy, 184, 189, 190
Teeth. *See* Dentition
TEF (thermic effect of food), 78, 79
Television, 226
Temperature, of body, 143
Temperature, of food
    in cooling and reheating, 268, 269
    esophageal spasm and, 424–425
    food-borne illness and, 257
Teratogenic, 195
Terminal illness, 497–505
    death, coping with, 497
    death process, 497–498
    diet in, 499, 500–503
    ethical and legal considerations in, 499,
        503–504
    general considerations in, 504–505
    nutrition assessment in, 499
    palliative care in, 498–499
Term infant, 204–206
Testosterone, 302–303
Tetany, 91, 115–117
Tetracycline, 318
T4 (thyroxine), 126
Theophylline, 318–319
Thermic effect of food (TEF), 78, 79
Thermogenesis, adaptive, 75

Thiamin. *See* Vitamin B_1
Thiaminase, 98
Thickeners, 266
Third-space losses, 155
Thirst, 147–148
Throat, disorders of, 424
    HIV/AIDS and, 487
Thrombus, 377
Thrush, 487
Thymus gland, 461
Thyroid gland, 126, 127
Thyroid stimulating hormone (TSH), 126
Thyroxine (T4), 126
Tissue (body)
    anabolism and catabolism in, 62
    carbohydrate intake and, 38
    epithelial, 88, 89
    fetal, 184
    growth and maintenance of, 6
    lubrication of, 50
    nutrient depletion in, 315–316
    scar tissue, 60
    vitamin A and, 88
    water in, 142
T-lymphocytes, 461
Tobacco use, in pregnancy, 191
Toddlers, 217–220
Tolerable upper intake levels (ULs), 24
Tolerance level, 265
Toothpaste, 221
Total parenteral nutrition (TPN), 285, 286–289
    in cancer, 462
    choline deficiency and, 102
    minerals and, 129, 130, 131
Toxicity
    of botanicals, 295–296, 298–299
    of breast milk, 195
    of chemicals, 195, 265–266
    food intoxication, 258–259, 261
    of metals, 265, 296
    of minerals or vitamins. *See specific mineral or*
        vitamin
TPN. *See* Total parenteral nutrition
Trace minerals, 120–134
Transcellular fluid, 143
Trans configuration double bond, 51, 52
Trans fatty acids, cholesterol and, 379–380,
    390–391
Transferrin, 123, 126
Transfusions, 157
Transitional milk, 207
Transition feedings, 287, 289
Transplant, kidney, 408
Trauma
    metabolic stress and, 472–476
    stress response to, 472
Travel
    diarrhea and, 430
    HIV and, 492
Triceps skinfold, 14
Trichinella spiralis, 261
Trichinosis, 261
Triglycerides, 45, 46
    renal disease and, 415
Triiodothyronine (T3), 126
Trousseau's sign, 117

Trust, infancy and, 203, 204
Tryptophan, 97
TSH (thyroid stimulating hormone), 126
T_3 (triiodothyronine), 126
Tube feeding
　in cancer, 462
　in cystic fibrosis, 444
　enteral, 281–285
　gastric surgery and, 429
　in infancy, 211
Tuberculosis, 487
Tubule, 403
Tumors, 449
Tumor suppressor genes, 450
Turgor, of skin, 155
Twin studies, of obesity, 337
Type 1 diabetes, 349–350, 351. *See also* Diabetes
　　mellitus
Type 2 diabetes, 350–351, 378, 381. *See also*
　　Diabetes mellitus
Typhoid fever, 262
Tyramine, 319–320

Ulcerations, oral, 461
Ulcerative colitis, 433, 434
Ulcers, 247, 429
　peptic, 429, 430
　stress and, 470
ULs (upper intake levels), 24
Ultrasound bone densitometer, 16
Undernutrition, 6
　brain development and, 8
　growth and, 63–64
Underwater weighing, 16
Universal precautions, 486
Unsaturated fats, 47–48
Upper intake levels (ULs), 24
Uremia, 407, 415
Ureter, 413
Uric acid stones, 414
Urinary calculus, 414
Urinary system
　dehydration indicators, 244
　in infancy, 204
　infections of, 416
　in older adulthood, 239
　urinary pH, drugs and, 322
Urinary tract infections (UTIs), 416
Urine acetone, 350
Urine output, 151, 152
　assessment of protein in, 473
　death and, 498
　drug effects on, 322
　kidney stones and, 414
　water imbalances and, 156, 157
Urine test, in diabetes mellitus, 350
USDA (U.S. Departments of Health and Human Ser-
　　vices), web site, 19
Usual body weight, 343
Uterine cancer, 451, 456
Uterine involution, 194
UTIs (urinary tract infections), 416

Vaginitis, 355
Valerian, 298, 299
Valeriana officinalis, 298, 299

Vascular disease, peripheral, 377
Vasopressin, 148
Vegetables
　calcium from, 113–114
　cancer and, 451, 453, 455, 456, 459
　cardiovascular disease and, 380, 383
　childhood and, 217, 218
　consistency modifications of, 277
　diet specifications for. *See specific diet*
　exchanges for, 25–26, 41, 66, 67, 364
　gluten in, 173
　goitrogens in, 127
　lactose intolerance and, 167–168
　minerals in, 121, 132–134
　older adulthood and, 243
　oxalic acid in, 416
　as protein source, 67
　recommendations for, compliance with, 242
　soyfood guide, 385
　vitamins in, 104–105
Vegetarianism, 67–68
　childhood and, 220
　Food Pyramid for, 70
　iodine deficiency and, 127
　iron absorption and, 123–124
　renal disease and, 409
　vitamin B_{12} deficiency and, 101
Veins, intravenous feeding, 285–289
Ventilation, 476–477
Ventilator weaning, 477
Very low-density lipoproteins (VLDL), 380
Vibrio cholerae, 208
Viral infections. *See also* HIV
　diabetes mellitus and, 354
　food-borne, 256, 259, 261, 492
Viral load tests, 484
Virus, 261
Visible fats, 48–49
Vision
　eye disease, antioxidants and zinc in, 93
　in older adulthood, 238
　vitamin A and, 88
Vital signs, death and, 498
Vitamins, 87–105. *See also* Vitamin deficiencies;
　　specific vitamin
　absorption of, 171
　adolescence and, 225
　atherosclerosis and, 375, 376
　breast-feeding and, 194
　cancer and, 453, 454–455
　cardiovascular disease and, 380
　choline and, 101–102
　classification of, 87
　diabetes mellitus and, 365–366
　fat soluble, 49, 87, 88–94, 95
　function of, 87
　hypermetabolism and, 474, 476
　infancy and, 205, 211, 214
　as medicine, 102
　metabolism of, interfering factors in, 314–315
　older adulthood and, 242–244
　postoperative healing and, 421
　pregnancy and, 184, 186
　RDAs for, 87
　recently emphasized, 101
　renal disease and, 411

sources of, 95, 103–105
stress and, 470
water soluble, 94–103
Vitamin A, 88–90, 95
　absorption, metabolism, and excretion of, 88
　bone loss and, 242
　cancer and, 89, 453
　deficiency of, 89, 95, 186
　function of, 88–89
　hypermetabolism and, 476
　infancy and, 211
　pregnancy and, 184
　preservation of, 89
　pulmonary disease and, 477
　RDAs for, 89
　sources of, 89, 103–105
　toxicity of, 89–90
Vitamin B_1 (thiamin), 94, 97–98, 103–105
　deficiency of, 97, 437
Vitamin B_2 (riboflavin), 94, 97, 98, 103–105
Vitamin B_3 (niacin), 94, 97, 98–99, 103–105
　niacin equivalents, 98
Vitamin B_6 (pyridoxine), 97, 99, 103–105
　atherosclerosis and, 375, 376
　deficiency of, 99, 315
Vitamin B_{12} (cyanocobalamin), 97, 100–101, 103–105
　atherosclerosis and, 375, 376
　deficiency of, 101
　infancy and, 205, 214
　nutrient absorption and, 313
　older adulthood and, 243
Vitamin C, 94–97, 103
　absorption, metabolism, and excretion of, 94
　cancer and, 453, 456
　cardiovascular disease and, 380
　deficiency of, 96
　function of, 95
　hypermetabolism and, 476
　infancy and, 214
　interfering factor for, 97
　iron absorption and, 123
　postoperative healing and, 421
　pulmonary disease and, 477
　RDAs for, 96, 102
　smoked meat and, 104
　sources of, 96, 104–105
　stability and preservation of, 96–97
　toxicity of, 97
　ulcers and, 247
Vitamin D, 90–92, 95
　absorption, metabolism, and excretion of, 90
　breast cancer and, 454
　calcium and, 112, 113
　cardiovascular disease and, 384
　deficiency of, 91, 95
　dietary reference intakes for, 91
　function of, 90–91
　infancy and, 205, 214
　older adulthood and, 242–243
　osteoporosis and, 116
　phosphorus and, 117
　renal disease and, 409–410
　renal function and, 403, 406
　sources of, 91, 104–105
　stability and interfering factors for, 91
　toxicity of, 91–92

Vitamin deficiencies, 95, 103. *See also specific vitamin*
  alcoholism and, 437
  in childhood, 89, 91, 100
  conditions mimicking, 96
  in infancy, 210
  in older adulthood, 242–244
  in pregnancy, 194
Vitamin E, 92, 95
  absorption, metabolism, and excretion of, 92
  cancer and, 454–455
  cardiovascular disease and, 380
  deficiency of, 92, 95
  function of, 92
  infancy and, 211, 214
  older adulthood and, 242
  preservation of, 92
  RDAs for, 92
  selenium and, 130
  sources of, 92, 104–105
  toxicity of, 92, 93
Vitamin K, 92–94, 95
  absorption, metabolism, and excretion of, 93, 314–315
  deficiency of, 94, 95
  function of, 93–94
  infancy and, 205–206, 214
  older adulthood and, 242–243
  postoperative healing and, 421
  RDAs for, 94
  sources of, 94, 104–105
  stability and interfering factors for, 94
  toxicity of, 94
  warfarin and, 315
VLDL (very low-density lipoproteins), 380
Vomiting
  cancer client and, 460–461, 462
  terminally ill and, 502

Waist circumference, 330
Waist measurement, 16, 19
Waist-to-hip ratio (WHR), 19
Warfarin, 313, 315, 318
Warfarin sodium, 94
Waste products. *See* Excretion; Feces
Wasting, 459. *See also* Malnutrition
  HIV/AIDS and, 490
Water balance, 144
  chronic obstructive pulmonary disease and, 477
  electrolyte effects on, 144–147
  hormonal control of, 149
  plasma protein effects on, 147
  regulatory process in, 147–148
Water, bodily, 141–157
  absorption, metabolism, and storage of, 143–144

acid-base balance in, 148–150
balance. *See* Water balance
bioelectrical impedance test and, 16
distribution of, 142–143
function of, 143
imbalances in, 155–157
in infancy, 154, 156, 206, 211
losses of, 151–155, 332–333
in older adulthood, 244
pregnancy and, 187, 188
sources of, 151
Water, for drinking
  absorption, metabolism, and storage of, 143–144
  cancer and, 455
  fluoridation of, 127–128
  infants and, 151
  kidney stones and, 414
  lead contamination in, 122
  older adulthood and, 243, 244
  pulmonary disease and, 477
  RDAs for, 150–151
  sodium intake and, 392
  sources of, 151
Water intoxication, 144
Water soluble vitamins, 87, 94–103. *See also specific vitamin*
  older adulthood and, 243–244
  pregnancy and, 186
  renal disease and, 411
Weakness, in terminally ill, 502
Weaning
  in infancy, 212–213
  from ventilator, 477
Web sites
  on aspartame, 37
  diet analysis, 22–23
  as information source, 20, 21–22
  for USDA, 19, 20
Weight. *See also* Obesity; Overweight
  age and, 227
  at birth, 204, 211
  of bodily water, 143
  energy requirements and, 79, 80
  ethnicity and, 227
  height-weight tables, 18, 327–328
  HIV/AIDS and, 490
  measurement of, 14, 327–330
  percent body fat and, 328–329
  percent reasonable, 328
  pregnancy and, 187, 188
  usual body weight, 343
Weight control, 327–343. *See also* Obesity; Overweight
  in adolescence, 225–227
  energy imbalance and, 331–333
  fad diets in, 337

goal setting for, 338
in older adulthood, 342
reduced body mass and, 342–344
scientific method and, 331
screening in, 337
terminology and classification of, 327–330
Weight cycling, 333
Weight loss
  advantages of, 338
  behavior modification for, 339–340
  cancer and, 460
  of fat versus water and protein, 332–333
  fluid balance and, 154
  goals for, 338
  maintenance of, 341–342
  methods for, 338–340
  obesity and, 333
  in older adulthood, 245–246
  rate of, 343
  screening for, 337, 343
  success rates in, 333
Wernicke-Korsakoff syndrome, 97–98, 437
Wernicke's encephalopathy, 97
Wet beriberi, 437
Wheat flour substitutions, 175
Wheat grain, 40
WHO (World Health Organization), 484, 485
Whole grains, 40–41
WHR (waist-to-hip ratio), 19
WIC (Supplemental Feeding Program for Women, Infants, and Children), 189
Wilson's disease, 130, 313
Wine, coronary heart disease and, 384
World Health Organization (WHO), 484, 485
Wounds, 502

Xerophthalmia, 89
Xerostomia, 238, 502
X-ray
  in barium enema, 277, 278
  dual-energy x-ray absorptiometry, 16

Yin and Yang beliefs, 30
Young adulthood, 235–236
Yo-yo dieting, 333

Zinc, 128–129, 133
  deficiency of, 96, 247
  eye disease and, 93
  hypermetabolism and, 476
  infantile diarrhea and, 217
  older adulthood and, 247
  postoperative healing and, 421
  pregnancy and, 187
Zingiber officinale, 297, 299